A Textbook of Children's and Young People's Nursing

A Textbook of Children's and Young People's Nursing

E Alan Glasper
Professor, Child Health Nursing,
University of Southampton School of Nursing
and Midwifery, Southampton, UK

Jim Richardson
Principal Lecturer, Child Health Nursing,
University of Glamorgan, Pontypridd, Wales, UK

Edinburgh London New York Oxford Philadelphia St Louis Sydney Toronto 2006

CHURCHILL
LIVINGSTONE
ELSEVIER
An imprint of Elsevier Limited

First published 2006
  Reprinted 2007

ISBN-13: 978–0–443–07401–1
ISBN-10: 0–443–07401–1

British Library Cataloguing in Publication Data
A catalogue record for this book is available from the British Library

Library of Congress Cataloging in Publication Data
A catalog record for this book is available from the Library of Congress

Notice

Medical knowledge is constantly changing. Standard safety precautions must be followed, but as new research and clinical experience broaden our knowledge, changes in treatment and drug therapy may become necessary or appropriate. Readers are advised to check the most current product information provided by the manufacturer of each drug to be administered to verify the recommended dose, the method and duration of administration, and contraindications. It is the responsibility of the practitioner, relying on experience and knowledge of the patient, to determine dosages and the best treatment for each individual patient. Neither the Publisher nor the Editors assumes any liability for any injury and/or damage to persons or property arising from this publication.

The Publisher

Working together to grow
libraries in developing countries

www.elsevier.com | www.bookaid.org | www.sabre.org

ELSEVIER   BOOK AID International   Sabre Foundation

ELSEVIER your source for books, journals and multimedia in the health sciences
www.elsevierhealth.com

Printed in China

Senior Commissioning Editor: Ninette Premdas
Project Development Manager: Katrina Mather
Project Manager: Anne Dickie
Design Direction: Stewart Larking
Cover Images: Rachel EA Haggarty

The
Publisher's
policy is to use
**paper manufactured
from sustainable forests**

Contents

Contributors. ix
Foreword. xiii
Preface. xv

Section 1   Essentials of children's nursing 01

1   Historical perspectives of children's nursing 03
E Alan Glasper, Ruth M Mitchell

2   Working with children and their families 18
Anna L Hemphill, Annette K Dearmun

3   Contemporary child health policy: the implications for children's nurses 33
E Alan Glasper, Susan Lowson

4   Cultural aspects of children's nursing 54
Jim Richardson

5   The psychological preparation of children for hospitalisation 61
E Alan Glasper, Rachel E A Haggarty

6   Family-centred care 77
Lynda Smith, Valerie Coleman, Maureen Bradshaw

7   Assessing and planning care in partnership 89
Anne Casey

8   Public health, primary health care and the development of community children's nursing 104
Mark Whiting

9   Family responses to ill health and admission to hospital 114
Sarah Dowle, Sally R Siddall

10   Communicating with children and their families 127
Janet Matthews

11   The dynamic child – children's psychological development and its application to the delivery of care 146
Helen E Rushforth

12 Physical growth and development in children 164
Janet Kelsey, Gill McEwing

13 Preparing the family for stressful life events, child life and the role
of therapeutic play 197
Gary Mountain, Sue Fallon, Barbara Wood

14 The evidence base for children's nursing practice 211
Peter Callery, Sarah Neill, Sue Feasey

15 Involving children in healthcare research 222
Jennifer Allison, Rosemary King, E Alan Glasper

16 Ensuring quality and the role of clinical audit 242
Janice Watson

17 The management of acute pain in children 256
Alison Twycross, Joanna Smith

18 Children and surgery 278
Linda Shields, Ann Tanner

19 Protecting children: the role of the children's nurse 297
Catherine Powell, Lorraine Ireland

20 Ethics in children's nursing 309
E Alan Glasper, Jim Richardson

21 Legal aspects of child health care 317
Louise M Terry, Anne Campbell

22 Assessing children's health needs over the telephone: using NHS
Direct as an exemplar 330
Felicity Thompson, Rosalyn Moore, Susan Bourner

23 The role of Paediatric Emergency Assessment Units 346
Penny Aitken, E Alan Glasper, Maureen Wiltshire

24 Emergency department management of sick children 353
Julie Flaherty, E Alan Glasper

Section 2 Knowledge and skills for practice 369

25 Children with complex motor disability 371
Jackie Parkes, Sonya Clarke

26 Caring for children with body fluid and electrolyte imbalance 389
Agnes B Kanneh

27 Caring for children with genitourinary problems 405
Kevin McFarlane

28 Respiratory illness in children 423
Janet Kelsey, Gill McEwing

29 Caring for children with gastrointestinal problems 445
Julia M Winter

30 Caring for children with cardiovascular problems 460
Barbara V Novak

31 Caring for children: the role of the immune system in protecting against disease . . . 476
Maureen R Harrison

32 Caring for children and adolescents with malignant disease 490
Beth Sepion

33 Caring for a child with neurological dysfunction 507
Joanna Smith

34 Caring for children with diabetes and other endocrine disorders 535
Philomena Morrow

35 Caring for children with orthopaedic disorders 558
Brian Silverwood

Section 3 Health problems and health promotion 579

36 Prevention of childhood injuries 581
Jo Sibert, Donna Mead, Jim Richardson

37 Information is the key to empowerment 591
Tom C A Hain, E Alan Glasper

38 Inherited conditions and the family 607
Maggie Kirk, Emer Parker

39 Health problems of the neonate 623
Mary Brophy, Clare Barrow

40 Health problems during infancy 637
Kathy Scanlon, Anna-Lisa Sorrentino

41 Health problems in early childhood 665
Arija Nikola Parker

42 Health needs of middle childhood 686
Susan Hooton, Diane Scott

43 Child and adolescent mental health: the nursing response 700
Michael Cooper

Section 4 Caring for children with special needs 721

44 Chronic illness and the family 723
Barbara Elliott, Peter Callery, Julie Mould

45 Caring for children with critical illness 739
Marion Aylott

46 Care of the child requiring palliative care 770
Jayne Price, Marisa McFarlane

47 Children with learning disabilities 784
Victoria Jones, Ruth Northway

Index 795

Contributors

Penny Aitken
Sister, Paediatric Emergency
Assessment Unit, Child Health
Directorate, Southampton General
Hospital, Southampton, UK

Jennifer Allison AAS RN RSCN
Senior Nurse Manager
Wellcome Trust Clinical Research
Facility, Southampton General Hospital
Southampton, UK

Marion Aylott BSc (Hons) MA
RGN RM RSCN
Lecturer Child Health Nursing, School
of Nursing and Midwifery, University of
Southampton, Southampton, UK

Clare Barrow BSc Neonatology
A19 RN Rm 405
Advanced Neonatal Nurse
Practitioner, NICU Singleton Hopsital,
Swansea, Wales, UK

Susan Bourner RGN BSc (Hons)
Project Manager NHS Pathways
Development Team,
Paignton, Devon, UK

Maureen Bradshaw RGN RSCn
MSc DipN CertEd (FE)
Children's Nursing Lecturer, School of
Nursing and Midwifery, University of
Sheffield, Sheffield, UK

Mary Brophy MSc RSCN RN RNT
ENB405 ENB 998
Child Health Lecturer, School of
Health Sciences, University of Wales,
Cardiff, Wales, UK

Peter Callery BA (Hons) RGN
RSCN MSc PhD
Professor, Children's Nursing,
University of Manchester School of
Nursing, Manchester, UK

Anne Campbell BA (Hons) MSc
RGN RSCN DN RNT
Senior Lecturer in Children's Nursing,
Division Faculty of Health, South Bank
University, Whipps Cross University
Hospital, London, UK

Anne Casey MSc RSCN FRCN
Editor and Advisor, Royal College of
Nursing, London, UK

Sonya Clarke PGCert BSc (Hons)
RGN RN(Child)
Teaching Fellow, Queen's University
Belfast, Belfast, Northern Ireland, UK

Valerie Coleman MA BSc RSCN
RGN Cert Fd (FE)
Children's Nursing Lecturer, School of
Nursing and Midwifery, University of
Sheffield, Sheffield, UK

Michael Cooper
School of Nursing and Midwifery,
University of Southampton,
Southampton, UK

Annette K Dearmun PhD BSc
(Hons) RSCN RGN DN DNE RNT
ITGE
Principal Lecturer Practitioner/Senior
Nurse, Children's Services, Oxford
Brookes University/Oxford Radcliffe
Hospital

Barbara Elliott BNURS MSc RGN
RSCN RHV NDNcert PGCHE
Lecturer, Faculty of Health and Social
Care, University of Hull, Hull, UK

Sarah Dowle RGN RSCN DipN
(Paediatric Intensive Care) BSc
(Hons)
Advanced Paediatric Nurse
Practitioner, Paediatric Unit, Diana,
Princess of Wales Hospital, Grimsby,
UK

Sue Fallon RGN MA RSCN PhD
Lecturer in Paediatric Oncology
Nursing, University of Leeds,
Leeds, UK

Sue Fensey RGN RCCN BA MSc
Head Nurse for Children's Medicine,
Oxford Radcliffe Hospitals NHS Trust,
Oxford, UK

Julie Flaherty MA BSc (Hons) DPPN
Cert Ed RSCN RGN ENB HA
Children's Consultant Nurse
Salford Royal Hospitals NHS Foundation
Trust, Department of Emergency
Medicine, Greater Manchester

E Alan Glasper
Professor, Child Health Nursing,
University of Southampton School of
Nursing and Midwifery, Southampton,
UK

Rachel E A Haggarty RGN RSCN
Sister, Children's Surgical Unit, Child
Health Directorate, Southampton
General Hospital, Southampton, UK

Tom C A Hain
Helpful Health Trust, Winchester, UK

Maureen Harrison MSc BSc CertEd RGN RSCN RNT
Lecturer in Child Health, School of Nursing and Midwifery, University of Southampton, Southampton, UK

Anna L Hemphill MSc BSc (Hons) RSCN RGN CTHE Dip Management
Senior Lecturer, Child Health Nursing, Oxford Brookes University, Oxford, UK

Susan Hooton RSCN RGN BSc (Hons) MA RNT
Quality Assurance and Enhancement Manager, Greater Manchester Strategic Health Authority, Manchester, UK

Lorraine Ireland SRN RSCN BSc (Hons) RNT PGCEA
Lecturer in Child Health Nursing, School of Nursing and Midwifery, University of Southampton, Southampton, UK

Victoria Jones BA (Hons) PGCE RNLD
Senior Lecturer Learning Disability Nursing, School of Care Sciences, University of Glamorgan, Pontypridd, Wales, UK

Agnes B Kanneh MSc BSc (Hons) PGCEA RCNT FETC RSCN RM RGN ENB402
City University, St Bartholomew School of Nursing, London, UK

Janet Kelsey
Institute of Health Studies, University of Plymouth, Drake Circus, Plymouth, Devon, UK

Rosemary King RGN Dip HE, RN(Child)
PGC Mechanisms & Management of Allergic Disease, PGC Research Methods in Healthcare Children's Research Sister, Wellcome Trust Clinical Research Facility, Southampton General Hospital, Southampton, UK

Maggie Kirk PhD BSc (Hons) RGn DipN
Professor of Genetics Education and Associate Head of School, School of Care Sciences, University of Glamorgan, Pontypridd, Wales, UK

Susan Lowson
Nurse Advisor to the Ombudsman, Office of the Health Service Ombudsman, London, UK

Gill McEwing
Senior Lecturer, Children's Nursing, Institute of Health Studies, University of Plymouth, Plymouth, UK

Kevin McFarlane RSCN B ed Masters Child Health RSCN
Lecturer, School of Nursing, Dundee University, Ninewells Hospital, Dundee, UK

Marisa McFarlane RGN RSCN BSc (Hons)
Paediatric Macmillan Nurse, Royal Belfast Hospital for Children, Belfast, Northern Ireland, UK

Janet Matthews RGN RM RSCN RNT MSc Nursing
Senior Lecturer, Napier University, School of Community Health, Edinburgh, UK

Donna Mead
Professor and Dean, Child Health Nursing, University of Glamorgan, Pontypridd, Wales, UK

Ruth M Mitchell RSCN RGN SCM RCNT DipCNE RNT Cert Ed MSc
Lecturer, Child Health, Faculty of Health and Life Sciences, Napier University, Edinburgh, UK

Rosalyn Moore RGN RNT Bsc (Hons) MA
National Leader for Quality and Learning, NHS Direct, Wakefield, UK

Julie Mould RGN RSCN BSc MSc
Lecturer/Practitioner, Faculty of Health and Social Care, University of Hull, UK

Philomena Morrow BSc (Hons) Nursing MSc Nursing Dip Nursing RGN RSCN
Nurse Lecturer, University of Belfast, Belfast, Northern Ireland, UK

Gary Mountain MA BA (Hons) RGN RSCn RCNT RNT
Senior Child Health Lecturer, School of Healthcare Studies, The University of Huddersfield, Huddersfield, UK

Sarah Neill MSc PGDE BSc (Hons) RGN RSCN
Senior Lecturer in Children's Nursing, Centre Healthcare Education, University College, Northampton General Hospital, Northampton

Ruth Northway PhD MSc (Econ) RNCD CertEd FRCN
Professor of Learning Disability Nursing, School of Care Sciences, University of Glamorgan, Pontypridd, Wales, UK

Barbara V Novak MSc (Comp Phys) B Ed (Hons) RSCN RN RM RNT
Lecturer in Applied Biological Sciences, City University, St Bartholomew's School of Nursing, London, UK

Arija Nikola Parker BA (Hons) RGN RSCN PGCE
Senior Lecturer, Division of Children's Nursing, University of Central Lancashire, Preston, UK

Emer Parker BSc (Hons) Psych RGN RSCN Cert Ed (FE)
Senior Lecturer, Genomics Policy Unit, University of Glamorgan, Cardiff, Wales, UK

Jackie Parkes PhD BNurs (Hons) RSCN RGN NONCert
Senior Lecturer, University of Belfast, Belfast, Northern Ireland

Jayne Price RGN RN (Child) MSc BSc (Hons) PGDipEd
Senior Teaching Fellow, School of Nursing and Midwifery, Queens University of Belfast, Belfast, Northern Ireland, UK

Catherine Powell PhD BNSc (Hons) RGN RSCN RHV
Lecturer in Child Health Nursing/Honorary Child Protection Nurse Specialist, School of Nursing and Midwifery, University of Southampton, Southampton, UK

Jim Richardson
Principal Lecturer, Child Health Nursing, University of Glamorgan, Pontypridd, Wales, UK

Helen Rushforth PhD BA(Hons) RSCn RGN RNT Nurse Teacher (Recorded)
Senior Lecturer, School of Nursing and Midwifery, University of Southampton, Southampton, UK

Kathy Scanlon BSc (Hons) DPSN PGDip Health Ethics RGN RM RSCN RNT
Senior Lecturer in Children's Nursing, Division of Children's Nursing, University of Central Lancashire, Preston, UK

Diane Scott SRN RSCN BSc MSc
Nurse Consultant, Child Health
Directorate, East Lancashire Hospitals
NHS Trust, Burnley, UK

Beth Sepion
School of Nursing and Midwifery,
University of Southampton,
Southampton, UK

Linda Shields PhD FRCNA
Professor of Nursing Practice and
Education, Faculty of Health and
Social Care, University of Hull, Hull, UK

Jo Sibert
Professor Of Child Health, University
of Cardiff, Cardiff, Wales, UK

Sally R Siddall RN RCNT RSCN
BA (Hons) MSc
Lecturer in Health Sciences,
Department of Health Sciences,
University of Hull, Hull, UK

Brian Silverwood RGN RSCN
ENB 998 N49 870
Orthopaedic Ward Manager, Sheffield
Children's Hospital, Sheffield, UK

Anna-Lisa Sorrentino BSc
(Hons) RGN RSCN ENB998 PGCE
Lecturer/Practitioner, Division of
Children's Nursing, University of
Central Lancashire, Preston, UK

Joanna Smith MSc BSc (Hons)
RNT RSCN RGN
Lecturer, Child Health, School of Child
Health, University of Leeds, Leeds, UK

Lynda Smith RGN RSCN BA
(Hons) MA Ed
Lecturer, Children's Nursing, School
of Nursing and Midwifery, University of
Sheffield, Sheffield, UK

Ann Tanner NHlth Sc (Hlth Prom)
Registered Nurse, Children's Theatre,
Royal Brisbane Children's Hospital,
Brisbane, Australia

Louise Terry PhD LLB RIIBMS
Senior Lecturer, Faculty of Health,
Southbank University, Essex, UK

Felicity Thompson RGN RCNT
Msc
Director of Clinical and Patient
Services, Hampshire Ambulance
Service NHS Trust, Hampshire, UK

Alison Twycross RGn RMN RSCN
MSc DMS CertEd(HE)
Principal Lecturer in Children's
Nursing, St George's University of
London, London, UK

Janice Watson RGN RSCN Bsc
(Hons) Msc
Lecturer, Child Health Nursing, School
of Nursing and Midwifery, University of
Southampton, Southampton, UK

Mark Whiting MSc B Nursing
RGN RSCN Dn HV PGDipEd RNT
Senior Lecturer in Community
Children's Nursing, Division Faculty
of Health, South Bank University,
Whipps Cross University Hospital,
London, UK

Maureen Wiltshire RSCN RGN
Dip HE
Sister, Paediatric Emergency
Assessment Unit, Child Health
Directorate, Southampton General
Hospital, Southampton, UK

Julia Winter MSc BSc RNT RSCN
RGN
Joint Programme Lead/Senior
Lecturer Children's Nursing, Oxford
Brookes University, Oxford, UK

Barbara Wood EdD RGN RSCN
Dip Nursing RNT RCNT
Principal Lecturer, School of Human
and Helth Sciences, University of
Huddersfield, Huddersfield, UK

Foreword

In the recent past, there has been a growing appreciation of the needs and rights of children and young people in our society. This change is being fuelled by a number of factors such as the ratification of the United Nations Convention on the Rights of the Child (1989) and the advent of the UK's Children Act (1989). Roles such as that of the children's commissioners have been created to foster the ability of children and young people to be heard and for their concerns and wishes to be taken seriously. These functions are a continuing catalyst for all in society to consider children and young people to be seen as equal fellow-citizens. These processes are dynamic and further improvements in legislation and policy formation will ensure continuing progress.

All professionals working with children and young people are in a position to work towards satisfying their clients' needs and rights. Every professional encounter is an opportunity to help children and young people to be heard and respected as unique individuals. These principles should form the core values of health care work with children, young people and their families.

This textbook has been produced by a wide range of children's and young people's nurses working in a variety of settings. Its objective has been to ensure that rights are embodied in every topic. A recurrent theme has been the need to ensure that children, young people and their families are received respectfully and that health care needs are identified and satisfied through health care professionals working in a collaborative spirit with these children, young people and families.

Peter Clarke,
Children's Commissioner for Wales, UK.

To
The memory of Chris Baker
A dedicated children's and young people's nurse
1953–2004

Preface

This comprehensive textbook of children's and young people's nursing has been written by some of the UK's most experienced nurses working within this developing field of health care practice. The National Service Frameworks for Children and Young People and Maternal Care in the UK envisage a therapeutic environment which values children and young people as full citizens deserving the optimum care that society is able to offer. We hope, through the pages of this textbook, to reinforce the reality that the wealth and success of a society has to be invested in the health of all its children and young people.

It is important to stress that this textbook is built upon the efforts of many generations of children's and young people's nurses who have developed the evidence base for this often underestimated and numerically small field of nursing. As readers will see, the fight for the registration of children and young people's nurses in the UK has its origins in the Victorian era. Although direct entry pre-registration preparation for the field of children's and young people's nursing eventually disappeared in all countries of the United Kingdom except Scotland, the fight to reintroduce it was continued. This culminated in the reintroduction of initial pre-registration education of children's and young people's nurses by the UKCC (now NMC) in 1989. Since then the importance of children's and young peoples nursing has grown with its popularity reflected in the fact that for every training place available within UK universities there are eight applicants.

Early pioneers in the field are to be thanked for their achievement in securing recognition for nurses educated to work with children, young people and their families. One such, Mrs Woods, is remembered for her memorable dictum, *'sick children require special nursing and sick children's nurses require special training'*. This has been a guiding principle in the production of this textbook. One of the earliest children's hospitals in the UK, London's Great Ormond Street, in 1852 adopted the mission statement "The Child First and Always". This textbook aims to be loyal to this inspiring maxim and we have no reservation in adopting the same philosophy. We hope that this book will assist in re-emphasising the primacy of children's and young people's rights and best interests.

Twenty-first century health care of children and young people demands nurses who are fully educated in care provision which recognises that the professional health care team whole is greater than the sum of its individual uni-professional parts. Therefore, a strong element of this book is its emphasis on the contribution of all health care professionals to the care of children, young people and their families.

We know that all nurses working within the field of children's and young people's nursing practice are in a climate of dynamic change; for example, expanding roles with inter-professional role blurring and the growing appreciation of the rights of children and young people to participate in their own health care. As a consequence, the role of the children's and young people's nurse is dynamic. It follows naturally that it is the child, young person and family who lie at the very heart of this field of nursing.

The issue of what children's and young people's nurses call themselves is as dynamic as the development of their role and society's growing appreciation of the needs and rights of children and young people. So dynamic, in fact, that naming conventions have moved on during the period of preparation of this textbook. As a result, you will find a variety of terms in the text such as children's nurse, child health nurse etc. At the time of publication the preferred term is that of the title of the book: children's and young people's nurse.

This textbook has been written for this generation of nurses. We have endeavoured to give the reader exemplars of how knowledge can be successfully used in practice. We have utilized an innovative approach to the arrangement of reader information and each chapter has an accompanying

PowerPoint presentation on the book's unique website which will present additional material (often in the form of colour slides) to enhance the learning opportunities for readers. This textbook is a celebration of the art and science of children and young people's nursing.

We hope you find this book and its companion website helpful and if you wish to comment on any aspect of its content do not hesitate to contact us by writing to the publishers – we will be pleased indeed to have your comments.

Alan Glasper & Jim Richardson, 2005.

Section One

Essentials of children's nursing

1   Historical perspectives of children's nursing 3
2   Working with children and families 18
3   Contemporary child health policy: the implications for children's nurses 33
4   Cultural aspects of children's nursing 54
5   The psychological preparation of children for hospitalisation 61
6   Family-centred care 77
7   Assessing and planning care in partnership 89
8   Public health, primary health care and the development of community children's nursing 104
9   Family responses to ill health and admission to hospital 114
10   Communicating with children and their families 127
11   The dynamic child 146
12   Physical growth and development in children 164
13   Preparing the family for stressful life events 197
14   The evidence base for children's nursing practice 211
15   Involving children in healthcare research 222
16   Ensuring quality and the role of clinical audit 242
17   The management of acute pain in children 256
18   Children and surgery 278
19   Protecting children: the role of the children's nurse 297
20   Ethics in children's nursing 309
21   Legal aspects of child health care 317
22   Assessing children's health care needs over the telephone 330
23   The role of paediatric emergency assessment units 346
24   Emergency department management of children 353

Chapter One

Historical Perspectives of Children's Nursing

E Alan Glasper, Ruth M Mitchell

ABSTRACT

The primary aim of this chapter and its companion PowerPoint presentation is to consider the historical perspectives of children's nursing, in the UK, since its inception in 1852. To do this, the origins of children's nursing are explored in the context of the changing concepts of childhood. Details of the fight for registration in the latter part of the 19th century, and of the evolution of children's nursing in the 19th and 20th centuries, provide the reader with an account of key developments. The final section includes an overview of the educational provision necessary to equip practitioners with the necessary knowledge and skills to care for children and families and the current issues in children's nursing that inform the curriculum.

Learning Outcomes

- Consider the origins of children's nursing in the context of the changing concepts of childhood.

- Understand the fight for registration and the subsequent evolution of children's nursing.

- Explore the developments in nurse education designed to ensure that children's nurses are fit for practice and purpose.

- Examine some of the key challenges facing child health nurses in the 21st century.

Introduction

Children in our present society are given 'rights' that were not accorded to children in previous generations. In Victorian times it was often said that children should be 'seen but not heard'. In today's society, children have rights under the United Nations Convention on the Rights of the Child (United Nations General Assembly 1989). This sets out the basic human rights that all children are entitled to without discrimination. The Convention is underpinned by four guiding principles, which are those of non-discrimination (Article 2), the best interests of the child (Article 3), survival and development (Article 6) and participation (Article 12). The British government ratified the document in 1991 and, by so doing, committed itself to protecting and ensuring children's rights and agreed to hold itself accountable before the international community. Although in itself it is not a legal statute, the United Nations Convention on the Rights of the Child can be used to support the rights of children. Legislation, which builds on the Articles contained in the Convention on the Rights of the Child, seeks to offer further protection to one of the most vulnerable groups within our society.

The Children Act (1989), which applies in England and Wales, is based on the principle that the child's welfare is the paramount consideration and that effective interventions should be in place to ensure the safety and well-being of children who are at risk of harm. It states that children should, wherever possible, be brought up and cared for within their own family, with both parents playing a full part in their lives, without resorting to legal proceedings. Only in situations where there is fundamental disagreement between parents, or concerns about the child's welfare, will the Courts make orders about a child's place of residence and contact arrangements. The Act emphasises the rights of children to be kept informed about issues that affect them.

The Children (Scotland) Act (1995), which applies in Scotland, is based on the following key principles:

- Each child has a right to be treated as an individual.

- Each child who can form his or her views on matters affecting him or her has the right to express those views if he or she wishes.

- Parents should normally be responsible for the upbringing of their children and should share that responsibility.

- Each child has the right to the protection from all forms of abuse, neglect or exploitation.

- In decisions relating to the protection of a child, every effort should be made to keep the child in the family home.

- Any intervention by a public authority in the life of a child should be properly supported by services from all relevant agencies working in collaboration.

WWW

Check out the UN convention on:
- http://www.unicef.org/crc/fulltext.htm

With the introduction of the Human Rights Act (DoH 1998) some of the rights set out in the European Convention for the Protection of Human Rights and Fundamental Freedoms (1950) became part of British law. Many rights are set out in the Act but of particular relevance to children's nurses, and indeed to all health professionals, are:

- the right to life: Article 2

- the right not to be subjected to degrading treatment: Article 3

- the right to a fair hearing: Article 5

- the right to respect for private and family life: Article 6

- the right not to suffer discrimination in relation to any of the other basic rights: Article 14.

The Human Rights Act, which is central to the right to self-determination by children and young people, includes their right to consent to or refuse treatment (Lowden 2002). However, the Children Act (1989) and the Children (Scotland) Act (1995), although providing legislation that relates to the care of children and their upbringing and protection from harm, do not go beyond establishing their right to be involved in decision making about their welfare. The Human Rights Act enables action to be taken if it is proved that children's rights have been infringed (Power 2002).

PowerPoint

Access the companion PowerPoint presentation and look up the following web pages and consider the extent of the material on children's rights:
- http://www.unhchr.ch/html/menu3/b/k2crc.htm
- http://www.hmso.gov.uk/acts/acts1998/19980042.htm

Children in our society are without a political voice and, until recently, played no significant role in the political processes that impact and influence their lives.

The recent appointment of Children's Commissioners in Wales, Northern Ireland and Scotland is a response to the need to address the rights of children. England delayed the appointment of a children's commissioner after lengthy discussions about the proposed role and powers. The role was felt to fall short of the United Nations international guidelines. In the interim, Margaret Hodge, the Minister for Children in England, held responsibility for children's services, childcare and the protection of the under fives as part of her portfolio. Al Aynsley-Green was appointed Commissioner for Children in England in March 2005. The appointment of Peter Clarke in Wales, Nigel Williams in Northern Ireland and Kathleen Marshall in Scotland ensures that children in these countries have an advocate in all matters that affect them, either directly or indirectly. Part of the role of the Commissioner is to monitor all proposed legislation to ensure that the needs and best interests of children are met. They will also have a remit in relation to child protection (see Chapter 19). Undertaking and commissioning research is another strand of their work. This activity should contribute to the body of knowledge on which sound decisions can be made on matters affecting children.

WWW

Look up the following web pages and read about the role and remit of the recently appointed Children's Commissioners:
- http://www.crights.org.uk/commissioner/commissioner.html
- http://www.niccy.org/
- http://www.childcom.org.uk/english/index.html
- http://www.scottish.parliament.uk/news/news-04/pa04-008.htm

With rights come societal responsibilities and subsequently new challenges for nurses caring for children and their families in hospital and community. In the past, children were considered as individuals with needs, whereas in contemporary society they are considered to be individuals with rights. The two standpoints are not mutually exclusive. However, the task facing children's nurses today is very different from the task faced by those caring for children at the time of the inception of children's nursing in 1852.

The Changing Concepts of Childhood

The material that follows traces the origins of children's nursing in the UK in the context of changing concepts of childhood. Consideration will be given to the fight for registration for sick children's nurses and the evolution of children's nursing in response to greater understanding of the needs of children and their families. Consideration will be given to the educational provision that seeks to ensure that the children's nurses of tomorrow are equipped to provide high standards of care for children and families. Finally, an overview will be given of some of the challenges currently facing children's nurses in the UK.

Children's nursing has undergone a number of fundamental changes since its inception in the mid-18th century. The changes reflect developments within the nursing profession but also changes in societal views towards children themselves and to the needs of children and families. Reference to the sociological analysis of childhood provides substantial evidence of the ambivalent attitude of the British towards children (Scraton 1997). Indeed, this began to change in the time of the European Enlightenment when, rather than looking at children as poor and weak, whose survival was little valued, society increasingly recognised that children were its future and that their healthy survival was essential for the continuation of society (Seidler 1990). However, there is continued evidence of a lack of respect for children and their specific needs within society in general, and this attitude is even more evident in the NHS than in the general population.

It is generally agreed that the perspective from which they are considered influences perceptions about children and childhood. Writers on the subject rarely reach a consensus. Thomas, cited by Avery & Briggs (1989), highlights the difficulties of unravelling the concept of childhood by suggesting that historians and modern writers continue to write the history of adults' attitudes towards children rather than the history of childhood. This can still be seen in society today, when debates about what constitutes the best interests of children often centre on what adults define as 'best interests'.

One of the most influential writers on the subject of childhood is Aries (1962), a French historian. He and de Mause (1995) are referred to in many childcare texts. Aries' (1962) views are often misrepresented, as he did not consider the absence of a concept of childhood as detrimental to children. He noted that children in the Middle Ages mingled with adults and spent considerable time in their presence, working and playing. In his opinion the separation of adults from children occurred in the 17th century, with the start of education dominated by religion-based morality. Not all historians agree with this view and, in his writings, de Mause makes the dramatic statement:

The historical record points to childhood being a nightmare from which we have only begun to awaken. The further back in history one goes, the lower the levels of childcare, the more likely children are to be killed, abandoned, beaten, terrorised and sexually abused (de Mause 1982)

During the 18th century the needs of children were increasingly recognised and, by the 19th century, children were considered valuable and therefore in need of protection (Stone 1977). It was this change in attitude that led to the establishment of foundling hospitals and dispensaries for children. In the 20th century the individuality of the child has become more evident. Family life has become increasingly important. The status of the child has increased significantly with the introduction of the European Convention on the Rights of the Child in 1989 and the Human Rights Act (1998). In our society today children have the right to expect protection from harm and a right to self-determination. This is in stark contrast to the Victorian view of children, whom they considered should be seen and not heard. It has been suggested that changing perceptions of childhood over the years can be considered by considering the themes of play, art and literature (Watt & Mitchell 1995).

Children throughout history and in all cultures engage in some form of play through which they learn to make sense of the world of which they are part. They use imitation and experimentation to learn and experience essential social roles and values. Before the 17th century, little evidence exists for children's play although in the 4th century BC Aristotle – a proponent of play as a prerequisite to health – advocated that children under the age of 5 years should not work. He considered that to do so would be detrimental to their health and well-being. Singer (1973) suggests that it is likely that children did play but, as it was not considered an important activity, adults did not comment upon it.

According to Aries (1962) there were few attempts to portray childhood in art before the 12th century. This reflected society at that time and the place of children within it. In some of the early artwork images children were depicted as miniature adults. It was not until the 15th and 16th centuries that it became popular to portray children in a social context. The Dutch artist Rembrandt achieved popular acclaim for his work, which included portraits of individual children.

Activity

Go to the website below and work through the different sections of the exhibition 'The new child'. This exhibition from Berkeley, USA, depicts British Art and Origins of Modern Childhood 1730–1830.

- http://www.bampfa.berkeley.edu/exhibits/newchild/index.html

There is limited evidence of children's literature prior to the 18th century. *Orbis Sensualism Pictus* by Comenius, which was printed in 1658, is said to be the earliest illustrated book specifically designed for children. Much of the early children's literature was written to appeal to adults and often contained moral messages. *Der Stuwwelpeter*, is a good example of this. Heinrich Hoffman (1809–1894), a German psychiatrist, wrote and illustrated it in 1845 for his son.

Activity

Look at the following extract from *Der Struwwlpeter* and compare it with an extract from a contemporary children's storybook. Consider what messages the books convey to young readers.

The story of little suck-a-thumb
One day, Mamma said, 'Conrad dear,
I must go out and leave you here.
But mind now, Conrad, what I say,
Don't suck your thumb while I'm away.
The great tall tailor always comes
To little boys who suck their thumbs:
And ere they dream what he's about,
He takes his great sharp scissors out
And cuts their thumbs off, and then,
You know, they never grow again.'
Mamma had scarcely turn'd her back,
The thumb was in, Alack! Alack!
The door flew open, in he ran,
The great, long, red-legged scissor-man.
Oh! Children, see! The tailor's come
And caught out little Suck-a-Thumb.
Snip! Snap! Snip! the scissors go;
And Conrad cries out – Oh! Oh! Oh!
Snip! Snap! Snip! They go so fast
That both his thumbs are off at last.
Mamma comes home; there Conrad stands
And looks quite sad and shows his hands
'Ah!' said Mamma, 'I knew he'd come
To naughty little Suck-a-Thumb.'

Look up the following website and read more about some of the early children's books:
- http://www.sc.edu/library/spcoll/kidlit/kidlit/kidlit.html

The following website contains details of the original illustrations which Dr Hoffman included in the original version of *Der Struwwelpeter*.
- http://www.fln.vcu.edu/struwwel/struwwel.html

This brief overview of the changing concept of childhood provides some insight into the nature of children's lives in earlier centuries.

The Origins of Foundling Hospitals and Dispensaries

In Britain in the mid-18th century, many parents – faced with extreme poverty – abandoned their infants and children. They did so in the hope that they would be taken by adults who were in a better position to love, nurture and care for them (Schwartzman 1978). Interestingly, the mortality rate among children who remained with their natural families was higher than among those who were abandoned and subsequently taken in by other adults. This was because the original home conditions for many children were squalid, with poor sanitation, overcrowding and high levels of poverty (Kosky & Lunnon 1991). It is estimated that during the 1850s, 50,000 deaths occurred each year, of which over 21,000 were children less than 10 years of age.

Activity

Consider what other circumstances, faced by parents in the mid-18th century, might have contributed to their decision to abandon their children. Consider some of the possible consequences for the children by reflecting on what happened to children in Romania prior to the overthrow of the Romanian dictator, Nicolae Ceausescu.

Thomas Coram (1668–1751) was born in Dorset and spent much of his life at sea. After working in the ship-building business he moved to London, where by 1732 he was a successful merchant. The sight of abandoned infants and children appalled Thomas Coram and in response to what he what he saw he applied for and was granted a Royal Charter by George II to open the Foundling Hospital, in Hatton Gardens in London in 1741 (Franklin 1964). By taking abandoned infants and children into the Foundling Hospital, Coram wanted to prevent the murder of infants at birth and to stop the practice of parents abandoning their infants and children to die on the streets of London. The primary aim of the Foundling Hospital, which was not a hospital as we know it today, was the provision of care and education. The visionary work of Thomas Coram was widely recognised and many famous artists became patrons and governors of the hospital. Some of their artwork was displayed in the Foundling Hospitals during the 18th century. Today examples of the work of Hogarth, Reynolds and Gainsborough are now on view in the Foundling Museum, established in London in 1998.

There were many such hospitals and, as the name suggests, they were places to which children who were the illegitimate offspring of the poor or who had been abandoned by their parents were taken. Members of the public viewed the foundling hospitals with a high degree of suspicion, considering them to be places of death because of their high mortality rates. In 1756 the governors appealed to the House of Commons for financial assistance. Although granted, the assistance was conditional and required that the governors accepted all children offered to them. The number of sick and seriously debilitated infants and children arriving at the hospital increased dramatically. According to Franklin (1964), the indiscriminate admission of 14,934 babies over a 46-month period in the 1760s resulted in 10,389 deaths. The majority of the infants who died were under 6 months of age. Increasingly it was recognised that children who survived until their second birthday had a significantly improved chance of surviving childhood.

In the UK, the response to the growing problem of sick children involved the setting up of charitable dispensaries. Dr George Armstrong (1719–1789), a Scottish surgeon, is credited with the establishment of the first dispensary or 'ambulatorium' in Red Lion Square, London, in 1769. His work is an early example of ambulatory care and some today consider him to be the 'father of ambulatory care'. The main aim of dispensaries was to lower the toll of mortality among infants and children by providing advice and administering medicines to children of the poor, from birth to 10–12 years of age. This provision was designed to meet the needs of infants and children who, at that time, were often refused admission by most hospitals. Children were acknowledged to be susceptible to infection often as a result of poor nutrition.

As well as keeping children out of hospital, the work of Dr George Armstrong was based on the belief that to separate children from their families was to 'break their heart' (Miles 1985). Accounts about the dispensaries suggest that cost of hospital care was a factor for many parents. Armstrong shared the concern that the economic pressure of looking after a child in hospital would place an intolerable financial burden on many parents. However, the over riding view of Armstrong was that children should 'remain at home, however humble, surrounded and affectionately nursed by their dearest relations, and by those who feel a natural and earnest interest in their welfare' (Miles 1986a,b).

John Bunnell Davis founded the Universal Dispensary for Children in 1816. In 1823 it became the Royal Universal Dispensary, located in Waterloo Road in London (Franklin 1964). It was intended to provide a center-point of medical attention for the investigation of diseases in children and young people. Although initially teaching and home visits appeared to central to the work of the dispensary, these elements gradually ceased. Other cities throughout the UK opened dispensaries based on similar principles, for example in Manchester in 1829 and Liverpool in 1851. The figures from the Universal Dispensary for Children during the first 3.5 years after its introduction demonstrate a significant improvement on the statistics from the

foundling hospitals. It is reported that during this time 7820 sick infants were treated and 7030 cured, 300 vaccinated, 130 died and the remainder continued to receive ongoing care (Franklin 1964). Charles West, the founder of the Hospital for Sick Children, Great Ormond Street, worked for almost 10 years as the physician from 1842. John Bunnell Davis died at the young age of 44 but is credited with being one of the most important influences on British paediatrics, having established an early version of a school of medicine linked to the Universal Dispensary for Children that he founded (Franklin 1964).

Although dispensaries met with some success in reducing the mortality rate amongst infants and children, physicians were forming the opinion that specialist inpatient care was becoming increasingly necessary. In their first argument for such a provision they cited examples of the European cities where children's hospitals were already established. The number of children's hospitals in Europe had increased steadily throughout the 17th, 18th and 19th centuries, starting with the La Maison de l'enfant Jesus (which was an orphanage, although reported by some writers to be a foundling hospital; Guthrie 1960), which opened in 1679. This institution was subsequently converted to L'Hôpital des Enfants Malades in 1802 at the Rue de Sevres in Paris. Other European cities that opened hospitals include St Petersburg in 1834, Vienna in 1837, Budapest in 1839 and Moscow in 1842. However, the mortality in such places was a cause for concern. The high mortality rate reported in L'Hôpital des Enfants Malades was attributed to infectious diseases and the scarcity of nurses with the necessary knowledge and skills (Lomax 1996). Around this time, Louis Pasteur's work on microorganisms was gaining momentum and the knowledge and understanding of microorganisms and cross-infection steadily increased (Craig 1977). Pasteur (1822–1895) provided the impetus for microbiology and contributed to the development of the first vaccines.

● Seminar discussion topic

In your study group, discuss the following questions:
1. What are the fundamental differences between a foundling hospital and a modern children's hospital?
2. Why did it take so long for the concept of a children's hospital to spread worldwide?

After your discussion go the following website and read the article by Retureta et al (2003) about foundling and children's hospitals in other parts of the world:
- http://www.int-pediatrics.org/Volume%2013/133hist.htm

The Establishment of Children's Hospitals

In London in 1850 it was estimated that children under the age of 10 years occupied approximately 3% of available hospital beds but that the deaths in the same age group accounted for 50% of all deaths in London (Franklin 1964). In 1851, a public meeting approved the idea of establishing a children's hospital and the Hospital for Sick Children, in Great Ormond Street, opened in 1852 with ten beds (Arton 1982). In 1858 the purchase of a second house adjacent to the original provided much needed additional accommodation and the number of children who could be admitted rose to 75. The novelist Charles Dickens, a close friend of Charles West – the founder of the Hospital for Sick Children, Great Ormond Street – was himself a strong advocate of the idea of a children's hospital and his depiction of the nurse Sairey Gamp in his novel *Martin Chuzzelwit* (Dickens 1984) has been credited with providing ammunition that undermined the early working-class domiciliary nursing movement in favour of a medically dominated, nurse subservient workforce (Rafferty 1995). Queen Victoria, who subscribed to the project, subsequently became its patron (Arton 1982) and Lord Shaftesbury (1801–1885), the factory reformer and philanthropist, was another supporter of the venture to build a children's hospital. The slogan used at the time of fundraising in the late 19th century was 'children's health, the nation's wealth'. Today, as the Hospital for Sick Children, Great Ormond Street, plans new and exciting developments, the centrality of the child continues to be reflected in its mission statement 'the child first and always'.

During his time at the Universal Dispensary for Children, West had had the opportunity to visit the homes of sick children and was aware of the acute problems, such as overcrowding and lack of ventilation, that made the home environment unsuitable for many of the children. Before establishing the Hospital for Sick Children, Great Ormond Street, he also visited the National Children's Hospital in Dublin, the first hospital in Britain entirely dedicated to the care of sick children.

Activity

Consider the aims set out by Charles West in 1852 for the Sick Children's Hospital, Great Ormond Street (Miles 1986a, b), and reflect on how they compare with the aims of the Alder Hey Children's Hospital, Liverpool, at the beginning of the 21st century.

The Sick Children's Hospital, Great Ormond Street
- To provide for the reception and maintenance and medical treatment of children of the poor during sickness and to furnish them with advice, that is, the mothers of those who cannot be admitted into the hospital.
- To promote the advancement of medical science generally with reference to the diseases of children and, in particular, to provide for the more efficient instruction of students in this department of medical knowledge.

- To disseminate among all classes of the community, but chiefly among the poor, a better acquaintance with the management of infants and children during illness by employing and training of women in the special duties of children's nursing.

Alder Hey Children's Hospital (2003)
- Aim: To provide a comprehensive, high-quality child health service that promotes the integration of hospital and community care in a family-centred, friendly and safe environment.
- Guiding principles:
  - A range of services will be provided to meet all child health needs with the least possible delay.
  - Parents will be involved with professionals in the planning and provision of care.
  - Parents shall be encouraged to stay with their children in hospital at all times.
  - Recreation, play activities and education will be provided according to individual needs.
  - Opportunities for development and training will be provided to ensure highly motivated, well-trained and educated staff.
  - Equal care and consideration will be given to all our patients so that their privacy, dignity and beliefs are respected at all times.
  - Children and parents will be told the name and status of any person caring for them.
- http://www.alderhey.com/RLCH/home.asp

The aims outlined by West in 1852 formed the basis for other similar institutions throughout the UK. They reflected a change in emphasis from reducing mortality to a stronger focus on teaching. This shift in emphasis acknowledged that specially trained children's nurses would be vital in the overall efficiency of care of sick children. By 1888 it was estimated that there were 38 hospitals for sick children in the UK (Franklin 1964). Many general hospitals dedicated wards to the care of sick children. The newly founded children's hospitals, in common with adult hospitals, were voluntary hospitals that relied entirely on public money for support.

Activity

Access the companion PowerPoint presentation and, using the map available at the website, identify the location of children's services throughout the UK (include children's hospitals and children's wards within District General Hospitals).
Suggested website:
- http://coursework.org.uk/essentials/ukmap.html

The Growth of Children's Hospitals

Many hospitals were established during the 19th and early 20th centuries. One such was the Royal Manchester

Children's Hospital, which was founded in 1829 as a dispensary and became a six-bedded hospital in 1855. Like many other early children's hospital, the demands on the hospital were great and in 1873 it moved to its present site to the north of the city centre. Booth Hall Infirmary, now known as Booth Hall Children's Hospital, opened in 1909 but its designation as a children's hospital came 6 years later in 1915 and Royal Patronage was granted in 1923.

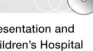

PowerPoint

Access the companion PowerPoint presentation and look at the website for Manchester Children's Hospital for further details of its history and planned developments:

*   http://www.cmht.nwest.nhs.uk

Nottingham Children's Hospital, originally referred to as the Free Hospital for Sick Children, was founded in 1869. The aims of the hospital included the reception, maintenance and provision of medical treatment to children less than 10 years of age. The hospital moved to a new site shortly after its opening and, in 1978, moved again to its present site as part of the University Hospital, Queens Medical Centre (Crothall 1978). Like many children's hospitals across the UK, it has an informative website detailing information about its history and current initiatives and future plans.

PowerPoint

Access the companion PowerPoint presentation and look at the website for Nottingham Children's Hospital:

*   http://www.mss.library.nottingham.ac.uk/isad/uhc.html

In Oxford, plans are in place to build a new children's hospital as part of the John Radcliffe Hospital. The new children's hospital will be linked to the new John Radcliffe Hospital and will provide centralised services for children.

PowerPoint

Access the companion PowerPoint presentation and look at the website for Oxford Children's Hospital:

*   http://www. chox.org.uk/plans/

Dr William Jackson Cleaver established the Sheffield Free Hospital for Sick Children in a rented property, Brightmore House, in 1867. Although the opening of the hospital met with some degree of opposition, the hospital accommodation was soon inadequate for the demands placed on it (Harvey 1976). Like so many other children's hospitals it moved to a new site a few years later.

The Southampton Children's Hospital, the only dedicated children's hospital in the Hampshire region, was established in 1884, initially as The Shirley Children's Hospital and Dispensary for Women. In reality, the hospital was little more than a small house in Church Street, Shirley – then an outlying village of Southampton. Although the hospital moved to larger premises in Winchester Road, Southampton, in 1912, it was not until 1920, when a new wing was built, that the name was changed to the Southampton Children's Hospital and Dispensary for Women. Although the General Nursing Council established the Register for Nurses in 1919, the Southampton Children's Hospital did not found its own school to train Registered Sick Children's Nurses (RSCN) until 1936. The nurses undertook a 3-year course leading to part 8 of the professional register. Probationers following the Registered Sick Children's Nursing course at the hospital had to work, attending lectures and studying in their own free time. The classroom was very small and the nurses were educated in the art and science of children's nursing by the resident Sister Tutor.

The RSCN course was suspended during the early years of the Second World War and recommenced in 1944, the same year that the hospital became the Southampton Children's Hospital. Although the hospital flourished after the inauguration of the National Health Service in 1948, the training of Registered Sick Children's Nurses was discontinued in 1960, after the General Nursing Council decreed that the hospital was too small to adequately train RSCNs. For a short time the Children's Hospital continued to offer training for Enrolled Nurses. The hospital was closed in 1974, transferring its children to the newly built east wing of Southampton General Hospital. Since then, children's services at Southampton have grown and, as in Oxford, there are plans for a separate children's hospital.

In Ireland, the Adelaide, Meath and National Children's Hospitals were all voluntary hospitals. The Meath was founded early – in 1753. In 1821 a group of doctors from Dublin founded the first hospital in Ireland – also the first in Britain – entirely devoted to the care of children. It was this hospital that Charles West visited before setting up the Hospital for Sick Children, Great Ormond Street. The Adelaide was founded in 1839 and opened a school of nursing in 1859, the year in which 'Notes on Nursing' was published. The three institutions amalgamated in 1998.

In Wales, the opening of a new children's hospital early in 2005 will replace a multisite service with services for children and their families at a central location. With a strong emphasis on creating a suitable environment for children and appropriate facilities for parents, the new hospital offers a wide range of specialist services to the children of Cardiff, south of Wales and beyond.

From 1860 to 1883, three children's hospitals opened in Scotland. The Hospital for Sick Children in Edinburgh opened in early 1860 and credit for the founding of this hospital is given to two members of the medical profession – Charles

Wilson and John Smith (Guthrie 1960). John Smith visited the Paris Children's Hospital and is reported to have stated:

There is no question whatever that it seemed inconceivable and altogether unaccountable what while almost every municipality on the continent of Europe possesses at least one, if not two, hospitals devoted to children's diseases, no such institution was to be found in the famous medical centre of Edinburgh (Birrell 1995)

The development of the Hospital for Sick Children was similar to the development of the Great Ormond Street hospital: it started with limited facilities and gradually acquired larger premises. Guthrie (1960), writing about the early days of the hospital, notes that when it was first opened children were, to some extent, still regarded as miniature adults, with little or no consideration given to the unique diseases from which they suffered.

PowerPoint

Access the companion PowerPoint presentation and look up the history of the Royal Hospital for Sick Children in Edinburgh and then view the silent film on childcare in the 1930s, in particular section 2:
- http://www.lhsa.lib.ed.ac.uk/images/hc/healthycity.html

The Aberdeen Children's Hospital opened in 1877 to provide services for children in the city of Aberdeen, the surrounding counties of Aberdeen, Kincardine, Banff, Moray and the islands of Orkney and Shetland. It moved to a site at Foresterhill in Aberdeen in 1929. A new children's hospital, built within the Foresterhill complex, opened early in 2004 and is one of the UK's newest children's hospitals.

The Glasgow Hospital for Sick Children, which later became the Royal Hospital for Sick Children, opened in 1883. It moved to its Yorkhill site in 1914 and is the largest children's hospital in Scotland.

PowerPoint

Access the companion PowerPoint presentation and view the archive material from the Royal Hospital for Sick Children in Glasgow, which provides an interesting account of nurses' training, working and living conditions 1883–1920.

Children's hospitals also opened in other parts of the world in the later part of the 19th century. Examples include the Children's Hospital of Philadelphia, which is the oldest hospital in the USA solely dedicated to the care of children. It was founded in 1895 during the Industrial Revolution.

Francis West Lewis visited the Hospital for Sick Children, Great Ormond Street and on his return to the USA decided to open a similar institution devoted to the care of sick children and to finding cures and treating illnesses and injuries specific to children. The innovative research programmes have led to developments such as fetal surgery techniques and the hospital is recognised to be a leader in its field.

PowerPoint

Access the companion PowerPoint presentation and look at the website for further information on the Children's Hospital of Philadelphia, which has detailed information about its contribution to developments in children's health care:
- http://www.chop.edu/consumer/index.jsp

Allan Campbell founded the Adelaide Children's Hospital in 1876. The hospital is now merged with the Queen Victoria Hospital and is the first fully integrated Women's and Children's Hospital in Australia.

In 1904, the Children's Memorial Hospital opened in Montreal, Canada. It was the first hospital in Montreal whose sole mandate was the provision of care for sick children. Five years after it opened a new hospital was built and in 1920 the hospital became part of a teaching hospital affiliated to McGill University; it is now part of the McGill University Health Centre. It is a multicultural, bilingual institution that serves an increasingly diverse community.

PowerPoint

Access the companion PowerPoint presentation and look at the website of the Children's Hospital of Montreal to explore the features of a multicultural/bilingual institution:
- http://www.thechildren.com

The Origins of Education and Registration of Children's Nurses

Undoubtedly, Charles West, the Founder of Great Ormond Street Children's Hospital, was a formidable individual. Before founding Great Ormond Street Children's Hospital, he worked in The Universal Dispensary for Children in London. He resigned when he failed to persuade the management of the need to expand the facilities to include inpatient beds. It was during his time in the dispensary that he came to the conclusion that dispensaries did not have all the necessary facilities to cope with the problems of children. In his opinion, the dispensaries served only to accentuate the need for specialist hospitals (Miles 1986a,b). Franklin, in his account of children's hospitals in the UK, pays this tribute to West, describing the way he dealt with children: 'the fractious or frightened child could not long resist the magic of his smile or the winning gentleness of his manner' (Franklin 1964). Charles West's book *How to nurse sick children* contains much of interest and he is very direct in his observation about what he considers to be the qualities of a sick children's nurse (West 1854). This book was published 5 years before *Notes on nursing* by Florence Nightingale. West's book formed the basis of the theoretical teaching at Great Ormond Street. Although only 52 pages in length, it was considered very comprehensive and for many years remained the mainstay of teaching within the hospital, continuing in print until 1907 (Arton 1982). It was recently reprinted by Great Ormond Street Children's Hospital.

Seminar discussion topic

Read this extract from West's book and discuss what qualities children's nurses need in order to be able to provide effective care for children and families in the 21st century.

Indeed, if any of you have entered on your office without a feeling of very earnest love to little children – a feeling which makes you long to be with them, to help them – you have made a great mistake in undertaking such duties as you are now engaged in: and the sooner you seek some other mode of gaining and honest livelihood, the better. I do not mean this unkindly, for you may be very good, very respectable women, and yet be very bad nurses. You may be feeble in health, and then you will be unable to bear the confinement and fatigue upon attending upon the sick; or you may be fretful in temper, and may find your greatest trial to consist in the difficulty of subduing it, and in being as thankful to God for all his daily mercies, and as friendly with those who you live amongst as you ought to be; or you may naturally have low spirits and a child's prattle, instead of refreshing, may weary you. Now if any of these things are really the case with you, I would advise you not to be a children's nurse, and especially not to be a nurse in the Hospital for Sick Children (West 1854).

In 1856, 2 years after the publication of his book, Charles West appointed a superintendent to oversee the training of pupil nurses. Catherine Jane Wood wrote the book entitled *A handbook for nursing*, which was considered an important adjunct to the original text written by West. Wood had many innovative ideas about how nursing should be organised and proposed patient allocation and an early version of the nursing process (Arton 1982).

Activity

Consider the following extract from West's book *How to nurse sick children*. How valid are the comments in the light of current knowledge about the care of sick children?

At the Children's Hospital you know it is customary, unless otherwise ordered by the doctor, to place a child on its admission in a warm bath. For this now there are several reasons in addition to the very evident one of ensuring the child's perfect cleanliness. The warmth of the water is grateful and soothing to its feverishness, and that is one advantage; but another is than when stripped for the bath the nurse has the opportunity of carefully examining the whole of the child's body and thus of seeing whether there is a any rash, or eruption as it is called, upon it, while the bath moreover helps to throw out any rash if it were about to appear.

Although part of the initial strategy, it was almost 26 years after the opening of Hospital for Sick Children, Great Ormond Street, before the first purpose-built training school for sick children's nurses opened under the tutelage of Catherine Jane Wood. She stated that 'sick children require special nurses and sick children's nurses need special training' (Wood 1888) and demonstrated great determination in her efforts to ensure that children received appropriate care. Often forgotten in the general discussion about the origins of nurse training is the fact that children's nurse training started almost 10 years before the training of adult nurses (Miles 1986a,b).

Florence Nightingale, on her return from the Crimea, was suffering from what many now believe to be post-traumatic stress syndrome. However, she and colleagues such as Mary Seacole were determined to professionalise nursing. Although Nightingale remained preoccupied with general nursing, she does make mention of the needs of children in her book entitled *Notes on nursing*, in which she states 'children; they are affected by the same things (as adults) but much more quickly and seriously' (Nightingale 1859). However, she saw no need for a children's hospital, although it is known that she corresponded with Charles West, possibly because she was considered the 'official voice of nursing' at that time. There is evidence from the archives of Hospital for Sick Children, Great Ormond Street, that West and Nightingale corresponded on matters such as the optimum way to nurse children. This is surprising in view of the fact that Nightingale's knowledge of children, sick or well, was considered to be scant. This pattern of prominent individuals seeking advice about children from nurses who do not hold the requisite qualification or knowledge continues to the current day.

Nightingale used money given to her by the State, in recognition of her contribution during the Crimean war, to develop a school of nursing. The Nightingale School at

St Thomas' Hospital in London contributed to the ascendancy of the generalist nurse with the subsequent denigration of other types of nursing, including children's nursing. The seeds of generic nurse preparation were sown and, like hydra's teeth of Greek mythology, have returned to haunt the profession in the years since.

The battle for training and a professional recordable qualification continued for many years. Florence Nightingale opposed registration and its introduction occurred only after her death in 1910 (Baly 1973). Baly describes how the Midwives Act, passed in 1902 and which mandated all midwives to undergo a period of formal training and to subsequently register with the Central Midwives Board, made the registration of general nurses an inevitability. The First World War slowed the progression towards registration but did not stop it. Mrs Bedford Fenwick, who was responsible for founding the British Nurses' Association, worked for more than two decades to develop a register and continued despite many obstacles, such as the introduction of Private Members bills during the war years. She, together with other colleagues, did not support the inclusion of children's nurses in the Registration Act (1919).

Conflict among the 'branches' of nursing was precipitated when the College of Nursing was founded in 1916. This organisation became the Royal College of Nursing; it was considered to be a rival group to the British Nurses' Association and had the backing of the medical Royal Colleges. The College of Nursing and the British Nurses' Association decided that nurses who had undergone training only in a children's hospital should not have their names included in the proposed register of nurses. There was also no attempt to include the names of children's nurses in the proposed supplementary register that was set up to include the names of male nurses, mental and fever nurses.

With little support from the nurses' organisations, staff in the sick children's hospitals took action. The matrons of the London children's hospitals produced a petition opposing the idea by the British Nurses' Association for a supplementary register without the names of children's nurses. The petition from the children's hospitals had the support of an eminent paediatrician from Great Ormond Street, Arthur Frances Voelcker. According to Twistington-Higgins (1952), Voelcker wrote in the petition that 'serious injury will be caused not only to children's nurses but to children's hospitals and the Empire'. He considered that to exclude the names of children's nurses from the supplementary register would be disadvantageous in terms of status, prestige and financial remuneration.

In 1919, the unified Nurses Registration Bill was presented to the House of Lords. In addition to the general part of the register, there were a number of supplementary parts, including one containing the names of nurses trained in the nursing of sick children. The supplementary part of the Register for sick children's nurses now remains part of the Register of Nurses in the UK (Barlow & Swanick 1994). The supplementary register was set up to recognise the specialist nursing required by children, although the records of the debate that preceded its establishment suggest that at least one Member of Parliament was keen to ensure that sick children's nurses should not masquerade as registered nurses! The Registration Bill, passed in December 1919, enabled the setting up of the General Nursing Council (GNC) for each of the countries in the UK. Initially, a caretaker GNC was formed until elections were arranged from amongst the registered nurses.

One of the remits of the GNC was to create the register of nurses. Those whose names appeared on the register were required to have completed a course of study of a designated length, to an agreed standard and in different areas of nursing. Arton (1988) reports on the opposition to the supplementary register by Bedford Fenwick, who believed that the supplementary register for children's nurses would be short lived. However, after 85 years of existence the future of the children's nurse appears to be assured.

Closer examination of the progress of registration for children's nurses, however, reveals it to be fraught with difficulties. Although the original idea was to ensure that nurses, practising in different disciplines, would be of equal qualification, the struggle to establish equity between the different parts of the register continues to the present day.

The Register opened on 27 July 1921 but the process of compiling it was slow because Mrs Bedford Fenwick insisted on scrutinising each individual application. The first sick children's nurse (RSCN no. 1) to be listed on the Supplementary Register was Evelyn Margaret Hughes, who registered on 28 October 1921 following a 3-year course at Birmingham Children's Hospital. Agnes Coulton (RSCN no. 96) was a member of the caretaker GNC, having trained at the Infirmary for Children in Liverpool. She became the Lady Superintendent of the East London Hospital for Children and was a member of the Registration Committee.

According to United Kingdom Central Council (UKCC) archives, of the 119 women who registered as a Sick Children's Nurse on the first published register, no fewer than 27 trained at the Hospital for Sick Children, Great Ormond Street. On 10 January 1923 the electorate for the forthcoming election for the GNC comprised all the registered nurses, as shown in Table 1.1. At that time a small victory for children's nurses occurred when Dr Addison, Minister for Health, was persuaded to include onto the GNC two nurses who had experience of caring for sick children.

Another remit of the GNC was to compile a syllabus of topics for examination. One of the criticisms of the English GNC was its generic focus, which from the perspective of sick children's nurses could be demonstrated in the content of the examination set in 1925.

Table 1.1 General Nursing Council Register in 1923 (from Arton 1987)

Type of nurse	Number
General nurses	10,887
Male nurses	24
Mental nurses	639
Sick children's nurses	191
Fever nurses	356
Total	12,097

Activity

The GNC examination (Arton 1992)

Read and consider the following questions:
1. Describe a case of acute nephritis. How would you nurse such a case? (Mention diet and nursing that might be ordered.)
2. Describe the nursing of a case of peritonitis.

In addition to completing the GNC examination, students were required to undertake a hospital examination before completing their training. A sample examination paper from the Hospital for Sick Children, Great Ormond Street, in 1931 has a clear child focus that is in stark contrast to the GNC questions above.

Activity

The 1931 Hospital for Sick Children examination paper

Read the following questions in the examination paper and compare and contrast them with examination questions in your current programme of study.
1. A child of five has developed an acute attack of asthma. Give the symptoms and nursing care of the immediate attack. What general steps would you take to prevent occurrences?
2. Give in detail the treatment of a child of four years suffering from:
   (a) scabies
   (b) threadworms.

Many of the issues that emerged at the time of the introduction of registration persisted in the years that followed. The ratification of the Supplementary Register created difficulties for RSCNs striving to maintain equal status with their colleagues on the General Register. Despite the recognition that sick children require specialist nurses, many hospitals insisted that, to be promoted to a Ward Sister post, the individual required a general nurse qualification in addition to the RSCN. The establishment of the Association of Sick Children's Hospital Nurses was an attempt by a group of matrons from Sick Children's Hospitals to further the interests of sick children's hospital nurses by enabling discussion on matters pertaining to the nursing of sick children. The over-riding principle of the Association of Sick Children's Hospital Nurses was that 'children's trained nurses should nurse sick children' (Duncombe 1979). The renaming of the Association of Sick Children's Hospital Nurses in 1953 to the Association of British Paediatric Nurses (ABPN) occurred in recognition that the initial title was too restrictive, focusing only on hospital-based nurses when in fact an increasing number of children were being cared for in the community.

PowerPoint

Access the companion PowerPoint presentation and look at the website for the Association of British Paediatric Nurses. Consider the contribution the association has made to children's nursing since it was founded in 1937:
- http://www.abpn.org.uk/

Between the mid-19th century and the inception of the NHS in 1948, considerable advances were made in the provision of community nursing. Community children's nursing services were first introduced during the latter part of the 19th century (Whiting 2000). The minutes of a meeting at the Nottingham Children's Hospital in the mid-1800s provides some of the earliest accounts of paediatric home care provision (RCN 1984/85). According to Hunt and Whiting (1999), a similar system operated from Great Ormond Street in the 1880s following an application to the Management Committee of the hospital. Similar accounts are found in the records from Liverpool Children's Hospital in 1910 (RCN 1984/85). According to Lomax (1996), there is limited information on the number of hospitals that employed nurses to visit children. Many hospitals found the expense of such schemes prohibitive and discontinued the service on these grounds. Great Ormond Street continued to provide a paediatric nursing service until the introduction of the NHS in 1948.

Following the introduction of the NHS, Rotherham is credited with the first appointment of a nurse involved exclusively in the care for sick children in the community in 1949 (Gillet 1954). Much of the work involved the care of children with acute infections such as pneumonia and bronchitis. Building on the success of Rotherham, other home care schemes emerged (While 1991). As early as the time of the Court Report (Department of Health and Social Security (DHSS) 1976) it was recognised that sick children required community care by nurses with the appropriate knowledge and skills. With the changing pattern of hospital care, including shorter admission stays and day surgery, growing numbers are currently being supported in the community. In addition, increasing numbers of children with complex and long-term needs are now being cared for at home (ACT and RCPCH 1997). In 1998 the Government made the decision to introduce community children's nursing teams to commemorate the memory of Diana, Princess of Wales. A qualified children's nurse with a community qualification leads each team. Known as Diana, Princess of Wales Community Child Nursing Teams, there are approximately 110 within the UK. The key aims of the initiative are to:

- support children with life-limiting illnesses and their families
- provide high-quality, seamless care
- involve other agencies
- bring different services together to meet a multitude of needs.

 Activity

Consider the above aims and explore the potential benefits of the service to children and their families.

Education of Children's Nurses

Inevitably, the educational programmes for children's nurses have evolved over the years in response to changing perceptions about children and childhood and the increased knowledge and understanding about children's needs in health and illness. The work of John Bowlby (1952, 1953a,b, 1960, 1971, 1988) and James Robertson (1955, 1968, 1970, 1989), among others, added considerably to the knowledge base about the needs of infants and children, and subsequently to the impact of hospitalisation on these groups. Bowlby (1907–1990) and Roberston (1911–1988) have had a profound influence on how infants and children are cared for in hospital and other settings. In his work, Bowlby provided a theoretical framework to explain the process of attachment (Bowlby 1953a) and separation (Bowlby 1953b). Although some criticised the theories of attachment and separation, the original work provoked further studies that have shown the accuracy of Bowlby's original work on the effects of separation (Alsop-Shields & Mohay 2001). Robertson, influenced by Bowlby's work, became very interested in the effects of hospitalisation on the behaviour of young children. He firmly believed in the need to change practices within children's hospitals and, to this end, produced a series of compelling films as evidence for his claims. His series of films included *A two-year-old goes to hospital* (Robertson 1953) and later – in 1969 – *John, 17 months, 9 days in a residential nursery* (Robertson 1969). Although professionals initially refused to accept these films, they stimulated a significant amount of discussion and debate.

As concern mounted about the welfare of children in hospital, the government response was to commission a report on the welfare of children in hospital, universally known as the Platt Report (Ministry of Health 1959). This report increased public awareness of the impact of separation on young children and led to the foundation, in 1961, of the organisation that became the National Association for the Welfare of Children in Hospital (NAWCH). This association became the Action For Sick Children (ASC) in 1990 when its role changed from being a pressure group to being an advisory one.

 Activity

Obtain a copy of the following article:
- Alsop-Shields L, Mohay H 2001 John Bowlby and James Robertson: theorists, scientists and crusaders for improvements in the care of children in hospital. Journal of Advanced Nursing 35(1):50–58.

To what degree do you consider the work of Bowlby and Robertson influences today's care of children in hospital?

 PowerPoint

Access the companion PowerPoint presentation and read the web pages describing the origins of Action For Sick Children and its ongoing contribution to the work with sick children and their families:
- http://www.actionforsickchildren.org

● **Seminar discussion topic**

Does Action For Sick Children still have a role in contemporary child health?

Throughout the years since its inception, children's nursing has faced many threats to its continuation, with many attempts from within the nursing profession to introduce a generic preparation for nurses in the UK. The publication of the RCN-commissioned report chaired by Lord Horder in 1943 (RCN 1946), just 5 years before the introduction of the NHS, made clear recommendations that sick children's nursing should become a post-registration qualification. Although never implemented, few doubt that this did a significant amount of damage to the continuation of the direct entry RSCN programme. Sir Alan Moncrieff, a paediatrician from the Hospital for Sick Children, Great Ormond Street, did much to mitigate the pernicious effects of the Horder Report when he addressed a meeting of the Association of Sick Children's Hospital Nurses in 1944 with a paper entitled *The future of the nursing of sick children*. Central to his message was the belief that 'paediatric nursing is not a specialty but general nursing at a special age period'. Price (1993) draws attention to the similarities between past discussions about children' nurses and the ongoing debate about the current child health qualification.

In England, the damaging effects of the recommendations of the Horder Report (RCN 1946) were profound and sustained. As a result, the direct-entry RSCN programme was phased out during the mid-1960s. Many RSCNs holding single qualifications found it difficult to further their careers without obtaining a second qualification, usually in adult nursing. The impact of nurses leaving to gain a second qualification proved detrimental to the recruitment and retention of staff in children's hospitals. To alleviate the situation, some of the larger teaching hospitals introduced a 4-year combined course leading to the qualification of SRN on completion of the first 3 years and RSCN on successful completion of the fourth year. However, an unexpected number of nurses leaving on successful completion of 3 years further exacerbated the issue of recruitment to children's nursing. To counter this difficulty, in 1968 several teaching hospitals introduced a new programme lasting 3 years and 8 months. This required students to complete the entire programme with one final examination from which, if successful, they received the award of SRN/RSCN and inclusion on Parts 1 and 8.

The 3-year programme in Ireland was discontinued in 1978 (Love 1998). In Wales, the first recognised courses for RSCN commenced in 1976 with limited post-registration courses. Accelerated courses were introduced in 1990 but were replaced by flexible pathways leading to registration and inclusion on Part 15 of the Register (Davies et al 2001). The Welsh Assembly acknowledged the need to employ additional children's nurses with the scheduled opening of the first Children's Hospital in Wales in 2005.

Only in Scotland did the 3-year direct entry continue. Combined courses leading to the award of RGN/RSCN were run in Scotland between 1950 and 1958. The programmes were 4 years and 3 months in length. The courses were subsequently discontinued in Scotland because of the high attrition rate. Just as the integrated schemes of training were discontinued in Scotland, in England they were gaining in popularity. In 1972 new comprehensive programmes were introduced in which all students gained experience in adult nursing, psychiatric nursing, obstetrics and community nursing.

The introduction of the United Kingdom Central Council and the four National Boards under the auspices of the Nurses, Midwives and Health Visitors Act (1974) led to significant changes in the education and registration of nurses. The culmination of the reforms resulted in the publication of Project 2000 (UKCC 1986), an examination of how nurse education should be changed to meet the predicted demands of society in the forthcoming century. Eve Bendall, a well-known and respected children's nurse and previous head of the School of Nursing at the Hospital for Sick Children, Great Ormond Street, became the Chief Executive of the UKCC and Sheila Barlow, Director of Nurse Education at the Hospital for Sick Children, Great Ormond Street, became Vice President of the Project 2000 working group. Her efforts resulted in the shaping of the new registration in which children's nursing (Part 15) was introduced as a discrete entity. The English National Board (ENB) approved the first 14 Project 2000 sites in England in the year between April 1989 and April 1990; 10 of these sites offered the new child branch programme leading to inclusion on Part 15 of the Register. The programmes embraced the new educational curriculum in which all nurses followed an 18-month common foundation programme irrespective of their chosen branch. It was anticipated that the new programmes would give all nurses equal status irrespective of their chosen branch and children's nurses were initially euphoric to the see their direct entry register returned to them. But the initial euphoria was short lived, as once again overt discrimination against children's nurses became apparent. In the new programmes, the adult nurse continues to be perceived as a 'general' nurse and children's nurses continue to experience difficulty undertaking shortened programmes such as the one leading to registration as a midwife. Employment overseas remains somewhat problematic for children's nurses. The changes in educational provision increase the opportunities for children's nurses who wish to work in Europe, but with the proviso that it must be a country where there is a reciprocal qualification (Smallman 1998). The lack of equity between branches, to the disadvantage of all but adult nurses, continues to be demonstrated by the adult bias of many common foundation programmes (UKCC 1999).

The publication of the UKCC (2001) document *Fitness for practice and purpose* reopened the debate about the education of children's nurses. Central to the debate is the question of genericism versus specialism (Glasper 1995). In the generic approach to nurse education, students would be required to undertake a general programme followed by a period of specialist preparation following initial registration (Barr & Sines 1996). Those in favour of genericism argue that children's nursing is a specialism and that education should therefore take place at the post-registration level. However, to suggest that children's nursing is a specialism is to fail to recognise the generic nature of the children's nursing curriculum (Glasper 1995). Those opposed to genericism share the view expressed by Moncrieff (1944) that children's nursing is not a specialty but general nursing at a special age period.

For many years there has been inequity between the branches and, with relatively few registered nurses on Parts 8 and 15 of the Register, they have become a vulnerable group (Glasper 1995). According to the Nursing and Midwifery Council (NMC) statistical analysis, of the 645,508 individuals on the Register (Table 1.2) only 36,314 are children's nurses (NMC 2004). It should be noted that a percentage of these might hold dual qualification.

Table 1.2 Geographical Breakdown of the Register (NMC 2004)

Country	Number on register	Percentage of register
England	470,536	72.89
Northern Ireland	20,968	3.25
Scotland	54,527	8.45
Wales	29,665	4.60
Overseas	28,974	4.48
Postcode not known	40,838	6.33

Gibson et al (2003) acknowledged that there is evidence in literature to support the continuation of a children's nursing qualification and considered the need to make a distinction between generalist and specialist nursing to distinguish children's nursing from all other branches of nursing. To do so, competencies required by generalist children's nurses are first identified and then additional competencies are identified. The competencies cover areas such as knowledge, abilities, values and qualities. Gibson et al contend that the development of these standards provides clear statements of what is required for a children's nurse to practice effectively. They suggest that this information can form the basis for identifying whether children's nursing is indeed a distinct and separate entity (Gibson et al 2003). The debates relating to the future of children's nursing will undoubtedly continue but it is important to stress that each year the evidence base for children's nursing interventions increases.

Summary

The role of historical investigation gives healthcare researchers not only a window to the past but also a vehicle to make judgements about the future. The work of the RCN in promoting the History of Nursing Society is commendable and provides all nurses with the opportunity of learning from the past. Not to do so, to cite Plato, is folly, as those who do not are doomed to repeat the lessons of history.

References

ACT and RCPCH 1997 A guide to developments of children's palliative care services. Report of a joint working party. Royal College of Paediatrics and Child Health, London

Alsop-Shields L, Mohay H 2001 John Bowlby and James Robertson: theorists, scientists and crusaders for improvements in care of children in hospital. Journal of Advanced Nursing 35(1):50–58

Aries P 1962 Centuries of childhood. Jonathan Cape, London

Arton M 1982 Children first and always. Nursing Times 78(40):1687–1688

Arton M 1987 The caretaker general nursing council and sick children's nursing 1920–1923. RCN History of Nursing Bulletin 2(1):1–7

Arton M 1988 The supplementary register for sick children's nurses. Accident or design 2(4):24–28

Arton M 1992 Development of sick children's nursing 1919–1939. MPhil thesis, University of Bath

Avery G, Briggs J (eds) 1989 Children and their books. Clarendon Press, Oxford

Baly ME 1973 Nursing and social change, 3rd edn. Routledge, London

Barlow S, Swanick M 1994 Supplementary benefits. Paediatric Nursing 6(3):16–17

Barr D, Sines D 1996 The development of the generalist nurse with the pre-registration education in the UK: some points for consideration. Nurse Education Today 16:74–77

Birrell J 1995 A most perfect hospital. Edinburgh Sick Children's NHS Trust, Edinburgh

Bowlby J 1952 Maternal child care and mental health. World Health Organization, Geneva

Bowlby J 1953a Child care and the growth of love. Penguin, Harmondsworth

Bowlby J 1953b Attachment. Penguin, Harmondsworth

Bowlby J 1960 Separation anxiety. International Journal of Psychoanalysis 41:89–113

Bowlby J 1971 Attachment, vol 1. Penguin, Harmondsworth

Bowlby J 1988 A secure base: parent–child attachment and health human development. Basic Books Inc., New York

Children Act 1989 HMSO, London

Children (Scotland) Act 1989 HMSO, London

Craig J 1977 A short history of the Royal Aberdeen Children's Hospital. University Press, Aberdeen

Crothall L 1978 Let's begin with the children. Nottingham Children's Hospital, Nottingham

Davies A, Earles C, Eaton N et al 2001 Educating children's nurses in Wales. Paediatric Nursing 13(6):21–24

Department of Health and Social Security (DHSS) 1976 Fit for the Future (the Court Report). The Report of the Committee on Child Health Services. HMSO, London

Dickens C 1984 Martin Chuzzlewitt. Oxford University Press, London

Duncombe MA 1979 A brief history of the Association of British Paediatric nurses 1938–1975. Association of British Paediatric Nurses, London

Franklin AW 1964 Children's hospitals. In Poynter FNL (ed) The evolution of hospitals in Britain. Pitman Medical, London

Gibson F, Fletcher M, Casey A 2003 Classifying general and specialist children's nursing competencies. Journal of Advanced Nursing 44(6):591–602

Gillet JA 1954 Children's nursing unit. British Medical Journal 4863:684–685

Glasper EA 1995 The value of children's nursing in the third millennium. British Journal of Nursing 4(1):27–30

Guthrie D 1960 The Royal Edinburgh Hospital for Sick Children. Churchill Livingstone, Edinburgh

Harvey P 1976 Up the hill to Western Bank, history of the Children's Hospital Sheffield, 1876–1976. The Centenary Committee, Sheffield Children's Hospital, Sheffield

Hoffman H 1845 Der Struwwlpeter. Kindlers Literaturlexikon. [English version 1994 The Struwwelpeter. Munich in association with Ragged Bears Ltd, Singapore]

Human Rights Act 1988 HMSO, London

Hunt M, Whiting M 1999 A re-examination of the history of children's community nursing. Paediatric Nursing 11(4):33–36

Kosky J, Lunnon R J 1991 Great Ormond Street Hospital and the story of medicine. The Hospitals For Sick Children in association with Granta Editions, London

Lomax E 1996 The control of contagious disease in nineteenth-century British paediatric hospitals. The Society for the Social History of Medicine 7(3):383–400

Love H (1998) The Royal Belfast Hospital for Sick Children: a history 1948–1998. Blackstaff Press, Belfast

Lowden J 2002 Children's rights: a decade of dispute. Journal of Advanced Nursing 37(1):100–106

de Mause L (1982) Foundations of psychohistory. Creative Roots, New York

de Mause L (ed.) 1995 The history of childhood: untold story of child abuse. Jason Aronson, Northvale, NJ

Miles I 1985 A suitable case for treatment. Nursing Times May:48–50

Miles I 1986a The emergence of sick children's nursing. Part 1: sick children's nursing before the turn of the century. Nurse Education Today 6:82–87

Miles I 1986b The emergence of sick children's nursing. Part 2: the emergence of sick children's nursing. Nurse Education Today 6:133–138

Ministry of Health 1959 Committee of the Central Health Services Council. Report of the Committee on the Welfare of Children in Hospital (The Platt Report). Ministry of Health, London

Moncrieff A 1944 The future of the nursing of sick children. The Association of Sick Children's Hospital Nurses. Great Ormond Street Archives, London

Nightingale F 1859 Notes on nursing: what it is and what it is not. Duckworth, London (reprinted 1970)

Nursing and Midwifery Council (NMC) 2004 Statistical analysis of the register, 1 April 2002 to 31 March 2003. NMC, London

Power K 2002 Implications of the Human Rights Act 1998. Paediatric Nursing 14(4):14–19

Price S 1993 Children's nursing, lessons from the past. Nursing Standard 7(50):31–35

Rafferty AM 1995 The anomaly of autonomy: space and status in early nursing reform. International History of Nursing Journal 1(1):43–45

Royal College of Nursing (RCN) 1946 Report of the Nursing Reconstruction Committee (Horder Report). RCN, London

Royal College of Nursing (RCN) 1984/85 Changing provision for sick children and diseases in childhood in Liverpool since 1850. RCN Bulletin 6. RCN, London

Robertson J 1953 A two-year-old goes to hospital. A scientific film record. Concord Film Council, Ipswich, Suffolk

Robertson J 1955 Young children in long-term hospitals. Nursing Times September 23:63–65

Robertson J 1968 The long-stay children in hospital. Maternal and Child Care 4:161–166

Robertson J 1969 John 17 months, 9 days in a residential nursery (film). Tavistock Institute for Human Relations, London

Robertson J 1970 Young children in hospital, 2nd edn. Tavistock, London

Robertson J 1989 Separation and the very young. Free Association Books, London

Schwartzman HB 1978 Transformations. Plenum Press, New York

Scraton P (ed.) 1997 Childhood in crisis. UCL Press, London

Seidler E 1990 An historical survey of children's hospitals. In: Granshaw L, Porter R (eds) The hospital in history. Routledge, London

Singer JL 1973 The child's world of make-believe. Academic Press, New York

Smallman S 1998 Children's nursing in Europe. Paediatric Nursing 11(11):6

Stone L 1977 The family, sex and marriage in England 1500–1800. Harper and Row, New York

Twistington-Higgins T 1952 Great Ormond Street 1852–1952. Odhams Press, Watford

United Kingdom Central Council (UKCC) 1986 Project 2000: a new preparation for practice. UKCC, London

United Kingdom Central Council (UKCC) 1999 Fitness for practice. UKCC, London

United Kingdom Central Council (UKCC) 2001 Fitness for practice and purpose. UKCC, London

United Nations General Assembly 1989 Convention on the rights of the child. UNICEF, Geneva

Watt S, Mitchell R 1995 Historical perspectives. In: Carter B, Dearnum A (eds) Child health care nursing. Concepts, theory and practice. Blackwell Science, Oxford

West C 1854 How to nurse sick children. Longman, Brown, Green and Longman, London

While A 1991 An evaluation of a paediatric home care service. Journal of Advanced Nursing 90(12):1413–1421

Whiting M 2000 1888–1988 100 years of community children's nursing. In: Muir J, Sidey A (eds) Textbook of community children's nursing. Balliére Tindall/Royal College of Nursing, London

Wood CJ 1888 The training of nurses for sick children. The Nursing Record December 6:507–510

Chapter Two

2

Working with Children and Families

Anna L Hemphill, Annette K Dearmun

ABSTRACT

The primary aim of this chapter and its companion PowerPoint presentation is to introduce ways of assessing the psychosocial needs of children and families and provide some tools that the health professional can draw on when working collaboratively with families. The assessment strategy is underpinned by a family systems approach and by Erikson's (1963) developmental model.

Learning Outcomes

- Recognise the value of working with the family as a system.
- Appreciate the theoretical concepts underpinning this approach.
- Develop the knowledge base underpinning a psychosocial assessment of the child and family.

Introduction

Since the 1980s there has been a sea change in the nature of children's nursing, from a focus on giving direct, 'hands on' care to working in a partnership with the family, providing support in the family's management of the care of the child and the impact that this has on their lives. There is a growing awareness that this facilitation can be more effective if the needs and resources of the family as a whole are understood (Whyte 1992).

Consideration of the family as the unit of care has been demonstrated for over a decade, in the work of American and Canadian writers (Friedemann 1989, Friedman 1998,

Wright & Leahey 1994). More recently, this concept of family nursing entered the British literature through the work of Whyte (1992, 1996, 1997). Although a family-centred approach to the care of the sick child is not new to children's nursing, the family was traditionally seen in relation to its ability to care for the child. In other words, the family was viewed as the context of the child. A family systems approach is a new orientation in that the focus of care is on the needs of the whole family. This demands an understanding of family dynamics in relation to a given situation, and the whole family becomes 'the client' (Friedemann 1989).

Consider the needs of the family in the scenario below.

Scenario

Richard, aged 18 months, sustained a head injury in a road traffic accident at the age of 1 year and has been in hospital and ventilated since then. He is to be discharged home. He has two siblings, a newborn baby brother and a 4-year-old sister who is just about to start school. Richard's father has recently started up his own furniture business and his grandmother, who lives locally, has just had a hip replacement.
- What are the stresses on this family?
- What are the strengths and resources?
- What would a health professional need to understand in order to devise a realistic, workable plan of care?

To work with this family in an effective, supportive and empowering way it would be necessary to understand how the family functions on both a practical and an emotional level. This understanding might be gained by spending time with the family and getting to know the individual family members. However, without a clear psychosocial assessment strategy, the family's needs might not be fully explored and important factors that could influence the family's coping might be missed.

Throughout this chapter, a systematic approach to the psychosocial assessment of child and family is advocated. This approach can be used in any setting and is valid for all children and families, including those requiring relatively short-term acute care, for example a child hospitalised for a tonsillectomy, and those requiring longer-term support, for example a child with cystic fibrosis.

The first part of this chapter explores the principles and beliefs underpinning the family systems approach. This is followed by a discussion of the value of psychosocial assessment. Finally, the elements of assessment are discussed, including relevant theory and practical application.

What is a Family?

Activity

- Think about the different types of family.
- Now do the activity on the Evolve website.

It is generally accepted that the family is the basic unit of society. However, many assumptions are made about what constitutes a family. At face value 'the family' might seem to be a very straightforward concept, readily understood but rarely contemplated. However, although families have internalised values and traditions, they do not exist in isolation but are influenced and determined by society and cultural norms. It is important to remember that, as such, they take many diverse forms and are open to many interpretations. In essence, the family is who it identifies itself to be, and therefore a family assessment should start by asking the family 'who is in this family?'.

Understanding the Family as a System

Thinking about the family as a system is a helpful way of understanding how families function. Family systems theory underpins the approach to psychosocial assessment taken in this chapter. First postulated by Von Bertalanffy (1968), it provides the theoretical underpinning to family therapy and this in turn has formed the fundamental basis for understanding the family within family nursing (Wright & Leahey 1994). The family is seen as a system of humans in interaction with one another (Jones 1993). It is open, in that interaction occurs with the environment outside it and influences both the family system and the environment. Change in one part of the system, for

example a child becoming ill, will influence interactions throughout the system.

Wright & Leahey (1994) have identified five concepts that provide a theoretical foundation for understanding the family as a system. The following explanation draws heavily on their work. Overall, it can be seen that communication and feedback mechanisms are important in the functioning of the family (Whyte 1997):

- **Concept 1: A family system is part of a larger supra-system and is also composed of many subsystems.** The family is part of larger supra-systems, for example its local community. Within the family there will be important subsystems, for example, the parental subsystem and the sibling subsystem. Family systems have emotional boundaries that help to establish what is inside the system and what is outside it.

- **Concept 2: The family as a whole is greater than a sum of its parts.** The family's wholeness is more than just the addition of another member. You can understand an individual better by understanding the way his or her family works.

- **Concept 3: A change in one family member affects all family members.** For example, the illness of a child impacts on all roles and relationships within the family: the mother's role, the father's role, their relationship, the sibling's roles and their relationship to their parents and to the sick sibling.

- **Concept 4: A family is able to create a balance between change and stability.** There is always change within families as individual members develop and change. Families adjust continually to incorporate these changes and maintain some stability. At times, family life can be dominated by change, for example when a family moves to a different country or when a family member dies. At other times stability seems to dominate.

- **Concept 5: Family members' behaviour is best understood from a view of circular rather than linear causality.** This is illustrated in the following scenario

Scenario

Mary is a 3-year-old girl who has begun to wet the bed again after the birth of her sibling. When she wets the bed her mother gets angry and slaps her.

From the perspective of *linear causality*, the child wetting the bed causes the mother to slap her: event A causes event B.

However, from the perspective of *circular causality*, the mother's anger and slap in turn affects the child's bedwetting – the child becomes more anxious and therefore more likely to wet the bed again. Thus the cycle continues: event A affects event B, which in turn affects event A and so on.

From the perspective of circular causality, each person mutually contributes to interactions. This is an empowering rather than blaming perspective in that no one individual is viewed as causing negative situations/problems.

These concepts are further illustrated on the Evolve website, where the family system is influenced by the introduction of an additional family member.

In summary there are there are three important concepts (Whyte 1997)

- change/stability
- circularity
- boundaries.

Undertaking a Psychosocial Assessment of the Family

Assessment is not just about gathering information it is also about establishing a relationship with a family and conveying concern about them as individuals and as a unit. The two core beliefs underpinning the family nursing approach are that:

- the central nursing function is to empower the family
- the family is capable of identifying its own needs and devising ways of meeting them.

The assessment can be a process of discovery for the family as well as for the practitioner. It prompts the family to think and talk about aspects of the family that they might not have discussed together before. Gaining an understanding of the family system will help the practitioner and family to identify ways of managing the family's problems.

The form of assessment discussed here would be helpful to anyone working with children and families. Experience from teaching and practising this form of assessment as part of a multidisciplinary course suggests that it has value for a range of practitioners working in community and acute settings who aim to take a holistic view of the child and family.

The approach is strongly influenced by Wright & Leahey's (1994) work on family nursing but also draws on Erikson's (1963) work on psychosocial development. It includes assessment of:

- family structure: using genograms and ecomaps as assessment tools (Wright & Leahey 1994)
- family development: including using an understanding of the family life cycle (Carter & McGoldrick 1989) and individual psychosocial development (Erikson 1963)
- family functioning: including problem solving, values and beliefs, communication, emotional life and alliances

and boundaries (Bentovim & Bingley Miller 2001, Whyte 1997).

Each of these aspects will be addressed later in the chapter.

Throughout the process, the practitioner works with the family and helps it to identify its problems and mobilise its own coping resources (Whyte 1997).

Guidelines for Effective Practice

The practitioner shares his or her understanding that the health problem of the child is likely to have an effect on the whole family and that the practitioner is therefore interested in the health of the whole family. When undertaking an assessment it is important to transmit acceptance of the family as it is and to phrase questions in a way that is not discriminatory or value laden.

Reflect on your Practice

How do you ask questions when you are undertaking assessment? Look at the following question:
- 'What does your husband do?' (i.e. 'What is your husband's occupation?')

What expectations, judgements and assumptions are conveyed in this question? How could you rephrase the question to remove these?

This question could be conceived to be judgemental on a number of counts. It implies that matrimony and employment of the husband are the only acceptable states. It does not allow for the fact the mother might be unmarried, widowed, divorced or in a same-sex relationship. Perhaps it is important to reflect on the reason for wanting to know about 'the husband'. If the intention is to gain knowledge about possible social support it might be more helpful to ask an open question that has the potential to elicit important information about the other significant family members. For example, 'Does anyone else help you to look after John?'

Assessment of Family Structure

GENOGRAMS AND ECOMAPS

These give information about the internal structure of the family and of its wider context. When assessing family structure the creation of a genogram (family diagram or family tree) is a valuable place to start an assessment for several reasons because it:

- summarises information about a family in a short period of time and in a simple way

- provides a vehicle for gaining insight into family development and functioning
- offers new insights to the family and can be a catalyst for change
- engages children, parents and adolescents in the assessment process.

A genogram broadly follows the conventions of a genetic chart. Usually at least three generations of a family are recorded, each generation occupying a separate horizontal level on the chart (Fig. 2.1).

Activity

Create a genogram for your family:
- Represent males by a square and females by a circle.
- Represent marriage or common-law relationships by a horizontal line joining the partners.
- Denote children by a vertical line dropping down from this horizontal; they should be represented in birth order, eldest to the left.
- Record the name and age of the individual within his or square/circle.

A variety of symbols are used to convey information. Those in common use are shown in Fig. 2.2.

TIPS FOR CREATING A GENOGRAM

The following helpful hints for constructing genograms have been informed by Levac & Leahey (1997):

- Define the extent and nature of the information required because this will determine the number of generations to be included in the genogram. If the concern is to identify support available within the family and/or if the child's health problem is influenced in any way by the grandparents then a three-generational genogram will be useful. When the child/family has minor health needs then a two-generational genogram might suffice. The practitioner should be guided by the family and include those whom the family feels are significant.

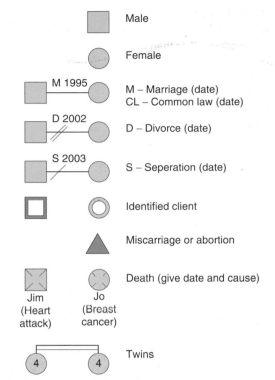

Fig. 2.2 • Common symbols used in genograms.

- Consider ways in which the child and family can be involved in the process. To maximise the value of the genogram as a vehicle to initiate conversation and establish rapport it is important to engage the family in the exercise. This can be achieved via a number of strategies:
  - begin by asking simple and concrete questions, e.g. age, occupation, hobbies, health, school, favourite games
  - when the family appears comfortable, move the discussion to more complex issues, e.g. sibling relationships or parental concerns. If there is a step family it will be relevant to ask questions about custody and contact with the non-custodial parent

Fig. 2.1 • A genogram of the Taylor family.

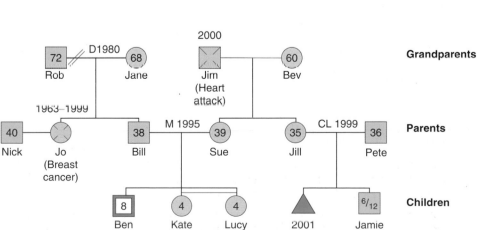

- if appropriate, ask family members how an absent family member might answer the questions
- overtly value each family member
- encourage the child's active participation by taking into account his or her developmental age, asking the questions at an appropriate level and interpreting non-verbal as well as verbal responses
- evaluate the contribution of young people – their inhibitions might prevent them from participating directly and it might be necessary to ask other family members about them.
- Observe the family's non-verbal communication throughout the process and take note of how family members express themselves as well as of the actual content (what is said).

ECOMAPS

Further insight into the family support network can be gained by creating an ecomap. An ecomap depicts the family members' interactions with the wider community. The family genogram is placed in the centre of a circle. Individuals, groups and institutions to whom the family relate are shown around the outside of the circle. Lines are drawn between family members and these outside contacts to show the nature of the relationship. Several lines represent strong connections, single lines represent weaker connections and slashed lines represent stressful relationships. Arrows can be used to illustrate the direction of flow of energy and resources. An ecomap for the Taylor family is shown in Fig. 2.3.

 Activity

Consider this ecomap for the Taylor family (Fig. 2.3) together with the information about the family below:

Bill, Sue, Ben, Lucy and Kate are placed in the central circle. Sue gains support from her mother, from her friend and neighbour Nicola, and from her health visitor. She finds her relationship with her sister stressful and demanding. Both Sue and Bill go to church regularly and place a strong value on their life within the church. Bill has strong connections with work. He coaches a boys' football team on Saturday morning. Ben enjoys going along with him to play. Lucy and Kate are twins.

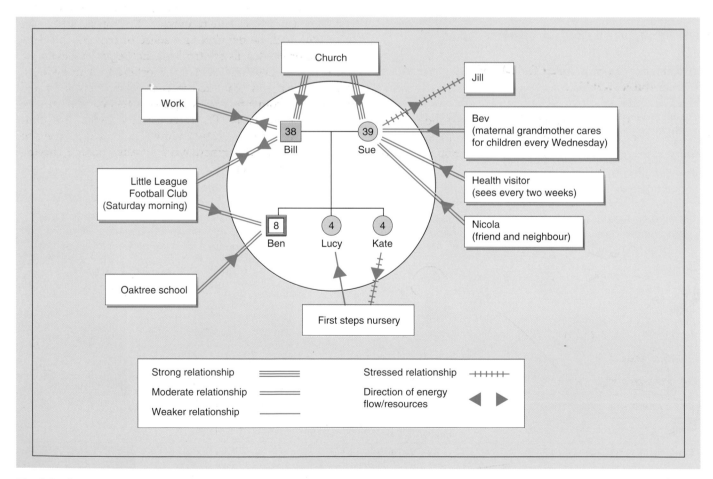

Fig. 2.3 • An ecomap of the Taylor family.

They go to nursery where Lucy has settled in well but Kate still finds it stressful and is reluctant to leave Sue.

In summary, genograms and ecomaps enable the practitioner to gain awareness of the internal structure of the family and of its wider context. It also provides the opportunity to begin to assess demands on the family, sources of stress and support available to the family.

Assessing Child and the Family Development

Consideration of the psychosocial development of the child and family will give insight into the stresses and challenges faced by individual family members and by the family as a whole. It is important to consider the usual developmental changes that all individuals and families experience over time because these influence and will be influenced by any health problem. In addition, the way in which a child copes with a situation will be influenced by past developmental experiences.

Two theories can help with this:

- Erikson's (1963) theory of the psychosocial development of the individual
- family life cycle theory.

PSYCHOSOCIAL DEVELOPMENT OF THE INDIVIDUAL

Erikson's (1963) theory is still widely accepted and used to aid understanding of children's behaviours and emotions. He presents eight stages of psychosocial development covering the whole lifecycle (Table 2.1).

The individual is faced with particular developmental tasks at each age-related stage. These tasks are a response to:

- the individual's physical and cognitive maturation
- societal demands
- cultural expectations.

Erikson refers to the individual's experience of working through the task as a crisis. Crisis in this context refers to normal stresses rather than extraordinary life events. The crisis requires the individual to make a fundamental shift in perspective. This experience is characterised both by the individual's increased vulnerability and by his or her heightened potential. The tasks are expressed as a pair of alternative orientations or 'attitudes' towards life, the self and other people. Ideally, the individual achieves a healthy balance between these. For example, in relation to the first stage (0–1 year) – trust versus mistrust – the infant would emerge with a generally optimistic view of life, trusting that his or her needs would be met. The infant would also have some awareness of danger, that some people/situations were not to be trusted.

The ages at which individuals experience each developmental stage are likely to vary. Furthermore, the stages are not discrete – they tend to overlap. So, for example, the infant will still be developing a sense of trust at the time when he or she learns to stand up and begins to develop a sense of autonomy. It is also important to acknowledge that each stage is grounded in those that precede it and that issues from previous stages of development can be revisited at any time. The developmental stages of children are discussed in detail below. The stages relating to adulthood are described within the accompanying PowerPoint presentation.

Table 2.1 Erikson's Eight Stages of Psychosocial Development

Stage	Age	Personality strength
1. Trust versus mistrust	0–1 years	Hope
2. Autonomy versus shame and doubt	1–3 years	Will
3. Initiative versus guilt	3–5: play age	Purpose
4. Industry versus inferiority	6–11: school age	Competence
5. Identity versus role confusion	Adolescence	Fidelity
6. Intimacy versus isolation	Young adulthood	Love
7. Generativity versus stagnation	Middle adulthood	Care
8. Integrity versus despair	Old age	Wisdom

PowerPoint

Access the companion PowerPoint presentation and read more about the adult stages of psychosocial development.

Stages 1 to 5 of Erikson's Theory of Psychosocial Development

1. Trust Versus Mistrust: Age 0–1 Year

The foundation of the development of a healthy personality is the establishment of basic trust. Erikson defines this as: 'An essential trustfulness in others as well as a fundamental sense of one's own trustworthiness' (1968 p 96).

The baby's relationship with a mothering figure is central to his or her development of trust. Consistency and dependability are important qualities in the parent. If the baby's physical and psychological needs are sensitively met, i.e. the baby is fed when hungry, reassured when frightened and comforted when in pain, then he or she will learn to trust that needs will be met. This leads to the development of a generally optimistic outlook. Erikson termed this the ego quality of 'hope'.

This understanding of this stage of development is commensurate with the perspective of those who understand attachment as a vital process within the first years of life. Klein (1940), a child psychoanalyst, identified processes of splitting and projection to be the predominant unconscious defence mechanisms used by young children to avoid pain. Splitting is the process of dividing feelings into different elements, such as good and bad. Projection is the process of locating feelings in others rather than oneself. A baby projects feelings onto the mother to rid him- or herself of the feelings, but also in the hope that the mother will contain the feelings and take on board what the baby cannot, and therefore help the baby experience the feelings as bearable.

This is one of the basic processes that provide the foundation for the development of attachment. Two different scenarios can be used to illustrate this process.

Scenario

Robert feels angry and cries. His mother picks him up, cuddles and reassures him. She 'copes with' the bad feelings. The baby feels better. The mother has contained the feelings. The baby begins to trust that he is safe. A secure attachment is developing.

Scenario

Roberta feels angry and cries. The mother hears and feels angry too. She shouts at the baby. The baby's feelings are not contained by the mother. The baby begins to mistrust her mother and herself. An insecure attachment is developing.

It is important, then, that the parent is able to enter the internal world of the baby, to imagine the world from the baby's point of view and use this empathy to respond to the baby's feelings. The baby can then view the world as a safe place. Erikson writes of a favourable ratio between trust and mistrust. It is important that babies have some sense of mistrust if they are to be alert to danger and recognise those who are not trustworthy. If, however, the baby develops an overriding sense of mistrust, of both self and others, the child – and later the adult – might be withdrawn, suspicious and lacking in self-confidence. Related to this, those who have insecure attachments to their primary carers can find it difficult to empathise with the feelings of others and might lack self-esteem.

2. Autonomy Versus Shame and Doubt: Age 1–3 Years

The neurological and muscular development of the young child facilitates the development of autonomy. Toddlers can walk, explore and 'get into everything'; they are also able to talk, and particularly to say 'no'. At this age they are also able to become continent. A central theme at this stage is 'holding on and letting go'. This does not apply only to bowel control but more globally to the child's struggle for autonomy and self-control. This is reflected in the child's behaviour in many ways. The toddler might cuddle into their mother then aggressively push away from her, they might hoard treasured toys one day then throw them out of the window the next (Erikson 1963). They are primarily trying to exercise a choice (Crain 1988) and to exert their will.

The task is to develop a healthy balance between a sense of autonomy, or self-control, and a sense of shame and doubt, that is, of being 'not good enough'. The child's sense of autonomy comes from within; the sense of shame and doubt comes from the child's social world, through his or her experience of social expectations and regulation. Children need to be able to exert their will while being aware of their capacity for evoking a negative response and of the need to comply with social rules.

Parenting a toddler can be challenging and experienced as a battle of wills (Miller 1993). The aim in relation to Erikson's tasks is to help children learn social behaviour without crushing their will – their desire for free choice (Stevens 1983). Giving children manageable responsibilities, for example, clearing their plate from the table or putting rubbish in the bin, then thanking them respectfully for doing it, will build their confidence in their abilities. Conversely, overcontrolling or critical responses to children's efforts to do things for themselves, or shaming them when they lack self-control (e.g. wet their pants), can lead to feelings that they are not good enough and doubts about their self control and independence.

3. Initiative Versus Guilt: Age 3–5 Years

At this age, children explore what kind of a person they are going to be. They are interested in sex roles, differences and relationships. They consider 'Will I grow up to be a mummy or a daddy?'. They rival the same-sex parent for the love of the other. Girls might transfer affections from their mother to their father, whereas boys compete with their father for their mother's affections. They imitate their parents and want to be like them and do what they do. They are also interested in adult roles and might declare ambitions to be a fireman, nurse or spaceman.

Through play, children learn about taking the initiative, forming and carrying out goals and competing. Their play is imaginative and used to explore roles and act out fantasies. For children to become socialised their drive to take the initiative needs to be tempered by inhibition, so that they learn not to impinge on the rights of others. They develop a conscience (a super ego), so that if they transgress social rules they feel guilty. Again the aim is to achieve a balance. An over-riding sense of guilt can result in overobedience, conformity and an inability to act out what is desired, so that the individual's emotional self might become hidden. In later years this can result in an inhibited and self-restricted personality (Stevens 1983).

To support children through this stage, Erikson (1963) suggests that parents ease their authority and foster children's desire to 'help' by involving them as equals in interesting projects. Their ambition is then channelled into socially useful activities.

1. Industry Versus Inferiority: Age 6–11 Years

The process of learning dominates this stage. This occurs in many settings: school, home, on the street, in clubs and from peers. The child's developing cognitive skills, including operational thinking, memory, problem solving and ability to separate fact from fiction, all facilitate learning and development of social skills.

Children of this age want to engage in tasks and activities and to carry them through to completion. They strive for the sense of competence that their industry can bring them, whether it is by scoring a goal or completing a painting. Their role models are those who know things and how to do things (Erikson 1968), for example, teachers and sports stars. They learn to cooperate with others, to compete and to follow the rules. Children often play within same-sex groups.

Feelings of limitless ability need to be checked by an awareness of one's genuine limitations if optimal development is to occur (Kroger 1996). Children become aware of being judged by their performance. The hurt of failure in class or at play is a common experience and the danger of this stage is that feelings of inadequacy can come to dominate the way children see themselves. These feelings can prevent a child from trying for fear of failure. Unresolved conflicts from previous stages can influence experience so, for example, children who developed more doubt than autonomy in the second stage might be unsure of themselves as they try to master new tasks (Crain 1988).

Erikson (1968) emphasises that parents and teachers play a crucial role in fostering either industry or inferiority. Praise and reward for a job well done will build the child's sense of competence; criticism will undermine it.

5. Identity Versus Role Confusion: Adolescence

The central psychosocial task for adolescents is to achieve a unique identity. This involves gaining a clear sense of who they are, what they believe in and the social and occupational roles they wish to pursue (Erikson 1968). Trust, autonomy, initiative and industry all contribute to the young person's identity, which has been forming throughout childhood. Identity formation reaches a crisis in adolescence when young people have to separate from their parents and commit themselves to a set of values, a sexual identity and a vocation (Kroger 1996).

The rapid physical growth and changes of puberty, and the accompanying sexual and aggressive drives, make this a turbulent time when 'trust in the body is shaken' (Wong 1995) and it is hard to know who you are. The following behaviours are typical and normal for young people going through the process of discovering who they are:

- risk-taking behaviour, e.g. smoking, drinking, using drugs, dangerous sports
- healthy assertion and rebellion, e.g. pushing parental boundaries, staying out late
- transferring dependency onto peers and/or a best friend
- trying out new roles, e.g. within religious or political movements
- some rejection of society's norms
- changeable mood, i.e. risking expressing what they feel
- peers alongside parents setting standards
- 'hanging out' with peers
- mobilising energy into action
- deviant self-image they can respect
- privacy and secrecy.

James Marcia (1966) elaborated on Erikson's description of this stage of development through his research on the identity formation process. He identified four identity statuses as described by Miller (1993):

1. **Identity diffusion.** The individual has not yet experienced an identity crisis, nor has he or she made any commitment to a vocation or set of beliefs. There is no indication that he or she is actively trying to make a commitment.

2. **Identity foreclosure.** The individual has not experienced a crisis but nevertheless is committed in his or her goals

and beliefs, largely as a result of choices made by others (often parents).

3. **Moratorium.** The individual is in a state of crisis and is actively searching in an attempt to arrive at a choice of identity.

4. **Identity achievement.** The individual has experienced a crisis, has resolved it on his or her own terms and is now firmly committed to an occupation, ideology and social roles.

Those experiencing one of the first three statuses have not formed an independent identity. They are therefore likely to exhibit some of the following features of role confusion:

- intense attachments: typically, difficulty in detaching themselves from parents, particularly the parent of the opposite sex (Marcia 1979)
- dependency on and imitation of parents: common in those with identity foreclosure
- solitary activity: particularly those with identity diffusion
- overobedience to parents
- unexpressed emotion
- anxiety over puberty
- no idealised future roles
- frustration.

Problems associated with role confusion include anxiety, depression and problems with independence.

As with all the stages of development, individuals will progress through the stages over different periods of time. Some individuals will achieve an identity by late adolescence, others in their early twenties and others might live with role confusion for many years and come to address identity issues later in their adult life.

The Value of Psychosocial Developmental Assessment

When trying to understand a child's feelings and psychosocial needs it is helpful to look at both the way the child is now and at his or her developmental history. The following case study illustrates how this aspect of assessment can be useful.

Scenario

Ben is coming into hospital to have a tonsillectomy. Ben is 8 years old and lives with his parents, Sue and Bill, and his younger twin sisters, Lucy and Kate, who are 4 years old (see the genogram of Ben's family in Fig. 2.1). Ben attends primary school, where he enjoys art and playing football, both of which his parents say he is very good at.

Ben's current behaviour

At his preadmission assessment visit, Ben's parents report difficult behaviour that they are struggling to manage, particularly aggression. Ben has anger outbursts during which he might kick furniture or throw things. He doesn't listen, especially when disciplining is involved. He is very active and always on the go or fiddling. At home he rarely sits still for long, except when he's playing on his play station, which he can play for an hour or more. Homework is a difficult time and it is hard to get Ben to do it. His parents have found that sitting next to him and encouraging him from start to finish works. Ben finds it difficult to wait for anything and wants it immediately. He does have friends but finds it difficult to share and compromise.

Developmental history

Ben was born of a planned pregnancy. Sue describes him as being a wriggly, noisy baby who cried a lot. She found him hard to soothe. She breastfed him for 3 months before bottle feeding him. She thinks she had postnatal depression (PND) that was not identified. She found the first 2 years very difficult and felt anxious at times about going out with Ben on her own and embarrassed at not being able to control Ben in front of others. Ben achieved his developmental milestones satisfactorily and attended nursery when he was two and a half.

Review of Ben's development in relation to Erikson's psychosocial stages of development

This assessment can be used to consider Ben's development in relation to the psychosocial tasks.

- *Trust versus mistrust:* from this initial assessment we know that Sue had PND and found her relationship with Ben difficult when he was a baby. Research suggests that mothers with PND find it more difficult to contain their baby's feelings (Goldberg 2000). It is therefore possible that Ben's development of a sense of trust might have been negatively affected. This could have contributed to his anxiety regarding getting his needs met immediately and might have left him lacking self-confidence/esteem.
- *Autonomy versus shame and doubt:* at this stage Sue reports feeling anxious about managing Ben's behaviour, particularly in public. Her doubts in relation to parenting Ben at this stage might have led to rather unclear boundaries. This could explain why Ben does not seem to have achieved a strong sense of self-control. His difficulty in complying with social rules suggests he has doubts about his ability to control himself and the world around him.
- *Initiative versus guilt:* Ben would have been at this stage when his twin sisters were born. His parents have not specifically mentioned Ben's experience of this stage but a nurse might be curious about how he reacted to the changes the birth of his sisters had on the family.

- *Industry versus inferiority:* strengths relating to this current stage include Ben's enjoyment of art and football and the related positive feedback he gets from parents and peers. He seems to have some difficulty starting and sticking at tasks he perceives as challenging, e.g. homework. This might be because his doubts about his ability (stemming from the earlier stage, autonomy versus shame and doubt) have made it difficult for him to risk trying for fear of failure.

Activity

Implications for Ben's care when in hospital

Think about the psychosocial needs revealed within the above scenario. When Ben comes into hospital for his tonsillectomy, what particular interventions might you use to support Ben and his family?

- Can you think of other interventions that might support Ben?

From this assessment, several interventions can be drawn out which may be supportive to Ben, when caring for him.

Provide boundaries by being clear regarding what you expect Ben to do and by being consistent in your approach.
Aim: to build trust

Give Ben praise and positive attention, particularly when he is faced with new situations or tasks, for example, when having anaesthetic cream applied or when needing to eat and drink postoperatively.
Aim: to build self-esteem

Keep Ben amused with activities he enjoys, such as art.
Aim: to encourage socially acceptable self-expression and build self-esteem

Use behaviour management techniques that encourage Ben to take control such as choices and consequences. For example, 'If you have your bath quickly now there will be time for me to play a game with you before bedtime; if you choose not to have your bath yet there won't be time for a game. Which would you rather do?
Aim: to build Ben's sense of self-control and autonomy

Encourage Ben to show his sisters around the ward when they visit.
Aim: to strengthen his relationship with his sisters and to build his self-esteem

Encourage Ben to phone, e-mail or write to his friends.
Aim: to strengthen peer relationships

It would be helpful to discuss the potential of these interventions with Ben's parents, to check whether they feel they are appropriate given their knowledge of Ben.

Psychosocial Development of the Family

When undertaking an assessment and supporting a family, consideration of the family's experience of changes as it has developed over time will enhance understanding of its strengths and current sources of stress.

Every family will follow its own unique developmental path, although all families experience changes over time as people enter and leave the family system. Typically, these include events such as birth, raising children, children leaving home, retirement and death.

FAMILY LIFE CYCLE THEORY

Family life cycle theory is grounded in the work of Erikson (see above). The family life cycle is a dynamic process of change that includes all the events, and periods of time between events, experienced by a family. Duvall (1977) described this family life cycle using an eight-stage model. Carter & McGoldrick (1989) built on this work to consider three generations of a family system as it moved through time. They recognised that family stress is often greatest at the times of change that mark the transition from one stage to the next within the family, because these are the times when the greatest emotional demands are made on the family.

PowerPoint

Access the companion PowerPoint presentation and look at Table 1, the stages of the family life cycle.

This life cycle model describes an intact American middle-class family. Carter & McGoldrick (1989) recognise that many trends within contemporary Western society affect change in family life cycle patterns. There is a decreasing birth rate, many couples are choosing to have their children when they are older, and life expectancy is increasing. Women's roles have changed, particularly in relation to work, and dual income households are becoming the norm in many countries. Cohabitation outside marriage, single-parent households, divorce and remarriage are all increasing. Carter & McGoldrick have considered the particular emotional challenges presented by divorce and remarriage. These are discussed within the PowerPoint presentation. Other factors that affect the life cycle include the culture of the family and the economic, political and social context in which they live.

PowerPoint

Access the companion PowerPoint presentation and read about the emotional challenges presented by divorce and remarriage.

Carter & McGoldrick's six-stage model can be criticised for being normative or overgeneralised. Nevertheless, it is helpful to have a model to identify the emotional tasks that need to be undertaken. The practitioner can then consider how the unique developmental path of the individual family might have influenced the emotional tasks it faces. When considering the challenges facing a particular family it is helpful to bear in mind that the family's experience might be considerably more complex than the model suggests. For example, the family could include adolescent children from a previous marriage and a young child from the current cohabiting partnership. The practitioner would then have to consider tasks from the two life cycle stages (families with young children and families with adolescents) and the developmental issues for the reconstituted family.

PowerPoint

Access the companion PowerPoint presentation and look at Table 3.

Carter & McGoldrick's Six Stages in a Family Life Cycle

Stage 1: Leaving Home, Single Young Adults

The task for young adults is to separate from their family of origin and establish an independent identity 'without cutting off or attaching reactively to an emotional surrogate' (Friedman 1998). Friedman (1998) explains that men and women typically face different challenges at this stage due to the way they are socialised. Both need to achieve a balance between autonomy and attachment in relationships and at work. Men have generally been encouraged to seek their identity through self-expression and therefore are more likely to struggle with attachment and commitment. Women have generally been encouraged to define themselves in terms of their relationships with others, their struggle is therefore more likely to relate to issues of autonomy.

Stage 2: Joining of Families, the New Couple

The new couple marks the beginning of a new family; it also represents the joining of two families. The partners bring beliefs from their experience of growing up in their own family. The task of the new couple is therefore to decide which beliefs, traditions and rules it is going to adopt from their families of origin, and which it is going to develop for itself. The members of the couple need to develop a new relationship with each set of parents, which is supportive yet protects the autonomy of their partnership. They will also need to make decisions regarding if and when to have children.

Stage 3: Families with Young Children

This is generally recognised to be the most stressful life transition (Friedman 1998). The parents have to adjust their relationship to make space for the child(ren). There are the extra demands of meeting the child's needs while continuing to meet one another's personal needs. Childrearing, financial and household tasks can all be sources of stress. This stage often coincides with parent's heavy involvement in career development and with financial resources being stretched. Juggling work and childcare is likely to present financial and emotional challenges.

Stage 4: Families with Adolescents

The central developmental task of this stage is to balance freedom with responsibility as teenagers mature and become increasingly autonomous. This requires renegotiation of boundaries and demands that parents begin to 'let go' of the adolescent while still providing for his or her dependency needs. For the parents, reduction in the dependency of their child(ren) and the adolescent's questioning of values and life style can refocus their attention on their marriage and career issues, and this phase is usually a time of exploration and refocusing. The ageing of grandparents can bring a change from receiving support from them to needing to support them.

Stage 5: Launching Children and Moving On

This phase can be a lengthy one, with many exits from and entries into the family. Increasingly, young adults are choosing to live at home with their parents, often for economic reasons. Consequently, the anticipated empty nest can be delayed by several years. There is a need to review and restructure the marital relationship once day-to-day parenting responsibilities cease. Parents and children need to renegotiate their roles so that they relate to one another as adults rather than parent and child. Parents might also need to adjust to include their child's partner and possibly grandchildren within the family. The responsibility for caring for the older generation can make considerable demands on the couple, both practically and emotionally, and might include coping with the death of parents.

Stage 6: Families in Later Life

This stage begins with the retirement and lasts until both spouses have died. It can span 20 to 30 years and the central process during this time is to accept the shift of generational roles. Tasks during this stage include adapting to new social roles, such as being grandparents, supporting the older generation and coping with loss. Stressors or losses commonly experienced by ageing people and families include economic, housing, social, work and health losses (Friedman 1998).

In summary, a sound knowledge of family development can help a practitioner to think about and assess the stresses experienced by the family. In many cases it helps to look beyond the immediately obvious stresses associated with the family's current circumstances, for example anxiety over the child illness, and to consider other issues that are concerning the family and which need to be acknowledged when helping the family find realistic ways of managing its situation.

Assessing Family Functioning

The seminal work of Epstein et al (1978) – the McMaster model of family functioning – underpins the assessment of family functioning as described by family nursing writers such as Friedman (1998), Whyte (1997) and Wright & Leahey (1994). The following suggestions for assessing family functioning draw on the work of these writers, and also on Bentovim & Bingley Miller's (2001) work on family assessment. This later work is particularly useful because the writers take the family's ability to meet the needs of children as a central focus within their approach.

The aim of functional assessment is to observe how family members interact and influence each other. In this way, individual family members' behaviour can be understood within the context of the family. It is important to assess the family's strengths as well as its difficulties. Recognition of strengths by the practitioner and, most importantly, by the family members themselves, is helpful because these strengths can be a major resource when working to resolve problems.

ASPECTS TO ASSESS

Problem Solving

One of the practitioner's goals is to support the family in solving its problems. It is therefore beneficial to have some insight into the family's problem-solving style and its ability to solve its own problems. A discussion of the way in which the family has managed past problems can give the practitioner and family insight into this. It is helpful to consider both practical and emotional problems.

- **Practical problem solving:** relating to how practical tasks are achieved within the family. For example, if parents both work then ascertaining what they did when their child had chickenpox and had to be off school would give the nurse insight into who takes responsibility for solving problems and also whether the family relies on those within the family (extended family) at times of need or seeks help outside the family.

- **Emotional problem solving:** sometimes problem solving is on an emotional level, an example of this is coping with jealousy between siblings.

 Activity

Alice is Jim's younger sister, she is 1 year old and, since her birth, Jim had displayed outward signs of aggression and jealousy.
- Think about questions you could ask to find out how the parents coped with this

The parents' explanation will give insight into how the problem is understood and whether they agree about solutions to emotional problems within the family. It might also give insight into how the parents control their children's behaviour.

Beliefs and Values

A family belief system is the family's way of knowing and understanding the world. It is made up of all the shared assumptions, values, myths and traditions that guide the family's behaviour

 Reflect on your Practice

Think about your own family:
- Note down any family myths, values and traditions. You might like to think particularly about beliefs in relation to health, education or children.
- How were these beliefs expressed?

For example, in relation to health one family might believe that the best way to manage illnesses is to allow the body to heal itself supported by homeopathic remedies, and thus family members will rarely go to their GP. Another family might believe that it is always safest to get professional advice and will visit the GP regularly, often with minor illnesses.

Beliefs are handed down through families from one generation to the next, and can be a very powerful influence on the way a family copes with stresses. Carter & McGoldrick (1989) conceptualise the flow anxiety in a family as being vertical and horizontal. Vertical, or transgenerational, stresses are the beliefs and patterns of functioning that flow through the generations. These interact with the horizontal stresses experienced by the family in the 'here and now' as a result of both predictable life cycle stresses, such as the birth of a baby, and unpredictable events, such as the baby having a congenital facial disfigurement. In this situation, if, for example, physical beauty is highly prized and a source of power within the family through the generations, then the baby's appearance will create more intensive stress than would have been the case if less importance was attached to physical attractiveness.

Family Communication

Communication affects all aspects of family life. The way a family communicates influences the self-esteem of family members and the children's development, particularly in relation to verbal and reading skills. Special care must be taken when working with families with a different first language to your own. It is important to appreciate the cultural expectations regarding communication within the family.

Effective communication requires messages to be clearly expressed and to be received and responded to. In families with communication strengths as identified by Bentovim and Bingley Miller (2001):

- People can express themselves clearly, directly and openly.
- Verbal messages will be matched by non-verbal communication (facial expression, body language) and by tone of voice.
- Family members listen and respond to what others say.
- All family members participate in conversations.
- The family can talk something over and move it on.

Families in which there are communication difficulties might exhibit some of the following problems as identified by Bentovim and Bingley Miller (2001)

- Communications are unclear or inhibited, e.g. whispered or poorly articulated.
- There is a mismatch between what is said and the tone of voice and/or non-verbal messages that accompany it. For example, 'I'm fine' might be said in an angry tone and accompanied by a glare and the slamming of a door as the person exits the room. This type of communication is ambiguous and confusing.
- People do not listen to or acknowledge what others communicate, or respond in inappropriate ways.
- In conversations, one or more family members dominate and others find it difficult to participate or are excluded.
- When the family tries to talk something over it tends to get stuck or it might return to the same topic repeatedly.

Most families will exhibit some strengths and some occasional difficulties. In families in which difficulties dominate it will be difficult for the family members to resolve problems together.

The Emotional Life of the Family

This is not easy to assess but it is important because it colours the whole way that life is experienced within the family. It is useful to consider how feelings are expressed within the family and also, less tangibly, how it might feel to be in the family.

In families in which emotional expression is a strength, a wide range of feelings will be expressed, the intensity of feelings will be appropriate to the situation referred to, and family members recognise each others' feelings and respond to them appropriately. In families in which emotional expression presents difficulties, expression of feelings might be generally discouraged, or certain feelings might not be expressed, for example, anger. The intensity of feelings expressed might not seem to match the situation, being either heightened and possibly overwhelming, or diminished and flat. Feelings expressed by others will not always be responded to helpfully. Physical or psychological symptoms can be a way of expressing feelings in families who have difficulties communicating.

When considering how it might feel to be in the family it is helpful to think about the overall feel of the family and the way family members treat one another. The family atmosphere might be generally warm, safe and reasonably relaxed, allowing family members to express themselves freely. Families with some difficulties are more likely to have a tense atmosphere. Where painful or negative emotions dominate, the family atmosphere might feel chaotic, dangerous or panicky. The way that family members treat one another might be mostly supportive and understanding of one another. In families with difficulties in the way they treat one another, family members will not feel valued or expect support from one another and attacking, undermining or rejecting relationships might be observed.

Alliances and Boundaries

Within the family system are subsystems that consist of a relationship or alliance between two or more people. These can be thought of as teams with particular functions (Bentovim & Bingley Miller 2001). It is useful to identify the important subsystems within the family and to consider how well they work, their strengths and difficulties, to identify any relationships that might require particular support.

The couple subsystem: in a family with two adults, the quality of their relationship and the way in which the couple meet one another's emotional and sexual needs will influence all other relationships in the family. In families with difficulties there might be lack of support or warmth within the couple relationship and dissatisfaction with it might be expressed as hostility or open conflict.

The parental subsystem: the task of the parents is to nurture and socialise their children. How well they do this will depend on how well they work as a team. Parents with reasonable strengths will cooperate and support one another, sharing parenting tasks. Difficulties occur when parents disagree about how to deal with the children, undermine one another or are unable to negotiate and compromise.

The sibling subsystem: children's psychosocial development is influenced by their relationship with their siblings. If relationships are affectionate and supportive they can be a source of strength. It is normal for siblings to quarrel and compete for parental attention but difficulties arise if there is continual fighting and rivalry or if children ignore one another.

The boundaries between the different subsystems can be useful to consider. Clear yet permeable boundaries allow flexibility while maintaining the distinct functions of the subsystems (Minuchin 1974). So, for example, in a family with clear intergenerational boundaries, the parents act as parents and the children act as children most of the time. In a family where this boundary is diffuse the child might be given adult responsibilities and power in decision making (Wright & Leahey 1994), or might even take on a parental role in relation to a child-like parent.

The balance between being able to be an independent individual and having a secure sense of belonging is also important. Family members might become overdependent on one another. This enmeshment can make it difficult for young people to act independently or to separate from some members of the family. Alternatively, when boundaries are rigid, individuals might become isolated and disengaged from the family.

In summary, the interaction of family members and the influence they have on each other and the family as a whole are key components of assessment. Family functioning is not something that can be assessed in one sitting. Assessment involves judgement and it is important that this is based on what has been learned from the family. Furthermore, it needs to be specifically described using evidence gained from talking with and observing the family.

Summary

Drawing on the evidence base, this chapter has argued the value of working with the family as a system and has offered some suggestions of how this could be implemented in practice. When conducting a psychosocial assessment of a child and his or her family, a systematic approach that considers the child's development within the context of the family, and the family structure, development and functioning will give a broad understanding of family strengths and problems. Some practitioners might have the confidence and competence to undertake a more detailed assessment of specific areas of family functioning. The framework presented within this chapter is designed to provide a tool to think with rather than to be prescriptive. Assessment should be a continuous process, rather than a single event, and although the initial gathering of information about the family is important, reflection and analysis of that information is essential to understand family strengths and difficulties. This, in turn, will determine the level of support required to maintain or restore equilibrium within the family.

References

Bentovim A, Bingley Miller L 2001 The family assessment: assessment of family competence, strengths and difficulties. Pavilion Publishing, Brighton

Carter B, McGoldrick M 1989 The changing family lifecycle, 2nd edn. Allyn & Bacon, London

Crain WC 1988 Erikson and the eight stages of life. In: Crain WC Theories of development: concepts and applications. Prentice Hall, London

Duvall E 1977 Marriage and family development. Lippincott, Philadelphia

Epstein NB, Bishop DS, Levin S 1978 The McMaster model of family functioning. Journal of Marriage and Family Counselling 4:19–31

Erikson EH 1963 Childhood and society, 2nd edn. Norton, New York

Erikson EH 1968 Identity: youth and crisis. Norton, New York

Friedemann ML 1989 The concept of family nursing. Journal of Advanced Nursing 14:211–216

Friedman MM 1998 Family nursing: theory and practice, 4th edn. Appleton & Lange, Norwalk, CT

Goldberg S 2000 Attachment and development. Arnold, London

Jones E 1993 Family systems therapy. John Wiley, Chichester

Klein M 1940/1975 Mourning and its relation to manic-depressive states. In: Klein M The writings of Melanie Klein, vol 1. Hogarth, London

Kroger J 1996 Adolescence as identity synthesis. Erikson's psychosocial approach. In: Kroger J Identity in adolescence: overview of major theorists, 2nd revised edn. Routledge, London

Levac AM, Leahey M 1997 Children and families: models for assessment and intervention. In: Fox J (ed) Primary healthcare of children. Mosby, Baltimore, MD

Marcia JE 1966 Development and validation of ego identity status. Journal of Personality and Social Psychology 3:551–558

Marcia JE 1979 Identity status in late adolescence: description and some clinical implications. Identity Development Symposium, Gronigen, the Netherlands

Miller PH 1993 Theories of developmental psychology, 3rd edn. WH Freeman, New York

Minuchin S 1974 Families and family therapy. Tavistock, London

Stevens R 1983 The life cycle. In: Stevens R Erik Erikson: an introduction. Open University Press, Buckingham

Von Bertalanffy L 1968 General system theory: foundations, development, applications. Brazillier, New York

Whyte D 1992 A family nursing approach to the care of a child with a chronic illness. Journal of Advanced Nursing 17:317–327

Whyte D 1996 Expanding the boundaries of care. Paediatric Nursing 8(4):10–23

Whyte D 1997 Explorations in family nursing. Routledge, London

Wong DL 1995 Growth and development of children. In: Campbell S, Glasper EA (eds) Whaley and Wong's nursing care of infants and children, 5th edn. CV Mosby, St Louis

Wright LM, Leahey M 1994 Nurses and families: a guide to family assessment and intervention, 2nd edn. FA Davis, Philadelphia

Further Reading

Allmond BW, Buckman W, Gofman HF 1979 The family is the patient. CV Mosby, St Louis

Cramp C, Tripp S, Hughes N, Dale J 2003 Children's home nursing: results of a national survey. Paediatric Nursing 15(8):39–43

Department of Health (DoH) 1991 Welfare of children and young people in hospital. HMSO, London

Department of Health (DoH) 2003 Getting the right start: National Service Framework for Children and Young People and Maternity Services, Part 1: Standard for Hospital Services. HMSO, London

Thornes R 1993 Bridging the gaps. Action for Sick Children, London

Chapter Three

3

Contemporary Child Health Policy: the Implications for Children's Nurses

E Alan Glasper, Susan Lowson

ABSTRACT

The primary aim of this chapter and its companion PowerPoint presentation is to investigate the relationship between child health policy and changes in the pattern of care delivery by children's nurses in the UK since 1959. Although it is not possible to cover all reports or indeed contemporary policy from other countries, a comprehensive range of published reports that demonstrate the complexities of child health policies is reviewed and the success or otherwise of government reforms is discussed. The role of the Health Service Ombudsman is outlined.

Learning Outcomes

- Recognise the impact of child health policy on changes in care delivery for children and their families.
- Appreciate the role of children's nurses in the translation of policy into practice.
- Recognise the barriers to policy recommendations in contemporary healthcare settings.
- Understand that policies can be a powerful weapon for family advocacy.
- Appreciate the role of the complaint process in the clinical governance agenda.
- Recognise the learning opportunities that arise from complaints.
- Understand the role of the nurse in complaint investigations.
- Recognise the effect of the bereavement process in complaint management.

Introduction

The publication of the now famous government white paper *Welfare of children in hospital* (Committee of the Central Health Services Council 1959) was a wake-up call for those healthcare workers involved in the care of sick children in hospital. The knowledge and confirmation that children could be harmed by early psychological traumas provided the necessary stimulus for a growing interest in the adverse events of childhood. The work of John Bowlby and James Robertson (Bowlby 1951, Robertson 1962) had been highly influential in bringing to the public domain the negative effects on development that could occur following a child's stay in hospital. Many of the subsequent policy recommendations reiterated the central tenet of the 1959 welfare document now universally known as the Platt report after its chairman Sir Harry Platt. It would be naïve to suggest that all policy documents published since then have taken a proactive stance, as many have been reactive to events or practices that actually harmed children and their families during the process of care. Current practice is therefore the prime beneficiary of the cumulative successes or otherwise of the implementation of the various policies and reports published since 1959. To suggest that health care for sick children is at an optimum level would be imprudent, and this is exemplified through the necessity for periodic public enquiries when and where poor practice flourishes. Child health policy reviews will therefore continue to play an important part in the evolution of optimum child health care.

The Role of Health Policy

The role of health policy is primarily concerned with maintaining or improving the health of individuals or groups within society. Increasingly, such policies are generated at local, national and international forums for the benefit of all. Despite this, it must be acknowledged that there are gross inequalities in health status among childhood populations both within and outside the UK.

Scenario

Louise is a second-year child branch student who, at a meeting of her weekly learning group, reveals that a number of children have been admitted to her ward suffering from chest infectons. These sick children are predominately from lower socio-economic groups.

Health Inequalities

A report published in 1955 by a joint committee of The Institute of Child Health, The Society of Medical Officers of Health and The Population Investigation Committee (University of London 1955) acknowledged that children from disadvantaged, lower socio-economic, manual labouring families had a higher admission rate to hospital with infections. Overcrowding was cited as a causative agent and was additionally linked to the high level of readmissions in the same group of children. Of historical interest is the reporting of 10% of all admissions being cared for in adult wards and 33% being admitted to wards that allowed no visitors. The final summary point in this report states 'It is too soon to attempt an assessment of the effects of hospitalisation' (University of London 1955 p 3).

Nearly half a century later, Utting (1997) revealed that approximately 15,300 children spent periods of more than a month per year as hospital in-patients. He particularly highlighted the vulnerability of certain categories of children, such as those with disabilities and emotional or behavioural difficulties. Carter (2002), in stating that children's nurses cannot be complacent about the negative effects of healthcare inequality on children, perhaps reinforces the reality that children's nurses can never be mere bystanders in the determination of health and social policy. To this end, children's nurses are helping in the process of setting and implementing policy, and are not simply following it. Utting's report was commissioned after continuing revelations of wide spread abuse of children living away from home, but especially those living in children's homes. The thrust of Utting's report for the NHS was to establish methods of monitoring and safeguarding the welfare of children in hospitals and other NHS settings.

How do Governments Respond to Policy Reviews?

The way in which, for example, the NHS responds to such reports is illuminating and the Utting report (Utting 1997) can serve here as a case in point of how the process works in practice (NHS Executive 1998). The Utting report, under the chairmanship of Sir William Utting, made over 150 recommendations. In response to the report, the government created a ministerial taskforce to advise it on how to respond appropriately to these recommendations. The ministerial taskforce duly reported to the government, which in turn translated some of the key findings into an action plan. This in turn was developed into a Health Service Circular, which was sent for action to, among others all the chief executives of the NHS Trusts in England. (It is important to stress here that Scotland and Wales commission their own policy documents, whereas the Northern Ireland Assembly has thus far primarily followed the English precedent. As a general rule of thumb, UK child health policies are transferable across the four countries of the UK.) The changes, which primarily related to who might or might not work with children, had to be implemented by 1 April 1999. As with other similar reports, the wording used by the NHS Executive was 'Ministers expect' and in this example Regional Offices of the NHS required written confirmation by 31 March 1999 that action had been taken to comply with this circular.

Other reports do not carry the weight of a Health Service Circular and it is for this reason that the reports outlined in this chapter have had mixed success in changing policies towards children requiring health care. For example, the famous Black Report (DHSS 1980) – commissioned by Labour Secretary of State, David Ennals – was predicated on the inability of the NHS to alleviate ill health among the poorest and disadvantaged sectors of society: the reality is that the greatest improvements in health since the foundation of the NHS have been among the upper socio-economic groups. The working party, under the chairmanship of Sir Douglas Black, an eminent and respected physician, uncovered significant weaknesses in the way that health services were delivered. Black's account recommended sweeping changes, particularly in the child health domain. Among other measures, he advocated increases in child benefit, infant care allowances and free school meals. However, the incoming Conservative government, led by Margaret Thatcher, was not persuaded by the findings and it was to be a further 20 years before the report was taken seriously (Ham 1999).

Black remained a strong supporter of the NHS until his death in 2002 (Tucker 2002) and, eventually, the gauntlet he threw down was picked up by Sir Donald Acheson, the former Chief Medical Officer, whose report – published in 1998 (Department of Health (DoH) 1998) – confirmed that health inequalities still existed. For example in the case of breast feeding – widely acknowledged to be the healthiest option for infants – Acheson revealed a striking difference between those mothers in the upper socio-economic groups and those in the lower.

WWW

Read the Acheson report online:
* http://www.official.documents.co.uk/documents/doh/ih/ih/htm

Seminar discussion topic

Analyse a local, national or international child health policy. In your learning group, discuss if the recommendations are met in your workplace. Are there variations in the way policy recommendations have been implemented?

UK Policy Variations

The individual countries within the UK can commission a report after specific problems arise within the child health arena. The Carlile review (National Assembly for Wales 2002) is cited here as an example of how an individual country responds to a crisis within its own children's services.

WWW

The full transcript of the Carlile review can be accessed on the National Assembly for Wales internet site:
* http://www.wales.gov.uk

THE CARLILE REVIEW (2002)

Welsh Assembly Minister for Health, Jane Hutt, commissioned the Carlile review after allegations of child sexual abuse within NHS child and adolescent inpatient facilities in Wales. Hutt's mandate to appointed chairman Lord Alex Carlile of Berriew was to make recommendations so that proper safeguards could be put in place whenever and wherever a child had contact with the NHS in Wales.

Lord Carlile made 150 recommendations based on his enquiry. His emphasis on child health nurses is interesting. For example, recommendation 93:

We recommend that urgent measures be pursued to increase college places for registered children's nurses including the encouragement of mature nurses to develop their skills and opportunities through training (National Assembly for Wales 2002 p 141)

Carlile places much emphasis on education and training, believing that all staff who come into contact with children

should be taught to recognise the signs of sexual, physical and emotional abuse.

Activity

Access the Carlile review from the PowerPoint presentation.
* How does it apply to you? If you live in Wales, have the recommendations been implemented? What messages does this report have for other countries?

The Welfare of Children in Hospital (1959)

The welfare of children in hospital, published in 1959 (Committee of the Central Health Services Council 1959), was the first of many reports specifically aimed at alleviating the psychological traumas perpetrated on children during a hospital stay. The main background to the commissioning of the report, chaired by Sir Harry Platt (a famous orthopaedic surgeon), was the growing public concern over the way children were cared for in hospital. The numbers of academic papers suggesting that a stay in hospital could be detrimental to a child's psychological development forced the pace of change and formed a platform upon which the subsequent report would be based. The report was commissioned on 12 June 1956 and the final report was sent to Lord Cohen of Birkenhead, Chair of the Central Health Services Council, on 28 October 1958. The reason given for the delay in reporting was the sheer enormity of the task facing Platt's committee, which included one children's nurse, Miss MW Janes SRN, SCM, RSCN. The primary term of reference given to the committee by the Central Health Services Council was:

To make a special study of the arrangements made in hospitals for the welfare of ill children – as distinct from their medical and nursing treatment – and to make suggestions which could be passed on to hospital authorities.

Over the two and a half years of the study, the Committee met 20 times to collate the written and verbal evidence. The antecedents of the report have already been covered but suffice to say that the work of Bowlby and Robertson was crucial. Of considerable interest is the revelation within the report that the Central Health Services Council had issued no fewer than three memoranda to hospital authorities to allow daily visiting for children. The failure of some hospitals to implement this recommendation is as pertinent today as it was then and reflects the status and perceived importance of 'topdown' government reports.

Activity

Consider the reasons why some reports related to children are ignored or poorly implemented.

PowerPoint

Access the companion PowerPoint presentation and read the full text of the Platt report.

The Platt report had profound and lasting effects on the welfare of children in hospital not only in the UK but also much further afield in countries such as Australia, New Zealand, Canada and The USA. The report made 55 recommendations, the majority of which can be summed up by one (recommendation 52):

> *Nurses (and all members of the child health care team) need training not only in the special aspects of disease in children but in the factors that influence the development of the normal child. Part of this training should take the form of practical experience in the care of well children both in nursery schools, etc. and in their homes. The emotional needs of children in hospital should be stressed in refresher courses for ward sisters.*

The last point was perhaps an acknowledgement that ward sisters were the gatekeepers who could facilitate or inhibit change. It is therefore ironic that in recommendation 10 Platt sows the seed of the demise of the RSCN direct-entry qualification when he states 'The Sister in charge of the ward should be RSCN as well as SRN'. Platt was not to know that the direct-entry single RSCN qualification was to disappear from England by the early 1960s, leading to shortages in the number of nurses holding a sick children's nursing qualification. If one could travel back in time to have a 1-to-1 with Sir Harry Platt, one could point out to him that the care a sick child receives is only as good as the nurse who delivers it.

Activity

Conduct a SWOT analysis of the Platt report and debate the strengths, weaknesses, opportunities and threats that it posed to health care practitioners in the 1960s.

Scenario

Louise is gaining experience in a children's medical unit where some of the nurses do not possess a children's nursing qualification.

Professional Conversation

" Harriet is a registered children's nurse on Part 15 of the Nursing and Midwifery Council's Professional Register. "

Issues affecting skill mix on the children's medical unit

I have been qualified for 4 years and I am really pleased that I decided to undertake a direct-entry children's nursing course. Some of my colleagues who trained some years ago have told me that this option was never open to them and that they had to undertake general nursing first. A few of these colleagues were actually seconded from the children's medical unit to undertake a post-registration children's nursing course. They said that more post-registration child branch places were made available by the workforce confederations in response to policy documents that stated that children should be cared for by people with specific training in the care of sick children. During coffee recently, one of the adult branch-registered nurses who works on my unit confided to me that she felt uncomfortable working with some of the sicker children because she did not feel that she had the right skills to do so.

- What do child health policy document recommendations have to say about skill mix?

Fit for the Future (1976)

Fit for the future (Committee on Child Health Services 1976) became known as the Court report, after the chairman of the committee, Professor Donald Court. Among the committee members was Miss Barchard, the Chief Nursing Officer of The Hospital for Sick Children, London. A health visitor was also part of the committee: Miss Bickerton, who subsequently became Professor of Public Health Nursing at The University of Western Sydney in Australia. By the time this report was commissioned – in 1973 – more attention than before was being focused on children. Donald Court introduces *Fit for the future* with a quotation from the novelist Katherine Mansfield:

> *By health I mean the power to live a full, adult, living breathing life in close contact with what I love – I want to be all that I am capable of becoming.*

This emphasis on letting children grow to their full potential reflected the growing recognition of the harmful effects that a period of ill health could have on a child's development. Although Court reiterates much of the earlier Platt report, as indeed do subsequent policy documents, the emphasis here is on preventing illness among children. Highlighted again is the stark reality that children born into lower socio-economic groups were dying unnecessarily from preventable 19th century reasons. In the section of the report on nurses, Court gives the number of RSCNs registered with the General Nursing Council as of March 1975 as 20,514. He uses this as evidence of the continuing shortage of children's nurses, adapting a line first used by Catherine Jane Wood, an early matron of London's Hospital For Sick Children: 'sick children should be nursed by nurses who have been trained to do so'.

Activity

Compare the numbers of children's nurses on the register of the Nursing and Midwifery Council (NMC) today. What inferences can you make?

Despite its size, the Court report gives a simple and clear set of recommendations, which can be summarised as:

We want to see a child- and family-centred service, in which skilled help is readily available and accessible, which is integrated in as much as it sees the child as a whole, and as a continuous developing person. We want to see a service that ensures that this paediatric skill and knowledge are applied in the care of every child whatever his age or disability, and wherever he lives, and we want a service that is increasingly orientated to prevention.

According to Court (Committee on Child Health Services 1976 p 368), all of this could be achieved through an integrated child health service.

Where are the Children?

Where are the children? (CCHS 1987) was the first of a number of important reports published by the organisation Caring for Children in the Health Services (CCHS). Founded in 1985, CCHS is a consortium of UK agencies made up of:

- the Royal College of Nursing of the United Kingdom (RCN)
- the British Paediatric Association (BPA), now the College of Paediatrics and Child Health (CPCH)
- Action for Sick Children, formerly the National Association for the Welfare of Children in Hospital (NAWCH)
- the National Association of Health Authorities and Trusts (NAHAT).

The CCHS has proved to be an influential body in improving the quality of child health services across the UK. *Where are the children?* was predicated on four standards that were first proposed by NAWCH (now called Action

for Sick Children) as part of its 10-point Charter for Children in Hospital.

WWW

Visit the Action for Sick Children website:
- http://www.actionforsickchildren.org/index2.html

PowerPoint

Access the companion PowerPoint presentation and compare the NAWCH 10-point Charter for Children in Hospital with the ASC Millennium Charter. In what ways do they differ?

The Four Standards Selected by CCHS

1. Children shall be admitted to hospital only if the care they require cannot be equally well provided at home or on a day basis.

2. Children shall be cared for with other children of the same age group.

3. Children in hospital shall have the right to have their parents with them at all times provided this is in the best interests of the child. Accommodation should therefore be offered to all parents and they should be encouraged to stay.

4. Children shall enjoy the care of appropriately trained staff, fully aware of the physical and emotional needs of each age group.

This first report from CCHS was motivated by concerns that various government recommendations related to children were being only slowly implemented. The NAWCH Charter had coalesced the recommendations of the Platt Report into 10 key standards and CCHS selected four of these to investigate. These related to where children were cared for and whether children were cared for with other children of a similar age by appropriately trained staff in the presence of parents or relatives.

Summary, Findings and Recommendations of *Where are the Children?*

An analysis of the data collected from the Regional Health Authorities showed that the proportion of children staying in hospital overnight was not decreasing and that paediatric community services had, like with day-case surgery, progressed only sluggishly. The pioneering work of Southampton paediatric surgeon John Atwell and paediatric community nurse Peggy Gow (Atwell & Gow 1985) demonstrated that, in fact, a large proportion of operations could be carried out safely and effectively as day surgery. Importantly, the report reinforced the essential ingredient in day-case surgery for children, that of a team of paediatric community nurses.

Activity

1. Investigate the role of the paediatric community nursing team in your area. Is it linked to day-case surgery?
2. The main finding of *Where are the children?* was that basic information about children and where they were cared for was lacking. Investigate how information about children is documented in your own clinical area. Has this improved since the publication of this report? Read below the four standards selected by CCHS below and answer the posed questions.

   - Standard 1: Children shall be admitted to hospital only if the care they require cannot be equally well provided at home or on a day case basis.

   What evidence is available to show that this has improved since this report was published in 1987?
   - Standard 2: Children shall be cared for with other children of the same age group.

   At the time of this report the data kept by hospitals was inadequate to ascertain if this standard was always met. Is this standard met in your hospital?
   - Standard 3: Children in hospital shall have the right to have their parents with them at all times.

   Is every parent asked if they wish to stay on your ward? What refreshment, sleeping and bathroom facilities do you have for your parents who stay overnight with their children?
   - Standard 4: Children shall enjoy the care of appropriately trained staff.

   Are children cared for on your ward by nurses who hold a children's nursing qualification or who have had training in the special needs of children? When children go home do they have the services of a paediatric community nursing team?

Seminar discussion topic

Of interest in this 1987 report is the recommendation that sisters of children's wards hold a children's nursing qualification. It should be noted that this report was published nearly two years prior to the full implementation of Project 2000 which led to the reintroduction of the direct entry children's nursing qualification for Part 15 of the Nursing and Midwifery Council register. The authors of this report were undoubtedly conscious of the advocacy role of qualified children's nurses, hence the emphasis on ward sisters holding the appropriate qualification. Additionally however is the reality that the post registration route to prepare children's nurses prior to the advent of Project 2000 was inadequate to provide the numbers necessary.

Other Reports from CCHS

PARENTS STAYING OVERNIGHT IN HOSPITAL WITH THEIR CHILDREN (CCHS 1988)

In this report, CCHS studied the success or otherwise of numerous recommendations that children in hospital have the right to the care and comfort of their parents during the process of the admission. A central tenet of these recommendations is the provision of unrestricted visiting and overnight accommodation for parents. This report concentrates on how parents/guardians fare during the process of staying with their children in hospital. In fact, there were wide variations of parental provision in hospital wards across the country, ranging from 20% to 87%. The 'accommodation' available for parents ranged from proper beds or reclining chairs, to mattresses on the floor and, at the extreme, upright wooden chairs.

The main objective of the report was to stimulate enhanced provision for the families of sick children. The report working party recognised that parents were crucial to the care of their children during periods of ill health. Furthermore, it was acknowledged that parents undertake many nursing duties during a child's admission, and that the role of the paediatric nurse changes from direct deliverer of care to facilitator and teacher. To best maximise the parental contribution to care it was accepted that the welfare of parents was important.

Scenario

Louise is admitting a 9-month-old infant who requires an overnight stay. The mother is worried that her 5-year-old son will miss her if she stays in hospital with the baby.

Reflect on your Practice

- What advice might Louise give to the mother regarding her dilemma?
- Which child is more at risk from separation anxiety?

Activity

Consider your own ward or unit and the success or otherwise of *Parents staying overnight in hospital with their children* in changing attitudes towards parents who wish to stay with their sick children in hospital:

- What type of bed is allocated to a parent?
- Where is the bed in relation to the child?
- What toilet and catering facilities are available for resident parents?
- Can all parents or guardians stay if they wish (including fathers)?
- Are parents informed of facilities for overnight accommodation before admission?
- Visit the websites of children's hospitals in North America and investigate parental provision. How do they compare with your own ward or unit?
- What are Ronald Macdonald Houses? (see http://www.ronaldhousecle.org/guest/)

JUST FOR THE DAY (CCHS 1991)

This far-reaching report was undertaken to accelerate the introduction of day care for children. The underlying philosophy was that admitting children as day patients was an excellent way of maintaining the integrity of the family while at the same time avoiding an overnight stay for the child in hospital. However, it is important to note that, in recommending day care services for sick children, CCHS was cognisant of the need to ensure that such services were fully planned in such a way as to avoid exacerbating family stress. Day care for children had been growing since the publication of *Fit for the future* (Committee on Child Health Services 1976) 15 years earlier, which strongly supported day-case surgery in particular. In *Just for the day*, CCHS was endeavouring to establish national protocols for the delivery of day-care services through the development of quality standards. These standards covered the whole of the family experience, from the preadmission period through to the postdischarge care at home. The project working party, chaired by Lady Lovell-Davies of NAWCH, had two members who were experienced children's nurses. The data collected as part of this work was exhaustive and, in addition to receiving evidence from the Royal Colleges, the professional and voluntary sectors, no less than 230 submissions were received and discussed at the monthly meetings of CCHS.

The Mission Statement Formulated by the Project Team

Most children, when they are sick, are cared for by their families within their own homes, with the help of GPs and community nurses. Children are more emotionally vulnera-ble than adults and should be admitted to hospital only if the care they require cannot be provided equally well at home, because hospitalisation can be a distressing and difficult experience. An admission should always be child centred, based on a partnership between the family and healthcare team. Children should not be nursed alongside adults. When hospital care is necessary, children should not be admitted overnight if an equivalent level of care can be provided on a day basis. Such admissions involve parents in additional responsibilities and entail careful preparation and support of the family, and efficient communication between the hospital and primary and/or community services. The planning and delivery of care should recognise the multicultural nature and diverse needs of the population and make provision accordingly (CCHS 1991 p 5).

Activity

- Is this mission statement formulated by the CCHS team still pertinent today?
- How does your clinical area perform in relation to this statement?

Main Recommendations

The conclusion of the project working party was that whenever and wherever a child is admitted for day-case treatment a planned package of care should be adopted based on 12 discrete standards relating to:

- overall planning
- preadmission preparation
- the provision of a designated day-case area
- the provision of specific written information
- not mixing children with adults
- designated staff
- staff skilled in day-case work
- organisation of patient care to ensure discharge within the same day
- buildings and equipment that comply with safety standards for children
- a child-friendly environment
- specific documentation
- paediatric community nursing provision after discharge.

Activity

- Does your unit meet these standards set in 1991?
- Does your unit or hospital offer preadmission preparation for families? (See Chapter 5 and companion PowerPoint presentation.)

BRIDGING THE GAPS (CCHS 1993)

In this report, which was to spotlight ambulatory care for children as a growing discipline, Rosemary Thornes, on behalf of CCHS, conducted an exploratory study of the interface between primary and specialist care for children within the health services. In particular, the study concentrated on the quality of care provided to children as they moved through the different sectors of the health service. The data that generated the evidence was collected from one Regional Health Authority (Wessex) that agreed to act as a case study for CCHS. The background to this report lay in the frequent accounts of dissatisfaction expressed by the families of sick children, and by professionals, about the inadequacies of the interfaces between hospital and home and the different health agencies within the community at large. During the 9 months of the study the primary aims of the project team were to analyse the failures in care delivery that occur at the point of transfer, to develop principles of care that could be expressed as standards by the differing agencies and to collect examples of good practice to aid in the suggestions for improvement. The report detailed nine key principles, each with detailed suggestions on how best they could be implemented (CCHS & Thornes 1993 pp 19–27):

1. Knowledge and information should be shared between professionals and families, so that the parents and children, when they are able, are in a strong position to take part in planning and decision making.

2. There should be equity in access to, and quality of, services. Particular care should be taken to ensure that vulnerable families receive appropriate services.

3. Consultation, tests and treatment should be provided as close as possible to each child's home. If a child has to travel to a distant hospital, attention should be paid to practical help for the family.

4. Referrals to specialist services, especially those provided by community health agencies, can be made by a range of health professionals who should work to agreed criteria to ensure that care is integrated.

5. The boundary between primary and specialist care, and thus the point of referral, varies from place to place according to the facilities available in the primary setting. The important criterion is for all concerned to accept an agreed standard of care and to ensure that the child is in the right place to receive it.

6. The boundary between care in hospital and at home, and thus the point of referral back to primary carers, should vary from place to place according to the facilities and expertise available in the primary care team and the home. The important criterion is for all to work to a recognised standard of care and to ensure that the child's family has appropriate support to provide it.

7. The steps taken to ensure continuation of the pattern of care should be made explicit to families, so that the parents know who is managing their child's clinical care at every stage and where to go for clinical help.

8. Parents should be quite clear about the care they are expected to provide and at what point to seek clinical help.

9. Communication should be organised in such a way that the professional managing a child's care has sufficient, timely information to continue the care.

Activity

- *Bridging the gaps* was published in 1993. For each of the nine principles above, consider how well your health service performs now.
- Read Charles-Edwards & Glasper 2002.

Evidence-Based Practice

The strength of a modern child health policy report is determined to a greater or lesser extent on the evidence offered by the reports authors in seeking to implement or effect change. In *Bridging the gaps*, the report author, Rosemary Thornes, cites evidence taken from a series of interviews with children and their parents. Additionally, data were collected from NHS managers and staff throughout the study area. In this way the researchers attempted to develop a multidisciplinary view, including a patient (family) perspective. In gathering qualitative and quantitative data from different disciplines the report was able to analyse failures as well as successes in care.

THE CHILDREN ACT 1989

The Children Act. An introductory guide for the NHS Health Publication Unit (DoH 1989) was written as a guide to staff working with children in the NHS. Although the topic of child abuse and neglect will be covered in detail in Chapter 19, it is worth noting this policy document as one of the most important published by a health service. The language used in this report is much more precise and the word 'duty' figures prominently in the text. The main principle of the Act is that, wherever possible, children should be brought up and cared for within their own families but – and importantly – children should be safe and protected by effective intervention if they are in danger.

THE WELFARE OF CHILDREN AND YOUNG PEOPLE IN HOSPITAL (1991)

Still an industry standard for the care of children in hospital, this report, which was written as a guide (DoH 1991), coalesced many of the previous reports, including those by Platt and Court. Perhaps it was hoped that the status of 'guide' rather than 'report' would enhance compliance with government recommendations. Sadly, a number of tragedies, but principally that of the Allitt case (Glasper & Campbell 1994), would show the extremes of failing to comply with the good practice recommendations of this document. Of interest in this guide are the terms 'advised' and 'should', the former obviously carrying more weight than the latter. To illustrate this, one of the key recommendations of this 'welfare document' is the statement that 'at least two registered sick children's nurses (RSCNs or Project 2000 child branch) should be on duty 24 hours a day in all hospital children's departments or wards' (DoH 1991 p 33). However, this was only advised and has been a contentious issue ever since. This guidance document was an attempt by the DoH to make health districts improve the quality of children's health care. Not all were successful in doing so.

Activity

Read *The welfare of children and young people in hospital* (DoH 1991) and examine the number of recommendations that are 'advised' or 'should' – compare your own unit's compliance with these recommendations.

CHILD HEALTH IN THE COMMUNITY (1996)

Published some 5 years after *The welfare of children and young people in hospital* (DoH 1991), *Child health in the community* (NHS Executive 1996) was intended to be a companion document reflecting major changes in the way children were managed during illness. Additionally, it highlighted the reality that, for most of the time, most children are cared for in their own homes. This was a reflection of a greater emphasis on preventive measures to avoid illness and therefore hospital admission. This report takes a broader perspective than earlier reports and begins to acknowledge that parenting skills are of paramount importance to the overall health of children. Concerns about falling levels of parenting within families is reflected and cited as one reason for the increase in emotional and behavioural disorders among children. Failure to break the cycle of deprivation when young people start families of their own before they have the skills to do so is highlighted and addressed in this far-reaching report. As in the CCHS report *Bridging the gaps* (CCHS & Thornes 1993), *Child health in the community* gives details of how services for children should be targeted and emphasises the importance of good working relationships between hospital and community staff and the value of closer collaboration with other agencies responsible for the welfare of children, including

the voluntary sector. In this respect, *Child health in the community* begins to move the emphasis of care away from simply those children in hospital. As with its companion 'welfare' document *The welfare of children and young people in hospital* (DoH 1991), *Child health in the community* uses the terms 'advise' and 'should'.

Activity

During your community placements, investigate through discussion with the paediatric community team whether practice is based on the recommendations of this report?

CHILDREN FIRST. A STUDY OF HOSPITAL SERVICES (1993)

As part of its remit to examine the economy, efficiency and effectiveness with which the NHS uses public resources, the Audit Commission conducted *Children first. A study of hospital services* (Audit Commission 1993). For the first time the effectiveness of treatment regimens and the need for children to be treated in hospital were questioned in the light of the Platt report of 1959 and other subsequent publications There was a tacit acknowledgement that reports pertaining to the welfare of children had too often not been fully implemented. Crucially, the Audit Commission report did not seek to reiterate the findings of other studies and reports but rather to investigate why these were not being met in some institutions. *Children first* states six main principles of caring for children in hospital:

1. child- and family-centred care
2. specially skilled staff
3. separate facilities
4. effective treatments
5. appropriate hospitalisation
6. strategic commissioning.

It also identifies the barriers preventing the achievement of good practice. Importantly, the report gives suggestions of how these might be overcome.

In summary, the Audit Commission report advises health agencies to adhere to the guidelines contained within *The welfare of children and young people in hospital* (DoH 1991).

Activity

- How does your unit measure compliance with national child health policy standards?
- What audit tools are used to gather data for this activity?

THE CARE OF SICK CHILDREN. A REVIEW OF THE GUIDELINES IN THE WAKE OF THE ALLITT INQUIRY

This document (RCN 1994) was published in the wake of the Allitt inquiry (Clothier et al 1994), which reported the deaths and injuries among hospitalised children caused by enrolled nurse Beverly Allitt. Recommendation 10 of the 13 made in the Allitt inquiry report recommends that the DoH should take steps to ensure that the policy document *The welfare of children and young people in hospital* (DoH 1991) be more closely observed. This is similar language to that used by the Audit Commission in its *Children first* report, published the year before in 1993. The purpose of the RCN guidelines in the wake of Allitt was to bring pressure to bear on purchasers and providers to improve the services offered to sick children by complying with DoH recommendations. The RCN publication reiterates and presents in a digestible format the recommendations of earlier reports, and in particular the need for sick children to be cared for by appropriately qualified staff, pointing out that over half the children in hospital were being cared for by nurses not holding a paediatric nursing qualification. Additionally, Grantham and Kesteven General Hospital, which employed Allitt, was criticised for having a poor appointments procedure (Dyer 1994). Beverly Allitt was reported to be suffering from a disease known as Munchausen syndrome by proxy, although this has subsequently been hotly debated.

● Seminar discussion topic

Read and discuss in your learning group the paper:

● Morley CJ 1995 Practical concerns about the diagnosis of Munchausen syndrome by proxy. Archives of Disease in Childhood 72:528–530

CHILD HEALTH RIGHTS: IMPLEMENTING THE UN CONVENTION ON THE RIGHTS OF THE CHILD WITHIN THE NHS. A PRACTITIONER'S GUIDE (1995)

Child health rights: Implementing the UN Convention on the rights of the child within the NHS. A practitioners' guide (British Association for Community Child Health (BACCH) 1995) was published to bring to the attention of all who work with children the mechanisms for the implementation of the UN Convention. This convention on the rights of the child was adopted by the General Assembly of The United Nations in November 1989. It came into force in the UK in January 1992 and its primary aim is to provide a comprehensive set of principles and standards to guide and inform planning and practice for children and young people up to 18 years of age. The BACCH publication attempts to show how it is possible to implement the Convention at local level. A number of other reports on children's rights have been published since and the second report to the UN (DoH 1999) gives details on progress made.

 WWW

Read a digestible précis of the UN Convention:
● http://www.unicef.org/crc/

LISTENING TO CHILDREN: CHILDREN, ETHICS, AND SOCIAL RESEARCH (1995)

Listening to children. Children, ethics, and social research (Alderson 1995) was published as concerns about the ethical aspects of research using children were being increasingly articulated, although the events at Alder Hey and Bristol were yet to hit the newspaper headlines. The whole topic of ethics and children's rights will be covered in a subsequent chapter but Alderson's contribution to the debate must be recognised. In this report, commissioned by Barnardos, Alderson identifies 10 key topics relating to research ethics:

1. the purpose of the research
2. researching with children – the costs and hoped for benefits
3. privacy and confidentiality
4. selection, inclusion and exclusion
5. funding
6. review and revision of the research aims and methods
7. information for children, parents and other carers
8. consent
9. dissemination (of the research findings)
10. impact on children.

 Activity

● Identify a research project in your own unit. Are all these 10 principles being adhered to?

 Reflect on your Practice

As a nurse working in a children's unit where research is carried out, are you accountable even if you are not directly involved?

GOVERNMENT RESPONSE TO THE HOUSE OF COMMONS HEALTH COMMITTEE REPORTS ON CHILDREN AND YOUNG PEOPLE (1997)

The official government response to the House of Commons Health Committee reports (DoH 1997a) is in many respects an endorsement of the original reports and of many of the other reports covered thus far.

Key Points

The government welcomed the reports as making a substantial contribution to the debate about child health:

- The response acknowledges that children are different.
- Care should encompass the needs of the whole child, with mental health especially highlighted.
- Fragmentation (between agencies) should be reduced, echoing *Bridging the gaps* (CCHS & Thornes 1993)
- Endorses *The welfare of children and young people in hospital* (DoH 1991).
- Endorses *Child health in the community: a guide to good practice* (NHS Executive 1996).

Although it is beyond the scope of this chapter to consider all aspects, one of the responses to the House of Commons reports highlights the slow development of paediatric community nursing services (House of Commons Health Committee 1997). This point is picked up by Whiting in a subsequent chapter, who discuss the development of a children's community nursing service, highlighting the benefits in terms of a reduction in the length of stay, a reduction in admissions and enhanced family satisfaction.

Activity

Read Chapter 8 by Whiting and review the level of community nursing services in your local area. How does the service operate?

THE CHILDREN'S CHARTER (1998)

The children's charter (DoH 1996) was launched as part of the UK government's commitment to accountability in public services. It made a number of innovative pledges to children and their families. These pledges were based on good practice generated through years of published child health policy.

Activity

- Obtain a copy of *The children's charter* and determine how many of the pledges are honoured in your own area of practice.
- Are copies of the charter freely available to children and their relatives in your clinical area?

A BRIDGE TO THE FUTURE (1997)

The tragic death of a child named Nicholas Geldhart in December 1995 was the precursor to the posing of fundamental questions about the national provision of paediatric intensive care facilities for children across the country. In the aftermath of the negative publicity surrounding this unfortunate child's death, the Chief Nursing Officer's taskforce recognised that demand for paediatric intensive care services for children was growing year on year. Crucial to the debate was the stark reality that there were insufficient paediatric intensive care nurses. The gold-standard qualification to equip paediatric nurses with the skills and knowledge to care for critically ill children was the English (Scottish or Welsh) National Board for Nursing and Midwifery course (ENB) 415. (These validating agency boards no longer exist). Additional intensive care courses and – importantly – student salaries were fully funded in the wake of *A bridge to the future* (DoH 1997b). To complement this initiative, new paediatric intensive care units were built and equipped. Unlike previous reports, huge amounts of money were invested in achieving improvements to a service that was found to be deficient and politically highly sensitive.

YOUTH MATTERS. EVIDENCE-BASED BEST PRACTICE FOR THE CARE OF YOUNG PEOPLE IN HOSPITAL (1998)

Youth matters (Viner & Keane 1998), coordinated through the consortium CCHS, aimed to raise awareness of the plight of young people in hospital. The report revealed that only 8% of health authorities contained adolescent provider units in their hospitals. Glasper & Cooper (1999) contrast the prominent position of young people in society with their invisibility in a hospital setting, where they have such a low profile despite the fact that in morbidity terms they continue to be one of the most vulnerable groups in society. This report asked all Health Authorities to conduct a detailed survey to determine what provision should be made for young people in hospital.

Despite a lack of progress following the publication of youth matters, Viner participated in a subsequent policy initiative on behalf of the Royal College of Paediatrics and Child Health, the Royal College of Psychiatrists and others in producing *Bridging the gaps: health care for adolescents (2003)*.

Activity

- Was this survey undertaken in your health area?
- Conduct your own survey in your own hospital or unit. Are you satisfied with the level of adolescent provision?
  The facilities for young people in hospital remain poor.

Activity

Access this policy at http://www.rcpsych.ac.uk/publications/cr/council/cr114.pdf. In your learning group debate the ramifications of this latest adolescent policy.

THE ROYAL LIVERPOOL CHILDREN'S INQUIRY (2001)

The Royal Liverpool children's inquiry (DoH 2001a) (available online at: http://www.rlcinquiry.org.uk/), chaired by Michael Redfern QC, was initiated after a storm of public protest broke out after revelations that deceased children's body parts had been removed at the Alder Hey children's hospital without parental consent. Prior to the publication of this report, Glasper & Powell (2000, 2001) had highlighted the vagueness of the law pertaining to post-mortems, in which some doctors exceeded their mandate. The whole issue of the scandal of Alder Hey revolved around informed consent and the lack of it. Redfern's report has made it clear that consent procedures must be tightened to ensure that a person must have all the information necessary to make an informed decision.

WWW

Read the report online and consider your own field of practice:
- http://www.rlcinquiry.org.uk/

THE BRISTOL INQUIRY (2001)

The report of the pubic inquiry into children's heart surgery (DoH 2001b) (available online at: http://www.bristol-inquiry.org.uk) revealed that the UK health service was badly in need of reform. The inquiry, chaired by Professor Ian Kennedy, was commissioned after it was revealed that success rates for children's heart surgery at the Bristol Royal Infirmary were less than in comparative centres elsewhere in the UK. The inquiry found that much of the criticism levelled at health professionals by parents was the result of a lack of information. Additionally, the report demanded that children in hospital must be cared for in an appropriate, safe environment by competent staff trained in caring for children. Glasper (2001) points out that a plethora of similar reports have made recommendations for prospective change in the health service and yet have achieved less than anticipated.

WWW

Read the report online. How is information given to children and parents in your clinical area?
- http://www.bristol-inquiry.org.uk

THE VICTORIA CLIMBIE INQUIRY

The death of 8-year-old Victoria Climbie precipitated a national inquiry chaired by Lord Laming, which was eventually published in 2003 (Laming 2003). Although this will be fully covered in Chapter 19, it is important to recognise that in the aftermath of this inquiry it became widely accepted that child maltreatment had become one of the major causes of morbidity in children. Profound changes in policy within all health and social care environments relating to child protection were subsequently introduced in an attempt to prevent such a tragedy from happening again. Powell (2003) highlights the need to ensure that child protection services are commensurate with the scale of the problem in the UK. Children's nurses play a crucial frontline role in the recognition of child maltreatment and this report and its policy recommendations are therefore essential reading.

WWW

Read the report online:
- http//www.victoria-climbie-inquiry.org.uk/finreport/finreport.htm

THE NATIONAL SERVICE FRAMEWORK FOR CHILDREN

The final installment of the national service framework (NSF) for children, young people and maternity services was published in September 2004 (DoH 2004) as part of the government's commitment to children exemplified in its Green Paper, *Every child matters* (DfES 2003). This sets out proposals for reforming the delivery of services for children, young people and families, augmenting existing measures to ensure that children at risk of harm and neglect are protected and enabled to develop their full potential.

The NSF sets new standards for children and young people across health and social care boundaries in England. Although many elements of health and social care services for children and young people were the subject of much criticism in the Bristol (DoH 2001b) and Victoria Climbie inquiries (Laming 2003) – the primary antecedents to the NSF – this policy document breathes new life into the old adage that the wealth of a nation is invested in the health and welfare of all its children. This will be achieved through the introduction of 11 auditable standards, which are predicated on best evidence-based practice in the care of pregnant women, children and young people. The NSF is presented in three parts:

- Part 1 is concerned with setting standards for well children and young people, and is aimed at keeping them safe and healthy through the provision of optimum life chances.

- Part 2 sets standards for sick children and young people in the community and hospital and for those with mental health problems, disabilities and complex health needs.
- Part 3 addresses maternity services.

In a way that is perhaps reminiscent of the main finding of the Black report (DHSS 1980), which was commissioned by the previous Labour government in 1979, and of *Tackling health inequalities* (DoH 2003), the introduction to the NSF by John Reid, the Labour Secretary of State for Health, reinforces the reality that inequalities in health and social care still impact on children and young people. His emphasis on child poverty, and on the effect this has on children and young people, forms the backdrop to the whole NSF, commencing perhaps with standard 11 of the report 'maternity services'.

It is known that much ill health and disease in adulthood has its origins before, during and after pregnancy. It is therefore fitting that this NSF standard should highlight the importance of improved preconception care and the role of health promotion in the future well-being of children and young people. The standards of the NSF cover many of the parameters of childhood, such as tackling the growing burden on health of obesity through recommendations to improve school meals and encouraging children to take 60 minutes of exercise daily. This must be tempered with the reality that many school playing fields have been sold for land development. School playing fields are now protected under Section 77 of the School Standards and Framework Act 1998, which empowers the Secretary of State to protect such fields in England from disposal or change of use, and this is an example of how the NSF has the potential to bridge all components of society in the promotion of optimum health for all children and young people. Although the government envisages that the full implementation of the NSF will take up to 10 years, it has stressed that the NHS and local authorities charged with its implementation will be frequently assessed by the Health Care Commission, the Commission for Social Care Inspection and OFSTED to ensure that they are compliant and making progress. Additionally, and of interest to nurses, is the work of the Association of Chief Children's Nurses (ACCN), which regularly posts exemplars of good practice related to the NSF on its website (http://www.accnuk.org)

The right start: the national service framework for children, young people and maternity services (DoH 2004, available online at: http://www.doh.gov/childrenstaskforce), the first part of the NSF to be published, was launched as part of the government's commitment to raising standards across the NHS and Social Services departments. In particular, this component of the whole NSF sets rigorous standards for children in hospital, grouped around three main themes:

- child-centred hospital services
- quality and safety of care provided
- quality of setting and environment.

To give robustness to these standards, the Healthcare Commission intends to ensure compliance through inspections. Those hospitals failing to meet these and the other NSF standards will be given appropriate advice on what they need to do to raise standards of care.

 Activity

Visit the NSF website (or access it from the PowerPoint presentation) and consider how the compliance to the standards will be audited by the Health Commission, one of whose statutory functions is to monitor and review the implementation of standards set out in the national service frameworks.

IN SUMMARY

This part of the chapter has not been able to consider every report concerning sick children. In the Carlile review (National Assembly for Wales 2002), for example, it was acknowledged that 65 guidance documents with respect to child protection alone were issued to the NHS between 1971 and 2001. The volume of reports commissioned about children in society indicates that much still needs to be achieved.

Getting it Right – Dealing with Complaints

From one of our most recently constructed hospitals complaints have been made that there were not sufficient nursing conveniences, that nothing was at hand, that everything had to be sought. Where this is the case the hospital administration must be both inefficient and costly (Florence Nightingale 1863)

Complaints are a fact of life. No organisation or profession can avoid them and it is not desirable to ignore or belittle them. Some are trivial, a few obsessive or malicious but most, if well handled, can have very positive outcomes. Complaints in the health service often indicate ways in which practice or procedures can be improved or highlight matters that really concern children, families or carers.

If a family makes a complaint about any aspect of their child's care, nurses not only need to be involved in the investigation of that complaint but must also reflect back on accurate record-keeping and records of any communication that they have had with the child or carers and multidisciplinary colleagues. If an aspect of care is not documented, how can there be any evidence that that care has taken place? Often a complaint is made several months after an issue has occurred and it would be difficult for any nurse to recall details of a particular case. Consequently, the nurse is reliant on what is documented.

The clinical governance agenda is a vital element of ensuring that complaints are seen as part of a Trust strategy and complaints are used to indicate improvements to services across the whole organisation. If procedures have changed, complainants appreciate being informed of the changes. Consideration needs to be given by Trusts as to the most effective way to encourage staff to change unacceptable practice.

CRITERIA FOR INVESTIGATING COMPLAINTS

For an investigation under the NHS complaints procedure, a complaint must be about NHS services received by an individual patient. Anyone making a complaint under the procedure is entitled to:

- A full and complete explanation of what happened and why, given in a language the complainant can understand.
- An apology if there was an error or omission on behalf of the staff.
- If an error or omission has occurred, the complainant should be given information about the action that the organisation has taken or is proposing to take to try and prevent it happening again.

Complaints should be dealt with quickly and accurately. Ideally they should be made as soon as possible after the incident has occurred. It must be within 6 months of the incident or within 6 months from the time that it came to the complainant's notice, providing that not more than 12 months have elapsed since the original incident. Occasionally, as a result of bereavement or prolonged illness, a Complaint Manager may need to decide whether a complaint should be investigated if it is outside these time limits.

Stages of the Complaints Procedure

The stages in the complaints system are currently:

- local resolution
- the convening decision
- the independent review panel
- the Health Service Commissioner (the Ombudsman).

In April 2004, the convening decision, which formerly had been undertaken within the NHS Trust, was moved to the Commission for Healthcare Audit and Inspection (CHAI/ the Healthcare Commission).

Local resolution is an essential stage of the complaint process. This is the stage at which nurses must become involved and take note of when families are becoming anxious or distressed or clearly need to sit down and talk through concerns. How local resolution is handled is for the individual organisation to decide. Staff need to be empowered and trained to act on concerns the moment they received them. The sooner a complaint is responded to the more likely it is to be resolved. Families often just want to be heard and to express their anxieties and it is at this stage that the Patient Advice and Liaison Service can be of great benefit.

Family advocates – Patient Advice and Liaison Service (PALS) – are available to help families. The service is free to all patients, families, carers and friends and they can speak in confidence to trained staff; information will not be disclosed unless permission is given. If it is thought necessary to protect a child from serious harm or injury then a decision needs to be made as to the way forward.

PALS can:

- provide a listening ear
- help sort out any problems by liaising with staff
- support families in making their concerns heard
- guide families through the hospital complaints process if they wish to make a formal complaint
- link families to information and support services.

 WWW

The PALS team at Great Ormond Street Hospital has implemented this service successfully. Visit their website:
- http://www.goshkids@nhs.uk

An oral response can be given to an oral complaint. However, written complaints must receive a written response. A range of individuals can provide this response, often it is a Complaints Manager but sometimes the healthcare professionals themselves will prepare a response for the Complaints Manager, and this will then be collated into a full response for the Chief Executive to sign. This is an important stage for nurses to be involved; they have often been working closely with the families and are able to provide their version of the story. It is important to understand the full picture from beginning to end and to hear that story from all the individuals involved. People's perceptions can be very different and it is important to receive a balanced perception of everybody's view.

A recommended way to look at the complaint is to actually highlight the questions that the complainant has raised in a letter and then to look at the response and consider whether those particular issues have been answered. The initial letter may well be followed up by a local resolution meeting. It is important that this meeting involves all of the healthcare professionals involved, particularly the nursing staff who can often provide necessary information in an understandable language for the family. PALS can often be involved at this stage by supporting the family or ensuring that an advocate is available to be there with the family at this local resolution meeting if that is helpful. Talking the issues through and taking time to explain procedures or issues that have been raised can be extremely helpful to the family.

The final letter at the end of local resolution must advise the complainant of his or her rights. A complainant has the right to request an independent review and needs to indicate by letter which issues he or she considers have not been addressed at local resolution. The request is then passed to the CHAI, which, since April 2004, has acted as Convener. CHAI's role as convener is to:

- Assess the correspondence and evaluate whether the complainant has received a full explanation, which covers all the outstanding issues identified.
- Assess if an apology is required and, if so, whether it has been given.

Finally, if something has gone wrong, CHAI – as convener – must decide whether it is clear from the correspondence what steps have been taken to try to prevent it happening again. It is at this stage that it is essential for the convener to take clinical independent advice if the complaint involves clinical issues. It is essential at this stage that the appropriate healthcare professionals are asked for advice, for example, nurses, midwives, dieticians or pharmacists. There are then three options:

- to refer the request back to local resolution
- CHAI to agree to undertake an independent review
- to fast-track a complaint to the Ombudsman's office.

If CHAI agrees that an independent review panel should be held, then it will first write the terms of reference for the panel. These will be based on the issues that remain outstanding from local resolution.

Complainants have a right to go to the Health Service Commissioner (the Ombudsman) if their request for an independent review panel is refused or if they remain dissatisfied at the end of this part of the process. The Ombudsman considers the request and decides whether to investigate. As a result, the Ombudsman has become the last resort for a complainant who remains dissatisfied after exhausting the initial two stages of the NHS complaints procedure. The Health Service Ombudsman's

powers and duties are set out in the Health Service Commissioner's Act 1993. Jurisdiction was initially confined to the classic Ombudsman territory of maladministration (in the NHS) but was extended in 1996 to include clinical complaints and complaints about family health service practitioners.

WWW

Visit these websites to view these Acts:
- http://www.hmso.gov.uk/acts/acts1993/ Ukpga_19930046_en_2.htm
- http://www.hmso.gov.uk/acts/acts1996/96005--b.htm

The positions of Parliamentary Commissioner, or Ombudsman, came into being in 1967; that of Health Service Ombudsman in 1973. The two offices are always held by the same person, who is appointed by the Queen and answerable to Parliament. The Ombudsman is independent of government and the NHS and is not a member of the medical profession.

If it appears that an investigation may be warranted then the Ombudsman may request that the organisation supplies information about how the complaint was handled and any further information that may help to make a final decision. The Ombudsman is interested to see that the correct procedure has been followed. For example, was appropriate clinical advice taken? If the Ombudsman decides to investigate, all the parties involved in the complaint process are interviewed and a report is written and published.

An example of a letter copied to the Ombudsman following an investigation is given below. The letter was sent to the Acute Trust involved in the complaint:

It was also important to us that we receive an apology for what had happened, but it was your policy to refuse point blank to apologise, and adopt the stance that our complaint was not justified. With the publication of the Ombudsman's report, this can now be seen to be an error of judgement on your part, and it has been clearly shown that our complaint was justified. The matter has now entered the public domain through the media, which will do nothing to enhance the reputation of the Health Authority or the hospital in question.

WWW

General information about the Ombudsman and copies of reports can be found on the following website:
- http://www.ombudsman.org.uk

You are thoroughly recommended to look at these published reports. They provide a valuable learning tool for any healthcare professional.

KEY FACTORS LEADING TO COMPLAINTS INVOLVING NURSING PRACTICE

Communication

Communication – or lack of it – is often a major issue in any complaint. In the medical context, the fundamentals of communication are information that can be understood, a clear explanation, reassurance and seeking consent where necessary. Nearly all complaints that the Ombudsman sees involve poor communication. It is widely recognised that what a doctor or nurse believes he or she said might be very different from a child or carer's perception of the same discussion. The importance of documenting such a discussion cannot be over emphasised.

Families who are distressed or vulnerable often fail to hear what is being said to them. It is therefore important to repeat information. Poor communication occurs between nurses and families, nurses and doctors or other healthcare professionals, and nurses and other wards/departments, particularly when patients are transferred from one ward to another. Handover is often extremely poor. This is a stage where often reassessment of the patient is needed to establish a relationship with the patients/carers and ensure all information is clarified.

The simple act of showing family members around a ward, introducing them to staff and being friendly and approachable seems simple but too often staff get this very wrong.

Disappointment

Families do very often have an unrealistic expectation of what can be achieved for their child. This is only natural; it is often their only coping mechanism. However, staff must manage this situation and clear explanations of what is available and what is achievable need to occur. An honest approach to families, particularly in obtaining their consent, is absolutely essential; telling families that there is a 90% chance of success is totally unacceptable. Parents will cling to the 90%, not thinking that there is a possibility that they may be in the 10%.

The disappointment caused by an unpleasant environment or rude staff might seem a minor issue. But it can easily develop into something much more serious that could have been avoided if staff had noticed that the problems were arising:

At the outset of this complaint when my family and I attended a meeting, my brother was asked in a very aggressive manner what it was we wanted to achieve by this complaint. It was our hope then, and continues to be, that we would achieve something positive, that would bring to your attention a problem within the hospital, and that with the new procedures your service would improve. We are unable to change what hap-

pened to our mother, but we can achieve something positive in her memory.

Basic Care

Nurses occasionally get fundamental basic care very wrong and inadequate assessment of a patient or implementation of documented care just does not occur. Consider the following scenarios:

Scenario

A robust assessment of a patient's skin is not available in any documentation and when the patient develops a sore on their ear on being intubated the family is not only extremely distressed but takes it as evidence of poor risk analysis of the patient.

Involving a dietician or a tissue viability nurse to give expert advice to a child and family often does not occur, even when these professionals are available within an organisation. These experts often have time to talk through the problems that may occur with the family.

Cot sides being left down on beds for a child to fall out are another example of lack of risk analysis.

There are many different examples of when healthcare professionals got the fundamentals of care wrong:

The quality of nursing documentation, in particular with regard to the recording of communications with the family, were particularly poor. Concerns were raised about care planning and management of Mrs K's pressure areas and blisters, the lack of leadership of her care process and poor integration between the palliative care specialist nurses and the ward staff.

The care afforded to Mrs A fell well below standard, there was sparsity of record keeping with little evidence of nutritional assessment and fluid intake and output. There was no formal risk assessment or any record of subsequent treatment.

If Only

Many families punish themselves with the 'if only syndrome':

- If only my child hadn't ridden his bike to school . . .
- If only my child had been seen more quickly in the emergency department . . .

- If only my child had gone to the intensive care unit sooner . . .

- If only I had noticed the rash sooner . . .

Many families need to be helped through this stage of distress but many repeat it constantly in the complaint process and expert attention is needed to move the family on.

Bereavement

Many complaints involve families who are also coping with their bereavement process. If the complaint has involved the death of a child, families sometimes feel that continuing the complaint process almost keeps the child alive for them; that while they are talking about the child they still feel able to cope. However, if the complaint process is closed, how do these families cope?

Bereavement is defined as the normal human reaction to loss and, as a result, medical situations other than death can result in a feeling of loss and bereavement:

- loss of a body part
- loss of body image
- loss of senses
- loss of function
- relative admitted to care.

People react differently to loss. Some of the more common reactions that are associated with complaints handling are:

- anger
- guilt
- shock, numbness and disbelief
- denial
- bargaining
- acceptance
- depression (Gunn 2001).

An obvious note of anger runs through many of the complaints that have been published and families sometimes seem to need to try to blame a particular individual for what has happened. A particularly moving account of a family working through its bereavement is given below in this anonymised quote from a family's letter:

Many people have asked me what was the point as at the end of the day it won't bring Mum back. The investigation has meant justice for Mum and has allowed us to start grieving for her instead of being so fixated by what happened. The work you have done has given a semblance of sense to what happened as it led to changes, and it has also given Mum the dignity taken from her during her stay in hospital. The consultant cardiologist works at the private hospital I work at and took time out to talk to me, and give me his true feelings about what happened. He reassured me that the changes were realistic. He said the nature of the complaints procedure was 'confrontational' and he had been unable to speak freely before then. It is a shame that we couldn't all work together to sort things out.

Complaints in the NHS often stem from stressful events at a time when people feel vulnerable and scared. They may at times be unreasonable but must still be assessed objectively. Complaints can also be stressful for NHS staff, who might well feel that they did their best in difficult circumstances and that the only outcome is for them to be criticised. It is essential that complaints departments are managed by experienced staff who are able to support both the complainant and staff.

MANAGING COMPLAINTS ON THE FRONT LINE

The only sustainable option for those in public services is to create a climate of openness. Openness is the only means of establishing public confidence in the Health Service and in the competence of its professionals (Sir Michael Buckley, Health Service Ombudsman, 1997–2002)

It is essential that all staff within a health organisation are trained to handle complainants and complaints. It should be an essential part of induction for all staff.

Handling Complaints Well

NHS organisations get it right when:

- handling complaints is part of daily clinical practice
- the approach to investigation is sound
- the response is open and complete and action follows.

What Should NHS Staff Do?

Remember that people want:

- to be acknowledged
- to be taken seriously
- an understandable explanation
- an apology
- to be reassured that it will not happen to anyone else.

The investigation needs to involve the appropriate staff and to be prompt and professional. An honest and open response is the only answer. It is also essential that the response is written in lay language. The response should be open and complete, connected to the clinical governance framework and communicated to both complainant and staff and the next steps explained, particularly if there has been a change of procedure as a result of the complaint.

The Complaint Pathway (Fig. 3.1)

Ensuring lessons are learnt from complaints in clinical practice (Figs 3.2 and 3.3) is important:

It may seem a strange principle to enunciate as a first requirement in a hospital, that it should do the sick no harm (Nightingale 1863)

It is essential that complaints management is seen as part of the clinical governance agenda and that when staff are reporting to Trust Board's on their quality agenda that complaints are also reported alongside serious incidents, quality audit and quality improvement programmes. They are a superb learning tool for all healthcare professionals and should be used in that way to enhance the clinical governance agenda and enhance the level of practice within an organisation. It is also essential that performance is linked with learning and that organisations such as the Nursing and Midwifery Council (NMC), CHAI and the National Institute for Clinical Excellence (NICE) all regularly collaborate about the issues of concern and review clinical practice.

OUTCOME OF THE COMPLAINT

Evaluation

Look at a complaint and consider the following questions:

- Would the person evaluating the complaint have been satisfied with the answer?
- Could responses have been improved?
- Were lessons learned?
- Was action required?
- Did action occur?

It is essential that complaints are reported on and that nurses are aware of any complaints that have occurred in

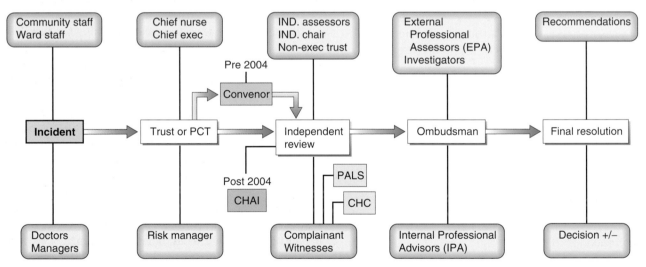

Fig. 3.1 • Complaint pathway.

Fig. 3.2 • Linking performance and learning.

Fig. 3.3 • Linking performance and learning.

their environment. There is no point in being immediately defensive about a complaint – all complaints must be considered from the perception of the family or child. Nurses need to consider the level of documentation and record keeping that they have made, take an opportunity to look through a care plan of a patient and see if they could really follow a patient's journey throughout their stay. Is it really possible to assess the level of care that the patient received? Were communication sheets recorded as to the level of conversation that occurred with either the child or the family? If things have gone wrong in the process of the care of the patient, has that been shared with colleagues and used as a learning tool?

ESSENCE OF CARE

The NHS plan (DoH 2000) reinforced the importance of getting the basics right and of improving the patient experience. The *Essence of care* launched in February 2001 (DoH 2001c) provides a tool to help practitioners take a patient focused and structured approach to sharing and comparing practice. It has enabled healthcare personnel to work with patients to identify best practice and to develop action plans to improve care. In July 2002, work began to develop further benchmarks, focusing on communication between patients and carers and healthcare personnel. The benchmarks cover nine areas of care:

1. continence and bladder and bowel care
2. personal and oral hygiene
3. food and nutrition
4. pressure ulcers
5. privacy and dignity
6. record keeping
7. safety of clients with mental health needs
8. principles of self-care
9. communication.

The benchmarks are relevant to all health and social care settings. Therefore the *Essence of care* is presented in a generic format so that it can be used in, for example, primary, secondary and tertiary settings and with all patient or carer groups, including paediatrics. Great Ormond Street Hospital has implemented the *Essence of care* and adapted it to their patients and families.

WWW

Visit the website and obtain a copy:
- http://www.doh.gov.uk/essenceofcare

Published Cases

It is essential for nurses to read complaints and really consider different familes' perceptions of healthcare professionals and the image that they portray.

● Seminar discussion topic

Read the published cases and discuss them amongst colleagues. The following case is an example to all nurses: Mrs A was admitted to hospital to have her baby delivered. She had given birth to her first child a year before by emergency caesarean section. The consultant obstetrician told Mrs A that there was no reason why she would not be able to have a normal vaginal delivery and did not warn her of any attendant risks. However, during her confinement Mrs A's uterus ruptured, thereby depriving her baby daughter of oxygen. The baby died of consequential brain damage a few days later. Mr and Mrs A asked whether any of their daughter's organs had been retained following the post-mortem. Hospital staff told them that wafer-thin samples of tissue might have been retained for research purposes. However, another hospital – which had subsequently undertaken the post-mortem – told Mr and Mrs A that their daughter's brain had been removed for further examination and disposed of by way of their clinical incineration process.

The Ombudsman found that it was reasonable for Mrs A to have been offered a normal vaginal delivery and that at the time of her treatment it was normal for obstetricians not to mention the very small possibility of risk involved. However, she was highly critical of the failure of relevant staff at the hospital to seek urgent medical help and the of decision by midwives to prescribe a drug – Syntocinon – which was contraindicated in women who had had previous Caesarean births and was against the hospital's ward guidelines. She also criticised weak management control and the hospital's failure to offer Mr and Mrs A any form of bereavement counselling until nearly 3 years after their daughter's death. The Ombudsman criticised the handling of Mr and Mrs A's complaint and found that the Trust had failed to be open and honest with them about the gross failures evident in this case. She described the clinical advice to the convener as flawed and unsound and considered that the convener should have sought advice from a demonstrably more independent source. The Ombudsman also found that the first Trust had failed to advise Mr and Mrs A of the likelihood that their daughter's brain would be removed at the post-mortem and then misled them as to what might actually have happened. She criticised both Trusts for the lack of effective liaison over the post-mortem.

Both Trusts accepted the criticisms made in the Ombudsman's report and apologised to Mr and Mrs A for the shortcomings identified. All of the Ombudsman's recommendations were accepted and the first Trust agreed to undertake an investigation into the Senior Midwife's actions and to refer her to the NMC. The second Trust advised the Ombudsman that it was no longer routine practice to remove organs from a body without specific agreement from relatives and that a new standard operating procedure on the post-mortem examination of neonatal, postnatal and child deaths had been introduced.

References

Alderson P (1995) Listening to children. Children, ethics, and social research. Barnardos, London

Atwell J, Gow MA 1985 Paediatric trained district nurses in the community: expensive luxury or economic necessity? British Medical Journal 291:227–229

Audit Commission (1993) Children first. A study of hospital services. HMSO, London

Bowlby J 1951 Maternal care and mental health. World Health Organization monograph. Series No. 2. WHO, Geneva

British Association for Community Child Health (BAACH) 1995 Child health rights, implementing the UN convention on the rights of the child within the National Health Service. A practitioner's guide. BAACH, London

Caring for Children in the Health Service (CCHS) 1988 Parents staying overnight in hospital with their children. NAWCH, London

Caring for Children in the Health Service (CCHS) 1991 Just for the day. NAWCH, London

Caring for Children in the Health Service (CCHS) 1987 Where are the children? NAWCH, London

Caring for Children in the Health Service (CCHS), Thornes R 1993 Bridging the gaps. Action for Sick Children, London

Carter B 2002 Health inequalities: a blight on children's lives and futures. Journal of Child Health Care 6(1):4–6

Charles-Edwards I, Glasper EA 2002 Ethics and children's rights: learning from past mistakes. British Journal of Nursing 11(17):1132–1140

Clothier C, MacDonald CA, Shaw DA 1994 The Allitt inquiry: independent inquiry relating to the deaths and injuries on the children's ward at Grantham and Kesteven General Hospital during the period February to April 1991. HMSO, London

Committee of the Central Health Services Council 1959 The welfare of children in hospital (Platt Report). HMSO, London

Committee on Child Health Services 1976 Fit for the future. HMSO, London

Department for Education and Skills (DfES) 2003 Every child matters. The Stationery Office, London

Department of Health (DoH) 1989 The Children Act. An introductory guide for the NHS Health Publications Unit. HMSO, London

Department of Health (DoH) 1991 The welfare of children and young people in hospital. HMSO, London

Department of Health (DoH) 1996 The patient's charter – services for children and young people. HMSO, London

Department of Health (DoH) 1997a Government response to the reports of the House of Commons Health Committee on health services for children and young people, session 1996–97: The specific health needs of children and young people (307-1); Health services for children and young people in the community, home and school (314-1); Hospital services for children and young people (128-1); Child and adolescent mental health services (26-1). DoH, London

Department of Health (DoH) 1997b A bridge to the future, nursing standards, education and workforce planning in paediatric intensive care. Report of the Chief Nursing Officer's task force. DoH, London

Department of Health (DoH) 1998 Independent inquiry into inequalities in health report (chairman Sir Donald Acheson). The Stationery Office, London

Department of Health (DoH) 1999 Convention on the rights of the child. Second report to the UN on the rights of the child by the United Kingdom 1999. Executive Summary. DoH, London

Department of Health (DoH) 2000 The NHS plan: a plan for investment, a plan for reform. The Stationery Office, London

Department of Health (DoH) 2001a The Royal Liverpool children's inquiry: summary and recommendations. The Stationery Office, London

Department of Health (DoH) 2001b The report of the public inquiry into children's heart surgery at the Bristol Royal Infirmary 1984–1995. Learning from Bristol. DoH, London

Department of Health (DoH) 2001c Essence of care. DoH, London

Department of Health (DoH) 2003 Tackling health inequalities. A programme for action. Online. Available at: http://www.doh.gov.uk/healthinequalities/programmeforaction [accessed 20 September 2004]

Department of Health (DoH) 2004 The right start: the national service framework for children, young people and maternity services. Online. Available at: http://www.doh.gov/childrenstaskforce

Department of Health and Social Security (DHSS) 1980 The Black report: inequalities in health. HMSO, London

Dyer C 1994 Inquiry into serial killer criticises hospital's response. British Medical Journal 308(6927):491

Glasper EA 2001 Nurses must enhance care in the wake of Bristol. British Journal of Nursing 10(15):966

Glasper EA, Campbell S 1994 Beyond the Clothier inquiry. Nursing Standard 8(23):18–19

Glasper EA, Cooper M 1999 Hospitals need specialist inpatient adolescent units. British Journal of Nursing 8(9):549

Glasper EA, Powell C 2000 Children deserve better. British Journal of Health Care Management 6(1):3

Glasper EA, Powell C 2001 Lessons of Alder Hey: consent must be informed. British Journal of Nursing 10(4):213

Gunn C 2001 A practical guide to complaints handling. In the context of clinical governance. Churchill Livingstone, Edinburgh

Ham C 1999 Health policy in Britain, 4th edn. Macmillan, Basingstoke

House of Commons Health Committee 1997 Third report: health services for children and young people in the community, home and school. The Stationery Office, London

Lord Laming 2003 The Victoria Climbie inquiry: report of an inquiry by Lord Laming. The Victoria Climbie Inquiry. Online. Available at: http://www.victoria-climbie-inquiry.org.uk/finreport/finreport.htm

National Assembly for Wales 2002 A review of safeguards for children and young people treated and cared for by the NHS in Wales. Too serious a thing. The Carlile review. The National Assembly of Wales, Cardiff

NHS Executive 1996 Child health in the community: a guide to good practice. DoH, London

NHS Executive 1998 Health service circular, children's safeguards review: choosing with care. HSC 1998/212. DoH, London. Online. Available at: http://www.open.gov.uk/doh/coinh.htm

Nightingale F 1863 Notes on hospitals, 3rd edn. Longmans Green and Co., London

Powell C 2003 Lessons to be learnt from the Victoria Climbie inquiry. British Journal of Nursing 12(3):137

Robertson J 1962 Hospitals and children, a parent's eye view. Victor Gollanez, London

Royal College of Nursing (RCN) 1994 The care of sick children. A review of the guidelines in the wake of the Allitt Inquiry. RCN, London

Royal College of Paediatrics and Child Health (RCPCH) 2003 Bridging the Gaps: Health Care for Adolescents. RCPCH, London

Tucker A 2002 Sir Douglas Black. The Guardian (Public health) Saturday 14 September 2002

University of London 1955 An account of hospital admissions in the pre-school period. Joint Committee of The Insitute of Child Health, Society of Medical Officers of Health and Population Investigation Committee. University of London, London

Utting W 1997 People like us: the report of the review of safeguards for children living away from home. The Stationery Office, London

Viner R, Keane M 1998 Youth matters: evidence-based best practice for the care of young people in hospital. Action For Sick Children, London

Chapter Four

4

Cultural Aspects of Children's Nursing

Jim Richardson

ABSTRACT

The primary aim of this chapter and its companion PowerPoint presentation is to explore the ideas of culture, its importance and how these ideas can be applied in everyday practice. By paying due regard to cultural factors when nursing children and families, we can help to ensure that nursing care is personalised and sensitive. Practical strategies for integrating ideas of culture into children's nursing will be introduced. An important element of the chapter is to encourage readers to consider how their own cultural expectations and assumptions might affect their professional decision making and actions.

Learning Outcomes

- Explore aspects of your own personal culture and the impact these might have on your professional interactions.

- Express what culture means as a term and appreciate the importance of taking culture into account in children's nursing work.

- Recognise what aspects of children's, and their families', responses are determined by their cultural background.

- Identify strategies for using ideas of culture in everyday children's nursing activity.

What is Culture?

It seems difficult to pin down precisely what we mean by 'culture', although the term is in frequent use. The word contains shades of meaning that include 'race' or 'nationality'; we now talk of multicultural Britain and transcultural nursing. Equally, culture can be taken to mean the creative product of a society such as literature, music, etc.

An examination of what idea of culture this chapter is offering should help to clarify terms from the outset. The Nursing Council of New Zealand (2002 p 3) defines culture quite simply: 'culture refers to the beliefs and practices common to any particular group.'

Helman (2000 p2) expands on this:

Culture is . . . a set of guidelines . . . which an individual inherits as a member of a particular society and which tells him/her how to view the world and learn how to behave in relation to other people. It also provides him/her with a way of transmitting these guidelines to the next generation.

Helman (2000) goes on to explain that culture can be seen as an acquired lens through which we see the world. This is a useful analogy because culture can be seen in this way as a sort of filter through which our experience of the world passes and which helps us to interpret it.

From these definitions some characteristics of culture can be teased out:

- Culture is learned, therefore, acquired. Children primarily learn their culture within the family and immediate community. Later, school life and peers contribute to the growing cultural sense of the child. In fact, it might be said that it is beliefs deriving from culture that dictate how we respond to children and our child-rearing practices.

- It is logical, then, that culture is passed from generation to generation. Some aspects of culture seem to change readily between generations (we don't tend to think or behave exactly as our parents or grandparents do!). On the other hand, once we have learned and internalised our cultural norms we might well be quite resistant to any change in these.

- Culture is dynamic – it changes while being passed between the generations (the generation gap). It might also change in response to the time, place and conditions within which a cultural group live.
- Culture helps us to identify the group to which we belong. By extension, it can help us to identify groups to which we do not belong. This can provide a potential source of sense of solidarity within our group but can also be the origin of friction between groups.
- Culture helps to identify core beliefs. This can include religious belief and spiritual responses. This aspect can be fundamentally important to people during periods of change, stress or crisis, for example, when a child is sick. This aspect of culture can also determine how people interpret health and ill-health, the causes of ill-health and which treatments should be used.
- Culture helps to define our core values. Culture influences us in how we judge what is 'right' and what is 'wrong' for example.
- Culture has a role to play in the development of our life habits and customs – the way we behave and dress, as well as the food that we eat, are determined by culture. How many of us, in times of stress or tiredness, prefer to eat familiar comforting food from our childhood?
- Culture gives us a pattern for living, it can give us a template for how to respond to crises and difficulties in everyday life.
- Culture is important to us because it dictates how we interpret and respond to the world around us. Without particularly reflecting on this, it can dictate our judgements on the views and actions of others. We tend to regard our own way as correct and might view others as being wrong on the basis of this. For professional people like children's nurses this tendency might seriously affect the quality of our relationships with those we work with.
- Culture is thoroughly internalised. Having learned our culture in childhood, it is an integral part of ourselves and largely subconscious. When we encounter new situations we tend to see them through our cultural 'lens' and make rapid judgements, sometimes without much further thought.

These definitions can be seen to be broad. They indicate that culture is a feature of a wide variety of different groups (Wilkins 1993). One of the bugbears of using cultural ideas in nursing in the past has been the tendency to see culture as being confined to ethnicity. Of course, ethnic groups can be seen as cultural groups but so too can a range of other groups who share beliefs, values and customs. By extension, it is easy then to say that cultural issues concern us *all*. If we confine our inquiry about cultural aspects to other ethnic groups then we run the risk of not considering our own cultural responses.

If we continue in the vein of considering culture broadly we create the opportunity of seeing a range of cultural groups that we might not otherwise see.

 Activity

Suggest a range of cultural groups that might not necessarily be based on ethnicity.

If we look at groups based on shared beliefs, values and customs on the list you compiled during the above activity we might find:

- Groups based on age, e.g. the elderly and youth might be seen as cultural or subcultural groups because, although they largely share a world-view with society as a whole, they also have distinctive, slightly different perspectives from the majority.
- Groups based on regional origin, e.g. those originating from the north or the south of England, those from the Midlands and those from the south west all carry with them distinct characteristics of groups from their home region. This is clearly illustrated when someone moves from their home region and is struck by the strange habits of the natives of their new home area.

It might even be argued that some of the perceived differences in beliefs and behaviours between men and women are based on cultural norms.

 Activity

- Stretch your imagination a little further and try to think of other areas that could be defined as cultural. An interesting perspective from the point of view of the children's nurse might be a suggestion that subcultures might be formed within the healthcare field.
- Consider, with a view to the definitions of culture given earlier, to what extent children's nurses might form a (sub)cultural group.

If we accept that nurses form a cultural group with a body of shared beliefs, values and customs then, by extension, children and their families do not belong to that group. It will often be observed that 'experienced' mothers, that is mothers whose child's health concerns have brought them into frequent contact with healthcare professionals, often seem to have learned the 'rules' of the culture of the healthcare world, including its language. One parent of a child in hospital observed to me that you could always tell 'experienced' mothers on a hospital ward; they are the ones who always have a packet of biscuits in their handbag!

It makes sense that parents unfamiliar with the healthcare context might find themselves bemused by the unspoken expectations and rules of the healthcare encounter. It is well documented that implementation of child and family care has been complicated by parents feeling uncertain about quite what is expected of them and not being clear about the unwritten 'rules' (Darbyshire 1994, Coyne 1995, Valentine 1998).

Activity

- Think of a family you have cared for who is deemed by healthcare professionals to be 'difficult'.
- To what extent do you think that cultural factors, e.g. beliefs, values and customs common to a group,might have been implicated in this situation?

Examples like this illustrate how cultural misunderstandings or lack of insight can hamper collaborative work or even, in extreme cases, form the basis of conflict situations. From this it can be seen how important culture can be as a factor in the everyday work of children's nurses (Andrews 1995).

Much of what you will read about cultural aspects of health care will appear to contradict this broad reading of what culture is. Many authorities will interpret culture as almost being synonymous with ethnicity. So when commentators describe Britain as being a multicultural society they often mean a multiethnic society. It must be emphasised that the broad reading of what culture is does not negate in any sense the importance of ethnicity in health and social care.

Ethnicity is a significant aspect of cultural care issues and caring for children from different ethnic groups often raises very clear cultural questions (Whiting 1999).

www

Find more material about ethnicity and health on the Department of Health website:
- http://www.dh.gov.uk

One of the problems of considering cultural aspects of culture in children's nursing is that it can often seem very abstract, and this is often not helped by the complex, sometimes even obscure, language used to describe cultural concepts (Ahmann 1994).

Considering some of these ideas in more detail can be useful in illustrating how facets of cultural thinking can be useful in the everyday, practical world.

ETHNOCENTRISM

Although this word appears fearsome it simply describes the situation where we consider our own personal cultural

world-view to be correct in all its detail. As we learn our culture from an early age – an important fact for children's nurses to bear in mind – it tends to be a deeply ingrained part of us. We do not usually consciously consider it when we are making judgements about our experiences. In this way our culture can be compared with Helman's lens, through which we filter everything that happens to us and colours our reaction to these experiences. Anyone who wears glasses will be aware of how quickly you become unaware of the glasses themselves when viewing the world around you.

Activity

Think of a situation in which you have disapproved of something that someone else has said or done. Can you think of why you reacted in this way?

Because the cultural lens, or yardstick, against which you measure your experiences is often virtually subliminal it can form the basis of the 'gut reaction'. Think of how you would feel if you went to eat at a friend's and were offered an unfamiliar or exotic food, such as snake, to eat. Your reaction would be based on your cultural concept of appropriate food to eat, which you learned in childhood. Of course, some of us are more daring and adventurous than others so you might enjoy the opportunity to sample snake! This same kind of 'it's not my way' reaction can occur to any aspect of other people's behaviour.

A few years ago I was involved in caring for the child in the following scenario:

Scenario

Five-year-old Rachel is being cared for following a traumatic fracture of her left femur. She is confined to bed on balanced traction. She is disorientated by what is happening and is often quite tearful. Her mother breastfeeds her in the morning and when she is settling to sleep in the evening. Many of the nurses on the ward are quite shocked by this.

Activity

- Consider why the nurses might be feeling shocked in this situation?
- What might be the effect of their reacting in this way?

You can see that it is difficult sometimes to be clear as to quite why we react to situations in the way that we do – this is culture in action.

Ethnocentrism could be argued to be a part of all of us and will lead to us responding positively to those with whom we share a culture (Sprott 1994). The other side of the coin is that we can respond negatively to people whose culture orientation leads them to behave or to value things that we do not. Clearly, we do not always demonstrate our reactions to others – nurses traditionally strive not to be judgemental – but it is all too easy for our reactions – positive or negative – to be communicated through channels such as body language. If we disapprove of someone's behaviour, which is based on their cultural orientation, and they become aware of our disapproval then that could have a seriously negative effect on our working together if this occurs in a professional setting. Equally, we might be led to condone behaviours that are culturally acceptable to us but that are not entirely constructive. Alcohol use among young people is widely acceptable within that age group within this community and is often talked of in a 'jokey' fashion.

Ethnocentrism is a natural part of us but it is particularly important for children's nurses to reflect on how it leads us to respond and behave in our work with children and families. Children are especially vulnerable to cultural disapproval because they are learning their family's and community's culture (Chevannes 1997). During this learning process their cultural self might be fragile and vulnerable to the disapproval or scorn of others. Cultural disrespect is potentially damaging. In this way, it can be seen how ethnocentrism can form the basis for prejudice, be it positive or negative. The process of reflecting on our cultural reactions based on ethnocentrism can help to improve our personal self-awareness and help avoid many harmful effects.

www

A range of materials relating to cultural factors in children's nursing along with some exercises can be found on the Royal College of Nursing's website at:

* http://www.rcn.org/resources/transcultural

Scenario

Three-month-old Matty, who was born at 34 weeks gestation and had a very stormy start to his life, was recently discharged home into the care of his parents and big sister. He has come to outpatients with his mother and 6-year-old sister, Adele. Adele is bored and frustrated with the wait and has just been involved in a noisy disagreement with another child. Her mother reacts strongly and smacks her several times on the legs.

Activity

* How do you feel about children being smacked by their parents?
* To what extent would you think that your views are culturally based?
* What kinds of messages do you give to those you disagree with on this question?

Any discussion about such matters is likely to generate a deal of heat. It could be suggested that this is because such views are often determined by cultural values. The perspective we adopt in relation to such issues is ethnocentric; anyone agreeing with us is right and anyone disagreeing is wrong. Such automatically and unthinkingly assumed polar positions are unhelpful. It could be said that self-awareness is largely cultural self-awareness.

STEREOTYPING

Stereotyping is a close cousin of ethnocentrism. It can be defined as assuming cultural characteristics of a person (without asking them!) based on our perception of the group that they belong to. An example of this might be when a nurse first meets the father of a child in his or her care. The father is wearing a turban. What does the nurse think? If the reaction is stereotypical it might run something like this:

Oh, Mr S— is a Sikh. I have nursed Sikh people before, they like to do A, B and C and they don't like D, E and F.

Although these assumptions might be correct, they could equally well be quite wrong. People within cultural groups will naturally have individual and subgroup variations. Even within cohesive groups we do not share identical beliefs, values and customs. You need only listen to the sorts of debates that go on around the time of national elections to appreciate this. It is unhelpful to 'pigeonhole' people on the basis of assumed characteristics. The only way to know about people's culturally determined beliefs and habits is to ask them!

CULTURE SHOCK

Another feature of our cultural understandings being learnt early in life, deeply ingrained and often subconsciously acted on is that we can rely on shared understandings and assumptions when we are within our cultural group. This is a comfortable, secure position to be in. However, if we move outside our group then we can no longer rely on these mutual interpretations. This can feel very disorientating. You might have noticed this when on holiday abroad; it is irritating when people do not do as you expect them to, for example, queue in an orderly fashion in a post office! A South-East Asian refugee to the United States expressed his feeling of culture shock as feeling like a goat in a herd of cows! This is a vivid illustration of how culture shock can make you feel almost visibly different from those around you. Our shared understandings within our own cultural group include many unwritten rules. Everyone in that environment understands and feels comfortable with these conventions; anyone new to the context is likely to feel discomfited.

It could be argued that the parents of a sick child experience a degree of culture shock when they come into contact with the hospital environment and healthcare professionals. Parents, and patients, often find it difficult to know what is expected of them and the rules that healthcare professionals expect them to abide by. This situation is not helped when children's nurses assume that parents have this knowledge and understanding. More open communication and clarity would go some way towards alleviating the discomfort and stress of culture shock.

Cultural Assessment

To be able to use all of these ideas in relation to culture it will be useful to examine a framework of cultural assessment. There are several of these (e.g. Tripp Reimer et al 1984, Giger & Davidhizar 1995, Purnell & Paulanka 1998) and they generally do not vary greatly in terms of content. However, some are more practical than others in terms of clarity and ease of use in practice. Giger & Davidhizar (1995) offer a framework with six dimensions:

1. communication
2. space
3. social organisation
4. time
5. environmental control
6. biological variation.

Giger & Davidhizar believe that each of these dimensions describes an area of human life that is universal, i.e. shared by all cultures, although there might be significant variation between cultural groups. Taken together, these universal dimensions illustrate the major culturally determined differences between people. Therefore, if we use them as a system of assessment for cultural differences then we should identify and capture those issues in the care encounter that require culture sensitivity and understanding.

COMMUNICATION

Communication is generally agreed to be a central part of the children's nurse's function. Communication is starkly illustrated as an issue when the nurse and patient/family speak different languages. However, it can be just as important when factors such as professional jargon or language that is too complex for the child to understand are used. Often, non-verbal communication is particularly challenging between people from different cultural backgrounds. Gestures carry different meanings in different groups and cultural norms, such as the use of eye contact, can vary a good deal. For some, avoiding eye contact, particularly with authority figures, is seen as simply polite; others would interpret this as shifty behaviour.

SOCIAL ORGANISATIONS

How we relate to each other as individuals and groups is strongly culture related. As they grow, children learn how to relate to their elders and parents. This can take the form of small children learning 'good manners', although what constitutes good manners changes over time and between cultural groups. That children should be 'seen and not heard' is not a value promoted in Western cultures today, but it is still a guiding principle for some groups. Similarly, some adults look askance on children behaving exuberantly in a public place, whereas for some groups it is to be positively encouraged. The respective roles adopted by men and women within communities and family groups are also determined largely by cultural norms.

TIME

This dimension is important in children's nursing because it takes children a good deal of effort to understand this abstract notion. Small children can struggle with the idea of 'tomorrow' or 'at 2 o'clock'. Some groups value punctuality whereas some are very much less concerned with this. Some cultures have a future orientation (study hard for your exams and you'll get to university then you'll get a good job) and others are more past oriented (what do you want to go to university for? No one in our family ever has done so before). Others again might be present oriented and see the future as impossible to predict, whereas the past is gone and irrelevant. Each of those positions can influence how children and families react to misfortune or ill health.

ENVIRONMENTAL CONTROL

The variation between groups in terms of how they perceive their ability to affect events in their environment and lives is contained in this dimension. This will affect how they interpret the reason for events, e.g. why a child becomes unwell, what causes this and what should be done about it. Therefore, it will dictate what should be done if a child has, for example, a fever; perhaps nothing will be done – just wait and see – perhaps a drug (e.g. paracetamol) will be given, perhaps the child will be taken to a doctor or to consult a folk healer.

BIOLOGICAL CONTROL

This is a very important dimension for nurses because it links to the variations seen under the environmental control category. Factors related to our place and group of origin are aspects of our cultural beliefs and customs in relation to life events. Rituals and required behaviours in the face of difficult challenges are affected by differences between cultures and these are often reflected in religious belief and practice. Dietary aspects also appear in this category – the foods we prefer and the effects we believe foods have on our bodies and health.

 Activity

> Running through these categories, make a list of factors you and your family/community consider to be important in each dimension, e.g. for the time dimension, do you consider punctuality to be important? Why?

Taking all of these factors together we can begin to get a picture of how complex, subtle and difficult to reveal and analyse cultural factors can be. However, it is not a hopeless picture! There are several approaches to working with cultural aspects in child health care. One is the promotion of cultural safety through self-awareness. This is an attractive idea because, as children's nurses, we seek to ensure the safety and well-being of the children and families in our care. In the past, culture was often not emphasised as a factor in nursing care and the potential for care to be culturally unsafe was considerable. This would occur when the beliefs, values and customs of children were ignored, or even worse scorned. Cultural safety is an orientation with an element of reaction to some previous attempts at developing transcultural nursing models. Some of these, although well meaning, tended to emphasise differences between groups by examining what were sometimes exotically different groups (e.g. the weaning habits of Tibetan yak herders). These also ran the risk of stereotyping people (e.g. all Tibetan yak herders wean their babies at the same age and in the same way). Cultural safety does not concentrate on learning a shopping list of factors that identify a cultural group. Rather, within this framework the children's nurse works to achieve an understanding of her/his own cultural values. This reflection would also

consider the nature of power within the nurse–child/family relationship. Obviously, if the nurse is basing professional and personal judgements on personal values, and also holds power in relation to the child and family, then the results could at best be non-constructive and at worst destructive.

Cultural safety consists of a set of ideas that have been evolving for some time in the social sciences and nursing. It is perhaps at its most developed in New Zealand. The context in New Zealand is particular; it is a postcolonial nation where the majority is descended from white European immigrants and the significant minority from the original inhabitants – the Maori. The last three decades of the 20th century saw a wide-ranging debate in New Zealand as to why outcomes for the Maori are worse on almost every dimension – and particularly in health – than for New Zealanders of European origin. The conclusion reached was that cultural oppression was a significant factor in this situation and solutions sought. The key features of cultural safety are (Nursing Council of New Zealand 2002 p 7):

> *The effective nursing or midwifery practice of a person or family from another culture, is determined by that person or family. Culture includes, but is not restricted to age or generation; gender; sexual orientation; occupation and socioeconomic status; ethnic origin or migrant experience; religious or spiritual belief; and disability.*
>
> *The nurse or midwife delivering the nursing or midwifery service will have undertaken a process of reflection on his or her own cultural identity and will recognise the impact that his or her personal culture has on his or her professional practice. Unsafe cultural practice comprises any action which diminishes, demeans or disempowers the cultural identity and well-being of an individual.*

Cultural safety in this system is based on each nurse gaining a knowledge and understanding of his or her own cultural values rather than trying to learn aspects of the culture of other groups (which runs the risk in any case of being stereotypical).

Cultural safety can be said to be achieved when each child/family receives care that is based on all that makes them individual and unique. This can only be defined by those who are receiving that care.

It is not a major leap to appreciating that if this is achieved then the respect, trust and effective communication will be in place on which to base a constructive helping relationship. The Nursing Council New Zealand (2002) proposes a series of stages in learning to integrate culture into care:

● Cultural awareness: simply understanding that people differ on the basis of learnt beliefs and values.

● Cultural sensitivity: acknowledging that these differences are legitimate and gaining awareness of one's own cultural norms and how these might affect others.

● Cultural safety: the care delivered is culturally safe as defined by those receiving care.

Clearly, this represents a theoretical framework that could be further legitimated by testing through research. However, it does offer a number of very thought-provoking insights. It emphasises that culture will be an issue in most caring encounters and that skill in working with cultural aspects will be fundamental for all nurses.

 WWW

Read more about the idea of cultural safety on the website of the Nursing Council of New Zealand:
● http://www.nursingcouncil.nz

Summary

Culture can be argued to be a significant factor in nursing work and there have been several approaches for nurses to develop their knowledge and skills in this arena. Culture is defined widely as being a characteristic of the beliefs and practices of a wide range of groups, which might include:

● age or generation
● gender
● sexual orientation
● occupation and socio-economic status
● ethnic origin or immigrant experience
● religious or spiritual belief
● disability.

Taking cultural aspects into account is especially important for children's nurses because of the special and particular nature of children. Because culture is a learnt phenomenon that occurs during childhood, then children will be active learners of their own culture at the time of the care encounter. As a person's individual culture is incompletely learnt until later in childhood, then the child might be at risk of confusion and distress if disrespect is shown towards his or her culturally determined beliefs, values and customs. As active learners of culture, children might also be confused by encountering cultural norms that are at variance with those they are in the process of learning at home and within their community. Failure to take culture into account might result in a discriminatory, insensitive and inappropriate attempt at care, which is bound to fail.

References

Ahmann E 1994 'Chunky stew': appreciating cultural diversity while providing health care for children. Pediatric Nursing 29(3):320–324

Andrews MM 1995 Transcultural perspectives in the nursing care of children and adolescents. In: Andrews MM, Boyle JS (eds) 1995 Transcultural concepts in nursing care, Lippincott, Philadelphia JB

Chevannes M 1997 Nursing care for families – issues in a multicultural society. British Journal of Nursing 6:161–167

Coyne I 1995 Parental participation in care: a critical review of the literature. Journal of Advanced Nursing 21:716–722

Darbyshire P 1994 Living with a sick child in hospital: the experiences of parents and nurses. Chapman & Hall, London

Giger JN, Davidhazar RE 1995 Transcultural nursing, 3rd edn. Mosby Year Book, St Louis

Helman CG 2000 Culture, health and illness, 4th edn. Butterworth Heinemann, Oxford

Nursing Council of New Zealand 2002 Guidelines for cultural safety, the treaty of Waitangi and Maori health in nursing and midwifery education and practice. Nursing Council of New Zealand, Wellington

Purnell LD, Paulanka BJ 1998 Transcultural healthcare. FA Davis, Philadelphia

Sprott JE 1994 One person's 'spoiling' is another's freedom to become: overcoming ethnocentric views about parental control. Social Sciences and Medicine 38(8):1111–1124

Tripp-Reimer T, Brink PJ, Saunders JM 1984 Cultural assessment: convert and process. Nursing Outlook 32(2):78–82

Valentine F 1998 Empowerment: family centred care. Paediatric Nursing 10(1):24–27

Whiting L 1999 Caring for children of differing cultures. Journal of Child Health Care 3(4):33–37

Wilkins H 1993 Transcultural nursing: a selective review of the literature 1985–1991. Journal of Advanced Nursing 18(4):606–612

Chapter Five

5

The Psychological Preparation of Children for Hospitalisation

E Alan Glasper, Rachel E A Haggarty

ABSTRACT

Historical and contemporary work identifies that children have fears and anxieties when they are admitted to hospital. After examining the rationale for such anxieties and potential consequences, this chapter concentrates on the various ways in which professionals can help children prepare for and cope with their hospital experience. The role of parents/carers is also identified and questions raised as to the specific needs of children with learning difficulties, communication impairment and chronic illness. Finally, the importance of ongoing staff education is noted

Learning Outcomes

- Appreciate why hospitals/healthcare institutions may be a source of anxiety for sick children.

- Explore a typical preadmission programme and discuss the pros and cons of such preparation.

- Describe the full range of interventions and distraction techniques used by children's nurses to allay anxiety preadmission and preprocedurally.

- Understand the ways in which parents/carers can contribute to the preparation of children for hospital/ procedures, and consider the educational support that parents/carers require.

- Describe how emergency admissions/non-attendees to programmes can be prepared for hospital interventions.

- Consider the specific preparation needs of children with learning difficulties, communication impairment and chronic illness.

- Recognise the importance of ongoing education for healthcare professionals involved in preparing children and families for hospitalisation.

Introduction

This chapter considers issues surrounding the emotional well-being of the sick child, and the psychological preparation of children for hospitalisation. Saile et al (1988 p 109) define psychological preparation as:

> . . . *any planned strategy used by a professional or trained helper on a child or his family with the purpose of reducing anxiety related to medical procedures, decreasing pain, accelerating the healing process and making it possible for the child to cope adequately with the procedure.*

The latter half of the 20th century, and indeed the first few years of the 21st, saw growing recognition within paediatric nursing of the potentially harmful effects that may result from children's hospitalisation. A range of initiatives have been implemented to minimise such harmful effects, including parental participation in care, play specialists, shorter inpatient stays, preadmission preparation programmes and the development of more 'child friendly' hospital environments. It is therefore important that the child health practitioner has a sound understanding of these issues, and of the historical background to these initiatives.

Historical Perspectives

The original founders of the UK children's hospitals, which were built during the reign of Queen Victoria, were primarily motivated by the alleviation of the physical elements of illness during childhood. Children's nurses of the past might not always have embraced the concept of family-centred care in the same way as contemporary nurses; this was perhaps a reflection of the poor understanding of the psychological aspects of health and illness prevalent at that time. Despite this, the maxim of the first of these Victorian edifices, the Hospital for Sick Children in London, is 'the child first and always' (Glasper & Charles-Edwards 2002). Indeed, during the 18th century, Dr George Armstrong is credited as being highly influential in delaying the opening of tertiary inpatient facilities for children in London, suggesting that children and their parents should not be separated as doing so would break the child's heart (Miles 1986). He believed that parents would not be able to look after their children in hospital because of economic pressures (Glasper & Lowson 1998). However, in reality the appalling sanitary conditions, the overcrowding and the general poverty prevalent at that time ensured that the little care available in the home was also often of a poor quality (Kosky & Lunnon 1991).

It should be remembered that the early children's hospitals were built in the pre-Nightingale era and before the professionalisation of nursing. The Nightingale tradition subtly changed the dynamics of the children's hospitals, and military principles developed by Nightingale in the Crimea began to be applied. The move away from essentially lay care and the development of professional paediatric nursing had some disadvantages, namely the gradual exclusion of parents from the direct participation in care. So although there is evidence from historical drawings of the first ward at Great Ormond Street that parents were able to be with their children in hospital and participate in their care, the military changes eventually resulted in the establishment of strict visiting hours, with parents prohibited from visiting at a time convenient to them. Some hospitals allowed parents to visit only once a week or less often.

Bed rest for children until the advent of antibiotics was long and continuous and the screams and incessant crying bouts that accompanied each weekly visit convinced the nursing staff that parents were generally a hindrance rather than a help. Eventually, parents were perceived to be such an infection risk that some hospitals abandoned visiting altogether. Relatives were therefore often excluded because they were likely harbingers of disease and, perhaps more importantly, potential disturbers of the smoothness of long-established ward routines. The visiting times in many children's hospitals were severely restricted. In the Southampton Children's Hospital, for example, at least up until the outbreak of the First World War, visiting was allowed from 2 to 4 p.m. daily, except Sundays. As the century progressed, it became confined to 1 hour on Wednesday and Sunday afternoons, and then in 1947 was banned completely. Visiting was recommenced in 1950 on a limited basis and parents had to wear face masks. Indeed, looking at the UK as a whole, of the 1300 hospitals in Britain in 1951 that admitted children, only 300 allowed daily visiting (usually limited to 30 minutes) and 150 prohibited visiting altogether (Robertson 1989). The white-coated doctors and the starchly uniformed nurses who were so confident about the rightness of traditional practice often intimidated parents and were inaccessible for discussion. There was little in the curricula of either profession on the emotional aspects of childhood and it was not until after the Second World War that the real detrimental effects of early hospital admission became widely recognised.

There were, however, some enlightened paediatricians who had begun to make observations on the detrimental effects on personality development of institutional care. Sir James Spence, Professor of Child Health at the University of Newcastle's Royal Victoria Hospital, began to allow mothers to stay in hospital with infants and young children although he did not extend this service to older children (RCPCH 2000).

The recognition that psychological trauma might be perpetrated on children during their hospital stay came about slowly, and in the UK owes much to the work of John Bowlby and James Robertson. Their work was instrumental in providing the precursors necessary for the creation of a much more family focused approach to the care of hospitalised children.

THEORY OF ATTACHMENT

John Bowlby was a London-based psychiatrist who developed a particular interest in developmental psychology. He described the concept of attachment as a tendency of the young to stay in close proximity to the primary care giver, usually the mother in the first instance, and to be comforted by her sight, sound and touch (Gleitman 1986). Bowlby commenced volunteer work with maladjusted children in a residential setting and his lifetime interest in attachment was stimulated through his experience of working with an affectionless teenager who had no familiarity with a permanent mother figure (Bretherton 2002). The century of childhood nursing practice in which parental roles had virtually disappeared was about to change in the light of his work.

Bowlby was heavily influenced by the science of ethology, the study of animal behaviour and in particular the work of Konrad Lorenz, who first postulated the theory of imprinting in young greylag geese chicks (Gleitman 1986, the PSI Café 2002). The process of imprinting is believed to occur in many animals but is graphically evident in animals such as geese or ducks when, shortly after hatching, the chicks form a strong attachment to whatever moving object they see in their line of vision. In the wild this is normally the mother but Lorenz and others substituted natural mothers with moving inanimate objects, such as rubber boots worn by the researchers. Once imprinted, the chicks follow the object wherever it goes throughout their early life.

Bowlby believed that a similar process occurred in human babies and he referred to this as attachment (Rutherford 1998). The crux of Bowlby's theory is that all human infants need to attach to their mothers (or primary caregiver) if they are to develop into healthy, well-adjusted adults. Furthermore he described the concept of 'bonding' as the mother's emotional attachment to the child (Rutherford 1998, Taylor et al 1999). This important process is put at risk by any form of separation between mother and infant. In 1951 Bowlby published a World Health Organisation monograph entitled *Maternal care and mental health* (Bowlby 1951) in which he began to articulate the adverse effects on personality development of inadequate maternal care. From this date the tide began to turn, albeit slowly.

Two famous quotations from the WHO monograph still have a resounding impact on contemporary health care, despite the fact that they were published over half a century ago:

It is essential for mental health that the infant and young child should experience a warm, intimate and continuous relationship with his mother (or mother substitute) in which to find satisfaction and enjoyment.

Motherlove in infancy and childhood is as important for mental health as are vitamins and proteins for physical health.

At the same time that Bowlby was developing his ideas about human attachment, a number of other researchers began a series of primate experiments to investigate attachment under controlled laboratory conditions, studies that continue to this day. Harry Harlow and fellow researchers at the primate laboratory at the University of Wisconsin carried out perhaps the best known of these experiments (Harlow 1958). Harlow demonstrated that nurturing was more important than sustenance when motherless infant monkeys raised in cages with surrogate mothers made of wire or soft cloth chose to spend the majority of their time with the cloth version despite the wire version having embedded within it a feeding bottle. It is important to stress that these monkeys grew into totally dysfunctional adults who were unable to function in primate society. There is no doubt that these studies reinforced Bowlby's assertion that bonding was a testable hypothesis.

If Harlow's work complemented that of Bowlby, it also revealed the inadequacies of the experimental monkeys when they in turn became mothers. These maternally deprived monkeys proved to be either indifferent to their offspring or outright abusive. It is salutary to note that continued research within the field of maternal deprivation using infant monkeys is coming under greater scrutiny and criticism (Maternal Deprivation Experiments 2002). However, although many now condemn the use of monkeys for the study of maternal deprivation it is sad to reflect that there are children today in many parts of the world who are cared for in suboptimum conditions, often without the benefit of a primary care giver. The situation of the orphanage and hospitalised children in Romania, which became apparent to the outside world only after the overthrow of Nicolae Ceausescu in 1989, is a timely reminder of how appallingly treated children are in some parts of the world, particularly in the aftermath of war (Glasper 1999).

Importantly, Bowlby's theories have been much criticised by other academic researchers, such as Rutter (1981), who believe that Bowlby's emphasis on the constant presence of the mother is overexaggerated, and also that other primary caregivers (most notably the father) also had vital roles. Wolkind & Rutter (1985) argued that infants are capable of 'multiple attachments', and furthermore that these relationships are not necessarily dependent on the amount of time spent with child, but rather on the quality of the interaction. Nevertheless, the concept of attachment and bonding remains the basis for good practice in the care of infants.

MATERNAL DEPRIVATION

As part of Bowlby's work to underpin his theory of attachment, he recruited James Robertson as a research associate to record filmed observations of young hospitalised and institutionalised children who had been separated from their mothers. Among these famous films was *A two-year-old goes to hospital*, which followed 'Laura' through her admission and vividly displayed the adverse effects of maternal separation (Thurtle 1998). Subsequent analysis of these data allowed Bowlby and Robertson to further refine and articulate the stages of separation anxiety that occur during maternal deprivation (Robertson 1970):

- **Protest:** This stage can last from a few hours to a few days. The child has a strong conscious need of the mother and the loud crying exhibited is based on the expectation built on previous experience that the mother will respond to his cries. During this stage of the maternal deprivation sequence the child will cry noisily and look eagerly towards any sound that might be the mother.

- **Despair:** This stage succeeds protest and can best be compared to clinical depression. It is a sign of increasing hopelessness and despondency. The child becomes less active and vocal; in the past this was interpreted by the nursing staff as a sign that the child was settling into the ward.

- **Denial/detachment:** In this the final stage of maternal deprivation the child represses his or her longing for the mother and begins to lose his or her attachment. The child appears, at least superficially, to have settled into the hospital routine and will respond positively, if shallowly, to kind adults who take an interest in him or her. Importantly, the child will react badly to brief reappearances of the mother, as for example during the weekly visiting periods, giving rise to the fallacy that parents actually made matters worse. There is no wonder that generations of children's nurses dreaded 'Sunday afternoon visiting'.

Activity

Obtain and view one of the Robertson videos, e.g.
A two-year-old goes to hospital
- How does this scenario compare with your experience today? Clearly there are improvements, but are there any areas of similarity?

Robertson's films were to play a crucial role in improving the conditions under which children were cared for in hospital. His work fuelled concern among the public, which was instrumental in compelling the government of the day to launch a White Paper, chaired by Sir Harry Platt, to investigate the plight of children in hospital. The seminal report *The welfare of children in hospital* was published in 1959 (Committee of the Central Health Services Council 1959) and it was to fundamentally change practice. Although the Platt report showed the way, subsequent reports began to tackle specific areas of childcare in hospital (Thurtle 1998 p 231 and see Chapter 3).

PowerPoint

Access the companion Chapter 1 PowerPoint presentation and look at the Platt report in full. Does this report still have messages for 21st century children's nurses?

Much of the credit for innovatory change must be attributed to the National Association for the Welfare of Children in Hospital (NAWCH), which is now called Action for Sick Children (ASC). NAWCH was originally founded in 1961 as Mother Care for Children in Hospital. With the support of James Robertson, this parental pressure group thrived and began to campaign for the full implementation of the Platt report. Soon, regional groups were convened all over the UK, which eventually amalgamated in 1963 and became the NAWCH in 1965 (ASC 2002). It is important to stress that although the Platt report was adopted as an official Ministry of Health policy, in the same way that subsequent Department of Health publications are, hospitals were not legally obliged to implement the recommendations. The gauntlet fell to NAWCH, which has since campaigned with considerable success as an advocate for sick children and their families.

Many generations of parents have expressed feelings of helplessness and inadequacy during their child's admission to hospital, when nurses took over care completely. It would be naïve to believe that this situation changed in the immediate aftermath of the publication of the Platt report, as this unhappy state of affairs continued for many years afterwards in some children's units. However, some children's hospitals began to respond to the White Paper in a positive way. The essential message of the document was that hospitals should take steps to reduce separation of parent and sick child (initially only mothers). This was to be achieved by introducing open and unrestricted visiting, providing parental accommodation and avoiding unnecessary hospital admissions. This would ultimately result in a move towards day surgery, but this did not happen immediately.

Daycare Services

Politicians of all political parties have described the health services for children as a potent investment in the country's future. Ambulatory care, of which daycare is a central component, provides the minimum of disruption to the family unit, as a result of shorter hospital stays, and is a potentially powerful weapon in the prevention of psychological trauma caused by an inpatient admission. Many hospitals now have purpose-built day units for children. Such units cater for children undergoing minor surgery, medical therapy, investigative procedures or observation (Ireland & Rushforth 1998). Day units function in a variety of ways; some keep patients for a full day before discharge and others only half a day. For day units to run optimally, a paediatric community nursing service is vital to provide an essential link between hospital and home (Atwell & Gow 1985). Without the provision of such services, the management of children undergoing daycare is fraught with difficulties.

Importance of Psychological Care

Smith (1986) believes that emotional factors might be an even greater source of concern than the child's physical condition during a hospital admission. Although improvements have occurred since the publication of the Platt report, it is important not to be complacent. The many practical tasks and physical needs required by the child and family can, due to time constraints, all too easily dominate the day. It can therefore be easy to lose sight of the child's psychological needs. In a seminal quote, Jolly (1976 p 1532) recorded the words of a 6-year-old child:

They looked at my throat and they looked at my ears. They looked at my heart but they didn't look at me.

Fear of the unknown, fear of physical harm and pain, loss of control and identity, uncertainty about what is expected of them and separation from security and family routine are identified by Visintainer & Wolfer (1975) as five key potential threats to a child on admission to hospital. Anecdotal evidence suggests that, 30 years later, these fears are no less real. Anxiety may be displayed in some by, for example, regressive behaviour, tearful/fearful mood, sleep disturbance or changes to eating pattern. Everyone, to a greater or lesser degree, will have concerns, questions and apprehensions when they are admitted to hospital; a child is no exception. In addition to this, the way in which children interact with the world and attempt to understand and interpret what they see and hear is influenced enormously by their age and stage of development (Piaget & Inhelder 1969) (see Chapter 11).

Professional Conversation

James, a 15-year-old boy with a learning disability, is being prepared for surgery. James clearly understood the concept of the faces pain scale, but then added:

That's all well and good, my physical pain right now is zero but what about a scale on which I can rate my emotions that right now are in a complete scramble?

In contrast to the well-established practice within paediatric nursing of measuring pain, it is interesting to note, as highlighted by James' comments, how rarely nurses explicitly seek to 'measure' children's emotional states. A notable exception is seen in the work of Ellerton & Merriman (1994), who used an 'anxiety faces scale', similar to the well-established 'faces' pain tools, to measure children's emotional anxiety. However, both scales are vulnerable with regard to their accuracy and it is – arguably – important to consider more objective means of measuring anxiety as well.

The link between physiological change and a person's psychological status has been recognised and researched (Hyland & Donaldson 1989). One such early study detected changes in urinary excretion in connection with anxiety responses (Wilson 1981). Additionally, seminal work by Brain & Maclay (1968) showed a higher incidence of complications, such as infection and haemorrhage, in a control group whose mothers were not resident during a child's stay compared with an experimental group whose parents were present. These studies support the fact that disease and illness are not purely a biological phenomenon. However, contemporary research tends to measure anxiety more by behavioural change and attitudinal scales; unfortunately there is a paucity of recent work exploring the physiological manifestations of anxiety.

Activity

Search the literature for different anxiety assessment scales:
- How well do you think these measure anxiety, and how appropriate are they for use with children?
- Create your own emotional rating scale.

Scenario

Ollie is 7 years old and his mother is concerned that he is having lots of time off school with frequent sore throats. She arranges for Ollie to be seen by her local family practitioner, who refers him to the local outpatient department.

Preparing Children for a Hospital Admission

On the premise that emotional needs might be as great, if not greater, than a child's physical needs during a hospital admission, a number of different strategies have been developed to help children and their families cope with hospital admission.

Family preparation for day and inpatient surgery is thought to be important in reducing the psychological effects of hospitalisation. Modern child healthcare services require integration between hospital and community. The service should provide for the child as a whole and should meet the social, emotional, spiritual needs of children and their families as well as their physical needs. The growth of paediatric preadmission programmes throughout the UK represents one facet only of this integrated service. Since the publication of the Platt report, paediatric nurses have developed a reputation for endeavouring to improve the care of their patients and families. Attempting to protect children from the stresses of hospital admission may be partially facilitated through the provision of preadmission programmes. Although the evidence base for the efficacy of these programmes has yet to be firmly established, the Commission for Health Audit and Inspection (CHAI, formerly CHI) has developed an audit tool for NHS Trusts to use to measure compliance to the standards of hospital services developed under the auspices of the National Service Framework for Children. One of the paediatric benchmarks that CHAI will audit is related to preparation, and preadmission clubs are specifically cited as examples of best practice.

Activity

Access the companion PowerPoint presentation and read the National Service Framework online.
- How does this document help children's healthcare professionals to better meet the emotional needs of children?

PREPARATION PROGRAMMES

Preadmission preparation programmes offer the child and family the opportunity to visit the hospital to be familiarised with the environment and personnel. At the same time, practical issues can be discussed and the child and family informed about anticipated specific events (Gaughan & Sweeney 1997). Such programmes are conducted either in outpatient departments, when children come in with the family for initial consultation, or in the main hospital at a set time, usually a week before admission. The changes found historically in children's behaviour after hospitalisation underpins the growth of such formal preadmission programmes. A study by Fassler (1980) indicates that a combination of emotional support and information appertaining to the admission appears to be an effective method of reducing preoperative anxiety. Keeton (1999) noted that children who had attended a preparation day settled more quickly in their surroundings and were more relaxed and happy than those who had not. Current work by Keeton is exploring whether preadmission programmes reduce stress and anxiety of family responses at anaesthetic induction in children undergoing day surgery.

PowerPoint

Access the companion PowerPoint presentation and follow the preadmission programme slides.

Scenario

Following Ollie's outpatient appointment, the ENT surgeon has indicated that he requires a tonsillectomy. He is scheduled for surgery within the next 3 months. Before his admission, he and his family receive an invitation to attend the preadmission programme.

The most common type of programme in the UK is conducted in hospital, often at weekends. One of the first preadmission programmes in the UK was developed at the Queen's Medical Centre in Nottingham in 1982. The format established at Nottingham has been emulated in a number of other children's units. Invitations to the programmes are posted to patients with all the other information prior to admission. The programmes often consist of a PowerPoint or video/DVD presentation followed by a visit to the ward/unit to which the child will be admitted. Additionally, children and their carers may have the opportunity of visiting the anaesthetic room, where they can see first hand where they will receive their anaesthetic and – importantly – be reassured that their parent/carer will be allowed to go with them on the day. Therapeutic play programmes and biscuits and juice for the children usually

complete the morning's programme. While the children are playing, the parents have coffee and time for 'question and answer', and conversation with other parents, which can yield invaluable peer support. Many children's units give the children a play-pack at the end of the programme consisting of a paper theatre hat, paints, name band, mask and badge, plus a cotton theatre gown which parents are asked to return on admission. Many members of theatre staff participate enthusiastically in preadmission programmes with positive effect (Bonner 1986). The role of the skilled play specialist is another essential element of preadmission preparation, but not to the exclusion of the skilled paediatric nurse. A major benefit of the programmes is that they facilitate interaction between hospital staff and parents/carers, who are encouraged to ask programme workers about their child's admission.

Scenario

Ollie's family is in a position to attend the preadmission programme and join other children one Saturday, 2 weeks before admission

The contents of such programmes are developed primarily from professional values and beliefs together with parental opinions, obtained by means of interviews and questionnaires (Gaughan & Sweeney 1997, Glasper & Stradling 1989). There is invaluable information to be learned by asking and involving the children about their feelings, beliefs and needs, a perspective endorsed by the recently published National Service Framework for Children (DoH 2003). The Commission of Patient and Public Involvement in Health (CPPIH), created in January 2003, will undoubtedly also encourage this.

Fradd (1986) argues that preadmission programmes are an 'undoubted success'. However, not all claims of success can be supported by documentary evidence. Although the principles of such programmes may be seen as positive, one needs to look closely at their content, structure and mode of delivery (Murphy-Taylor 1999). Communication is crucial for effective psychological care and may be considered as the key to its achievement. For example:

- What to say?
- What not to say?
- How to say it?
- When to say it?
- Who should say it?
- Where it should be said?

One significant issue in this respect is that preadmission preparation programmes appear to attempt to teach children of various ages and cultures via a common group programme, thus not allowing or acknowledging individuality, cognitive ability, existing knowledge or previous experience. Such limitations have been recognised by Eiser (1988) and Saile et al (1988). Many misconceptions and fantasies may occur if not handled appropriately by a skilled practitioner. Other limitations include the length of time between preparation programme and actual admission. It could be argued that during the gap between the preparation programme and admission, the child will forget the information or have too much time to worry and panic.

Ward visits offer the opportunity for each child and family to meet, on a one-to-one basis, the staff who will nurse them, and offer an excellent chance to offer personalised, individual preparation; a situation many ward staff make good use of. If, however, a tour of the clinical area is not an appropriately prearranged part of the preadmission programme, families might arrive on the ward unexpectedly. They may be exposed to a busy, noisy atmosphere with people rushing back and forth, seeing other children with beeping monitors attached and 'tubes sticking out of them'. They may be kept waiting while an appropriate member of staff is found to welcome them. The parents in particular may feel uncomfortable in this situation 'taking the nurse away from urgent duties' (Taylor 1991). Although this may be a reality to which they will be exposed in the future, it is not an ideal first impression.

It is noted, though not always clearly highlighted, that – relatively speaking – a minority of children admitted to hospital attend preparation programmes (Gaughan & Sweeney 1997). This could be for a number of reasons. Parents might not be able to spare an extra day from work or family commitment and finances for transport may be limited. Their own beliefs that such preparation is either unnecessary (particularly if their child has been admitted before), or that it could increase their or their child's fear may also prevent them from attending. Interestingly, more under 5s are admitted to hospital than any other age group (Atwell 1997), yet they are not always included in preparation visits (Ellerton & Merriman 1994). Consideration too is needed for those children admitted as an emergency. Thus it is necessary that health professionals look at alternative methods of preparation both prior to and during the admission.

FURTHER KEY ISSUES IN PREPARATION

Play

Children learn through play; it is a natural part of life. Time set aside to play gives the child an ideal opportunity to find out about their hospital experience. In doing so their fears may be allayed and their abilities to cope enhanced. Webster (2000) refers to key policy documents, namely

ASC (2000) and the Children Act (DoH 1989), and identifies the recognition in these documents that play preparation allows the child an age-appropriate opportunity to be involved in decisions that are to affect their lives. A knowledge of how children may perceive their internal anatomy, coupled with an understanding of children's cognitive development is clearly essential before embarking on any preparation programme (see Chapter 11). Each child's needs will be unique.

Activity

Find out about the detailed literature available to complement that provided by hospitals on the website of the National Association of Hospital Play Staff:

- http://www.nahps.org.uk

There may be different classifications of different types of play. In a helpful recent paper, Mathison & Butterworth (2001) suggest that play be divided into three types – educative, normative and therapeutic:

- The essence of **educative play** is to give information. This may be in the form of personal letters to the child, indicating in a child-centred way what to bring to hospital. It also includes use of books, pictures and diagram for parents and children to read together to learn more about their hospital admission.

- **Normative play** is 'everyday' play that is offered within the hospital environment to bridge the gap between home and hospital. It offers comfort and security, a sense of familiarity and normality. Frustrations and fears may also be expressed, thus helping the child to gain a feeling of control and confidence in his/her new and potentially threatening environment. It is important to consider that due to their illness and potentially alien environment, the child may need permission, encouragement and assistance to play.

- **Therapeutic play** centres on what the child is about to actually experience or has previously experienced, and uses play to convey information both from the child to the carer, and from the carer to the child (see also Chapter 13). In respect of preparation, when discussing certain procedures involving parts of the anatomy with younger children (especially if they cannot see, hear or touch the relevant part) it is necessary to use things the children *can* see, hear, touch and relate to concretely, for example anatomical dolls.

Scenario

Ollie's father watches with interest as the nurse uses a doll to explain to Ollie what is going to happen when he attends for surgery and finds this helpful as a tool to ask further questions for himself.

Dolls

The use of dolls is a popular tool in preparing children for specific events. For example Zaadi dolls (Glasper & Thompson 1993), both male and female, are anatomical models developed specifically for children in hospital. These cloth-covered rag dolls have three layers, which peel apart using 'velcro' fastenings to expose the vital organs (note: the dolls have several faces and it is important that the sleeping face is in place before the doll is opened). The body parts are detachable. They can be catheterised and injected, and generally allow the child a visual and tactile experience to support their thoughts and understanding. Calico dolls (Matthews & Silk 1992) also allow the child an opportunity to explore and learn by vision and touch. The simply made cloth dolls can have a variety of procedures simulated upon them, e.g. skin testing and 'drawing blood' (via plastic tubing attached to a cannula and bag of coloured water). These dolls can also be drawn upon, which can help children to demonstrate where their pain is (Ballentine & Gow 1998). These dolls also have the potential to allow parents/practitioners a visual way of supporting their verbal explanation about a procedure.

Activity

Access the companion PowerPoint presentation to see slides of these dolls.
- Use the pattern to make a calico doll yourself.

As part of her research to investigate children's knowledge of their internal anatomy, Gaudian (2000) created her own life-sized anatomical rag doll. The internal parts, each made in different-coloured fabric for easy identification, were large enough for the children to compare with their own bodies. She demonstrated that their knowledge of anatomy and physiology was more readily recalled by these three-dimensional prompts than by giving a child a two-dimensional picture to draw on. This suggests the value of such dolls in maximising children's questioning and understanding, and also helping to assess children's existing knowledge accurately before giving explanations.

'Play people' hospital toys are excellent, as are 'doctors and nurses' sets, which contain stethoscopes, auroscopes and fake syringes. It is interesting that dressing up in traditional hospital clothing continues to be popular with children despite the fact that nursing and medical staff no longer wear such uniforms in many children's units. With such toys, as well as standard teddy bears, dolls, paints and plasticine, the child has the opportunity to act out any fears, anxieties or aggressions. Children will often mirror their own experiences through a favourite toy. An observer, be it parent or professional, can gain valuable insight into the child's understanding, potential misconceptions and current feelings, and thus tailor care even more uniquely.

Distraction

Distraction is associated with helping the child cope during a specific event. The purpose of distraction is not purely to divert the child's attention or simply to provide entertainment during a medical or nursing procedure but, more importantly, to use personal, focused and developmentally appropriate play to maximise their coping strategies (Webster 2000). The professional should offer relevant information, assess the child's understanding, guide manageable goals, allow the child some choice and control and ensure emotional support with praise and reward throughout and after the event. The key to distraction is to understand it not as the removal of pain or distress directly, but rather to make the treatment more bearable by taking the focus away from the unpleasant event onto something more interesting or enjoyable (Salantera et al 1999). It may therefore be seen as a powerful intervention to help children cope with stress points/stressful procedures such as venesection/cannulation. Indeed, Willock et al (2004) give consideration to the experience of venepuncture and note the work of Doellman (2003), who describes a wide range of distraction and other supportive interventions that nurses can undertake to help children cope with this stressful procedure. Willcock et al also cite the work of Hodgins & Lander (1997), which categorises the different coping strategies displayed by different children. These range from looking away and wanting to focus on other events, to seeking support (e.g. a hand to hold), to wanting to watch the whole procedure. However, such interventions must be individualised: consider two 3-year-olds, one clinging to her parents and the other actively exploring and interacting inquisitively with the professional.

Individualised care is undoubtedly vital in planning how best to support children through hospital events. Ill-prepared and ill-supported experiences can clearly produce negative effects and distress, as well as a poor ability to cope in the future with similar or associated events.

Activity

List a selection of distraction methods and the age groups and situations where they might be appropriate.

To prepare children effectively for hospital events, it is clearly important to have a concept/knowledge of the fears a child may have when hospitalised. The seminal work of Visintainer & Wolfer (1975) describes this in terms of five key potential threats (see p 65). In their study they used four variables when preparing children for specific events:

- a control group

- a group that received supportive care

- a group that was given a single session of preparation on admission

- a group that was prepared immediately before each stressful procedure (stress-point preparation).

Within each group, the children's anxiety response was measured using behaviour upset scales, ease of postoperative fluid intake, medication on recovery, pulse rate and time of first voiding. The group with the optimal outcome was the one that had received stress-point preparation at six key points:

1. admission

2. shortly before a blood test

3. late in the afternoon the day before surgery

4. shortly before pre-med

5. before transfer to theatre

6. upon return from recovery room.

The children and parents were given 'information, instruction, rehearsal and support from a single nurse who was present at these critical times'. Even for younger children (2–6 years), single preparation was significantly more highly rated than consistent support, suggesting that giving information to such young children can do much to mitigate preoperative stress. However, it must be noted that replications of Visintainer & Wolfer's work have been unable to demonstrate findings of the same quality.

It is positive to note that, although limited, studies are still investigating preparation for specific events. Unlike Visintainer & Wolfer, one such study (by Holden et al in 1997) showed that there were no differences statistically in the distress experienced by toddlers and young children (and their parents) when a nasogastric tube was passed, whether they received detailed or routine preparation. All were equally unhappy during the procedure. However, Holden et al found a significant difference for older children and adolescents, who showed a more positive response and outcome when prepared for the event as mentioned above.

Giving Information

It is apparent that the stress of hospital can be alleviated by giving children and their families information before, during and after anxiety-provoking experiences. For many ages of children, verbal explanation alone will be insufficient because of their immature verbal and comprehension skills. The methods discussed (therapeutic play, story books, games, role play and puppet shows) will need to be utilised. When giving information verbally the choice of words and supportive explanation become important. For example, how appropriate is it to refer to an X-ray machine as a camera (Ballentine & Gow 1998)? Or, when taking blood and

cannulating, to say that it is like 'a small scratch' or 'a butterfly on your hand'? Such things might be said with the good intention to soothe and reassure, but could cause children confusion, anxiety and fear of butterflies when they are discharged home! Nurses are often required to translate medical jargon but they also need to consider whether their words and descriptions require greater thought as well (Jolly 1976; see also Chapters 11 and 37).

A further point in respect of giving information is that it is imperative to be sure that it has been understood if it is to be of positive benefit. The best way to assess this, after assessing prior knowledge and having given the relevant information, is by asking questions of the child and parent, encouraging them to ask questions, and observing their interactions in play and conversation. It is also important to go back at a later point to reinforce and re-evaluate. The child and family may feel they should know what to expect so they may not ask for information. If they don't ask it is important not to assume they know. An interesting study by Kiely (1989) found that 80% of parents interviewed about preparation thought they had been given enough information. However, this was not reflected in further interviews when their knowledge was assessed.

We must also be aware that too much information can increase rather than decrease stress (Acharya 1992). As a means of coping, information may be blocked out. When stressed, e.g. learning about the need for an operation, information may be misinterpreted and can be easily forgotten (Taylor et al 1999).

Such considerations might have influenced the work of Sutherland (2003), who sought to explore the value of preparation for cardiac surgery for adolescents in the home environment as opposed to the hospital. This intervention was positively evaluated by those who received it, although the failure to use a matched control makes it impossible to say for certain that this approach is always preferable. Crucially, the opportunity to talk to a knowledgeable practitioner who had the skill to listen well and give information with sensitivity was viewed as the greatest benefit of this approach.

Caress (2003) discusses in depth the many facets of successful communication of information. She considers the benefits of giving information, and raises questions and offers suggestions as to where the information may be given, how it may be given and who is giving and receiving it.

Using Written and Visual Material to Prepare Children for Admission

Hain and Glasper (see Chapter 37) show that written and illustrated material can be effective in relieving the stresses of hospitalisation. The use of highly specific information is important to produce accurate expectations in families attending hospital. To this end, a number of books have been written for children about hospital. They can be read as part of a general educational strategy or can be used by parents and others prior to a child's admission. Some are better than others and should be read discerningly by nurses and play specialists before being recommended/made available. At best, they can be perceived as an aid only, but they do fulfil a role as part of an overall preparatory package. Children's books and the use of story telling has been exemplified by Robinson et al (2002), who highlight the health benefits of story telling to address complex issues.

WWW

Go to the following website. Could this North American website be used for children in the UK?

- http://kidshealth.org/index.html

Nicklin (2002) has demonstrated that information needs to be accurate, have provenance and be appropriate for the readership if ambiguity is not to compromise the intentions of the material. The growth in the use of the world-wide web via home computers now gives an increasing number of people the advantage of instant access to material. Although it is often stressed that information is the key to empowerment, not all the information available on the internet is of the highest quality. This is also true of written material produced by health professionals, who are as likely to use 'gobbledegook' as anyone else; there is little point in writing for families if, in turn, they cannot read or understand the information presented.

Other issues to consider include the availability of information in different languages and Braille or on audiotape and the need for professionals to be aware that using family members as translators can raise a confidentiality dilemma. In recent years, it has become customary for many children's units to send out written material in the mail, usually with the letter of admission. Like the books discussed above, this written material can be of varying quality. Some of it attempts to communicate with the parent and some with the child, some do both.

WWW

Read the new booklet from Queens Medical Centre in Nottingham. Compare this with what is available in your area of work:

- http://www.qmc.nhs.uk/WhatsHappening/ ChildrensBooklet.htm

Parents interviewed in studies frequently request leaflets giving details of hospital facilities, personnel and routine, and facts about specific medical or surgical conditions (Kiely 1989). It appears that few leaflets actually offer suggestions to parents regarding how to prepare their child psychologically for hospital. Parents in Southampton received such information very positively when a leaflet containing recommendations for preparation was produced (Stone & Glasper 1997) (see also Chapter 37). Murphy-Taylor (1999) also found a desire among parents for more information, and suggested that specific information sheets about individual operations could be included in the mail-out to parents. In this way children could be prepared for surgery through the parents, who are best placed to achieve this.

WWW

Go to the following website and click on the information pages. Is the description of glue ear helpful for children and parents/carers?

- http://www.ich.ucl.ac.uk/

The development of a centre for health information and promotion (CHIP) in Southampton, linked to the outpatient department, offered a valuable resource for families. Such initiatives recognise the importance of empowering families through giving them information (Glasper et al 1995). Perhaps greater links between such services and ward areas are also required to maximise their potential.

Some hospitals have produced video, DVD films or PowerPoint presentations, which can be given to parents and children. Such programmes have been found to be so effective that they are increasingly being developed and used throughout the UK. The complexity of educational material for children is such that healthcare professionals are increasingly using multimedia as a vehicle of delivering material. Children are now very computer literate and McPherson et al (2002) have described how a multimedia package has helped in the delivery of asthma education for children.

The cost of producing professionally edited videotapes is prohibitive for most units, and these products date very quickly. PowerPoint presentations are easier and cheaper to produce and have the added advantage that they can be updated periodically with little difficulty. The flexibility of a PowerPoint presentation is the most effective method of addressing parental concerns about a child's forthcoming hospital admission. PowerPoint slides are easy to produce and can be scanned or imported directly from digital cameras. They are very simple to update and a consistent format can be adopted, perhaps of sequential digital photographs covering the hospital stay from admission to discharge. Ideally, everyone involved in writing the presentation should follow a set script, although the preparation of such is always difficult. In lieu of an agreed script, some units follow an informal approach that takes cues from the PowerPoint slides.

Some hospitals, for example the Hospital for Sick Children in Toronto, have developed very sophisticated virtual tours of clinical areas, which are available for parents and children to view through the hospital website.

Hospital-based television programmes may also have a general effect in raising the awareness of preparing children for hospital.

www

Go to the following website and take a virtual tour. Discuss this in your learning group:
- http://www.sickkids.on.ca/

OTHER CONSIDERATIONS IN PARENTAL PREPARATION

Parents are seen as prime informants and interpreters, the people with the most in-depth knowledge about the child. They therefore have a vital need themselves for information and support (Whiting1993). As discussed earlier, the work of Visintainer & Wolfer (1975) shows favourable parental response to preparation. Parents were more able to cope themselves and thus more effective at supporting their child. Siblings and the wider family also have needs and can also contribute to a child's care, provided education and support from health professionals is available.

The trend to shorter inpatient stays and more day surgery has increased the need for parents to be responsible for both the child's emotional and physical care. Darbyshire (2003) looked at mothers' experiences of their child's recovery both in hospital and at home, and makes important observations regarding the considerable challenges that parents face in caring for their sick child on discharge. One hopes that such work will allow professionals the opportunity to develop preparation programmes and information to suit the client's true needs. Such observations about parental responsibility are also echoed in much of the literature on day surgery (Ireland & Rushforth 1998). It is therefore important that preparation focuses on all stages of the illnesses trajectory, from admission right through to discharge and beyond.

Battrick & Glasper (2004) highlighted the importance of seeking the opinion of the consumers. Such consumer surveys invariably demonstrate that parents are in favour of information. However, whereas some hunger for that information others may avoid it (Miller 1979). In the absence of information, but with their own fears and anxieties, a parent may say nothing to the child and the first the child knows of an admission is walking through the portals of the hospital. Given that parents' informed consent should ideally be sought before any preparation/explanation is given to a younger child, parental refusal to allow the child to be informed about aspects of his or her care places the healthcare professional in a challenging ethical situation to ensure that the child's rights are upheld.

● Seminar discussion topic

A parent doesn't want to tell their child they are coming to hospital/about to undergo surgery. Why might the parent feel like this? As the paediatric nurse and professional advocate for that child and family, how would you approach this situation? (See also Chapter 20)

Just because a certain fact or experience worries an adult it doesn't mean it will worry a child. Both parents and professionals should take care not to impose their fears upon a child. Adults, like children have different coping strategies. The benefits of parents may be immeasurable in helping a child cope with a stressful event but, paradoxically, an anxious parent is likely to increase the anxiety in their child. This is clarified further by Glasper & Thompson (1993) in their elaboration of 'emotional contagion'.

Emotional contagion, i.e. the transmission of anxiety from an adult to a child, is a major source of concern to those individuals planning any form of supportive programme. Most children depend on emotional support from their parents for help in coping with anxieties. The simplest anxiety is that produced by contagion. This is exemplified by a child who becomes frightened when in close contact with frightened adults. If those whose role is one of protection become frightened themselves, this fear can be transmitted to the child. It may be hypothesised that parents who are frightened are less able to contribute to the psychological welfare of a child who is undergoing a stressful procedure.

In some early work, Campbell (1957) discussed how emotional states in mothers can be communicated to their children. Her investigation, conducted in a well baby clinic, showed that significantly more infants of mothers who received anxiety-arousing instructions cried before immunisation injections than infants of mothers who received neutral instruction. It is thus important to prepare parents as well as children for stressful events to avoid parental anxiety being mirrored in children. Some parents can become frightened about the welfare of their child and sometimes their reaction appears out of proportion to the event at hand. The quality of interaction between an authoritative person, such as a nurse, and a hospitalised child's parent can lower the parent's level of stress and produce changes in the parent's definition of the situation. This in turn can have a demonstrable effect on the child's level of stress, producing a change in his or her social, psychological and physiological behaviour. Children's nurses must learn to recognise the natural resource they have at their disposal in the form of parents and guardians. They must be perceived as partners in the traditional nurse–doctor–patient relationship.

It must be recognised that parents/carers are trying to understand and absorb, in a matter of hours and days, information that professionals have spent years learning. They are expected to trust relative strangers with the life of their child. Professionals need to listen to them, acknowledge their fears and offer factual and practical information with sensitivity and understanding. Parents often fail to ask for advice or help with the daily care needs of their child because they believe the nurse to be too busy in dealing with more important tasks. It is crucial that nurses offer their time to listen to the child and family.

Gibson's (1991) definition of empowerment is one all professionals should emulate:

Recognising, promoting and enhancing people's ability to meet their own needs, solve their own problems and mobilise their own resources in order to feel in control of their own lives.

◆ Scenario

After surgery, Ollie returns home the following day and although he makes an uneventful physical recovery he sleeps less well and remains 'clingy' for several days (see Chapter 8).

Preparation in the Community: Emergency Admissions and Non-attendees

By the age of 5 years, 25% of children will have had a stay in hospital, and one-third of these admissions will be caused by accidents (see Chapter 24). Indeed, half of infants aged under 12 months, and a quarter of older children, will attend an A&E over a 1-year period (DoH 2003). Hospitalisation is, therefore, not an uncommon childhood experience. Brett (1983) has indicated that preparation should begin in the classroom and feature as a component of general education.

The needs of children vary with age. It has been suggested that children's fears change with age and cognitive development. Miller (1979) has stated that preschool children are especially frightened of noises, strange persons or events. Schoolchildren's particular fears may be of bodily injury, disease and separation. Vernon et al (1960), in a classic study, collected data that support the hypothesis that children between the ages of 6 months and 4 years of age are the most likely to be upset following hospitalisation. This would suggest that preparation might begin in nursery school or play group. Many nurseries and primary schools have 'hospital play corners' that allow children the opportunity to explore and learn through 'role play'.

Families, like individuals, are unique, each with their own needs, but all appear to profit from a modicum of preparation. Any preparation will be intimately concerned with stress inoculation. Meng & Zastowny (1981) have likened stress inoculation to medical inoculation and indicate that preparatory programmes should achieve this goal. Stress inoculation can be carried out successfully in school classroom situations and the benefit of this approach is that all children can be prepared for the eventuality of being admitted to hospital. School-age children are more likely than preschool children to cope positively with hospitalisation. This is because they are more able to reason, describe and verbalise their feelings than younger children. The school classroom may, therefore, be an excellent environment in which to teach children the skills necessary to cope with hospitalisation. Hospitals in many areas offer schools fairly in-depth and interactive education sessions, both in the hospital setting and with hospital personnel visiting the schools themselves.

● Seminar discussion topic

James Robertson, a staunch NAWCH member, stopped the school-wide preparatory programmes because he believed they may cause unnecessary fear and anxiety in children concerning separation, bodily mutilation and the pain of operations. Debate this stance in your action learning group.

Dedicated paediatric areas in emergency departments, with appropriately qualified staff, can clearly provide a more conducive environment for a child. Teddy bears feature highly as a tool for learning. A 'well teddy clinic' in the Emergency Department at the Royal Belfast Hospital for Sick Children proved a great success in helping to allay the fears of children and parents requiring emergency care (Burton 1994). Similarly, a 3-day teddy bear community project in Kentucky offered valuable learning for all involved (Santen & Feldman 1994).

Universal preparation for all children facilitated through preschool or school-based programmes may not be the whole answer. Young children are susceptible to fantasy and misunderstanding, and anxiety may even be provoked if ideas of separation from home and family are introduced unnecessarily, leading some critics to question the appropriateness of such blanket preparation. Any preparation for hospital must be carried out accurately and sensitively, with due importance being given to the age and level of cognitive development of the child. The role of the primary healthcare team should also be considered when planning preparatory programmes for children and families. In a typical year, a preschool child will see the GP around six times, and a school-age child two or three times (DoH 2003). It is obvious, therefore, that GPs, health visitors and school nurses are in a good position to supply information about hospitals, especially for elective admissions.

Preparation in the outpatient department has also received attention (Achayra 1992). It is the belief of the authors and their play specialist colleagues that, if handled and organised well, education here – as with formal preparation programmes – can form a firm basis of support and knowledge for the child and family before their ultimate admission to a hospital ward. First impressions are powerful and lasting. In any year, one in eleven children will be referred to an outpatient department (DoH 2003).

Children with Specific Preparation Needs

Much of the literature with regard to preparation refers to the well and acutely ill child. Particular consideration needs to be given to the children with chronic illnesses, learning difficulties and communication impairment. It might be assumed that a child who regularly attends hospital is better informed than he or she actually is. The practitioner also needs to assess carefully the child's previous experiences, as these will undoubtedly influence his or her behaviour and emotional needs each time they are subsequently admitted to hospital. It is easy to think that everyone else has explained a routine or aspect of care, or indeed that the child and family know what to do, say or feel.

Although much is written about the benefits of preparing the well child for a future period of hospitalisation, it should be stressed that children with chronic conditions and their families may have different and potentially more lasting and serious psychological reactions (Ogden Burke et al 2001). Preparation for such children may be difficult, particularly if the family has experienced prior negative events. The focus of Ogden Burke's study is on using family-centred strategies for coping with stress-point interventions by nurses (SPIN). For children with chronic illness, recognition that others have similar problems, and perhaps the setting-up of peer health groups at ward level and in the community, can offer valuable support. As part of preparation, families in Nottingham are often introduced to another family whose child has had the same surgery (Crawford & Raven 2002).

It is still important for nurses to explain their intended actions, even to children with limited verbal responses who might still be experiencing anxiety and fear. The professional and parents/carers must be aware of children's non-verbal communication and endeavour to interpret and address their needs. The focus may then be on helping them to cope with a potentially frightening experience.

Burgess (2001) offers an interesting perspective on the complementary therapies guided imagery and infant massage as distraction therapy. There was particular emphasis upon such techniques being used to support the child through episodes of pain. Savins (2002) explored the value of art therapy with children in pain and it has also been recognised that music has therapeutic benefits. Music therapy can build a bridge between two worlds – perhaps between those with sight and hearing and those without, and between those with command of speech and those yet to master such skills – in essence, it is a means of non-verbal communication and expression of emotion. Complementary and alternative therapies can help relationships be built and pathways of trust and communication opened. This is clearly a sound basis for preparing and supporting children through new experiences.

The psychological preparation of children whose special needs, e.g. cerebral palsy, result in global developmental delay is beginning to receive attention. Crawford & Raven (2002) offer a multifaceted approach to preparing such children for gastrostomy insertion, which uses many of the interventions previously discussed. They use Minnie and Mickey Mouse dolls, similar to the Zaadi and calico dolls, to allow the child and parent to insert, remove and play with appropriate related pieces of equipment. It was felt important that the characters chosen should not be associated with a particular class, culture or race, or create the image/stereotype of a 'normal' child. Preparation began in the home and continued for some several weeks before hospitalisation and surgery. Another technique used for one particular child in their study was music and massage, which were found to aid relaxation. Also worth highlighting was the introduction of various textures and pressures to the child's abdomen, with the idea that the child could begin to get used to a sensation that later would be associated with their new gastrostomy. This, the mother reported, became a significant and valuable part of her child's care.

Essentially, children with complex needs require no less and no more support and information than any other child in respect of what is offered in preparation for hospital or events within it. The difference will be that professionals need to find out about the specific illness/disability and then tailor and adapt the tools and resources they use to communicate effectively. Interaction with the multidisciplinary team and specialist services will undoubtedly offer valuable information and support. Whoever they are and whatever their circumstances, the children should all be given appropriate opportunities and stimulation, time to respond, to endeavour to share their perspective and develop their strengths and abilities; above all to be respected as unique individuals.

Activity

What are the specific preparation needs of the following groups of children?
- Those with global developmental delay.
- Those with communication difficulty e.g. blindness, deafness.
- Those with a chronic illness.
- Adolescents.
- What specific information is available in the children's nursing literature to guide practitioners in preparing these specific groups of children? Is there any evidence regarding its efficacy?
- Give examples of your own ideas of other interventions that may address such children's needs (see also Chapters 43, 44 and 47).

Practitioner Perspectives

When children are in hospital, the nurse must adopt the role of facilitator and coordinator to all their needs. Continuity and documentation of preparation and information given is imperative if confusion by duplication is to be avoided (Rushforth 1999). Communication is vital, particularly between the nurse and the play specialist, whose skill and knowledge of child development and the therapy of play is of paramount importance. Active participation by the children and families should be encouraged with regard to planning and evaluating their preparation and emotional needs. Praise and rewards by health carers and family members will increase self-esteem and reinforce positive behaviour. Even children who cry or shout should receive acknowledgement that they have done well and tried their best.

Taylor (1991) identified a situation when a child had interactions with 25 people in a 3-hour period. This may be difficult for anyone to assimilate when well, let alone when 4 years old, unwell and most likely feeling somewhat vulnerable. Nurse-led ventures/clinics could be said not only to allow increased professional development and skill for the nurse but, perhaps more importantly, give greater opportunity for trust, security and coping by the child because of an environment in which there is continuity of action, care and management by one or a small number of people (Lawton & Rose 2003). There is a close link here with the concept of primary and named nursing.

It could be argued that clinical psychologists are under-utilised in respect of preparing children for hospitalisation. Their role could perhaps be expanded further within the mutidisciplinary team. For example, they could contribute to the formation of protocols of care and advise literature for professionals/carers in respect of the child and families preparation for hospitalisation and emotional needs.

A small-scale study by Rushforth (1996) looked at nurses' beliefs, knowledge and practice regarding children's ability to understand concepts of health and illness. It concluded that nurses' knowledge about a child's conceptual ability, and beliefs in cognitive immaturity, may be adversely influencing practice. Staff education is obviously indicated in this respect, and so too is the need for all those involved in the health care of children to be reminded of how the hospital might be seen through the child's eye (Haggarty & Rushforth 1999).

One tool to achieve this is the video *A child's eye view* (Haggarty & Rushforth 1996, 1999). The video, recorded at the eye level of a young child, offers an audiovisual encounter of the sights, sounds and experiences of a hospital, offering examples of good and bad practice. The video acts as a catalyst for the viewer to consider what the child might be seeing, hearing and feeling, and how he might react; the video is accompanied by a teaching booklet.

Evaluation data demonstrated a very positive picture with regard to the video as a learning tool. Practitioners felt that their 'habituation' of seeing the hospital world through professional eyes had been challenged and that viewing the video had allowed them to revisit the care situation with 'new eyes', those of the children themselves (Haggarty & Rushforth 1999).

Activity

Obtain and view the video *A child's eye view*. While watching the video, keep note of:
- what you see
- what you hear
- what you are thinking
- how you will act when next with a child.

Summary

It is important that paediatric practitioners are constantly aware of the psychological well-being of the children in their care, and that they take every opportunity to maximise the child-centredness of their approach and of the environment in which children are nursed. Such care should be part of the professional's daily routine, not an after-thought or added extra. In particular, the carer (parents and professionals) needs to remember to give children permission to express their emotions and also to negotiate care, with informed consent, to give choices, praise and reward. All details regarding assessment of need, preparation given and outcome for the child should be clearly documented, available for all involved with the family, and appropriately evaluated and modified as the child indicates.

Further development is required to consider the role of a specific person for a child's psychological preparation from assessment of health need through treatment to settling back to normal routine at home. It is important to stress that further work is also needed to look at the specific needs when preparing children with learning difficulties, communication impairment and chronic illness. Information for families about why and how to prepare their child for hospital and how such literature may be disseminated also needs to be expanded.

To conclude this chapter, it would be difficult to find better words than those of Mellish (1969), who pointed out that successful preparation for surgery depends on the attitude of many people, including the surgeon, anaesthetist, and nurses and that:

> . . . the criteria for surgical success should not only be measured by intact wounds but also by intact emotions.

Dedication

Rachel Haggarty wishes to dedicate this chapter to the memory of Ben Voller:

When you reached out, I was privileged to be there for you and to be able to hold your hand.

References

Achayra S 1992 Assessing the need for pre-admission visits. Paediatric Nursing 4(9):20–23

ASC 2002 Online. Available at: http://www.actionforsickchildren.org/about_history.html

Atwell J 1997 Paediatric surgery. Arnold, London

Atwell J, Gow M 1985 Paediatric trained district nurses in the community: expensive luxury or economic necessity? British Nursing Journal 291:227–229

Ballentine M, Gow D 1998 The value of play in ambulatory settings. In: Glasper EA, Lowson S (eds) Innovations in paediatric ambulatory care. Macmillan, London

Battrick C, Glasper EA 2004 The views of children and their families on being in hospital. British Journal of Nursing 12(6):36–44

Bonner ML 1986 Can my friend go with me? Nursing Times October:75–76

Bowlby J 1951 Maternal care and mental health. WHO monograph, series 2. WHO, Geneva

Brain D, Maclay I 1968 Cited in Bielby E 1984 A childish concept. Nursing Mirror 159(18):26–28

Bretherton I 2002 Online. Available at: http://attachment.edu.or/bio.html

Brett A 1983 Preparing children for hospitalisation – a classroom teaching approach. Journal of School Nursing 53(9):561–563

Burgess C 2001 Complementary therapies: guided imagery and infant massage. Paediatric Nursing 13(6):37–41

Burton R 1994 How to bear the pain. Child Health April/May:251–254

Campbell EH 1957 The effects of mothers' anxiety on infants' behaviour – a dissertation presented to the Faculty of the Graduate School of Yale University. Unpublished doctoral thesis

Caress AL 2003 Giving information to patients. Nursing Standard 17(43):47–54

Committee of the Central Health Services Council (the Platt report) 1959 The welfare of children in hospital. HMSO, London

Crawford C, Raven K 2002 Play preparation for children with special needs. Paediatric Nursing 14(8):27–29

Darbyshire P 2003 Mothers' experience of their child's recovery in hospital and at home: a qualitative investigation. Journal of Child Health Care 17(4):291–309

Department of Health (DoH) 1989 The Children Act. An introductory guide for the NHS Health Publications Unit. HMSO, London

Department of Health (DoH) 2003 Getting the right start: national service framework for children, young people and maternity services. DoH, London

Doellman D 2003 Pharmacological vs non pharmacological techniques in reducing venepuncture psychological trauma in pediatric patients. Journal of Infusion Nursing 26(2):103–109. Cited in: Willock J, Richardson J, Brazier A et al 2004 Peripheral venepuncture in infants and children. Nursing Standard 18(27):43–50

Eiser C 1988 Do children benefit from psychological preparation for hospitalisation? Psychology and Health 2:133–138

Ellerton M, Merriam C 1994 Preparing children and families psychologically for day surgery: an evaluation. Journal of Advanced Nursing 19:1057–1062

Fassler D 1980 Reducing preoperative anxiety in children – information versus emotional support. Patient Counselling & Health Education 2(3):130–134

Fradd E 1986 Learning about hospital. Nursing Times 82(3):28–30

Gaudian C 2000 Children's knowledge of their internal anatomy. In: Glapsper EA, Ireland LM (eds) Evidence-based child health care. Macmillan, Basingstoke

Gaughan M, Sweeney E 1997 Take heart: setting up a pre-admission day. Paediatric Nursing 9(1):22–23

Gibson C 1991 A concept analysis of empowerment. Journal of Advanced Nursing 16(3):354–361

Glasper EA 1999 An evaluation of five years' work in Romania. Paediatric Nursing 11(8):32–35

Glasper EA, Charles-Edwards I 2002 The child first and always: the registered children's nurse over 150 years. Part one. Paediatric Nursing 14(4):38–42

Glasper EA, Lowson S 1998 Ambulatory care – the scope of practice. In: Glasper EA, Lowson S (eds) Innovations in paediatric ambulatory care: a nursing perspective. Macmillan, London

Glasper EA, Lowson S, Manger R, Phillips L 1995 Developing a centre for health information and promotion. British Journal of Nursing 4(12):693–697

Glasper EA, Stradling P 1989 Preparing children for admission. Paediatric Nursing July:18–20

Glasper EA, Thompson M 1993 Preparing children for hospital. In: Glasper EA, Tucker A (eds) Advances in child health nursing. Scutari, London

Gleitman H 1986 Psychology, 2nd edn. WW Norton, Ontario

Haggarty R, Rushforth H 1996 A child's eye view. Video and teaching package. Department of Teaching Media, University of Southampton

Haggarty R, Rushforth H 1999 A child's eye view. Paediatric Nursing 11(10):27–30

Harlow HF 1958 The nature of love. Address of the President at the sixty-sixth annual Convention of the American Psychological Association, Washington DC, 31 August. Online. Available at: http://psychclassics.yorku.ca/Harlow/love.htm

Hodgins M, Lander J 1997 Children's coping with venepuncture. Journal of Pain and Symptom Management 13(5):274–285. Cited in Willock J, Richardson J, Brazier A et al 2004 Peripheral venepuncture in infants and children. Nursing Standard 18(27):43–50

Holden CE, Macdonald A, Ward M et al 1997 Psychological preparation for nasogastric feeding in children. British Journal of Nursing 6(7):376–385

Hyland M, Donaldson M 1989 Psychological care in nursing practice. Scutari Press, London

In Defense of Animals 2002 Maternal deprivation experiments. Online. Available at: http://www.vivisectioninfo.org/deprivation/

Ireland L, Rushforth H 1998 Paediatric day care and it contribution to ambulatory care nursing. In: Glasper EA, Lowson S (eds) Innovations in paediatric ambulatory care. Macmillan, London

Jolly J 1976 Preparing children for hospital. Nursing Times 72:1532–1533

Keeton D 1999 Pain, nausea and vomiting: a day surgery audit. Paediatric Nursing 11(5):28–32

Kiely T 1989 Preparing children for admission to hospital. Nursing 3(33):42–44

Kosky J, Lunnon RJ 1991 Great Ormond Street and the story of medicine. Granta Editions, London

Lawton LC, Rose P 2003 Changing practice in invasive procedures: the experience of the Krishnan Chandran Children's Centre. Journal of Child Health Care 7(4):248–257

Mathisen L, Butterworth D 2001 The role of play in the hospitalisation of young children. Neonatal, Paediatric and Child Health Nursing, 4(3):23–26

Matthews M, Silk G 1992 Young children, priority one. Kwanis, Melborne. Cited in: Ballentine M, Gow D 1998 The value of play in ambulatory settings. In: Glasper EA, Lowson S (eds) Innovations in paediatric ambulatory care. Macmillan, London

McPherson A, Foster D, Glazebrook C, Symth A 2002 The asthma files; evaluation of a multimedia package for children's asthma education. Paediatric Nursing 14(2):32–35

Mellish PWR 1969 Preparation of a child for hospitalisation and surgery. Pediatric Clinics of North America 16(3):543–554

Meng A, Zastowny T 1982 Preparation for hospitalisation: a stress inoculation training program for parents and children. Maternal-Child Nursing Journal 11(2):87–94

Miles I 1986 The emergence of sick children's nursing. Part 1. Sick children's nursing before the turn of the century. Nurse Education Today 6:82–87

Miller S 1979 Children's fears – a review of the literature with implications for nursing research and practice. Nursing Research 28(4):217–223

Murphy-Taylor C 1999 The benefits of preparing children and parents for day surgery. British Journal of Nursing 8(12):801–804

Nicklin J 2002 Improving the quality of written information for patients. Nursing Standard 16(49):39–44

Ogden Burke S, Harrison MB, Kaufman E, Wong C 2001 effects of stress-point intervention with families of repeatedly hospitalized children. Journal of Family Nursing 7(2):128–158

Piaget J, Inhelder B 1969 The psychology of the child. Routledge and Kegan Paul, London

RCPCH 2000 Online. Available at: http://www.rcpch.ac.uk/publications/recent_publications/Advocacy/advocting.pdf

Robertson J 1970 Young children in hospital. Tavistock, London

Robertson J 1989 Separation and the very young. Free Association Books, London

Robinson S, Hughes K, Manning K 2002 Children's books: a resource for children's nursing. Paediatric Nursing 14(5):26–31

Rushforth H 1996 Nurses' knowledge of how children view health and illness. Paediatric Nursing 8(5):23–27

Rushforth, H 1999 Practitioner review. Communicating with hospitalised children: review and application of research pertaining to children's understanding of health and illness. Journal of Child Psychology and Psychiatry 40(5):683–691

Rutherford D 1998 Children's relationships. In: Taylor J, Woods M (eds) Early childhood studies. Arnold, London

Rutter M 1981 Maternal deprivation reassessed, 2nd edn. Penguin, Harmondsworth

Saile H, Burgemeier R, Schmidt L 1988 A meta-analysis of studies on psychological preparation of children facing medical procedures. Psychology and Health 2:107–132

Salantera S, Lauri S, Salmi S, Helenius T 1999 Nurses' knowledge about pharmacological and non pharmacological pain management. Journal of Pain and Symptom Management 18(4):289–299

Santen L, Feldman T 1994 A huge community project. American Journal of Maternal-Child Nursing 19:102–106

Savins C 2002 Therapeutic work with children in pain. Paediatric Nursing 14(5):14–16

Smith RM 1986 Anesthesia for infants and children, 3rd edn. CV Mosby, St Louis

Stone K, Glasper EA 1997 Can leaflets assist parents in preparing children for hospital? British Journal of Nursing 6(18):1054–1058

Sutherland T 2003 Comparison of hospital and home based preparation for cardiac surgery. Paediatric Nursing 15(5):13–16

Taylor D 1991 Prepare for the best. Nursing Times 87(31):64–65

Taylor J, Muller D, Wattley L, Harris P 1999 Nursing children: psychology, research and practice, 3rd edn. Stanley Thornes, Cheltenham

The PSI Café 2002 A psychology resource site. Online. Available at: http://www.psy.pdx.edu/PsiCafe/KeyTheorists/Lorenz.htm

Thurtle V 1998 Multi-disciplinary care of the sick child in the community. In: Taylor J, Woods M (eds) Early childhood studies. Arnold, London

Vernon DT, Schulman JL, Foley JM 1966 Changes in children's behaviour after hospitalisation. American Journal of Diseases of Children 111(6):81–93

Visintainer M, Wolfer J 1975 Psychogical preparation for surgical pediatric patients: the effect on children's and parents' stress responses and adjustments. Pediatrics 56(2):187–201

Webster A 2000 The facilitating role of the play specialist. Paediatric Nursing 12(7):24–27

Whiting M 1993 Play and surgical patients. Paediatric Nursing 5(6):11–13

Willock J, Richardson J, Brazier A et al 2004 Peripheral venepuncture in infants and children. Nursing Standard 18(27):43–50

Wilson H 1981 Behavioural preparation for surgery: benefit or harm? Journal of Behavioural Medicine 4:79–102. Cited in Salmon P 1992 Anxiety and stress in surgical patients. British Journal of Hospital Medicine 48(9):531–533

Wolkind S, Rutter M 1985 Separation, loss and family relationships. In: Rutter M, Hersov L (eds) Child and adolescent psychiatry. Blackwell Scientific, Oxford. Cited in Taylor J, Muller D, Wattley L, Harris P 1999 Nursing children: psychology, research and practice, 3rd edn. Stanley Thornes, Cheltenham

Chapter **Six**

6

Family-centred Care

Lynda Smith, Valerie Coleman, Maureen Bradshaw

ABSTRACT

The primary aim of this chapter and its companion PowerPoint presentation is to translate the concept of family-centred care into everyday practice for nurses working with children and their families.

Learning Outcomes

- Understand family-centred care as a concept in children's nursing.

- Understand and appreciate the use of the practice continuum tool in children's nursing practice.

- Use negotiation, empowerment and reflective skills in the delivery of family-centred care.

- Appreciate the challenges of delivering family-centred care in practice.

- Understand the professional and legal implications of using a family-centred approach to care.

Glossary

Concept:
The way a particular subject is viewed and how it is classified. These views can vary from person to person, which is why family-centred care is difficult to define, because different individuals consider different aspects of family-centred care to be important.

Continuum:
A continuum is a continuous whole rather than something that has a defined beginning and end. In this instance, continuum means that there is no start or

finish point, that families can be on the continuum at any point and move along it in any direction.

Framework:
Identifies and outlines the elements that explicitly belong to a subject, in this instance family-centred care. A number of frameworks describe the different elements or attributes of family-centred care.

Philosophy:
An explicit statement of one's beliefs and values. Family-centred care is an explicit statement about the values and beliefs of children's nursing practice, in relation to the children and families in our care.

Self-efficacy:
Individuals believe that 'they are capable of performing a given activity' (Tones & Tilford 2001, p 104). In terms of family-centred care, nurses can help families to develop self-efficacy beliefs by negotiating short-term goals related to the care of their children and by providing the appropriate support to enable the families to achieve. Achievement is likely to result in families believing that they are capable of performing this negotiated care and other aspects of their children's care.

Introduction

Family-centred care is a multifaceted concept that has evolved over the past 50 years and remains a significant concept for children's nursing in the 21st century. The concept embraces caring for the child in the context of the family and therefore nurses recognise the central role of the family in the child's life.

Today's healthcare culture, however, continues to present many challenges in translating family-centred care theory into practice. The focus of this chapter is to clarify and enhance understanding of family-centred care as a theoretical construct and to discuss how this can be applied in everyday clinical practice using the practice continuum tool, which was developed for this purpose. This is supported by a toolkit of skills that will enable nurses to practice family-centred care effectively.

Understanding Family-centred Care as a Concept

Different definitions and theoretical frameworks have been used to explain the evolving concept of family-centred care. These definitions and frameworks are all still reflected to some extent in the family-centred care approaches that are currently used by children's nurses in practice. This is because some children's nurses, using their professional judgement, will select the most appropriate family-centred care framework to meet the needs of individual children and their families. Conversely, other children's nurses have not adopted contemporary theoretical family-centred care frameworks for implementation in practice and their approach to care is based on earlier theories. This may be due to choice or because of a lack of knowledge, skills or willingness to adopt new ways of working in practice. Bruce & Ritchie (1997) identify a need for skill development in areas of communication that involve negotiation and the sharing of information with children and their families. These areas of communication are defining characteristics of contemporary family-centred care theoretical frameworks.

This situation, concerning the use of different family-centred care frameworks in practice, can be confusing, making family-centred care potentially one of 'nursing's most amorphous concepts' (Darbyshire 1994) and 'rather ad hoc and unpredictable' (Callery 1997). Dunst & Trivette (1996) argue that to improve family-centred care practice nurses need to understand the characteristics of using different approaches in their nursing care. Therefore it is essential to have an awareness and understanding of functional, holistic, hierarchical and continuum family-centred care theoretical frameworks.

Due to the evolving nature of the concept of family-centred care, different definitions have underpinned the development of these different theoretical frameworks.

Reflect on your Practice

- How are families involved in their children's care on your clinical placement?
- Define family-centred care based on this reflection.

Your definition is likely to reflect one of the definitions provided by others to underpin the different family-centred care theoretical frameworks that exist. An early definition was:

Family-centred care provides an opportunity for the family to care for the hospitalised child under nursing supervision . . . The goal of family-centred care is to maintain or strengthen the roles and ties of the family with the hospitalised child in order to promote normality of the family unit (Brunner & Suddarth 1986 p 66)

This definition suggests that the nurse supervises care and plays a rather passive role with the family and no active role with children. It identifies the opportunity for families to be involved in the care of the hospitalised child and seems to recognise the importance of addressing the psychological needs of the child with regard to promoting normality of the family unit. This definition was largely congruent with societal values and beliefs – and the care of sick children (which predominantly took place in the hospital setting) – up to the early 1980s. However, children are now cared for at home whenever possible and hence family-centred care is likely to have a different meaning, because the context of care has changed. An overarching contemporary definition of family-centred care is:

The professional support of the child and family through a process of involvement, participation and partnership underpinned by empowerment and negotiation (Smith et al 2002 p 22)

This definition recognises that family-centred care is not an *ad hoc* approach to care but that it requires the nurse to make use of professional knowledge and skills to support the child and family, participating in care in both hospital and community settings. It offers different dimensions to family-centred care (involvement, participation and partnership), which are 'each in their own way relevant and provide an opportunity for families to be involved in the care of their child, preferably to an extent of their own choosing through negotiation with nurses' (Smith et al 2002 p 22). In other words, family-centred care does not have to be the same for every family and it may change for individual families at different times during a child's healthcare journey. The implications of this are that it is acceptable for family-centred care to be either nurse-led or family-led, making it significantly different from the earlier definition offered by Brunner & Suddarth (1986), which relied on nursing supervision. The contemporary definition also suggests that an outcome of family-centred care is the empowerment of children and their families, demonstrating its congruence with contemporary health policy in the 21st century, which advocates for child and family empowerment (Department of Health (DoH) 1999, 2000, 2003).

WWW

Read *Getting the right start: national service framework for children standard for hospital services* (DoH 2003) online:

- http://www.doh.gov.uk/nsf/children/
standardhospserviceindex.htm

This emphasises the need to work in partnership with families and to involve them in decision-making.

Scenario

Gemma, a second year student nurse, starts her clinical placement on a children's medical ward. She is keen to learn about family-centred care and asks her mentor lots of questions.

Professional Conversation

"

Helen, a registered children's nurse on Part 1 of the Nursing and Midwifery Council's Professional Register, is Gemma's mentor.

Issues affecting the use of family-centred care theoretical frameworks for nursing practice on different children's wards

I have been qualified for 3 years now. When I worked as a staff nurse on the children's surgical ward we usually asked the families to continue to give 'basic care' to their children in hospital, just like they would at home. I don't think they always wanted to do it but most families would comply, especially when they saw other families doing the care. We wanted them, for example, to feed their children, help with hygiene needs and to play with the children. The families were all treated the same with regard to involving them in caring for their children, except of course if the child was very ill and it was better for the nurse to do all the care then. Sometimes we had to teach the child or the family how to do some of the nursing or medical care to enable them to care for the child on discharge home. This all took time and some of my colleagues used to be rather impatient and judgemental with families who were slower to learn than others.

I started working on the medical ward about 3 months ago. Family-centred care is very different here, because we really do seem to give individual care to the different families. We listen to what the child and different family members have to say and information-giving is a two-way process. After all, the family are the experts on their child. The families still give 'basic care' to their children but we negotiate with them so that they can choose what care they want to participate in and when. We also assess their learning needs and teach them accordingly either to adapt their skills or to learn new ones. In fact, the children and families are much more involved altogether on this ward. The families really do participate in the decision-making process about their children's care and many do work in partnership with us.

Helen is distinguishing between using a functional framework on the children's surgical ward and using a framework on the children's medical ward.

In practice, using a functional framework results in a lack of collaboration between the nurse and family. In other words, families are understood in terms of having a functional value and they become resources to be effectively used and managed by nurses (Darbyshire 1993). The nurse using a functional framework takes on the role of gatekeeper and decides what care the family can participate in (Hutchfield 1999). Families are allowed to continue performing tasks that they would usually perform at home in hospital to help the nurse and to make them feel useful (Darbyshire 1993, Nethercott 1993). Although some families might be involved in more technical aspects of the child's care, that depends on their willingness and ability, as assessed by nurses (Nethercott 1993). The power very much resides with the nurse when this functional approach to family-centred care is used.

The holistic approach to family-centred care had its origins within the framework developed by Shelton et al in 1987, which identifies a framework of elements all linked together by a strong thread of communication (Shelton & Smith Stepanek 1995). It has a fundamentally different underlying philosophy to the functional approach (Smith et al 2002):

✳ *It is an approach that requires nurses to shift from a professionally centred view of health care to a collaborative model that recognises the family as central to a child's life (Ahmann 1994, p 113)*

The holistic approach is grounded in respect for and cooperation with the family (Hutchfield 1999). It is underpinned by the principle that there should be an exchange of complete and unbiased information between the family and professionals (Shelton & Smith Stepanek 1995). The approach recognises that all families have some strengths. Nurses can help families to recognise these strengths and build on them to participate in the provision of optimum care to their own children. Families are more likely to take the lead in care and to work in partnership with nurses when this approach is used, as opposed to the nurse-led functional approach.

Hierarchical frameworks may also be used to underpin the practice of family-centred care. The evolvement of the concept of family-centred care has seen a move from parental involvement to parental participation through to partnership working, and finally to family-centred care. It could be that one concept has replaced the other during the evolvement of the concept of family-centred care, but Cahill (1996) suggests that there is a hierarchical relationship between the concepts. Hutchfield (1999) proposes that involvement, participation and partnerships are precursors and depicts them at the lower levels of a hierarchy that has family-centred care at the highest level. The differences between the levels of participation are clearly explained. Nurses, through accurate assessment and negotiation with children and families, are able to use the framework to identify the appropriate level of care for individual families and may then facilitate the family engaging in care at this level. Reassessment may result in families staying at the same level or moving up a level on the hierarchy (Darbyshire 1994).

Seminar discussion topic

Advantages and disadvantages of functional, holistic and hierarchical family-centred care theoretical frameworks
There are advantages and disadvantages of using all these theoretical frameworks.

The functional framework may be judged to be appropriate because families with a sick child will prefer nurses to lead the care and to be told what to do. However, families can be disempowered by this approach, in which the power remains with the nurse as the gatekeeper.

Holistic frameworks are positive because the family members are valued and respected as individuals. The family can negotiate its participation in care and is empowered to work in partnership with the nurse. Conversely, some families may feel they have too much responsibility in care and on occasions they could do 'with a break'.

The hierarchical framework is really positive because 'it recognises that families want to participate in the care of their children in hospital at a level of their own choosing' (Smith et al 2002 p 29). Conversely, the hierarchical framework suggests that families move up the hierarchy and that there is not the option to return to a lower level of participation in care.

Another criticism of hierarchical frameworks is that nurses only use them to negotiate levels of care for families and not to find out about family experiences of living with a sick child in hospital (Darbyshire 1994).

To conclude, there are pros and cons to all these frameworks.

Family-centred Care: The Practice Continuum Tool

This tool has been developed specifically for use in clinical practice. On the continuum (Fig. 6.1), families are facilitated to move in either direction at any time according to individual family and nursing needs. The practice continuum tool can be used for the delivery of family-centred care in any clinical setting involving families both in hospital and in the community.

The practice continuum tool acknowledges the key elements identified by the literature. Thus it comprises parental involvement, participation, partnership and

No involvement	Involvement	Participation	Partnership	Parent-led
Nurse-led	Nurse-led	Nurse-led	Equal status	Parent-led

Fig. 6.1 ● Family-centred care: the practice continuum tool. Smith, L, Colemen, V, Bradshaw, M (eds) (2002) Family-centred Care: Concept, Theory and Practice. Palgrave, reproduced with permission of Palgrave Macmillan.

parent-led care. 'No involvement' is also included to encompass the full spectrum of care that may be experienced by the child within the context of his or her family. The practice continuum tool was synthesised from available research and theoretical material, as well as practice experience, and therefore incorporates all the elements of the theoretical frameworks already discussed.

Children's nurses should be familiar with the terms contained within the tool but because these terms are sometimes used interchangeably to mean the same thing, and because using the practice continuum tool provides practitioners with a dialogue through which to articulate family-centred care in a meaningful and achievable way, it is important to understand what we mean by the following terms:

- **Nurse-led care, no family involvement:** this may occur in situations where the family is not able or willing to be involved for a particular reason for a period of time. This is still family-centred care because the nurse still uses a family-centred focus in care delivery in the family's absence.

- **Nurse-led care, family involvement in care:** this may occur when the family is involved in some basic care, such as feeding, hygiene and/or emotional support. The nurse takes the lead in care management at this stage.

- **Nurse-led, family participation in care:** a good rapport is established, which is collaborative in nature, and the family participates in chosen aspects of nursing care following negotiation. The nurse continues to oversee care management and where necessary teaches relevant care skills to the child and/or family.

- **Equal status, family partnership in care:** this is exemplified by the change in the nurse's role to becoming more of a supporter and facilitator. As families become more empowered they resume their role as primary care givers and the relationship with the nurse is much more equal in nature.

- **Parent-led care, nurse-consulted care:** the family is now expert in all aspects of the child's care. There is a mutual, respectful relationship with the nurse, who is used in a consultative capacity from time to time. Although this is expressed explicitly as parent-led care, the implicit notion is that children are involved in their care and can lead their care in some instances.

No matter where the family is on the practice continuum, it is family-centred care; family-centred care is not only achieved by reaching an 'end stage'. Parents negotiating with the nurse choose where they wish to be on the continuum. For some this may be a progression along the continuum, particularly for those families with a child with an ongoing illness, whereas others may prefer to be involved differently, providing normal childcare and emotional support only.

By being actively involved in the process rather than passive recipients of the nurse's interpretation of family-centred care, families may be less disappointed with their experience as highlighted by research into this area (Darbyshire 1994, Neill 1996). Additionally, nurses may feel less pressured by this approach than by literature that has continually highlighted shortcomings in their ability to embrace family-centred care in a way that is acceptable to the parents. By communicating effectively with families, nurses can focus on their specific needs in relation to family-centred care rather than adopting a blanket approach to it (Smith et al 2002).

The strength of the practice continuum tool is its ability to respond to individual need day by day/shift by shift as the child and family's situation changes. Hence nurses facilitate forward and backward movement along the practice continuum tool as the child's condition changes or as family circumstances dictate. Ongoing evaluation is very much a part of the nurse's caregiving role and therefore incorporating such an explicit approach to family-centred care should not be onerous and will facilitate communication between different nurses caring for the family.

One of the criticisms of parents experiencing family-centred care is lack of continuity between nurses as shifts change and staff approaches to the parent's involvement are different (Dearmun 1992).

PowerPoint

Access the companion PowerPoint presentation for guidelines on using the practice continuum tool.

Activity

Use the scenario on the Evolve website *Family-centred care in practice* and position the child/family on the continuum.

TOOLKIT OF SKILLS

To be able to use the practice continuum tool, or any other theoretical family-centred care framework, children's nurses need to have a toolkit of skills to empower families to negotiate their way through the interfaces of different health care environments. Good communication and teach-

ing skills are essential for the successful implementation of family-centred care.

Communication Skills

Without good communications skills, assumptions may well be made about what families will do for their children in hospital and in the community.

> ### Reflect on your Practice
>
> Think of some examples of good practice in family-centred care that you have observed.
> What communication skills did the nurse use?

You probably mentioned skills like listening, explaining, clarifying, using open-ended questions and negotiating. Communication frameworks that enable skills like these to be used should be chosen to facilitate nurses and families working collaboratively together to care for children. The LEARN model framework (Berlin & Fowkes 1983) promotes interaction between the nurse and family, encouraging active listening by both parties, and acknowledges perceptual differences and similarities with regard to problems and negotiation about the child's care. LEARN is an acronym:

L = Listen
E = Explain
A = Acknowledge
R = Recommend
N = Negotiate.

The Nursing Mutual Participation Model (Curley, cited in Ahmann 1994) requires asking open-ended questions to find out how the child and family feel that they can best participate in care. Families usually know their own child best and therefore professionals should not make independent decisions about involving them in care. Casey (1995) suggests that person-centred nurses are skilled practitioners who are willing to share their knowledge and expertise and to listen to families. Families may well become disempowered if decision-making is taken out of their control and they are put in a position where they are expected to undertake aspects of their child's care that they are not competent to do or are not happy about doing.

Empowerment

> ### Reflect on your Practice
>
> Identify a situation in which either a family or yourself was disempowered.
> What were the inner and outer manifestations of this disempowerment?

Disempowerment engenders such feelings as being: out of control, confused, anxious, angry and frustrated over not being heard by healthcare professionals. These are obviously very strong negative feelings, which need to be avoided, and hence there is a need for collaborative working in family-centred care to empower families.

Empowerment is a reciprocal social process that helps people to participate with competence (Coleman 1998) and to assert control over factors that affect their lives (Gibson 1991)

Professional Conversation

Helen, a registered children's nurse on Part 1 of the Nursing and Midwifery Council's Professional Register, discusses the empowerment of families with Gemma, a student nurse.

Issues affecting family empowerment on a children's ward
It took me a long while to really understand what empowerment was all about. It wasn't until I started working on this ward that it began to make sense. This was because we are encouraged to get to know the children and their families quite well (even those that are only in a short time) and really build up a trusting relationship with them. This makes it easier to negotiate with them and to agree on their participation in chosen aspects of their child's care. Families also seem more receptive to our teaching and information giving because we have taken time to listen to them and to find out about them as a family unit. It's really good when the families become competent in doing negotiated aspects of their child's care. The families grow in confidence and then are usually ready to learn to do other aspects of the child's basic or nursing care.

Helen is describing empowerment both as an outcome and a process.

EMPOWERMENT OUTCOMES

Children and their families have to take some power and control over their own situation to be able to reach empowerment outcomes. This does not mean having power over others. Instead, it signals that a family has taken some of the power from health professionals so that it can make decisions itself about the child's healthcare and/or give nursing care to the children. In their study of the families of children with middle ear infections, Wuest and Stern (1991) found that empowerment outcomes were domain specific. The families did not achieve an effective management of care outcome and stay there because new events in their child's healthcare journey would result in them mov-

ing along the continuum to adopt more passive behaviours until further competencies were developed for empowerment in new domains. However, these families developed an increasing repertoire of management strategies, which they used in different domains of their child's care to achieve empowerment outcomes. This suggests that an empowerment outcome increases family confidence and that it is also a regenerative process. Empowerment outcomes may be achieved in physical, social and/or psychological domains, or an outcome of empowerment may 'simply' mean that children and their families develop a sense of psychological well-being, promoting feelings of being in control of the situation in which they find themselves instead of being powerless or disempowered (Coleman 2002).

THE EMPOWERMENT PROCESS

The empowerment process is described as being a four-stage process (Gibson 1995, Kieffer 1984, Tones & Tilford 2001)

- Stage one: the entry stage is triggered by a specific incident, which leads to the discovery of the personal reality of the situation.

- Stage two: critical reflection to search for and identify the root cause of that reality to be able to move forward. Mentor and peer relationships are seen as being important during this stage.

- Stage three: this is a self-development stage, which may involve examining the implications of actions and may result in individuals wanting to 'take charge' of a situation.

- Stage four: this stage involves developing plans of action, gaining participatory competence in care, taking power from professionals and holding on to it.

During the four stages of the empowerment process a caring relationship should evolve between nurse and family, within which there is building of trust, connecting, mutual knowing and creating to promote self-esteem, self-confidence and self-insight (McWilliam et al 1997) to empower children and families.

Conversely, Gibson (1995) described how mothers of chronically ill children with neurological problems had achieved empowerment outcomes without facilitation from nurses. The mothers in this particular study were empowered in an intrapersonal process to have their voices heard in decision-making and to participate with competence in their children's care. This process was triggered by their frustration on realising that no one was listening to them. A study by Valentine (1998) found that although nurses had the necessary knowledge to empower families, they needed to develop the skills to do it and an empowering environment to practice in.

Activity

Read Gibson (1995) and Valentine (1998).
- How do the findings of these studies relate to your workplace?
- Consider the recommendations of the studies for your workplace.

Scenario

Gemma discusses her written reflective account of a very positive experience of being involved in the empowerment of a child and family, with her mentor Helen.

Gemma describes how a child and family achieved empowerment outcomes and the process used to develop competencies. The nursing process was used to provide a systematic framework for practice and three key stages of an empowerment process in children's nursing emerged (Coleman 2002):

1. Relationship Building

During the continuing nursing assessment the child and family were listened to and there was a sharing of perceptions and knowledge with the nurse. The nurse explored family strengths, as opposed to weaknesses, to promote self-efficacy beliefs to achieve empowerment outcomes. An assessment was made of issues that the child and the family considered to be problems so that these could be addressed along with the nurse-perceived problems. Using appropriate communication skills, the nurse built up a trusting relationship within which there was respect and valuing of the child and family. This relationship helped the nurse and family to journey together through the four stages of an empowerment process.

2. Facilitating Participatory Experiences to Develop Competencies

This was a planned process to enable the child and family to develop competence in negotiated aspects of care. Initially, short-term goals were agreed between the nurse and family to promote self-efficacy beliefs. The family was initially helped to adapt the care usually undertaken at home by the parents to the hospital situation, before being taught and facilitated to do some nursing care appropriate to their situation. The participatory experiences had physical, social and psychological dimensions. The child was also offered opportunities for empowerment, by being given choices at an appropriate developmental level about play and who should give him his medicine. Other children with

continuing care needs will also be taught how to do specific physical nursing skills.

3. Information Giving to Empower Families

Information is fundamental to the empowerment of children and families. It is a two-way process with nurses and families sharing information. Information is conveyed to children and families in many different ways including:

- verbal information on an individual basis
- NHS Direct
- written literature including leaflets, books and posters
- other media including videos, television and the internet
- play activities to educate children
- support groups.

A planned approach to information giving is essential to enable children and families to use it to take some control of their situation. Conversely, information may be disempowering if it is given in an *ad hoc* manner, which for example may result in too much information being given at the wrong time (Coleman 2002).

Reflect on your Practice

Identify one situation when information giving was empowering and another one when information giving was disempowering.
How did information giving differ in these two situations?

Empowerment in a family-centred care approach is often associated with children with continuing care needs, whose care is parent-led. However, children and families experiencing day care or acute care may also be empowered to some extent in all the positions identified on the practice continuum tool.

Activity

Discuss in your learning group how participatory experiences to empower children and families may differ according to the following contexts of care:
- day care
- acute care
- continuing care.

Negotiating Care with Children and Families

Negotiation is a recurring theme in the literature on family-centred care. Research in this area repeatedly reminds nurses that negotiation either does not happen or that there is not the willingness or skills for it to happen (Blower & Morgan 2000, Casey 1995, Dearmun 1992, Evans 1994, Kawik 1996, Neill 1996).

To facilitate negotiation, nurses need to be equipped not only with the skills to implement it in practice but also a means of incorporating it into everyday practice so that it becomes an everyday part of their role with children and families.

To start this process nurses need to reflect on their current practice and evaluate the extent to which they do currently negotiate care with children and families. Self-awareness and analysis of our own practice enables care delivery to develop and remain dynamic offering the highest possible quality of care to children and their families. For student nurses and qualified nurses reflective practice has become accepted as a way of challenging and preventing routinised practice.

 Scenario

'But we're doing it already'
Gemma is attending a study day on family-centred care. In the session the group of child branch students are discussing their experiences of family-centred care. The group discuss how families are involved in the care of their child. A frequent comment was 'We always ask them if they want to be involved and encourage them to participate'.
The lecturer facilitating the study day asks 'Is this negotiated care'?
You might find it useful to read the research by Callery & Smith (1991).

The scenario highlights a common response to what constitutes how parents become involved in the care of their child. Sometimes parents are not asked and it is just assumed they will participate in the care of their child (Kawik 1996, Neill 1996).

What therefore constitutes negotiation needs to be clarified if nurses are to incorporate the concept into their day-to-day practice. Simply, Gourlay (1987) would see negotiations being about meeting people's needs. In this case not only the nurses' needs but those of the child and family. Expectation and assumption should not therefore play a part in the process, rather it is an acceptable agreement between those involved. This involves a relationship where both parties feel equally able to be involved and have their point of view heard. This can be difficult to achieve, as families often feel at a disadvantage, being in an unfamiliar, potentially stressful environment and needing to be empowered to fully participate. How nurses enable families to overcome these barriers is the key to successful negotia-

tion. Equally, nurses need to feel enabled and empowered to undertake the negotiation.

Encouragement and expectation implies that the involvement is very much on the nurse's terms. Although it might, at face value, seem not unreasonable that a parent would want to be involved in the care of his or her child, non-negotiation does not facilitate different styles of coping and adjustment, the type of support the parents need, informed decision-making on which to base their input or even the acknowledging that some parents need respite from some of the care demands placed upon them.

The practice continuum tool enables facilitation of the involvement in care by parents or child at a level they have negotiated with the nurse. The following framework, adapted from *Negotiation of care* (Smith 2002), offers nurses a step-by-step approach to planned negotiation. In following this approach the nurse needs to utilise verbal, non-verbal and written communication skills that are an explicit part of the nurse's role. The LEARN framework (see earlier) will help.

At the start of any relationship, to minimise the potential for misunderstanding, there needs to be some discussion involving the boundaries and expectations (such as nurses assuming parents will always want to be involved or parents not being sure what their role is or can be). Most clinical areas will have a philosophy or mission statement and information booklet about their ward/unit or department that can be shared to start the negotiation process. This introduces the notion that there are opportunities for involvement that will be discussed.

ASSESS

In any negotiation process you need to discover each other's needs. The emphasis here is primarily on the family's needs as it adapts to the diagnosis, treatment, prognosis of the child and the demands that will be placed on the different family members. This, coupled with a strange environment, for many make it essential that the nurse uses a range of communication skills with the family (e.g. listening, open-ended questions, silence, paraphrasing to check understanding).

PLAN

There needs to be an understanding of what is on offer. In what ways can the family be involved? How this can be facilitated? Everyone needs to be aware of this to avoid differences between staff at changeovers for example.

This will also help identify any points that aren't acceptable and reduce the risk of assumptions being made about each other's role.

Record what has been agreed so that everyone is aware of the plan that is being developed.

Underpinning planned negotiation is the empowerment of all participants, as discussed earlier in the chapter. As you are planning with the level of involvement at this stage with the family, are you considering the family's information or teaching needs, because these will impact on their decision-making ability and hence their involvement?

IMPLEMENT

Summarise the agreement and check understanding.

How will the agreements be implemented? (Are there any teaching or support implications needed to facilitate implementation?)

Consider how the negotiated care will be documented.

These issues are important because nurses are responsible and accountable for the care delivered. These are discussed in relation to family-centred care later in the chapter.

EVALUATE

Review the agreements. In the same way we evaluate the child's ongoing care, the family's involvement may need to change. Knowing that if something doesn't work it can be changed enhances the trusting relationship between nurse and family. Confidence in the process is more likely to reduce the potential miscommunication between parties and lead to a more positive experience for all.

Using a framework linked to the systematic approach to nursing care that nurse's use on a daily basis should enable negotiated care to become a reality and not just another 'add on' to the day's work that doesn't always happen for many families.

The Challenges of Delivering Family-centred Care

Scenario

Gemma is gaining experience on a children's ward working alongside Helen, her mentor. Gemma has been introduced to the concept of family-centred care in school but linking this theory to ward practice seems less than straightforward to her. She discusses some of her reflections on this issue with Helen at her intermediate interview.

There is potential for family-centred care to be confusing because it can mean different things to children and parents, student and qualified nurses, or other healthcare professionals. The way individuals think of and define things like 'family' or 'care' can vary enormously. Their diverse understanding, assumptions and values may have been shaped by things like personal life experiences thus far and general or professional education. So when it comes to actually practising family-centred care, one of the challenges for children's nurses is to keep abreast of the breadth and depth of the evolving concept through personal commitment to their own continuing development. Unless children's nurses really do internalise and value the concept, in practice it won't come out of their mouths and fingertips in what they say and do with children and families (Bradshaw 2002). Also, in the light of current literature, nurses have the extra challenge of teasing out what family-centred care is in terms of their own particular ward or unit, so that they and other healthcare professionals connected to it understand, share and value the philosophy. Then comes the challenge of acquainting children and families with the philosophy and using it to underpin all subsequent interactions with them.

Getting family-centred care theory implemented in practice is not always easy or straightforward. It appears to require a 'bottom-up' approach whereby children's nurses working on the 'shop floor' really believe the concept to be valuable, desire to see it underpinning practice and adjust and align their professional behaviours so that they are congruent with this goal. If such goals are not to be thwarted, then appropriate managerial support is vital. The 'top-down' approach to implementing family-centred care can be equally helpful when nurse managers lead from the front and demonstrate their commitment to it by making clear their expectations that it will be fully implemented and audited in the clinical areas.

Activity

Consider your own healthcare trust and find out:

- What commitment to family-centred care does the healthcare trust demonstrate?
- What commitment to family-centred care does the senior nursing management demonstrate?
- What commitment to family-centred care does your ward/unit nursing staff demonstrate?
- What commitment to family-centred care do other members of the multiprofessional team demonstrate?
- How do families especially those whose first language is not English become aware of family-centred care and recipients of it?

For each of the above questions, what written, verbal and non-verbal local evidence do you have to support your findings?

Family-centred care involves nurses negotiating choices and desired amounts of involvement or participation in care

...en and their families. This involves much skill ...ctivity on the part of the nurse. Nurses have tradi- ...ly been seen as the experts who assumed responsibil- ...for orchestrating patient care in line with medical prescriptions and institutional requirements. However, if care is to be truly family-centred, then recognising family expertise in care is vital. When nurse and family meet for the first time, they come together as experts but in different things. The family is often expert on things like getting the child to sleep, knowing what foods to tempt the reluctant eater with, what kind of play captures the child's imagination or distracts him or her, and how best to comfort him or her when upset. The children's nurse is an expert in meeting the ill child's nursing needs. The challenge for children's nurses is to work harmoniously with the family and to engineer pooling of all expertise in order that it may be a powerful force in meeting the child and family's needs.

The way nursing documentation is set out and therefore recorded can itself either hinder or enhance family-centred care. It needs to be developed in such a way that it is a good prompt and makes the elements of family-centred care philosophy overt and an expected requirement.

Activity

With regard to family-centred care, try to look critically at the nursing documentation on your next new ward before anyone has a chance to explain it to you.
- Who do the documents require you to talk to?
- Whose thoughts and concerns do they require you to record?
- What do they require you to do and for whom?
- Will anyone else be contributing to care and if so what?
- What do the child and family think about care and progress so far? How do you know?
- Are the child and family involved in documentation? What advantages or problems might this raise?
(Bradshaw 2002)

Scenario

The staff on Gemma's ward largely seem to value the principles of family-centred care. However, she notices that when other professionals visit children and families on her ward, or when children have to visit other departments, then this doesn't always seem to be the case.

Helen explains that as yet family-centred care is not necessarily a multiprofessional or interprofessional philosophy. From the child and family's point of view, if the professionals that they encounter are not being guided by the same philosophical framework, 'then there is much poten-

tial for what families actually receive and the way they receive it to be disjointed and confusing' (Bradshaw et al 2003). As a result, trust relationships between health professionals and families can be damaged and this itself can impinge on the child's therapeutic progress. One strategy currently being explored to help overcome this is interprofessional shared learning, whereby different professionals are exposed to the same evidence-based education, the idea being that the ensuing discussions, critical analysis and interprofessional debate (in this instance on family-centred care) will lead to the different professionals understanding, valuing and practising the philosophy in a corporate, overt way that is therapeutic for children and families.

Professional and Legal Issues

For the nurse, family-centred care creates a range of professional and legal issues that need to be addressed. Nurses undertaking family-centred care owe a specific duty of care not only to the child but also to the parents, siblings and other family members. Negligence results when this duty of care is breached. Nurses delegating care to participating parents should provide them with adequate information and teaching, and ensure that they have the ability to perform the necessary care in a reliable and responsible way (Foxcroft 2002). To discharge the duty of care it is also important to identify when the child is able to make healthcare decisions and participate in care.

Activity

Find out what legal and other guidelines there are to inform you about children's rights and ability to consent, make healthcare decisions and to participate in care.

Nurses should use these guidelines to inform their professional judgement to decide whether a child has sufficient understanding and intelligence to participate in family-centred care, ensuring 'that the child is treated appropriately and that adequate care is provided so that the child does not suffer harm' (Foxcroft 2002 pp 156–157). The nurse also has a duty to supervise family-centred care, ensuring that the family is sufficiently competent to undertake that care before being allowed to act alone.

Nurses are accountable to their employer, to children/families by way of the law and to the Nursing and Midwifery Council (NMC). The NMC Code of Professional Conduct (2002) states that:

1.4 You have a duty of care to your patients and clients, who are entitled to receive safe and competent care (NMC 2002 p 3)

4.6   You may be expected to delegate care delivery to others who are not registered nurses or midwives . . . You remain accountable for the appropriateness of the delegation, for ensuring that the person who does the work is able to do it and that adequate supervision or support is provided (NMC 2002 p 7)

Nurses must adhere to this code in family-centred care nursing practice. Care plans should be negotiated, agreed and documented with the family so that all concerned are clear as to each person's role in the care of the child. The documentation includes, parental agreement to participation in care, teaching undertaken, parental confidence to do certain tasks and planned review of care dates.

Summary

Contemporary health policy in the 21st century continues to highlight family-centred care as an essential concept for children's nurses. The need to work in partnership with families and involve them in decision-making must be supported by children's nurses with the appropriate skills to facilitate this. The practice continuum tool as a framework for the practice of family-centred care will enable nurses to implement this concept in a variety of healthcare settings. Understanding the challenges, the legal and professional implications of family-centred care can only enhance the delivery of quality care.

References

Ahmann E 1994 Family-centred care: shifting orientation. Pediatric Nursing 20(2): 113–116

Berlin EA, Fowkes WC 1983 A teaching framework for cross-cultural health care. Western Journal of Medicine 139(6):934–938

Blower K, Morgan E 2000 Great expectations? Parental participation in care. Journal of Child Health Care 4(2):60–65

Bradshaw M, Coleman V, Smith L 2003 Interprofessional learning and family-centred care. Paediatric Nursing 15(7):30–33

Bradshaw M 2002 Implications and challenges for family-centred care. In: Smith L, Coleman V, Bradshaw M (eds) Family-centred care: concept, theory and practice. Palgrave, Basingstoke, pp 47–61

Bruce B, Ritchie J 1997 Nurses' practices and perceptions of family centred care. Journal of Pediatric Nursing 12(4):214–222

Brunner L, Suddarth D 1986 The Lippincott manual of paediatric nursing, 2nd edn. Harper and Row, London

Cahill J 1996 Patient participation: a concept analysis. Journal of Advanced Nursing 24:561–571

Callery P, Smith L 1991 A study of role negotiation between nurses and the parents of hospitalised children. Journal of Advanced Nursing 16:772–781

Callery P 1997 Caring for parents of hospitalised children: a hidden area of nursing work. Journal of Advanced Nursing 26(5):992–998

Casey A 1995 Partnership nursing: influences on involvement of informal carers. Journal of Advanced Nursing 22:1058–1062

Coleman V 1998 What is the meaning of empowerment and do nurses use it to promote the health of children with a chronic illness. Unpublished Masters dissertation, Sheffield Hallam University

Coleman V 2002 Empowerment: rhetoric, reality and skills. In: Smith L, Coleman V, Bradshaw M (eds) Family-centred care: concept, theory and practice. Palgrave, Basingstoke, pp 85–113

Darbyshire P 1993 Parents, nurses and paediatric nursing: a critical review. Journal of Advanced Nursing 18:1670–1680

Darbyshire P 1994 Living with a sick child in hospital: the experiences of parents and nurses. Chapman and Hall, London

Dearmun A 1992 Perceptions of parental participation. Paediatric Nursing 4(7):6–9

Department of Health (DoH) 1999 Saving lives: our healthier nation. The Stationery Office, London

Department of Health (DoH) 2000 The NHS plan, a plan for investment, a plan for reform. DoH, London. Online. Available at: http://www.nhs.uk/nhsplan

Department of Health (DoH) 2003 Getting the right start: national service framework for children: standards for hospital services. DoH, London

Dunst C, Trivette C 1996 Empowerment, effective help giving practices and family centred care. Pediatric Nursing 22(4):334–337

Evans M 1994 An investigation into the feasibility of parental participation in the nursing care of their children. Journal of Advanced Nursing 20:447–482

Foxcroft L 2002 Professional and legal issues. In: Smith L, Coleman V, Bradshaw M (eds) Family-centred care: concept, theory and practice. Palgrave, Basingstoke, pp 148–170

Gibson C 1991 A concept analysis of empowerment. Journal of Advanced Nursing 16:354–361

Gibson C 1995 The process of empowerment in mothers of chronically ill children. Journal of Advanced Nursing 21:1201–1210

Gourlay R 1987 Negotiations for managers. Health Services Manpower review. University of Keele

Hutchfield K 1999 Family centred care: a concept analysis. Journal of Advanced Nursing 29(5):1178–1187

Kieffer CH 1984 Citizen empowerment. A developmental perspective. Prevention in Human Services 2(2/3):9–36

Kawik L 1996 Nurses and parents' perceptions of participation and partnership in caring for a hospitalized child. British Journal of Nursing 5(7):430–434

McWilliam C, Stewart M, Brown J et al 1997 Creating empowering meaning; an interactive process of promoting health with chronically older Canadians. Health Promotion International 12(2):111–123

Neill S 1996 Parent participation. British Journal of Nursing 5(2):110–117

Nethercott S 1993 Family centred care: a concept analysis. Professional Nurse September:794–797

Nursing and Midwifery Council (NMC) 2002 Nursing and Midwifery Council Code of Professional Conduct. NMC, London

Shelton T, Smith Stepanek J 1995 Excerpts from family centred care for children needing health and developmental services. Pediatric Nursing 21(4):362–364

Smith L, Coleman V, Bradshaw M (eds) 2002 Family-centred care: concept, theory and practice. Palgrave, Basingstoke

Smith L 2002 Negotiation of care. In: Smith L, Coleman V, Bradshaw M (eds) Family-centred care: concept, theory and practice. Palgrave, Basingstoke, pp 114–130

Tones K, Tilford S 2001 Health education: effectiveness, efficiency and equity, 2nd edn. Nelson Thornes, Cheltenham

Valentine F 1998 Empowerment: family centred care. Paediatric Nursing 10(1):24–27

Wuest J, Stern P 1991 Empowerment in primary health care: the challenge for nurses. Qualitative Health Research 11(1):80–99

Additional Reading

Coleman V, Smith L, Bradshaw M 2003 Enhancing consumer participation using the practice continuum tool for family-centred care. Paediatric Nursing 15(8):28–31

Useful Websites

http://www.actionforsickchildren.org – contains useful information for families and healthcare professionals on major topics in children's healthcare.

http://www.doh.gov.uk/nsf/children/gettingtherightstart – contains the document detailing the National Service Framework for Children setting out the standard for hospital services.

http://www.familycenteredcare.org – American-based institute providing a resource for health professionals through training, information dissemination, policy and research initiatives.

Chapter Seven

7

Assessing and Planning Care in Partnership

Anne Casey

ABSTRACT

Assessment is the basis for planning and delivering nursing care to children, young people and families. Whether it is a comprehensive, holistic review of a child's health needs and problems, or a rapid, focused check on some aspect of his or her condition, assessment provides the information needed to agree with the child and family what needs to be done, when and by whom. Clinical reasoning skills are required for the nurse to interpret assessment data and identify appropriate actions, using evidence where possible. Information and knowledge management skills are required to support accurate recording and use of information about assessment and care and to enable children, young people and their families to participate fully in the care process.

All aspects of care, from assessment to evaluation, are affected by the context in which the care takes place and in particular by the attitudes and values of the nurse and the care team. Working in partnership requires a specific focus for nursing assessment, planning and evaluation which is different to traditional disease focused models.

Learning Outcomes

- Appreciate the importance of accurate and detailed observation and assessment (and recording of same).
- Identify and select from a range of assessment approaches for different children and clinical situations.
- Undertake, with supervision, holistic assessment of the infant/child/young person as a basis for planning general nursing care.

- Use assessment data to make initial judgements about the child and family's need for general nursing care, to be validated by an experienced nurse.
- Describe how assessment findings and clinical evidence inter-relate when planning care.
- Incorporate reassessment and evaluation of outcomes in the care plan.
- Recognise the complex nature of clinical reasoning and the roles of the child, family, nurse and multiagency team in assessment, planning and evaluation of care.

The Nature of Assessment

In any walk of life, assessment is the basis for making decisions about what to do. Unless an action is completely spontaneous, it is usually preceded by the person gathering together relevant facts, thinking about them to make sense of the situation and then weighing up the possible alternatives for what to do next. During and after the action, further thought is given to whether the choice of action was the right one: is this having the effect I expected it to? What else could I try? Perhaps I jumped to the wrong conclusion about what was wrong?

Assessment is both a process and a result: assessing the level of oil in the engine might give a result of 'its getting low' and a plan to top up next time I'm passing the service station. Of course, if I then notice a patch of oil under the car I revise my initial assessment result to 'there could be a leak' and plan to go straight to a repair centre.

In health care, the process of assessment attempts to answer the question 'What is (probably) going on here?' With some degree of certainty about what is happening, it is possible to make a plan that will address the problem. But there is much more to assessing and planning care than simply discovering the problem and deciding what to do. This chapter explores assessment and care planning in the context of child/family/nurse partnerships to provide insights into these complex interpersonal and clinical processes that are the cornerstones of clinical practice. Recording, communicating and evaluating planned care are also considered, with an emphasis on the clinical and information governance responsibilities of the nurse. The chapter does not cover assessment for the specific purpose of investigating, diagnosing and treating medical conditions; Barnes (2003) is the recommended text for nurse practitioners undertaking what were traditionally medical roles. Assessment of and planning for community and population child health needs are also not covered here (see Chapter 8).

Assessment and Planning in Context

THE CLINICAL PROCESS

When first learning about something as complex as nursing, it helps to use diagrams or models that simplify the situation but demonstrate how things relate and where they fit in the real world of practice. Conceptual models and process models are used in nursing and other disciplines to clarify concepts important to the discipline and define relationships between them. The 'nursing process' was one such model introduced to the UK in the 1970s to help nurses focus on each individual patient and his or her needs, rather than on the medical condition and 'what we always do for patients with x'. It is clear that health professionals other than nurses use a similar process and that parents and children follow the same basic steps when managing illness at home. This 'clinical process' as it applies to nursing is outlined in Fig. 7.1 to help you visualise the practical steps that are taken in the care and treatment of children and young people.

The first step in the process is prompted by any one of a number of 'triggers': a mother notices a rash on her baby's face, the community nurse visits a sick child at home, the teenager walks into the school drop-in centre, a 4-hourly temperature measurement is due and so on. The steps of assessing, planning, implementing and evaluating can take

seconds in an emergency and months or years, for example, in the case of a child who has sustained a severe head injury. Although the model suggests a straight line, where one step neatly follows the one before, the process is anything but linear. Observing a bruise will lead to a plan for further assessment; when teaching a child about his asthma he may reveal concerns about exercise, which will prompt assessment and a different plan; assessment may lead to a decision to take no further action and so on. The three pillars of assessment (listening, observing and measuring) are constant activities throughout the care process. Planned assessments such as hourly monitoring of pain level and ad hoc or opportunistic assessments such as noticing a change in one child while attending to another, become the basis for changes to planned care, new assessments and new plans.

It can be helpful to distinguish between initial or **generalised assessment** of the kind that would be carried out at a first contact or admission in a non-emergency situation and **focused assessment**, where attention is directed at a specific state, behaviour, concern or situation. The goals of an initial assessment are to identify:

1. Immediate and ongoing care needs related to the reason for the visit, contact or admission.
2. Other issues/areas of concern.
3. Health promotion needs and opportunities.

It is important to establish a baseline of assessment data that can be used to agree care aims, monitor progress and evaluate outcomes.

Results of initial assessments are used to plan for and to provide care, support, information and education and to communicate with/refer to other professionals. Generalised and focused assessments are discussed later in this chapter after an introduction to clinical reasoning and exploration of the contextual factors that affect both the process and outcome of assessment (and the rest of the care process).

CLINICAL REASONING

A process model of the kind described above has limitations: one criticism of the nursing process is that it emphasises patient problems (it is sometimes referred to as a 'problem-solving process') and therefore is unsuited to health promotion and 'well person' elements of nursing roles. Although it clearly shows how a nurse could provide individualised, planned care, the process focuses on 'doing' steps, and thus hides the clinical reasoning that is required to sift through the available assessment data and to weigh up the evidence to make good clinical decisions.

Another way of looking at the same process is to consider the cognitive processes that underpin assessment, planning and evaluation, rather than the action steps. 'Clinical rea-

Fig. 7.1 • The clinical process.

soning' is a general term covering the cognitive processes of diagnostic reasoning (also known as clinical judgement) and clinical decision making. Higgs (2000) provides an excellent overview of clinical reasoning in the health professions. Knowing about these clinical and cognitive processes can help direct your approach to care and will inform your practice in helping children, young people and families to carry out assessments themselves and make decisions about what actions to take in the light of their own findings.

Activity

Imagine that you woke up this morning with a slight pain in your knee that has worsened during the day. List the things you might ask yourself or do to try to establish what the problem is. What knowledge have you drawn on to inform your 'diagnostic reasoning'?

Figure 7.2 shows how the data that are collected by listening, observing, measuring and communicating with other professionals are sifted and sorted to select what is relevant and then analysed to reach a conclusion on whether the situation is normal for this child, a problem, a risk and so on. If there are insufficient data to reach a conclusion, a further decision is required: what more data do I need? To make good clinical judgements, the person doing the assessment draws on existing knowledge and past experience, and uses cognitive skills such as pattern recognition ('I've seen this kind of thing before') and ruling out by hypothesis testing ('It can't be infection because there's no fever') to reach conclusions. These assessment 'conclusions' are known in some nursing literature and practice as nursing diagnoses.

In the US and many other countries (and to a small extent in the UK) nurses use the concept of nursing diag-nosis to describe and communicate to others the primary focus of nursing care. A nursing diagnosis is 'a clinical judgement about individual family or community responses to actual or potential health problems/life processes' (North American Nursing Diagnosis Association (NANDA) 2003). It is usually expressed as a diagnostic statement and reflects some aspect of the child and family's response to a health issue or problem, as distinct from the medical diagnosis of the problem.

One of the benefits of reaching a firm conclusion is that this can be discussed openly. Your initial conclusion about what is making a child cry, for example, could lead you to take certain actions, which might be totally inappropriate unless you confirm your 'diagnosis' with the child. A fully expressed nursing diagnosis contains not only the diagnosis but also the cause or 'related factors' and the assessment data that support your conclusion ('defining characteristics' of the diagnosis) (Carpenito-Moyet 2004). 'Pain in the arm related to the splint rubbing' requires very different action from 'pain in arm related to fracture'.

Deciding what action to take (clinical decision making) uses different knowledge and cognitive skills than judging whether there is a need for action, as Table 7.1 illustrates. Based on the 'diagnosis', and when appropriate, goals or expected outcomes can be discussed and agreed with the child and family so that everyone is clear about what can be expected. Knowledge from research and other evidence (see Chapter 14), and personal experience of what works in this kind of situation, inform cognitive decision-making processes such as narrowing of options and weighing-up pros and cons. Possible actions need to be balanced against available resources to arrive at an agreed plan of what is to be done, by whom and when.

CONTEXT FOR CARE

Patient care and the clinical process do not take place in isolation. No matter how good the assessment is and how well planned the care, there are many other factors that influence whether the child's and family's expectations of care are achieved and their experience of nursing and healthcare is a positive one. The context of care, from the interpersonal relationships between family and staff to the prevailing political climate, heavily impact on the quality of the services and care provided. Figure 7.3 illustrates the multitude of factors that have an influence on the care process, many of which are addressed in the chapters in Section 1 of this book. At different times and in different situations the impact of the various factors will be different but four of them are particularly important in nursing:

- Interpersonal: relationships and interactions between and among the child, the family and the clinical team.

Fig. 7.2 • Clinical reasoning in assessment.

Table 7.1 Differences in Making Clinical Judgements and Clinical Decisions

	Cognitive processes – examples	Knowledge used
Making clinical judgements: reaching a conclusion about what is (probably) going on	Collation of data/cues Data analysis Pattern recognition Hypothesis generation and evaluation Dealing with uncertainty	Previous experience of this child or similar situations, patterns, etc. Knowledge of effects of disease, surgery etc. on child and family Research evidence and patient 'stories' of what it is like to be a child, parent, family member in this situation
Making clinical decisions: deciding what to do – choosing a course of action (in relation to goals)	Critical thinking/weighing up research evidence Identifying and evaluating options Setting priorities and managing constraints: time, resources, crises	Knowledge about what has worked for this child in the past Previous experience of what works in similar situations Evidence, guidelines, protocols for the best approach to take

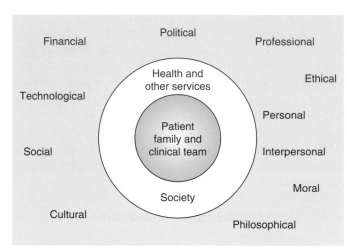

Fig. 7.3 • Context of care: influences on the care process.

- Financial: availability of and ease of access to specific services and resources, e.g. equipment, staff, time.
- Philosophical: the ethos of the team that pervades all aspects of care delivery.
- Ethical: recognition of rights, equity, etc.

Partnership Principles Applied to Assessing and Planning Care

In Chapter 6, Lynda Smith, Valerie Coleman and Maureen Bradshaw described parental involvement in care as moving along a continuum from nurse led to parent led. Other conceptual models of nursing use similar constructs to help explain aspects of the relationship between nurses and patients, for example, Orem's view of the patient as totally dependent through to self caring (Orem 2001). These kinds of models and terms such as 'nurse led', 'patient centred', 'child friendly' represent particular philosophies: ways of thinking and then acting that directly influence the child's and family's experience of care. Even the language we use implies a particular way of thinking and acting. You might hear the term 'non-compliant' applied in a situation, for example, where a teenager with diabetes is admitted to hospital. 'Non-compliance' suggests that heavy-handed sanctions will be needed to get the patient to manage diet, exercise and insulin properly. If the teenager is described instead as 'making choices that can put her at risk' then the management approach is more likely to be one that reflects an understanding of adolescent needs.

▶ Reflect on your Practice

Interpersonal context

How could interpersonal relationships between members of a clinical team (an aspect of the interpersonal context) influence the quality of your nursing care? For example, what would happen if the nursing team does not feel able to question medical staff decisions?

▶ Reflect on your Practice

Philosophical context

Nurses often provide information to the child and family about the child's condition or treatment, reflecting a view of children and families as passive recipients of healthcare. What view would you be reflecting if instead of providing information you helped the child to find out where to get information for herself?

The term 'partnership' is widely used in health and social care to represent the ideal or preferred relationship between agencies and between professionals and clients. In the nursing care of children and families it has come to mean a changing, negotiated, shared responsibility for care between child, family and nurse, with support and teaching provided (including teaching of nurses by the child and family). Family involvement in care may be a result of the negotiation of care responsibility but is not necessarily so. Conversely, nursing involvement in care may not be what the child and family want: respite care at home for the child with complex needs may be better provided by a social care assistant with specific training. A key principle of partnership working is that responsibility does not have to be shared equally: the extent to which the child, family member and nurse are ready for and able to contribute to the partnership dictates changes in responsibility – for the child towards independent self-care and for some parents towards leading and delegating care. In some situations, the nursing team may only be able to offer limited services so the burden of care remains with the family.

Partnership complements other constructs valued by nurses caring for children and young people such as 'child-centred care' and respect for children's rights, particularly the right to be informed and to have a say in decision making (see Chapters 10 and 18). There is very little evidence of how children and parents view partnership working (as distinct from research into their views on involvement or participation in care), and little to indicate whether true partnerships are possible in a context where professionals have more power and there are limited resources. In Coyne's (1995) study, parents reported difficulties with lack of information, non-negotiation of roles, and feelings of anxiety and loneliness when caring for their child in hospital.

Evidence-based Practice

Negotiated roles

Kirk (2001) investigated whether there was any negotiation of caring roles between professionals and parents of children with complex needs:

From the parents' perspective, their initial assumption of responsibility for the care of their child was not subject to negotiation with professionals. Prior to discharge, feelings of obligation, their strong desire for their child to come home and the absence of alternatives to parental care in the community were key motivating factors in their acceptance of responsibility from professionals (Kirk 2000 p 593).

Professionals had concerns about whether parents were given a choice and the degree of choice they could exercise in the face of professional power. As parents gained experience in caring for their child, and as their relationships with professionals developed, role

negotiation started to happen. Kirk concluded that professional expectations of parental involvement probably acted as a barrier to negotiation of roles and that parental choices were initially constrained by their feelings of obligation.

Applying a partnership approach to assessment alters the goals that were listed on page 90, which now become:

- With the child and family, to identify:
  - their immediate and ongoing care needs related to the reason for the visit, contact or admission
  - other issues/areas of concern
  - health promotion needs and opportunities
  - their experience and expectations of care and services
  - their readiness and preferences in relation to participation in care and decision making
- To establish a baseline (as before).

Traditional, profession-centred models of care still exist where the mother, not the child or young person, is asked about the child's condition and progress. The clinician interprets the assessment information and informs the parent what needs to happen next. However, in most services it is accepted that the children and young people themselves are the best source of information and that seeking their views and involving them in decision making and self-care are beneficial not just in terms of outcome but in making their whole experience of health care more positive.

Evidence-based Practice

Who knows best?

A study by Waters et al (2003) explored differences between adolescent and parental reports of physical, emotional, mental and social health and well-being. Over 2000 young people (with and without chronic illness) and their parents were involved in the study. All the adolescents were much less optimistic about their health and well-being than their parents. There were significant differences in their reports of general health, mental health, frequency and amount of pain and the impact on the family of their health problems.

Child Conversation
Kate aged 11 years with asthma.

Kate: *Once I started doing it myself [the asthma diary] I could see much better how I was doing. I could tell the nurse how much Ventolin I'd needed and sometimes we could see what was making it worse. Once we decided for* *me to try taking Ventolin before going outdoors or for PE when it was cold outside.*

Kate's mum: *She was better at keeping the diary than me, at least at first. Now she only uses it when she's having problems and that helps her see what needs doing.*

Using the communication tools that are most familiar to children and young people, such as mobile phones and the internet, goes some way to improving the child friendliness of services. Although these approaches are still being evaluated, it is possible to envisage young people with diabetes, for example, managing their condition at home with internet-based decision support, e-mail advice and mobile phone text reminders for medication times. But there is still a significant shift needed in the way professionals view the child and young person's world, particularly the child/young person with a chronic condition or disability. More locally delivered services and better use of technology will support moves from a world where the child/young person and the family must adapt their lives to fit around the condition and its management to a world where the condition and its management are adapted to their lifestyles. With more children's nurses as part of the primary care team supporting children and families at home there will hopefully be greater attention focused on assessment and intervention in relation to the safety and suitability of the child's environment, his or her access to community services and the appropriateness of those services. Simple solutions like having appointments outside of college hours seem obvious but there are very few clinics that consider the needs and lifestyles of children and young people.

Before moving on to the practice of assessment and care planning, it is appropriate to summarise the clinical process as it can look when informed by partnership and other nursing values/philosophies (Table 7.2). Listening to and respecting the child/young person's and family's views and involving them in decision making is not a luxury that only applies in long-term care situations; it is a fundamental right that applies equally in emergencies, in ambulatory and short-stay settings – everywhere that children and young people receive health care.

Assessment and Planning in Practice

Having considered the process of assessing and planning, the context in which it occurs and the ways in which values and philosophies influence the process, it is now time to address the important question of how to assess and plan care. In this section the focus for nursing assessment is discussed, and assessment approaches and tools introduced. The section concludes with examples of approaches and tools to support evidence-based care planning.

A growing thread throughout health and social care in the UK is the single, shared patient record as a necessary requirement for ensuring continuity in an age when many different disciplines and services may be providing care for one child. This theme will be picked up in the final section of the chapter; recording, communicating and auditing care. A single record suggests a single assessment and one care plan for the child, something that many professionals believe would get rid of many of the communication failures and frustrations that parents and children experience.

Table 7.2 Partnership in the Care Process	
Assess	Ask the child, ask the parents/carer Invite the child, parents/carer to observe and measure Observe and measure Confirm your impressions and conclusions with the child and parents/carer, especially their view of the priorities
Plan	Agree appropriate goals with the child and parents/carer Discuss possible actions and assist them in making choices Agree initial plan for what needs to be done, who will do it, when and how Plan for regular shared review of the plan, care responsibilities and teaching and support needs
Implement	Perform direct care as planned (child, parent/carer, nurse) Facilitate learning and information sharing Provide support and supervision Monitor progress and reassess as planned (child, parent/carer, nurse) With consent, refer to other professionals and coordinate care
Evaluate	Invite the child, parents/carer to observe and measure outcomes and report their experience of care Review and reflect on the care process from child and family perspective and from the professional nursing perspective

THE FOCUS OF ASSESSMENT

Even when single, shared patient records are a reality, nurses will still be responsible for the nursing elements of assessment and planning. But what are these, where do you start and how much do you cover? The obvious starting point is to identify those aspects of the health care of children and young people for which nurses are responsible. To some extent these are dictated by Health Service managers through role and job descriptions and can change over time and between settings. But the profession itself, in consultation with the public and other professional groups, defines the core focus of nursing work. The regulatory and professional bodies set standards for practice and education that specify what nurses are educated to do and how they will practice. The Royal College of Nursing (RCN) defines nursing as providing clear directions for assessment and for the way in which care is provided (RCN 2003).

Professional Conversation

What is nursing? Extracts from Defining nursing (RCN 2003).

Nursing is . . .

- The use of clinical judgement in the provision of care to enable people to improve, maintain, or recover health, to cope with health problems, and to achieve the best possible quality of life.
- The purpose of nursing is to promote health, healing, growth and development, and to prevent disease, illness, injury, and disability. When people become ill or disabled, the purpose of nursing is, in addition, to minimise distress and suffering, and to enable people to understand and cope with their disease or disability, its treatment and its consequences. When death is inevitable, the purpose of nursing is to maintain the best possible quality of life until its end.
- The specific domain of nursing is people's unique responses to and experience of health, illness, frailty, disability and health related life events in whatever environment or circumstances they find themselves.
- The focus of nursing is the whole person and the human response rather than a particular aspect of the person or a particular pathological condition.

Applying and expanding this definition in the client group of children and young people results in a number of different areas of responsibility for nursing, which in some cases could all apply at once:

- protecting
- living with disability
- living healthy lives
- preventing accidents and illness
- managing/living with health problems, including mental health problems.

In this last area, the nursing focus is on the child's/young person's (and family's) experiences of the health problem and its management. Nursing assessment covers the physiological, physical, psychological, social and spiritual effects they may experience, including effects on development and family life. Nursing care is primarily focused not on the disease, injury or disability itself but on the symptoms, limitations, feelings, behaviour, lifestyle changes and so on experienced by the child and the concerns or problems that the family may have in providing care for their child.

Traditional, disease-focused models of nursing assessment are very common and illustrate the need for improved understanding of the unique contribution of nursing. Reductions in medical staff numbers and advances in health technology mean that more and more nurses are taking on what were previously medical roles, from technical tasks to investigation, diagnosis and treatment of disorders. Evidence suggests that with appropriate education and training nurses can provide safe, high quality clinical services (see Redshaw & Harvey 2002). But the unique contribution that nursing care makes to improving the experiences and quality of life patients and families needs to be recognised so that when nurses do take on new roles overall quality is not compromised.

It is impossible to totally separate the specific focus and contribution of nursing: nurses' work encompasses aspects of many other disciplines from play therapy to prescribing, and often substitutes for parental 'work' – the continual care, protection, comfort, distraction and encouragement that parents provide to their children. However, a clear understanding of those situations that are the primary responsibility of nurses and those that are a collaborative responsibility helps to ensure that nurses meet the requirements of their professional role (Carpenito-Moyet 2004).

Evidence-based Practice

Nursing or medicine?
In 1997, Mason & Webb found that nursing records reflected children's medical/physical needs and care but that much practice was focused on psychosocial needs. When nurses were provided with a nursing framework for assessment their clinical judgements were no longer described in terms of the primary medical diagnosis but reflected the family-centred nursing model, including:
- continuity of usual care by parents
- support for family members
- impact of illness and hospitalisation
- participation by parents in nursing and medical care.

As part of their collaborative role with medicine, nurses do include aspects of illness/injury management in their assessments such as:

- assessing any risks for complications of treatment
- monitoring treatment progress
- assessing the child/family ability to carry out treatment plans.

In collaboration with mental health and social care professionals working with children in need and their families, nurses may undertake diagnostic assessments related to development, behaviour, parenting capacity, family functioning and so on (see Hockenberry et al 2003 for examples of physical, developmental and family assessment techniques). As nursing specialist roles expand and more nurse-led services develop, assessments now incorporate tests and investigations relating to the child's medical condition. Combining nursing and medical or other discipline focused assessment is time consuming and complex but marks the difference between the nurse with an expanded role and the nurse as 'doctor substitute'.

Evidence-based Practice

Combining nursing and medical roles

Although there is a great deal of research on diabetes care in children, there is a concern that nursing practice may be mostly guided by 'biomedical models'. Marshall et al (2002) argue that 'psychosocial constructs have an important role in the development of self-management of chronic illness in children' and that care in children should focus on family-centred approaches based in the community. They conclude that paediatric diabetes nurse specialists are pivotal in facilitating family-centred care based on personal models of child and family interventions, whilst also addressing the physiological, developmental and treatment issues.

GENERALISED ASSESSMENT FRAMEWORKS

Discussion of the focus of nursing assessment concludes with a very practical question around scope – how wide ranging should your questions be and what observations and measurements should you make? The concept of holism is an important one in nursing: you will not discover how a diagnosis of epilepsy has affected a child's life if your assessment consists of taking the child's temperature, measuring blood pressure and weight and asking when the last fit occurred. However, it will not be appropriate to ask broader questions when the child is already under the care of the epilepsy specialist nurse and you are doing an assessment prior to a CT scan. The breadth and depth of nursing assessments need to be adapted to the child and family situation, the clinical context and – to some extent – the resources available for subsequent action. There would be no point conducting a full assessment of the social and financial impact of weekly hos-

pital treatment if there is no alternative and the family won't be eligible for disability allowances or income support.

Scenario

A child is admitted to the day ward for minor surgery under general anaesthetic. As she had attended the clinic the week before, her height and weight are already noted. After greeting the child and mother and introducing herself, the nurse records the child's temperature, pulse and respirations, asks whether she has had a cough or cold in the previous few days and when she last had something to eat or drink. Having checked that the consent form is signed, the nurse asks whether the mother or child have any questions about the procedure.

This scenario is a good example of the clinical situation alone dictating the assessment. The nurse is using knowledge of what is important for ensuring a safe anaesthetic procedure, but is not using knowledge from nursing theory and research of what the child and the mother might be experiencing or other concerns and needs they may have. This is the crux of good nursing assessment:

- using knowledge from different sources (including from personal experience)
  ↓
- combining it with the results of holistic and focused assessment in order to
  ↓
- apply the knowledge appropriately to the individual child and family in order to
  ↓
- discover (and confirm with them) their care needs.

Professional Conversation

" Meena is a third-year children's nursing student. "

Theory into practice with caution

We'd been studying Piaget's developmental stages and what they mean in terms of preparing children for surgery. So when I knew I'd be admitting a 4-year-old boy I thought carefully about what his understanding would be at that age about his body and the surgery and being in hospital. I was prepared with simple pictures of tubes going into the tummy and so on but he waved me away and seemed annoyed that I hadn't used the words gastrostomy, abdomen, etc. One of the staff nurses explained he'd been in and out of hospital since birth and had a better understanding of his condition than many of the nurses. It made me realise that although applying theory in practice was important, I needed to use it to inform what I thought and did for each individual patient, not to make assumptions about what their actual needs were.

The following list summarises the scope of nursing assessment and also suggests a logical prioritisation of assessment topics.

1. Risk to life of child and risk of harm to child.

2. Communication – abilities, means, aids, language etc.

3. Fears and anxieties – immediate concerns addressed.

4. Systematic and ongoing assessment – generalised, focused, changes, progress.

5. Preferences and needs related to participation in decision making and care.

The first priority must obviously be risks to life and risk of harm. Second, there must be a means of communicating and establishing a relationship with the child/young person and the parents/carer (see Chapter 11). When communication is possible, fears, anxieties and immediate concerns need to be identified and addressed. Appropriate, systematic assessment can then be carried out, including identification of other risks such as potential environmental threats or stress related to family disruption.

A number of frameworks are available to help the nurse to decide what topics to cover in generalised assessment, from activities of living (Roper & Tierney 2000) to Gordon's 'functional health patterns' adapted for use with children and young people (Hockenberry et al 2003). Outside the UK, Gordon's (2002) work is one of the most widely used frameworks because it supports comprehensive, patient-centred assessment. The eleven health patterns (Box 7.1) can be used to develop and organise locally developed assessment tools or to test them for holism. A good example of the benefit of such a framework is the issue of complementary and alternative therapies. Assessing activities of living would not usually elicit a family's interest in or use of herbal medicines, for example. Gordon's 'health perception/health management pattern' category directs the nurse to enquire about health beliefs and use of other therapies.

Generalised assessment tools based on this kind of framework give structure to assessments and reinforce the philosophy and values on which they are based. Whatever the clinical context, there will be a core set of items relevant to every child, young person and family such as their understanding of the situation and their special needs. As care needs emerge and a relationship is established, the child and family's preferences and readiness for participation in care and decision making and their information, learning and support needs can be identified.

Depending on the clinical context, specific assessment items will be prioritised, for example, respiration, hydration, skin integrity and pain level in intensive care; self-care, self-image, feeding regime and educational needs in the head injury rehabilitation unit. Some of these areas will

Box 7.1

Functional health patterns: a framework for holistic nursing assessment (Gordon 2002)

- Health perception/health management pattern
- Nutrition/metabolic pattern
- Elimination pattern
- Sleep/rest pattern
- Activity/exercise pattern
- Cognitive/perceptual pattern
- Self-perception/self-concept pattern
- Role/relationship pattern
- Sexuality/reproductive pattern
- Coping/stress tolerance pattern
- Value/belief pattern

Reflect on your Practice

Choose a clinical area that you have worked in and list the topics that you recall being the focus of nursing assessment. Consider your list in the light of Fig. 7.4 and the functional patterns in Box 7.1. Would you add anything to your list?

be assessed using validated tools like the ones introduced in the next section and in other chapters in this book. It would not be possible to publish all possible frameworks that might be appropriate for the many different health and nursing needs of children and young people. However, it is possible to list a set of principles for evaluation of those that are presently available, or to underpin the development of new ones. Most importantly, frameworks for comprehensive nursing assessment of children and young people must support the identification of health issues that require nursing intervention or referral to other team members. They should also:

- be child- and family-centred: consider the child's/young person's rights, responsibilities and relationships within the family and society

- be holistic: covering physiological, physical, social, psychological and spiritual aspects of the developing child/young person

- reflect partnership values: including consideration of child and family preferences related to care, and their involvement in care and decision making

- be practical to use

- be acceptable to children/young people and families

- have a nursing focus: address the effects of the health issue and its management (not the diagnosis and treatment alone).

Although nursing assessment has a specific focus, as with all aspects of children's healthcare, team approaches to assessment should be considered. Many aspects of the child's care are managed by the whole team and joint or shared assessment approaches are becoming the norm. The national (English) standard approach to assessing children in need and their families is one example of an agreed multi-disciplinary assessment framework with practice guidance that makes it clear which professionals are responsible for the different aspects of assessment and management (Department for Education and Skills 2005). It is important that nursing elements of assessment are included in joint assessment frameworks so that issues related to the child and family experience of the health problem are identified and addressed.

TOOLS AND METHODS FOR FOCUSED ASSESSMENT

Unlike generalised frameworks, most assessment tools measure just one aspect of the child's health status. Assessment tools can improve the quality and accuracy of assessments; their usefulness will depend on their purpose, content and practicality. As Harris (2002) points out, the development and evaluation of assessment tools is complex. Any measurement instrument needs to be reliable and valid: it should return consistent results when used repeatedly to measure the same thing and it should measure what it is supposed to be measuring. Signs and symptoms such as raised body temperature, weight loss and ulcerated lips are relatively easy to measure and quantify. However, most aspects of the child and family's responses to health problems and their management (i.e. nursing concerns) are subjective, variable and multifaceted, making them difficult to recognise and even more difficult to 'measure'. Some paediatric and child health assessment instruments have been well researched, notably pain assessment scales (see Chapter 14), quality of life measures (Schmidt et al 2002) and growth and development (Royal College of Paediatrics and Child Health (RCPCH) 2000).

Systematic reviews have been published summarising the best available evidence for use of different measurement tools (e.g. Duce 1996, Eiser & Morse 2001). There are many examples in the literature of tools developed at local level to address clinical problems where assessment is known to be poor, for example, self-harm risk assessment (Marfe 2003) and skin assessment (Rogers 2003). Although clinically relevant, much of this work is still exploratory and unvalidated so should be applied in other contexts with caution.

Taking instruments that have been developed for research and using them in the clinical setting is also problematic, not least because research measurements tend to

be at a level of detail that is impractical and unnecessary in the clinical situation. It is possible to adapt tools validated for use with adults, as children's cancer nurses found when they introduced oral assessment scoring (Gibson & Nelson 2000). As a general guide, any tool that is adapted from another setting or client group must first be validated for use with your client group in your clinical setting.

Evidence-based Practice

Transferability of assessment tools

Gharaibeh & Abu-Saad (2002) looked at the cultural validity, reliability and children's preferences of three pain assessment tools among Jordanian children. They found that the scales were valid and reliable but that there were gender differences in preference for particular scales, explained by the researchers as part of the socialisation process within the Arab culture.

Criteria to be considered when choosing an appropriate assessment tool or device are summarised in Box 7.2. Those that do not meet the criteria should be used with caution, as indeed should any measurement tool: the evidence from measurements should be combined with observations and child/parent reports if an accurate assessment is to be made.

Before moving on to planning in partnership, there are several summary points to be made about assessment. First, admitting a patient is not the same as assessing a patient, and assessment is not just a form-filling exercise (Harris 2002). Second, there is no point doing a 'once only' generalised assessment: ongoing review is essential to monitor changes and the success or otherwise of nursing interventions. Finally, without a nursing framework to guide the focus of assessment, care will focus solely on the medical-physical needs of patients (Mason & Webb 1997).

Parent Conversation

Georgina is the mother of 17-month-old William.

Relying on measurement tools

The nurse in A&E used an ear thermometer and said his temperature was normal. I knew he wasn't well. His temperature had been very high at home; he was pale, his head felt hot but his hands and feet were cold. She didn't seem to hear me saying that his temperature was on the way up again.

Box 7.2

Criteria for choosing an assessment tool or device

- Developed for the purpose: the aspect of the child/family's state, behaviour, feelings, etc. that you are wanting to measure/assess.
- Tested and validated in this age group.
- Tested and validated in this clinical context, e.g. in children with same or closely related condition.
- Culturally appropriate.
- Appropriate for and acceptable to the specific child/young person and family, e.g. the child's cognitive level.

PLANNING CARE

Whether or not a formal care plan is written down, some level of planning takes place before any action is taken. Based on assessment findings (and on what they are hoping to achieve if goals have been set), the planners identify available options and make decisions about what needs to be done. Chapter 14 goes into detail about how evidence can be used to inform such decisions, not withstanding the influence of resource availability, patient and family choice or other context of care factors. The plan of care is a communication tool and makes clear to all concerned who will be doing what, when and how. It can be as simple as a checklist or as complex as a step-by-step statement of a procedure with timed goals and expected outcomes: the detail and complexity of the plan depends on the communication need. A plan in the child's home that will be used to inform a bank nurse providing respite care will need to be very detailed; a plan for a child seen in A&E with a fever may consist of a standard form with four actions to be ticked by whoever completes them (and space to write additional, individualised actions if required).

Care plans may be based on standard plans or pathways of care. Standard care pathways that have been developed using evidence and expert opinion are one way of implementing evidence-based practice. Care pathways (also known as integrated care pathways) set out detailed steps for the management of patients with a particular problem or undergoing a specific procedure. Ideally, they are developed by the multidisciplinary team and reflect standardised care and treatment as well as expected progress (National Electronic Library for Health 2003). To date, care pathways have been mainly implemented in hospitals where care is more predictable but standardised approaches to care in home and school settings may be just as appropriate in some circumstances. As computer records and systems spread throughout the health service, 'e-pathways' will enable evidence-based standards to be better individualised and for individual differences to be analysed to provide improved evidence (de Luc & Todd 2003).

Evidence-based Practice

The integrated care pathway as an audit tool

Staff in a paediatric oncology unit aimed to improve care for children with fever and neutropenia by introducing an integrated care pathway. Guidelines for neutropenia were examined and a retrospective analysis of notes undertaken to study what was happening before a pathway was introduced. Following the introduction of the pathway, audit findings revealed variances in practice and identified areas for improvement such as referral to dieticians, types of investigations ordered and time taken to administer the first dose of antibiotics, particularly at night. Evidence from the audit was used to amend the pathway and improve practice (Selwood 2000).

SUPPORTING DECISION MAKING

Those planning care will be any combination of health professionals, the child/young person and family members. A key role for the nurse working in partnership to plan care is to support decision making by the child/young person and family. The first step is to assess their decision making preferences, not an easy task but one that acknowledges them as equals and establishes that their experiences and perspectives are valued and will be taken into account.

Activity

Think about your own most recent consultation with a doctor:

- How involved were you in the decision about what action to take?
- How involved would you have preferred to be?
- Having thought about this last question, choose your preference for that particular encounter from the bullet list below:
- I would prefer to make the decision myself with information only.
- I would prefer to make the decision myself considering the doctor's view.
- I would prefer the doctor to make the decision but considering my views.
- I would prefer the doctor to make the decision.

Having been involved in the decision about what to do, you are more likely to adhere to the course of action than if someone else has decided for you. As long ago as 1977, a doctor writing in the *Lancet* suggested that if doctors 'were willing to let go of the notion that they are responsible for controlling their patients', then patients who wanted to could 'make informed decisions on the basis of their own values' (Slack 1977). Not all parents and children will want to participate in decision making but the danger is in assuming that they do not wish to and ignoring their right to be heard.

Chapter 10 deals with the issue of consent and whether children are really given choices. This question of 'who decides?' applies to all kinds of care decisions, from whether to proceed with a heart–lung transplant to what to have for breakfast. Alderson & Montgomery's (1996) seminal text addresses the challenges of healthcare decision making with children and parents. At the level of day-to-day practice it is the values and attitudes of nurses and other team members that influence whether partnership in decision making is a reality. In addition, healthcare professionals need to have the confidence and be equipped with skills and tools with which to:

- assess preferences (which may change)
- assess competence (which will change)
- provide information without persuasion
- 'teach' decision-making strategies
- record and communicate decisions
- support child and family when they have made their decision (even if you don't agree with it).

EVALUATION AND OUTCOMES

Evaluation of the effectiveness of care for an individual child (and family) is an important part of nursing care. It needs to take place throughout the care process, with continual reassessment of their responses to interventions so that these can be changed or discontinued if they are ineffective or no longer needed. Initial assessment identifies health problems or issues that need addressing at the beginning of a care programme or episode; outcome evaluation identifies the extent of change in the health problem or achievement of goals related to the health issue.

A number of issues are related to the identification of what have been termed 'nursing sensitive patient outcomes' (those outcomes that are influenced by nursing care). The same difficulties that are faced when assessing less concrete aspects of the child's state, behaviour, feelings, etc. also apply in evaluation. The child and family's own reports of their experience and satisfaction with care are the most important evaluation evidence. However, nurses should supplement this evidence with outcome measures suited to the clinical setting and, where possible, derived from standards or benchmarks. Children and families will not know what should have been done in every case, for example they may accept as normal that the child did not eat during a short stay in hospital. This is an unacceptable outcome when measured against the national (English) benchmark: 'The amount of food patients actually eat is monitored, recorded and leads to action when cause for concern' (NHS Modernisation Agency 2003).

It may be difficult to differentiate the outcomes that are the result of nursing from those that result from interventions by others (including the child and family's own actions). However, it is important to consider 'nursing sensitive patient outcomes' for two main reasons: to monitor and improve effectiveness and to justify resources. Nurses do things for, with and to patients; they act on the results of assessments and decide what is an appropriate course of action. If they don't evaluate the results of their actions (i.e. measure outcomes) they cannot know whether they made the right decision nor learn what works to provide evidence for future practice.

Nursing staff salaries cost a great deal and the more senior the staff the greater the cost. Unless nurses can demonstrate that they contribute to improved outcomes for children and families, their value to health services may not be recognised and posts not funded. Recent evidence that patient safety and outcomes are significantly affected by skill mix of nursing staff show how measures of adverse outcome can be used to justify higher ratios of qualified to unqualified staff (Yang 2003). When new services such as community children's nursing teams or specialist practitioner posts are established, evidence collected about outcomes will be critical for ensuring the long-term viability of these services.

Evidence-based Practice

Nurse staffing and patient outcomes

Lower adverse outcome (measured as patient falls, pressure ulcers, respiratory and urinary tract infections, and patient/family complaints) were related to a higher proportion of experienced registered nurses in a study of over 1300 medical–surgical inpatients in Taiwan. Variations in the workload of nurses were found to be the most powerful predictor of nosocomial infections with hours of care provided to the patient the best predictor of adverse patient outcome (Yang 2003).

Much of the evidence we have about effectiveness and outcomes can be derived from intervention studies. For example, a study of the efficacy of tepid sponging to reduce fever in children (Sharber 1997) used simple outcome measures of fever reduction and signs of discomfort (crying, shivering, goosebumps). Petryshen et al (1998) used stability of physiological measures such as pulse and respirations as well as length of stay to evaluate the effectiveness of developmental care in very low birth weight babies.

Nursing interventions are directed at a number of child and family's responses to health problems and their management, from symptoms and behaviours through to their feelings and knowledge about their condition and how they cope with self-management at home and school. Table 7.3

Table 7.3 Outcomes Relevant to Nursing and Suggested Measures

	Measurement
Child/young person: outcome – change in . . .	
. . . symptom, e.g. pain, nausea	Symptom diary Score/scale
. . . condition/state, e.g. of wound, nutritional state	Description Measurement, e.g. weight
. . . activity, e.g. mobility, eating, school attendance	Self-report against targets Diary
Child and/or parents/carer: outcome – change in . . .	
. . . behaviour/skill	Self-report Observation
. . . understanding/attitude, e.g. improved acceptance of . . .	Self-report Satisfaction with information giving Observation
. . . feelings	Self-report Stress and coping measures Anxiety/depression scales
. . . quality of life/general well-being	Self-report Quality of life measures
Service and child/family/carer outcome	
Reduced length of stay/avoidance of admission	Individual comparisons, e.g. 'managed at home this time' Admission and length of stay statistics
Better provision of equipment/supplies at home	Self-report – satisfaction Monitoring of phone calls
Improved coordination of care	Number of staff visiting

lists the kinds of outcome that may be the result of effective nursing interventions with examples of measures that might be useful in outcome evaluation and in audits of quality.

Recording and Auditing Practice

INFORMATION MANAGEMENT

As this chapter has shown, the clinical process involves a number of steps and all of these steps generate information about the child's and family's needs and preferences, care decisions that are made, things that are planned and done and results or outcomes of what was done. Much of this information needs to be communicated and recorded and some of it will need to be used for other purposes such as audit and service planning.

Recording, storing, communicating and using information is known as information management. The goal of information management is to ensure relevant information is in the hands of those who need it, at the time they need it, and in a format that they can understand and use. Patients, parents, staff and managers need information so they can make sense of the situation and make decisions about what to do. The child's healthcare record is the main tool for managing this information. Every professional who comes in contact with the patient needs to be able to make timely decisions about what care is needed and how best to deliver that care. If it is to be an effective information tool, the record should support this process of clinical decision making. The *Essence of Care* benchmark for record keeping, now part of the clinical governance framework for the NHS in England, states that 'all records must be legible, accurate, signed with designation stated, dated, timed, contemporaneous, be able to provide a chronology of events and use only agreed abbreviations' (NHS Modernisation Agency 2003). These 'patient-focused benchmarks' set standards for progress towards single, life-long, patient held records that are secure and support high-quality, evidence-based care.

The purposes of the record dictate its format as well as its content. A key purpose of records is communication between disciplines, which suggests that moves towards a single record, used by all professionals and possibly held by the child or parent, will help to achieve 'fitness for purpose'. Another function is to serve as a secondary source of data: for audit, research and as evidence for legal or other enquiries.

Evidence-based Practice

Parent-held records

In the UK, parent-held child health records have been used for many years. In a study of parents' and professionals' views, Charles (1994) found that almost all respondents in both groups liked the record and most professionals believed it improved communication with parents. Parents reported that the record helped them remember important advice and enabled them to play a more active role in their child's health care. The study also showed that over two-thirds of parents had made entries in the parent-held record and the records were more complete than traditional clinic cards.

CONTENT OF THE RECORD

NMC guidance on record keeping is at a very general level, stating only that the record should 'identify problems that have arisen and action taken to rectify them' and 'provide clear evidence of the care planned, the decisions made, the care delivered and the information shared' (NMC 2002). It is left up to each professional to decide what is appropriate to record and the level of detail that is necessary. In some areas, groups of professionals have reached a consensus on what should be in the record and developed standard formats that at least provide a guide for those using them. One example is the parent-held child health record, which has been used in community settings across the UK for many years. As the NHS moves towards computerised records, the structure and to some extent the content of records will become standardised. Nurses need to be able to identify what it is important to record about nursing care and how that should be structured in electronic records.

WWW

The development of electronic records is an area of rapid change. For information about this topic and on the standards and specifications for nursing content of electronic patient records go to the websites of the health service information departments such as:

- http://www.connectingforhealth.nhs.uk
- http://www.isdscotland.org

A good way to decide whether the content of your records is adequate is to ask the question 'can those coming after me find out from the record what they need to know to continue the care of this child?' This tests the fitness of the record for the purpose of communication to support continuity of care. A second question that tests the quality of the record for all other purposes is 'can those who need to know find out from the record what we found on assessment, what we did and the results of our actions?' Working in partnership implies that the content of the record will reflect not just the nurse's view but the assessments, plans actions and evaluations of the child/young person, parents and other members of the team.

Data to support audit, management and research can be obtained directly from these records or collected using specific data collection tools. One of the benefits of computerising patient records is that these will provide structured data that can be more easily aggregated and analysed. There will still be a need for other forms of data collection, for example the patient record won't tell you how many staff were available on a particular day or which nurses have specialist qualifications, important information when evaluating the quality of your service.

INFORMATION GOVERNANCE

An important part of information management is information governance, a quality framework that brings together legal requirements and professional guidance around record keeping, confidentiality, access to records, data quality, etc. The key principles of information governance are that information is:

H = held securely and confidentially

O = obtained fairly and efficiently

R = recorded accurately and reliably

U = used effectively and ethically

S = shared appropriately and lawfully.

Good practice requires the nurse to ensure that children, young people and parents/carers are informed of what is recorded about them and who has access to that information so that they can choose whether to restrict access to the information in the record or withhold information they do not wish to be shared. This is even more important as electronic records are introduced in all health care settings making access easier.

Summary

New skills in information and knowledge management are being developed by nurses concerned to ensure that children and families have control over information and knowledge, that they can make sense of what is happening and participate knowledgeably in decisions. The nurse's role is shifting from one of information provider to one of supporting children, young people and families to access, understand and use information themselves, increasing their independence and their capacity for self care. With these skills and the increasing expectations and skills of the children and young people themselves, true partnerships may become the norm, rather than an ideal that is perhaps seldom achieved.

References

Alderson P, Montgomery J 1996 Health care choices: making decisions with children. Institute of Public Policy Research, London

Barnes K (ed.) 2003 Paediatrics: a guide for nurse practitioners. Butterworth-Heinemann, Edinburgh

Carpenito-Moyet LJ 2004 Nursing diagnosis: application to clinical practice, 10th edn. Lippincott Williams and Wilkins, Philadelphia

Charles R 1994 An evaluation of parent held child health records. Health Visitor 67(8):270–272

Coyne IT 1995 Partnership in care: parents' views of participation in their hospitalised child's care. Journal of Clinical Nursing 4(2):71–79

de Luc K, Todd J 2003 E-pathways: computers and the patient's journey through care. Radcliffe Medical, Oxford

Department for Education and Skills 2005 Common assessment framework. Online. Available at: http://www.everychildmatters gov.uk [accessed 26 May 2005]

Duce SJ 1996 A systematic review of the literature to determine optimal methods of temperature measurement in neonates, infants and children. NHS Centre for Reviews and Dissemination 1:124

Eiser C, Morse R 2001 Quality-of-life measures in chronic diseases of childhood. Health Technology Assessment 5:4

Gharaibeh M, Abu-Saad H 2002 Cultural validation of pediatric pain assessment tools: Jordanian perspective. Journal of Transcultural Nursing 13(1):12–18

Gibson F, Nelson W 2000 Mouth care for children with cancer. Paediatric Nursing 12(1):18–22

Gordon M 2002 Manual of nursing diagnosis, 10th edn. Mosby, St Louis

Harris R 2002 Physical assessment of patients: the Byron physical assessment framework. Whurr, London

Higgs J 2000 Clinical reasoning in the health professions, 2nd edn. Butterworth-Heinemann, Oxford

Hockenberry M, Wilson D, Winkenstein M et al 2003 Wong's nursing care of infants and children. Mosby, St Louis

Kirk S 2001 Negotiating lay and professional roles in the care of children with complex health care needs. Journal of Advanced Nursing 34(5):593–602

Marfe E 2003 Assessing risk following deliberate self harm. Paediatric Nursing 15(8):32–34

Marshall M, Fleming E, Gillibrand W et al 2002 Adaptation and negotiation as an approach to care in paediatric diabetes specialist nursing practice: a critical review. Journal of Clinical Nursing 11(4):421–429

Mason G, Webb C 1997 Researching children's nurses' clinical judgements about assessment data. Clinical Effectiveness in Nursing 1:47–55

National Electronic Library for Health 2003 Care pathways. Online. Available at: http://www.nelh.nhs.uk/management/mantop/0302Care Pathways.htm [accessed 6 December 2003]

NHS Modernisation Agency 2003 Essence of Care benchmarks: support for clinical governance. Online. Available at: http://www.cgsupport. nhs. uk/PDFs/articles/Essence_of_Care_2003.pdf [accessed 17 March 2004]

North American Nursing Diagnosis Association (NANDA) 2003 Nursing diagnosis: definitions and classification. NANDA, Philadelphia

Nursing and Midwifery Council (NMC) 2002 Guidelines for records and record keeping. NMC, London

Orem D 2001 Nursing: concepts of practice. Mosby, St Louis

Petryshen P, Stevens B, Hawkins J et al 1998 Comparing nursing costs for preterm infants receiving conventional vs developmental care. Neonatal Intensive Care 11(2):18–24

Redshaw M, Harvey M 2002 Working together: neonatal nurse practitioners in practice. Acta Paediatrica 91(2):178–183

Rogers D 2003 Skin assessment: improving communication and recording. Paediatric Nursing 15(10):20–23

Roper N, Tierney A 2000 The Roper, Logan, Tierney model of nursing based on activities of living. Churchill Livingstone, Edinburgh

Royal College of Nursing (RCN) 2003 Defining nursing. RCN, London

Royal College of Paediatrics and Child Health (RCPCH) 2000 Growth reference charts for use in the United Kingdom. RCPCH, London

Schmidt LJ, Garratt AM, Fitzpatrick R 2002 Child/parent-assessed population health outcome measures: a structured review. Child: Care, Health and Development 28(3):227–237

Selwood K 2000 Integrated care pathways: an audit tool in paediatric oncology. British Journal of Nursing 9(1):34–38

Sharber J 1997 The efficacy of tepid sponge bathing to reduce fever in young children. American Journal of Emergency Medicine 15(2):188–192

Slack W 1977 The patient's right to decide. The Lancet 296:240

Waters E, Stewart-Brown S, Fitzpatrick R 2003 Agreement between adolescent self-report and parent reports of health and well-being: results of an epidemiological study. Child: Care, Health and Development 29(6):501–509

Yang KP 2003 Relationships between nurse staffing and patient outcomes. Journal of Nursing Research 11(3):149–158

Chapter Eight

8

Public Health, Primary Health Care and the Development of Community Children's Nursing

Mark Whiting

ABSTRACT

This chapter will examine the historical development, current arrangements for and possible future provision of primary healthcare nursing services for children in the UK.

Learning Outcomes

- To develop an awareness of the origins and history of approaches to public health within the United Kingdom

- To develop an knowledge of and insight into the historical development of nursing services for children in non hospital settings in the United Kingdom

- To develop insight into the range of primary health care services provision for children in the United Kingdom

- To develop knowledge in relation specifically to the provision of community children's nursing in the United Kingdom

Introduction

Before starting the chapter proper, it is important to provide a brief explanation of the term 'primary health care' as it has been interpreted here. Primary health care can be defined as:

The provision of health services to individuals and populations within non-hospital settings.

However, this definition is contestable on a number of points. First, although it could be argued that health/illness protection, health promotion and public healthcare are exclusively components of primary health care, the counterargument might be offered that all three of these activities also take place on a very regular basis within hospital settings.

The second area of contention relates to the interface points between hospital and non-hospital services provision, for instance Accident and Emergency departments, outpatient clinics, short-stay assessment wards, minor injury units, 'walk-in' centres, ambulatory care facilities, hospital-at-home schemes, each of which might arguably be considered to be part of either primary care or secondary care.

This chapter will not specifically set out to provide a clear resolution to these areas of debate, however, when appropriate, discussion within the chapter will incorporate an exploration of both wider public health/health promotion perspectives and will also consider issues pertaining to the interfaces between in hospital and out-of-hospital provision.

Historical Considerations

The emergence of both primary health care and coordinated approaches to public health in the UK is generally traced to the 19th century, that is, to the second half of the Industrial Revolution. In 1800, around 80% of the British population lived in rural communities, in villages, hamlets and the countryside; within 100 years, almost three-quarters of the population lived in towns and cities (Briggs 1983, Gregg 1976). This had major implications for family life, including significant changes to the care and welfare of children as the nature of rural/village/community existence was transformed. Blair et al (2003) graphically illustrates the consequences of this for the children of the working classes:

Mothers needed to work up to and straight after childbirth to bring in sufficient income, but the Industrial Revolution had separated the world of work from the world of home, so children were often abandoned to the care of someone else from an early age (Blair et al 2003 p 88)

This 'someone' was often a young aunt or even an older sibling and, as Lomax (1996 p 2) acknowledges, at that time '. . . the concept of state or even charitable intervention in family to enhance the welfare of children was frowned upon'. It might be argued that such a view prevails even to the present day! However, Blair and colleagues (2003) suggest that as the 19th century progressed a number of factors came together to enable a more coordinated public health response. These included:

- The emergence of philanthropic approaches towards the poor and needy.
- The need for 'self-preservation' for the middle/upper classes as it became widely recognised that diseases such as cholera and smallpox, often endemic in the growing cities, were no respecter of social class.
- Utilitarian approaches to social policy/welfare reform.
- The need for a healthy, well-fed productive workforce.

The mass migration of the population from the countryside into the larger towns and cities led to major problems of overcrowding, and in particular to problems of waste disposal and sanitation. Overcrowded and poor conditions provided the ideal environment for the spread of infectious disease and, during the early part of the 19th century, in response to concerns about potential or actual epidemics, a number of local Boards of Health were established by the Privy Council. Fears of a cholera epidemic lead to the creation of a consultative Board of Health in June 1831 and, later that year, to the establishment of the Central Board of Health under the aegis of the Privy Council. Within the year, nearly 1200 local Boards of Health were established by order of the Council but, just as quickly, as the threat of the cholera epidemic receded, the central and local Boards were dissolved in 1832. However, conditions of public health and, in particular, sanitation remained a concern of the Poor Law Commissioners. Their work, and perhaps most significantly, Edwin Chadwick's 1842 report *A survey into the sanitary condition of the labouring classes in Great Britain* (with its detailed and graphic accounts of how the insanitary conditions in which the poor were forced to live was a major factor in the spread of disease) led directly to the establishment of The Royal Commission on the Health of Towns.

The Royal Commission set to work immediately, following-up Chadwick's report and undertaking an investigation of sanitary conditions in 50 English towns. The findings of the Royal Commission investigation led to directly to the publication of the first Public Health Act in 1848.

 WWW

Read a more detailed account of the history leading up to the Public Health Act in the National Archives at:

- http://catalogue.pro.gov.uk/leaflets/ri2180.htm

Perhaps the most widely recognised event from this period of public health history relates to Dr John Snow who, in 1854, plotted the pattern of occurrence of deaths from cholera in the Golden Square area of Soho, London. As a direct result of Snow's work, the spread of disease was linked directly to water supplied from the water pump in Broad Street. Snow himself removed this pump and, within 7 days, the cholera outbreak was officially declared as over. Snow's action demonstrated that the spread of this particular disease could be prevented by replacing a contaminated water supply with an alternative source of clean water.

 WWW

Further details of Snow's work can be found on the website of the Royal Institute for Public Health at:

- http://www.riphh.org.uk

Thus the public health movement of the 19th century involved a combination of health services provision (at both local and governmental levels), social reform (at both local and governmental levels) and investigation into the causes, effects and distribution of disease (epidemiology).

A Hospital for Children

In 1739, over 100 years before the Public Health Act of 1848, Thomas Coram had established the Foundling Hospital in an attempt to provide care for the growing number of babies (often illegitimate children of the poor/working classes) abandoned on London's streets. Coram's initial attempts to secure funding from the government and the Anglican Church were rejected, but with perseverance and the help of charitable funding, he established a hospital that rapidly became overwhelmed with admissions (Franklin 1964, Kosky & Lunnon 1991, Lomax 1996). Government financial support was eventually forthcoming, although Lomax (1996 p 4) suggests that State intervention was, in part, responsible for the discrediting of the hospital, leading to accusations that by agreeing to accept all children arriving at its doors, it encouraged 'irresponsibility and immorality'.

www

For a more detailed account of the work of Thomas Coram go to:
- http://www.coram.org.uk/heritage.htm

The Foundling Hospital was primarily concerned with providing protection and education for children. Its support of the medical or health care needs of children was somewhat of a secondary consideration. By contrast, the work of Dr John Bunnell Davis, who established a children's dispensary in London in 1816, set out to both treat children (on what would now be described as an outpatient basis) and also 'serve to train parents in the better care of their offspring' (Lomax 1996 p 5). When Davis died in 1824, the work of the dispensary went through a period of decline until the arrival, in 1839, of Dr Charles West, who worked at what was now referred to as the Royal Universal Dispensary for 10 years while simultaneously striving to convert the dispensary into an inpatient hospital. Although this particular aspiration floundered, Charles West is often credited with being almost single-handedly responsible for the establishment of the first Hospital for Sick Children in Great Ormond Street, London, in 1852. West's pioneering endeavour was then followed by a period of 50 years of intense activity in building and establishing children's hospitals throughout the UK. By 1900, there were over 30 children's hospitals and upwards of 50 children's convalescent homes. In addition, many general hospitals had formally dedicated one or more wards exclusively for the care of children (Lomax 1996).

This dramatic growth in the provision of hospital care for children occurred largely as a result of charitable intervention and voluntary funding. Many of the hospitals or wards therein bore the names of the benefactors whose contributions had made the building and staffing of the institutions possible. In addition, 'private' payments for care afforded to children within the hospitals contributed significantly to the hospitals' income and thus to the provision of care to those who could not afford to pay, but who might be considered as 'interesting cases'.

Lomax (1996) suggests that, in addition to providing inpatient and outpatient services, many of the children's hospitals also established private home-nursing services, particularly when they first opened. However, such initiatives were often short-lived, partly because of the expense but also because of resistance from the hospital medical staff and hospital administrators. Charles West, however, considered this to be an essential element of the service provided by Great Ormond Street and, in the mid-1870s, made formal proposals to develop a private domiciliary nursing service to the hospital's management committee:

> *Some consideration took place on the reference in Dr West's paper to the training of nurses proposed by the Lady Superintendent in visiting hospital out-patients at their own homes, under the regulations suggested by Dr West and coincided in by the Lady Superintendent. The majority of the Medical Officers were in favour of the plan being made trial of for 6 months, but the lay members of the committee were unanimously opposed to the extension of the work of the hospital beyond the walls (The Hospital for Sick Children 1874)*

www

For a more detailed history of the Hospital for Children, Great Ormond Street see:
- http://www.ich.ucl.ac.uk/150/whole_story.html

It was another 14 years before the persistence and persuasion of Dr West and Dame Catherine Wood, the Lady Superintendent of the hospital, led to the establishment of the Great Ormond Street private domiciliary nursing service in 1888 (Whiting 2000). Elsewhere in the country, those children's hospitals that continued to provide a domiciliary outreach service did so on a private, fee-paying basis only.

Nursing Children in the Community

The provision of non-fee-paying nursing support of children in the community did, however, begin to develop towards the end of the 19th century from two distinct sources: district nursing and in the forerunner of current health visiting service, the Sanitary Reform Associations. In addition, school-nursing services for children began to emerge in the final decade of the century.

DISTRICT NURSING

It is generally accepted that the roots of our present district nursing service lie in the pioneering work of William Rathbone, in Liverpool, who in 1859 engaged the services of a hospital-trained nurse to help care for his dying wife at home. Rathbone was very aware of the appalling living conditions of the overcrowded city of Liverpool and, following his wife's death, he asked the nurse to continue in his employment and provide care to the sick poor people, including children, in the city (Rathbone 1890). By 1874, a National Association for 'Providing Trained Nurses for the Sick and Poor in London and Elsewhere' had been founded (Kratz 1982). In 1887, Queen Victoria's Jubilee Institute for Nurses was established as the first formally organised district nursing scheme. In 1928, this became the Queen's

 WWW

Look at the photographic archive of the Queen's Nursing Institute on the Welcome Trust website:
- http://medphoto.wellcome.ac.uk/

Institute for District Nurses and the institute assumed responsibility for the training of district nurses (Baly 1987). During the next 50 years, district nursing services expanded steadily, being organised on a local basis by either voluntary agencies or local authorities (Stocks 1960). The National Health Service Act of 1946 first placed formal responsibility upon local health authorities:

> . . . for securing the attendance of nurses on persons who require nursing in their own homes (NHS Act 1946 part III section 25)

The predominant focus of the work of district nurses was the care of the adult patient. In general, children who required symptom relief/management at home were cared for by their parents with support from the general practitioner, and only occasional input from the district nurse, whereas those who were acutely unwell and whose condition merited closer medical attention were admitted to hospital. In addition, many children with chronic or long-standing illness spent long periods as hospital inpatients, often many miles away from their families in long-stay or rehabilitation facilities.

Successive studies of district nursing practice over the last 40 years have shown that children form only a small part of their caseload (Hockey 1966, McIntosh 1975, OPCS 1982). Jackson (1978), describing the development of a community nursing service aimed specifically at children in Gateshead, commented that although children had formed a significant part of the early district nursing caseload, the increasing sophistication of paediatric practice meant that more children were admitted to hospital and thus the numbers of children cared for by district nurses diminished steadily. The Court Committee (DHSS 1976 p 81) observed that although the district nurse syllabus included some detail on the special needs of children and their families, the time allocated was 'inevitably minimal'.

HEALTH VISITING

As with district nursing, the history of health visiting can be traced to the middle of second half of the 19th century.

The same circumstances that had prompted William Rathbone's philanthropic activities in Liverpool led to the establishment of the Manchester and Salford Sanitary Reform Association in 1852 (Hale et al 1968, While 1985). This was one of a number of initially small-scale efforts that developed in several of the larger cities. Although the Association was founded in 1852, it was not until 1862 that a fulltime visitor was first appointed. The role of the visitors was principally one of teaching and counselling, rather than of practical nursing. At this time, no previous nursing experience was deemed necessary for the visitors, whose title changed to 'health visitors' around the turn of the century. The first health visitor training school was established, with considerable guidance from Florence Nightingale, in Buckinghamshire in the 1890s. A requirement for visitors to have previously undergone nurse training was introduced in Manchester at around the time the 'health visitor' title was first introduced.

The Statutory Rules and Orders of the Local Government Act (1929) made provision for a qualification and standard training for health visitors. The National Health Service Act of 1946 required that all health visitors must be qualified as such. As with district nursing, the National Health Service Act placed responsibility on the Local Health Authorities to provide a health visiting service. The Act stated:

> It shall be the duty of every local health authority to make provision in their area for the visiting of persons in their homes by visitors to be called 'health visitors' for the purpose of giving advice as to the care of young children, persons suffering from illness and expectant or nursing mothers, and as to the measures necessary for the spread of infection (NHS Act 1946 part III section 24 [1])

The work of the health visitor is, however, principally located in the areas of health surveillance and health education, and not in the care of children with discrete nursing needs:

> The professional practice of health visiting consists of planned activities aimed at the promotion of health and the prevention of ill-health (Council for the Education and Training of Health Visitors (CETHV) 1977)

The Court Committee (DHSS 1976) discussed the role of the various members of the primary health care team in caring for the sick child in the community and concluded that although mothers might seek advice on the care of a sick child from the health visitor, only rarely did health visitors undertake any practical nursing care with children. The Committee had recommended the appointment of specialist Child Health Visitors (section 17.25) with joint responsibility for the promotion of health and the management of paediatric nursing problems in the community. However, considerable doubt was expressed at the time (Sartain 1977) – and subsequently (While 1986) – over the wisdom of attempting to combine preventive and curative roles in this fashion, the principal fear being that curative work would take precedence. Health visitors themselves have commented that despite the fact that their work is concentrated in the care of the under fives, there is a reluctance to take on a more acute, disease-centred role (Jones 1988, Ledger 1988).

SCHOOL NURSING

The contribution of the school nurse to the care of the sick child merits brief consideration at this point. Strehlow (1987) has reviewed the history of the school nursing services in some detail. Although a number of nurses were appointed during the latter years of the 19th century, services were very limited indeed. The first formally organised school nursing services were established in response to the report of the Interdepartmental Committee on Physical Deterioration, published in 1904, which found that 60% of potential army recruits were unfit for military service as a result of a catalogue of health problems, in particular issues concerning undiagnosed/treated chronic illness and the poor nutritional and overall health status of the young men coming forward to enlist for military service.

School nursing services have historically focused predominantly on aspects of child health, including screening and surveillance, and health promotion. The one area of practice that is exceptional to this relates to the field of 'special education', i.e. those settings that have focused their attention on children with particular health problems, such as epilepsy, physical and/or learning disabilities, schools for 'delicate' children and those for children with visual and auditory impairments. The Warnock review of 1978 (Department of Education and Science (DES) 1978) provides a useful review of what is referred to as 'special education for the handicapped'.

Perhaps the two most significant developments in the provision of education for children with health-related problems are, first, the Education Act of 1944, which resulted in the alignment of widely disparate education provision for such children with the new education arrangements for all children within the UK, and second (which followed on from the Warnock Report itself) the integration of children with 'special educational needs' within the mainstream of education provision.

COMMUNITY CHILDREN'S NURSING

District nursing, health visiting and school nursing each provide a piece of the complex historical jigsaw of community nursing provision for children although, as can be seen from the discussion above, none of the these services are specifically configured to provide care for children with nursing needs outside of hospital settings. A children's nurse writing in the *British Medical Journal* in the mid-1980s observed:

> *There is an increasing muddle over who does what in the community . . . but because paediatric community nursing is not apparently regarded as a speciality in its own right, some of the work is being done by district nurses, some by health visitors and some by midwives. This cannot be sensible and perhaps accounts for the fact that often the wrong children are kept at home and the wrong ones admitted to hospital (Davies 1985 p 547)*

This is perhaps not entirely surprising. Throughout the early to middle part of the 20th century, the predominant view of paediatric clinical staff (doctors, nurses and therapists) was that the most appropriate (the best) place to care for the sick child was in hospital. It is interesting to note, that with the introduction of the National Health Service in 1948, the Great Ormond Street Private Community Nursing Service was required by law to disestablish and the service closed in 1949.

At around this time, the pioneering work of John Bowlby (1951), a psychiatrist, and James Robertson (1956), a psychoanalyst and social worker, brought the whole question of hospital care for children into sharp relief. Their work led directly to the realisation that hospitalisation, or other forms of disruption to family/home life, particularly for young children (under the age of five), for long periods or for repeated episodes of care, had the potential to adversely influence the psychological well-being of the child.

As the 1950s drew to a close, the recommendations of the Ministry of Health *Report on the welfare of children in hospital* (Ministry of Health 1959: the 'Platt report') heralded a fundamental shift in attitudes to the care of the sick child with its two key recommendations:

1. *Greater attention needs to be paid to the emotional and mental needs of the child in hospital, against the background of changes in attitudes towards children, in the hospital's place in the community, and in medical and surgical practice. The authority and responsibility of parents, the individuality of the child, and the importance of mitigating the effects of the break with home should all be more fully recognised (paragraphs 6–14).*
2. *Children should not be admitted to hospital if it can possibly be avoided (paragraph 17).*

In recommending this new approach to caring for children, the Platt Committee identified the need for the care of children outside of hospital to be supported by the development of home nursing schemes for children:

> 3. *Special nursing facilities for looking after sick children at home should be extended (paragraphs 18–19).*

The report's authors made specific reference to recently established services in Paddington, Birmingham and Rotherham. However, although the committee's recommendations undoubtedly had an immediate and dramatic effect on the services provided for children and their families within the hospital setting, the impact on the community was almost undetectable. Indeed, it was not for another 10 years after the publication of the report that a single additional paediatric community nursing service was established and, during this period (as noted above), the contribution of district nurses and health visitors to the nursing care of children was very limited indeed.

Those services that had been identified by the Platt Committee were largely concerned with the care of children experiencing acute, episodic illness (Gillett 1954 (Rotherham), Lightwood 1956 (Paddington), Smellie 1956 (Birmingham)). However, in 1969, two new approaches emerged. In Southampton, a paediatric community nursing service was established to support the work of a newly established Day Surgery Unit, with the nurses providing community follow up for children undergoing a range of surgical procedures (Atwell et al 1973). By contrast, the service established in Edinburgh in the same year was based in the Children's Outpatient department and concentrated on the outpatient nursing care of children with 'long-term disability' (including diabetes mellitus and coeliac disease) and on those with congenital abnormalities (including cleft lip) (Hunter 1974). In Edinburgh, further developments soon followed both for children who required follow-up of short-term problems and also for those with cystic fibrosis (Hunter 1977).

Some 7 years after the initiatives in Southampton and Edinburgh, the Court report (DHSS 1976), the specific focus of which was community child health services, offered a further endorsement of the Platt report recommendations relating to the development of paediatric community nursing. Once again, these recommendations appeared in large part to fall on deaf ears. Indeed, by 1984 there were still only a smattering of services across the UK and it was not until the late 1980s that there was a significant expansion in what was beginning to be referred to across the UK as 'community children's nursing'.

Activity

Read a more detailed account of the historical emergence of community children's nursing in Whiting (2000).

Further consideration to the current provision of community children's nursing will be provided later in the chapter, but it is important to set that provision within the broader, overall context of child health services and public health care provision and it is to those areas that attention will now be directed.

Primary Health Care and Primary Health Care Teams

A succession of reorganisations of the NHS during the 1970s resulted in the emergence in the early 1980s of the Primary Health Care Team (PHCT) as the dominant model/focus of community nursing activity. A typical PHCT was based in a health centre, and its work was concentrated on the caseload of one or more general medical practitioners (GPs). The team usually included a GP, district nurse, health visitor and practice nurse, although these were often joined by a community midwife and occasionally by other members of the nursing workforce and a range of allied health professionals.

In 1986, a major review of community nursing was undertaken on behalf of the Department of Health and Social Security by Julia Cumberledge. This review endorsed the by now well-established PHCT model, although neither the specific nursing needs of children nor the emerging practice discipline of community children's nursing featured in any significant part in the review's recommendations.

It was perhaps hardly surprising, therefore, that when the United Kingdom Central Council for Nursing, Midwifery and Health Visiting (UKCC), in part in response to the Cumberledge recommendations, brought forward proposals for the reform of community nursing education in the early 1990s the nursing needs of children barely merited a mention (UKCC 1991). Two years later, as the proposals for the reform of community nursing education were incorporated into the Council's rather more extensive Post-registration Education Project (UKCC 1993), the needs of children were recognised but were included in a rather intriguing suggestion to develop a new education programme concerned with the '. . . general nursing care of children which relates to the practice of school nursing and of paediatric nursing' (UKCC 1993 annexe 3 p 1). In the consultation process that followed, school nurses and community children's nurses made strenuous representation to the UKCC. Eventually common sense prevailed and final proposals for the new discipline of specialist community health nursing included separate education pathways leading to qualification as either a school nurse or a community children's nurse as well as for six other community nursing disciplines (UKCC 1994) (Box 8.1).

The programmes of education in specialist community health nursing reflected a growing recognition in the early

Box 8.1

Specialist community health nursing pathways (UKCC 1994)

- General practice nursing
- Community mental health nursing
- Community mental handicap nursing
- Community children's nursing
- Public health nursing – health visiting
- Occupational health nursing
- Nursing in the home – district nursing
- School nursing

1990s of the potential role of all community nurses within the field of public health. The 1994 UKCC report demanded both a clear focus on public health and health promotion within the programmes and required that such themes played a key role within the minimum one-third of the programme that would be based on shared learning across the community nursing disciplines.

This strong emphasis on public health and health promotion had its roots in the World Health Organization's 1978 'Alma Ata' declaration of its goal of 'health for all by the year 2000' and the European review of the global targets, which was published by WHO in 1985.

WWW

Read the 'Alma Ata' document at:
- http://www.who.int/hpr/NPH/docs/declaration_ almaata.pdf

By the time the UKCC recommendations were published, the social policy context in the UK had been set out by the Department of Health (DoH), initially in the publication *Promoting better health* (DoH 1988), which set out the key philosophical underpinning of the public health agenda, and then in the rather more strategic *The health of the nation* (DoH 1992), which set the broad policy context for the promotion of health by identifying five key areas of work (Box 8.2) and setting key targets for health improvement within each area.

In more recent years, this policy has been updated and developed (DoH 1998a, 1999a) with a renewed emphasis upon the need to tackle issues of inequality (DoH 1998b)

Box 8.2

Target areas: *The health of the nation* (DoH 1992)

- Accidents
- Coronary heart disease and strokes
- Mental illness
- Sexual health
- Cancer

and, with the Sure Start programme, to make sure that children have a good start in life (DoH 1999b). Nurses have remained at the forefront of this area of health policy, with aspects of children's health being given a high priority in much of the current debate about public health (Her Majesty's Treasury/DoH 2004). Specific concerns relating to obesity, smoking and sexual health in childhood have taken centre stage in much of the current debate.

A Public Health Role for the Community Children's Nurse?

The Cumberledge report (DHSS 1986) recommended that all nurses working in specialist roles outside the hospital setting should be based in the community. However, the justification for such an approach was not made at all clear and was certainly out of step with developments in the provision of community children's nursing (CCN) services. At this time (as before and since), community children's nursing was made up of a heterogeneous mix of services, some based in health centres or community clinics, and some based in hospital children's wards or outpatient departments. A number of teams provided care to children based on traditional medical specialties such as oncology or respiratory care, others took on a more generic role. Much of the work of community children's nurses cut across organisational boundaries between hospital- and community-based services. Indeed, although the recommendation of the Cumberledge report to establish 'neighbourhood nursing teams' based on populations of approximately 25,000 failed to materialise, the late 1980s

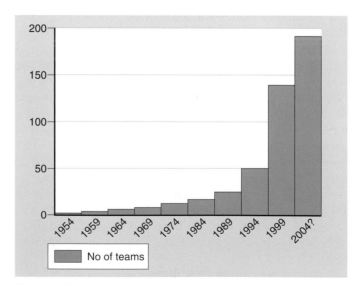

Fig. 8.1 • Growth in the provision of community children's nursing services in the UK (1954–2004).

and early 1990s saw a dramatic expansion in the provision of community children's nursing (Fig. 8.1), with most teams serving a typical District Health Authority based population of around 250,000 (within which there were between 45,000 and 60,000 children) and with many teams working very closely with the one or two children's wards in the local District General Hospital. As more teams were introduced, a range of differing models of service provision began to emerge, including ambulatory care, hospital-at-home care and specialist services based around tertiary centres, each added a new dimension to the complex array of community children's nursing services which featured by the turn of the century.

In general, local teams have developed in response to local demands, and no one model of service provision has yet become clearly established as the preferred model of service delivery. The work of the community children's nursing teams varies, often depending on the needs and/or demands of their local populations. However, there remain very significant variations in the *modus operandi* of the teams within the UK, as different teams respond to the demands of children/families with a range of nursing need (Box 8.3).

Box 8.3

Range of nursing need for which community children's nursing services might be provided

- Children who are acutely unwell
- Children who have been involved in accidents
- Children who have undergone surgery
- Children with chronic illness
- Children with physical disabilities
- Children with life-threatening/life-limiting illness
- Children who require palliative care
- Children who are learning disabled
- Children with emotional or behavioural disturbance
- Children with mental ill health

The work of the community children's nurse is very much focused on the needs of individual children and their families. Whereas health visiting and school nursing are population-based services and arguably 'every child has either a named health visitor or a named school nurse', community children's nursing services operate on a referred-child model, so whereas a typical community children's nursing team provides a service to a child population of around 50,000, at any one time only a fraction of that population constitutes part of the community children's nursing caseload.

The scenarios below provide illustrative examples of how the community children's nurse might engage in opportunistic promotion of health at an individual level.

Scenarios

David

David, aged 13, has diabetes. Over the course of the last year his weight has increased, moving him from the 75th to the 90th centile. During a home visit, the community children's nurse takes the opportunity to talk to David and his mother about both exercise and diet, and to set these in the context of the possibility of the whole family adopting a more healthy life style.

Assad

Assad is 4 years old and has been referred to the community children's nursing team for removal of sutures from his face following a fall. During the visit, the community children's nurse observes that Assad's 1-year-old brother is beginning to pull himself to a standing position and walk around furniture. There are no stair gates, fire guards or electrical plug socket covers in the house and the nurse is concerned about the generally chaotic nature of the home. She provides Assad's mother with an information leaflet about home safety and successfully engages her in a long conversation about avoiding childhood accidents. She is able to refer the family to the local health/social services accident prevention team, who provides a variety of home safety equipment on a loan/low-cost basis. The nurse makes some summary notes in Assad's Personal Child Health Record and notifies the family health visitor of the outcome of her visit.

Jenny

During a visit to Jenny, a 14-year-old with cystic fibrosis, Jenny's mother expresses concern to the community children's nurse that Jenny is beginning to engage in a sexual relationship with her boyfriend. The nurse knows the family well and has acted as 'key worker' to Jenny for several years. Together, the nurse and mother are able to discuss the situation with Jenny. They provide some initial advice and Jenny agrees to visit the family planning clinic with her mother.

Jack

Jack, aged 3, is about to return to his day nursery following an initial diagnostic admission and treatment for acute lymphoblastic leukaemia. His mother asks the community children's nurse whether she might be able to prepare the staff and children at the nursery for Jack's return. The nurse and mother speak together to all of the staff at the nursery about aspects of infection control and avoidance of possible risk.

As noted above, health visitors and school nurses have a much more wide-reaching role in promoting health within the child population as a whole. Recent public health policy statements (DoH 2004, Her Majesty's Treasury/DoH 2004, Skills for Health 2004) have provided a clear sense of direction for all health professionals working with children, with major policy initiatives focused on sexual health, reduction in teenage pregnancy rates, obesity, smoking, drugs and alcohol. The extent to which the community children's nurse might embrace a wider public health role within such areas remains to be seen. However, CCNs have established a very clear public health role in working with children and young people who are already experiencing health-related problems. Such work should be recognised and valued in the context of the overall public health agenda for children. Clearly, all nurses working with children have a role in health promotion.

References

Atwell J, Burns JM, Dewar AK, Freeman NV 1973 Paediatric day case surgery. The Lancet ii 895–897

Baly M 1987 A history of the Queen's Nursing Institute. Croom Helm, Beckenham, Kent

Blair M, Stewart-Brown S, Waterston T, Crowther R 2003 Child public health. Oxford University Press, Oxford

Bowlby J 1951 Maternal care and mental health. Monograph Series No. 2. World Health Organization, Geneva

Briggs A 1983 A social history of England. Weidenfeld and Nicolson, London

Chadwick E 1842 A survey into the sanitary condition of the labouring classes in Great Britain. Published on behalf of the Poor Law Commissioners. Reproduced in full in Flinn MW (ed.) 1965 Report on the sanitary condition of the labouring population of Great Britain by Edwin Chadwick. Edinburgh University Press, Edinburgh

Coram Family 2004 Coram family heritage. Online. Available at: http://www.coram.org.uk/heritage.htm [accessed July 2004]

Council for the Education and Training of Health Visitors (CETHV) 1977 An investigation in the principles and practice of health visiting. CETHV, London

Davies A 1985 Paediatric trained district nurse in the community (letter). British Medical Journal 291:247

Department of Education and Science (DES) 1978 Report of the Committee of Enquiry on Special Educational Needs (the Warnock report). HMSO, London

Department of Health (DoH) 1988 Promoting better health. HMSO, London

Department of Health (DoH) 1992 The health of the nation. HMSO, London

Department of Health (DoH) 1998a Our healthier nation. TSO, London

Department of Health (DoH) 1998b Independent inquiry into inequalities in health (Chairman D Acheson). TSO, London

Department of Health (DoH) 1999a Saving lives – our healthier nation. TSO, London

Department of Health (DoH) 1999b Sure Start. Health Services Circular HSC 199/02. TSO, London

Department of Health 2004 Choosing health: making healthier choices easier. TSO, London

Department of Health and Social Security (DHSS) 1976 Fit for the future. The report of the Committee on Child Health Services (the Court report). HMSO, London

Department of Health and Social Security (DHSS) 1986 Neighbourhood nursing – a focus for care. Report of the community nursing review (Chairman J Cumberledge). HMSO, London

Franklin AW 1964 Children's hospitals. In: Poynter FNL (ed.) The evolution of hospitals in Britain. Pitman Medical, London

Gillet JA 1954 Children's nursing unit. British Medical Journal 20th March:684–685

Gregg P 1976 Black death to industrial revolution: a social and economic history of England. Harrap, London

Hale R, Loveland MK, Owen GM 1968 The principles and practice of health visiting. Pergamon Press, London

Harrison S 1977 Families in stress. Royal College of Nursing, London

Her Majesty's Treasury & Department of Health 2004 Securing good health for the whole population (Chairman D Wanless). TSO, London

Hockey E 1966 Feeling the pulse. Queen's Nursing Institute, London

Hunter MHS 1974 A programme of integrated hospital and home nursing care for children. Paper presented to the annual conference of the National Association for the Welfare of Children in Hospital. NAWCH, London

Hunter MHS 1977 Paediatric hospital at home care: 1. Integrated programmes. Nursing Times Occasional Papers 10th March:33–36

Institute of Child Health 2002 The whole story: the history of Great Ormond Street Hospital for Children. Online. Available at: http://www.ich.ucl.ac.uk/150/whole_story.html [accessed July 2004]

Jackson RH 1978 Home care for children. The Journal of Maternal and Child Health March:96, 98, 100

Jones M 1988 Health visiting: the time has come to define the job more clearly. Nursing Times 84(3):11

Kosky J, Lunnon RL 1991 Great Ormond Street and the history of medicine. Hospitals for Sick Children, London

Kratz C 1982 District nursing. In: Allen P, Jolley M (eds) Nursing, midwifery and health visiting since 1900. Faber and Faber, London

Ledger P 1988 Feasibility study for weekend and evening health visiting. Health Visitor 61(3):71–72

Lightwood R 1956 The home care of sick children. The Practitioner 177:10–14

Lomax EMR 1996 Small and special: the development of hospitals for children in Victorian Britain (Medical History, Supplement No. 16). Welcome Institute for the History of Medicine, London

McIntosh JB 1975 An observation and time study of the work of district nurses. University of Aberdeen, unpublished PhD thesis

Ministry of Health 1959 The welfare of children in hospital: report of the committee (the Platt report). HMSO, London

OPCS 1982 Nurses working in the community. HMSO, London

Rathbone W 1890 Sketch of the history and progress of district nursing from its commencement in 1859 to the present day. Macmillan, London

Robertson J 1958 Young children in hospital. Tavistock, London

Royal College of Nursing (RCN) 2004 Directory of community children's nursing services. RCN, London

Royal Institute for Public Health 2004 The John Snow Society. Online. Available at: http://www.riphh.org.uk [accessed July 2004]

Sartain B1977 Views from Hampshire HA. Nursing Times 23rd June:944–947

Skills for Health 2004 National occupational standards for the practice of public health. Skills for Health, Bristol

Smellie JM 1956 Domiciliary nursing service for infants and children. British Medical Journal 1:256

Stocks B 1960 A hundred years of district nursing. Allen & Unwin, London

Strehlow MH 1987 Nursing in educational settings. Harper and Row, London

The Hospital for Sick Children 1874 Medical committee minutes, vol 6: special meeting of the joint committee – March 18. Hospital for Sick Children Great Ormond Street, London

United Kingdom Central Council for Nursing, Midwifery and Health Visiting (UKCC) 1991 Report on proposals for the future of community education and practice. UKCC, London

United Kingdom Central Council for Nursing, Midwifery and Health Visiting 1993 (UKCC) Consultation on the Councils proposed standards for post-registration education. UKCC, London.

United Kingdom Central Council for Nursing, Midwifery and Health Visiting 1994 (UKCC) The future of professional practice – the Council's standards for education and practice following registration. UKCC, London.

While AE 1985 Health visiting and health experience of infants in 3 areas. University of London, unpublished PhD thesis

While AE 1986 The value of health visitors. Health Visitor 59(6):171–173

Whiting M 2000 1888–1988: 100 years of community children's nursing. In: Muir J, Sidey A (eds) Textbook of community children's nursing. Bailliere Tindall, Edinburgh

World Health Organization (WHO) 1978 Declaration of Alma Ata. WHO, Geneva. Online. Available at: http://www.who.int/hpr/NPH/docs/declaration_almaata.pdf [accessed July 2004]

World Health Organization (WHO) 1985 Targets for health for all. WHO, Copenhagen

Chapter Nine

9

Family Responses to Ill Health and Admission to Hospital

Sarah Dowle, Sally R Siddall

ABSTRACT

Children are admitted to hospital for a variety of reasons. Regardless of reason for admission, the child and family will be apprehensive and feel vulnerable away from their normal environment. This chapter explores why children are admitted to hospital, how the family might have coped up to this point and how a child's ill health can affect both child and family. Social and psychological responses to an admission to hospital are examined and the reader is encouraged to participate actively in the review of this material and application to the clinical environment. Empowerment of the child and family through utilisation of clinical nursing skills and therapeutic communication are reviewed.

Learning Outcomes

- Discuss the difference between the number of sick children and the number of hospital admissions.

- Detail the various coping strategies commonly utilised by families who have sick children.

- Explore parental reactions/responses to sickness in their child.

- Consider the nature and implications of hospital admissions – planned versus unplanned.

Introduction

Childhood is a journey of new experiences, some good, others not so good. Children cannot be viewed simply as small adults – they have special and changing needs, making vary-ing demands at different stages of their life. Therefore, mere consideration of their age and developmental level is not sufficient in recognising these unique diverse needs. Ill health can be regarded as undesirable and yet also allows the child to develop a coping strategy for being ill. Respect of how a child's life experiences affect his or her ability to cope with illness, and indeed how these experiences ultimately affect the child's future development requires consideration. The experienced illness and the actual event of 'being ill' should be viewed as part of a learning process – the illness can be adapted, fought, accepted or rejected (Douglas 1993). The development of psychological coping mechanisms complements the evidence that illness enhances the maturing immune system to help manage further episodes of ill health (Hall & Elliman 2003).

The child's family, notably the parents, are usually the first to recognise illness and to act on the changing verbal and observational cues gained from knowing their child so well. It is important to remember that the majority of sick children will not require hospitalisation, or even a visit to their own GP, but will be managed by a range of skills and advice gained from previous experience and from others. Recognition of the potential difficulties and coping mechanisms utilised by healthy families and their children requires consideration. The child and family often regard admission to hospital as a serious consequence of ill health, therefore setting the scene for the child and family to be apprehensive, fearful and anxious. Hospitalisation has long been recognised as being a potentially stressful time for children and families alike (Darbyshire 1994). Health professionals on the admitting ward may well consider the child's illness to be relatively 'minor' in terms of morbidity and sometimes fail to anticipate or recognise the family's overwhelming concern. Unfamiliarity with both the situation and the organisational boundaries –

the need for compliance, disruption to the family unit and the overall impact these variables have on the family – must be considered throughout.

This chapter seeks to investigate the decision process that leads to a child being admitted to hospital and looks at how the child and family might react in this situation. It will consider both planned and unplanned hospital admissions and consider the socialisation process associated with ill health.

Statistics

Perhaps the most useful activity to set the scene for this chapter is to establish how sick children are managed by the family and by the health services. This will provide an understanding of ill-health episodes families experience with their children and also the ratio of primary and secondary care episodes. What will be more difficult to extract is how many children become ill and yet do not see a GP or are referred to the hospital. It will also be useful to see if there are any trends in age groups of children being referred to the GP or hospital:

- In England and Wales children under 16 years comprise 20% of the population (Office for National Statistics Census 2001).
- 19% of consultations with GPs and 15% of practice nurse consultations are with the 16-year and under age group (McCormick et al 1995, General Household survey 2001/02).
- The most common childhood system affected is respiratory – accounting for 27.6% of consultations (Health Committee 1997).
- 90% of all episodes of acute childhood illnesses at home are reported to be managed without recourse to health professionals (Department of Health 2003).
- One in 10–15 children will be admitted to hospital between birth and the age of 16 (Department of Health 2003).
- 70–90% of health care takes place within the family – this includes the care of all family members, not just children (Kleinman et al 1978, Scambler 1997).
- A random sample study found that 26% of respondents with at least one severe symptom chose not to consult a doctor (Hannay 1991).
- A subsequent study established that nearly 50% of mothers (sample size 52) identified illness symptoms in their child yet did not seek medical intervention (Cunningham-Burley & Irvine 1991).
- In 2001/02 16% of health service expenditure was spent on children under 16 years of age. On average, £259 is spent on each child aged between 5 and 15 per year, and £1,172 on each child under 5 years of age, including births. This can be compared with £3,315 per year spent on adults over the age of 85 (Office for National Statistics 2005.)

Activity

Consider the statistics outlined above in your learning group:
- What is the most important consideration for nurses in caring for sick children in the community or the hospital setting in terms of age at time of illness?
- Consider the range of nursing skills parents are likely to have as a result of such regular exposure to child ill health.

Coping Strategies Commonly Utilised by Families with a Sick Child

It is suggested there are three inter-related and overlapping arenas in which health care takes place – the 'popular' sector (or family wisdom), the 'folklore' sector (involving cultural and personal beliefs about health care) and the 'professional' sector (Kleinman 1980). It is important for the children's nurse to understand and recognise the importance of these care arenas, as families will usually arrive in the hospital setting with a range of knowledge and interventions taken from the first two sectors that can assist, support and direct the nurse during the admission and planning process. Families are integral to the care and support of their children therefore the impact of any health care intervention must be considered within this context. An understanding of the theories seeking to explain how families cope and interact under stress is essential and several theories have been postulated and subsequently applied to children's nursing (Crawford 2002).

FAMILY WISDOM

Much research has been undertaken exploring how parents cope with their sick child, particularly in relation to the provision of care (Helman 1994, Oakley et al 1994). It is important to remember that families have to experience an ill-health situation to learn how to handle the consequences. Advice and help are readily offered and sought from within immediate family and friends. Some of the advice may be sound and 'evidence based' (e.g. the more a child sleeps, the better he or she grows), whereas other help may be more dubious and based on 'old wives tales' (e.g. feed a cold, starve a fever) (Seabrook 1986). Either way, if the child is seen to improve, it is unlikely that external help will be sought such as from the health visitor or GP. This then sets up an 'encyclopaedia' of knowledge that is held by the family and used again as needed.

Helman's work (1995) utilises the 'germ theory', whereby people regard an illness being caused by 'invading germs' and describe the illness in terms of hot/cold and wet/dry symptoms. Once identified in these terms, a visit to the doctor enables the parent to articulate their concern. Research investigating mother's understanding of the causation of illness has revealed significant and useful data for children's nurses to consider. Pill & Stott (1982) found 11 categories of illness causation; 5 of these were deemed to be external, and therefore out of the parent's control, and the other 6 were internalised, and therefore within the parent's control (Table 9.1). The factors in the first column perhaps lead the parent to believe that the responsibility for the illness and subsequent management are the responsibility of others, whereas the factors in the second column require an acceptance of responsibility and therefore an agreement to some positive action by the parent to alter the cause of illness.

Activity

- Do you think nurses and doctors work on a similar view in defining the cause of a child's illness so that an effective plan of care, including relevant health promotion/education, can be devised?
- Is there a risk of stereotyping people by using this approach, because of their dress; personal hygiene; personality?

Evidence-based Practice

On your own and in your learning group:
- Reflect on methods used within your family to help manage illness.
- Did they work?
- Can you establish if they are evidenced based by today's approach to a similar situation?
- Consider the value of the following 'folklore' advice:
  - 'Don't wash your hair when you are having a period'
  - 'Salt in the bath water helps to heal skin wounds'
  - 'Make children sick by getting them to drink salt water if they say they have taken a noxious substance'
  - 'Put vinegar on a bee sting, bicarbonate of soda on a wasp sting'

An opposing view is that the development of professional and statutory services has served to erode the need for families to rely on their own family knowledge and skills in caring (Graham 1984). For example, SureStart is an excellent new multiagency (non-statutory) service where parents can seek out a range of advice and guidance and are actively encouraged to do so (Department for Education and Skills and Department for Work and Pensions 2005). The availability and 'free at the point of delivery' health service can serve to reduce the importance of creating the encyclopaedia of family knowledge. The emergence of a 'blame culture' might also have challenged the reliance on family wisdom, resulting in a reduction in the number of parents taking responsibility for healthcare decisions.

Sociological research examining the domestic management of children's healthcare tends to relate to the mother (Pitts & Phillips 1991, Helman 1994, Broome et al 1998). There is further useful analysis of several studies within the last 14 years considering the child and family's response to acute illness in children (Youngblut 1998). Nurses need to familiarise themselves with different cultures and how culture can also influence the family's decision to seek its own solution or to utilise health professionals.

Socioeconomic conditions may also influence decision making. Limited access to health centres, chemists and hospitals because of transport and/or cost can serve to delay the decision to seek medical help. The provision of health care within the family is often related to the family income. The mother often acts as housekeeper and carer and therefore recognises the need to provide sufficient resources to meet each role effectively. However, if the 'carer' needs outweigh the 'housekeeper' needs in terms of resources, time and cost, then the family/mother will go without essential provisions. This compromise can lead to conflict within and outside the family (Graham 1984).

Single-parent families invariably have less income than dual-income families, and sometimes less access to other family members and so less emotional and practical support (Blackburn 1991). This can influence the management of a child's illness, with the parent visiting the GP more frequently for reassurance and guidance, or not visiting a

Table 9.1 Categories of Illness Causation (Adapted from Pill & Stott 1982)

External causative factors	Internal causative factors
Environmental: the weather, pollution, pesticides	Type of person you are, e.g. more nervous/unhappy
Heredity and susceptibility	Being 'run down'
Individual susceptibility	'Way of life'
Germs, bugs, viruses, infection	Diet
Stress, worry	Hygiene Neglect, not looking after yourself properly

GP because of the cost of travel and lack of companionship to share the concerns of the health status of a child. Stereotypes of the 'overconcerned' parent or 'negligent parent' can arise in these instances, and yet there is a sound rationale for why this behaviour might arise.

Activity

- What is meant by 'hot' and 'cold' illnesses as expressed by many Asian cultures? How are each type generally managed?
- Consider the cost, in economic and practical terms, for a parent with three children under the age of 5, living on a farm, to travel to town or health center to seek advice, equipment and/or treatment for a sick child?

Activity

On your own and subsequently in your learning group:
- Explore your town, supermarket, pharmacist and health center, and collect a range of available leaflets on helping the sick child. Do they seem to be written for the parent's needs?
- Scan the supermarket shelves to see the range of medicines that are available to families. How are they packaged? Child friendly, colourful, etc. Do they offer easy-to-read instructions, dosage preparations and age restrictions?

COMMUNITY SUPPORT

Families have a further range of support to help them in deciding which is the best course of action for their ill child, for example accessing the local pharmacy for advice or just a scan of products that may help (Birchley 2002). Many weekly and monthly family-type magazines contain useful healthcare advice, as do the daily papers. Searching the internet for advice is also done on an increasingly regular basis.

www

Visit the *Guardian* website and search through the health sections to see the diversity of health advice available:
- http://guardian.com

Visit a common search engine such as Google:
- http://www.google.com

and find out how many hits there are for the medical condition of:
- toothache
- diarrhoea
- conjunctivitis.

Look at the first five English 'hits' for each condition and see how helpful they might be to someone wanting to manage this condition without recourse to a healthcare professional.

As a result of the explosion in internet usage, many government agencies, in particular the Department of Health (DoH), have set up websites to support the enquiring mind. Several innovative health services have also been created to utilise this latest technology. One such service is NHS Direct. It offers both a telephone service and an internet site (DoH 1997, National Audit Office 2002).

Activity

In your learning group: discuss what use any of you have made using NHS Direct.
- Who do you believe it is aimed at?
- Do you know the telephone number?
- Where is your local NHS Direct call centre based?
- Have any of you visited this centre to establish what they do? Would it be useful to ask your course tutor to arrange such a visit?

Read the article by Hall (2003) about the NHS Direct and children's care.

www

Visit the NHS Direct online website and seek out the advice for 'tummyache' in children:
- http://www.nhsdirect.nhs.uk

Seminar discussion topic

In your learning group:
- Discuss how useful a site like NHS Direct is for anxious parents, concerned children and other child carers such as grandparents and child minders.
- Spend 10 minutes exploring the Internet to see what other government 'online' support services there are for people, particularly the child and family. Make a list of these and share them with your colleagues for future use.

Seminar discussion topic

In your learning group, select one of the following 'support networks' that you wish to explore in more detail:
- evidence-based home care
- 'folk lore' remedies
- pharmacy support
- available health education leaflets
- NHS Direct.

Investigate one of these and write up what advice is available for parents to help their sick child and whether the advice is something nurses would undertake in their role in a ward or community setting.

PRIMARY CARE SUPPORT

All children have a right to regular health support and health checks during childhood (Hall & Elliman 2003). The midwife takes a full responsibility for newborn babies up to

28 days and a named health visitor shares and then assumes this responsibility 28 days after birth (Statutory Instrument 1992 No. 635). This health promotion/education role enables parents, and children, to learn about healthy choices and safe ways of dealing with everyday situations, from preventing accidents to managing illnesses. The health visitor will refer health concerns to the family's GP as necessary and make other referrals to other practitioners if felt appropriate; for example social services, speech therapy and child development centres.

Additionally, teams of appropriately qualified nursing staff working in the child's home, school and community settings can provide health care. These teams can consist of school nurses providing health promotion and education within the school setting, offering health interventions, support for children with long-term illnesses and the empowerment of child and family in maintaining the integrity of the family unit.

Likewise, community children's nursing teams (CCNs) provide a link between the secondary and tertiary services and the primary care provision (DoH 1996, Kelly 1998). They typically provide ongoing care interventions for children with known illnesses or following discharge from hospital for routine or emergency health care.

Activity

One of the roles of the midwife following delivery is to help establish the feeding needs of the child with the mother/parents.
- What sort of advice will be given during this time that will provide parents with an insight as to how to cope should they have concerns about their baby's feeding routine in the future?

Activity

A health visitor undertakes a routine hearing check on a 9-month-old baby:
- What teaching and learning is likely to take place for the baby's parent(s) in attendance?
- How is this likely to help the parent(s) at a later time in terms of coping strategies if the child becomes unwell?

Evidence-based Practice

Consider the standard immunisation schedule available to all children. Create a list of these:
- Identify the knowledge required by a parent in order to have informed choice and provide informed consent for these vaccinations.
- Who provides this information? Where would you seek such knowledge for yourself?

Immunisation

Immunisation is the use of a vaccine to protect against a specific disease. Vaccines act on preventing disease in one of three specific ways:

1. Administration of a live bacteria or virus which has been attenuated so it does not cause the disease.
2. Administration of the dead bacteria/virus.
3. Administration of part of the bacteria/virus.

Vaccines also contain substances to enable them to work effectively (DoH 2002).

The fundamental aim of an effective immunisation programme is to reduce the incidence (i.e. the number of people acquiring the disease in the population as a whole) of a specific disease, with the ultimate aim of eradication where possible. It is important, however, to remember that some diseases will never be eradicated either because there is a 'carrier' population (i.e. people who are able to carry a disease but who themselves remain unaffected) or because of the specific mode of transfer/activity (e.g. tetanus is carried in the soil spores). Indeed, despite improvements in hygiene, nutrition, health care and public immunisation programmes, some diseases continue to cause serious complications and fatalities (DoH 2002). Equally, there are dramatic success stories: before the introduction of the measles vaccination in 1988; an average 250,000 cases/year were noted, resulting in 85 deaths. By 1999, a significant reduction to 2438 cases/year, with two deaths was evident (DoH 2002).

www

In view of the media interest in the measles, mumps and rubella (MMR) vaccination; visit the following website:
- http://www.mmrthefacts.nhs.uk

Consider the advantages and disadvantages of the vaccination as it is currently offered:
- Identify the knowledge you would require as a parent considering MMR vaccination for your first child.
- As a health professional consider how you would promote the uptake of the immunisation programme.

Activity

Consider, with rationale, the skill mix of children's nurses employed in a community children's nurse team. For example, should there be a member of the team with additional skills and knowledge in adolescent care?

Parsons' Sick Role

There is a well established, although regularly challenged, functionalist theory on how society might expect someone to behave when 'sick' in order to protect the individual and society (Bury 1997). This theory was originally described by Talcott Parson in 1951, and was used by many health practitioners and employers at that time to determine whether the individual was 'sick' or 'ill' (Parson, 1951). Medical support and employment support would then be offered according to this analysis.

 ## Activity

- Define the difference between being 'sick' and being 'ill'?

 ## PowerPoint

Access the companion PowerPoint presentation and look at Parson's sick role and then list the two components deemed essential for being 'sick'.
- Can these be easily applied to children?
- How can this theory be supported where children have a permanent disability or are terminally ill?
- Do you see evidence of 'medical dominance' in this theory? If so, what are the implications for such a view?

 ## Scenario

You have woken up this morning with 'bad back' and feel generally unwell. You have taken an anti-inflammatory drug and ring your ward to say you will be unable to come in for your late shift that day.
- Do you think the staff will believe you?
- Do you feel the need to sound weak and ill over the telephone?
- Do you think the nurse receiving your call will ask/expect you to go to see your doctor for further support?

You go to your GP, who offers to sign you 'off sick' for 2 weeks.
- Would you decline the advice because of your need to keep your course theory and practice hours up to date?
- If you do reject the advice, would you expect your GP to be sympathetic or dismissive of your decision? In other words, might your GP subsequently disbelieve your bad back?

Does any of the above fit in with Parson's sick role theory?

Research has established that children are often socialised to deal with an illness relative to the environment they are in (Mayall 1996). At home, parents may actively discourage children from staying home from school and do not let them fulfil the 'sick role' by expecting them to do their homework. This may reflect the parents' coping strategy of hoping the illness is 'make-believe' or not serious, or fulfilling their role as 'constructive agents within the family' (Mayall 1996 p 82). Conversely, at school, children might have to negotiate their illness by seeking help at school breaks and after school. Injuries are more likely to occur in the playground, with the teacher seeing children as 'the objects of their socialisation and curriculum work' (Mayall 1996 p 82). Parents who accept their child's illness will implement the 'sick role' by renegotiating school attendance and workload.

Seminar discussion topic

School children are still heard to refer to the school nurse as the 'nit nurse':
- How far from the truth is this?
- Why do you think children still use this terminology?
- Seek out journal/internet, Nursing and Midwifery Council (NMC) and DoH information about the evolving role of the school nurse.

Doctors are not the only health professionals who expect a degree of conformity to the health advice they give to a child or parent; nurses can also make judgements on parents who perhaps challenge the advice they are given or appear to dismiss it.

Professional Conversation

 A mother rings the ward to seek advice on her 5-year-old child who was discharged from your ward yesterday following a routine tonsillectomy. She is concerned that her daughter is 'still not wanting to eat'.

Your advice is to try soft foods that her daughter normally likes and to give her plenty of fluids.

The mother states she has tried this to little avail. You ask her if her daughter has any pain and if her prescribed pain relief is effective. The mother says she has not given any because she sees no need – her daughter is not saying she is in pain. You suggest she gives her some anyway. The mother says she can see no need to do this.

You suggest that the mother contacts her own GP or rings the ward back the following day if there is still no improvement. The mother says she does not really think this will be necessary and thanks you for your time and says goodbye.

- What are your thoughts on the mother's behaviour – is her child 'sick' or not?
- Are you tempted to think the daughter cannot be too ill if the mother is reluctant to try out the care you offer?
- Is this 'Parson's non-conforming sick role theory by proxy'?
- What would you do once the call ended?

The information and activities so far have highlighted how vital it is that children's nurses seek out the knowledge parents and child already hold about the particular illness that necessitates hospital care and, specifically, what management has already been offered. Without these initial enquiries there may be a wide discrepancy between the professional care being offered and how the parent or child perceives this care. Parents might also need to be supported in their own previous understanding so they can also reflect on their skills, knowledge base and application. This may serve to positively reinforce their skills and ability or redirect these. Either way, continued empowerment of the family would result.

Activity

Access the companion PowerPoint presentation *Childhood illness and the family* and complete the various activities. Share your thoughts with your peer group and ask clinical staff for their views and experiences in some of these areas.

Parents, children and the wider family experience many mixed emotions when admission to hospital is decided on. This is in part due to the nature of admission, planned or unplanned (see later). However, most admissions are unplanned and these usually create the greatest upheaval for all concerned (Kendrick et al 2000, Young & McCubbin 2002). The next section explores the range of common emotions experienced by those involved.

Psychological Reactions

Many parents feel both relieved and guilty about their child's imminent admission to hospital. Their relief is based on the reassurance that their child will be cared for by people with the skills and resources to do so effectively; their guilt is because they are anxious that perhaps the care they had offered up to that point was inappropriate or had merely delayed the inevitable admission. They may also feel disappointed or angry because the health advice they might have already sought led them to believe their child was not as ill as they now fear he or she is.

It is imperative that the admitting nurse seeks to establish the nature of the parents' key concerns in these respects. Positive support can then be quickly provided and evaluated. However, appreciation of the parents' role as advocates for their child can mean that the health professional views the parents' concern as paramount, rather than seeking to determine the lived experience of the 'sick' child. This can then restrict the child's own understanding and involvement in decision making if their own perception of what it is like to be ill is unspoken (James 1998).

Scenario

Danny, a 2-year-old boy, is rushed to the local A&E department having suffered a convulsion at home. Both his parents witnessed this and had never seen this before in their son.

On admission, it is established that Danny has a temperature of 40.2° C and the staff plan their care around the likely event that this is a febrile convulsion. This care involves removing the blanket Danny was wrapped in, plus a jacket, jumper, dungarees, a vest and nappy. They quickly explain to parents the importance of letting Danny cool down so to help prevent a further seizure.

- What do you imagine Danny's parents will think when they see this action and hear the rationale for it?
- Might they feel they are partly responsible for Danny maintaining this high temperature because of the clothes he was dressed in?
- Might they feel inadequate as parents and people?
- How does this parental effort of keeping Danny warm when ill fit with a lay person's views on managing fever?

For further reading on managing a fever, read Harrison (2000).

The above scenario explores the possible effects on child and parents when an acute illness occurs. Health staff need to recognise the limitations of parental knowledge if a particular event has never happened before. It is possible to see how much knowledge can be gained in a very short space of time by the parents witnessing actions and listening to the explanations and rationale for these. Consequently, the majority of parents would be able to recognise and anticipate the changed care approach should a similar situation occur again. This also explains why many childhood illnesses are managed effectively in the community and family home.

Nurses also need to consider how parents manage the continuing ill-health needs of a child with a long-term health problem. Using the above exploration of how parents develop a skill and knowledge base, one might assume the parents of a child with a long-term health need are better equipped and skilled to deal with both minor and major health changes (Kirk 2001). However, it is pertinent to reflect on the nature of many of these conditions and the potential for them to be 'life-limiting' or 'life-threatening'. In these situations, parents often prepare themselves by considering the latest illness as being potentially fatal.

Reflect on your Practice

Imagine the feelings of parents of a young boy with cerebral palsy who is admitted with a chest infection for ongoing management. He has been unwell at home now for 5 days, with GP support. His parents are skilled in offering basic suction, chest physiotherapy and adapting his medicine regime to suit his needs.

- How are the parents likely to feel once the GP has decided that hospital care is now the most appropriate way forward?
- How are they, as parents, likely to feel in a physical sense, having been sharing the care between them for such a long time and with broken nights sleep and neglecting their own basic needs?
- Reflect on how often nurses encourage such parents to stay and help because they know the parents can handle their child's physical needs better than they are likely to do. Is it in everyone's best interest to use this strategy of care?
- Dwell on the information parents might have been given when they were first aware of their son's physical disability in terms of:
  - Parents: 'what might cause our son's early death?'
  - Doctor: 'a serious chest infection'.
- How can nurses address this diversity of needs for these parents?

A further issue to be considered was raised in the above 'Reflect on your practice' box. Many families have become adept at utilising medical equipment, pharmacological knowledge and symptom analysis that might easily match or surpass those of the health professionals they come into contact with. These families — and this might include the siblings and the sick child him- or herself – are used to risk assessment and high-level decision-making situations and so feel marginalised if the health professional dealing with the imminent hospital admission uses inappropriate language (e.g. simplifying technical jargon or offering patronising comments that are meant to be supportive). Likewise, the health professional might feel intimidated by the apparent wealth of knowledge and skill being shared and demonstrated by the child and family. The days when the medical world was secret, superior and only accessed by those qualified to do so are gone. Yet paternalism in the health service still exists and can undermine such families and also prevent other families reaching this level of medical/nursing competency if it is not challenged or eliminated (Dickinson & Dignam 2002). Family-centred care must begin at the time of the decision made to admit the child, not when he or she arrives on the ward.

Activity

Read Sarah O'Neill's article *Acute childhood illness at home: the parents' perspective* (O'Neill 2000):
- Make a list of the areas you consider to be important your developing knowledge base and clinical application.

Another important aspect of a sudden, or planned, admission to hospital is how the child's siblings deal with the sit-

uation. Seminal work in the 1990s explored the effects on siblings when a sick child was admitted to hospital or had a long-term illness (Eiser 1990). It was found that many siblings lost self-esteem, confidence and identity and felt socially isolated. These problems can be expected to be more evident where a sibling has a chronic illness but is not uncommon in a sudden acute illness. Siblings should always be included in the planning of a hospital admission wherever possible and the outpatient clinic is an ideal area for planned preparation to include this type of advice.

Unexpected admissions are different and families often choose to deal with the 'breaking of bad news' at a time they best believe they can support their other children. However, some siblings are left feeling vulnerable and excluded if this is delayed for any length of time, such as waiting for the end of the school day. Nurses have a role in supporting the parent with this type of decision making.

It is important to have useful and easily obtainable information in a variety of formats and languages to help parents in the preparation for hospital care – for themselves, the affected child and his or her siblings. Recent innovations include preparation for hospital by hospital staff visiting children in their own homes before admission, so involving the wider family and answering a range of questions that might be thought of in the safety of the home but lost in the sterility of the hospital environment (Sutherland 2003). The national curriculum also enables some discussion about ill health and the caring professions. This can lead to innovative use of hospital visits or health professionals visiting the classroom. A range of leaflets, videos (e.g. Action for Sick Children) and books (Lansdown 1996) are available in public libraries and from outpatient clinics to further support the needs of the child and family (Adams et al 1991, Carney et al 2003). The internet is another source of useful but not always accurate information, in that it might not reflect the British approach or support the services that are available in other English-speaking countries.

Activity

Check the health library, public libraries and internet for booklets and leaflets exploring the needs of the child and family when hospital admission is decided upon:
- Do they offer a good insight into how families can be prepared and prepare each other?
- Does your own children's unit offer locally created leaflets? Check these out as well.

www

Visit:
- http://www.childrensward.net (click on teddy bear in top left hand corner to enter site)
- http://www.rcseng.ac.uk/services/publications/publications/pdf/children_hospital.pdf

These are just two sites of many to offer help. However, they were not easy to find and this may be a problem for enquiring parents and family members.

A key aspect, which is of the utmost importance to any children's nurse, is the need to be skilled in understanding and applying the diverse nature of childhood growth and development. Parents are often familiar with how their child's behaviour changes during periods of ill health. There is increasing evidence to suggest even short periods of hospitalisation can result in transitory changes in behaviour (Rennick 1995). However, admission to hospital can further these changes, known as 'regression', and parents may not be skilled or competent at recognising these, sometimes believing their child to be deviant or 'attention seeking'. Regression can be explained as the concentration required by the child to cope with a strange environment and illness, this can be such that it leads to the child adopting everyday practices that they may have 'grown out of'. These include activities such as feeding and drinking using different implements (i.e. a bottle instead of a beaker), a reduction in vocabulary, crawling instead of walking, reverting to wanting a nappy again, or bed wetting. All these and many more activities require little concentration by the child; they are well-learned behaviours whereas the behaviours that replaced them may still require concentration to accomplish them. There is increasing evidence that even short periods of hospitalisation can result in transitory changes in children's behaviour and psychological status (Rennick 1995). Regression is usually self-limiting to the length of the illness or hospital stay but has often been viewed, by family members and health staff, as 'attention seeking' ploys. This view must be rejected and explanations and useful strategies for dealing with these offered as they happen and preferably in anticipation of them occurring.

Activity

- Relate your own experiences of 'regression' while ill to your study group.
- If you left home to start your nursing career, or a previous career; what special items did you want to pack to take with you? Why?
- Do you take any special mascots with you into exams? Why?

The following areas are important considerations in the effective management of both child and family when hospital admission is being considered.

Age of Child and Developmental Status of the Child

As we have ascertained, children have special health needs necessitating constant attention and support from their families/carers. Increasing emphasis on child- and family-centred care advocates the involvement of parents in the overall management of their child, impacting on both the quality and role of those delivering care (Audit Commission 1993).

As discussed earlier in this chapter, an essential skill of any children's nurse is the need to be accomplished in understanding and applying knowledge of childhood growth and development. There is much in hospitals that is unfamiliar, perturbing and frightening to a child; the more one can be prepared for an event, to counter the fear of the unknown, the better one copes (Landsdown 1996). Diversity in a child's behaviour can frequently be accounted for by the parents, who will have greater knowledge of how their child reacts in stressful situations and during periods of ill health.

The age and developmental level of children, previous experience of ill health and hospital, and the parents' emotional status are likely to determine the effectiveness of the preparation (Landsdown 1996). When one considers the psychological implications of hospitalisation one must also respect the increasing volume of evidence associating heightened parental anxiety with increased child anxiety (Rennick 1995). Indeed, parent-initiated preparation and interventions to reduce anxiety are reported to influence children's adjustment to and acceptance of medical procedures and hospitalisation (Rennick 1995). Deciding how much children can understand is not easy; one of the reasons this is such a complex skill is the limitation on children's language skills. Even to adults, with complex cognitive skills and understanding, the world can be a bewildering place. Landsdown (1996) suggested that young children use fantasy and magical thinking to reduce tension, resolve conflict and fill gaps in their knowledge. On this basis then, it is suggested younger children are more likely to have misconceptions about the cause of their illness and therefore have less effective coping strategies. The majority of hospital admissions, for either planned or unplanned admissions, involve children under the age of 4.

Activity

1. Consider the key principles of preparation for
   and
2. Identify key areas likely to cause distress in:
   - a preverbal child
   - an adolescent.

A good grasp of child development theories is essential if the child is to have a positive experience within a negative situation.

Nature of Hospital Admissions – Planned Versus Unplanned

Planned Admissions

These can be arranged for medical or, more commonly, surgical needs. Outpatient care will usually have preceded the admission and the waiting list for surgical admissions is considerably shorter than in the adult population. There is often a converse picture of hospital admission in these situations. The healthcarers need to have a healthy child on admission and then proceed to make the child 'clinically ill' by the planned procedure. However, to help offset this, the child and family are aware of the need for admission and can plan ahead, asking relevant questions and so being empowered in advance. A range of services exists to support the imminent admission, so maintaining a degree of control within the family group and hopefully ensuring the integrity of the family dynamics is achieved.

Activity

- Identify the numbers of children admitted as planned and unplanned in your local unit.
- If possible, establish the age ranges for each category of admission.

Use your local hospital's audit officer to assist you in this exercise.

Unplanned Admissions

These were considered earlier in the chapter. However, in light of the work undertaken in the above Activity, it becomes apparent how different an unplanned admission is and the likely effects on parents, sick child and siblings can differ.

Far more children will experience a hospital stay as a result of an unplanned admission than a planned one. The skills of the nurse lie in determining the likely reactions exhibited by the family and supporting them effectively.

RESPONSES TO EITHER TYPE BY CHILD/FAMILY, INCLUDING SOCIAL CONSEQUENCES FOR EITHER TYPE OF ADMISSION

Studies done during the last 30 years have identified that the occupational (social) class status of families has a direct link to hospital experiences of children. Work done by Earthrowl & Stacey (1977) indicates that children from social classes C2 to DE would have experienced more emergency admissions than children from AB to C1 (the middle classes), whereas planned admissions saw the reverse of this incidence. This suggests that nurses must

therefore have a working understanding of the effects of occupational class in relation to health and the experiences of illness. The Black report (Department of Health and Social Security (DHSS) 1980) and subsequent studies (Davy Smith et al 1994, Townsend et al 1988) suggest that poverty is a key indicator on the likely health status of individuals and families.

Regardless of the occupational class of the family, however, is the knowledge that children are very reliant on their parents for security, direction and approval. An ill child will be even more dependent on such support and cues from the parent. However, the illness in a child will have a major effect on how the parent copes and this may be indicated by distress, anger, denial or relinquishing of normal parenting role. The child may subsequently feel let down by the parent and lose some degree of trust in the decision-making skills previously taken for granted.

Seminar discussion topic

Review Erik Erikson's eight stages of development (Erikson 1950) (these can be found in any good child development text and an overview is given in Chapter 2). Consider the first five stages in light of the above parental reactions when their child needs hospital admission.

The 'trust versus mistrust' stage is a particularly important stage to consider:

- Why do you think this stage is the most important in terms of the child's age and cognitive reasoning skills?
- How can children's nurses use the theory underpinning each of these first five stages to support the child's need to know what is happening?

A recent study found differing types of satisfaction/dissatisfaction with information sought as to diagnosis (Starke & Möller 2002). It was established that parents sought information for one of two reasons – to control the professional intervention or to provide sufficient information to others.

Additionally, the publishing of the report investigating the care of babies and children with complex needs at the Bristol Royal Infirmary identified malpractice, by way of a range of individual and system failures, resulting in a drive for reform of the medical profession (DoH 2001). Anachronistic modes of professional practice were identified, with parents having little or no involvement in ongoing discussions about the care of their children (DoH 2001). The prominent role of parents was a distinctive feature of the inquiry: their empowerment throughout this case may also be viewed as contradictory, as arguably their grief was exploited in pursuit of an agenda of reform. The response to the Bristol Inquiry has been remarkable in its unanimity, being welcomed by the government, endorsed by leading medical organisations and approved by representatives of families whose children underwent surgery in the Unit. It would seem the media have broadcast, without reservation, reports demanding that the 'club culture' of the medical profession must be relinquished in favour of a new culture of external regulation with imposed standards and performance indicators (DoH 2001). Consideration of the wider implications of the inquiry, including long-term damaging effects on medical practice, public confidence with the medical profession and relationships between doctors and patients must be sought.

www

Visit:

- http://www.bristol-inquiry.org.uk

This site enables you to see the background to the inquiry and the findings of the report. Although the inquiry was specific to children with complex needs, the findings can be disseminated across all areas where children receive health care.

Seminar discussion topic

In your seminar group, read Chapter 17 of the Bristol Royal Infirmary Inquiry (parents' experiences; DoH 2001) and consider how the findings from this chapter can be applied to your own nursing experiences and future care planning.

The release of the Kennedy report (DoH 2001) resulted in early publication of part of the government's National Service Framework (NSF) for Children (DoH 2004). This publication has argued that the fundamental principle is the intention to place patients at the centre of care delivery. Integral to this is the need for quality assurance, including patient safety and children's rights. Identification of clear national standards supported by the National Institute for Clinical Excellence (NICE) and independently monitored by the Commission for Health Audit and Inspection (CHAI; formerly the Commission for Health Improvement (CHI)) are central to delivery of equitable care.

The full National Service Framework for Children, Young People and Maternity Services is now available and supports the need for clear and accessible information being made available to children and their families in health and illness, home and hospital (Department of Health 2004).

www

Visit:

- http://www.doh.gov.uk/childrenstrusts
- http://www.dh.gov.uk/PolicyAndGuidance/Health AndSocialCareTopics/ChildrenServicesInformation/fs/en
- http://www.doh.gov.uk/nsf/children/gettingtherightstart (downloadable pdf document)

View these sites and seek out your local NHS Trust's efforts being made to implement the NSF standards.

Reflect on your Practice

When you need to wash your hands following completion of a procedure, do you typically wash them:

- in the sluice
- at the nurses station
- in view of the parents and children?

Which approach is the most likely to reassure the interested family and onlooker?

Having dwelt on this activity, are you likely to reconsider your usual practice to offer greater confidence to the families in your clinical area?

Choice of Ward and Informed Choice/Consent

Nowadays, many NHS Trusts have specific accommodation for young people (National Association for the Welfare of Children in Hospital 1990). However, this is not yet universal and there are various clinical and management approaches to offering adolescent accommodation. The most common is identifying an area within a paediatric unit, although there are some 'stand-alone' units with clinical support from both the paediatric and adult services. There are no specific guidelines as to age group or clinical speciality so a range of protocols exists (National Association for the Welfare of Children in Hospital 1985).

Seminar discussion topic

- An adolescent area within a paediatric ward should receive girls who are seeking to have a termination of pregnancy or to give birth to a baby.
- Adolescent areas should receive all young people who have attempted suicide/parasuicide/self-harm.

Discuss these two statements, offering rationale to support your views. Consider the skill mix of staff in this discussion:

- Explore your local provision to establish the views held in these two specific examples.
- Consider whether other similar situations might prompt moral or ethical consideration.

Evidence-based Practice

In your local NHS Trust:

- Find out who provides young people with the information needed to know whether admission to a children's area or an adult area is an option.
- Whose role should it be?
- Is there a medium available to provide such information before admission to hospital?
- Does your local children's unit know of children under the age of 16 being cared for in adult areas?

Summary

In conclusion, it can be seen that there is a diversity of knowledge and skills to be considered when receiving children into hospital. Historical, social, psychological, economic, ethical and moral views are all intertwined and need to be engaged by the admitting nurse, or the community nurse, managing an episode of ill heath in a child. The need for good anticipating skills, an ability to 'stand back' from the immediate needs of the child to establish a dialogue with both child and family is essential if therapeutic communication, sensitive application of the nursing process and a trusting relationship are to develop and survive.

The age of the child, the size of the family, the occupational class and previous family experiences of ill health must all be embraced by the nurse to complement the care already provided and empower the family members to retain and develop, where necessary, skills in the care and management of their child.

References

Adams J, Gill S, McDonald M 1991 Child health: reducing fear in hospital. Nursing Times 87(1):62–64

Audit Commission 1993 Children first: a study of children's services. The Stationery Office, London

Birchley N 2002 Parental management of over-the-counter medicines. Paediatric Nursing 14(9):24–28

Blackburn C 1991 Poverty and health: working with families. Open University Press, Buckingham

Broome ME, Knafl K, Pridham K, Feetcham S (eds) 1998 Children and families in health and illness. Sage Publications, London

Bury M 1997 Health and illness in a changing society. Routledge, London

Carney T, Murphy S, McClure J et al 2003 Children's views of hospitalization: an exploratory study of data collection. Journal of Child Health 7(1):27–40

Crawford DA 2002 Keep the focus on the family. Journal of Child Health Care 6(2):133–146

Cunningham-Burley S, Irvine S 1991 In: Pitts M, K Phillips (eds) The psychology of health: an introduction. Routledge, London

Darbyshire P 1994 Living with a sick child in hospital. Chapman and Hall, London

Davy Smith G, Blane D, Bartley M 1994 Explanations for socio-economic differentials in mortality: evidence from Britain and elsewhere. European Journal of Public Health 4:131–144. Cited in: Field D, Taylor S (eds) 1998 Sociological perspectives on health, illness and health care. Blackwell Science, Oxford

Department for Education and Skills and Department for Work and Pensions 2005 SureStart, www.surestart.gov.uk

Department of Health (DoH) 1996 Child health in the community: a guide to good practice. Stationery Office, London

Department of Health (DoH) 1997 The new NHS: modern, dependable. Stationery Office, London

Department of Health (DoH) 2001 The report of the public inquiry into children's heart surgery at the Bristol Royal Infirmary 1984–1995. Learning from Bristol (the Kennedy report). DoH, London

Department of Health (DoH) 2002 Immunisation: the safest way to protect your child. Stationery Office, London

Department of Health (DoH) 2003 Getting the Right Start: National Framework for Children's Services Standard for Hospital Services. Stationary Office & www.doh.gov.uk/nsf/children/gettingtherightstart

Department of Health (DoH) 2004 National service framework for children, young people and maternity services. Department of Health, London http://www.dh.gov.uk/PolicyAndGuidance/HealthAndSocialCareTopics/ChildrenServices/ChildrenServicesInformation/ChildrenServicesInformationArticle/fs/en

Department of Health and Social Security (DHSS) 1980 The Black report: inequalities in health. HMSO, London

Dickinson AR, Dignam D 2002 Managing it: a mother's perspective of managing a pre-school child's acute asthma episode. Journal of Child Health 6(1):7–18

Douglas J 1993 Psychology and nursing children. Macmillan Press, Basingstoke

Earthrowl B, Stacey M 1977 Social class and children in hospital. Social Science and Medicine 11:83–88. Cited in: Black N, Boswell D, Gray A et al 1984 Health and disease: a reader. Open University Press, Buckingham

Eiser C 1990 Psychological effects of chronic disease. Journal of Child Psychology and Psychiatry 31:85–98

Erikson EH 1950 Childhood and society. WW Norton, New York

Graham H 1984 Women, health and the family. Wheatsheaf, Brighton

Hall DMB, Elliman F (eds) 2003 Health for all children. Oxford University Press, Oxford

Hall KA 2003 NHS Direct and children's A&E services: a case review Paediatric Nursing 15(5):36–39

Hannay J 1991 In: Pitts M, Phillips K (eds) The psychology of health: an introduction. Routledge, London

Harrison MR 2000 Nurses' management of fever in children: rituals or evidence based practice? In: Glasper EA, Ireland L (eds) Evidence-based child health care. Macmillan Press, Basingstoke

Health Committee 1997 Health services for children and young people in the community: home and school. Third report. The Stationery Office, London

Helman CG 1978 'Feed a cold, starve a fever': folk models of infection in an English suburban community and their relation to medical treatment. Culture, Medicine and Psychiatry 2:107–137

Helman CG 1994 Culture, health and illness, 3rd edn. Butterworth-Heinemann, Oxford

James A 1998 Children, health and illness. In: Field D, Taylor S (eds) 1998 Sociological perspectives on health, illness and health care. Blackwell Science, Oxford

Kelly P 1998 The role of the community children's nurse in enhancing the primary-secondary care interface. In: Glasper EA, Lowson S (eds) Innovations in ambulatory care: a nursing perspective. Macmillan, London

Kendrick D, Young A, Futers D 2000 The diagnosis and management of acute childhood illness: is there a role for health visitors? Journal of Advanced Nursing 32(6):1492–1498

Kirk S 2001 Negotiating lay and professional roles in the care of children with complex health care needs. Journal of Advanced Nursing 34(5):582–592

Kleinman A 1980 Patients and healers in the context of culture. University of California Press, Berkley

Kleinman A, Eisenberg L, Good B 1978 In: Helman CG (ed.) 1994 Culture, health and illness, 3rd edn. Butterworth-Heinemann, Oxford

Lansdown R 1996 Children in hospital: a guide for family and carers. Oxford University Press, Oxford

McCormick A, Fleming D, Charlton J 1995 Morbidity statistics from the general practice 1991–2. HMSO, London

National Association for the Welfare of Children in Hospital (NAWCH) 1985 Too young or too old – how and where should adolescents be nursed? NAWCH, London

National Association for the Welfare of Children in Hospital (NAWCH) 1990 Setting standards for adolescents in hospital. NAWCH, London

National Audit Office 2002 NHS Direct in England. The Stationery Office, London

O'Neill SJ 2000 Acute childhood illness at home: the parents' perspective. Journal of Advanced Nursing 31(4):821–832

Oakley A, Hickey D, Rigby AS 1994 Love or money? Social support, class inequality and the health of women and children. European Journal of Public Health 4:265–273

Office for National Statistics 2001 Census 2001 www.statistics.gov.uk

Office for National Statistics 2005 General household survey (2001/02)

Parson T 1951 The social system. Free Press, New York

Pill R, Stott N 1982 Concepts of illness causation and responsibility: some preliminary data from a sample of working class mothers. Social Science and Medicine 16:43-52. Cited in: Currer C, Stacey M (eds) Concepts of health, illness and disease. Berg, Oxford

Pitts M, K Phillips 1998 The psychology of health: an introduction. Routledge, London

Rennick JE 1995 The changing profile of acute childhood illness: a need for the development of family nursing knowledge. Journal of Advanced Nursing 22:258–266

Scambler G (ed) 1997 Sociology as applied to medicine, 4th edn. WB Saunders, London

Seabrook J 1986 The unprivileged. In: Currer C, Stacey M (eds) Concepts of health, illness and disease. Berg, Oxford

Starke M, Möller A 2002 Parent's needs for knowledge concerning the medical diagnosis of their children. Journal of Child Health Care 6(4):245–257

Statutory Instument 1992 No. 635 The National Health Service (General Medical Services) regulations

Sutherland T 2003 Comparison of hospital and home base preparation for cardiac surgery. Paediatric Nursing 15(5):13–16

Townsend P, Davidson N, Whitehead M 1988 Inequalities in health: the Black report/the health divide. Penguin, Harmondsworth

Young RT, McCubbin M 2002 Family stress, perceived social support and coping following the diagnosis of a child's congenital heart disease. Journal of Advanced Nursing 39(2):190–198

Youngblut JM 1998 Integrative review of assessment models for examining children's and families' responses to acute illness. In: Broome ME, Knafl K, Pridham K, Feetcham S (eds) Children and families in health and illness. Sage Publications, London

Communicating with Children and their Families

Janet Matthews

ABSTRACT

This chapter aims to ensure that the reader clearly understands the impact of communication on child development, daily living and health. The development of communication from conception to adolescents is outlined, and the implications for those who work with children of different ages and their families are high-lighted. Research, which explores health professional, child and family interaction, is reviewed, taking into account children's rights. Issues related to communi-cating with young people who are long-term recipients of health care, and with their parents, are discussed. Communication exercises and focused reflection on communication in practice will facilitate the develop-ment of self-awareness, knowledge and skills. Signposts to other chapters and recommended reading as a guide for further study are posted throughout the chapter.

Learning Outcomes

- Outline the development of communication from birth to adolescence.

- Discuss factors that have an impact on communication with children and families in the context of health care.

- Discuss communication strategies that facilitate family coping when communicating a serious diagnosis.

- Use relevant literature and research to identify good practice when working with children and families when the child has a life-limiting illness or disability and communication barriers.

Introduction

From the moment of birth, the child instinctively attempts to communicate with adults (Fig. 10.1). Communication is vital to the ongoing development of the child and to the ful-filment of his or her needs. If nurses are to promote child development, health and family integrity, they must learn how children and families communicate and develop the skills required to communicate effectively with children of all ages and their families. Providing clear, understandable information helps the child and family cope with alterations in health by enabling them to maintain control in the healthcare context. This chapter is designed to help nurses fulfill this role.

Development of Communication Skills from Conception to Adolescence

Infants begin life with a rich innate structure which changes in their understanding of persons – themselves and others – and is transformed through interpersonal exchanges. By the end of infancy they appreciate that they are psychological beings and among other psycholog-ical beings, different from others, yet neither alone nor unique in the world (Metzoff & Moore 1998 p 62)

BEFORE WE ARE BORN

Research studies (Zigler & Stevenson 1993) make it clear that, even before birth, babies can hear. Zigler & Stevenson

Fig. 10.1 • Engaging with mother 10 minutes after birth.

cite an earlier study by Spence & DeCasper (1986) that demonstrated the ability of newborns to select a tape recording from one of three children's storybooks. By sucking in a different pattern, the infants selected the recording that their mother had read aloud repeatedly before they were born.

 WWW

Find out more about more about DeCasper's research:
• http://www.uncg.edu/psy/tempfaculty/decasper/ intro.html

NEWBORN IMITATION

Heimann (1998) emphasised that, as the result of several studies in the 1970s, neonatal imitation is now described as a 'robust phenomenon' that can be observed from the minute of birth. The ability to imitate social gestures is believed to be due to the innate social motivation to interact, especially in a face-to-face position (Heimann 1998). Kugiumutzakis (1998) states that neonatal imitation takes place within the neonate–maternal 'intersubjective companion space'.

Children do not learn to speak unless they are exposed to human language and reinforcement in the form of adult pleasure at their achievements (touch, smiling, play, reciprocal communication, praise) and correction (Bruce 2001, Zigler & Stevenson 1993) (Fig. 10.2). According to Murray (1998), infants are remarkably sensitive to the quality of communication and seem to understand the significance of different types of communication. Two-month-old infants

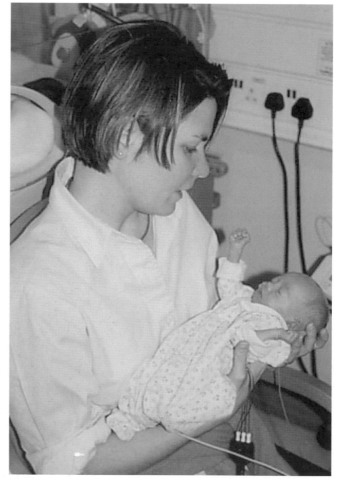

Fig. 10.2 • Face to face.

demonstrate signs of let-down and disengagement when a happy mother suddenly becomes still and expressionless. Sustained reciprocal engagement with an adult seems to play a key role in development.

First Sounds

The speed of language acquisition has been described as a mystery by linguists, who still cannot fully explain 'the apparent ease with which almost all babies acquire essential structure of one or more languages in their first three years' (Whitehead 2000 p 1)

The real mystery is that if children do not develop language skills when very young, it will be more difficult when they get older. Unlike animals, children are born with the biological mechanism to enable them to articulate words and the mental processing ability that enables them to isolate speech from other sounds, process and reproduce this information (Zigler & Stevenson 1993). Newborns are particularly receptive to the human voice (Zigler & Stevenson 1993). At 2 months old, the infant will respond differently to its mother's voice distinguishing between different sounding words (Zigler & Stevenson 1993). The infant's inner drive, increasing adoration and desire to communicate is reciprocation of the love and adoration communicated by the adult, which draws the infant out into the world of language (Matthews 1994, Whitehead 2000). In the early stages, older siblings also contribute to the development of the young infant (Fig. 10.3).

In the first few months of life the immature sound-making skills of the infant are constantly changing, making it difficult to identify what a word is. However, their early sounds are not random – crying begins at birth, cooing by the end of the first month and babbling begins at around 6 months (Oller 1980). It is believed that the repetitiveness of one syllable 'ba ba ba' exercises and thus aids the development of the muscles required in articulation. Furthermore, the tone and pitch of babbling seems to differ in keeping with the tone and pitch of the language to which the child is exposed (Zigler & Stevenson 1993). Initially, babbling can mask deafness but it will diminish if the infant cannot hear feedback. If deafness is not detected early the child will have more difficulty learning to speak. Deaf infants who are signed to from an early age develop sign language at a similar pace to the hearing child who is learning to speak. Early assessment and intervention by a speech and language therapist is very important.

PowerPoint

Access Part 2 (Eyesight, speech, language and hearing difficulties) of the companion PowerPoint presentation *Communication with children and families*. This provides website links to valuable information for children, families and health professionals. It also contains information on the role of speech and language therapists.

Fig. 10.3 • Older siblings contribute to the development of a young infant.

The speed of language acquisition is variable and individual to each infant and context. Many studies cited by Whitehead (2000) show that a true word (one that is repeated spontaneously in the same context) can be produced from 9 months of life, although this usually takes place between 12 and 18 months. The first early word sounds are personal to the infant and recognised by the carer as a statement of interest or a specific request. Single words (e.g. 'dink' or 'joo') are used to transmit the meaning of a sentence 'come and give me a drink of juice'. The words are often combined with actions (e.g. banging something), which communicates urgency and determination (Zigler & Stevenson 1993). Parental understanding of the meaning and the context of early words is vital to the child's continuity of development and this must be taken into consideration when engaging with the family, especially in the context of health care.

MAKING SENSE OF THE WORLD: 1–2 YEARS

The speed and complexity with which infants combine words varies and is generally based on their need to get things done, to involve others or to make a comment. Emphasis in first sentences is usually placed on the main object requested, e.g. 'book ma ma read'.

Communication increasingly becomes a means of exploration and development of personality. Children then use language to share their new experiences with us. Language enables children to think in a symbolic way, which is the principle underpinning learning words using pictures in books and surroundings. Symbolic language is very important for children who have communication difficulties associated with deafness or blindness (Whitehead 2000). Sign language and touch are essentially symbolic, enabling children who are hearing or sight impaired to make sense of their experiences, observations and feelings as they interact socially with others.

EXPLORING THE 'BIG WIDE' WORLD: 2–5 YEARS

By the age of two, children have become talkers or signers and communication enables infants to explore who they are (Bruce 2001) and where they fit in the bigger picture. Between two and four years of age children start to improve their grammar, sorting out singular and pleural differences and past tense by adding 's' and 'ed' (Whitehead 2000, Zigler & Stevenson 1993). Whitehead (2000) states that spontaneous errors created as the child tries to correct early words, e.g. mouses and goed, are evidence of the ability of a child's mind to process and produce the rules of language.

In the preschool years, children start to use joining words ('because', 'and', 'if') as they begin to understand cause and effect, sequencing of events, trial and error (Whitehead 2000). Their increasing ability to use words like 'why', 'how', 'where', 'who' and 'what' is essential to their cognitive development.

Edwards (1998) emphasises that other 'relational motivations', which develop from an early stage, take interaction beyond the boundaries of attachment as the child begins to engage in meaningful reciprocal communication within small groups. The child's vocabulary increases to include words that enable him or her to share feelings and to explore how others are feeling.

Dunn (1998) conducted longitudinal research that measured the child's ability to correctly interpret the emotions (happiness, anger, fear, sadness) related to various situations.

Evidence-based Practice

Naturalistic observation of 50 2-year-olds interacting with their mothers and older siblings at home was undertaken (Dunn 1998). The results indicated that children had a greater understanding of others at 40 months old if the following observations had been made when they were 24 months old:
- frequently observed talking to family members about their feelings and engaging in cooperative interaction with their siblings including participation in social pretend play
- exposed to greater emotional intensity, intimacy and frequency of the interaction
- their mothers were more likely to engage in frequent controlling behaviour with older siblings.

The results suggest that personal experience and interest in how parents interact with siblings plays a key role in the development of emotional understanding.

Further observation of the children over the next few years revealed that, between 33 and 47 months:
- talk about feelings to siblings quadrupled
- talking to mothers declined.

This study reflects the speed at which children develop the capacity to interact with others who, unlike a mother, may not always respond sensitively to them.

THE PRIMARY SCHOOL YEARS: 5–12 YEARS

Once the child starts school, language development is increasingly influenced by the wider social, cultural experience and literacy. The use and understanding of words such as 'perhaps', 'probably', 'scarcely', 'hardly' demonstrate the child's early understanding of probability, possibility and uncertainty (Whitehead 2000). Increasing diversity of experience influences social and moral development characterised by the child's attitude and behaviour towards others. Studies by Braten (1998) support the theory that children who have been the recipients of affective care when they have been distressed will respond caringly to others in distress. Studies show that children who have been victims of neglect or physical abuse are more likely to demonstrate indifference, fear or aggression (George & Main 1979, Klimes-Dogan & Kistner 1990, Main & George 1985; all of which are cited in Edwards 1998).

Childhood influences are not always positive and as a result children learn to use swear words, foul language and give verbal abuse, presenting a challenge to their families, teachers and healthcare providers. A study by Wilson et al (2003) showed that children between 2 and 4 years commonly told lies to cover up wrong-doing or to control another person's behaviour (Wilson et al 2003). Children tell lies about their health to avoid going to school or undertaking daily chores. They lie to conceal an illness or injury due to fear of painful interventions, e.g. tetanus injection, which could have serious implications.

The prevailing characteristics and attitudes in the family become the basis of unwritten rules, which are part of the child's primary socialisation. The child can learn dysfunctional values and ways of communicating with others, which negatively affect the development of all members of the family (Friedman 1992). Dysfunctional communication in families may affect how the child and family communicate with health professionals. Families who have closed dysfunctional patterns of communicating will have more difficulty coping, which may delay psychosocial recovery (Townley & Welton 2000).

Scenario

Brian is a second-year student nurse on placement on an acute medical paediatric ward. In his peer reflective group he describes an incident that caused him great concern.

'Last week a 5-year-old boy was admitted for investigations of failure to thrive. He seemed to be allergic to so many things. On the handover I was allocated to look after him. I was warned that he was rude and abusive and that his mother and father were also troublesome.'

'The nurse in charge suggested I speak to them only when spoken to and generally watch my back. I was really anxious when approaching the family but I saw the boy had a book on Manchester United football club so I asked him who his favourite player was and we had a good chat. He was cheeky at times but I discovered that he had a good sense of humour. His mother really appreciated the time I had spent talking to her son, which enabled her to go out for a cigarette. Other students also got on well with the family. The mother and child continued to be rude and abusive to the registered nurses and doctors.'

Reflect on your Practice

Identify and discuss the issues outlined above. In a similar situation how would you react?

The 'company-they-keep' hypothesis emphasises that adults who engage with children from an early age must recognise that they play a part in the development of prosocial or anti-social behaviour towards peers, which may continue throughout life (Edwards 1998). Modelling positive behaviour for the developing child is also the responsibility of all those who work with children.

THE TEENAGER: 13–ADULTHOOD

The ongoing development of good communication skills throughout the adolescent years is problematic if the acquisition of language and literacy are not well established at this point. David Bell, Her Majesty's Chief Inspector of Schools, stated:

Far too many young people reach the end of their compulsory schooling with inadequate basic skills (Ofsted 2003)

The maturity of the adolescent is closely related to levels of communication. Problems with self-esteem may be the result of a whole range of issues related to schooling and family life. General lack of confidence and unhappiness about the changes associated with the onset of puberty also impact on the quality of interaction with the teenager.

Activity

Study Fig. 10.4. How is this 12 year old girl in her bedroom feeling?

'Just leave me alone please'

'I want to watch my favourite TV programme without being pestered by my big brother'

'Why does everyone assume I am sad when I just want some space to myself?'

Consider the danger of observing but not listening to her.

Family communication patterns will either exacerbate or buffer adolescent stressors (Collins & Russell 1991). Saetermoe et al (1999) refer to several research studies that demonstrate that communication problems within the family affect health and well-being. Aggressive behaviour in children emerged as strongly linked to parental conflict (Davis et al 1998). Lanz et al (1999) conducted a large study that revealed that children from separated or divorced families had more problems communicating with their parents and

Fig. 10.4 • What is being communicated?

peer groups than adopted adolescents from intact families. Lanz et al (1999) concluded that male and female adolescent self-esteem is related to how well parents interact with each other.

Health professionals should remember that adolescent physical and emotional transitional stress can be exacerbated by traumatic experiences that impact on the young person's maturity, beliefs, attitudes, health, behaviour and communication. Morrison & Anders (2001) claim that there is little evidence to support the myth of adolescence as a period of 'storm or stress'. Most adolescents maintain close and supportive relations with their parents and 'embody parental values rather than oppose them' (Morrison & Anders 2001 p 69). It would appear that adults are too quick to label the 'terrible' teenager (Fig. 10.5). Can teenagers be blamed for behaving badly if that is what we expect of them?

The Value of Play as a Communication Tool

Children often find it difficult to talk about their fears, frustrations and uncertainty to strangers. Play helps break down barriers with smaller children and enables them to express their feelings (Ellis 2000) and to reduce tension, anger, frustration, conflict and anxiety, which are mainly due to perceived loss of control and self-esteem (Haiait et al 2003).

Techniques are used to enable children to project what they want using painting, puppets, drama and story telling (Fig. 10.6). Transferring ownership of emotions and feelings to a character seems to enable children to communicate powerful feelings, which would normally be too difficult to acknowledge due to embarrassment, loyalty or fear (Herpert & Harper-Dorton 2002).

Fig. 10.5 • Teenage sibling fun or fury?

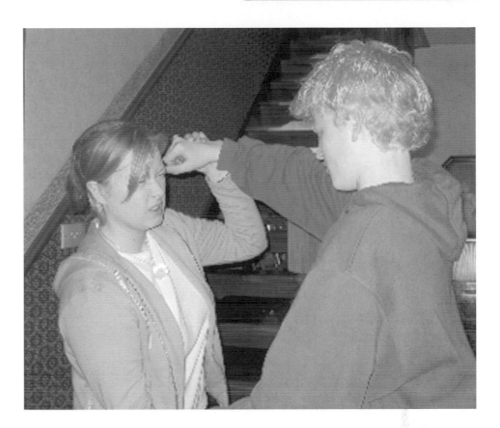

When a child is filling the gaps in story telling, caution must be taken in interpreting what is projected from reality and what is based on make believe.

Sometimes we see the world in fewer dimensions than children and all too often we reduce their imagination, creativity and energy into something that we feel comfortable with (Carter 2002 p 83)

Play is an effective means of preparing children for admission to hospital and for medical or surgical procedures. Demonstrating interventions on a doll or a teddy enables a child to take part and ask questions. The equipment becomes familiar and misconceptions are dispelled, which can reduce anxiety (Ellis 2000) as the child gains control in the process of play (Haiait et al 2003). It is within the guided framework of play that children are more likely to paint, write or talk about their emotions and experiences related to their illness, injury, treatment and hospitalisation (Haiait et al 2003) (Fig. 10.7). Play enables nurses, and other health professionals, to connect with child patients and to help them to feel at ease and secure, which is the basis of closeness and trust in a child's relationship (Haiait et al 2003). To communicate effectively with children, taking account of their cognitive development, play must become an essential part of a nurse's toolkit.

Understanding Health and Illness

In the early 1980s, Bibace & Walsh (1980, 1981) outlined the stages of cognitive development and the relevance to healthcare professionals. It is not until the preoperational stage of development (2–6 years) that children attempt to understand why things happen, often assuming that illness is magically passed through close contact with another sick person. As cognitive development progresses (6–12 years), more concrete operational patterns of thinking enable children to use cause and effect as a basis of their understanding (if you go out in the cold without a coat you will get the cold). Children grasp that the illness is inside their body before they can comprehend how external factors can cause illness internally (Vacik et al 2001). In the formal operational stage, adolescents begin to understand body systems and how physical and psychological processes can result in illness (Vacik et al 2001).

Although Piaget mapped cognitive development into age groups, he repeatedly stressed the importance of sequence over rate. Bibace & Walsh (1980, 1981) point out that a child's understanding is limited because memory, attention, bodily sensations and perception are still in the process of development (see Chapter 11 for further information on cognitive development).

Determining an individual child's understanding and perception of illness is critical for effective communication to take place. Over the last 20 years, there has been growing

I feel safe with my mum and Dad

Fig. 10.6 • Expressing feelings through painting.

evidence of the need for adults to provide clarity when answering children's questions about medical equipment, illness and treatment (Abbot 1990, McGrath and Huff 2001, Pidgeon 1981, Ritchie et al 1984, Tates et al 2002). If age-appropriate strategies are used, children can learn more about their illness, increasing compliance. Children as young as 4 years old have been taught how to effectively manage certain parts of their illness (Vacik et al 2001) (Fig. 10.8).

McGrath & Huff (2001) conducted a study of preschool children playing with medical equipment. They discovered that most of them had a very 'unsophisticated' understanding of the use of the equipment but were keen to ask questions and learn. Two children whose older relatives had been in hospital made a good attempt at explaining surgery and the circulatory system:

> . . . *when the people are asleep. You get a very sharp knife and cut their tummy. That's how they get things out (McGrath &Huff 2001 p 458)*

> . . . *actually you need blood inside you because it flows around our heart and if we didn't have blood we'd die (McGrath & Huff 2001 p 458)*

Worryingly, the children who did not engage in play had had previous experience of hospital (self or sibling) and either did not want to talk about hospital or about a related, unpleasant experience. The 'naive confidence' demonstrated by the other children was replaced by 'fearful descriptions' (McGrath & Huff 2001 p 460). This would suggest that they had developed misconceptions due to lack of understanding of their hospital experience. All of the children in the study demonstrated a readiness to use their imagination to fill the gaps when information was lacking (McGrath & Huff 2001).

Effective communication with children can dispel misconceptions and anxieties, ultimately improving their healthcare experience (Fig. 10.9). Nursing staff must explain that preparing the child for admission to hospital promotes recovery. Special dolls, storybooks, videos should be made available for use at a preadmission play clinic or at home. However, such techniques are not appropriate for use with older children (see Chapter 5 for further information on pre-admission visits).

Communicating with Young People in a Healthcare Context

Two studies have highlighted positive and negative aspects of interaction between health professionals and families. In the first study, funded by their local health authority, Elliot & Watson (2000) conducted 21 semi-structured group interviews involving over 200 children aged between 4 and 16 years. They ascertained the children's views on various aspects of health care and the services provided. Children expressed valuable views with as much authenticity and meaning as could be expected from an adult group.

Evidence-based Practice

Elliot & Watson (2000)
- Doctors tended to automatically address parents or other adult carers, regardless of the child's age.
- Some doctors did not speak to them at all, even during an examination.
- They doubted a doctor's ability to find out what was wrong with them by asking only their parents, who did not know all of their problems.
- When they were allowed to speak, some doctors dismissed or trivialised their complaints.
- Doctors used language children could not understand.
- Doctors did not always keep their promises.
- Generally, doctors were perceived as important people who had curative powers and who were authoritarian and judgemental at times.

Fig. 10.7 • Painting and communicating in hospital.

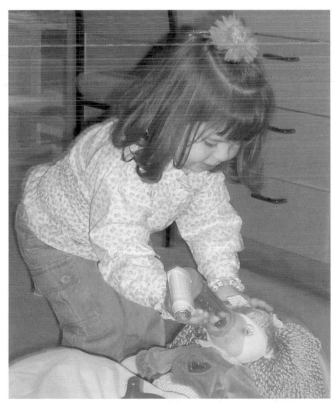

Fig. 10.8 • Two-year-old giving dolly a nebuliser.

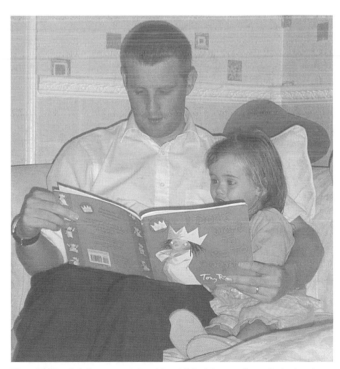

Fig. 10.9 • A father prepares his child at home for admission to hospital.

- Doctors had a negative image of older children, viewing younger children as small and sweet and not old enough to be trusted.
- Nurses listen more than doctors and are more approachable because they were perceived as less powerful.
- They valued the opportunity to talk to a trusted knowledgeable person in confidence about matters they might not be able to discuss with parents and friends.
- They wanted more information and confidential advice relevant for children and young adults.

In the second study, quantitative analysis of 106 videotaped interactions was used to describe the patterns of communication that emerged during GP parent and child interviews (Tates et al 2002).

Evidence-based Practice

Tates et al (2002)
- Parents generally viewed their child's health as their responsibility so the interview was conducted as if the child was absent.
- GPs did take into account the child's age and understanding (the child was asked what the problem was in only 35 out of 104 interviews).
- Some parents restricted child participation by interfering in GP–child interaction.
- Lack of participation on the child's part was not due to lack of understanding.
- Only 5% of children were given information on diagnosis and treatment directly.

The research by Tates et al (2002) corroborates the concerns of the young people highlighted by Elliot & Watson (2000). It is clear that although some GPs did attempt to consider the child's understanding and engage the child in discussion, this was an exception rather than a rule. Mayall (1996 p 275) states that, from the literature, the child's 'position within medical encounters is doubly dependent on parental and medical staff behaviour'. Therefore it is the responsibility of the adults in the interaction to provide a developmentally sensitive environment in which children are given the opportunity to be active participants in a healthcare context (Tates et al 2002).

WWW

- http://www.dh.gov.uk/assetRoot/04/06/72/51/ 04067251.pdf
  Take time to consider implications of Department of Health (DoH) (2003) *Getting the right start: National Service Framework for Children: standards for hospital services.* Pay particular attention to:
  - Chapter 2 Standards for hospital services for children: paragraphs 2.8 and 2.21–2.23 Quality of setting and environment

- Chapter 3 Child-centred services: paragraphs 3.10–3.35 Treating children and families with respect.
- http://www.dh.gov.uk/PolicyAndGuidance/Health AndSocialCareTopics/ChildrenServices/ChildrenServices Information/ChildrenServicesInformationArticle/fs/en? CONTENT_ID=4089111&chk=U8cln

Take time to consider implications of Department of Health (DoH) (2003) National Service Framework for Children, Young People and Maternity Services. Follow leads to part 1 and 2. Identify and discuss relevance to communicating with children and their families in the context of health care.

Children's Rights

In attempts to protect children it is easy to assume that they are incompetent and too foolish to know what is best for them:

> *The complexity of this issue can lead clinicians to take the easier option of assuming adults are competent and children are not (Brook 2000 p 33)*

The more pragmatic, balanced approach places the onus on the family and institutions to, on their behalf, ensure children's well-being until they become adults, when they will be able to speak for themselves (Fulton 1996).

WWW

Compare and contrast the principles in the Declaration of the Rights of the Child 1959:
- http://www.unhchr.ch/html/menu3/b/25.htm
  with the Articles in the United Nations Convention on the Rights of the Child 1989:
- http://www.unicef.org/crc/crc.htm
  Note the change of approach to children's rights and consider its relevance to communication with children today.

The Convention on Rights of the Child (United Nations General Assembly 1989) precipitated a shift of opinion among academics and professionals, who now believe that children are able and should be encouraged to participate and negotiate in their health care, education and social welfare (Elliot & Watson 2000, Mayall 1996).

WWW

The part adults play in ensuring children's' rights are not infringed is clearly documented in the United Nations Convention on the Rights of the Child. Visit the website and read the articles, with particular reference to 3, 5, 12 and 13. Consider the implications of each for communicating with the child and family in a healthcare context:
- http://www.unicef.org/crc/crc.htm

Health professionals need to work with each child on an individual basis so that they can determine the level of involvement the child wants and feels comfortable with. However, this takes time, which is often lacking (Brook 2000).

The Children Act (DoH 1989) states that parents no longer have rights over their children; instead, parents have responsibilities towards their children and must have regard to their children's views when making any major decision affecting them. Practitioners should ensure that when working with children they listen to each child, provide appropriate information and take account of the child's wishes and feelings (DoH 1989).

www

Take time to follow links relevant to communication at this website:

- http://www.hmso.gov.uk/acts/acts1989/ Ukpga_19890041_en_1.htm

How are children's views considered in the Children Act (DoH 1989) and the Children Act Scotland (DoH 1995)?

- http://www.hmso.gov.uk/acts/acts1995/ Ukpga_19950036_en_1.htm

Adults have a legal and moral obligation to ensure children have access to truthful information and the opportunity to share their views in what is still an adult-shaped world in which children are relatively powerless (Elliot & Watson 2000).

There is sufficient evidence to suggest that when children are involved in this way they are more willing to cooperate and have better healthcare outcomes (Alderson & Montgomery 1996, de Winter et al 1999, Tates et al 2002). This particularly applies to children and adolescents who require long-term health care and, as a result, are more likely to have a clearer understanding of their own health and illness.

Communicating with Children and Adolescents Who have Life-limiting Illness or Disability

PowerPoint

Access Part 3 (The healthcare context) of the companion PowerPoint presentation *Communication with children and families.*

From the literature reviewed, recurring issues related to interaction between adolescents who have prolonged healthcare needs and health professionals have emerged (Beresford & Sloper 2003, Couriel 2003, Elliot & Watson 2000, Jacobson & Wilkinson 1994, Lask 2003, Morrison & Anders 2001, Runeson et al 2000). Their collective findings fall into three categories.

Evidence-based Practice

Collective findings from Beresford & Sloper 2003, Couriel 2003, Elliot & Watson 2000, Jacobson & Wilkinson 1994, Lask 2003, Morrison & Anders 2001, Runeson et al 2000:

Organisational and team issues
- Duration and frequency of contact, continuity affects openness and effectiveness of communication.
- Communications skills of health professionals.
- Lack of consistency in information giving/approach can lead to loss of trust.
- Insufficient time to give information required.
- Information overload – failure to grasp certain key points.
- Differing approaches and conflict within a team (overinvolvement to perceived aloofness) confuse adolescents.

Attitude and approach
- Perceived negative attitude of health professionals – patronising.
- Ability to understand information is underrated.
- Exclusively focusing on the condition due to perceived lack of interest in wider impact of illness on daily life.
- Different rules of behaviour and expression of feelings and attitudes between adolescent and health professionals.
- Perceived powerfulness of doctor – powerlessness of adolescent.
- Wrong assumptions with regard to doctors' and adolescents' knowledge, expectation of treatment, course and outcome of the illness.
- Emergence of intense painful emotions (tear, helplessness, anger, despair), which may be reciprocated by health professionals.
- Complete disregard for opinions and feelings of adolescence.

Right to and need for increasing independence
- To be able to choose who is present (parent, medical students).
- Need to be given precedence (over parents).
- Need recognition of ability to effectively communicate own history.
- Need to be treated respectfully as opposed to being patronised or ignored.
- Health professionals need to emphasise the adolescent's right to confidentiality.
- Respect and showing interest in adolescent interests.
- Discrepancies between what health professionals assumed to be the needs of the older children and what the children believed themselves.

These pertinent issues impact on adolescent's self-esteem, their understanding of healthcare needs and adherence to treatment regimes, which impacts on the course and outcome of their illness or injury. Health professionals perceived lack of holistic interest in them and their fear of loss of privacy meant that they have difficulty in raising personal

Fig. 10.10 • Can't talk about it.

or sensitive issues with health professionals (Elliot & Watson 2000) (Fig. 10.10).

There is a widely held view that the limitations of chronic illness and disability affect the behavioural, psychological and social well-being of children and adolescents. However, several research study results (comparing children and adolescence with their healthy peers) refute this view. It is important to note that the results of the studies cannot always be generalised due to the small sample size, although they do inform nurses of the possibly of both positive and negative impact of the illness on the child and adolescents

✚ Evidence-based Practice

Subjects: impact compared with healthy peers/siblings

- Yarcheskie et al 1987: adolescents with cystic fibrosis – did not feel more lonely.
- Vera et al 1997: adolescent girls with insulin-dependent diabetes mellitus – no difference in social interaction or social anxiety.

- Pendley et al 1997: adolescent cancer survivors – no difference in overall popularity, social anxiety or loneliness.
- Forero et al 1996: adolescents with asthma – reported more feelings of loneliness.
- Saetermoe et al 1999: when compared with healthy siblings, disabled adolescents had less involvement in family interactions and the interactions were less meaningful. They also had less control in conversation.
- Noll et al 1993: adolescents with cancer – similar levels of self-esteem.
- Meijer et al 2000: adolescents with a range of chronic illness – engaged in lower levels of social activities but this could not be contributed to function limitations, although pain was a factor for boys. Some girls and boys displayed less adequate social skills and lower levels of social activities

The conclusion drawn from the largest study reviewed (98 chronically ill adolescents) was that adolescents with chronic illness are socially well-adjusted when compared with healthy peer group. This is probably because they have developed coping mechanisms during the course of their illness (Meijer et al 2000). It is therefore vital that health professionals do not make assumptions but assess each young person as an individual by engaging them in meaningful interaction (see Chapters 44–47 for further information on caring for children with special needs).

Communicating with Parents

Communicating effectively with parents of sick children is essential because their concerns about their child's health generate stress. Mothers have stated (Neill 2000, Young et al 2002) that when their child is ill they need:

- to be reassured that they have done the right thing for their child

- information on their child's illness and treatment

- respect and recognition of their competence to care for their child.

Instead, parents report dissatisfaction with medical staff who allegedly make them feel stupid and a nuisance for asking too many questions.

Parents with low levels of education are less likely to challenge professional judgements related to the health of their children (Spencer 2000). But disadvantaged parents are perceptive to the negative attitudes of staff members. When doctors dismiss parents' concerns regarding the health of their children, the parents' perceived powerlessness renders them unable to act on their own judgements, which in some cases has resulted in unexpected infant death (Spencer 1984). Mothers' concerns must be taken seriously because they describe their baby's health and happiness in terms of alertness and responsiveness to their environment (Mayall 1996), which are the first assessments undertaken by health professionals in the process of recognition of the sick child.

Parents feel that health professionals are more powerful in the hospital setting (Callery & Smith 1991, Sartain et al 2001). Darbyshire (1994) reports that parents feel frustrated when health professionals in hospital don't hear what they are trying to say. Although nurses strive towards partnership with parents in hospital, a more balanced approach is better achieved in the home (Sartain et al 2001). A study by Kirk (2001) highlighted that although professionals felt that parents exercised greater parental power in the home, many parents found 'being assertive' difficult even in the home.

Seminar discussion topic

Espezel and Canam (2003 p 34) state:

The parent–nurse relationship is considered to be a cornerstone of quality paediatric nursing . . . However while family centred care is promoted philosophically by policy makers and nurse leaders . . . how is the espoused view enacted in practice?

In their research paper, Espezel & Canam examine parents' experience of interacting with nurses when their child is in hospital. Critically review the article (publication details in the Reference list) and discuss with your colleagues. Attempt to answer the question highlighted above.

To inform your discussion, see Chapter 6 on partnership and family-centred care.

Communication between parents and healthcare providers may be influenced by their perceptions of who owns the child in hospital. Shields et al (2003) questions whether health professionals are aware of this.

Activity

Read Shields et al (2003) and visit the following website:
- http://www.blackwell-synergy.com/ doi/abs/10.1046/ j.1365-2648.2003.02521.

Nurses, who are placed at the communication interface, should urge their colleagues not to take control away from the family. Concerns related to the rights of the child and family should impact on interventions such as the development of a good working relationship, communication skills and determining the accuracy, relevance and meaning of information needed by families (Herpert & Harper-Dorton 2002), regardless of social status or the nature of the child's illness.

COMMUNICATING A SERIOUS DIAGNOSIS

The most difficult time for the parents is when they are facing a diagnosis that informs them that their child is developmentally delayed, has an illness or disability that will place restrictions on one or many aspects of their daily life or has a life-threatening illness. Although hearing such a diagnosis brings the realisation that their lives as a family are going to change forever, it also brings relief. Parents have reported that being provided with the information enabled them to feel in control again (Fisher 2001), to establish a new type of normality (Bartolo 2002) and to restore order amidst chaos (Starke & Mollier 2002). Studies (Fisher 2001, Starke & Mollier 2002) identified that communication problems generated feelings of uncertainty, which included:

- use of specific medical words or phrases
- being given information too quickly or not quickly enough
- the information was inaccurate or explanations incomprehensible
- overwhelming need to know but difficulty getting answers.

Parents reported having to trap a professional in a room and demand information (Fisher 2001), whereas Starke & Mollier (2002) stated that at times parents needed to limit or modify information received if they felt they could not cope with it.

Only 23 of the 44 parents interviewed were satisfied with the information received at the time they were told by the physician that their daughters had Turner syndrome (Starke & Mollier 2002). As a result, parents lacked confidence in the health professional's ability to ensure their child would get the best treatment. Parents (mostly mothers) sought information from the internet or from other agencies (Fisher 2001) so that they could explain the child's problems to others (Starke & Mollier 2002).

The quality of information given when communicating a serious diagnosis is crucial because those who are deeply shocked and distressed are unable to take it in (Young et al 2002). Bartolo (2002) emphasises the need for a balancing act because the parents need the professional to be frank and honest but also to show compassion. Switching the focus from negative outcomes to acknowledge positive coping strategies and their child's progress will foster hopefulness.

 www
- http://www.skillscascade.com/badnews.htm

ONGOING COMMUNICATION

When assessing what 'works best' for a family, nurses must maintain 'open and ongoing communication'. Parents need to talk about their child's symptoms but also the 'whole' experience which includes their many 'rough spots' (Woodgate & Degner 2003). In the early stages education is important to enable parents to take on more technical roles beyond the normal domain of parenting (Slade 2000). Tasks that seem straightforward to the nurse can be daunting to the parent and should not be rushed. Clear and effective communication is essential so that the parents know exactly what preparation is required for the task, each step of the procedure, and what to do in the event of something going wrong. What they need most is genuine encouragement and feedback on their progress so that growing confidence is based on competence to perform a new skill.

Scenario

Hilary is a third-year student nurse on placement on a short stay ward. In her reflective journal she records an incident that took place the week before.

'Last week a mother of a child with complex needs told me how upset she was when she was not invited to join the other Mums' introductory tour of the ward facilities. She felt most of the nurses on the ward avoided her. She was horrified to come back from a short break to find her child very distressed because a doctor had attempted – and failed – to insert an intravenous cannula in her son's arm; the doctor claimed she was too busy to wait for the child's Mum.'

'She is an excellent mother and appears to know far more about her child's disability than any of us, but nobody is taking this into account.'

Reflect on your Practice

How does Hilary's experience compare with your experiences of caring for children with special needs? How can you prevent similar occurrences happening in your area of work?

As the emphasis on equality and supporting inclusion increases, nurses need to consider their role in meeting the needs of children with special or complex needs and their families.

WWW

Take time to explore the role of nurses and other health professionals in promoting health, supporting inclusion at both these government websites:
- http://www.scotland.gov.uk/library5/health/phsi-00.asp
- http://www.scotland.gov.uk/library5/health/phsin-00.asp

Consider the work of the Learning Disability Task Force at:
- http://www.dh.gov.uk/assetRoot/04/07/47/27/04074727.pdf

The following NSF papers are specifically relevant to communicating with children and their families:
- http://www.dh.gov.uk/assetRoot/04/06/10/47/04061047.pdf

Parents appreciate health professionals who are honest about their professional limitations (Coyne 1997, Fisher 2001, Kirk 2001, Kirk & Glendinning 2002, Stewart et al 1994), especially when the parents are the experts on their children. Professionals who acknowledge and respect parents as experts interact within a different style of doctor–parent relationship (Kirk & Glendinning 2002). Parents needed their expertise to be acknowledged and failing to do so resulted in additional stress (Coyne 1997, Fisher 2001, Kirk 2001, Kirk & Glendinning 2002, Stewart et al 1994). From Fisher's literature review (2001) it is clear that health professionals have the potential to create uncertainty, disrupting normality. They should be aware of the fragility of the parental coping mechanism. There is a consensus that professional interaction should be informed by a sensitive understanding of what parents feel about their role and what they believe to be their needs (Coyne 1997, Fisher 2001, Kirk 2001, Kirk & Glendinning 2002, Stewart et al 1994). They need someone to 'be there' as an easily accessible source of support and information with whom they feel comfortable about sharing their anxieties. They need professional advocates who will help them to obtain the services their child needs (Kirk & Glendinning 2002). From the point of diagnosis, developing and maintaining trust in the health professionals caring for their child was really important to parents (Kirk 2001).

IMPARTING EXPERT INFORMATION

Imparting information is essential for parents to make decisions. Alderson (1993) cites several examples of professionals who have communicated information to parents in a sensitive, caring and clear way. Being kept informed of what is happening helps parents adapt a more positive attitude towards staff (Palmer 1993). Dale (1996) presents a list of communication guidelines, taken from an extensive literature review of communication techniques, which were shown to increase understanding and improve doctors' communication skills.

Guidelines for Practice (Dale 1996)

- Start by assessing the parent's emotional state.
- Be sympathetic considerate and caring.
- Invite the parents to present their own ideas, expectations and questions.
- The message should be:
  - clear, straightforward, direct
  - simplified using shorter (non-medical) words and sentences.

- To help recall use:
  - primary effects
  - explicit categorisation
  - repetition.
- To help understanding:
  - where possible avoid technical jargon and include explanation
  - help the parent to ask questions about information received.
- Use trained translators when working with parents from ethnic minority groups.
- Write down or give written information.
- Check understanding at regular intervals and hold a follow-up meeting to check understanding and retention.

Dale (1996) believes that one barrier to professional communication is that professionals may believe they have told the parents everything and assume they understand, making no attempt to find out if the message has been received and understood.

LISTENING

Listening is of major importance to the parent of a child with special or long-term healthcare needs but it is reported frequently as an area of weakness (Dale 1996). Parents worry about taking up the professional's valuable time or feel frustrated if the professional cannot offer solutions to problems. Professionals may feel compelled to interject, offer interpretations and solutions when it is not appropriate or find it difficult to gauge what is the appropriate time to respond or be silent. Either party may feel anxious or uncomfortable in silence (Dale 1996).

Active listening is achieved by adapting an open posture, maintaining eye contact and an appropriate facial expression. Kagan & Evans (1995) state that in certain situations using short verbal/non-verbal responses will be appropriate. In other situations a more active approach is needed – the listener seeks further information by asking appropriate questions, clarifying or paraphrasing, demonstrating empathy and understanding. The timing of questions or reflective statements is very important so that communication is not disrupted inappropriately (Kagan & Evans 1995). Active listeners make sure they do not lose their concentration. It is essential that nurses practice active listening skills and use reflection to adapt their skills for different situations. Active listening lets the parents, child and young person know they are important and central to the decision-making process. Listening is a supportive intervention, which facilitates coping enabling the family to remain in control and participate in partnership with the professional.

PROBLEM SOLVING

Finding solutions to problems can overwhelm the parent who has a child with a life-limiting illness or disability. Dale (1996) states that guided problem solving helps the parent to find the solution to a problem, which is often a personal concern. Negotiated problem solving involves parents and professionals striving towards a joint decision to a problem, which is of concern to both parties. Dale (1996) states that negotiation requires a high level of trust, openness, honesty, assertion and cooperation between the parties involved, and a willingness to recognise the importance of the other's view point and wishes in reaching an agreement. It may be necessary for the professional to concede, especially if disagreement occurs early in the relationship-forming process. In the interim, building trust and openness with the family is essential. The ability to compromise is essential for reaching an acceptable middle-ground decision, which is a step in the right direction.

When conflict situations are not recognised, levels of adherence to treatment regimes may fall as an expression of protest or due to lack of appreciation of the benefit (Lask 2003). Acknowledging differences and respecting autonomy validates parents' right to express their opinion and to disagree with others, however wise, senior or powerful they may appear (Lask 2003). Accepting the possibility of conflict within the therapeutic relationship promotes early recognition and resolution (Lask 2003).

Communicating with Siblings

Crises emerge throughout the course of a child's life-limiting illness. These can force the parents to put their healthy children on hold, enforcing prolonged periods of separation. Siblings become distressed if they have not been given information that helps explain the change in their parents behaviour (Mackenzie1997). They may think they are in some way responsible (Langton 2000). The siblings of children with chronic illness have an increased risk of developing behavioural or mental health problems, showing signs of attitude change and low self-esteem (Williams et al 2003). It is therefore important that, when communicating with the family, the parents are encouraged to:

- focus on all of their children
- keep in contact and spend time with their other children
- keep siblings informed of what is happening and how their brother or sister is responding to treatment
- involve siblings in decision making
- bring siblings into the hospital and help prepare them for the visit.

At times, the siblings may elect to stay away and not get involved, which may be their way of coping with the crisis. Parents need to be supported in deciding what is the right level of involvement. To do this nurses must work at developing a rapport and trusting relationship with the siblings (Fig. 10.11).

Bereavement

Communicating with families who are facing bereavement is complex as parents often find it difficult to express their feelings and emotions, which may be negative or confusing. In a study by Laakso & Paunonen-Llmonen (2001), many mothers – following the death of their child – did not share their feelings and experiences of grief because they felt that staff did not have the ability to meet their needs and that information was insufficient and ambiguous. It is essential that nurses continue to be accessible and approachable, maintaining open and honest communication (Mackenzie 1997). Professionals are often at a loss as to what to say. Fostering a sense of hope seems inappropriate but is vital and should be based on the family's ability to cope, support each other and come to terms with their loss (Mackenzie 1997).

Health professionals need to help parents identify what level of information the dying child and other children can cope with, and help them to work out and rehearse what they want to say:

We worry that children have neither the emotional maturity to cope nor the breadth of experience to understand about death. We worry that we will not be able to contain our own emotions or find the right words (Cardranell 1994 p 33)

Cardranell (1994) points out that children as young as four are aware of death and that by the time they are 8 years old all children know that we all die. Children will detect emotional tension or anxiety in the non-verbal cues of adults around them, which can be misinterpreted, causing distress. Cardranell (1994) concludes that children have the right to know the truth about what is going to happen to them, especially as older children are able to work it out for themselves. They need to be able to share their thoughts and fears about death, be allowed to ask questions about death and dying and be involved in making decisions about stopping treatment or dying at home or in hospital.

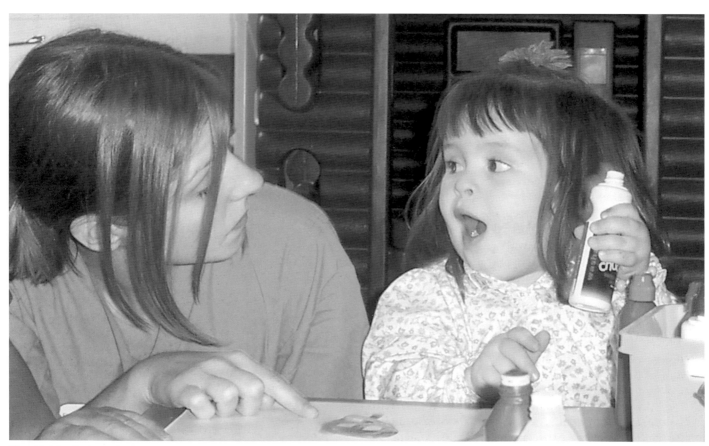

Fig. 10.11 • An intensive care nurse plays with a sibling.

Even with good support this may be too difficult for some parents to accomplish in full and they should be commended for doing their best. Sometimes children recognise this and in attempting to protect their parents will, if given the opportunity, share their feelings with a nurse who they trust. Confidentiality is a major concern for older children, who may not want their parents to know how they are feeling. However, some parents may decide that they do not want any talk of prognosis (Goodall 1994). While their wishes must be respected it is important that all parties are made aware that the nurse cannot lie or collude with attempts to withhold the truth (Goodall 1994).

It is helpful for families to know that nurses and other health professionals are emotionally involved but they must control their grief, avoid intrusion and establish a level of involvement or exclusion that is based on what the child and family needs. Nurses need to enable the family to stay in control, and should commend their ability to cope. Laasko & Paunonen-Llmonen (2001) emphasised the need for education and reflective practice to improve the quality of bereavement care.

Summary

The development of communication from conception to adolescents depends on interaction with the family in the preschool years. As the breadth of the child's experience extends beyond the boundaries of home, the development of communication and attitudes is also influenced by teachers, other children and other adults besides the parents. Children's nurses must take this seriously. When communicating with children, nurses must ascertain the level of understanding of each child. Play can be used to build up a relationship while facilitating a child's understanding of interventions. Parents play a key role in supporting their child through the assessment process. Nurses play a part ensuring that the rights of the child are not infringed by reminding both parents and other health professionals that they must engage with older children and listen to what they have to say when assessing and planning their care.

In the context of health care, parents' views must be taken seriously because they know their child best and have valid concerns when their child becomes ill. Complete disregard for parental views is dangerous practice and can lead to the death of a child. The parents of a child with long-term healthcare needs are the experts. They need the help of clinical experts who will use active listening and supportive problem solving, especially in times of crisis. Gaining information by listening to children and their families and providing regular, comprehensible information in a sensitive manner enables the family to stay in control and cope with crisis, even the death of a child.

References

Abbott K 1990 Therapeutic use of play in the psychological preparation of preschool children undergoing cardiac surgery. Issues in Comprehensive Pediatric Nursing 13:265–277

Alderson P 1993 Children's consent to surgery. Open University Press, Buckingham

Alderson P, Montgomery J 1996 Health care choices, making decisions with children. Institute for Policy Research, London

Bartolo PA 2002 Communicating a diagnosis of developmental disability to parents: multi-professional negotiation framework. Child: Care, Health and Development 28(1):65–71

Beresford BA Sloper P 2003 Chronically ill adolescents' experiences of communicating with doctors: a qualitative study. Journal of Adolescent Health 33:172–179

Bibace R, Walsh M 1980 Development of children's concepts of illness. Psychology and Health 4:175–185

Bibace R, Walsh M (eds) 1981 Children's concepts of health, illness and bodily function. Jossey-Bass, San Francisco

Braten S 1998 Intersubjective communication and understanding: development and pertubation. In: Braten S (ed) Intersubjective communication and emotion in early ontogeny. Cambridge University Press, Cambridge

Brook G 2000 Children's competency to consent; a framework for practice paediatric. Nursing 12(50):31–35

Bruce T 2001 Learning through play; babies, toddlers and the foundation years. Hodder and Stoughton, London

Callery P, Smith L 1991 A study of role negotiation between nurses and the parents of hospitalised children. Journal of Advanced Nursing 16(7):72–81

Cardranell J 1994 Talking about death – parents and children. In: Hill L (ed) Caring for dying children and their families. Chapman and Hall, London

Carter B 2002 On 'irafs' and other amazing things . . . Journal of Child Health Care 6(2) 82–83

Collins WA, Russell G 1991 Mother–child and father–child relationships in middle childhood and adolescence: a developmental analysis. Developmental Psychology 11:99 136

Couriel J 2003 Asthma in adolescence. Paediatric Respiratory Reviews 4:47–54

Coyne I 1997 Chronic illness: the importance of support for families caring for a child with cystic fibrosis. Journal of Clinical Nursing 6:121–129

Dale N 1996 Working with families of children with special needs: partnership and practice. Routledge, London

Darbyshire P 1994 Living with a sick child in hospital: the experience of parents and nurses. Chapman and Hall, London

Davis BT, Hops H, Alperst A, Sheeber L 1998 Child responses to parental conflict and their effect on adjustment: a study of triadic relations. Journal of Family Psychology 12(2):163–177

de Winter M, Baerveldt C, Kooistra J 1999 Enabling children: participation as a new perspective on child-health promotion. Child: Care, Health, and Development 25:15–25

Department of Health (DoH) 1989 The Children Act 1989. HMSO, London. Online. Available at: http://www.hmso.gov.uk/acts/acts1989/Ukpga_19890041_en_1.htm

Department of Health (DoH) 1995 The Children Act Scotland. HMSO, London

Department of Health (DoH) 2003 Getting the right start: national service framework for children: standards for hospital services. Online. Available at: http://www.dh.gov.uk/assetRoot/04/06/72/51/04067251.pdf

Dunn J 1998 Siblings, emotions and the development of understanding. In: Braten S (ed.) Intersubjective communication and emotion in early ontogeny. Cambridge University Press, Cambridge

Edwards CP 1998 The company children keep: suggestive evidence from cultural studies. In: Braten S (ed.) Intersubjective communication and emotion in early ontogeny. Cambridge University Press, Cambridge

Elliot E, Watson A 2000 Children's voices in health care planning. In: Glasper A, Ireland L (ed.) Evidence-based child health care: challenges for practice. Macmillan Press, Basingstoke

Ellis J 2000 Games without frontiers. Nursing Times 96(26):32–33

Espezel HJE, Canam CJ 2003 Parent–nurse interaction: care of the hospitalized child. Journal of Advanced Nursing 11(1):34–41

Fisher HR 2001 The needs of parents with chronically sick children: a literature review. Journal of Advanced Nursing 36(4):600–607

Forero R, Bauman A, Young L, Booth Nutbeam D 1996 Asthma, health behaviours, social adjustment and psychosomatic symptoms in adolescence. Journal of Asthma 33:157–164

Friedman MM 1992 Family nursing theory and practice, 3rd edn. Appleton and Lange, Norwalk, CT

Fulton Y 1996 Children's rights and the role of the nurse. Paediatric Nursing 8(10):29–31

Goodall J 1994 Thinking like a child about death and dying. In: Hill L (ed.) Caring for dying children and their families. Chapman & Hall, London

Haiait H, Bar-Mor G, Schobat M 2003 The world of the child: a world of play even in hospital. Journal of Pediatric Nursing 18(3):209–214

Heimann M 1998 Imitation in neonate, in older infants and in children with autism: feedback to theory. In: Braten S (ed.) Intersubjective communication and emotion in early ontogeny. Cambridge University Press, Cambridge

Herpert M, Harper-Dorton KV 2002 Working with children, adolescents and their families. Blackwell, London.

Jacobson LD, Wilkinson CE 1994 Review of teenage health: time for a new direction. British Journal of General Practice 44:420–424

Kagan C, Evans J 1995 Professional interpersonal skills for nurses. Chapman and Hall, London

Kirk S 2001 Negotiating lay and professional roles in the care of children with complex health care needs. Journal of Advanced Nursing 34(5):593–602

Kirk S, Glendinning C 2002 Supporting expert parents: professional support and families caring for a child with complex health care needs in the community. International Journal of Nursing Studies 39(6):625–635

Kugiumutzakis G 1998 Neonatal imitation in the intersubjective companion space. In: Braten S (ed.) Intersubjective communication and emotion in early ontogeny. Cambridge University Press, Cambridge

Laakso H, Paunonen-Llmonen M 2001 Mothers' grief following the death of a child. Journal of Advanced Nursing 36(1):69–77

Langton H 2000 Negotiating care. In: Langton H (ed.) The child with cancer: family-centred care in practice. Ballière Tindall, Edinburgh

Lanz M, Iarfrate R, Rosnati R, Scabina E 1999 Parent–child communication and adolescent self esteem in separated, intercountry adoptive and intact non adoptive families. Journal of Adolescence 22:758–794

Lask B 2003 Patient–clinician conflict: causes and compromises. Journal of Cystic Fibrosis 2:42–45

Mackenzie H 1997 The terminally ill child: supporting the family anticipating loss. In: Whyte DA (ed.) Explorations in family nursing. Routledge, London

Matthews J 1994 Helping children to draw and paint in early childhood. Children and visual representation. Hodder and Stoughton, London

Mayall B 1996 Children, health and the social order. Open University Press, Buckingham

McGrath P, Huff N 2001 'What is it'? Findings on a preschoolers' responses to play with medical equipment. Child Care, Health and Development 27(5):451–462

Meijer SA, Sinnema G, Bijstra JO, et al 2000 Peer interaction in adolescents with a chronic illness. Personality and Individual Differences 29(5):799–813

Metzoff AN, Moore KM 1998 Infant intersubjectivity: imitation, identity and intention. In: Braten S (ed.) Intersubjective communication and emotion in early ontogeny. Cambridge University Press, Cambridge

Morrison J, Anders TF 2001 Interviewing children and adolescents. Skills and strategies for effective DSM-IV diagnosis. The Guilford Press, New York

Murray L 1998 experimental perturbations of mother–infant communication. In: Braten S (ed.) Intersubjective communication and emotion in early ontogeny. Cambridge University Press, Cambridge

Neill SJ 2000 Acute childhood illness at home: the parents' perspective. Journal of Advanced Nursing 31(4):821–832

Noll RB, Bukowski WM, Davies WH et al 1993 adjustment in the peer system of adolescents with cancer: a two year study. Journal of Paediatric Psychology 18:351–364

Ofsted (2003) Adult basic skills development hampered by poor quality teaching skills. Online. Available at: http://www.ofsted.gov.uk/publications/index.cfm?fuseaction=pubs.displayfile&id=3410&type=pdf

Oller DR 1980 The emergence of the sounds of speech in infancy. In: Yeni-Komshian G, Ferguson C (eds) Child phonology, vol 1. Academic Press, New York

Palmer SJ 1993 Care of sick children by parents: a meaningful role. Journal of Advanced Nursing 18:185–191

Pendley JS, Dahlquist LM, Dreyer Z 1997 Body image and psychosocial adjustment in adolescent cancer survivors. Journal of Pediatric Psychology 22:29–43

Pidgeon V 1981 Function of preschool children's questions in coping with hospitalization. Research in Nursing and Health 4:229–235

Ritchie JA, Caty S, Ellerton M 1984 Concerns of acutely ill, chronically ill and healthy preschool children. Research in Nursing and Health 4:229–235

Runeson I, Hermerén G, Elander G, Kristensson-Hallström I 2000 Children's consent to treatment: using a scale to assess degree of self-determination. Pediatric Nursing 26(5):455–458, 515

Saetermoe CL, Farruggia SP, Lopez C 1999 Differential parental communication with adolescents who are disabled and their healthy siblings. Journal of Adolescent Health 24(6):427–432

Sartain SA, Maxwell MJ, Todd PT et al 2001 Users views on hospital and home care for acute illness in childhood. Health and Social Care in the Community 9(2):108–117

Shields LK, Kristensson-Hallström I, Kristjánsdóttir G, Hunter J 2003 Philosophical and ethical issues: who owns the child in hospital? A preliminary discussion. Journal of Advanced Nursing 41(3):213–222

Slade A 2000 Impact of treatment on the family. In: Langton H (ed.) The child with cancer: family-centred care in practice. Ballière Tindall, Edinburgh

Spence MJ, DeCasper AJ 1986 Prenatal experience with low-frequency maternal speech sounds influences newborns' perception of female voices. International Conference on Infant Studies, Los Angeles, April

Spencer N 2000 Poverty and child health, 2nd edn. Radcliffe Medical. Oxford

Spencer NH 1984 Parents' identification of the ill child. In: MacFarlane JA (ed.) Progress in child health. Churchill Livingstone, Edinburgh

Starke M, Mollier A 2002 Parents' need for knowledge concerning the medical diagnosis of their children. Journal of Child Health Care 6(4):245–257

Stewart MJ, Ritchie JA, McGrath P, Thompson D, Bruce B 1994 Mothers of children with chronic conditions: supportive and stressful interactions with partners and professionals regarding caregiving burdens. Canadian Journal of Nursing Research 26(1):61–82

Tates K, Meeuwesen L, Bensing J 2002 'I've come for his throat': roles and identities in doctor–parent–child communication. Child: Care, Health and Development 28(1):109–116

Townley M, Welton S 2000 Coping mechanisms. In: Langton H (ed.) The child with cancer: family-centred care in practice. Ballière Tindall, Edinburgh

United Nations General Assembly 1989 United Nations Convention on the Rights of the Child. UNICEF, Geneva. Online. Available at: http://www.unicef.org/crc/crc.htm

United Nations General Assembly 1959 Declaration of the rights of the child. UNICEF. Geneva. Online. Available at: http://www.unhchr.ch/html/menu3/b/25.htm

Vacik HD, Nagy MC, Jessee PO 2001 Children's understanding of illness: student's assessments. Journal of Pediatric Nursing 16:6

Vera L, Nollet-Clémencon C, Vila G et al 1997 Social anxiety in insulin-dependent girls. European Psychiatry 12:58–63

Whitehead M 2000 The development of language and literacy. Hodder and Stoughton, London

Williams PDW, Williams AR, Graff JC et al 2003 A community-based intervention for siblings and parents of children with chronic illness or disability: the ISEE study. The Journal of Pediatrics 142(3):386–393

Wilson AE, Smith MD, Ross HS 2003 The nature and effects of young children's lies. Social Development 12(1):21–44

Woodgate RL, Degner LF 2003 A substantive theory of keeping the spirit alive: the spirit within children with cancer and their families. Journal of Paediatric Oncology Nursing 20(3):103–119

Yarcheskie A, Mahon NE, Kraynyak-Luise B, Baker CD 1987 Testing the validity of categories in a theoretical perspective on chronic illness. International Journal of Nursing Studies 24:249–260

Young B, Dixon Woods M, Findlay M, Henry D 2002 Parenting in a crisis: conceptualising mothers of children with cancer. Social Science Medicine 33:1835–1847

Zigler EF, Stevenson MF 1993 Children in a changing world. Development and social issues, 2nd edn. Brooks/Cole Publishing, Pacific Grove

Chapter Eleven

The Dynamic Child: Children's Psychological Development and its Application to the Delivery of Care

Helen E Rushforth

ABSTRACT

This chapter offers an overview of psychological developmental theory and its application to children's nursing practice. Particular emphasis is placed on cognitive development, and the work of Jean Piaget, Lev Vygotsky and other contributors to the field is critically appraised. Implications for children's nursing practice are articulated by exploring the application of the different psychological developmental theories to children's understanding of health and illness concepts. The chapter then considers language development and personality development, again exploring the implications of these theories within children's nursing.

Learning Outcomes

- Recognise the importance of an understanding of the role of cognitive developmental theory within children's nursing.

- Gain enhanced insight into the ways in which children conceptualise health, illness and their internal bodies, and be able to use this information to offer enhanced explanations to children and families.

- Gain an appreciation of children's language and personality development, and be able to articulate the ways in which these theories can also contribute to the care given by the children's nurse.

- Develop insight into the critical appraisal of psychological theory and its application to care delivery.

Introduction

The purpose of this chapter is to offer readers an overview of key theories in children's psychological development, and to consider these in terms of their relevance to children's nursing practice. Particular emphasis is placed on cognitive developmental theory, as this appears to have the most direct relevance for care delivery. To illustrate this, an exploration of the ways in which children conceptualise health and illness is offered as a key example of the application of theory to practice. Consideration is also given to the related areas of language and personality development, which also have important implications for the delivery of child health care.

A range of developmental theories is explored within this chapter, and readers are encouraged to critically consider the appropriateness of each as a tool to guide their future professional development. Perhaps the most important guiding principle in selecting an appropriate theory to underpin practice is to consider the congruence of the theories offered with other contemporary notions of childhood, children's rights, and child healthcare delivery. Increasingly, recognition is being made of children's potential to be 'active participants' in their health care, rather than passive recipients. Arguably, therefore, it is particularly appropriate to question the continued dominance of many theories, particularly in cognitive development, which cast children in a primarily dependent role. If developmental psychology is to continue to have meaning for the healthcare practitioners of the 21st century, then it must reflect contemporary views of childhood in other domains.

The Nature–Nurture Debate

For any student considering developmental psychology, the nature–nurture debate is a key concept that underpins the work of almost all the major contributors. Thus an understanding of the nature–nurture concept is a useful starting point. Santrock (1999 p 21) defines nature as 'an organism's biological inheritance' and nurture as 'environmental experiences'. Therefore, the nature perspective would argue that a personality characteristic, such as moral behaviour for example, will develop naturally over time irrespective of external influences. By contrast, the nurture perspective would take the position that morality is a phenomenon that is learned, and thus is dependent on external stimuli.

In reality, of course, there are few who would argue that any aspect of child psychological development is entirely attributable to one or the other perspective, and it is increasingly acknowledged that the acquisition of any human characteristic is inevitably a synthesis of both inherited and environmental influences. So when a particular psychologist is described as being a nativist (nature, e.g. Piaget) or empiricist (nurture, e.g. Carey), this does not mean the psychologist believes the characteristic is *entirely* attributable to nature or nurture, but rather that he or she believes one or the other to be the *dominant* influence within that area of child development. Thus it is helpful to see nature–nurture not as an either/or concept but rather as a continuum. And indeed, although some theorists come very much from one or other end of the continuum, others sit far closer to the midline (and are often referred to as the interactionists or constructivists, e.g. Vygotsky). These psychologists suggest a more equal contribution of both nature *and* nurture to a particular aspect of development.

Cognitive Development

Although developmental psychology considers a variety of important domains, there is little doubt that the topic with the greatest influence for the child healthcare practitioner is that of cognitive development. From the outset it is important to acknowledge the dominance within this field of Jean Piaget (1896–1980); his profound influence on our understanding of childhood cannot be overestimated. However, although Piaget's invaluable contribution to developmental psychology is both acknowledged and valued, it is important to question the appropriateness of the domination of some of his assertions within the theory and practice of child healthcare delivery. Consequently, this chapter balances the Piagetian perspective with the views of other cognitive developmental psychologists, particularly Lev Vygotsky (1896–1934), thereby offering alternative tools to guide practice, which may be more congruent with other contemporary views of childhood.

PIAGETIAN PERSPECTIVES

Piaget was a prolific author whose worked spanned most of his very long and active life as a psychological theorist. Most students with some insight into Piaget's work will be familiar with his four stages of psychological development, a summary of which is offered below (derived from Bee & Boyd 2003, Meadows 1993, Piaget 1929, 1930, Piaget & Inhelder 1969, Santrock 1999, Shaffer & Bjorklund 1999, Taylor et al 1999).

Sensory Motor Stage: from Birth to Around 2 Years

Piaget identifies this first stage as characterised by the links formed between the infant and the environment as the infant comes to understand the relationship between actions, sensation and movement. Piaget divided the stage into six subsections (for more detail see Piaget & Inhelder 1969 pp 4–12). These stages characterise the infant's development from being primarily reflexive/reactive (stage 1) through processes of trial and error, experiment and reinforcement (stages 2–5), to finally being able to actively understand and manipulate aspects of his or her world (stage 6). In other words, the infant has a gradually increasing awareness of the relationship between action and effect.

Piaget saw a key concept within this stage as something he called 'object permanence'. This means that for the younger infant 'out of sight' is also 'out of mind'. In contrast, older infants (Piaget argued from around 8 months) realise that an object exists even when it cannot be seen. Also, throughout this first stage the child is described as egocentric, i.e. 'the child's initial universe is entirely centred on his [sic] own body' (Piaget & Inhelder 1969 p 13).

Preoperational Stage: from Around 2 Years to Around 7 Years

Piaget viewed the next two stages as a vital period of transition. At the beginning of this second stage, Piaget argued that the child's behaviour is characterised by actions; by its end the child will have reached the level of operations, summarised by Santrock (1999 p 203) as 'internalised sets of actions that allow the child to do mentally what was done physically before'. Piaget regarded achieving this as of pivotal importance and saw the preoperational period as dominated by organisation and preparation towards becoming 'operational' (Piaget & Inhelder 1969 p 96). Consequently, the stage tends to be characterised negatively, by what children are not yet able to do, rather than what they can. Examples include their perceived inability to classify objects into groups, to think logically and to engage in moral reasoning. A key skill not yet achieved is that of conservation, i.e. the ability to realise that something might 'stay the same' despite a change in appearance. For example, a preoperational child would think the amount of juice in a short, fat glass becomes 'more' when poured into a tall, thin glass (see also Channel 4 Television 2001, Santrock 1999 p 208).

Also within this stage is a continued focus on the child's egocentricity, characterised particularly by the inability to be able to see the world from another's point of view or to distinguish another's point of view from their own (both visually and intellectually). Closely linked to this is Piaget's belief that these children could not conceptualise a world beyond their direct experience, i.e. what he or she had actually seen or experienced. Practically applied, it can be seen how such beliefs can limit perceptions of the preoperational child's abilities in a whole variety of conceptual domains. Piaget also noted that these children display animism, the attribution of 'life' to non-live objects.

Concrete Operational Stage: from Around 7 Years to Around 11 Years

Piaget saw this stage as characterised by children becoming 'operational', and thus being able to do many of the activities that they were working towards in the preoperational stage. He argued that operational children are capable of logical, systematic thought, and able to 'conserve' concepts such as number, mass, length, weight and volume. They are also able to classify and seriate objects/items, and to understand logical relationships between them. However, Piaget felt at this 'concrete' stage that children could only understand problems related to direct experience; they are not seen as capable of abstract or hypothetical thought or the manipulation of variables.

Formal Operational Stage: from Around 12 Years Onwards

Piaget used the term 'propositional operations' to describe this final stage. He regarded these skills as congruent with preparation for adolescence, with the child able to think in abstract terms and capable of 'the handling of hypotheses and reasoning with regard to propositions removed from concrete and present operation' (Piaget & Inhelder 1969 p 131). Thus young people are able systematically to explore the solutions to an abstract or hypothetical problem, including everything from algebra to decisions concerning their future! An important extension of this is described as 'reflective abstraction'; self-awareness in relation to one's own strategies and thoughts.

These four stages are the centre-piece of Piaget's theories of childhood but many other important concepts also exist within his works. Those with particular relevance for child health practitioners can be summarised as follows:

- The way in which children think is fundamentally different from the way in which adults think.

- Development is fundamentally reliant on the concept of maturation, i.e. developmental pace is predetermined, and the teacher cannot accelerate this process.

- The child's understanding derives from self-directed actions upon the physical world. Thus, the teacher's role

is limited to constructing learning opportunities, and it is primarily through the child's independent interaction with the world that learning takes place.

- The child develops in a series of 'discrete stages' like 'caterpillar, chrysalis, butterfly', as opposed to a continuous development such as 'kitten to cat'.

(See also, Bee & Boyd 2003, Santrock 1999, Shaffer & Bjorklund 1999, Taylor et al 1999.)

Within Piaget's theories three key concepts underpin a child's emergent understanding of the world (derived from Meadows 1993, Piaget 1929,1930, Piaget & Inhelder 1969, Santrock 1999, Vacik et al 2001):

- **Scheme** or **schema**: the cognitive structure whereby the child organises his understanding of a particular concept.

- **Assimilation**: new information is incorporated into the child' existing schema, i.e. that which the child already knows.

- **Accommodation**: existing understanding ceases to be sufficient to make sense of the world. The schema is reorganised to understand the world in a new way.

To illustrate these somewhat abstract concepts, it might be helpful to consider an example. Imagine for a moment the child seeing a picture of a zebra for the first time.

- If the child already has a **schema** for horses, he or she might very well suppose that the zebra is another type of horse.

- This then would be **assimilation**: the child has taken the new information and incorporated it into his or her existing schema.

- However, through education and/or experience, the child will learn that the new animal is not a horse but actually something rather different, i.e. a zebra. Therefore the child develops a new schema for the zebra (and perhaps a wider schema for African animals). Thus a change in the child's understanding of the world has taken place, i.e. **accommodation**.

- Successful accommodation was viewed as essential to ongoing cognitive development, and enabled the child to achieve what Piaget called **equilibrium**.

- However, the risks inherent within the process are that from time to time **misunderstanding** will occur, e.g. instead of accommodation, the child happily goes on to describe an animal as a 'stripy horse'.

Reflect on your Practice

Before reading further, think about the following situation. Suppose you are admitting Jack, a 5-year-old child, to hospital for a course of intravenous antibiotics due to pneumonia:

- Consider Piaget's views on cognitive development. In what ways might your care of Jack be influenced if you assumed all of Piaget's assertions to be true?
- Think particularly about what explanations you might give to Jack regarding the treatment and care he will receive?
- Do you feel entirely comfortable with the approach you would take, or is there some conflict with your current experience and understanding of hospitalised children?

Influences of Piagetian Theory on Contemporary Practice

Piagetian theories influenced the delivery of child health care throughout much of the latter half of the 20th century and many of his views continue to be profoundly influential. For example, in the care of infants, Piaget's theory of 'object permanence' suggests that under about 8 months a child does not realise an object still exists when it cannot be seen, a theory applied not only to inanimate objects but also to people. Thus it has been argued in some centres that younger infants will not be unduly distressed when separated from their parents. So although unrestricted parental visiting is now more or less universally accepted within child health care, the parents of infants continue to be excluded in some care settings from anaesthetic rooms, recovery rooms and a variety of other procedures, on the grounds that this age group of children won't be unduly distressed by parental absence.

For the 'pre-operational' child, assumptions are often made about what the child is or is not able to understand about an illness, procedure or investigation. A Piagetian perspective would assume that children under the age of about seven were incapable of conceptualising their internal anatomy, and thus suggests that it may be pointless to attempt any realistic explanation of an internal procedure. As will be discussed in detail later, such guidelines were heavily influential during the 1970s and 1980s. A Piagetian stance would also contend that other misconceptions are inevitable and cannot be overcome until a child reaches a certain point of maturation. Examples include 'immanent justice' (Santrock 1999), which is the belief that pain or injury is a punishment, and 'overgeneralising contagion', e.g. believing cancer is 'catching'.

Even as the child becomes 'operational', assumptions continue to be made. As Piaget asserts that the concrete operational child cannot hypothesise, look meaningfully into the future or make decisions based on abstract concepts, it is often suggested that, until mid to late adolescence, a child cannot make an informed decision about what might be in his or her 'best interests'. Such beliefs have historically limited children's opportunities of having any meaningful involvement in decisions regarding their care, and arguably continue to do so in many care settings even today.

Thus it can be seen how important it is to gain an accurate picture of the extent to which Piaget's beliefs represent 'truth'. If there are doubts about some aspects of his theory, then such doubts must inevitably be extended to the application of Piagetian principles to care delivery. It is therefore important both to review the literature that takes a more critical view of Piaget's work and also to consider different theoretical perspectives that might offer alternative tools to guide contemporary practice.

Critiquing Piaget

The 1970s and 1980s were characterised by a series of challenges to Piaget's perspective on child development, with a whole range of authors suggesting that Piagetian theory unreasonably limited our beliefs in children's abilities and that, in reality, children were capable of far more, in a variety of domains, than Piaget gave them credit for.

In respect of the preoperational child, various studies have demonstrated the ability of young infants to visually recognise their parents and distinguish them from strangers (see Taylor et al 1999 pp 25–26). Similarly, Santrock (1999) and Bee & Boyd (2003) describe studies where infants demonstrate learning at just a few weeks old, far younger than Piaget would have accepted that these infants could proactively manipulate their environment. In one example, Santrock (1999 p 153) cites the work of Rovee-Colyer (1987), who took infants at just a few months old and tied their foot to a ribbon that moved a mobile. Weeks later, when placed under the mobile, the infants will once again kick in an attempt to move the mobile, despite no ribbon being in place.

Similar critiques of Piagetian theory are found in respect of the preoperational child. For example, in his study of egocentricity, Piaget devised a test known as the 'three mountains experiment' (Piaget & Inhelder 1956). The child was shown a three-dimensional model of three differently coloured mountains, positioned so that clearly different views of the mountains were visible from each of the four sides of the model (see Piaget & Inhelder 1969 or Santrock 1999 p 205 for more detail). The child was given a series of four two-dimensional drawings representing the view from each side of the model, and asked to 'work out' which drawing represented the view of a doll positioned on the opposite side of the model to the child. The fact that most children under seven were unable to do this was central to Piaget's persistent belief in their egocentricity; their inability to see the world from another's point of view.

Yet in contrast, Donaldson (1978), one of Piaget's foremost critics, constructed another experiment where children were far more successful, using an intersection of two walls in a 'cross shape' (see Donaldson 1978 pp 21–22 or Taylor et al 1999 p 58 for more detail). Two policeman models were positioned in such a way that they could see behind most of the walls but not all. In this study, children who got the three-mountain test wrong were frequently able to position a naughty doll so that the policemen was unable to see her; clearly they had to understand what the world looked like from the doll's perspective to do this. Perhaps the key difference, Donaldson suggests, is that this experiment 'made sense' to the child and so was more readily understood. Clearly if children below seven *are* able to see another's point of view there are major implications for beliefs regarding their egocentricity.

Activity

Gaining evidence of children's ability to see the world from another's perspective may be simpler even than Donaldson suggests:

- Take a favourite toy belonging to a child as young as three and position it facing the wall. Ask the child what the toy can see?
- Now move the toy to face in different directions in the room, and ask the same question.

Many 3- and 4-year-old children will happily tell you what the toy can or can't see. Yet these children are up to 4 years younger than those Piaget claimed were still egocentric.

In another of her critiques of Piaget's work, Donaldson also challenged some of his conservation experiments. For example, Piaget had conducted a study where children are asked to view two identical rows of sweets and say whether the rows are the same. The experimenter then repositions the sweets in one row so they are further apart, but leaves the same number. When re-questioned in Piaget's study, many under sevens insisted the row where the sweets have been moved now contained 'more'. Yet when Donaldson (1978) replicated the study using a 'naughty teddy' to move the sweets, significantly fewer children got the answer wrong than in the control group, which exactly replicated Piaget's study. Donaldson argued this was because the answer 'still being the same' now 'made sense', unlike the Piagetian version in which many children assumed the answer must now be different. Indeed, central to Donaldson's (1978) theories about Piaget was a recurrent theme that his experiments were designed in such a way that the children were often set up to fail, and that as a consequence children's abilities at a given age/stage were at significant risk of being underestimated.

For the concrete operational child, again, numerous studies challenge Piaget's perspectives. One particular study with clear healthcare implications is by Alderson (1993). She interviewed 120 children, many of whom fell into Piaget's concrete operational age group, and demonstrated the ability of several of these children to make carefully considered and informed choices about non-essential surgery.

It is beyond the scope of this chapter to illuminate the dozens of similar examples of experiments that call into question many of Piaget's findings (see Bee & Boyd 2003, Berger 2001, Berk 1996, 2001, Donaldson 1978, Santrock 1999 for more details). It is important to stress, however, that it is not Piaget's fundamental assertions about the systematic way in which children develop cognitively that are necessarily being challenged; his model continues to offer extremely valuable insight into the sequential ways in which children develop. Rather it is the nativist domination in his theories that has become the key focus of his critics, i.e. the:

- inevitability of constraints imposed by age and maturation
- protracted timescale taken to reach each developmental stage
- impossibility of accelerating the developmental process by education
- minimal credence given to the influences of experience, society and culture
- fact that, translated into practical terms, such beliefs have the potential to limit opportunities – given to younger children in particular – to understand their world and make sense of their experiences.

However, if these critiques of Piaget's work cast doubt on his theories in this way, then there are also inevitably important implications for many of the traditional applications of his theory to care delivery. Thus it may no longer be safe to assume that a 4-month-old baby can go for surgery alone and not be adversely affected by parental separation before he or she is asleep. Similarly, it might be unsafe to assume that a 4-year-old cannot understand an explanation of his or her heart surgery, or that a 9-year-old is unable to contribute meaningfully to a decision to undergo leg lengthening. It is therefore vital that such assumptions are carefully considered in light of the research that casts doubt on aspects of Piagetian theory, and also in the light of the views of alternative theorists, who may offer a more positive interpretation of younger children's cognitive development.

CAREY: 'NOVICE TO EXPERT SHIFT' THEORY

One of the key theorists who offers a very different view to that of Piaget is Carey (1985). In her 'novice to expert shift' theory, Carey – writing from an empirical perspective – argued that there is nothing fundamentally different about the way in which children and adults think and come to an understanding of the world. She argued that it is knowledge, not maturation, that is the key. Where only a little knowledge of a topic exists, thinking is 'novice', and thus it is likely that a concept will be misinterpreted or only partially understood. By contrast, the expert thinker has a great deal of knowledge of a topic, and thus sophisticated understanding exists. Crucially though, Carey argued that both children and adults are capable of 'novice' and 'expert' levels of understanding simultaneously, depending on how much they know about a particular topic.

For example, Carey cites 3-year-old dinosaur 'experts' who can tell you not only the names of all the dinosaurs but their eating habits, habitat, chronology and relative size. She similarly recognises young computer experts and chess players. Equally possible is novice thinking by adults when learning about a new topic for the first time, as evidenced for example by game-show contestants attempting to draw their internal anatomy! Thus, Carey argues that whereas children are far more likely to be 'novice' thinkers on a range of topics because their overall knowledge level is inevitably less, there is nothing about childhood thinking *per se* that limits children's understanding. Thus a child as young as three may well be able to develop a sophisticated understanding of a topic provided the knowledge is imparted at an accessible level and pace.

What emerges when comparing Piaget's nativist perspective and Carey's empirical perspective is a polarity between their two views, which regard either maturation or learning as very much the dominant forces in child development. It is the interactionist perspective, however, that offers the possibility of bridging this nature–nurture gap. Thus the theories of Lev Vygotsky (1896–1934) perhaps offer the most useful tool for healthcare practitioners in seeking developmental theory to underpin their practice (Holaday et al 1994, Rushforth 1999, Shayer 2003).

VYGOTSKY AND THE 'ZONE OF PROXIMAL DEVELOPMENT'

Vygotsky (1978) was working in Russia at a similar time to Piaget but his early death (aged just 38) and delayed translation of his work hindered his wider recognition for many years. Importantly, unlike Carey, his views were not in opposition to those of Piaget, and indeed contemporary authors have argued that there are rather more similarities than differences in their work (Shayer 2003). Like Piaget, Vygotsky believed in the importance of maturation and biological processes but he saw the interplay between these processes and the child's social world as being of prime importance. He saw thought processes as uniquely human and derived from children's early exposure to language, and from social and cultural influences conveyed to the child by both family and teachers. Indeed, the nature of the role of 'the teacher' is perhaps one of the key differences between Piagetian and Vygotiskian perspectives.

Central to Vygotsky's work was his notion of the 'zone of proximal development', which he defined as:

The distance between the actual developmental level as determined by independent problem solving and the level of potential development as determined through problem solving under adult guidance or in collaboration with more capable peers (Vygotsky 1978 p 86)

In other words, he saw the actual developmental level as the point of maturation that the child has already reached, but also recognised that at any given point in time the child had the potential for additional knowledge and understanding to be gained in that particular area of development. Thus the zone of proximal development looks at development 'prospectively', taking what the child knows as a starting point and using this to discern what the child is capable of achieving in the immediate future. Thus Vygotsky argued that you cannot determine any child's cognitive level without observing both what they already know and how they respond to instruction, hence the role of the teacher being so crucial (for more detail see Holaday et al 1994, Rushforth 1999, Santrock 1999 pp 214–215, Shayer 2003, Taylor & Woods 1998 p 159).

Translating Vygotskian Perspectives into Practice

The significance of Vygotsky's perspective in contrast to Piaget's is considerable because it offers the possibility of enhancing and accelerating the child's development by teaching. Unlike Carey, Vygotsky felt there were maturational limits on how far a child's understanding could develop at a given point in time. However, although these limits are in many ways congruent with the stages Piaget describes, in Vygotsky's theories the child can achieve understanding at a far earlier age than Piaget would suggest. Thus Vygotsky's theory offers teachers and health practitioners the possibility of considerably enhancing children's understanding through education.

Thus if a Vygotskian perspective rather than a Piagetian perspective influences our healthcare practice, the key difference is that a child's developmental potential is not persistently viewed in negative terms but rather in positive ones. Piagetian 'tools to guide practice' are framed in terms of what children are unable to understand (e.g. Taylor et al 1999 p 64). By contrast, a Vygotskian perspective encourages the practitioner to find out what the child already knows and then to use this as a basis for working with the child and family to help the child to reach an enhanced level of understanding (Gaffney 2000, Holaday et al 1994, Rushforth 1999).

Vygotsky's work was further developed by Bruner (1972), who used the analogous term 'scaffolding' to describe the role of teachers (both professionals and parents) within the 'zone of proximal development'. Bruner saw this human scaffolding as a 'supportive mechanism', which was gradually withdrawn as the child strengthens in his or her own knowledge and understanding. Bruner believed that any topic could be meaningfully conveyed at some level to any child, provided it was appropriately individualised and congruent with what the child already knew and understood.

Reflect on your Practice

Case study: Vygotskian perspectives

Consider again Jack, the 5-year-old child admitted to hospital described earlier. Now reconsider his care from a Vygotskian perspective:

- What differences emerge when compared with the earlier Piagetian perspective?
- Which approach to Jack's care are you more comfortable with and why?

Children's Conceptualisation of Health, Illness and their Internal Bodies

One example of applying cognitive developmental theory to practice is consideration of the ways in which children conceptualise health and illness concepts. The ways in which we interpret children's abilities in this domain has considerable potential to influence the quality of care they receive, their understanding of their illness and treatment, and the extent to which they can be actively involved in decisions pertaining to their care. A summary is offered here; for a more detailed consideration of this area see edited works by Bibace & Walsh (1981) and Siegal & Peterson (1999), and earlier work by the author (Rushforth 1999).

Since the middle part of the 20th century, numerous authors have researched children's ability to understand the concepts of health, illness and their internal bodies. The early 1960s through to the mid-1980s saw the publicataion of numerous studies suggesting that children's understanding of these concepts increased with age. Many studies also offered clear links with Piagetian theory, arguing the inevitability of the many misconceptions displayed by the younger children within the studies. However, the seminal work within the field was arguably that of Bibace & Walsh (1980, 1981), who offered a stage theory of children's conceptualisation of illness that was very closely aligned to Piaget's earlier described stage theory of cognitive development. Thus preoperational children (aged 2–7) were seen as having an illogical or magical understanding of illness, and concrete operational children (aged 7–11) were seen as having a limited but largely external understanding with limited awareness of internal biological processes. It was only the formal operational child (aged 11+) who was viewed as likely to have any detailed understanding of illness physiology (see Vacik et al 2001 for a fuller summary).

A similar stage theory was also published by Perrin & Gerrity (1981). The title of this study, 'There's a demon in my belly' (actually the child had been told he had oedema) clearly conveyed the typical misconceptions of younger children. Like Bibace & Walsh (1980, 1981) before them, Perrin & Gerrity (1981) argued that such misunderstandings are an inevitably consequence of cognitive immaturity.

However, the later 1980s and 1990s saw a gradual turning within the literature. A growing body of authors recognised that such studies, although offering useful tools in terms of understanding the way in which children conceptualise health and illness, were also misrepresenting younger children's potential to gain enhanced understanding of these health and illness concepts.

As early as 1980, and many years ahead of their peers, Kister & Patterson (1980) noticed that children who better understood 'contagion' were less likely to display 'imminent justice explanations' (the belief that illness was a punishment). Thus for the first time they acknowledged that enhancing understanding had the potential to reduce children's fears and misconceptions.

Also of interest at this time was the work of Burbach & Peterson (1986), who offered the first systematic review of the earlier literature, and again criticised the Piagetian dominance within the earlier work. Similarly Eiser (1989), a prominent UK researcher in the field, challenged the Piagetian dominance in her own earlier work and suggested the earlier discussed theory of Carey (1985) as an important alternative perspective.

One of the most important studies at this time was the work of Vessey (1988), who tested children's knowledge of their internal anatomy before and after instruction. She was thus the first author to clearly demonstrate the potential for children to achieve enhanced understanding of their internal bodies in response to instruction. Many other authors from this era also carried out studies that demonstrated children's greater understanding of health and illness concepts. These included Bird & Podmore (1990), Hergenrather & Rabinowitz (1991) and Longsdon (1991). It is important to state that these authors did not dismiss Piaget's theories outright, but they certainly challenged his assertions that children's potential to understand was limited by their maturation. All offered evidence of children demonstrating far more sophisticated levels of understanding than Piaget had previously given them credit for.

In reviewing these more recent studies, it is easy to see the parallels with Vygotsky's work, although it was only in Holaday et al's 1994 paper that this link was first explored explicitly. Since then, many authors have offered studies that demonstrate considerable understanding of health, illness and internal anatomy by even very young children (Elliott & Watson 2000, Gaffney 2000, Gaudion 1997, McEwing 1996, McGrath & Huff 2001, Schmidt 2001, Williams & Binnie 2002, Yoos 1994). However, what is interesting in many of these more recent papers is the balanced viewpoint often taken in recognising the contribution of the key theorists as complementary rather than in opposition. Thus, although Piaget's negativity in respect of younger children's understanding of the world is repeatedly challenged, the contribution of his stage theory to our understanding of childhood and cognitive development is readily acknowledged. Yet alongside this, the Vygotskian perspective that acknowledges children's potential to achieve enhanced understanding with careful teaching is also increasingly recognised. However, readers should be aware that some contemporary authors (e.g. Betz et al 2000, Taylor et al 1999, Twycross 1998, Williams 1995) continue to offer guidelines for practice that frame younger children's potential understanding in negative Piagetian terms. Whilst the evidence base to support any particular theorist is far from conclusive, any guideline for practice that suggests that certain groups of children cannot or will not understand particular health and illness concept should be viewed with caution.

It is also important to acknowledge within contemporary research in this area the fundamental importance of recognising children as individuals, thereby emphasising the importance of basing any explanation to a child on an understanding of what he or she already knows. This is particularly important in respect of the care of children with chronic illness, where there may be assumptions that knowledge levels are good because of previous experience. Yet seminal and contemporary work (Burbach & Peterson 1986, Crisp et al 1996) has repeatedly failed to demonstrate a clear link between illness experience and understanding of health and illness concepts. To make such assumptions therefore places the child at considerable risk, leading Ireland (1997) to advocate the 'gather, give, gather' model of explanation giving. In other words, find out what the child already knows, give the explanation and then (because we know how readily misunderstandings can occur despite good explanation) recheck the child's understanding to ensure that the explanation has been safely received.

As stated earlier, despite these recent studies, the evidence base is still far from perfect. In particular, researchers continue to study what children already know and to make assumptions about what they are capable of knowing. This view fundamentally opposes Vygotsky's assertion of the need to explore a child's response to instruction to recognise what he or she is capable of understanding. Thus, far more research like that of Vessey (1988) or Williams & Binnie (2002) is needed to address this deficit. This would help to create an evidence base that effectively guides future practitioners regarding the best ways of conveying information regarding health and illness concepts to the children in their care.

Reflect on your Practice

Case study: children's concepts of Illness

Suppose a 4-year-old girl tells you after her appendicectomy that the reason her tummy hurts is 'because I have been naughty':

- What might be the reasons for her beliefs?
- How can you help her to realise this is not the case, and understand the real reasons for what has happened and why?
- What theories are influencing your explanation giving?

Concepts of Health and Illness: Application to Care Delivery

APPLICATION: CONCEPTS OF ILLNESS

The potential to enhance children's understanding through information giving has relevance both for the acutely ill child admitted to hospital and also for the care of children with chronic illnesses. For the child undergoing a planned admission, this body of literature has considerable potential to greatly enhance hospital-based preparation programmes (for more detail on these, see Chapter 9). Even for emergency admissions, readily understandable explanations of illnesses and procedures are a crucially important aspect of care delivery.

Appropriate education for chronically ill children is central to helping those with conditions such as asthma, eczema, cystic fibrosis and diabetes become active participants in their care from an early age. Not only can it empower them to take control of their illness, it also enables them to make informed decisions about aspects of their treatment, as well as increasing their safety when they are among adults who have limited familiarity with their condition.

The Vygotskian (1962) principles of gathering information to find out what the child knows before any informative intervention takes place, as discussed above, cannot be overemphasised. As the school curriculum gradually introduces different approaches to biological and health education, knowledge levels within similar age groups are likely to be greater, but potentially more diverse, than ever. This arguably also further limits the usefulness of age-dependent stage theories. Furthermore, it is likely that within a class of up to 35 children, at least some will have misunderstood aspects of the teaching. Thus whilst giving an explanation to a child it may be necessary for misconceptions to be corrected before new knowledge can be explored. Despite children's clear potential to gain understanding at an enhanced level with appropriate instruction, misconceptions are, as noted earlier in discussion of Piagetian schemas, a very real risk within new learning. Thus children might be distressed by misunderstanding concepts we might take for granted, for example (see also Barnes 2003, Taylor et al 1999):

- **balloons**: analogous for bladders, lungs and stomachs, but children know that balloons can 'burst'

- **dye**: as in various radiographic investigations, but clearly having a potentially very different meaning

- **test**: a term widely used but again with a negative connotation for most children

- **bugs**: a term sometimes used by health staff to denote infection but which again is potentially frightening in a child's conception of sinister creatures

- **put to sleep**: if used to describe an anaesthetic could readily be misunderstood by a child whose pet has been 'put to sleep' by the vet; the concept of a 'special sleep' and an emphasis on waking up when the procedure is over is clearly vital.

Activity

Hannah, aged three, has come home from playschool having had a talk about hospitals, and has announced to her mother that: 'When we go to playschool tomorrow we are going to have our tonsils out and you can bring them home in a box'.

Considering the theories discussed so far, how did Hannah end up with this misconception, and in what way could this talk have been better organised to avoid this potential problem.

APPLICATION: CONCEPTS OF HEALTH

The implications of the children's concepts literature for the ways in which children conceptualise health are important. Given that contemporary health policy suggests that children as young as five need to be taught about drug abuse, for example (Travis 1998), it is vital that we consider ways of conveying messages to children about these complex concepts in ways they can understand. An approach that emphasises the typical 5-year-old's limited preoperational understanding is of little value here and it the work of authors such as Carey (1985) and Vygotsky (1978) that arguably offers better tools to guide those who construct health promotion campaigns for these age groups.

Even for older age groups of children the challenges of constructing effective health promotion campaigns can be considerable. Even the more contemporary work such as that of Oakley et al (1995) suggests that, whatever model

is used, conveying the longer-term adverse consequences of unhealthy behaviours to children and young people is extremely difficult. Indeed, Piaget's caution about the challenges even adolescents have in appreciating the longer-term consequences of actions might well be relevant here, although others would argue this is more to do with adolescent 'denial' than an inability to understand (see Santrock 1999). Nevertheless, it is arguably important that health promoters focus on the positive and short-term benefits of healthy choices within any health promotion campaign (such as weight loss increasing attractiveness to potential partners, for example) rather than the longer-term risks (such as death from heart disease 50 years hence).

WIDER APPLICATION OF THE CHILDREN'S CONCEPTS OF HEALTH AND ILLNESS LITERATURE TO CARE DELIVERY

Detailed consideration of how all aspects of the literature pertaining to children's conceptualisation of health and illness can be applied to practice is beyond the scope of this chapter. Specific areas that the reader might wish to further consider include the study of children's perceptions of pain (Gaffney 2000, Harbech & Peterson 1992, Rushforth 1999, Twycross 1998), children's competence to consent (Alderson 1993, Alderson & Montgomery 1996, Rushforth 1999) and children's understanding of death (Bluebond-Langer 1989, Smith & McSherry 2004).

Finally, it has been suggested – within both earlier work (Perrin & Perrin 1983, Rushforth 1996) and in a more recent study (Vacik et al 2001) – that healthcare practitioners often have an inadequate understanding of how children conceptualise health and illness. It is therefore possible that such a lack of understanding might in turn inhibit the quality of the communication and information-giving undertaken by children's nurses and other healthcare practitioners; gaining enhanced levels of knowledge within this domain therefore has the potential to considerably enhance care delivery.

Language Development

Many texts offer detailed accounts of the ways in which children develop language, breaking it down into the complex processes of phonology, morphology, semantics and pragmatics (Santrock 1999). The importance of these processes in helping children with specific problems cannot be overestimated but the greater priority for most healthcare practitioners working with children is an understanding of the psychological processes underpinning language development, and the extent to which these can be influenced by a period of illness or hospitalisation. Alongside this it is important that students have sufficient understanding of what constitutes normal language development if they are to be able to access expert opinion and help for a child whose linguistic development appears to be delayed.

THE EMPIRICIST PERSPECTIVE

Skinner (1957) took a view of language development that is congruent with the empiricist perspective. He believed that children's earliest language development was shaped from their meaningless infant 'babbling', through a process of reinforcement. This involves parents praising, reiterating and thereby reinforcing sounds that most closely approximate to actual words (e.g. 'ma ma ma' 'da da da'). This is seen alongside the process of 'imitation', suggesting that children's verbatim copying of words, phrases and sentences uttered by adults enables them to construct sentences themselves.

This view of language development, sometimes referred to as the behaviourist perspective, sees children very much as a 'blank slate', on whom language is imposed. However, as Berk (1996) points out, the 3- or 4-year-old child typically has a vocabulary of around 14,000 words, which he or she can use correctly to construct sophisticated and grammatically correct, or near correct, sentences. Thus, if the behaviourist perspective alone was responsible for language development, it would rely on parents and others engaging in the equivalent of extremely intensive language tuition processes. Many contemporary psychologists agree that the empiricist perspective alone is insufficient to explain young children's sophisticated language development.

THE NATIVIST PERSPECTIVE

Ironically published in the same year as Skinner's work, another seminal text (Chomsky 1957) proposed an opposing view of language development. Chomsky viewed children as far more active participants in the process of language acquisition. Although exposure to adult language was clearly important, he argued that they were effectively 'pre programmed' to learn language (Grieg 1998) via what he referred to as the language acquisition device (LAD). He saw this as a mental 'apparatus', which innately enables children to actively construct their vocabulary into grammatically sound sentence constructions.

Chomsky drew on the evidence of when children get things wrong to support his theory. For example, children who say they 'ridded' their bike, 'didded up' their shoes or 'maked a picture for Mummy' are using words they are unlikely to have been taught or even heard in that context. Rather, it appears that children have actively constructed the words by mistakenly interpreting or overgeneralising their grammatical understanding. For Chomsky, this was supportive of his view that a maturational process was primarily responsible for what he viewed as the unique human ability to construct language.

Perhaps one of the most persuasive arguments in support of Chomsky's perspective is the ease with which younger children can assimilate a new language or learn two languages simultaneously. However, critics of Chomsky's perspective have questioned whether it is realistic to suggest that children have an innate grammatical structure (Berk 1996), and argue that it would be unsafe to underplay the role of both parents and teachers in the development of meaningful language and purposeful communication.

THE INTERACTIONIST PERSPECTIVE

These views have led to a third, interactionist, perspective on language development. This viewpoint recognises both the inherent linguistic abilities of young children and the importance of education and social experience in informing and shaping these inherent processes. The perspective is supported by the work of Bruner (1983), who believes that a rich social environment is central to language acquisition, while at the same time acknowledging the importance of innate determinants of both linguistic and social behaviour. As an extension of this perspective, play is also seen as intrinsically linked to the language development process (Grieg 1998)

Vygotsky (1962) also acknowledged the fundamentally important contribution of both innate and social processes to language development. He further believed language was central to development of children's thought processes, with social exposure and language learning being gradually internalised by the child to become the human thought processes central to cognitive development. Thus, for Vygotsky, the acceleration of language learning was linked implicitly to accelerating cognitive developmental processes and children's abilities in a whole variety of other domains (Holaday et al 1994).

It is important that beliefs regarding links between linguistic and cognitive ability are not applied universally. There are significant numbers of children with little or no verbal language but highly sophisticated cognitive development (e.g. some children with cerebral palsy.) This can be at least partly explained by the observation that children's development of language comprehension occurs more rapidly than their ability to produce language (Berk 1996); the latter requiring additional cognitive and neuromuscular skills. However, there are also clear indications that children with delayed language development can struggle with a whole range of cognitive processes. For these children there appears to be a link between language and reasoning, and thus enhancing a child's language development through the provision of speech and language therapy can be the key that 'unlocks' other aspects of their cognitive development (Wood 1988). Furthermore, acceleration of language development, both comprehension and articulation, can enable many children to 'keep up' with their peers in mainstream education, when they would otherwise have lagged impossibly far behind.

PRACTICAL APPLICATIONS

In considering these perspectives on language development, a number of important considerations emerge for practitioners caring for younger children, particularly in hospital settings. These include the following two key perspectives:

- The importance of providing a **stimulating environment**, which maintains the child's exposure to social language. This is particularly important for children whose parents cannot be resident, for those requiring long-term admission and those requiring isolation. Infants with complex problems who spend many months in hospital, often in an incubator, are particularly vulnerable. Parents can be supported and encouraged in this provision of social language stimulation, and helped to understand the positive contribution they can make to their child's ongoing development. Indeed, recent work is attesting to the value of even 6-month-old infants being read to daily, and suggesting long-term benefits in cognitive and linguistic development (e.g. the 'Books build brighter babies' scheme run by BBC television and local libraries).

- The importance of knowing **normal developmental milestones** well enough to recognise a child whose language development may require additional support and intervention. More detail on this can be found in a range of texts of physical development and/or child assessment (e.g. Barnes 2003). Many children are helped enormously by speech and language therapy but a nurse might well be the first health professional to recognise that a child could benefit from such support, particularly if the family has had minimal contact with other health professionals. In the first instance, follow-up of such concerns are best made via the named health visitor (in the UK), who will know of current interventions. It is also useful to recognise that unless specific problems can be predicted due to a pre-existing condition, speech and language therapy does not normally commence until 3 years of age.

Reflect on your Practice

Sian, aged 3 years and 6 months, is admitted to your ward for routine surgery. She is the youngest of four children. During the admission process you observe that Sian is speaking only in single words, and also that these words are quite difficult for you to understand. You explore this concern with Sian's mother during the admission process but Sian's mother seeks to reassure you, saying:

'Oh, I'm not worried, I think it's just that her older brothers do all the talking and translating for her – she'll get there in the end.'

When you ask whether Sian's health visitor is concerned her mother says:

'Oh, I haven't seen her since Sian was about 12 months. If I don't know what I'm doing after four of them, then I never will!'

- Based on your experience and on your knowledge of speech and language development, are the mother's assumptions about Sian's language development correct?
- What actions should you take to ensure that your concerns are followed up?

Personality Development

As with other aspects of psychological development, the development of personality has been linked very strongly to the nature–nurture debate, focusing on the extent to which personality is innately inherited and predestined, and the extent to which it is shaped by society and environmental influences. Ultimately, here also one is left to conclude that both factors play a part. Innate determinants are clearly influential, as attested by studies of twins reared apart who display markedly similar personality traits (see Santrock 1999 for examples). However, experience undoubtedly also shapes personality, and two important theorists have contributed to these dimensions of our understanding of personality development, Erikson (1902–1994) and Freud (1856–1939). Although in many ways their work currently receives less recognition than that of the cognitive developmental theorists, they offer perspectives that greatly influence our understanding of many phenomena, such as infant attachment, child-rearing practices, moral development and sex role identification. There are consequently clear implications for child healthcare delivery.

ERIK ERIKSON

Erikson, like Piaget, offered a stage theory of development (Erikson 1950). Erikson's theories are fully summarised in Chapter 2 by Hemphill and Dearmun, but are discussed briefly here so that their place within developmental theory can be fully appreciated. Importantly, when compared with Piaget, Erikson's theories offer a far more holistic view of the individual. Furthermore, his stages were not restricted to childhood but rather reflected ongoing development throughout the lifespan, a psychological perspective that particularly gained popularity throughout the 1990s (e.g. Bee & Boyd 2003, Berger 2001, Berk 2001, Santrock 1999). Such a perspective is very important for practitioners who care for adults as well as children, and can even help child health practitioners' understanding of the parents and grandparents with whom they work.

Also in contrast to Piaget, Erikson's theory is readily accessible. It was published within a single volume *Childhood and society* (Erikson 1950) and later became available in a 'popular' paperback edition (Erikson 1965), which gave wide access to the lay public as well as the professional readership. The core of Erikson's work is his 'eight stages of man' (1965 Chapter 7 and see Table 2.1, p 23), which he sees as a series of conflicts thorough which the developing individual needs to pass. At any point in the process, a developmental conflict can have a negative effect on personality and future development. Importantly though, Erikson's stages cannot be seen as sequential. Although the age groups indicated are likely to represent the earliest point at which that stage becomes significant, the importance of each of the earlier stages is maintained to some extent throughout the lifespan, and is thus vulnerable at any point to deviation into the alternative path.

Activity

Turn to Chapter 2 (pp 18 to 32) and read Hemphill and Dearmun's summary of Erikson's stage theory before reading the rest of this chapter.

Links between Erikson's Work, other Developmental Theories and Care Delivery

1. Trust Versus Mistrust

As Hemphill and Dearmun describe in Chapter 2, trust is seen as the essential norm of babies' early experience, in the presence of food, sleep and other essential bodily functions. The infant's first real act of trust is 'to let the mother out of sight without undue anxiety or rage' (Erikson 1965 p 239), arguably based on a certainty that she will always be there to meet his or her needs. This may explain why the younger infant seems to derive positive comfort from parental presence, but not to protest strongly in its absence, in opposition to Piaget's notion of 'object permanence' – 'out of sight' and therefore 'out of mind'. Thus trust is seen to depend on the quality of the maternal relationship (later theorists would include the father and significant others). Although it is part of normal development to recognise the possibility that these support figures may not always be present (hence the protest on separation made by the older infant), prolonged parental separation can be seen to be intrinsically linked to development of 'mistrust', which Erikson would argue can even perpetuate into adulthood. It can thus be seen how closely Erikson's perspective links

with Bowlby's (1969) notion of 'attachment' and the need for the infant to have a close and continuous relationship with a 'mother figure' and significant others. It also links with the extensive work surrounding the harmful effects of hospitalisation by Robertson (1952) and others (see Chapter 5 or Taylor et al 1999 for a summary). The widespread belief in the importance of parental presence with children in hospital is testament to the value placed on these theories, and beliefs in the harmful effects of separation.

2. Autonomy Versus Shame and Doubt

As Hemphill and Dearmun explain in Chapter 2, the development of control within aspects of the younger child's world is seen as central to the development of autonomy. 'Shame and doubt' are seen as negative outcomes of this process. To use Erikson's own words:

> For if denied the gradual and well-guided experience of the autonomy of free choice (or if, indeed, weakened by an initial loss of trust) the child will turn against himself . . . (Erikson 1965 p 244)

From a nursing care perspective the negative consequences of lack of autonomy for the child will be inappropriate endeavours to gain control in any way possible. Examples could include such phenomena as inappropriate toileting behaviour (e.g. soiling or constipation) or, in an older child, more proactive processes of rebellion and even self-harm. Appropriate levels of autonomy are therefore vital for child health development, and these principles should be readily reflected in the care of sick or hospitalised children. Although many processes are essential to the child's well-being, choices such as 'which arm is used for a blood test', 'which parent accompanies them for a procedure' or 'whether something happens before or after breakfast', can all help to restore a sense of control for the child in what is often a very threatening and 'controlling' environment. The potential value of such choices to the child's well being cannot be overestimated.

Reflect on your Practice

Consider Cameron, a child admitted to hospital following a fractured femur. He is 4 years old and must stay on bed rest, on traction, for 5 weeks:
- What are some of the threats to Cameron's autonomy that exist as a result of this experience?
- What are the realistic choices Cameron can be given within his treatment and care delivery that can help to minimise the threats to his autonomy?

3. Initiative Versus Guilt

Initiative links in many ways to the notion of autonomy, and characterises development of understanding and the child's active construction of the world, concepts congruent with Vygotskian theory. Erikson sees initiative as fundamental to all learning processes. The child is seen as deriving pleasure from actively setting out to achieve certain goals, and indeed doing so. Key aspects of this stage, as detailed in Chapter 2 by Hemphill and Dearmun, are issues pertaining to psychosexual development. Here, important links with Freudian theory (which Erikson readily identified as influencing his work) can be seen; these will be discussed more fully in the next section.

'Guilt' is closely linked with initiative, in that the child will frequently overstep boundaries. He or she will encounter a range of negative emotions as a result of external, and increasingly internal, regulation of his or her inappropriate behaviour. This stage can thus also be very closely linked to the child's moral development (Santrock 1999). Erikson (1965 p 248) sees the consequence of these processes as the child becoming 'divided in himself' with internalised 'infantile' and 'parental' sets of guidelines emerging in parallel and influencing future aspects of behaviour. In the most extreme cases, children who encounter problems at this stage can require support from experts in child mental health. In contrast, however, most children show a more balanced adherence to 'both selves', requiring regular guidance but gradually achieving a sense of individual responsibility and 'self-regulation' as they progress through childhood.

4. Industry Versus Inferiority

This stage is seen as concurrent with the school age child and, as Hemphill and Dearmun describe in more detail in Chapter 2, reflects a central focus on learning and social development. These theories also have implications within the healthcare arena.

For many children, educational processes are continued in hospital settings and individualised programmes of learning are essential to ensure a child's self-esteem is not harmed by this different educational encounter. Also, some procedures that a child undergoes, such as 'bat ear repair', 'birth mark removal', 'hypospadias repair' or 'leg lengthening' will often have primarily social functions, including acceptance of children by their peers. Whereas some would justifiably debate the importance of changing 'societal acceptance of individual differences' rather than changing 'the individual who is different', the potential harm caused to children by teasing and bullying should not be under estimated. Thus although education of all children in accepting diversity is clearly vital, it is also important that in a fiscally dominated healthcare environment such seemingly 'non-essential' procedures are not lost to the private sector.

5. Identity Versus Role Confusion

This fifth (and final childhood) stage is characteristic of the adolescent and with the development of self-identity. As Hemphill and Dearmun explain in Chapter 2, adolescence represents a particularly turbulent time for the child.

Although the reality is that most adolescents 'make it', the potential negative outcome is 'role confusion', which can arise from any number of factors, e.g. uncertainty regarding sexual identity or orientation, uncertainty about future career paths, or coping with delayed physical development. In extreme cases such situations can have a profoundly negative effect on the individual's personality development. However, most adolescents normally experience some elements of 'role confusion', responding by what Erikson (1965 p 253) describes as 'overidentification, to the point of apparent complete loss of identity'. Such overidentification and associated peer pressure might be important influential factors in experimentation with drugs, smoking, alcohol and sexual activity. Thus the need for carefully targeted and insightful health promotion is paramount.

For adolescents who are sick, this can be a particularly difficult time to cope with illness. For many chronically ill children, social and physical development can lag behind that of their well peers, leading to teasing and feelings of alienation. Altered body image (e.g. hair loss in cancer) can also be particularly difficult for this age group to cope with. Even a brief hospital stay can be extremely traumatic, threatening privacy and dignity, new-found autonomy and the fragile sense of self-identity. Adolescent units are widely regarded as the ideal environment for this age group but, to date, most adolescents continue to be cared for in either paediatric or adult environments. Careful consideration must be given by healthcare practitioners to the psychological effects of hospitalisation in either setting and every effort made to minimise such harmful effects (see Taylor et al 1999).

Reflect on your Practice

Consider Lucy, an adolescent girl aged 13, recently diagnosed with leukaemia. She will require repeated hospital admissions and an extensive programme of chemotherapy:

- What might be some of the psychological challenges and risks Lucy faces during her period of illness?
- How can both hospital- and community-based practitioners help Lucy to minimise these risks and to emerge from her illness experience with a sense of 'identity' as opposed to 'role confusion'?

Activity

Smith & McSherry (2004) have published a concept analysis of children's understanding of spirituality, which is an important but often under recognised aspect of children's care delivery. They use Erikson's first five stages to frame their exploration of children's spiritual development:

- Based on what you now know about Erikson's theory, consider the different stages and how each might influence children's spiritual development. Then read the article and compare your thoughts and ideas with those offered by Smith & McSherry.

SIGMUND FREUD'S THEORY OF PERSONALITY DEVELOPMENT

Freud (1856–1939) belonged to a school of thought that is often referred to as psychoanalytic, in that it sought to explain individual differences in personality. Erikson represented the same school and his theories are more usually reported in texts after the earlier theories of Freud. Furthermore, Erikson regularly referred to Freudian theory in support of his own hypotheses about human development. However, whereas Erikson's holistic perspective remains widely respected, Freudian theory is often regarded as being somewhat eccentric and 'off beam', largely because of his beliefs around the domination of sexuality on personality development. Yet by relating Freudian theory to the previous consideration of Erikson's work, it can perhaps be seen that Freud's theory does retain some useful practical application for students of child development.

The Id, Ego and Superego

Freud (1938/1973, 1923/1974) (see also Berk 1996, Santrock 1999) recognised three facets of personality: the id, the ego and the superego:

- The id is the inherited component, biologically influenced and desiring immediate gratification of need.
- The ego is an emergent component, influenced by the environment. It regulates the id's desire for immediate gratification into socially acceptable channels.
- The superego is the final component, governing 'conscience'. It is therefore potentially in conflict with the desires of the id.

Parallels can thus already be seen with Erikson's notion of conflict within the different stages of development, which expand Freud's fundamental notions of the relationship between id, ego and superego in mediating individual desires.

Freudian Stages of Personality Development

Freud (1938/1973) further argued that there were five key stages of personality development (see also Santrock 1999, Berk 1996, Taylor et al 1999, Erikson 1965):

1. The Oral Stage (Birth to 1 Year)
This stage is dominated by the id, with the gratification of hunger being the primary drive that is satisfied by sucking

to take in nutrition. For Freud, lack of gratification of oral urges led to nail biting and thumbsucking, which he regarded as deviant behaviours. Lack of oral gratification has also been used to explain cigarette smoking and excessive eating by older children and adults.

However, 'non-nutritive sucking' of either a dummy/pacifier or fingers is seen as normal within infant development. Indeed, for an infant unable to feed orally, a pacifier is regarded as essential to maintain the sucking reflex. Furthermore, infants clearly derive a great comfort from sucking, which often extends well into childhood. It can be argued that denying the infant the opportunity to suck may be a contributor to the child developing parental 'mistrust' in Eriksonian terms, with consequent problems in the child's future personality development.

The importance of such beliefs is evidenced, for example, in the practice of 'sham feeding'. This historically allowed a child with a long-term gastrointestinal problem, which contraindicated oral feeding (such as tracheo-oesophageal fistula), to take in milk via the mouth and then collect it via an upper oesophageal stoma situated in the neck. This procedure is currently rare because it can be quite distressing for both child and parents. But the fact that it existed at all is testimony to the importance placed on oral stimulation in infant development.

2. The Anal Stage (1–3 Years)
In this stage Freud argued that pleasure was primarily gained from the processes of passing urine or having a bowel action. He argued that the role of the ego was to learn that the pleasure had to be appropriately channelled in time or place via the process of 'toilet training'. Thus for Freud a child 'potty trained' too soon may later develop obsession with order and cleanliness (hence the expression 'anally retentive'), whereas a child not properly trained at all is likely to demonstrate untidiness and an acceptance of mess and squalor.

Criticisms of Freudian theory include a rejection of his singular acceptance of the domination of anal pleasure at this point in life. Certainly, it would appear not only that oral pleasures continue but also that many other factors influence the child's experience of pleasure and his or her future personality development. However, in terms of Erikson's notion of autonomy, it can be seen that bladder and bowel function offers children powerful modes of exerting control over their parents or carers. Within normal development this might include the toddler who regularly 'needs a wee' in the middle of dinner (unless it is something he or she especially likes!) but it can also have more extreme manifestations. At a conscious or subconscious level constipation is seen as having significant psychological components for many children, and is frequently linked to other behavioural problems (Smith & Ward 2003). In terms of seeking attention, inappropriate passing of urine or faeces is also a good way for the desired attention to be achieved; remember a child who receives inadequate attention will often choose chastisement in preference to no attention at all.

Reflect on your Practice

Imagine you are caring for Matthew, a 4-year-old child who has been admitted with a history of severe constipation and soiling, which requires intervention under anaesthesia as well as laxative drug therapy. No physiological cause for the problem has been identified. His older brother, Jacob, has severe Down syndrome and his parents are currently considering separating:

- How might you consider Matthew's problems in Freudian and Eriksonian terms?
- What advice and support might his parents be given to help overcome the problem?

3. The Phallic Stage (3–6 Years)

This stage is perhaps the one that caused the greatest controversy when Freud's theories were first published. He argued that pleasure is now derived from genitally focused desires. He suggested that boys feel sexual desire for their mother but fear their father's disapproval. Consequently they end up identifying with the father and adopting the father's personality characteristics, behaviours and beliefs. For girls the reverse situation exists, i.e. paternal desire and maternal identification. Freud refers to these phases respectively as the oedipal phase and the Electra complex, and saw the resolution of this conflict as effectively the development of the superego and the individual's personality.

These theories have been widely and controversially used to describe a whole range of phenomena, including promiscuity, frigidity and deviant sexual behaviour. Evidence to support such beliefs remains minimal but many psychologists nevertheless retain some respect for aspects of Freudian theory. Links can be seen between the Eriksonian notion of 'guilt' and Freudian beliefs that morality and the conscience were products of the child's resolution of his or her desires for the opposite sex parent. However, although such extreme beliefs remain controversial, it would appear probable that, at some level, parental attitudes, behaviours and indeed relationships influence children's sexual development (Lips 1997).

For boys, Freud also described an important additional phenomenon he referred to as castration anxiety, which he saw as a fear of genital mutilation based on a belief that girls might have once had a penis that had been 'cut off' as a punishment. This theory is particularly pertinent for child health practitioners caring for boys who require procedures such as circumcision or hypospadias repair (hypospadias being a urethral opening not at the end of the penis; Atwell 1997). Boys with hypospadias, for example, often require repeated operations, and the psychological consequences of such experiences perhaps remain both under-recognised and under-researched.

4. The Latency Period (6 to Puberty)

For Freud, this stage was one in which sexual desire and instinct were repressed, hence the preference for friends of the same sex. Curiously, as the title 'latency' suggests, Freud believed little of importance would happen in the absence of sexual development. For Erikson, by contrast, this latency was put to good use in the notion of 'industry' as the child focuses on the processes of academic learning and ongoing social development.

5. The Genital Stage (Puberty Onwards)

This stage is characterised by the emergence of adult sexual desire, and all the repressed sexual desires of childhood can now be appropriately channelled into sexual relationships with partners. This forms an important part of Erikson's views of the adolescent's search for identity, although for Erikson it was balanced by recognition of other important factors in adolescent development. Nevertheless, sexual identity is recognised as a vital part of adolescent development and the perceived appropriateness or inappropriateness of various sexual activities would appear to be an ongoing and cyclic process within different cultures and generations. Currently, within Western society, views on sexual behaviour have been greatly influenced by the existence of effective contraception, and also more recently by the emergence of human immunodeficiency virus (HIV) (Lips 1997). Thus, although the 20th century saw a relaxation in attitudes towards sexual behaviour, there is an important need to convey responsibility around sexual behaviour and the risks of both pregnancy at young age and virus transmission. Child health professionals and schoolteachers are seen as having a pivotal role in the education of children and adolescents in the domain of sexual health.

Some Important Observations about 'Truth' and 'Understanding' in Developmental Psychology

When studying developmental psychology, including the range of seminal theories considered here, there are important observations to be made with regard to the difference between primary and secondary sources; recognition of these factors is important for any student of the subject. For example, when considering the work of Piaget it is usual for authors constructing a portrayal of his theory to use a whole range of secondary sources. The reason for this is that, for a significant proportion of his life, Piaget published virtually a book a year, and thus it is only at doctorate level that the student of Piaget can hope to comprehensively study his original work and synthesise from it an overview of his perspectives on child development. Even then they are likely to be reliant on someone else's translation of French into English! Furthermore, as Piaget grew older, his views and perspectives changed, and thus his assertions in the 1920s tend to differ somewhat from his perspective when he was still writing in the 1970s. But reliance on secondary sources is inevitably accompanied by a degree of risk in terms of the extent to which they truly represent what Piaget said; indeed it is probable that many texts have themselves used earlier secondary sources, and so on *ad infinitum*. (If you doubt this, one key original Piaget text borrowed for this chapter from a major university library had last been borrowed 13 years ago!) Consequently, the theory portrayed might have strayed somewhat from the original; distorted in the telling like a childhood game of 'Chinese whispers'. Thus the 'Piagetian perspective' on child development may be attributable as much to the speculation of others as to the work of Piaget himself.

In seeking to illustrate this point, the student seeking clear elucidation of the 'four stages of cognitive development', for example, is likely to have a long and difficult search through Piaget's original work. What one finds repeatedly is a range of developing ideas and debates (e.g. as in his 1929 *Children's conceptualisation of the world*). However, although Piaget (1929) is frequently cited as the source of the 'four stages' so widely quoted, these are at best implicitly contained within a series of observations he made of different children and their responses to various abstract questions. Even Piaget & Inhelder (1969), offered as a summary of Piaget's work 'so far', appears nearer to, but still someway off, the neat 'four-stage' theory with which we are familiar. By contrast, the student of Erikson's work will have no such challenges, being able to read the 'eight stages of man' within a single chapter of his original work (Erikson 1965).

What is important, then, is that all who cite the work of developmental psychologists – especially the seminal authors – must be sure always to acknowledge their sources, whether primary or secondary, and always try to use primary sources wherever possible. The importance of this is not only in seeking to minimise the 'Chinese whisper' effect but also in being able to openly acknowledge the inherent biases that different students of developmental psychology inevitably have. The author of this paper, for example, openly acknowledges and articulates her doubts about the appropriateness of many Piagetian theories to contemporary child health practice. But other authors will argue from a far more pro-Piagetian stance and in contrast might be much more critical of the work of Vygotsky or Erikson, for example.

Ultimately, then, it is up to each reader to make up his or her own mind based on the available information, opinion and evidence. The plea therefore within this chapter, is *not* for you to adopt 'wholesale' the theories and perspectives offered. Rather, it is that you read as widely and critically as possible, engage in debate with peers and professional colleagues, and take every opportunity to reflect upon the extent to which the different theories are borne out by current best evidence and practice experience. Only in this way can you make a fully informed decision about these theoretical perspectives and their practical application, and make judgements regarding which theories best inform contemporary healthcare practice and have the greatest potential to enhance care delivery.

Summary

This chapter has offered the reader a review of seminal and contemporary theories pertaining to children's psychological development. Particular emphasis has been placed on the importance of cognitive development, language development and personality development, as it is these aspects of psychological development that are seen as having particular relevance to the health care of children and families provided by the child healthcare practitioner.

In reviewing these theories, clear links can be seen throughout with the care that children and families receive. In particular, understanding of psychological theory can be seen as influencing communication with children, the quality of explanation giving, the quality of preparation and a minimising of the harmful effects of hospitalisation.

However, what the chapter has hopefully also offered the reader is an opportunity to reflect on the contrasting theories and theoretical perspectives that influence how psychologists, educators and healthcare practitioners view child development. In contrast to some aspects of care delivery, where best available evidence clearly supports a particular approach to treatment, aspects of psychological care are often subject to differences in opinion and ongoing debate. Thus, although few would debate the importance of minimising the potentially harmful effects of parent/child separation (for example), other aspects of psychological care remain a matter of opinion. Thus there is arguably an ongoing need for much more in the way of focused, applied research into many of the aspects of care delivery debated within this chapter.

This being said, it is hoped that the insight gained from studying this chapter will offer the student of children's nursing a useful guide to some of the key child developmental theories, and their potential application to children's nursing practice. Although physical care is infinitely more measurable than psychological care, the latter is arguably no less important in all but the most critically ill child. Thus if this chapter leads the reader to pause and consider the importance of these psychological perspectives within care delivery, then there is a very real chance that the insight gained could make a considerable difference to the quality of care which children and families receive.

References

Alderson P 1993 Children's consent to surgery. Open University Press, Buckingham

Alderson P, Montgomery J 1996 Children's services. What about me? Health Service Journal 106(5498):22–24

Atwell J 1997 Paediatric surgery, Arnold. London

Barnes K 2003 Paediatrics: a clinical guide for nurse practitioners. Butterworth Heinemann, Edinburgh

Bee H, Boyd D 2003 Lifespan development, study edn. Allyn and Bacon, Boston

Berger K 2001 The developing person through the lifespan, 5th edn. Worth Publishers, New York

Berk L 1996 Child development, 4th edn. Allyn and Bacon, Boston

Berk L 2001 Development through the lifespan, 2nd edn. Allyn and Bacon, Boston

Betz C 2000 California healthy and ready to work transition health guidelines: developmental guidelines for teaching health care self care skills to children. Issues in Comprehensive Pediatric Nursing 23(4):203–244

Bibace R, Walsh M 1980 Development of children's concepts of illness. Pediatrics 66(6):912–917

Bibace R, Walsh M (eds) 1981 Children's concepts of health, illness and bodily function. Jossey-Bass, San Francisco

Bird J, Podmore V 1990 Children's understanding of health and illness. Psychology and Health 4:175–185

Bluebond-Langer M 1989 Worlds of dying children and their well siblings. Death Studies 13:1–16

Bowlby J 1969 Attachment and loss, vol 1. Hogarth Press, London

Bruner JS 1972 The relevance of education. Allen and Unwin, London

Bruner JS 1983 Child's talk: learning to use language. WW Norton, New York

Burbach D, Peterson L 1986 Children's concepts of physical illness: a review and critique of the cognitive developmental literature. Health Psychology 5:307–325

Carey S 1985 Conceptual change in childhood. MIT Press, Cambridge, MA

Channel 4 Television 2001 The child as thinker. Part 4 of the 6-part series The child's world. Broadcast 10 January 2001. Channel Four Television, London

Chomsky N 1957 Systematic structures. Mouton, The Hague

Crisp J, Ungerer J, Goodnow J 1996 The impact of experience on children's understanding of illness. Journal of Pediatric Psychology 21(1):57–72

Donaldson M 1978 Children's minds. Fontana Press, Glasgow

Eiser C 1989 Children's concepts of illness: towards an alternative to the stage approach. Psychology and Health 3:93–101

Elliott E, Watson A 2000 Children's voices in health care planning. In: Glasper EA, Ireland L (eds) Evidence-based child health care. Macmillan, Basingstoke

Erikson E 1950 Childhood and society. WW Norton, New York

Erikson E 1965 Childhood and society, revised edn. Penguin, London

Freud S 1973 An outline of psychoanalysis. Hogarth Press, London (original work published 1938)

Freud S 1974 The ego and the id. Hogarth Press, London (original work published 1923)

Gaffney A 2000 Pain and Piaget: qualitative change with age in the content area about children's ideas of pain. The Irish Journal of Psychology 21:3–4, 194–202

Gaudion C 1997 Children's knowledge of their internal anatomy. Paediatric Nursing 9(5):14–17

Grieg A 1998 Play, language and learning. In: Taylor J, Woods M (eds) Early childhood studies. Arnold, London

Harbech C, Peterson L 1992 Elephants dancing on my head: a developmental approach to children's concepts of specific pains. Child Development 63:138–149

Hergenrather J, Rabinowitz M 1991 Age-related differences in the organisation of children's knowledge of illness. Developmental Psychology 27(6):952–959

Holaday B, LaMontagne L, Marciel J 1994 Vygotsky's zone of proximal development: implications for nurse assistance of children's learning. Issues in Comprehensive Paediatric Nursing 17:15–27

Ireland LM 1997 Children's perceptions of asthma: establishing normality. British Journal of Nursing 6(18):1059–1064

Kister M, Patterson C 1980 Children's conceptions of the causes of illness: understanding contagion and use of imminent justice. Child Development 51:839–846

Lips H 1997 Sex and gender: an introduction, 3rd edn. Mayfield Publishing, Mountain View, CA

Longsdon D 1991 Conceptions of health and health behaviours of pre-school children. Journal of Paediatric Nursing 6(6):396–406

McEwing G 1996 Children's understanding of their internal body parts. British Journal of Nursing 5(7):423–429

McGrath P, Huff N 2001 What is it? Findings of pre-schoolers responses to play with medical equipment. Child Care, Health and Development 27(5):451–462

Meadows S 1993 The child as thinker. Routledge, London

Oakley A, Bendelow G, Barnes J et al 1995 Health and cancer prevention: knowledge and beliefs of children and young people. British Medical Journal 310:1029–1033

Perrin E, Gerrity PS 1981 There's a demon in your belly: children's understanding of illness. Pediatrics 67(6):841–849

Perrin E, Perrin J 1983 Clinician's assessment of children's understanding of illness. American Journal of Diseases in Childhood 137:874–878

Piaget J 1929 The child's conception of the world. Routledge and Kegan Paul, London

Piaget J 1930 The child's conception on physical causality. Kegan Paul, Trench, Trubner and Co. New York

Piaget J, Inhelder B 1956 The child's conception of space. Routledge and Kegan Paul, London

Piaget J, Inhelder B 1969 The psychology of the child. Routledge and Kegan Paul, London

Robertson J 1952 A two-year-old goes to hospital (film). Cited in: Taylor J et al (eds) 1999 Nursing children: psychology, research and practice, 3rd edn. Stanley Thornes, Cheltenham

Rovee-Colyer C 1987 Learning and memory in children. In: Osofsky JD (ed.) Handbook of infant development, 2nd edn. Wiley, New York. Cited by: Santrock J 1999 Life-span development, 7th edn. McGraw Hill College, Boston

Rushforth H 1996 Nurses' knowledge of how children view health and illness. Paediatric Nursing 8(9):23–27

Rushforth H 1999 Practitioner review: communicating with hospitalised children. Journal of Child Psychology and Psychiatry 40(5):683–691

Santrock J 1999 Life-span development, 7th edn. McGraw Hill College, Boston

Schmidt C 2001 Development of children's body knowledge using lungs as an exemplar. Issues in Comprehensive Pediatric Nursing 24(3):177–191

Shaffer D, Bjorklund D 1999 Developmental psychology: childhood and adolescence. Brooks/Cole Publishing Company, Pacific Grove

Shayer M 2003 Not just Piaget, not just Vygotsky, and certainly not Vygotsky as an alternative to Piaget. Learning and Instruction 13(5):465–485

Siegal M, Peterson C 1999 Children's understanding of biology and health. Cambridge University Press, Cambridge

Skinner BF 1957 Verbal behaviour. Appleton Century Crofts, New York

Smith J, McSherry W 2004 Spirituality and child development: a concept analysis. Journal of Advanced Nursing 45(3):307–315

Smith L, Ward C 2003 Childhood constipation and encopresis. In: Barnes K (ed.) Paediatrics: a clinical guide for nurse practitioners. Butterworth Heinemann, Edinburgh

Taylor J, Woods M 1998 Early childhood studies. Arnold, London

Taylor J, Muller D, Wattley L, Harris P 1999 Nursing children: psychology, research and practice, 3rd edn. Stanley Thornes, Cheltenham

Travis A 1998 £5m extra for war on drugs. The Guardian, 28 April:2

Twycross A 1998 Children's cognitive level and perception of pain. Paediatric Nursing 14(1):35–37

Vacik HW, Nagy CM, Jessee PO 2001 Children's understanding of illness: students' assessments. Journal of Pediatric Nursing 16(6):429–437

Vessey J 1988 Comparison of two teaching methods on children's knowledge of their internal bodies. Nursing Research 37:262–267

Vygotsky LS 1962 Thought and language. MIT Press, Cambridge, MA

Vygotsky LS 1978. Mind in society. Harvard University Press, Cambridge, MA

Williams C 1995 Children's understanding of treatment in the A&E department. British Journal of Nursing 4(7):385–387

Williams J, Binnie L 2002 Children's concepts of illness: an intervention to improve knowledge. British Journal of Health Psychology 7(2):129–148

Wood D 1988 How children think and learn. Blackwell, Oxford

Yoos HL 1994 Children's illness concepts: old and new paradigms. Pediatric Nursing (US), 20(2):134–140

Chapter Twelve

12

Physical Growth and Development in Children

Janet Kelsey, Gill McEwing

ABSTRACT

This chapter will give the reader a broad understanding of the growth and development of children. Physical growth will be defined and methods of measurement discussed. Normal stages of child development are described and activities suggested to encourage the reader to make links with practice.

Learning Outcomes

- Define growth and development and understand how they can be assessed.

- Demonstrate an understanding of the anatomy and physiology of the newborn baby.

- Gain an overview of the development of the child from birth to adolescence.

- Be aware of the importance of assessing child development and the detection of deviations from normal.

Introduction

The physical development of the child is only one aspect of its whole development, which includes cognitive, social and emotional elements. Inherited attributes and environmental factors will affect physical development. These factors interact to cause effects on the child's development from conception to adulthood.

Activity
- Write down what you think is meant by the terms 'growth' and 'development'.

- Why might it be important to you as a nurse to have some understanding of the growth and development of children?

Babies and children vary considerably in exactly when and in what way they progress in all areas of development. It is not always appropriate to assign exact ages in months and years to stages of development, although an approximate age range is possible.

Factors Affecting Growth and Development

- Genetic/chromosomal factors: inherited rate of growth and individual differences.

- Racial factors.

- Endocrine system.

- Drugs.

- Illness: children grow more slowly during periods of illness but there might be increased growth to catch up after recovery.

- Nutrition: poorly nourished children grow more slowly and do not reach their full potential size; malnutrition can have a permanent effect on some parts of the brain and nervous system.

- Environment: the ability to practise skills, e.g. crawling, walking.

Other factors also govern growth and physical changes. Hormones are the most important of these (Table 12.1).

Table 12.1 The Hormones Involved in Growth and Physical Development

Gland	Hormone	Aspects of growth
Thyroid	Thyroxine	Normal brain development and overall rate of growth
Adrenal	Adrenal androgen	Involved in some changes at puberty, particularly the development of secondary sex characteristics in girls
Testes	Testosterone	Formation of male genitals before birth. Also triggers the sequence of changes in primary and secondary sex characteristics at puberty in the male
Ovaries	Oestradiol	Development of the menstrual cycle and breasts in girls. Less important than testosterone for secondary sex characteristics in boys
Pituitary	Growth hormone activating hormone	Rate of physical maturation Signals other glands to secrete hormones

Physical Growth

Physical growth and maturation is important for child development. Maturation is the:

. . . universal sequence of biological events occurring in the body and the brain that permits psychological function to appear, provided that the infant is healthy and lives in an environment containing people and objects (Mussen et al 1990)

Growth is defined as an increase in the size of and number of cells that results in an increase in size and weight of the whole, or any of its parts. In clinical practice, growth of the infant is generally measured by estimating the weight, length, head circumference and, in certain circumstances, skin-fold thickness.

PATTERN OF GROWTH

The most obvious thing about children's physical development is that they get bigger as they get older. Growth proceeds in a continuous pattern but is not smooth; the most rapid growth takes place in utero, the first 2 years of life and during adolescence (Fig. 12.1). However, acceleration and deceleration occur in response to illness and changes in nutrition or environment. As Fig. 12.1 shows, infants grow very quickly in the first year of life, adding 25–30 cm to their height.

Children gain weight at an equally rapid rate, doubling birth weight by the age of 5–6 months and tripling it by the end of the first year. The birth size of a normal infant is determined by the mother. Inherited factors, however, are one of the greatest influences affecting the final stature of the child. Although children tend to attain a stature between those of their parents, some children take after one parent, a grandparent or even a more remote member of the family.

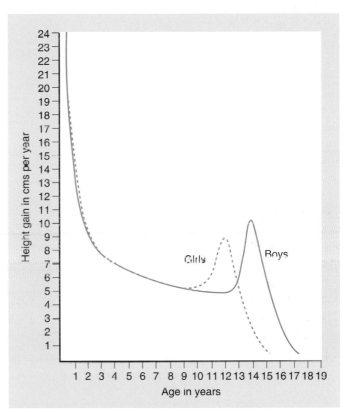

Fig. 12.1 • Rates of growth (adapted from Bee 1997).

MEASURING GROWTH

Length/Height

An infant's recumbent length is measured supine on a measuring board, placing the head firmly at the top of the board and the heels of the feet at the foot-board (Figs 12.2 and 12.3).

Height is the measurement taken when children are measured upright. Shoes should be removed and the child should stand as tall and straight as possible with the head in mid-line

Fig. 12.2 • Infant length.

Fig. 12.4 • Child height.

Head circumference Chest circumference Abdominal circumference

Head-to-heel length

Fig. 12.3 • Measurement of the head, chest, abdominal circumference and the recumbent length.

and the line of vision parallel to the floor. The most accurate measurement of height is gained by using a wall-mounted stadiometer (Fig. 12.4). It might be useful to remember that the height will be less when measured in the afternoon than in the morning. This effect can be reduced by applying modest upward pressure under the jaw or mastoid process.

Classic clues: height

The height of an infant increases by around 12 cm during the first 6 months of life. By the age of 1 year, the height has increased by almost 50% and by the age of 2 years an infant is about half as tall as he or she will be as an adult (Bee 1997). There is a rapid increase in size during the first 2 years, which then settles down to a slower and steadier rate: 5–7.5 cm in height per year and 3 kg in weight per year. Adolescence then brings a 'growth spurt', following which height and weight are slowly gained until adult size is achieved.

Weight

Infants should be weighed naked and preferably at the same time of the day. Older children can be weighed in light clothing without their shoes (Fig. 12.5).

Fig. 12.5 • Child weight.

Classic clues: weight

On average an infant gains 600–800 g in weight per month. An infant's weight at 6 months will therefore be almost double the birth weight. By the first year of life, weight has tripled.

Head Circumference

This measurement is important because the size of the skull is closely related to the size of the brain. It is usually recorded in children who are under 3 years of age or in cases where the growth of the brain/skull is under observation. It is advisable to use a paper disposable tape measure for this measurement as linen tape measures stretch and produce inaccurate results (Hockenberry et al 2003). The head should be measured around the point of greatest circumference, this is usually slightly above the eyebrows and pinna of the ears and around the occipital prominence at the back of the skull.

Classic clues: head circumference

The head growth of an infant is rapid. In the first 6 months the circumference increases by between 8 and 9 cm. By the first year there is an increase of 33% in the overall size of the head.

Surface Area

The child's surface area can be calculated once the height and weight of the child is known using the body surface area nomogram. This measurement is important for the prescription of some drugs.

Activity

Find a copy of the body surface area nomogram and calculate the body surface area for:
- a newborn weighing 3 kg and 50 cm in length
- a 6-year-old child weighing 20 kg and with a height of 115 cm.

Skinfold Thickness

Skinfold thickness is a quick and easy method of measuring subcutaneous fat that allows for the estimation of an individual's body fat.

The most common site for measuring skinfold thickness is the triceps; others include the subscapula, suprailiac, abdomen and upper thigh. The measurement is made by pinching the skin between two fingers and measuring the skinfold thickness using specially designed callipers (Fig. 12.6).

Bone Age

Bone age is a method of measuring skeletal maturity; the appearance of the epiphyseal centres is compared with standard charts. This is best achieved using the child's left wrist and hand, where the 20 bones can be judged against that recognised as the normal pattern of development.

Activity

Two groups of factors that strongly influence normal growth and development are heredity and environment. From your observations of children, give two examples from each group.

ASSESSMENT OF GROWTH

Centile charts have been developed using statistics of children's growth patterns. They give estimations of expected height, weight and head circumference for boys and girls at different ages. An infant usually has a similar centile at birth for head circumference and weight. Children of large parents tend to be towards the 90th centile and those of small parents tend towards the 10th, most will remain on these centiles for the rest of their lives. A common problem in the paediatric outpatient department is short parents who think that their child is not growing as expected because he or she is not as big as their peers. Plotting growth measurements confirms that the child's growth is normal and that the child's final size will be similar to that of the parents.

Fig. 12.6 • Skinfold thickness.

www

Go to:
- http://www.nelh.shef.ac.uk

Search for and read the growth reference charts, paying attention to the recommendations of the expert consensus group on the use of growth reference charts in the UK.

Some children resemble one parent more than the other in final size. If only their weights are recorded, they may appear to have faltering growth if father is small, or gaining weight excessively if father is tall. If weight is plotted against head circumference then they can be seen to be running in parallel, i.e. the whole of the child's size is approaching that of a particular parent.

Activity

Percentile charts provide a useful measure of normal growth. Different charts are available for boys and girls, for different age groups and for different cultures. Children may need to be assessed if they are above the 97th or below the 3rd centile. Some show height and weight measurements only, whereas others also show head circumference. To ensure that you understand the format of a percentile chart, look at a chart in your practice area and answer the following questions:
- What sex, age and measurements does it cover?
- Which percentiles does it show?
- Where on the chart would you find a child of abnormal growth?
- If Helen is 3.5 years and 98 cm tall, which percentile is she on?
- How many children fall below the 50th centile and how many above?
- John is on the 90th centile. Is he above or below the average for his age?

Activity

Plot the following weight, height/length and head circumferences on to growth charts from your practice area.

John (male)

Age	Weight (kg)	Head (cm)	Length (cm)
Birth (40 weeks)	3.5	34	51
6 weeks	5	38	56
20 weeks	7.25	42	66
36 weeks	9.75	46	72

Rebecca (female)

Age	Weight (kg)	Head (cm)	Length (cm)
Birth (37 weeks)	2.6 kg	34 cm	50 cm
4 weeks	4 kg	36 cm	52 cm
12 weeks	6.25 kg	41 cm	61 cm
40 weeks	9.25 kg	44.25 cm	68 cm

Growth charts give an early warning of some problems, such as obesity, which will be indicated by the child's weight starting to deviate upwards although the head circumference remains on the same centile.

Activity

Now complete some growth charts to demonstrate the probable recording for a child where there is:
- faltering growth
- obesity
- born of small parents.

CHANGES IN SHAPE AND PROPORTION

After 2 years, the rate of growth slows down and the child gains approximately 2.7 kg in weight each year until adolescence. Changes in proportion and shape take place at the same time. An adult's head is an eighth of his total height but in a 2-year-old the head is a quarter of the total body length. In addition to this, a 2-year-old has a large body and shorter legs in proportion to that of an adult (Bee 1997).

If a child is growing and his or her shape is altering then there must be changes occurring in the child's bones, muscles and fat. Bones increase in number, become longer and grow harder. Although bones are not all formed at birth, the newborn baby has virtually all the muscle fibres that will ever be needed. As a child grows, the muscle fibres get longer, thicker and less watery.

Development

According to the *Penguin dictionary* (Allan 2001), the definition of development is 'to bring out the possibilities of something, to acquire gradually'. It is the sequence of organic changes by which the fertilised ovum becomes the mature human being. An increase in complexity of the individual involves structure and function; the emerging of an individual's capacities through learning, growth and maturation. Maturation can be defined as an increase in competence and adaptability; a change in the complexity of a structure that makes it possible for that structure to work. Many of the debates about child development have centred on the nature versus nurture controversy. The former believe that human behaviour is guided by inborn factors and argues that differences are a result of heredity. Those who err towards nurture stress the importance of acknowledging the influence of a child's physical and social environment. According to them, individual differences are a result of the child's life experiences. The reality is probably somewhere in between. What is certain is that development is a complex process in which many variables play a part. We as nurses need to assess each child on an individual basis.

MEASURING DEVELOPMENT

Development is measured using developmental scales. It is divided into four major areas:

1. Physical: growth, vision, hearing, locomotion, coordination.

2. Cognitive: language and understanding.

3. Psychosocial: adapting to the society and culture to which the child belongs.

4. Emotional: control of feelings and emotions.

As with growth we need to have some idea of what is the norm. The charts by Sheridan (1975) and Frankenburg & Dodds (1967) (the Denver Developmental Screening Test) were developed to show what can be expected at key stages of development. Sheridan (1975) is a little didactic, she herself suggested that her charts should be used only by experienced professionals. The Denver scale is a little more flexible, allowing the assessor to accommodate the individuality of the child, although it is suggested that the user should be trained in the use of the scale.

Differences in Rate

There may be individual differences in the rate and timing of developmental progress, e.g. three perfectly normal infants may sit unaided at 5, 6 or 9 months. However, the sequence of developmental progress is always the same. A child may be consistently early, average or slow in development, e.g. a child whose bone development is slower probably walks later and eventually reaches puberty later.

The development of walking can be used to illustrate the factors that influence growth and development (Bee 1997):

- Newborn infants held with the sole of the foot on a table move their legs in a reflex walking action.
- By 8 weeks: infants briefly hold their head up if held in a standing posture.
- At 36 weeks: infants pull themselves up and remain standing by grasping furniture.
- At 48 weeks: infants walk forwards if both hands are held, or sideways if holding furniture.
- By 52 weeks: infants walk forwards if held by one hand.
- At 13 months: infants walk without help.

Factors Required for the Development of Walking

A complex set of changes in muscle, bone and nervous system:

- nutrition: for growth
- environment: in which to practice walking
- genetics: were the parents early walkers?

The child's ability to walk (or not) will also affect other areas of development such as social, emotional and intellectual.

Activity

From your experience of your own childhood, can you think of areas where the rate and timing of the development for certain skills was different between yourself and others. Make some notes about your ideas.

DEVELOPMENTAL ASSESSMENT

In the main, developmental assessments are performed by the child's health visitor and GP, although there might be occasions when a paediatrician will also perform them. These assessments include the evaluation of:

- locomotion or gross motor development referring to large muscle skills
- fine motor or manipulation skills: referring to small muscle skills
- hearing and speech
- vision
- social development, e.g. feeding, dressing and social behaviour.

To assess deviations from normal, it is first necessary to know about normal development. The development of a child between the ages of 0 and 18 months is very complex.

These are the major milestones and their approximate age of appearance:

- smile: 1–2 months
- laugh: 6 months
- sits (with support): 6 months
- sits (without support): 8–9 months
- crawls: 8–9 months
- stands/walks: 12 months
- pincer grip: 12 months
- delicate pincer: 18 months
- walks backwards: 18 months.

Activity

Watch a video showing different aspects of child development, find one at your university library or your local health promotion centre.

All aspects of development are interlinked. Skills are acquired sequentially; an example of this is the sequence of development of motor skills, which is often described as cephalocaudal, i.e. head (cephalo) to toe via the spine (caudal). So, initially, head control is developed before the baby is able to sit independently; this is followed by crawling and finally by control of the lower limbs for standing and walking. Each new skill usually appears at the most appropriate time to make use of information coming in to carry out activities to prepare for the next stage (Table 12.2).

It is important to know about child development to:

- teach and advise parents
- have reasonable expectations of the child
- be able to plan suitable activities and play
- be able to identify limits and capabilities
- be able to recognise deviations from the norm and be alert to regression (behaviour from an earlier stage of development), disability and abnormality.

Table 12.2 Interlinked Aspects of Development

Skill	Information	Activity	Next stage
Drawing	Holding pencil	Drawing	Writing
Running	Spatial awareness	Running	Football, dancing

Transition from Intrauterine to Extrauterine Life

This demands considerable effective physiological changes by the baby to ensure survival. Simultaneously, he or she has to make major adjustments in his or her respiratory and circulatory systems, as well as gaining control of his or her body temperature. The baby emerges to encounter, light, noise, cool air, gravity and tactile stimuli. Adaptation to extrauterine life involves the onset of respiration, circulatory changes and thermal adaptation.

ONSET OF RESPIRATION

Regular respirations begin 60–90 seconds after complete expulsion from the mother as a result of both chemical and thermal stimulation. Thermal stimulation is caused by the sudden cooling of the infant leaving the warm environment of the uterus (37.7°C) and entering the cold atmosphere of the outside environment (approximately 21°C). This cooling excites sensory impulses in the skin that are transmitted to the respiratory centre. In addition, low levels of oxygen, high levels of carbon dioxide and low pH initiate impulses that excite the respiratory centre. At term, approximately 100 mL lung fluid is present within the respiratory tract. Some fluid is expelled through the mouth, assisted by the pressure on the thorax during vaginal delivery; the remainder is absorbed via the pulmonary lymphatics during the first 24 h of life. The first breath requires a large pressure to open the terminal airways and overcome the initial stiffness of the lungs.

CIRCULATORY CHANGES

Separated from the placenta, the infant must make major adjustments within the circulatory system to divert deoxygenated blood to the lungs for reoxygenation. The transition from fetal to postnatal circulation involves the closure of the foramen ovale, the ductus arteriosus and the ductus venosus.

Fetal blood pressure (BP) is low as a result of low vascular resistance in the placental circuit. A systolic BP of around 76 mmHg is found at birth; this level rises to 96 mmHg by 4 weeks. Coughing, crying and straining raise the BP.

The Newborn Baby

MEASUREMENTS

The average measurements at the 50th centile are shown in Table 12.3. The weight of the infant at birth also correlates with the incidence of perinatal morbidity and mortality. At

Table 12.3 Newborn Measurements		
	Girls	**Boys**
Weight on 50th centile	3.4 kg	3.5 kg
Length on 50th centile	50 cm	51 cm
Occipitofrontal circumference on 50th centile	34.5 cm	35 cm

birth, head circumference head is usually 2–3 cm greater than the circumference of the chest.

APPEARANCE

- Head: one-quarter the body size (Fig. 12.7).
- Plump.
- Prominent abdomen.
- Lies in an attitude of flexion.
- Lusty cry used to evoke a response from attendants with a view to controlling environment.

THE SKIN

The skin has a film of vernix caseosa – a white sticky substance that is absorbed within a few hours and thought to have a protective function. The skin is thin and delicate; it is prone to blistering, infection and excoriation. Lanugo, downy hair, covers the skin and is plentiful over the shoulders, upper arms and thighs. Colour depends on ethnic origin.

Sebaceous glands are active late in fetal life and early infancy because of the high levels of maternal androgens. Plugging of the sebaceous glands causes milia. The epidermis and dermis are loosely bound to each other and very thin, friction such as removing sticky tape can separate the layers and cause blistering. The eccrine sweat glands (found mainly on the palms of the hands and the soles of the feet and forehead) are functional at birth and respond to heat and emotional stimulus. By the age of 43 weeks, palmar sweating can be used in pain assessment. The mature baby has many skin creases on its palms and soles; the nails are fully formed and adhere to the fingertips. Melanin levels are low at birth therefore the skin of the newborn is lighter than that it will be as a child, which means that young babies are more susceptible to the harmful effects of the sun. The hair is soft and silky; there may be lots or nearly none. The same is true for the eyebrows. The cartilage of the ears is well formed. The cord stump necroses and falls off within the first 10 days of life.

GENITALIA AND BREASTS

In both sexes the breasts may be enlarged in the period immediately after birth. They may also discharge clear fluid. This is due to the stimulation caused by maternal hormones; these effects subside in the first few weeks of extrauterine life (MacGregor 2000). There are nodules of breast tissue around the nipple. The testes are descended and the scrotum has plenty of rugae, the prepuce is adherent to the glans penis. The labia majora cover the labia minora.

THERMOREGULATION

Heat regulation is critical to the newborn baby's survival. The baby's capacity for heat production is adequate but several factors predispose to excessive heat loss. The newborn's large surface area increases the possibility of heat loss to the environment, although this is normally partially compensated for by their position flexion, which effectively decreases the amount of surface area exposed to the environment. The subcutaneous fat layer is thin, giving poor insulation. This also allows transfer of core heat to the environment and cooling of blood. The hypothalamus in the brain has the capacity to promote heat production in response to stimuli received to thermoreceptors. Babies cannot shiver, nor are they able to voluntarily increase muscle activity to generate heat. Infants do produce heat by non-shivering thermogenesis and that generated by the heart, liver, brain and skeletal muscles.

Fig. 12.7 • The newborn baby.

Noradrenaline (norephinephrine) is secreted by the sympathetic nerve endings in response to chilling and stimulates fat metabolism in brown adipose tissue (BAT); this is unique to the newborn baby. BAT has a greater capacity for heat production through intensified metabolic activity than ordinary adipose tissue. BAT is situated between the scapulae, around the neck, in the axilla, behind the sternum around the kidneys, trachea, oesophagus, adrenal glands and some arteries. However, this process does require energy, so the infant's oxygen requirement will increase. The regeneration of this tissue also requires good nutrition; a poor calorie intake will mean that the brown fat is not replaced and the infant will be less able to maintain body heat in a cool environment. Healthy, clothed infants will maintain their temperature provided the environmental temperature is maintained between 18 and 20°C, nutrition is adequate and movements are not restricted. The temperature of the newborn is 37.5°C, by the age of 13 years it has reduced to 36.6°C, this is because infants produce more heat per kilogram body weight than older children. The temperature regulatory system is immature in the newborn infant, rendering infants and small children susceptible to temperature fluctuations. Factors such as environmental temperature, increased activity, crying or infection can cause a rapid increase in body temperature in the infant.

EYES

At birth, the eyeball is too short for its lens therefore babies focus best at approximately 20 cm (Fig. 12.8). As the eyeball continues to grow, distance vision is achieved. The ciliary muscles are immature, limiting the ability of the eyes to accommodate and fixate for any length of time. Babies have been shown to demonstrate visual preferences for some colours

Fig. 12.8 • The eyes.

rather than others. No tears are present and eyes are easily infected. Corneal, papillary and blink reflexes are present.

HEARING

Once the amniotic fluid is drained from the external ear canal the acuity is similar to that of an adult. Babies can detect pitch, loudness and timbre of sound in addition to location and changes in complex sounds. The internal and middle ear is larger in proportion at birth and the external canal small. The mastoid process and the bony part of the external canal have not yet developed. The tympanic membrane and facial nerve are close to the surface and easily damaged.

RESPIRATORY SYSTEM

The respiratory system is developmentally incomplete. The lungs mature after birth and new alveoli continue to grow for many years. There are 20 million alveoli at birth, increasing to 300 million alveoli in the fully formed lungs of the adult (Meadow & Newell 2002). This means that infants and young children have a relatively small alveolar surface area for gaseous exchange. Airway resistance in children is high due to the small diameter of the respiratory tree. The lumen of the peripheral airways is narrow, which predisposes the infant to airway obstruction. The infant's breathing is mainly abdominal: the abdomen distends, the diaphragm contracts and the thorax expands. The chest wall is very compliant and therefore easily distorted, which can increase the work of respiration.

Babies are obligatory nose breathers and do not convert automatically to mouth breathing when nasal obstruction occurs. Respiratory rate is 30–60 per minute. Respirations are shallow and the pattern alters during sleeping and waking. Many term babies have periods of rapid breathing alternating with periods of breathing at a slower rate, or they may not breathe for periods of up to 15 seconds, this is normal as long as the colour and heart rate do not change significantly and the infant then begins to breathe again spontaneously (MacGregor 2000). Periods of apnoea, when breathing ceases for more than 20 seconds, are only common in babies under 32 weeks' gestation unless there is an underlying condition.

CARDIOVASCULAR SYSTEM

The heart rate is roughly 120–160 beats per minute and fluctuates with respiratory function, activity and sleep. It reaches a maximum at 1 month, after which there is a gradual slowing until adult levels at 12–16 years of age.

Peripheral circulation is sluggish and there may be mild cyanosis of hands and feet with mottling of skin when exposed.

Normal blood pressure ranges between 50/25 and 70/40 mm Hg. The amount of total circulating blood is 80 mL/kg or approximately 300 mL at birth. Haemoglobin (Hb) =15–2O g/dL; 70% is fetal Hb, which is replaced by adult Hb in the first 2 years of life. Mean cell volume (MCV)/100 L = 135 femtolitres = 10^{-12} g.

Breakdown of excess red blood cells in the liver and spleen predisposes to jaundice in the first few weeks. Prothrombin levels are low due to a lack of vitamin K. Colonisation of the intestine promotes synthesis of vitamin K. The white cell count is initially 18×10^9/L and reduces rapidly. Cardiac output is related to the heart rate and the stroke volume; as children have smaller hearts the stroke volume is reduced. The heart then needs to beat faster in order to oxygenate their body tissues.

RENAL SYSTEM

The newborn baby's kidneys weigh 23 g, this will have doubled by 6 months and trebled by the end of the first year (Sinclair 1991, cited in MacGregor 2000). The renal system is functional before birth but the workload is minimal. The infant is not able to concentrate or dilute urine very well in response to variations in fluid intake, and cannot compensate well for high or low solutes in blood. The ability to excrete drugs is also limited. However, the newborn can excrete amino acids and conserve sodium and glucose. The glomeruli are immature; they are resistant to aldosterone, which results in limited ability to concentrate the urine. This lack of ability to conserve or excrete water makes the baby vulnerable to dehydration. The glomerular filtration rate is 30 mL/min/m² at birth, 100 mL/min/m² at 9 months and reaches adult values at 1 year (Davenport 1996, cited in MacGregor 2000). Dehydration, hypotension and hypoxaemia all produce a fall in glomerular filtration rate so renal function becomes compromised very quickly in a crisis. Urine is voided by reflex emptying of the bladder. The first urine is passed either at birth or during the first 24 hours and then increases in frequency as the fluid intake increases. The specific gravity should be 1.020. After birth, the kidneys increase in size in proportion to body length, the weight doubling in the first 10 months as a result of tubular growth.

ENDOCRINE SYSTEM

The endocrine system produces limited quantities of anti-diuretic hormone from the posterior pituitary gland, thus making the infant more susceptible to dehydration.

The effect of maternal hormones may cause the labia to be hypertrophied and the breasts engorged.

GASTROINTESTINAL SYSTEM

This system is structurally complete but functionally immature. The teeth are usually still buried in the gums. Sucking pads in the cheeks give them a full appearance. Sucking and swallowing reflexes are coordinated.

The stomach's capacity at birth is approximately 10–20 mL, although this increases rapidly in the first few weeks of life up to 150 mL by 1 month. The cardiac sphincter is weak, making the baby prone to regurgitation or possiting and gastric emptying time is 2.5–3 h. Hydrochloric acid is present in the stomach at birth but, due to swallowing of amniotic fluid, the pH is nearly neutral. Acid secretion commences within 8 h of birth and digestion in the stomach is then reliant on the action of hydrochloric acid and rennin to cause the formation of curds by coagulating the casein in milk. Human milk contains e-fructose, a bacterium that raises the acidity of the gut inhibiting the growth of *Escherichia coli* bacteria. Adult levels of acid secretion are reached by the age of 10 years.

INTESTINE

The breakdown of most food occurs in the intestine. In the young infant the colon has a small volume and therefore results in frequent bowel movements. Food reaches the caecum in about 4 h. The breakdown of protein into large polypeptides is brought about by pepsin and hydrochloric acid. Subsequent breakdown into amino acids occurs by the action of the pancreatic enzymes, trypsin, chymotrypsin and polypeptides, and by enzymes derived from the small intestinal mucosa, such as enterokinase. Hence enzymes are available to catalyse proteins and simple carbohydrates but deficient production of pancreatic amylase impairs utilisation of complex carbohydrates. A deficiency of pancreatic lipase until 4–5 months of age reduces the infant's capacity to convert fat into fatty acids and glycerol. The gastrocolic reflex opens the ileocaecal valve so that feeding is often accompanied by emptying of the bowel and meconium, which is present in the large colon from 16 weeks gestation is normally passed within 24 h and totally excreted within 48–72 h. Meconium is blackish in colour, tenacious and contains bile, fatty acids, and mucous and epithelial cells. Following passage of the meconium, the stools change to brownish yellow, their frequency and consistency depending on the method of feeding. Breastfed babies stools are loose, bright yellow and inoffensive. Bottle-fed babies stools are paler, semi-formed and have a sharper odour, there is an increased tendency to constipation.

The liver occupies 40% of the peritoneal cavity at birth (MacGregor 2000). There is decreased activity of the enzyme glucuronyl transferase, which is needed to conjugate bilirubin resulting in physiological jaundice of the newborn. The liver also stores less glycogen leaving the infant susceptible to hypoglycaemia.

Absorption of Minerals and Vitamins

Vitamin B is absorbed from the terminal ileum. Iron, calcium, magnesium, sodium, potassium, ascorbic acid, folic acid and water-soluble vitamins are absorbed from the proximal small intestine.

Activity

Find out what advice is given to the parents of newborns regarding feeding. How does this relate to the absorption capabilities of the infant's stomach and intestines?

Reflect on your Practice

- Explain to a junior nurse or parent why newborn babies are at risk of jaundice.
- How do babies digest cows milk?

IMMUNOLOGICAL ADAPTATIONS

There are three main immunoglobulins: immunoglobulin G (IgG), immunoglobulin A (IgA) and immunoglobulin M (IgM). Infants are unable to produce their own immunoglobulins until 5 weeks old. IgG can cross the placenta so that at birth the baby's level is as high as the mother's. Breast milk, and especially colostrum, provide the infant with additional IgG. This gives passive immunity for the first few months of life, which gives the infant protection against most of the major childhood illnesses such as diphtheria, measles, poliomyelitis and rubella for about 12 weeks, provided the mother has antibodies to these diseases. The fetus can manufacture IgM and IgA but it takes 2 years to achieve adult levels. IgA protects against infections of the respiratory and gastrointestinal tract and eyes. The thymus gland, where lymphocytes are produced, is relatively large at birth and continues to grow until 8 years of age.

REPRODUCTIVE SYSTEM

Spermatogenesis does not occur until puberty. The total complement of primordial follicles containing primitive ova is present in the ovaries at birth.

SKELETOMUSCULAR SYSTEM

All muscles are present at birth, although the muscle tissue is 35% water. The long bones are incompletely ossified allowing for growth at the epiphyses. The bones of the skull are incompletely ossified essential for growth of the brain and moulding during labour. Moulding is resolved within a few days of birth. The posterior fontanelle closes within 6 weeks and the anterior fontanelle remains open for up to 18 months. This allows assessment of intracranial pressure by palpation.

In ventral suspension the head droops below the plane of the body (Fig. 12.9).

Pulled to sit there is marked head lag (Figs 12.10 and 12.11).

Fig. 12.9 • In ventral suspension, the head droops below the plane of the body.

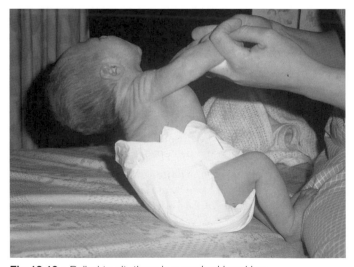

Fig 12.10 • Pulled to sit, there is a marked head lag.

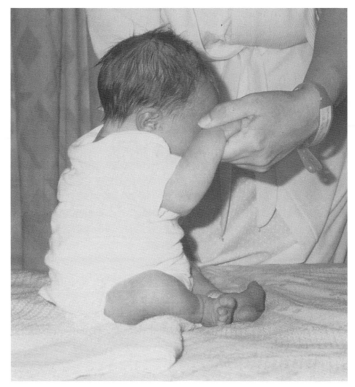

Fig 12.11 • Pulled to sit, there is a marked head lag.

NEUROLOGICAL SYSTEM

Compared with other systems this is very immature both anatomically and physiologically at birth. The most fully developed parts of the brain are the medulla (or hindbrain) and the midbrain. The least developed part is the cortex. This is no surprise when you consider the function of these areas of the brain and the abilities of the newborn/older child:

- The medulla is in the lower part of the skull and regulates sucking, breathing, heart rate, body temperature and muscle tone.
- The midbrain governs attention, sleeping, eating and eliminating. This part of the brain is similar to the brain of lower animals, i.e. the primitive reflexes are in control.
- The cortex governs perception, body movements, complex thinking and language. It follows that development of certain areas of the cortex sets limits on the development of the child's motor and perceptional skills.

The nerve cells or neurons of the brain are present at birth but the neurons of the cortex are not well connected. Over the first 2 years of life, the number and density of the dendrites, and speed of the synapses, increase rapidly, along with the size of individual neurons and the total weight of the brain (Bee 1997). At birth the spinal cord is not fully myelinated. Fibres that are not myelinated conduct slowly

and inefficiently. Myelination of the nerves leading to and from the brain is almost complete by the time the child is 2 years old. Myelination and growth of connective tissue continues until adolescence. After birth, brain growth is rapid, requiring constant and adequate supplies of oxygen and glucose. The immaturity of the brain renders it particularly vulnerable to hypoxia, biochemical imbalance, infection and haemorrhage. Temperature instability and uncoordinated muscle movement reflect the incomplete state of brain development and incomplete myelination of the nerves.

A neonate is equipped with many reflexes, the presence of which indicates normality and integrity of the neurological and skeletomuscular system. Reflexes are automatic physical responses triggered involuntarily by a specific stimulus. Many of these reflexes are still present in adults (e.g. the knee jerk, automatic eye blink when a puff of air hits the eye, and the involuntary narrowing of the pupil when exposed to a bright light).

The newborn infant also has a set of 'primitive' reflexes. These are controlled by the more primitive parts of the brain: the medulla and the midbrain. By about 6 months, when the portion of the brain governing more complex activities such as perception, body movement, thinking and language has developed more fully, these primitive reflexes begin to disappear, as if superseded by the higher-level brain functions.

Some primitive reflexes are essential for survival, such as the breathing reflex and the reflexes involved in eating. Infants who are touched on the cheek will automatically turn towards the touch and search for something to suck on; this is the rooting reflex (Fig. 12.12). The suck reflex is demonstrated when infants locate a suitable object that fits in the mouth and automatically begin to suck and swallow.

There are other primitive reflexes that do not have an obvious use. Infants who are confronted with a loud noise

Fig 12.12 • The rooting reflex.

or some kind of physical shock will throw their arms outward and arch their back; this is the startle reflex. The Moro reflex occurs when the baby suffers a change in equilibrium or sudden jarring, which causes tension and abduction of the extremities and fanning of the fingers, followed by flexion and adduction of the extremities and the infant may cry (Fig. 12.13). The step reflex can be demonstrated by holding the baby so the sole of the foot touches a hard surface, this causes a reciprocal flexion and extension of the leg simulating walking (Fig. 12.14). If you touch an infant on the bottom of the foot, the Babinski reflex will be demonstrated when the toes are first splayed out and then curled in. If you touch an infant on the palm of the hand, his or her fingers will curl around your hand and hold on tightly, this is called the grasp reflex.

These reflex patterns are interesting not only because they may be remnants from our evolutionary past but because their presence past the age of roughly 6 months may signal the existence of some kind of neurological problem. The Babinski reflex is used as a diagnostic tool by neurologists who suspect the existence of some dysfunction.

Fig. 12.14 • The step reflex.

1 Month to 2 Years

AGED 1 MONTH

After birth, the rate of weight gain and growth in length accelerates to reach a maximum velocity between 4 and 6 weeks. The velocity of growth then declines rapidly until 4–5 years. Weight has a similar growth curve to height. Other organs show variations in their growth curve.

Posture and Large Movement

When the baby is pulled to sit, the head lags until the body is vertical (Fig 12.15) when the head is held momentarily erect before falling forward.

Fig. 12.13 • Moro reflex.

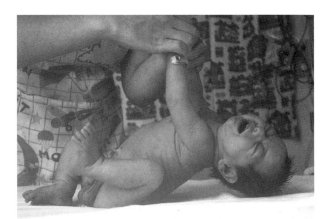

Fig 12.15 • When pulled to sit, the head lags until the body is vertical.

When held sitting, the back is one complete curve (Fig. 12.16).

In ventral suspension, the head is in line with the body and the hips are semi-extended (Fig. 12.17).

Vision and Fine Movement

- Pupils react to light.
- Turns head and eyes to light source.
- Follows pen torch briefly with eyes at 25 cm.
- Shuts eyes tightly when light is shone in them.
- Fixes and follows.
- Watches mother's nearby face when she feeds or talks to him with increasingly alert facial expression.

Hearing and Speech

- Startled by sudden noise.
- Stops whimpering and (usually) turns towards sound of nearby soothing voice, but not when screaming or feeding.
- Cries lustfully when hungry or uncomfortable.
- Guttural noises when content.
- Coos responsively to mother's talk from 5 to 6 weeks.

Social Behaviour and Play

- Sucks well.
- Sleeps most of the time when not being fed or handled.
- Expression still vague: more alert later, progressing to social smile and responsive vocalisations at 5–6 weeks. Hands are normally closed but fingers are grasped when palm is touched.
- Stops crying when picked up and spoken to. Turns to regard nearby speaker's face. Needs head support when being carried, dressed or bathed. Passive acceptance of bath and dressing routines gradually changes to an increasing awareness and response.

6-WEEK CHECK

The 6-week examination should include a physical examination and assessment of alertness, vision and motor function.

Vision

The infant turns to regard the speaker's face (Fig. 12.18). The infant holds gaze and follows to 90° – failure to do so

Fig. 12.16 • When held sitting, the back is one complete curve.

Fig. 12.17 • In ventral suspension the head is in line with the body and the hips are semi-extended.

Fig. 12.18 • 6-week check.

is not normal but may be due to distraction. Infants who do not follow should be rechecked at 8 weeks.

Motor Function

When placed prone, infant will lift their head for a few seconds. Infants who normally sleep prone are more advanced at this than others. Infants who fail this test should be retested 2 weeks later.

Other Assessments

The testes and hips should be assessed. It is difficult to detect a dislocated hip at 6 weeks as this should have been detected at birth. Normal infants will respond to sound by stopping crying, opening eyes widely or startle reflex.

AGE 6 WEEKS UPWARDS

Sleep

At 3–7 months infants sleep through the night with two or three short naps during the day. Rapid eye movement (REM) sleep is less frequent by 6 months and levels off at 25–30% total sleep time. There are four stages to sleep:

1. drowsiness
2. sleeping: easily wakened
3. sleep becomes increasingly deeper: heart rate stable, muscles relaxed, brain waves slow
4. deepest: difficult to rouse from.

A single night-time sleep contains all four stages arranged in cycles. The length of the sleep cycle gradually increases with age.

Skeletal System

The growth and development of bone consists of two processes, which occur at the same time: the creation of new cells and tissue and the consolidation of these tissues into a permanent form. The number of bones increases in the hand, wrist, ankle and foot. New centres of ossification in bones of hand and wrist are present at 5–6 months. These are useful for determining skeletal age. The length of the bones, particularly the long bones of the arms and legs, also increases to attain increase in height. Infant bones contain much more water than those of the adult, which makes them softer and more malleable (this ability to bend enabled the fetus to curl up inside the uterus). The bones of the skull are joined together as the fontanelles fill with bone; this process is usually complete by the age of 2 years. The ossification process takes place throughout infancy to

adulthood. Girls mature faster than boys. At birth, girls are 5–6 weeks ahead in level of skeletal maturity.

3 MONTHS

Posture and Large Movement

- Supine: prefers to lie with head in midline, limb movements smooth (Fig. 12.19).
- Pulled to sit: little or no head lag (Fig. 12.20).
- Held sitting: the back is straight except for lumbar region (Fig. 12.21).
- In ventral suspension: head held well above line of body (Fig. 12.22).
- Prone: lifts head and upper chest, uses forearms for support, buttocks flat (Fig. 12.23).

Fig. 12.19 • When supine, prefers to lie with head in midline, limb movements smoother.

Fig. 12.20 • Pulled to sit, there is little or no head lag.

Fig. 12.21 • Held sitting, the back is straight except for the lumbar region.

Fig. 12.22 • In ventral suspension, the head is held well above the line of the body.

Fig. 12.23 • When prone, lifts head and upper chest and uses forearms for support; the buttocks are flat.

Vision and Fine Movement

- Visually alert, responds to nearby human face.
- Turns head deliberately to look around.
- Follows hanging ball at 30 cm through 180°.
- Watches movements of own hands and demonstrates finger play.
- Recognises feeding bottle and makes eager movements as it approaches.
- Defensive blink present.
- Holds rattle for a few seconds but doesn't look at it at the same time.

Hearing and Speech

- Sudden loud noises still cause distress, eyes close tightly and the infant cries.
- Definite quietening or smiling in response to mother's voice.
- Vocalises happily when spoken to, can also vocalise when playing alone.
- Cries when uncomfortable or angry.
- Sometimes sucks or licks lips when food is being prepared.
- Demonstrates excitement when hears people approaching.

Social Behaviour and Play

- Intense gaze at mother's face when being fed.
- Reacts to familiar situations by showing excitement.
- Enjoys bathing.
- Responds with obvious pleasure when played with.

6 MONTHS

Posture and Large Movement

- Supine: raises head to look at feet, lifts legs into vertical and grasps feet (Fig. 12.24).
- When hands are held: braces shoulders and pulls self to sit (Fig. 12.25).
- Held sitting: head firmly erect, back straight. Can sit momentarily alone (Fig. 12.26).
- Held standing: bears weight on feet and bounces up and down.
- Can stand momentarily when holding on to furniture (Fig. 12.27).
- When placed prone: lifts head and chest well up, supporting him- or herself on extended arms (Fig. 12.28).

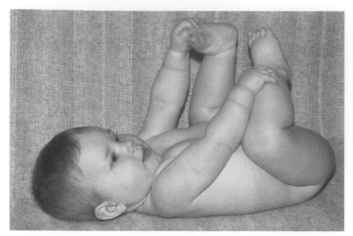

Fig. 12.24 • When supine, raises the head to look at the feet, lifts legs into the vertical and grasps the feet.

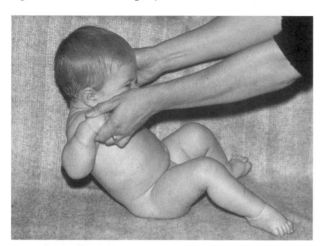

Fig. 12.25 • When the hands are held, braces shoulders and pulls self to sit.

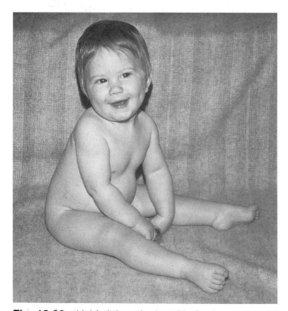

Fig. 12.26 • Held sitting, the head is firmly erect and the back is straight. Can sit momentarily alone.

Fig. 12.27 • When held standing, bears weight on feet and bounces up and down. Can stand momentarily holding on to furniture.

Vision and Fine Movement

- Visually insatiable, moves head and eyes eagerly when attention attracted.
- Shows interest and watches adult movements at a distance.
- Eyes move in unison.
- Immediate fixation on interesting small objects at 30 cm.
- Uses whole hand to palmar grasp and passes object from one hand to the other.
- When toys fall outside visual field: does not follow them.

Hearing and Speech

- Turns immediately to mother's voice.
- Vocalises tunefully to self and others
- Using single or double syllables: 'adah', 'goo', 'aroo'.
- Laughs and chuckles.
- Screams with annoyance.
- Demonstrates different responses to mother's tone of voice.

Fig. 12.28 • When placed prone, lifts head and chest well up, supporting self on extended arms.

Social Behaviour and Play

- Reaches out and grasps small toys.
- Takes everything to mouth.
- Plays with feet and hands.
- Puts hands around bottle and pats it.
- Shakes rattle deliberately to make sound.
- Manipulates objects attentively passing from hand to hand.
- Friendly with strangers but does show some anxiety if approached too quickly.

THE 8-MONTH CHECK (Fig. 12.29)

Mothers are asked if there have been any problems or illnesses since the last check. They are asked if the infant is making sounds and for details of the diet including whether the infant is chewing solids. Alertness and interest, weight and length are checked.

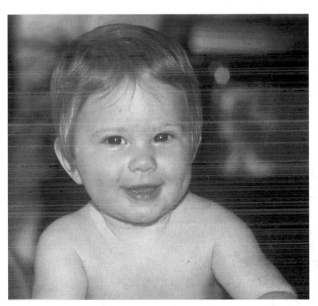

Fig. 12.29 • The 8-month check.

Vision

Near vision can be tested by placing a small pellet about 20 cm in front of the infant and seeing whether he or she reaches out for it. Distance vision is not usually tested at this stage.

Motor Function

- From the prone position: infants should get up on their wrists.
- When pulled from supine: they should be able to sit spontaneously for a minute or two.
- Children can normally sit without help at 8 months (Fig. 12.30); they should be able to take their weight on their legs when they are held standing.
- If a cube is placed in front of them, infants should grab it with their whole hand (Fig. 12.31) (test both left and right hands). Infants should transfer objects from one hand to the other.

Hearing

The distraction method is the hearing test used at this age. The distracter holds the infant's attention while the tester produces a sound. Careful attention to detail is essential

Fig. 12.30 • 8-month infants can sit without being held.

Fig. 12.31 • 8-month infants pick up and explore objects presented to them.

to produce reliable results. The most common reasons for failure to respond to sound are tiredness, lack of interest, distraction, ear wax, otitis media and lack of familiarity with the test sounds. Infants who fail this test should be retested 2 months later. At 8 months, infants normally respond to their own name.

1 YEAR (Fig. 12.32)

Posture and Large Movement

- Crawls on hands and knees, shuffles on buttocks or bear walks.
- Usually able to stand alone, may walk.

Vision and Fine Movement

- Looks in correct place for toys dropped out of sight.
- Recognises familiar people at 7 m distance.

Hearing and Speech

- Turns immediately to own name.
- Comprehends simple instructions associated with gesture, e.g. 'come to mummy'.

Social Behaviour and Play

- Drinks from a cup.
- Waves 'bye-bye', plays 'pat-a-cake'.
- Helps with dressing, e.g. holding out arm for sleeve.

Fig. 12.32 • 1 year.

18 MONTHS

Posture and Large Movement

- Walks competently, starts and stops safely.
- Walks upstairs with hand held.

Vision and Fine Movement

- Picks up small sweets, beads, etc. with delicate pincer grasp (Fig. 12.33).
- Beginning to show a preference for using one hand.
- Enjoys simple picture books, recognises objects.
- Builds tower of three cubes (Fig. 12.34), knocks it down.

Hearing and Speech

- Uses 6–20 words and understands more.
- Attempts to sing.

Social Behaviour and Play

- Holds spoon, gets food safely to mouth (Fig. 12.35).
- Takes off clothes but unable to dress self.

The physiological Changes of a Toddler

The physical appearance is squat with a pot-belly and slightly bowed legs (Fig. 12.36); by preschool children become more slender and graceful.

The rate of increase of head circumference slows with head and chest having roughly the same circumference by 1–2 years of age. In the second year the increase in head

Fig. 12.33 • 18 months.

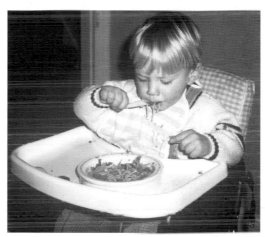

Fig. 12.35 • Social behaviour and play.

Fig. 12.34 • Vision and fine movement.

Fig. 12.36 • Physical appearance.

circumference is 2.5 cm. By 5 years the rate of increase has reduced to 1.25 cm a year. Between 12 and 18 months the anterior fontanelle closes (Hockenberry et al 2003).

Myelinisation of the spinal cord is almost complete by 2 years of age and brain growth is 75% complete. As specific areas of the brain develop, the child progresses developmentally, e.g. as the cortex develops then better control of the arms, legs and feet is gained.

During infancy, the capacity of the stomach increases to allow digestion of three meals a day and milk in the evening. Bowel movements have reduced to one or two a day, although bowel irregularity is common as the infant changes from a bland simple weaning diet to that of the family. Young children cannot control their bowel until they develop central nervous system control, although the tendency to defaecate after breakfast is often taken advantage of. Children have daytime control of their bowel movements from about 24–30 months old (MacGregor 2000).

The skin matures during early childhood, with the epidermis and the dermis becoming more tightly bound together thus the effectiveness of the skin as a barrier to infection and against fluid loss is improved.

The child's ability to maintain body temperature improves, with the capillaries constricting and dilating in response to cold and heat and shivering as an effective means of thermogenesis.

The volume of the respiratory tract increases but the internal structures of the ear and throat continue to be short and straight with the lymphoid tissue of the tonsils and adenoids large, which predisposes the young child to otitis media, tonsillitis and upper respiratory tract infections.

Metabolism

This is affected by an assortment of intrinsic and extrinsic factors. The basal metabolic rate (BMR) is highest in newborns. BMR closely relates to the proportion of surface area (SA) to the body mass, which decreases with maturity. The rate of metabolism determines caloric and protein requirements (Table 12.4). During illness, needs can be high.

There is an increased metabolic rate (about twice that of an adult) and an increased respiratory demand for oxygen consumption and carbon dioxide elimination.

Table 12.4 Recommended Daily Requirements of Calories and Protein

	Energy allowance (kcal/kg)	Protein (g)
0–6 months	108	13
6 months to 1 year	98	14

The proportion of energy intake used to build and maintain tissue changes as the child grows:

- birth: 40%
- 3 months: 40%
- 1–2 years: 20%
- 9–11 years: 4–10%.

Respiratory System

Overall lung growth has been measured in children using annual radiographs. Lung width and length follows a similar growth curve to overall height, with an adolescent growth spurt. Boys are on an average larger than girls in all lung dimensions.

The number of alveoli increases after birth reaching 90% at age 4 years. By the age of about 10 the increase in alveoli ceases and is followed by an increase in size. The total capacity of a child's lungs increases from 1.4 L in the 5-year-old child to 4.5 L at the time of puberty (MacGregor 2000). The ribs lie more horizontally in infants and contribute less to chest expansion. This results in infants and young children breathing diaphragmatically and respiration rate therefore is observed by watching abdominal movement rather than the movement of the chest.

The muscles are more likely to fatigue than those of adults and young children are more prone to respiratory failure. Anything that impedes diaphragm contraction or movement, e.g. abdominal distension, can contribute to the development of respiratory failure. The sternum and ribs are cartilaginous, the chest wall is soft and the intercostal muscles are poorly developed. In the event of illness, the infant's chest wall may move inwards instead of outwards during inspiration (retractions).

Smooth muscle is present throughout the lungs at birth and bronchospasm can occur even in the very young infant.

Lymphatics: B and T Cell Systems

The total amount of lymphoid tissue in the body (thymus, lymph nodes and lymphoid tissue of gut) increases throughout childhood.

 Activity

What childhood illness is a particular indicator of this growth and what common surgery is carried out?

Dental Eruption

Deciduous Teeth (Fig. 12.37)
- Incisors: 6–9 months
- Canines: 16–19 months
- 1st molars: 10–15 months
- 2nd molars: 16–27 months.

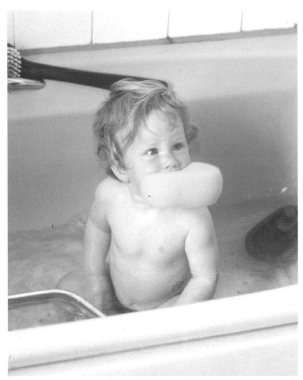

Fig. 12.37 • The pain and irritation of teething is relieved by biting.

Salivary Glands

These start to function at 2–3 months; hence this is when babies start drooling.

Activity

Think of the implications of malnutrition and understimulation on a young infant.

NORMAL OBSERVATIONS

Respiration

1–11 months: 30/min.

Heart Rate: 3 Months–2 Years

- Resting awake: 80–150 bpm.
- Sleeping: 70–120 bpm.
- Exercise or fever: up to 220 bpm.

Temperature

- 37.5°C.

Blood Pressure

Table 12.5 shows blood pressure by age.

Table 12.5 Blood Pressure (mmHg) by Age		
Age	**Girls**	**Boys**
3 months	89/51	91/50
6 months	91/53	90/53
12 months	91/54	90/56

General Trends in Height and Weight Gain during Childhood

WEIGHT GAIN

Table 12.6 shows weight gain by age.

Table 12.6 Weight Gain by Age	
Age	**Weight gain**
Birth to 6 months	Weekly 140–200 g
	Doubles by end of 4–7 months
6–12 months	Weekly 85–140 g
	Triples by end of first year
Toddlers	Yearly 2–3 kg Quadruples age 2.5 years
Preschoolers	Yearly 2–3 kg

HEIGHT

Table 12.7 shows height gain by age.

Table 12.7 Height Gain by Age	
Age	**Height gain**
Birth to 6 months	Monthly 2.5 cm
6–12 months	Monthly 1–5 cm
Toddlers	By age 2 years 50% adult
Preschoolers	Yearly gain 7.5 cm Birth length is doubled by 4 years

The Preschool Child

During this period the child grows 6–8 cm and gains 2 kg each year. The child has 20 deciduous teeth at 2.5 years.

THE 2-YEAR-OLD

- Walks, runs, stops and starts to avoid collisions.
- Squats to play and rise again (Fig. 12.38).
- Climbs on furniture to look out window or open door.
- Attempts to throw and kick a ball.
- Operates a sit-and-ride toy.
- Has difficulty with spatial awareness.
- Has strong sense of identity. Will resist things being done to them.
- Temper tantrums common.
- Holds a pencil like a rod and copies straight lines.
- Usually dry by day.
- Spontaneous engages in make- believe play (Fig. 12.39).

Fig. 12.39 • Spontaneously engages in make-believe play.

THE 3-YEAR-OLD

- Speech is well developed (girls better than boys).
- Understands sharing, turn taking.
- Is nimble and can judge distances.
- Jumps, stands briefly on one leg.
- Rides a tricycle and other toys (Fig. 12.40).

Fig. 12.38 • The 2-year-old.

Fig. 12.40 • 3-year-olds enjoy riding on toys.

- Motor skills well established, can climb stairs with alternate feet (coming down puts both feet on the same step).

- Is clean and dry and can self-feed.

- Can build a tower of eight or nine cubes.

- Holds a pencil using almost a mature grasp, copies circles, cuts with scissors.

- Can attempt to dress self, can pull on clothes over head, pull up pants but needs help with buttons (Fig. 12.41).

- Joins in active make-believe play (Figs 12.42–12.44).

THE 4-YEAR-OLD

- Self-care skills are developing, is willing to attempt to brush own hair (Fig. 12.45) and brush own teeth (Fig. 12.46).

Figs 12.42 • Joins in make-believe play.

- Holds a pencil in a mature grasp (Fig. 12.47) and copies circles and crosses as well as drawing an accurate body shape.

- Matches and names four primary colours.

- Gives full name, home address and sometimes age.

- Enjoys jokes, knows several nursery rhymes.

- Walks and runs skillfully and negotiates objects at speed without running into them.

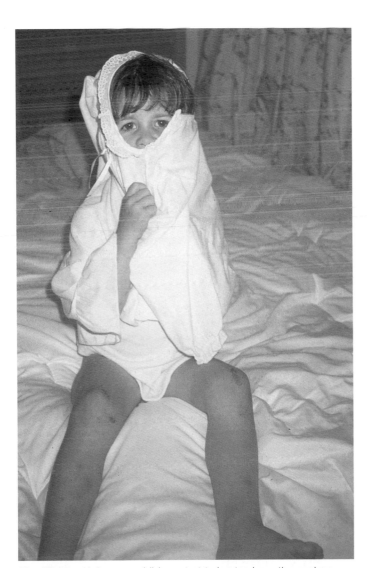

Fig. 12.41 • At 3 years, children start trying to dress themselves.

Figs 12.43 • Joins in make-believe play.

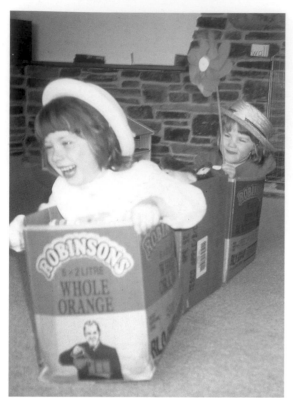

Figs 12.44 • Joins in make-believe play.

 Activity

The child's need for sleep varies at different ages:
- Find out how much sleep you would expect a 1-year-old and a 4-year-old to require?

Activity

Between the ages of 1 and 5 years growth slows considerably compared with the first year of life:
- What would be considered an average weight gain per year?
- What would be considered an average height gain?
- Birth weight is quadrupled by what age?
- Adult height is twice the child's height at what age?
- Brain growth is what percentage complete by 2 years?
- At what age should myelination of the spinal cord be complete?
- What age should the anterior fontanelle close?
- At what age would you expect a child to be:
  - dry by day?
  - dry by night?
- What energy (k/cal/g) and protein (g) requirements are needed for a 1–3-year-old daily?
- What would you expect the normal pulse, respirations and BP to be of a 4-year-old?
- At what ages would you expect to see a growth spurt in children?

Fig. 12.45 • A 4-year-old learning to brush her hair.

Fig. 12.46 • Learning to clean her teeth.

- Can balance (Fig. 12.48), hop and climb up and downstairs.
- Enjoys the company of and is aware of the feelings of other children.
- Looks forward to treats and has some concept of time.
- 'Lordosis' (pot belly) disappears.

Physical Growth from 5 Years to Adolescence

Physical changes are less obvious than 0–5 years. Children grow taller, change shape and acquire new skills. By the age of 5 years the child's height and weight are increasing steadily at the rate of 5 cm and 2–3 kg/year. Boys are on

Fig. 12.47 • Demonstrating a mature grip.

Fig. 12.48 • Demonstrating balance.

average 2.5 cm taller and 1 kg heavier than girls during early school years, however by 12 years of age girls are both taller and heavier than boys in their peer group.

- The 5-year-old is able to:
  - Draw a recognisable person or house, and write his or her own name.
  - Hop, skip, swing, jump, balance, climb, dance and throw a ball (Figs 12.49-12.51)
  - Ride a two-wheel bicycle.
  - Choose friends.
  - Undress and dress, except for laces and ties (Fig. 12.52).
  - Perform domestic and dramatic play alone or with friends (Figs 12.53 and 12.54).
- Age 6: swings by arms and skips with rope (Fig. 12.55).
- Age 7: 'walks the plank' (Fig. 12.56), uses a bat and ball (Fig. 12.57).
- Age 8–10: hopscotch, skipping games.

SKELETAL GROWTH

The growth of the trunk and extremities exceeds that of the head.

The centre of gravity lowers and body proportions become slimmer. Growth hormone stimulates longitudinal growth in a dose dependent manner, however other influences on growth are socio-economic, emotional and genetic factors. Problems are caused by ill-fitting shoes, chairs of the wrong height and carrying heavy loads, such as school bags.

The muscles are also immature and susceptible to damage.

Growth is reflected in limb length. Girls stop growing sooner than boys because of epiphyseal unity, which is under the control of oestrogen secretion. Boys' longer growth is reflected in their greater height and longer arms and legs. The extremities grow first, followed by neck, hip, chest, shoulder, trunk and depth of chest, hence the long-legged, gangly appearance of teenage boys with trousers and jumpers that never fit the limbs as well as the body.

TEETH

Children start to lose their deciduous teeth and permanent teeth appear at about the rate of four per year between the ages of 7–14 years.

Figs 12.49 • A 5-year-old learning sophisticated motor skills.

Figs 12.51 • A 5-year-old learning sophisticated motor skills.

Figs 12.50 • A 5-year-old learning sophisticated motor skills.

Figs 12.52 • Dress and undress except for laces and ties.

Figs 12.53 • Perform domestic and dramatic play alone or with friends.

Fig. 12.55 • Aged 6, swings by the arms and skips with a rope.

 Activity

Find out the sequence of teeth eruption for permanent dentition from a recommended textbook.

Figs 12.54 • Perform domestic and dramatic play alone or with friends.

Fig. 12.56 • Aged 7, greater strength and body control.

191

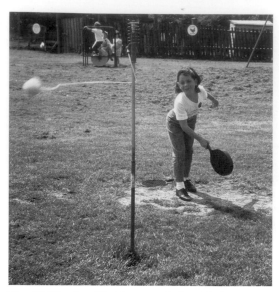

Fig. 12.57 • Aged 8–10, uses a bat and ball.

Fig. 12.59 • 5 years.

HEAD

- 6 months (Fig. 12.58).
- 5 years (Fig. 12.59).
- 10 years (Fig. 12.60).
- 13 years (Fig. 12.61).
- 16 years (Fig. 12.62).

The shape of the child's face changes from infancy to adulthood. Facial proportions change and the face grows faster in relation to the cranium. The frontal sinuses become visible on X-ray. When the permanent teeth erupt they force the shape of the jaw to change to accommodate them. In adolescence, both the jaw and the forehead alter, the jaw grows forward and the forehead becomes more prominent. This changes the overall shape of the face from a rounded appearance to one that is longer and more angular. The head and eyes are extra large in children, by the age of 8 years the child's head is 90% of its adult size. As facial remodelling continues and the jaw reaches adult size, there is hypertrophy of the laryngeal mucosa and enlargement of the larynx and vocal cords.

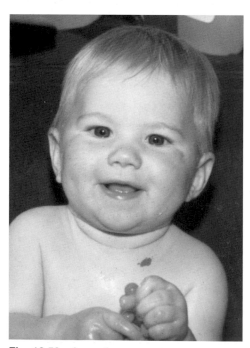

Fig. 12.58 • 6 months.

Fig. 12.60 • 10 years.

tolic BP rises at an accelerated rate during puberty, and pulse rate decreases. Blood volume, Hb, and red blood cell count rise more in boys than girls; by adulthood, women have one million fewer red cells per mL than men.

RESPIRATORY SYSTEM

The size and capacity increase; the respiratory rate decreases. Boys take in more air at one breath than girls, due to the increased chest and shoulder size.

Peak flow rate measures the maximum flow achieved in expiration after a maximum inspiration. Normal ranges of peak flow rates are:

- 5 years: 150 L/min.
- 10 years: 240 L/min.
- 15 years: 400 L/min.

SKIN

Oestrogen causes the skin of the female to develop a soft smooth, thicker texture. The sebaceous glands are particularly active and the eccrine and apocrine sweat glands become fully functional. Body hair takes on the characteristic distribution patterns and the texture changes.

Adolescence

Puberty is triggered by a chain of hormonal effects that bring on visible physical changes. The biology of puberty is triggered by hormonal influences and is controlled by the anterior pituitary in response to a stimulus from the hypothalamus (Fig. 12.63).

Fig. 12.61 • 13 years.

Fig. 12.62 • 16 years.

BODY MASS

Muscle growth follows that of bone and is therefore greater in boys.

CARDIOVASCULAR SYSTEM

This participates in the muscular growth spurt – its weight nearly doubles (this is more pronounced in boys). The sys-

Fig. 12.63 • The hormones produced in adolescence.

SEXUAL MATURATION OF GIRLS

The average age for appearance of breast buds is 10–11 years, with a range between 9 and 11½ years. The appearance of pubic hair usually follows breast development by about 2–6 months, although in about one-third of girls the appearance of pubic hair may occur first. There is often an increase in normal vaginal discharge associated with uterine development. Menarche usually occurs 2 years after the appearance of breast buds with a critical weight of 45 kg or 17% body fat required before menarche begins.

Development of the Breasts (Fig. 12.64)

- Stage one: Elevation of papilla.
- Stage two: Small area of elevation around papilla, enlargement of areolar diameter.

- Stage three: Further development of breast and areola with no separation of their contours.
- Stage four: Projection of areola and papilla to form a secondary mound (may not appear in all girls).
- Stage five: Mature configuration, projection of papilla only caused by recession of areola into general contour.

Growth of pubic hair follows the same pattern as for boys, with stage one having no pubic hair, through stages two and three when the hair goes from sparse and downy to more coarse and curly, and stages four and five when the hair becomes denser, curled and finally adult in quality, with spread of hair to the thighs.

Figure 12.65 shows the pubertal changes for girls.

Fig. 12.64 • Development of the breasts.

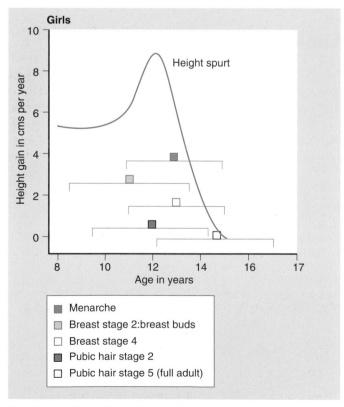

Fig. 12.65 • The pubertal changes for girls (Chimlea 1982 (cited in Bee 1997), Garn 1980, Tanner 1978).

SEXUAL MATURATION OF BOYS

Maturation begins in boys with an increase in the rate of growth of the testes and scrotum at about age 12 years of age. There is slow growth of pubic hair at about the same time and, approximately 1 year later, accelerated growth of the penis. Ejaculation occurs about 1½ years after the accelerated growth of the penis begins. Body and facial hair usually appear about 2 years after the beginning of pubic hair growth. The lowering of the voice occurs quite late in puberty. Some changes also occur to the male breast this includes an enlargement of the areola there may also be some enlargement but this usually disappears within a year or so.

Marshall & Tanner (1969) describe the developmental stages of genital development in boys as:

- Stage one: Prepubertal. No pubic hair – essentially the same as in childhood.
- Stage two: Pubertal. Initial enlargement of the scrotum and testes with reddening of the scrotal skin.
- Stage three: Penile lengthening, thinning of the scrotal skin, testicular enlargement which begins between 10½ and 14½ years with pubic hair spread sparsely over the entire pubis.
- Stage four: Glans enlargement, penile broadening, testicular enlargement, scrotal increase in size and

deepening of pigmentation with more abundant pubic hair but restricted to the pubic area.

- Stage five: Adult size and shape with spread of hair to inner thighs.

Spermatogenesis is active from the time of penile growth; and ejaculate can be produced from 1 year after its onset. Figure 12.66 shows the pubertal changes for boys.

WWW

Look at the following website for a PowerPoint slide show on pubertal processes:

- http://faculty.cua.edu/wagnerb/biologicalchanges.pps

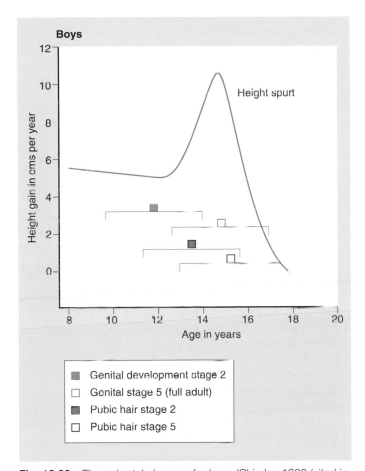

Legend:
- ■ Genital development stage 2
- □ Genital stage 5 (full adult)
- ■ Pubic hair stage 2
- □ Pubic hair stage 5

Fig. 12.66 • The pubertal changes for boys (Chimlea 1982 (cited in Bee 1997), Garn 1980, Tanner 1978).

THE ADOLESCENT GROWTH SPURT

The internal organs grow, including the lungs and heart, which increases physical endurance.

The lymphoid system, including the tonsils and adenoids, decreases in size, improving asthma, in some teenagers.

The growth of the skeletal system is reflected in limb growth. Boys' longer growth is reflected in their greater height and longer arms and legs.

Muscle mass increases in boys and girls. For girls, this peaks at menarche then slows; for boys it continues, resulting in a higher lean body mass in boys.

Adolescence is a time of continued brain growth. There is no actual increase in number of neurons but growth of the myelin sheath continues until at least puberty, thus enabling faster neural processing, which corresponds with the development of cognitive abilities.

The rate of growth may double during the pubertal growth spurt. The final 20–25% of linear growth is achieved; this can be as much as 12.5 cm in a peak year. Girls gain an average of 5–20 cm in height and 7–25 kg in weight; boys gain 10–30 cm in height and 7–30 kg in weight.

Both the growth spurt and onset of menstruation are occurring earlier now than they used to. Since 1850, the age at which menarche occurs has been declining in Western countries, probably the result of better nutrition, fewer diseases and good medical care. For example, in the US, girls first menstruated at 13–15 years; this is now 11–13 years. This means that girls are reaching the 'critical weight' of 45 kg, which must be attained before menstruation can begin, earlier than in former times.

Activity

What size do you imagine the knights of yesteryear were?

They were actually about the size of today's 12-year-old. A more recent example can be seen at La Scala opera house, which was built between 1776 and 1778 with seats that were 33 cm wide; this means of course that this must have been the average size of the bottom! In 1975 aircraft seats were 60 cm wide. (Do you know how wide they are today? Watch the TV commercials to find out.) What does this say about the size of our bottoms?

Activity

Look up the hormonal changes and sequence of sexual maturation at puberty in a recommended textbook and in Table 12.8.

Table 12.8 Timings for Hormonal Changes/Developments at Puberty

	Boy	Girl
Begins as early as	10½ years	7½ years
Begins as late as	16 years	11½ years
Average onset	12 years	10 years
Peaks	14 years	12 years

Suggested Areas for Observation of Children

The following is a list of placement areas where the theory of child development can be observed in practice. The list is not exclusive and you may visit other areas where you can observe children:

- child health clinics
- developmental screening
- home visits with health visitor
- school health checks
- practice nurses
- family centres
- mother and toddler groups
- play groups
- nurseries
- schools
- youth centres/organisations, e.g. Cub Scouts, Girl Guides, youth centres
- voluntary-sector child-oriented organisations, e.g. riding for the disabled, youth enquiry service, play centres, toy libraries.

When observing and interacting with children, consider their developmental progress using a developmental screening chart as a framework. Please use it simply as a guide to your observation, do not feel you have to test the child or check every item. Do not attempt any of the specific screening tests, such as hearing, physical examinations of the hips and testicles and checking of reflexes. Do not record any information that might compromise the confidentiality of the child (Nursing Midwifery Council 2002), e.g. name, address.

The following three activities can help to focus your findings when observing children.

Activity

Complete the following worksheet as a record of your findings.

Developmental observation exercise
- Practice area
- Age of child
- Gender
- Context of observation
- Background of child (if applicable)
- Social behaviour and play
- Hearing and speech
- Fine motor and vision
- Gross motor
- Feeding and nutrition (if applicable)
- Physical appearance
- Personality and demeanour
- Additional comments (e.g. reasons for any developmental issues)

Activity

If you have the opportunity, when out with the health visitor, weigh and measure three babies or young children and plot their heights and weights on the percentile chart . Be sure to ask the permission of the child's parents before you undertake this exercise.

Activity

The ways in which family life affects development are many. Through daily incidents and decisions parents affect their child's development in both positive and negative ways. Think of some examples in which parents can affect their child's development:
- Sean is 5 months old and cannot sit unaided
- Sue is 2 years old and screams when her mother dresses her. But she cannot cope on her own
- John is 6 and is slow in beginning to read
- Gill has just begun her periods and her body is changing
- Gary is 16 with no qualifications, out every night and surly

References

Allen R 2001 The Penguin English dictionary. Penguin Books, London

Bee H 1997 The developing child, 8th edn. Harper Collins, London

Frankenburg WK, Dodds JB 1967 The Denver developmental screening test. Journal of Pediatrics 71:181–191

Hockenberry MJ, Wilson D, Winkelstein ML, Kline NE 2003 Wong's nursing care of infants and children, 7th edn. Mosby, St Louis

MacGregor J 2000 Introduction to the anatomy and physiology of children. Routledge, London

Marshall WA, Tanner JH 1969 Variations in pattern of pubertal changes in girls. Archives of Diseases in Childhood 44:291

Meadow R, Newell S 2002 Lecture notes in paediatrics, 7th edn. Blackwell Science, Oxford

Mussen PH 1990 Child development and personality, 7th edn. HarperCollins College Division Row, New York

Sheridan M 1975 Children's developmental progress, from birth to five years: The Stycar sequences. NFER Publishing Company, Windsor

Chapter Thirteen

13

Preparing the Family for Stressful Life Events
Child life and the role of therapeutic play

Gary Mountain, Sue Fallon, Barbara Wood

ABSTRACT

Gaining a critical appreciation and understanding of the life world of children and their families within the health–illness experience is a central tenet of family-based health care. The intent of this chapter is to help readers develop their knowledge and understanding of how individual children, young people and their families perceive and adjust to the various life stressor(s) they experience along the health–illness continuum. Being in tune with how families perceive the stressor(s) they are experiencing provides for early recognition and the planning of interventions that monopolise on the resources and strengths available and promote family empowerment.

Learning Outcomes

- Identify the major categories of stress in children and young people.

- Discuss the aetiological processes of stress in children/young people and their family.

- Debate the short- and long-term impact of adverse life events on the child, young person and the family.

- Evaluate the effectiveness of some of the assessment models and/or frameworks available, which claim to predict the implications of adverse events on the family.

- Understand the roles and responsibilities of the children's nurse in providing structured psychosocial–emotional preparation and support for children/young people and their family.

- Appreciate the role of therapeutic play as a tool in helping children/young people understand and deal with particular stressful life events.

Introduction

Although stress in adults has been well researched, the existence and reactions of children and young people to life stressors – despite the accumulating evidence that they are frequently some of the most affected subsections of our society – have not been investigated. Accepting this point, it can be seen that in attempting to understand this complex topic we also need to take account of the interdependence of the individual within the family, the family system and the environment (Friedman 1998) and therefore individuals are best understood in the context of their family.

Stress is a constant aspect of daily living and is initiated by both positive and negative life events. Some form of stress is accepted as commonplace in our lives and perhaps ceases only at the time of death (Selye 1978). A number of suppositions are central to the theme of stress in children, young people and their families (Box 13.1).

At a simple level, the analysis of the impact of stress on children, young people and their families involves close examination of the following key elements: (a) the stressor(s)

Box 13.1

Summary of life's stressors in children and families

- Stress in its numerous variations can be perceived as normal; it is the individual's/family's perceptions that are important.
- Stress sometime places extraordinary demands on individuals and their families.
- Most individuals and their families adapt reasonably well to life's stressors.
- If individuals/families do not adapt reasonably well, negative outcomes (which can be short or long term) may follow.

involved and the stress responses invoked; (b) the resources available to individuals and groups when faced with stressful events; (c) the coping strategies that may or may not be called on to deal with the stress response; and (d) the outcomes. Other broader conceptual models may refer to some of the above as 'mediators' and 'moderators' of the relation between stress and outcomes, as well as of the reciprocal and dynamic relationships between these variables (Grant 2003). However, although this simplistic interpretation may seem plausible, a number of general issues and questions need to be considered.

First, children and their families can experience an infinite variety of categories, or even clusters of categories, of life stressors along a continuum ranging from ordinary 'hassles' to adverse and severe events or crises. There are events that many children would consider as unusually stressful. These might include:

- death of a parent or grandparent
- abuse
- disturbed family relationships
- birth of a sibling
- illness or accident involving the child or their parent
- parental unemployment
- change of school in particular starting secondary school (Sharman 1997).

Further lists of acute stressful life events and their impact on children are available, e.g. those detailed in Coddington's (1972) life events scales (cited in Clunn 1991). However, in a broad review of the literature findings, it is apparent that the most stressful events all appear to centre on tangible loss or circumstances that threaten loss (Hobfoll 1988).

Second, there is an array of related measurement problems. A critical review of the mass of available evidence-based literature found that research designs have adopted a wide variety of methodologies. Many of the designs make serious attempts to disaggregate a large number of stressful events and determine how they might be combined (reduced) into meaningful and useable subscales to try and predict cause and effect relationships. The stressor measures used in research studies have been found to combine neutral, negative and positive items; this could produce misleading findings. Aggregating stressors that are different in nature into a single measure could mask the impact of the different stressors on the individual. For example, economic deprivation would be associated with a range of additional specific stressful experiences, including conflict (exposure to abuse, marital conflict) and loss-based stressors (e.g. loss of role, death). However, studying each stressor individually demands complex statistical modelling techniques that would involve an array of parameters and a fragmented approach.

The number of potential outcome variables can be exceedingly large. It is necessary to study multiple outcome variables because they may be related not only to the nature of the stressor but also to its sequelae. Possible consequences are complex, which again makes measurement and prediction difficult. To complicate matters even further, sources of stress are closely related to an array of possible psychological and physical outcomes that are mediated by a mass of possible intervening factors such as age, gender, developmental level and the environmental context. Outcome measures can be further confounded or masked when the use of measures is eclectic. Thus it is easy to detect – even at this early stage – that studies will need to draw on sophisticated statistical modelling techniques when trying to disentangle cause and effect relationships.

Third, various factors might increase children's and young people's likelihood of exposure to stress or may moderate the effects of stress. The transition into adolescence is frequently cited as being characterised by an accumulation of stressful events and psychological challenges (Ge et al 1994). The salience and impact of certain social contexts such as the family, peers and school have a tendency to be singled out as having a significant influence on children and young people. Nevertheless we must remember that children are not simply passive recipients but also make an active contribution to their social worlds (Rudolph & Hammen 1999) and growth, maturation and expansion of environmental influences that occur with increasing age will inevitably change the nature of stressful experiences (Berk 2001).

Finally, just as there are an infinite number of stresses, so there is an array of coping strategies. Although these are likely to be less sophisticated than those used by adults, because of a relative lack of life experiences, they are perhaps just as resource intensive.

It is only possible here to start critically examining a small selection of the key life stressors children and young people experience and their underlying aetiological processes in the hope that the reader may be motivated to seek out further studies.

Life Stressors, Social Responses and Coping/Adaptive Strategies

Stressors are said to be the initiating or precipitating agents that activate the stress process and stress is the response or state of tension produced by the stressor(s) or by the actual/perceived demands that remains unmanaged (Friedman 1998 p 437). In reality, stress is a normal part of a child's or young person's life trajectory and encompasses common, developmental stressors of everyday life for which there may be fairly well-defined coping mechanisms (Santrock 2001) as well as unusual adverse events or crises. Apart from the well-known categories of major stressors or major life events, such as poverty, family instability, life-threatening illness and child abuse, it is crucial that we do not lose sight of the social context of modern everyday life that children and young people experience. It is within this context that children and young people may experience life's 'hassles'. These might be managed well or they might accumulate to such an extent that they present a significant threat to the child and/or family.

A useful model for understanding stress responses in children and young people is that presented by Moos (2002). This offers an 'integrated stress and coping framework' that can help the reader begin to understand the complex interplay between children and young people's acute and chronic life stressors and the variety of coping and adaptation strategies available. The framework comprises five main elements:

- The first (environmental system) reflects key life domains. These should be relatively stable conditions that include the family climate, ongoing life stressors and social resources.

- The second element is classified as the personal system, which includes the person's biogenetic characteristics and such personal resources as cognitive and intellectual abilities, social competence, self-confidence, self-esteem and personality.

- Element three includes the transitory conditions that children and young people may face, such as novel life events, which might in turn offer either new opportunities for learning and personal development or conversely dysfunction.

Moos (2002) states that these three sets of factors shape and indeed are almost precursors to, the child/young person's cognitive appraisal and coping skills (element 4) and, in turn, the child's/young person's health and well being (element 5) (for a full explanation of this model, see Moos 2002).

THE SCHOOL ENVIRONMENT AS A POTENTIAL MAJOR STRESSOR

From a very early age, the school environment is where a child or young person can directly and indirectly experience stress. The impact of the pressures and expectations within the school environment are certainly among the most frequently reported stressors by adolescents (de Anda et al 2000). Relevant stressors include fear of success or failure, test or performance anxiety and fears associated with the unrelenting academic pressure often imposed in today's

school environment. In a study by de Anda (2... from concerns about future goals, school-rela... show the highest recorded frequency in high sc... dents. The pressure of time, achievement and expec... in the form of tests, grades, homework and pressures... parents were reported as being stress factors that were... 'often' to 'very often' on a daily and weekly basis by ado... lescent respondents.

When the school environment imposes a significant continuing source of stress, children tend to avoid school altogether. These children almost become school phobic and appear to experience relatively significant emotional and physical effects even at the very thought of going to school. Unfortunately, such children can inadvertently become categorised as persistent truants and labelled as exhibiting behavioural problems.

Children can face other types of stress at school apart from those associated with scholarly activities. Bullying has become a significant social problem in contemporary school life. Kidscape (whose website can be found at: http://www.kidscape.org.uk) is a national charity that supplies sensitive advice for bullied children as well as providing individuals and organisations with the practical skills and resources necessary to keep children safe from harm. Kidscape (2003) feels that this kind of work is vital given the frightening statistics that:

- Each year 10–14 youth suicides are directly attributed to bullying.

- Bullied children are six times more likely to contemplate suicide than their non-bullied counterparts.

- 1 in 12 children are badly bullied to the point that it affects their education, relationships and even their prospects for work in later life.

THE LOSS OF A PARENT

The loss of parent, either through death or through separation/divorce, is a devastating loss that permanently changes the family dynamics. Although some children are well cared for when facing such stressors, other longitudinal studies show that even among adults who claim to have coped with the loss of a parent in childhood, certain life cycle events, such as marriage, can sometimes trigger a surge of maturational grief responses (Moos 1986). It is also now acknowledged that children whose parents divorce are exposed to multiple losses and adversities that may have a negative impact on the child's health, well-being and achievement in life many years later (Papalia et al 1999).

Separation and divorce – and the consequent single parenthood – inevitably bring changes in financial circumstances. Compared with children in 'intact' families, children in one-parent families are more likely to experience

and less support. They are
old responsibilities, more
hesion and less support,
99). Children suffering
se) may suffer higher
of illnesses including
problems, and are more
earlier age (Burges 1994, Jenkins
palia et al 1999). Longitudinal studies
children of separated or divorced parents have
at some of them are still experiencing problems ten
more years later (Papalia et al 1999).

PARENTAL PSYCHOPATHOLOGY AND CHILD ABUSE

Differences in what is termed the 'emotional tone' of the family can have profound effects on children (Mountain 2002). In particular, children who live in situations of neglect or abuse are more likely to experience disorganised/disorientated attachments to their parents, have negative, ill-conceived self-concepts, find it difficult to engage in social interactions and consequently have difficulty forming social relationships. These children may develop particular characteristics and personality traits that in turn make them less well liked. For example, there is an abundance of evidence to suggest a link between abuse and children's low self-esteem, emotional maladjustment, dependency, underachievement, depression, faltering growth, deliberate selfharm and other psychological distress in later life (Papalia et al 1999).

Many forms of mental health problem in parents have a direct impact on the quality and nature of parenting. Therefore nearly all types of mental health problems in parents have been linked to an increased likelihood of behavioural and emotional problems in children and young people (Graham et al 1999). Research on the children of depressed parents signals a clear causal relationship between depression in parents and problems of adjustment and depression in their children. Similarly, toddlers of depressed parents are more likely to exhibit emotional and behavioural disturbances, delayed language and cognitive developments (Steinhausen & Verhulst 1999).

ADOLESCENT LIFE STRESSORS

The period of adolescence (whenever this is said to commence) has traditionally been described as a particularly critical period of physical, psychological and social change for young people, often characterised by emotional and psychological stress and, indeed, clusters of crises. However, although contemporary studies concur with some of these

claims in some cases, they are not always generalisable to all adolescents. Indeed, in most cases adolescents are remarkably level-headed and well equipped to resolve many of the problems they encounter during this transitional period (Erwin 1998).

Nevertheless with the continuing rise of reported mental illness episodes and suicidal behaviours in adolescence (Stoleb & Chiribogo 1988), along with clear associations between stress and psychological symptoms (Jenson et al 1991), one can logically and safely conclude that for some individuals within this relatively large section of society certain life stressors can appear to have a significant and dramatic effect on their lives. According to Lau (2002), this can be partly explained by the fact that negative life events, especially if cumulative in nature, negatively affect adolescents' adjustment in various ways. Similarly, it must be remembered that the foundation for adolescence begins to be laid during early childhood (Jackson & Rodriguez-Tome 1995).

As well as exposure to violence, abuse and divorce, which we have already noted, other examples of adolescent life stressors include disciplinary action taken against them, incidence of rejection/humiliation by others, moves to new environments, terminations of friendships or relationships, and conflict with relatives or peers. Across the various stressors the various research studies have chosen to study, there is little evidence to detect patterns of specificity in any of them apart from the broad outcomes associated with sexual abuse (McMahon et al 2003). As noted earlier, it is well recognised that the nature of the family climate or environment is a key context that sets the stage for adolescent development and affects adolescent's reactions to life stressors (Moos 2002). In particular, the family and peers provide a source of social support that helps the young person facing life stressors to maintain his or her coping efforts. The *quality* of social support and peer relations (rather than the *number* of social supports) has been demonstrated to be associated with favourable mental health outcomes. A growing sense of group membership also appears to play a key protective role in negating the effects of life crises in adolescents (D'Attilio et al 1992, Morano et al 1993).

Given the centrality of the family environment, it may come of no surprise to learn that 50% of suicidal adolescents are found to come from broken homes – family environments characterised by divorces or single-parent structures. Adolescents who have experienced violence or sexual abuse are also at higher risk of negative mental health outcomes. Parents of suicidal adolescents tend to be more depressed, consume more alcohol, and have lower self-esteem and increased anxiety.

Gender differences have been found to exist. There is a tendency for female adolescents to report more sensitivity than boys to interpersonal stressors and to those related to peer values regarding dress and appearance (Coleman 1990). There is a dearth of research on the links between ethnic differences and life stressors. However, a few studies indicate that issues surrounding identity, including the impact of prejudice and stereotypes are additional stressors for young people from different cultural groups (Phinney & Alipuria 1990).

The notion of 'family stress' will now be examined briefly before moving on to explore the social resources and coping responses children, young people and family members may utilise to manage life stressors.

FAMILY STRESS

Boss (1988 p 704) claims that the family, as a group, is not coping if even one member manifests stress-related symptoms. If this stringent criterion is adopted then family stress can be seen as a natural and logical extension of individual stress applied to the family domain and, importantly, both the individual and family are of equal importance when examining the impact of life's stressors.

To paraphrase Hobfoll & Spielberger (1992), family stress is the state in which both family members and the family as a unit are challenged by the environment in a way that overtakes the individual or collective resources and threatens the well-being of individuals within the family, or the family as a whole.

Whereas Moos' (2002) framework has a tendency to be directed to individual stress, McCubbin & McCubbin's (1993) resiliency model is family-centred and focuses not only on the factors that produce crisis/non-crisis in families but also how family members adjust and how the family adapts during and after crisis.

A focus on stressors is key in virtually all theories of family stress but different theorists envisage different conceptions of the nature of those stressors. Traditionally, research has tended to focus on stressors being caused by pressures for change on the family system or the accumulation of demands for change. According to Hill (cited in Health Advisory Service 1995), a stressor consists of those life events or occurrences that are sufficient magnitude to bring about change in the family system.

Family stressors can derive from interpersonal, environmental, economic or sociocultural events or experiences (Friedman 1998) and they can be acute, chronic, major, minor and/or ongoing (Hobfoll & Spielberger 1992). The perception and interpretation of stressors is highly subjective and individual to each family unit. For example, what one family may perceive as challenging opportunities may be perceived as threatening and overwhelming by another.

Like stress responses in the individual, family life stressors can be accumulative or 'pile up' (McCubbin & Patterson 1983). Likewise, a family stressor event is only a stimulus that holds the potential for beginning the process of change of stress. Whether it does or does not depends on the family's response to the stressor (Boss 1988). According to Boss, family crisis differs from, but precedes, stress when stress is so significant that the family's resources are no longer adequate to maintain the structure. In families who face adversity, boundaries are not maintained, customary roles and tasks are no longer performed and individual members may no longer function at optimal levels. However, it should be noted that crises could result in families redefining themselves. A positive outcome arising from, say, the admission of a child to a paediatric intensive care unit, may result in a higher level of family functioning after recovering from the crisis event.

COPING

'Stress' and 'coping' are terms used ubiquitously in the literature without specific definition and consensus as to the meanings of the concepts. A useful definition of coping comes from Cohen & Lazarus (1979), who view coping as:

. . . a wide range of problem-solving efforts both externally orientated and intra-psychic used to manage, master, tolerate, reduce or minimise the environmental and internal demands and conflicts between them or exceed an individual's resources.

Analysis of the processes involved and resources available to individuals and their families has found coping to comprise individual, family and/or socially based strategies. We must also remember that a multicultural perspective on the subject is vital and that, cross-culturally, individual, family and socially based coping strategies are not only sometimes different but can often be in direct conflict with each other.

To achieve the goals of coping the child/young person needs to engage in a number of activities or tasks. However, just as there are an infinite number of life stressors so there are an infinite number of coping strategies and responses. Nevertheless, a number of protective factors seem to increase a child's capacity to cope with stress, these include (Spender et al, cited in Townley 2002):

- an easy temperament, e.g. some children make friends easily whereas others struggle with establishing relationships
- higher intelligence
- support from parents
- support from peers
- a sense of humour
- positive experiences at school
- support from other adults outside the immediate family

- religious faith
- a tendency to plan and set goals for life decisions
- positive experiences that help to neutralise the effects of adverse factors
- taking extra responsibility, which can lead to increase in self-esteem
- cognitive processing of experiences, i.e. the ability to find meaning in life experiences and learn from them.

Years of research appear to have failed to identify either higher-order or core categories of specific coping responses. Almost every activity can be considered to be a way of coping and each one has its body of research. These can be behavioural, cognitive or emotional in nature and include problem solving, information seeking, planning, negotiation, compliance, self and other blame, help seeking, social support, opposition, venting, selecting optimisation, compensation, rumination, disclosure and discussion, primary and secondary control, optimism and positive illusions to name but a few.

Additionally, individual predisposing factors influence a child's or young person's capacity to cope. These include age, gender, temperament, arousal, imagery and/or coping response styles, which in turn may influence both the perception of the problem and the ability to motivate resources or engage the support of others. Current research into coping tends to favour longitudinal designs, repeating measures over a short time or over several years, often including markers of the progress of stressful events. The criteria for measuring the outcomes of the coping process usually focus on the psychosocial, physical and functional status of the child or young person at a given single or multiple points.

Two points are worth noting at this stage. First, whereas some of the aforementioned coping strategies may be effective in dealing with stress in the short term, we also need to examine the predicted longer-term consequences of these strategies. Second, whereas it is hoped that many of the coping strategies children and young people employ are adaptive, maladaptive ways of coping exist, including catastrophising and panic, social isolation, blame of others, denial, withdrawal confrontation, aggressive behaviour and even substance misuse (de Anda et al 2000).

The Family Environment

Family support and structure are key influencing factors associated with children's and young people's ability to cope and adapt to life's stressors. Numerous research studies point to a strong correlation between parental functioning and competence and the family environment generally, and how children succeed or not with many life stressors.

In a chapter of this kind it is therefore important that we at least make some reference to the notion of family coping as opposed to individual coping. Boss defined family coping as 'the management of a stressful event by the family and by each individual in the family'. She goes on to assert that it is the cognitive and affective process by which individuals and their family system adjust to, rather than eradicate stress (Boss 1988).

In his Conservation of Resources Theory, Hobfoll (1988) claims that the role of resources is pivotal for families trying to cope with stressors. He defines resources as those things that people (or this case families) value or that act as a means of obtaining or protecting that which they value. The Conservation of Resources Theory suggests four principal resource categories:

1. object resources (e.g. transport and housing)
2. condition resources (e.g. good marital relationships)
3. personal resources (e.g. self-esteem)
4. energy resources (e.g. money and time).

The theory states that stress occurs with resource loss even if total resources available are not outstripped. Furthermore, loss of resources makes families more vulnerable because they have fewer resources available to deal with future stressors. Loss of resources can be cumulative, whereby resource loss sets up an adverse reaction where further loss is likely. Hence the family becomes less resilient and more vulnerable. Conversely, future gains are more likely to follow after resource gain, i.e. by successfully meeting the challenges of some life stressors, the family gains confidence and competence to address more stressful challenges heading its way.

A number of family resources have been identified as especially important in coping with stressful life events. Among these are:

- flexibility/adaptability versus rigidity
- cohesion versus separateness
- communication versus privacy
- boundary clarity versus boundary ambiguity.

A full explanation of each of these can be found in Hobfoll & Spielberger (1992 p 103).

An additional key resource the family has available outside of, but yet interconnected with, the family system is that of social support. Again, a review of the literature helps identify three major sources:

- support network resources
- supportive behaviour
- the subjective appraisal of support.

All three aspects of social support are important and have different causes and influences.

The Short- and Long-term Impact of Stress Caused by Life Events

If a child's mental health needs are not met, or are only partially met, when the child faces a stressful situation this might result in a particular physical or psychological problem or disorder. In a review of the literature on the association of environmental stressors on the psychological and physical health of children, Grey (1993) cited many studies that seem to suggest that there is a link between stress and the development of symptoms of a particular disorder or disease. For example she cites two small studies that suggest that major psychological stress may be one of the precipitating factors in the onset of leukaemia symptoms (Green & Swisher 1969, Miller 1982). The onset and exacerbation of diabetes and diabetic ketoacidosis have been associated with stressful life events in the year before their diagnosis and in the triggering of acute ketoacidosis in children (Fallon 1995, Johnson 1982, Stein & Charles 1971). There is also evidence to suggest that life stressors are also associated with the exacerbation of asthma (Johnson 1982). Recurrent abdominal pain has also been found to relate directly to increased stress levels (Wilson-Sharrer & Ryan-Wenger 1991).

Other studies also cited by Grey (1993) suggest a link between stressful life events and psychological problems, such as low self-esteem, poor school performance (Bedell 1977), maladaptive behaviour (Sandler & Block 1979), suicidal behaviour (Pfeffer et al 1979), teenage pregnancy (Coddington 1979), drug addiction (Duncan 1977) and psychiatric hospitalisation (Vincent & Rosenstock 1979). Buchanan & Tenbrink (1997) add that in adulthood the consequences of unmet mental health needs associated with stressful life events in childhood may result in poorer relationships with partners and own children, mental health problems and possible serious physical illnesses.

Sharman (1997) suggests that if parents are aware that stress can precipitate the onset of asthmatic or diabetic symptoms they may be able to prevent this by ensuring that the need for extra emotional support is anticipated and that the support is given. This is good preventive advice but, as further research has shown, stress alone is not the one single precipitator to illness and thus parents should not be made to feel guilty if a child develops symptoms or an illness that does have a tenuous link with increased stress. This point leads onto Grey's (1993) observation of the flaws of much of the research she reviewed. Her major criticisms were that there is difficulty in describing, and thus estimating, the magnitude of various stressful life events and that there is a glaring lack of data on intervening and

mediating variables that may modify the impact of stress on the development of illness. This observation is supported by McMahon et al's (2003) review of the literature, which concludes that apart from the major stressor of child sexual abuse there is very little evidence to uniquely link specific stressful life evens to the onset of specific physical or mental illnesses or diseases.

McMahon et al (2003) suggest that many different avenues of stressful experience can lead to the same outcome (equifinality) or that similar stressful conditions can lead to multiple outcomes (multifinality). They add that the outcomes of stressful situations depend on many systems that moderate or mediate the effect on a child's behaviour, such as family variables, larger contextual variables, environmental stressors and biological vulnerability.

Assessment and Appraisal of Stress in Children and Families within the Healthcare Context

Given the knowledge that hospitalisation and illness are major stressors for children and young people, how do we assess how stressed they actually are? Townley (2002) suggests that before any assessment the nurse must have an understanding of the normal developmental stages and mental health needs of children and young people. Hill (cited in Health Advisory Service 1995) suggests that mental health in children and young people is indicated by:

- The capacity to enter into and sustain mutually satisfying personal relationships.
- Continuing progression of psychological development.
- An ability to play and learn so that achievements are appropriate for age and intellectual level.
- A developing sense of right and wrong.
- The degree of psychological distress and maladaptive behaviour that is within the normal limits for the child's age and context.

There is a wide range of standardised inventories designed to measure individual child life stressors. Due to the number and diversity of potential life stressors in children and young people, as well as the wide range of contexts healthcare professional may find themselves in, it is difficult to recommend any one particular assessment scale. However, before assessment it would be useful for a children's nurse to be familiar with Coddington's (1972) work, if only to be aware of some of the most common social acute stressors, both positive and negative, that children might experience in addition to the stress that hospitalisation and illness may bring. Similarly the Stress Impact Scale (SIS) by Hutton and Roberts, reviewed by Drummond & Meier (1995), claims to measure the occurrence and effect of 70 potentially stressful events on adolescents.

Following on from the above, it is also important that the children's nurse is aware of some of the mental health risk factors, such as those related to home, family, school and peers, that may make a child more susceptible to develop mental health problems as a result of stress. The Mental Health Foundation (1999) suggests that these include:

- Risk factors in the child:
  - genetic influences
  - low IQ and learning disability
  - specific developmental delay
  - communication difficulty
  - difficult temperament
  - physical illness, especially if chronic/or neurological
  - academic failure
  - low self-esteem.

- Risk factors in the family:
  - overt parental conflict
  - family breakdown
  - inconsistent or unclear discipline
  - hostile and rejecting relationships
  - failure to adapt to child's changing needs
  - physical, sexual and/or emotional abuse
  - parental psychiatric illness
  - parental criminality, alcoholism or personality disorder
  - death and loss, including loss of friendship.

- Risk factors in the community:
  - socio-economic disadvantage
  - homelessness
  - disaster
  - discrimination
  - other significant life events.

Finally, the other baseline information the children's nurse must acquire prior to assessment relates to the stressors children experience that are specific to hospitalisation. Melamed et al (1988) details the common (most reported) features of hospital-related stressors in children.

Activity

Taking each of the components mentioned above, how might a 2-year-old respond to hospitalisation/illness and how might you help a 2-year-old overcome his or her responses?

www

Click on the following hyperlinks for useful good practice ideas in relation to preparing children for hospitalisation:
- http://www.actionforsickchildren.org/hospital1.html
- http://bch.org.uk/parents-carers/preparingyourchild.html
- http://gosh.nhs.uk/kidsandteens/kids/real-stories/html
- http://www.kidshealth.org/kid/fee-better/places.html

Not every child will experience all these stressors or respond to a stressor in the same way. The response will depend on the child's previous experience with the same or similar procedures, and on the parents' ability to prepare the child for the impending event and their skill to communicate effectively what this will involve. The practitioner's ability to prepare the child for the event in advance is essential. Also, instructions given to children should be appropriate to their level of understanding and ability to carry out those instructions (Melamed 1993).

ASSESSMENT TOOLS

When assessing psychological stress levels in children, nurses depend largely on their observation skills and the child's self report (Grey & Hayman 1987). Both methods are useful but both are also prone to major subjectivity. Observation of the child's behaviour can be limited by observer bias, the timing of the observation and where the observation takes place. Similarly, the child's self report can also be affected by a number of factors, such as the child's willingness and/or ability to communicate and cooperate, and how the child actually recalls and reports a particular stressful event. This indicates the value of and need for a multidisciplinary approach with assessment, utilising observation and self-report taking place over a period of time and in different situations before conclusions about a child's level of stress/anxiety are made.

Townley (2002) points out that for most nurses working in general children's wards it is inappropriate and impractical to carry out lengthy and detailed assessments of a child's full mental health status. He suggests that a quick assessment tool/framework for use in general ward situations would be more useful. The aim of this aspect of assessment is to establish the extent of the anxiety, unhappiness or distress that the stressor of illness and/or hospitalisation is causing the child. The nurse competently facilitating the expression of the reasons behind the child's feelings could achieve this. The nurse must not force the child to express his or her thoughts and feelings but must go at the child's pace. This process requires time, sensitivity and creativity.

Children often find it easier to communicate through play and art. Sharman (1997) suggests a wide range of play strategies to establish a therapeutic relationship with a child. These in turn would enable children to feel comfortable to then express their thoughts and feelings of what it is that actually worries them or makes them feel tense or stressed. This information will form the key basis of the information required for assessment.

All nurses working with children must also be able to work with their families. Increasingly, nursing research is pointing to the importance of child-centred care and family nursing (Friedman 1998, McCubbin & McCubbin1993), whereby the sick child is assessed but within the context of the whole family. Thus assessment and understanding of how the parents and other family members perceive and cope with stressors (i.e. the child's hospitalisation) is key to the understanding of how the child will behave and cope in that situation.

Activity

There is a wide range of family assessment tools with varying complexity and sophistication:
- Search the literature to find an example of a family assessment tool.
- Consider how this tool may possibly be adapted for application to your practice area.
- Consider the skills the practitioner may need and the adaptations that may need to be made to use this or similar assessment tools in your area of practice.

The items outlined above offer the practitioner a number of areas to consider when approaching an assessment of the older child's stressors and her/his capacity to cope (Spender et al, cited in Townley 2002).

Illness and Hospitalisation as a Major Source of Stress in Children

Success and a sense of competence in mastering challenging life experiences such as illness and hospitalisation contribute to a child's evolving self-concept (Harter 1983). To enable children and parents to cope with a situation that may be fully outside their experience, planning and rehearsing coping strategies congruent with their individual styles, beliefs and developmental capacities can be used. Indeed, successful coping with one stressful event increases a child's coping repertoire and confidence to address subsequent stressors (Lutz 1986). It has long been recognised that children and young people benefit tremendously from preparation and support before hospitalisation (Eisner 1990, Glasper & Thompson, Robertson 1995, While 1994). This recognition is supported in a number of studies (Adams et al 1991, Bielby 1984), which demonstrate that children who receive some type of preadmission preparation cope much better with hospitalisation, have fewer behavioural problems after discharge, spend less time as an inpatient and return to school more quickly than their counterparts.

For a child, more than for an adult, the prospect of a hospital admission can be very distressing and frightening. When admission is an emergency, time for preparation is extremely limited as the following conversation reveals.

Child Conversation
C J Wood, aged 12 years.

8.15 a.m. Saturday 28 July my whole world turned upside down. As I lay floating on top of the water the paramedics told me that they had to get me out of the pool and to hospital as quickly as possible. They kept telling me not to move, and my mum kept saying the same and telling me she loved me. As all of this was going on all I could think about was am I going to live? I was absolutely terrified.

As the paramedics lifted me onto the stretcher they told me that I must not move my head! As I was lying there I couldn't feel or move my arms or legs. The paramedics wrapped me in foil to keep me warm as we made our way to the ambulance.

I had never been in an ambulance before so I was a bit scared! I had to have an oxygen mask over my mouth. I kept complaining about my arms and legs because I couldn't move and there was so much pain. The paramedics didn't give me any information on what was going to happen in the accident and emergency department and although I didn't know what to expect, I thought something really bad was going to happen as everyone around me was whispering and my mum was crying but trying to be calm at the same time.

The paramedics rushed me into the accident and emergency department and I heard someone shout 'straight into resus'. I was lifted off the stretcher and on to a very hard, cold table. There were loads of doctors and a mass of faces looking down at me telling me not to move and that I was going to be OK.

The doctors didn't tell me that they were going to put a few injections into my arms, hands, feet and legs: they just went on and did it! I very frightened, I mean I didn't know what the injections were going to do to me or what they for! I wasn't used to any of this. The doctors never told me. That was what I was worried about the most. I didn't have a clue what was happening or what to think! The doctors kept telling me I was going to be OK but I didn't know what to believe.

My mum and dad came into the room. I wish they had been with me I wanted them beside me; they would believe me about the pain! I don't think they had been allowed in at first. I remember my dad was a dreadful colour and my mum was trying to be brave but was so upset. She obviously knew one of the nurses in the room as they were hugging each other.

After about 2 hours in the department I started to get feeling back into my legs. I thought to myself after all I'm going to be OK! But still nothing in my arms or hands. Overall I was in the department for 3½ hours. It felt like a lot longer.

My mum tried to explain things to me about what was happening, as the doctors seemed to have forgotten I was still there. They only spoke to mum and dad. I know I had a lot of pain but it was me who was hurting. Why wouldn't they talk to me?

It is highly likely that these traumatic memories and behaviours will be carried into future similar situations (Solnit 1984), and may persist well into adulthood (Sugar 1992).

Activity

As a children's nurse:

- What key issues is the child in the conversation above trying to communicate?
- What lessons can be learnt from this scenario for your future nursing practice?

www

Visit the following website for further children's accounts regarding their experiences in hospital:

- http://www.bch.org.uk

The appointment of a Minister for Children, and the future appointment of a Commissioner of Children, together with the Children's National Service Framework highlight the seriousness and importance of the rights of the child. These rights have been acknowledged within the last decade, but there are elements that remain solely within the domain of adults. Children's participation in healthcare decisions is well supported by Alderson & Montgomery (1996). Cohen & Emmanuel (1999) suggest that the need to involve and consult young people places a duty on governments and professionals to seek, and take full account of, the views of young people in the planning and delivery of services. Consultation with children is crucial. As Article 12 of the United Nations Convention on the Rights of the Child (UNCRC) states:

Parties shall assure to the child who is capable of forming his or her own views the right to express those views freely in all matters affecting the child, the views of the child being given due weight in accordance with age and maturity of the child (DoH 1999)

The process by which children are consulted must reflect a commitment by the healthcare team to respect the dignity, welfare and views at all times of that child (Balen et al 2000). Children being prepared for admission to hospital must be empowered to express their views, and they should expect due notice to be taken of those views. Parents and carers are tuned into their child's ability to express their views from birth. As healthcare workers, we must liaise closely with the parents/carers to ensure the child's views are acknowledged. In some instances, children are not able to speak for themselves in situations that may have an impact on their short- or long-term future, therefore as advocates for children we must have the opportunity to speak for them. As children's nurses, we are authentic representatives who should value the individuality and diversity of the child.

Activity

What are the first thoughts that enter your head when you hear 'consultation with children'? It is quite common for people to dismiss this as a right of children, and see it in an adult domain. What do you think might have influenced the way in which you answered this question? Now consider the various ways you may approach this in your practice area.

Findings by Eisner (1990) suggest that children from 2 years of age, have well-ordered ideas about what hospital is like and what happens there; information that is presumably gained from such sources as television, books and other people's accounts. Yet, despite this children are infrequently involved in choices about their care and treatments. Flatman (2002) suggests there are various ways of consulting with children, but considerations should include:

- communication: age-appropriate methods
- checking comprehension: using both visual and verbal clues
- motivation: value placed on interaction should be made clear, be meaningful for the child and offer tangible rewards
- accuracy of representation of children's views
- confidentiality
- parental concerns: informed about nature and intention of consultation and consent sought.

Whether a planned admission or an emergency admission, children respond better when they are supplied with basic information about what is going to happen to them (Ivory 1998). A report published by Rennick (2002) supports what children's nurses have known for a long time, namely that children who are admitted to hospital unprepared may have lingering psychological problems months after they return home:

Children who were younger, more severely ill, and who endured more invasive procedures had significantly more medical fears, a lower sense of control over their health, and on-going post-traumatic stress responses for six months (Rennick 2002 p 133)

Effective communication, which is jargon-free and appropriate to all involved, is essential for ensuring clarity with regard to who is providing what care and how they intend to do it (Heywood 2002). Marks (1994) suggests that aspects of care are generally discussed and planned separately, which leads to the increased risk of a fragmented view of the care pathway. If care is organised separately, children and carers could receive a disjointed care experience. However, if each element of care is planned as part of the whole, and the child and family are involved in all aspects of planning, then there is a greater chance of their perceived needs being met. Children and carers need clear information so that their choices and options can be increased. Kitson (1999 p 42), states:

Understanding the support network around patients, and their carers' capacity to cope both in the short and long term, are dimensions of care that need to be considered within the remit of continuity of care.

Active participation by children in preparation for hospital admission is a good way to reduce anxiety and increase compliance during any medical and nursing procedures. Useful pointers include:

- Tell children where they are going, what is going to happen to them and why.
- Be honest with children. Too much information can be overwhelming, stick to the essentials.
- Don't start preparing too soon, a few days is usually adequate.
- Use simple language and give clear explanations appropriate to the child's age.
- Encourage children to ask questions.
- Give child something to look forward to after their treatment.
- Let the children know it is OK to feel scared and encourage them to talk about their feelings.
- Let the children pack their own bag to instill a sense of involvement.

Each child will react differently to hospital admission. The following highlights a number of stress responses exhibited by children to hospitalisation:

- Separation anxiety: some children feel secure and safe as long as their parents are there, but this is not always possible and some children can react badly to the absence of a parent or carer. Regression in their behaviour may be noticeable, e.g. bed wetting, tantrums, refusal to eat, withdrawn, crying a lot.
- Older children may fear a loss of new skills, separation from friends/school, loss of privacy. They may even blame their parents and see hospitalisation as a form of punishment.
- Young adults may feel embarrassment over loss of privacy and independence, threatened, anxious over their separation from their peers and anxious about their illness.

Activity

Think of the times when you have felt low or anxious, or wanted to be alone, or perhaps when you have felt angry:

- Identify the factors in your life around that time that might have influenced the way you responded.
- Consider the children and young adults you come into contact with in your practice area. What are the factors they are exposed to that might lead to such responses?

Written and illustrated information is effective in relieving stresses associated with hospitalisation. Stone (1994) designed a leaflet – *Preparing your child for hospital: a parents' guide* – to educate parents on how to prepare their child for hospital admission. The parental survey demonstrated that the leaflet did help parents to prepare children for elective admission to hospital. Written information comes in many formats, from leaflets and books written specifically for children (e.g. Topsy and Tim) to excellent pages on the internet. Visual/audio material in the form of videotapes and children's hospital programmes are a good preparation.

Perhaps one of the most effective forms of preparation is play therapy. Play is an essential element in every child's life. It enables them to communicate and develop many other life skills and, as well as being fun, it can also be an emotionally balancing activity for the child (Barry 2000). Play is fundamental for a healthy childhood, but for a child who is being admitted to hospital or is in hospital it serves the further purpose of helping the child to adjust to its new circumstances. Children who are experiencing illness express their needs differently to adults and viewed as a language, play becomes a crucial tool in helping a child adjust to a period of time in hospital.

Play facilities aim to (GOSH/ICH, 2002):

- Provide a normal, reassuring experience and increase each individual child's ability to regain confidence, independence and self-esteem.

- Promote normal child development and help children regain skills lost through regression and the effects of illness and hospitalisation.

- Aid diagnosis and help the child understand illness and treatments, and participate in decision-making.

- Encourage families to be involved in the child's care and play and to relieve anxiety and anger by providing a creative outlet.

- Encourage and enable other members of staff to be involved in the child's play.

- Ensure the play environment is safe, stimulating and well maintained.

- Promote the value of play in hospital through training and education.

- Have fun!

Activity

Having read through the aims of play, give some thought to play activities that could promote well being in a child to be admitted to hospital or for a child already on your ward:
- Which of the activities do you feel that you currently engage in?
- Consider how you might extend these activities to assist other children.

www

There are some excellent examples of good practice in relation to the provision of play in the health care context at:
- http://www.addenbrookes.org.uk.html

Activity

Consider the many issues that have been discussed in this section and write a list of those about which it might be useful to have more information available for children and young people, parents and carers. Over the next few weeks, collect resources such as booklets and websites, which will help to increase the resources in your practice area.

Summary

This chapter set out to draw together contemporary authoritative sources, reflection, case study material and experiences to help advance the readers understanding of a complex and vast topic. It is worth noting that, despite rigorous and strategically planned literature reviews being undertaken, there is a definite absence of systematic reviews of the evidence on this theme, which can be used to inform our thinking.

Although stress in adults has been well researched and documented, much less is known about the existence and reactions of children and young people to life's stressors. Hopefully, what should have become apparent is that numerous methodological limitations abound that not only hamper generalisation of research findings but also could be cited as one of the main reasons for the relative dearth of studies focusing specifically on the subject. The problem is further compounded when attempts are made to broaden the critique to include the interdependence between the child, her/his family and the environment.

Children are subject to an array of stressors throughout their lives, from ordinary to severe, and, as with adults, those who are unable to develop appropriate coping or adaptation strategies are at greater risk of falling ill. The results of various studies point to an overarching theme; that particular stressors cannot be related to particular internal/external outcomes. Among the various stressors examined, the only consistent evidence for specificity focuses on the impact of sexual abuse. Even then, the outcomes of such studies must be interpreted with caution. This chapter focused on a limited selection of the key life stressors children and young people have been deemed to experience and, while avoiding pathologising the phenomenon, some of the underlying aetiological processes were offered for critical examination. It has been argued that it is almost impossible to compile a hierarchical order of stress categories or clusters. Nevertheless, it is clear that the most stressful events, regardless of the impetus appear to centre on loss or the threat of loss.

The overriding theme in terms of helping children cope/adapt to stressors points to the necessity of a stable, loving, supportive family unit. Longitudinal research is needed to evaluate the longer-term consequences of stress and coping on the child and family and the effectiveness of new and existing interventions for helping children and young people facing stress.

Family assessment is pivotal to family nursing. Just as an array of instruments is available to the healthcare professional to assess family needs, so too are there standardised inventories designed to measure individual life stressors. Instruments that are easy to administer and score will most likely be preferred and adopted by healthcare staff and family members. It is strongly recommended that readers gain a working knowledge of some of the instruments so that they can critically assess their reliability, validity and utility for practice. Unfortunately, most of the instruments critiqued may not be easily administered nor scored.

Children and young people are susceptible to the negative impact of acute/critical illness and hospitalisation. Real-life reflective accounts included in this chapter have hopefully served to illustrate the impact of associated stressors on the cognitive, affective and emotional domains of family functioning in such contexts. As well as requiring complex and comprehensive assessment, healthcare professionals need to know how the family uses existing support mechanisms, how family members clarify what they need and expect from each other – as well as from the health and social care system – and apply effective and appropriate interventions that help them cope with or at least adjust to the stress invoked reactions. Individual responses may vary tremendously, depending on a range of factors such as the quality and strength of the family relationships. Responses by individuals are complex entities with no single element that can explain the whole. Helping those children and families experiencing stress represents a major challenge to healthcare professionals. Some of the key features, it could be argued, include assessing the needs of the child and her/his family, detecting any adverse responses to stressors and assisting the child and family with the use of appropriate interventions. Allowing for cultural diversity when assessing and meeting the needs of children and families facing stress is a crucial way of demonstrating sensitivity and personalised care.

References

Adams J, Gill S, McDonald M 1991 Reducing fears in hospital. Nursing Times 87(1):624

Alderson P, Montgomery J 1996 Health care choices – making decisions with children. Institute for Public Policy Research, London

Balen R, Holroyd C, Mountain G, Wood B 2000 Giving children a voice: methodological and practical implications of research involving children. Paediatric Nursing 12:24–29

Barry P 2000 I go to the hospital to play, oh, and while I'm there I see the doctor. Online. Available at: http://www.nahps.org.uk/playprep.htm [accessed 24 September 2003]

Berk LE 2001 Child development. McGraw Hill, Boston

Bedell JR 1977 Life stress and the psychological and medical adjustment of chronically ill children. Journal of Psychosomatic Research 21:237–242

Bielby E 1984 A childish concept. Nursing Mirror 159(18):268

Boss P 1988 Family stress management. Sage, CA

Buchanan A, Tenbrink JA 1997 Recovery from emotional and behavioural problems. NHS Executive, Anglia & University of Oxford, Oxford

Burges L 1994 The developing person through the life span. Worth, New York

Clunn P 1991 Child psychiatric nursing. Mosby, St Louis, pp 110–111

Codddington RD 1972 The significance of life events as etiologic factors in the diseases of children. II. A study of a normal population. Journal of Psychosomatic Research 16:205–213

Coddington RD 1979 Life events associated with adolescent pregnancies. Journal of Clinical Psychiatry 40:180–185

Cohen J, Emmanuel J 1999 Positive participation: consulting and involving young people in health related work: a planning and training resource. Health Education Authority, London

Cohen F, Lazarus RS 1979 Coping with the stresses of illness. In: Stone GC, Cohen F, Adler NS (eds) Health psychology. Jossey-Bass, San Francisco

Coleman JC 1990 The nature of adolescence. Routledge, New York

D'Attilio JP, Campbell BM, Lubold P et al 1992 Social support and suicide potential: preliminary findings for adolescent populations. Psychological Reports 70:76–78

de Anda D, Baroni S, Boskin L et al 2000 Stress, stressors and coping among high school students. Children and Young Services Review 6:441–463

Department of Health 1999 Convention on the rights of the child. Second report to the United Nations committee on the rights of the child by the United Kingdom. Executive summary. The Stationery Office, London

Drummond RJ, Meieir ST 1995 Review of the Stress Index Scale. In: Conoley JC, Impara JC (eds) Mental measurements year book, 12th edn. University of Nebraska Press, Lincoln, NE, pp 994–995

Duncan DF 1977 Life stress as a precursor to adolescent drug dependence. International Journal of the Addictions 12:1047–1056

Eisner C 1990 Chronic childhood disease: an introduction to psychological theory and research. Cambridge University Press, Cambridge

Erwin P 1998 Friendship in childhood and adolescence. Routledge, London

Fallon S 1995 Hospital nursing care. In: Kelner CJH (ed.) Childhood and adolescent diabetes. Chapman & Hall, London

Flatman D 2002 Consulting children: are we listening? Paediatric Nursing 14(7):28

Friedman MM 1998 Family nursing: research, theory & practice, 4th edn. Appleton & Lange, Stamford

Ge X, Lorenz FO, Conger RD et al 1994 Trajectories of stressful life events and depressive symptoms during adolescence. Developmental Psychology 30:467–483

Glasper EA, Thompson M 1993 Preparing children for hospital. In: Glasper EA, Tucker A (eds) Advances in child health nursing. Scutari Press, London

GOSH/ICH 2002 The play service fact sheet. Great Ormond Street Hospital, London

Graham P, Turk J, Verhulst F 1999 Child psychiatry. Oxford University Press, Oxford

Grant K E 2003 Stressors and child/adolescent psychopathology: moving from markers to mechanisms of risk. In: McMahon SD, Grant KE, Compas BE et al (eds) Stress and psychopathology in children and adolescents: is there evidence of specificity? Journal of Child Psychology and Psychiatry 44(1):107–133

Green WA, Swisher SN 1969 Psychologic and somatic variables associated with the development and course of monozygotic twins discordant for leukaemia. Annals of the New York Academy of Science 164:394–408

Grey M 1993 Stressors and children's health. Journal of Pediatric Nursing 8(2):85–91

Grey M, Hayman LL 1987 Assessing stress in children: research and clinical implications. Journal of Pediatric Nursing 2(5):316–327

Harter S 1983 Developmental perspectives on the self esteem. In: P Mussen (ed.) Handbook of child psychology, 4th edn. Wiley, New York

Health Advisory Service 1995 Health Advisory Service child and adolescent mental health services: together we stand. HMSO, London

Heywood J 2002 Enhancing seamless care: a review. Paediatric Nursing 14(5):18–20

Hobfoll SE 1988 The ecology of stress. Hemisphere, Washington, DC

Hobfoll SE, Spielberger CD 1992 Family stress: integrating theory and measurement. Journal of Family Psychology 6(2):99–112

Ivory P 1998 Taking the scare out of hospital care for your child. Quest 5(3):1–6

Jackson S, Rodriguez-Tome H 1995 Adolescence and its social worlds. Lawrence Erlbaum, Hove

Jenkins R, Urstrun TB 1998 Preventing mental illness: mental health promotion in primary care. Wiley, Chichester

Jenson PS, Richters J, Ussery T et al 1991 Child psychopathology and emotional influences: discrete life events versus ongoing adversity. Journal of American Academy of Child and Adolescent Psychiatry 30:303–309

Johnson JII 1982 Life events as stressors in childhood and adolescence. In: Lahey BB, Kazdin AE (eds) Advances in clinical child psychology. Plenum, New York

Kidscape 2003 Online. Available at: http://www.kidscape.org.uk [accessed 24 September 2003]

Kitson A 1999 The essence of nursing. Nursing Standard 13(23):42–46

Lau BWK 2002 Does the stress in childhood and adolescence matter? A psychological perspective. The Journal of the Society for the Promotion of Health, 122(4):238–244

Lutz W 1986 Helping hospitalised children and their parents cope with painful procedures. Journal of Pediatric Nursing 1:24–32

Marks L 1994 Seamless care or patchwork quilt? Discharging patients from acute hospital care. Kings Fund Institute, London

McCubbin MA, McCubbin HI 1993 Families coping with illness: the resiliency model of family stress, adjustment and adaptation. In: Danielson C, Hamel-Bissell B, Winstead-Fry P (eds) Families, health, and illness: perspectives on coping and intervention. Mosby, St Louis, pp 21–63

McCubbin MA, Patterson C 1983 Family stress and adaptation to crises: a double ABCX model of family behaviour. In: Olson D, Miller B (eds) Family studies review yearbook. Sage, Beverly Hills, CA, pp 125–135

McMahon SD, Grant K, Compas BE et al 2003 Stress and psychopathology in children and adolescents: is there evidence of specificity? Journal of Child Psychology and Psychiatry 44(1):107–133

Melamed BG 1993 Putting the family back in the child. Behavioural Research Theory 31(3):239–247

Melamed BG, Siegel LJ, Ridley-Johnson R 1988 Coping behaviours in children facing medical stress. In: Field T, Schneiderman N, McCabe P (eds) Stress and coping. Lawrence Erlbaum, Hillsdale, NJ

Mental Health Foundation 1999 Bright futures: promoting children and young people's mental health. Mental Health Foundation, London

Miller MS 1982 Child's stress: understanding and answering of stress signals of infants, children and teenagers. Doubleday, Garden City, NY

Moos RH 1986 Coping with life crises. Plenum, New York

Moos RH 2002 Life stressors, social resources, and coping skills in youth: applications to adolescents with chronic disorders. Journal of Adolescent Health 30: 22–29

Morano CD, Cisler BA, Lemerond J 1993 Risk factors for adolescent suicide behaviour: loss, insufficient familial support, and hopelessness. Adolescence, 28:112

Mountain G 2002 Parenting in society: a critical review. In: Smith L, Coleman V, Bradshaw M (eds) Family centred care. Palgrave, Basingstoke

Papalia DE, Olds SW, Feldman RD 1999 A child's world: infancy through adolescence. McGraw-Hill, New York

Pfeffer SR, Conte IIR, Plutchick R, Jerrett I 1979 Suicidal behaviour in latency-age children: an empirical study. Journal of the American Academy of Child Psychiatry 18:679–692

Phinney JS, Alipuria LL 1990 Ethnic identity in college students from four ethnic groups. Journal of Adolescence 13:171–183

Rennick J 2002 Children's psychological responses after critical illness and exposure to invasive technology. Journal of Developmental and Behavioural Paediatrics 23(3):133–144

Robertson L 1995 The giving of information is the key to family empowerment. British Journal of Nursing 4(12):692

Rudolph KD, Hammen C 1999 Age and gender as determinants of stress exposure, generation, and reactions in youngsters: a transactional perspective. Child Development 70(3): 660–667

Sandler IN, Block M 1979 Life stress and the maladaptation of children. American Journal of Community Psychology (7):425–440

Santrock JW 2001 Child development. McGraw-Hill, New York

Selye H 1978 The stress of life. McGraw-Hill, New York

Sharman W 1997 Children and adolescents with mental health problems. Ballière Tindall, London

Solnit A 1984 Preparing. Psychoanalytic Study of the Child 39:613–632

Stein SP, Charles E 1971 Emotional factors in juvenile diabetes mellitus: a study of early life experiences. American Journal of Psychiatry 128:56–60

Steinhausen H, Verhulst F 1999 Risk and outcomes in developmental psychology. Oxford University Press, New York

Stoleb M, Chiriboga J 1998 A process model for assessing adolescent risk for suicide. Journal of Adolescence 21:359–370

Stone K 1994 Preparing your child for hospital: a parents' guide. Child Health 2(4):165

Sugar NF 1992 Toddlers' traumatic memories. Infant Mental Health Journal 16(4):259–270

Townley M 2002 Mental health needs of young people. Nursing Standard 16(30):38–45

Vincent KR, Rosenstock HA 1979 The relationship between stressful life events and hospitalised adolescent patients. Journal of Clinical Psychiatry 40:262–264

While A 1994 Day case surgery. Maternal Child Health 19(6):1846

Wilson-Sharrer V, Ryan-Wenger NM 1991 Measurements of stress and coping amongst school aged children with and without recurrent abdominal pain. Journal of School Health 61(2):86–91

Chapter Fourteen

14

The Evidence Base for Children's Nursing Practice

Peter Callery, Sarah Neill, Sue Feasey

ABSTRACT

Children's nurses are now expected to be able to provide the evidence base that underpins their clinical practice. This simple statement hides the complex nature of the processes involved in bringing together such evidence, given the vast wealth of published resources. The first part of this chapter aims to explore the sources of evidence available to children's nurses and how they can be used to develop the evidence base for a particular area of practice. This is followed by an exploration of the use of benchmarking to assess the quality of practice measured against the evidence. Inherent within these processes is the need to be able to critically appraise the evidence gathered. Every good research textbook includes general guidance on research critiquing but these texts do not generally explore issues specific to research involving children. These are explored in some depth in the next section of the chapter. Finally, the historical context of children's nursing research is discussed from which some of the emerging themes for future research are outlined.

Learning Outcomes

- Describe the sources of evidence that can contribute to development of interventions in children's nursing.

- Describe a hierarchy of evidence for interventions in children's nursing.

- Describe evidence required in implementation of interventions.

- Describe the use of benchmarking in children's nursing.

- Describe critical appraisal issues specific to research with children.

- Describe emerging themes in children's nursing research.

Introduction

The volume of research publications is daunting. Asthma, as the most common illness of childhood and involving children's nurses in community and hospital settings, can illustrate the volume and types of evidence used in children's nursing practice. Ovid Medline lists 7091 papers in English indexed under 'Asthma' 'limited to child (0–18 years)' in the period 1996 to July 2003. A systematic approach is therefore required if research is to be used to inform decisions about care. The evidence-based medicine movement has developed principles and procedures for searching and assessing research literature. Nurses can use the approach to base their own practice on evidence provided that there is recognition of the special features of children's nursing.

Formulating Questions

It is important to define the question that evidence is required to answer. The more clearly focused the question, the more likely that it will be possible to identify the most appropriate evidence available for the answer. Questions can be expressed in terms of four elements, using the PICO framework:

P = patient

I = intervention

C = comparison

O = outcome (Sackett et al 1997).

Craig (2002) illustrated how this framework can be used to identify and answer questions arising from practice in nursing. Her first example was a child who had developed a pressure ulcer on the back of her head when recovering from open heart surgery (Craig 2002). The question about the individual child: 'How can I prevent further pressure ulcers from developing in this child?' can be developed into a question to be answered by systematic review of randomised, controlled trials: 'In critically ill children, are constant low-pressure beds more effective than high specification foam mattresses in preventing pressure ulcers (defined here as constant discolouration of the skin, or partial or full thickness skin loss)?'(Craig 2002). This type of question is well suited to the PICO framework because it is concerned with a nursing action (the choice between a constant low-pressure bed and a foam mattress); that can be clearly associated with one consequence, formation of pressure ulcers. The direct link between cause and effect makes possible the use of experimental designs, including the randomised, controlled trial.

Evidence-based principles might suggest that all practice should be based on experimental research. However, even though experimental methods are well suited to pharmaceutical therapy, many drugs are not tested and therefore not specifically licensed for use in children (Conroy et al 2000). The limitations of the evidence base for treatment of children and young people is highlighted by the few studies that provide the basis for treating 40,000 people under the age of 18 years with major depressive disorder (Ramchandani 2004). Experiments to compare different treatments have not been conducted in children for various reasons. Some treatments are given to small numbers of children, which makes large-scale trials difficult to arrange or expensive. Ethical considerations can present difficulties in establishing trials to compare different treatments, particularly when alternative treatments are not available.

Not everything that nurses do can be tested by an experiment. Limitations of the PICO framework are illustrated by another of Craig's examples: a health visitor wants to understand why mothers feed infants with formula milk rather than breast feeding. The question is concerned with identifying information that could lead to an intervention to promote breast feeding. Craig (2002) suggested the question be formulated using the Patient and Outcome elements of the framework, excluding the Intervention and Comparison elements: 'What are the factors identified by mothers who live in deprived inner city areas that influence them to breast feed or to bottle feed using infant milk formula?'; a qualitative design would be required.

'Why?' questions such as this can be answered by understanding the world from the viewpoint of the people concerned. It is therefore best to take an open-ended approach, avoiding assumptions that may not be shared by the people who are to be studied. The types of question that are most

appropriately asked would therefore be concerned with how mothers make decisions about feeding their infants. There is a risk that the prior definition of patient (or, in this case, population) and outcome is based on assumptions about common characteristics of mothers and the definition of breast feeding as an outcome. The formulation of the question therefore requires reference to a theory of why mothers in deprived areas will have similar concerns about breast feeding.

The application of the PICO framework in children's nursing can be complicated by tensions between children's and parents' perspectives and interests. Children and parents may have different understandings of health problems and different goals for care. Questions about care may need to reflect differences between parents' and children's concerns and goals.

Activity

Think about your day-to-day practice and identify a problem that you need evidence to solve (e.g. 'What will prevent development of pressure ulcers in critically ill children?'):

- Try to turn your identified problem into a question that follows the PICO framework.
- What sort of evidence could provide the answer that you need?
- Is there a clear link between cause and effect and could an experiment be performed?

Complex Interventions

Nursing interventions in children's health care are often 'complex interventions':

Complex interventions in health care, whether therapeutic or preventative, comprise a number of separate elements which seem essential to the proper functioning of the intervention although the 'active ingredient' of the intervention that is effective is difficult to specify. If we were to consider a randomised controlled trial of a drug vs. a placebo as being at the simplest end of the spectrum, then we might see a comparison of a stroke unit to traditional care as being at the most complex end of the spectrum. The greater the difficulty in defining precisely what, exactly, are the 'active ingredients' of an intervention and how they relate to each other, the greater the likelihood that you are dealing with a complex intervention (MRC Health Services and Public Health Research Board 2000)

www

The full MRC document can be downloaded from the web as (you will need to download the free Acrobat Reader software to read it):

- http://www.mrc.ac.uk/pdf-mrc_cpr.pdf

Health visitors wishing to promote breast feeding will develop complex interventions. They might devise educational programmes whose 'active ingredients' include the quality of continuing relationships with mothers, information about the benefits of breast feeding and the method of communication, whether in groups or through individual contact.

Similar complexity can be seen in many nursing interventions. In hospital, nurses help children to cooperate with delivery of drug therapy by nebuliser, which requires the child to wear a mask. Community nurses explain how to use medication to control asthma at home. In each case the 'active ingredient' is difficult to identify: the manner in which the nurse forms a relationship with child and family, the content of the nurse's explanations, and the time and place at which the information is provided could all have important effects.

Identification and measurement of outcomes presents particular difficulties in children's nursing. Some outcomes are clear-cut, e.g. the formation of pressure ulcers, whereas others can be assessed only in relation to children's development, e.g. satisfactory growth, or require assessment by children themselves, e.g. assessment of quality of life.

Activity

Identify a complex intervention from your area of practice. List the possible 'active ingredients'.

Types of Evidence

Once the question has been identified, the next task is to identify the best evidence that will contribute to the answer. A systematic approach to literature searching is required to ensure that important evidence is not missed. A hierarchy of the different forms of evidence available can be used to identify the best evidence that is available. For example, studies can be organised in order of the strength of their design (Muir Gray 1997):

- I. Strong evidence from at least one systematic review of multiple, well-designed, randomised controlled trials.
- II. Strong evidence from at least one properly designed randomised, controlled trial of appropriate size.
- III. Strong evidence from well-designed trials without randomisation, single group, cohort, time series or matched case-control studies.
- IV. Evidence from well-designed, non-experimental studies from more than one centre or research group.
- V. Opinions of respected authorities based on clinical evidence, descriptive studies or reports of expert committees.

Categorisation of evidence usually follows the principle that the best evidence is to be found in studies that have minimised bias through design, for example by randomly allocating subjects to intervention and control groups to enable comparison of the effects of treatments. However, the design of a study does not guarantee the quality of the evidence (Wilson et al 1995).

WWW

More detailed categorisation of studies is presented and explained at the website of the Centre for Evidence-based Medicine:

- http://www.cebm. net/levels_of_evidence.asp#levels

Nursing interventions in asthma illustrate the use of evidence from studies of various designs and the contribution of qualitative research to the evidence base for children's nursing practice.

SYSTEMATIC REVIEWS

A systematic review of randomised, controlled trials of education in asthma concluded that:

Educational programmes for the self management of asthma in children and adolescents improve lung function and feelings of self control, reduce absenteeism from school, number of days with restricted activity, number of visits to an emergency department, and possibly number of disturbed nights. Educational programmes should be considered a part of the routine care of young people with asthma (Guevara et al 2003)

The review used a systematic method of searching the literature. The search terms used for Medline (1966–98), Embase (1980–98), and CINAHL (1982–98) were:

asthma OR wheez*

AND education* OR self management OR self-management

AND placebo* OR trial* OR random* OR double-blind OR double blind OR single-blind OR single blind OR controlled study OR comparative study.

Other databases and journals were also searched and 318 studies were identified. The quality of studies was assessed on the basis of the design, including whether allocation to the intervention or to the control group was known before each subject was included in the study. This criterion for quality was therefore concerned with potential bias: whether all the children in the population to be studied had an equal chance of being included in the sample. Once these criteria were applied, 45 of 318 identified studies were potentially eligible. However, 13 were excluded when other quality criteria were applied, leaving 32 trials totalling 3706 children and adolescents with asthma.

The stricter the criteria used for selecting studies eligible for inclusion in a systematic review, the fewer studies that will be included, so judgements about the criteria to be applied are important in designing such reviews. Guevara et al (2003) summarised the studies they reviewed:

Most were relatively small randomised controlled trials and enrolled children with severe asthma. Fifteen trials enrolled adolescents aged 13 to 18 years, and 12 enrolled children aged 2 to 5 years; no study stratified data on age. The educational programmes were diverse and targeted children, parents, or both. Most had programmes with multiple sessions and symptom based strategies.

The conclusions that could be reached by the review were therefore limited by the characteristics of the studies that were included. Guevara et al's review could make limited comments about: non-severe asthma, interventions at different ages, the types of education that is most effective and whether education should be directed at children, parents or both. The conclusion that education should be incorporated into the routine care of children with asthma is welcome but somewhat limited.

Guevara et al recommend further research, and here they are more specific. They suggest that:

Future studies should test alternative components directly to determine their relative effectiveness, for example, studies should focus on morbidity measurements and quality of life and directly compare strategies based on peak flow with those based on symptoms and compare strategies aimed at the individual with those aimed at the group.

These suggestions highlight the importance of understanding the intervention thoroughly. Guevara et al are essentially asking what might be the 'active ingredient' of education: is it directed at preventing the occurrence of acute episodes of illness or at improving quality of life? Is the active ingredient individualised education or education provided for groups? Their other question, 'Should education be based on symptoms or on peak flow measurement?' can be answered by another study from lower in the hierarchy of study designs. Forty asthmatic children (5–16 years) were asked to:

. . . perform peak flow measurements twice daily for 4 weeks by means of an electronic peak flow meter and to record values in a written diary. Patients and parents were unaware that the device stored the peak flow values on a microchip. Data in the written diary (reported data) were compared with those from the electronic diary (actual data) (Kamps et al 2001)

The authors reported that children's peak flow results were so unreliable that they should not be trusted:

The percentage of correct peak flow entries decreased from 56% to <50% from the first to the last study week (p < 0.04), mainly as a result of an increase in self-invented peak flow entries . . . Peak flow diaries kept by asthmatic children are unreliable. Electronic peak flow meters should be used if peak flow monitoring is required in children with asthma (Kamps et al 2001)

This illustrates how descriptive studies that add to understanding of how people behave in health care can make important contributions to developing evidence-based practice. (The 'p' value reported by Kamps refers to the probability that the difference was caused by chance, in most studies it is accepted that a result is statistically significant if there was a less than 5% (1 in 20) likelihood that the differences between two values could have been caused by chance.)

RANDOMISED CONTROLLED TRIALS

Randomised controlled trials (RCTs) have shown that nurses can make important differences to the health of children with asthma by educating them about self-management of their condition:

A prospective randomised control study of an asthma home management training programme was performed in children aged two years or over admitted with acute asthma. Two hundred and one children were randomised at admission to either an intervention group (n = 96), which received the teaching programme, or a control group (n = 105). A nurse-led teaching programme used the current attack as a model for the management of future attacks and included discussion, written information, subsequent follow up and telephone advice aimed at developing and reinforcing individualised asthma management plans. Parents were also provided with a course of oral steroids and guidance on when to start them . . . Subsequent readmissions were significantly reduced in the intervention group from 25% to 8% in individual follow up periods that ranged from two to 14 months (Madge et al 1997)

Madge et al's study demonstrated both the value and limitations of RCTs. The study showed that children educated by a nurse fared better, with less need for readmission and reduction in asthma symptoms. However, the problem of deciding what is the 'active ingredient' is evident. One nurse delivered the education – would other nurses have been as effective? The education was delivered as children were discharged from hospital. The authors followed-up children to assess the duration of the effect of education but this analysis was limited by the variation in the period of follow-up from 2–14 months. There is evidence that asthma attacks affect receptiveness to information in adults with asthma:

> 'strong cognitive/affective responses to attacks may motivate improved self-care and this represents a window of opportunity for self-care interventions' (Greaves et al 2002).

Was the education effective in Madge et al's study because it was delivered while the children were being discharged from hospital? In a qualitative study of parents' and children's perspectives on asthma it was reported that parents gave more emphasis to acute attacks than children and that they accepted some symptoms as tolerable provided that they did not result in an acute attack (Callery et al 2003). Could education at the time of an attack reinforce parental focus on acute attacks and hospitalisations rather than drawing parents' attention to controlling low-level symptoms that might affect children's quality of life? In addition to the educational intervention, the authors reported that parents were given oral steroids and instructions about their use. Were oral steroids one of the 'active ingredients' that resulted in improved outcomes for the intervention group? These questions arise because of the difficulty of separating different effects, or confounding variables, on the outcomes. The questions also indicate the importance of a thorough understanding of interventions and how they are seen by those involved, including children as well as parents and health professionals. Therefore descriptive studies, including qualitative studies are required to complement experimental studies in the development and evaluation of complex interventions.

Activity

Find research paper(s) that explore a problem relevant to your nursing practice:
- What type of evidence has been used to study the problem?
- What other types of design could be used to study this problem?

Researching Complex Interventions

Phases of development may be required to test complex interventions (MRC Health Services and Public Health Research Board 2000):

The first phase is preclinical and is concerned with developing the underlying theory for the intervention. Studies of educational interventions in asthma have been criticised for neglecting this phase, so that educational programmes have been developed without first identifying the theory that will guide practice (Clark & Gong 2000).

- Phase I – in which the components of the intervention are identified and assessed – commences once the theoretical framework has been identified. This phase is concerned with identifying the active ingredients.
- Phase II is an exploratory trial, or pilot study, that checks that an experimental study can be conducted.
- Phase III is the full trial.
- The final phase, IV, is concerned with long-term implementation: can others produce similar results with the intervention and maintain them over time?

The need for detailed developmental work before trialling interventions was highlighted in a report on diabetes education in childhood:

> This review recommends that a phase of programme development be undertaken involving a consultation process with adolescents with type 1 diabetes, their families, doctors, nurses, health economists and health psychologists. This consultation exercise would enable the establishment of possible interventions that are seen as plausible and potentially effective by patients and their parents, feasible and practical in the context of the NHS diabetes services and understood and accepted by doctors and nurses as key and integral parts of diabetes care. The interventions would also need to have the potential to be cost-effective and be based on sound behavioural principles. Such interventions, if subsequently demonstrated by commissioned research to be effective, would be much more likely to be implemented than ones developed without such a process (Hampson et al 2001)

Therefore a range of designs, including descriptive studies and qualitative studies, is required at different stages in the development of nursing interventions. Whereas this is true in all healthcare practice, it is particularly important in children's nursing. Studies must be designed to reflect the needs of children and not merely to apply concepts from adult health care to children. Evidence is required about children's perspectives, as well as the perspectives of adults involved in their care.

The evidence for children's nursing practice can therefore be complex and require skilled interpretation. Knowledge of both quantitative and qualitative research methods is required to assess evidence, particularly about complex interventions.

 WWW

You can keep up to date with the evidence base for practice by reading a good evidence-based journal such as *Evidence Based Nursing*, which uses rigorous procedures to identify and summarise the practice implications of new research publications. The website is:

- http://ebn.bmjjournals.com/

Benchmarking in Children's Nursing

Benchmarking is identified by the Department of Health (DoH 2000) as:

'A process through which best practice is identified and continuous improvement pursued through comparison and sharing'.

Benchmarking promotes evidence-based practice.

A 'comparison group' often consists of representatives from individual departments or directorates seeking to compare and improve practice plus individuals such as patient representation, multiprofessional colleagues and clinical experts. This group embarks on the benchmarking cycle (DoH 2001a) by deciding the area of practice to benchmark and agreeing what constitutes best practice using the best available evidence. A numerical scoring continuum is developed, including supporting statements that qualify numerical scores.

The clinical area representatives then score their own area and both the quantitative (scores) and qualitative (supporting statements) data are presented at subsequent comparison group meetings so that pockets of best practice are identified and shared, enabling lower scoring areas to action plan improvements.

The lack of 'higher levels' of research evidence to support the development of best practice statements results in the use of descriptive studies and professional consensus. However, this framework helps to promote better-informed professional consensus and acknowledges that multiple realities of best practice exist and are both socially constructed and situated (Bland 2001) and supports the use of research. This is significant because studies evaluating the strategies designed to promote evidence-based practice have not identified any 'magic bullets' (Oxman et al 1995) guaranteeing success. Acknowledging this, the Research in Child Health (RiCH) Group at the Royal College of Nursing (RCN) produced a 'Benchmark for evidence-based care' based on the research evidence for the structures and processes that seem crucial to getting evidence into practice. This informs the factors and standards within the benchmark that should enable the user to identify reasons for any lack of congruence between clinical practice and research plus gaps in the organisational infrastructure for implementing evidence-based practice (Feasey & Fox 2001).

 www

Read the research in *Child health benchmark for evidence-based care* at:

- http://www.man. ac.uk/rcn/ukwide/richnotice.htm

Any such lack of congruence will be most readily identified by the use of paediatric clinical practice benchmarks, such as those developed by the North West Clinical Practice Benchmarking Group established in 1994 involving seven hospital children's units. Its remit was to develop benchmarking as a quality improvement tool and standardise children's nursing practice.

Each of the benchmarks focuses on a single area of clinical practice, such as children's pain, and is broken down into a number of factors. For example, factor 1 is concerned with whether an individualised pain assessment tool exists, and factor 2 with whether pain is assessed and recorded (Bland 2001).

The *Essence of care* benchmarking toolkit, published by the DoH (2001a), is designed for use in all healthcare specialties and settings. The standards reflect the basics of care that were identified from complaints and patient/consumer and professional feedback as being highly significant to the patient experience but sometimes lacking. They are based on research evidence, national guidance and policies and consensus opinion amongst patient, professional and user groups. These benchmarks are therefore considered to be highly evidence-based and sufficiently flexible to enable application to the local situation during the 'agreeing best practice' stage of the benchmarking cycle (Jones & Evans 2003).

 www

Read the *Essence of care* benchmark (DoH 2001a) at:

- http://www.doh. gov.uk/essenceofcare/index.htm

Critical Appraisal Issues Specific to Research with Children: Ethical and Methodological Issues

Critical appraisal of research involves consideration of the ethical conduct of research as well as the rigour of the methodological process. When the subjects of the research are children, specific ethical and methodological issues need to be considered. In Western societies, children continue to be viewed as 'becoming' rather than 'being' a social person, an idea that results in notions of children as vulnerable, incompetent and dependent on adults (Christensen 1998). The resulting power differential between children and adults presents a range of different ethical issues that need to be considered in the critical appraisal process.

This section of the chapter will explore the ethics of conducting research with children including: guidelines for the ethical conduct of research with children, researcher role conflict for healthcare professionals, children as researchers, and the psychological impact of the research on child participants, with the intention of highlighting issues specific to researching with children for appraisers and planners of research.

ETHICS OF CONDUCTING RESEARCH WITH CHILDREN

The protective approach to children might initially provoke a reaction that excludes children from involvement in research, thereby protecting them from any potentially harmful effects – physical or psychological. This approach would result in less knowledge about children, excluding them from the benefits of research (Morrow & Richards 1996). Not to conduct research with children would therefore be unethical (Darbyshire 2000, Royal College of Paediatrics and Child Health (RCPCH) 2000).

It is therefore important to conduct research with and for children but to do so in such a way as to ensure their voluntary participation. Children, as well as adults, need to be able to make an uncoerced, informed decision before consenting to their participation in research. Even when children are not 'Gillick competent', i.e. of sufficient understanding and intelligence to understand fully what is proposed, opportunities need to be provided with sufficient appropriately formatted information to enable them to assent or dissent to their involvement (see Box 14.1 for definitions of consent, assent and dissent). Critical appraisal of research with children should therefore include consideration of how consent or assent was sought from children and their parents or guardians. For further discussion on the assessment of a child's competence to consent to research,

readers are referred to Alderson (1995), an overview of which is presented in Chapter 3.

It should be noted that ensuring uncoerced consent is particularly important, because coercion has serious possible effects on the validity of data gathered. This applies most particularly to qualitative research, which might result in children giving the responses they feel are wanted, but also in quantitative research where physiological measures of anxiety are used, as when participation in research is not voluntary, the participation itself may increase anxiety rather than any intervention being measured.

Activity

Find a research study involving children and identify:
- The procedures used to obtain consent to participation in the research from children and/or their parents.
- The extent to which children's competence to consent has been assessed prior to seeking consent.
- How the process for seeking consent could have been improved for your chosen research study.

GUIDELINES ON RESEARCH WITH CHILDREN

A number of published guidelines can be used as standards against which to measure an individual research project. However, the only guidelines written specifically for child health research in the UK to date are those from the RCPCH (2000), to which the DoH (2001b) research governance document also refers. These guidelines provide some direction for researchers (and those assessing research proposals for local research ethics committees (LRECs)) concerning the consent process and include consideration of acceptable areas to research with children. It should be noted, in accordance with the DoH (2001b) guidance, that LREC approval is required for all child health research projects.

Box 14.1

Definitions (from Broome & Stieglitz 1992)

Informed consent: an interactive process between subject and researcher involving disclosure, discussion and a complete understanding of a proposed research activity, and which culminates in the individual freely expressing a desire to participate.

Parental consent: all of the components of informed consent and should include consideration of the implications of research involvement for the child.

Assent: an interactive process between a child and researcher involving disclosure, discussion and a limited understanding of a proposed research activity, wherein the child freely expresses a preference for participation but has insufficient maturity to make a fully informed and autonomous decision.

Dissent: is an interactive process between a child and researcher involving disclosure, discussion and a limited understanding of the proposed research activity, wherein the child freely expresses an objection to the participation but has insufficient maturity to make a fully informed and autonomous decision.

WWW

Read the Royal College of Paediatrics and Child Health's guidelines (RCPCH 2000) online via the Archives of Disease in Childhood website:
- http://adc.bmjjournals. com/cgi/content/full/archdischild; 82/2/177

WWW

Read the Department of Health's research governance document online:
- http://www.doh.gov. uk/research/rd1/researchgovernance/ socialcare.htm

Any research critique should include consideration of whether the project was ethical to conduct with children as a sample or whether comparable research could have been conducted on adults instead.

These guidelines focus quite clearly on quantitative research, as they state that research is only worthwhile if the project

'involves a statistically appropriate number of subjects'.

Further guidance for qualitative research needs to be sought elsewhere. The reader is referred to the National Children's Bureau's (NCB 1996) guidelines for research, which provides detailed practical advice for researchers and therefore is also useful for those critiquing such research.

WWW

Read the National Children's Bureau's guidelines for research online:

* http://www.ncb.org.uk/research/guidelines.htm

Activity

Find a research study with a sample of children and analyse it using both the Royal College of Paediatrics and Child Health's guidelines and those from the NCB.

* How effective did you find each set of guidelines?
* What, if any, different issues did you identify from using one set of guidelines or the other?

RESEARCHER ROLE CONFLICT

Readers of research, and researchers themselves, also need to be aware of the potential for role conflict – when the researcher is a healthcare professional – between his/her role as a researcher who is present only to gather data from the child, and his/her role as a healthcare professional when issues concerning the child's ongoing health care emerge. For example, a child may tell the researcher during an interview about their dissatisfaction with their current treatment. The researcher may know about more effective treatment available or that the child's current treatment is no longer recommended practice. To ignore the needs of the child and continue with the interview would be unethical and would also indicate a lack of concern for the child that could damage the relationship between the researcher and the child and therefore reduce the extent, and validity of, the data collected.

CHILD PROTECTION AND CONFIDENTIALITY

Whenever healthcare professionals are involved with children child protection must be considered. This is no less the case when the activity concerned is research, presenting the researcher with a further role conflict. Researchers would normally offer guarantees of confidentiality and inform participants that their identity will not be disclosed in any research reports or to anyone other than the researchers involved. Yet where the respondent is a child, the NCB (1996) state clearly that confidentiality must be limited because:

Where a child or young person divulges that they or others are at risk of significant harm, or where the researcher observes or receives evidence of incidents likely to cause serious harm, the researcher has a duty to take steps to protect the child or other children.

Projects involving children should include consideration of the way in which children are informed of these limitations.

Activity

* Identify two other situations that might result in researcher role conflict.
* Discuss with your peer group how such conflict could be managed without undermining the ethical conduct of the research.

CHILDREN AS RESEARCHERS

Children are increasingly becoming involved in research as a part of the research team, including acting as interviewers, partly following the trend towards user involvement in research and partly to reduce the power imbalance that exists between an adult interviewer and a child. Traditionally, in adult qualitative research attempts are made to match interviewer and interviewee for age, social position, gender and ethnicity (Hood et al 1996, Mahon et al 1996) to avoid any power imbalance between researcher and subject. It is obviously difficult to match all children for age in this way, although adolescents have been engaged as interviewers (Alderson 1995). Ethical problems must be addressed in such circumstances, in particular, these centre around the child protection issues mentioned above: should child researchers be placed in a position where they may receive disturbing information from another child? Such research projects need to be assessed carefully on the basis of the appropriateness of the focus of the research, the methods used and the skills required of the researcher (Mahon et al 1996). Research reports should provide information on how such young interviewers are prepared for, supported through, and debriefed after the research.

PROTECTING THE CHILD FROM HARM

Monitoring the Impact on the Child

The RCPCH (2000) guidelines are very clear about the need to protect the child from unnecessary physical harm. They state that the decision concerning whether the research is allowed to take place should be based on an assessment of the balance of potential benefit against potential harm. In research involving physical procedures the degree of 'harm' involved is relatively predictable. The psychological impact on the child is less predictable, but it is well recognised that it may occur at the time or at a later date (Mahon et al 1996, NCB 1996). Research projects involving children should include strategies for the emotional support for children immediately after data collection and the provision of information about sources of help for the future. Throughout the research process, researchers need to monitor the child's non-verbal signs for any indication of unwillingness to take part or to continue with the research (Alderson 1995).

The Child's Comfort with the Research Process

The child's comfort with the whole process is likely to affect the consent process and the quality of the data collected. Children need to feel emotionally safe with any individual to be able to talk about their views or experiences or to submit to physical investigations. Appraisers of research should consider how children were put at their ease, for example through the use of ice-breaking techniques (Borland et al 1998). Children's understanding of what is involved in a project is affected by the way in which information is presented in terms of the content and the pace of information giving (Ireland & Holloway 1996). Qualitative research should also be critiqued for the flexibility provided in terms of the methods used to gather data. Whereas some children are content to talk, others might feel more comfortable drawing or taking pictures of relevant objects and places (Coyne 1998, Matthews et al 1998). Researchers in the social science field have emphasised the importance of using methods which interest and therefore engage children and which are within the child's ability (Boyden & Ennew 1997, Matthews & Tucker 2000).

Historical Overview of Children's Nursing Research: The Context for the Emerging Themes of the Future

Research in children's nursing and child health care is a relatively new field of enquiry. Alderson (1993) points out that research involving children only began seriously in the latter part of the 20th century. Traditionally, children have been seen as subjects to be acted upon by others (Christensen 1998) rather than individuals to be asked to participate in research in their own right. This should not be surprising given the social construction of childhood that has largely prevailed throughout the 20th and into the 21st centuries, which sees childhood as the precursor to adulthood rather than as a stage of life to be valued in its own right. However, as will be discussed below, ideas about children are beginning to change and this is influencing the way in which research is conducted in children's nursing and child health care.

During the 20th century children were studied using mostly experimental, observational and standard measurement techniques. This research has generally taken no account of the research subject's (child's) viewpoint (Alderson 1993). When research did focus on the child's experiences, this was primarily conducted through proxies, in research about rather than with children. Included here is much of the research on parent participation, for example: Algren (1985), Darbyshire (1994), Knafl et al (1988), Neill (1996a,b) or on partnership, for example: Casey (1993, 1995), Cleary (1992), Coyne (1995). Adults set themselves up as the interpreters of children's behaviour (Waksler 1991). Although much was learnt about adults' perceptions of childhood experiences through this research, nothing was learnt about the child's own experiences, from which knowledge services could be developed more in tune with the child's wants and needs.

Social perceptions of childhood are changing, albeit slowly. Children are gradually being given the opportunity to be listened to, not just heard. Hearing is merely the perception of sound whereas listening involves paying attention to what is being said. The United Nations Convention on the rights of the child (United Nations General Assembly 1989) includes two articles that focus specifically on children's rights to have their views taken into account.

- Article 12: Parties shall assure to the child who is capable of forming his or her own views the right to express those views freely in all matters affecting the child, the views of the child being given due weight in accordance with the age and maturity of the child.

- Article 13: The child shall have the right to freedom of expression; this right shall include freedom to seek, receive and impart information and ideas of all kinds, regardless of frontiers, either orally, in writing or in print, in the form of art, or through any other media of the child's choice.

WWW

The full text of the UN Convention on the Rights of the Child (1989) can be viewed online at:
- http://www.unicef.org/crc/crc.htm

It has taken some time to see these rights being operationalised at a national level in the UK:

- The DoH (2002) produced an action plan to guide the involvement of children and young people in the NHS entitled *Listening, hearing and responding*.
- A Children and Young People's Unit has been created to support cross-government work on child poverty and youth disadvantage.
- Consultation with children is currently underpinning the development of the National Service Framework for Children.

These initiatives reflect the emerging agenda for service user involvement in health care.

WWW

Read the DoH's (2002) action plan online:
- http://www.doh. gov.uk/scg/actionplaninvolveyoung2002. htm

Visit the Children and Young People's Unit website and find out about activities in progress and consider their relevance to your practice area:
- http://www.cypu.gov.uk

Visit the National Service Framework's website to find out about the latest progress in developing and implementing the NSF:
- http://www.doh.gov.uk/nsf/children.htm

What are you doing in your practice area towards the implementation of the NSF?

It is clear that children should have the right to contribute to research themselves, rather than through others and that changes in society are taking place which should support such research.

Research is emerging that does reflect both the changes in society's perception of children and the changes within children's nursing itself where the emphasis has moved from parent participation and partnership with parents to listening to children first and foremost. Research conducted with children as active research participants, which seeks their views on health and health care, has been increasing rapidly since the 1990s (e.g. Action for Sick Children 1998, Alderson 1993, Coyne 1998, Ireland & Holloway 1996, Pridmore & Bendelow 1995). Children have also begun to get involved as researchers, either as a member of the research planning team or as interviewers (Alderson 1995). Further research is still needed to explore both children's perspectives on child health and the ways in which children can be involved in research. It is also to be hoped that in focusing on the child, researchers will not forget that children live in families and that there is a need to explore the interrelationships between the adults and the children in families with respect to their influence on children and families' health and their perspectives on health care services. Finally, it should be remembered that whereas the discussion here has focused largely on qualitative approaches to research to generate a knowledge of children's perspectives, it should not be forgotten that such research will lay the foundations for more large-scale quantitative research. Quantitative approaches are also needed to test many treatment modalities. Little work has so far been conducted here, leaving practice based on custom and practice rather than a sound evidence base. This situation should be remedied in future research.

Summary

Guidance on research involving children indicates a general agreement that not to undertake research with children would be unethical because there would then be no evidence on which to develop relevant and effective services. Appraisal of research with children should include methods used to put the child at ease with the researcher as well as an assessment of methods used to obtain consent. Consent should be obtained from both the child and the parent or guardian. Where the child does not have sufficient understanding of what is involved and the implications of such involvement, the assent of the child should be sought. Strategies in place to manage the potential role conflict between the researcher as health professional and the researcher as data collector should be identified. Research involving interviews with children should be assessed against the NCB (1996) guidance concerning the limitations on confidentially for child protection issues. Appraisers also need to consider whether the potential impact of the child, physically and psychologically has been addressed. Finally, in reviewing the methodologies chosen in qualitative research with children, appraisers should be able to identify flexibility in the range of options provided for children to share their knowledge, views and experiences.

References

Action for Sick Children 1998 Pictures of healthcare. A child's eye view. Action for Sick Children, London

Alderson P 1993 Children's consent to surgery. Open University Press, Buckingham

Alderson P 1995 Listening to children. Children, ethics and social research. Barnardos, Ilford

Algren CL 1985 Role perception of mothers who have hospitalised children. Children's Health Care 14:6–9

Bland M 2001 North West clinical practice benchmarking group: principles, processes and evaluations. Nursing Times Research 6(2):581–593

Borland M, Laybourn A, Hill M, Brown J 1998 Middle childhood. The perspectives of children and parents. Jessica Kingsley, London

Boyden J, Ennew J 1997 Children in focus: a manual for participatory research with children. Swedish Save the Children, Radda Barnen, Stockholm

Broome ME, Stieglitz KA 1992 The consent process and children. Research in Nursing & Health 15:147–152

Callery P, Milnes L, Couriel J, Verduyn C 2003 Qualitative study of children's and parents' beliefs about childhood asthma. British Journal of General Practice 53:185–190

Casey A 1993 Development and use of the partnership model of nursing care. In: Glasper EA, Tucker A (eds) Advances in child health nursing. Scutari Press, London

Casey A 1995 Partnership nursing: influences on involvement of informal carers. Journal of Advanced Nursing 22:1058–1062

Christensen PH 1998 Difference and similarity: how children's competence is constructed in illness and its treatment. In: Hutchby and Moran-Ellis (eds) Children and social competence: arenas of action. Falmer Press, London

Clark NM, Gong M 2000 Management of chronic disease by practitioners and patients: are we teaching the wrong things? British Medical Journal 320:572–575

Cleary J 1992 Caring for children in hospital. Parents and nurses in partnership. Scutari Press, London

Conroy S, Choonara I, Impicciatore P et al 2000 Survey of unlicensed and off label drug use in paediatric wards in European countries. British Medical Journal 320:79–82

Coyne IT 1995 Partnership in care: parents' views of participating in their hospitalized child's care. Journal of Clinical Nursing 4:71–79

Coyne IT 1998 Researching children: some methodological and ethical considerations. Journal of Clinical Nursing 7:409–416

Craig JV 2002 Skills for evidence based practice: how to ask the right question. In: JV Craig, RL Smyth (eds) The evidence-based practice manual for nurses. Churchill Livingstone, Edinburgh

Darbyshire P 1994 Living with a sick child in hospital. The experiences of parents and nurses. Chapman & Hall, London

Darbyshire P 2000 Guest editorial. From research on children to research with children. Neonatal, Paediatric and Child Health Nursing 3(1):2–3

Department of Health (DoH) 2000 The NHS plan: a plan for investment, a plan for reform. The Stationery Office, London

Department of Health (DoH) 2001a The essence of care: patient-focused benchmarking for healthcare practitioners. DoH, London

Department of Health (2001b) Research Governance Framework for Health & Social Care. DoH, London

Department of Health (DoH) 2002 Listening, hearing and responding. Department of Health action plan. Core principles for the involvement of children and young people. DoH, London

Feasey S, Fox C 2001 Benchmarking evidence-based care. Paediatric Nursing 13(5):22–25

Greaves CJ, Eiser C, Seamark D, Halpin DMG 2002 Attack context: an important mediator of the relationship between psychological status and asthma outcomes. Thorax 57:217–221

Guevara JP, Wolf FM, Grum CM, Clark NM 2003 Effects of educational interventions for self management of asthma in children and adolescents: systematic review and meta-analysis. British Medical Journal 326:1308–1309

Hampson S, Skinner T, Hart J et al 2001 Effects of educational and psychosocial interventions for adolescents with diabetes mellitus: a systematic review. Health Technology Assessment 5(10):1–79

Hood S, Kelley P, Mayall B 1996 Children as research subjects: a risky enterprise. Children and Society 10(2):117–128

Ireland L, Holloway I 1996 Qualitative health research with children. Children and Society 10:155–164

Jones S, Evans K 2003 Essence of care in a children's hospital. Paediatric Nursing 15(3):42–43

Kamps AW, Roorda RJ, Brand PL 2001 Peak flow diaries in childhood asthma are unreliable. Thorax 56:180–182

Knafl KA, Cavallari KA, Dixon DM 1988 Pediatric hospitalization. Family and nurse perspectives. Scott, Forseman & Co., Glenview, IL

Madge P, McColl J, Paton J 1997 Impact of a nurse-led home management training programme in children admitted to hospital with acute asthma: a randomised controlled study. Thorax 52:223–228

Mahon A, Glendinning C, Clarke K, Craig G 1996 Researching children: methods and ethics. Children and Society 10:145–154

Matthews H, Limb M, Taylor M 1998 The geography of children: some ethical and methodological considerations for project and dissertations work. Journal of Geography in Higher Education 22(3):311–324

Matthews H, Tucker F 2000 Consulting children. Directions JGHE Study Guide. Journal of Geography in Higher Education 24(2):299–310

Morrow V, Richards M 1996 The ethics of social research with children: an overview. Children and Society 10:90–105

MRC Health Services and Public Health Research Board 2000 A framework for development and evaluation of RCTs for complex interventions to improve health. Medical Research Council, London

Muir Gray JA 1997 Evidence-based healthcare. How to make health policy and management decisions. Churchill Livingstone, Edinburgh

National Children's Bureau (NCB) 1996 Guidelines for research. NCB, London

Neill SJ 1996a Parent participation 1: literature review and methodology. British Journal of Nursing 5(1):34–40

Neill SJ 1996b Parent participation 2: findings and their implications for practice. British Journal of Nursing 5(2):110–117

Oxman AD, Thompson MA, Davis DA, Haynes RB 1995 No magic bullets: a systematic reviews of 102 trials of interventions to improve professional practice. Canadian Medical Association Journal 153(10):1423–1431

Pridmore P, Bendelow G 1995 Images of health: exploring beliefs of children using the 'draw-and-write' technique. Health Education Journal 54:473–488

Ramchandani P 2004 Treatment of major depressive disorder in children and adolescents. British Medical Journal 328:3–4

Royal College of Paediatrics and Child Health: Ethics Advisory Committee 2000 Guidelines for the ethical conduct of medical research involving children. Archives of Disease in Children 82(Feb):117–182

Sackett D, Richardson W, Rosenburg W, Haynes R 1997 Evidence-based medicine. Churchill Livingstone, Edinburgh

United Nations General Assembly 1989 Convention on the rights of the child. UNICEF, Geneva

Waksler FC 1991 Studying the social worlds of children: sociological readings. Falmer Press, London

Wilson MC, Hayward RSA, Tunis SR et al 1995 How to use clinical guidelines: what are the recommendations and will they help you in caring for your patients? (Users' guides to the medical literature, part 8). Journal of the American Medical Association 274:1630–1633

Chapter Fifteen

15

Involving Children in Healthcare Research

Jennifer Allison, Rosemary King, E Alan Glasper

ABSTRACT

The aim of this chapter and its companion PowerPoint presentation is to explore the research process and investigate the various issues involved when children participate in clinical research.

Learning Outcomes

- Recognise that conducting research with children is different.

- Examine elements of informed consent and assent.

- Appreciate the need for conducting research with children.

- Understand how research is conducted with children.

- Explore methods of actively involving children as researchers.

Introduction: Children are not Small Adults

Nurses, and indeed any professional wishing to be involved in research with children, must have a basic understanding of the fundamental differences between adults and children. Children are not small adults, so having an appreciation of what children really *are* will increase the likelihood of a successful outcome. Rates of physical and psychological change throughout childhood are so great that simply discussing 'the child' as one would 'the adult' is not sufficient. Further subgroups are necessary to describe childhood fully. Common divisions of childhood include: infant, child and teenager. These can

be divided more finely and have been discussed in other chapters (see Chapter 11).

The legal definition of a child in England, Wales and Northern Ireland is simply anyone under the age of 18 years (Department of Health (DoH) 2001a); in Scotland it is under 16 years (Age of Legal Capacity (Scotland) Act 1991). But the characteristics and diversity of childhood creates a far more complex picture. Children's unique qualities will impact upon every aspect of the research project and ultimately determine its success or failure. Most importantly, infants, children and teenagers are distinctive individuals and the nurse involved in research with children must continually assess and meet the needs of these young volunteers.

PHYSICAL AND PHYSIOLOGICAL DIFFERENCES

There are physical differences between children and adults both in terms of size and proportion. In relation to the rest of their bodies, newborns' heads are much larger than those of adults. Their brains and nervous systems are not fully grown or formed. There is rapid growth of the infant brain during the first year of life and even the structure of the infant skull changes, e.g. initial presence and then closure of fontanelles. Children's abdomens look large and distended, their arms and legs small. These differences in proportions result in higher body surface area in relation to height and higher basal metabolic rate (BMR). This in turn results in higher energy requirements. Growth is a unique facet of childhood and requires energy. Infants also need more calories per kilogram than adults to maintain normal function (MacGregor 2001). Children have faster heart rates, breathe faster and have lower blood pressure. Young children also suffer from illnesses that do not exist in the adult population: respiratory distress syndrome, bronchiolitis, croup and necrotising enterocolitis are just a few (Behrman & Kliegman 1998). The developing organ systems of children can respond to drugs very differently from fully developed adults. Adverse events may not be obvious initially. Long-term effects on growth and development become apparent only as the child grows (International Conference on Harmonisation (ICH) 2000).

The ICH *Guideline for good clinical practice*, first operational in 1997, provides crucial, basic standards for research practice (ICH 2002). A more recent document – ICH E11 (2000) –looks specifically at children's participation in medicinal product research. Issues regarding preterm neonates through to young adults are examined with guidance to minimise risk. With the potential for accidental or deliberate harm so great, the international community has created these guidelines for professionals who involve children and young people as research volunteers.

Unless exposed to teratogens in utero, infants are born as a 'clean slate'. They have not damaged their lungs with cigarette smoke or pollution. Their livers have not been subjected to abuse by alcohol; their arteries are not clogged with cholesterol plaques. Children metabolise most drugs at a much faster rate than adults and the potential for accidental damage is much greater. In addition, it is not uncommon for initial or phase I paediatric drug studies to produce recommended doses much higher than adult doses (Morland 2003).

Physical and physiological changes are numerous and continuous throughout childhood. These changes impact on all relationships. Knowledge and understanding of this dynamic process will allow the research nurse to have meaningful interaction with the child or young person based on age appropriate expectations.

www

Visit the European Agency for the Evaluation of Medicinal Products website for access to International Conference on Harmonisation (ICH) documents, including topic E11:
- http://www.emea.eu.int

DEVELOPMENTAL DIFFERENCES

Developmental changes occur alongside physical maturation. This is an ongoing, ever-changing process. It is accepted theory that children move along a continuum in an expected and orderly fashion, but the exact timing is unique for each child. Piaget, Erikson and Freud devised established theories of development. Each examined children's development but from different perspectives (Behrman & Kliegman 1998). Table 15.1 provides the basic components of their theories. For further information see Chapter 11.

Developmental stages will help determine the way a child responds and behaves. Young research volunteers can be expected to react in certain ways depending on these stages. Therefore, it is possible for the research nurse to anticipate the reaction prior to approaching the child. However, these stages of development should serve only as a guideline, it is also imperative to assess each child as an individual. Children of the same age can differ greatly and are constantly changing and developing. Being equipped to

Table 15.1 Summaries of the Different Theories of Child Development

Age	Piaget	Erikson	Freud
Birth–18 months		Trust versus mistrust	Oral stage
Birth–2 years	Sensorimotor		
18 months–2 years		Autonomy versus shame and doubt	Anal stage
2–6 or 7 years	Preoperational		
3–6 years		Initiative versus guilt	Phallic stage
6 or 7–11 years	Concrete operations		
6–12 years		Industry versus inferiority	Latency stage
12 years–adult	Formal operations		
Adult		Identity versus role confusion	Genital stage

Adapted from Behrman & Kleigman 1998 pp 18–19.

interact appropriately with children at all stages is vital to establishing a successful relationship with each child.

Alderson & Montgomery (1996) question traditional theories that used the obvious physical growth of children as a metaphor for maturation of mental and emotional abilities, resulting in a gradual increase in ability while assuming younger children remain unable to participate in decisions. They argue that the experience of the child has greater impact on ability than age. However, this view and traditional theories agree that children mature at uneven rates. Therefore, researchers must continually evaluate the individual and changing needs of young volunteers.

Scenario

Julia is a third year child branch student on placement in a Clinical Research Facility (CRF). Three year old Amanda arrives with her parents for a bronchoscopy. She requires this diagnostic procedure and will be part of a research study, as bronchial wash samples will also be taken. She requires anaesthetic cream for a cannula. Julia asks her if she would like to sit on the treatment table or in the chair on mummy's lap. Amanda points to the treatment table with a brightly coloured toy on the pillow. Why did Julia give her a choice? Would this have been different if Amanda was 6 months old, or 12 years old?

SOCIAL DIFFERENCES

An appreciation of the unique social environment of children further enhances the creation of a successful relationship with a young volunteer. The family unit is the socially accepted and identifiable model of childcare and socialisation (DoH 2003a). It is rarely permissible to involve children in research without involving the child's family. Building a trusting relationship with a child volunteer requires an equally strong relationship with the family. As is made clear later in this chapter regarding issues of consent, without parental consent it is impossible to proceed with the research project (DoH 2001a). Studies have shown that parental attitudes are most influential in a child or young person's decision-making process. As decisions become more complex, younger children appear more susceptible to parental influence (Broome & Richards 2003). Young children are totally dependant within the family unit, a situation rarely seen within other patient groups. The UK National Service Framework (NSF) for Children (DoH 2003a) recognises this and mandates 'children and young people should receive care that is integrated and coordinated around their particular needs, and the needs of their family'.

WWW

Search for the UK National Service Framework for Children online at the Department of Health website
• http://www.dh.gov.uk

PowerPoint

Access the companion PowerPoint presentation and look at examples of child-friendly information leaflets used in the Wellcome Trust Clinical Research Facility. How do these compare with information you have used on placements?

COMMUNICATION

Information is the cornerstone of the research process and is basic to the concept of informed consent, which will be discussed in detail later.

It is the duty of the research nurse to provide the necessary information to the family and the child. This can be achieved in a number of ways including printed materials, audiovisual format and discussions. Regardless of the method used, all information must be age appropriate and formatted in a way easily understood by the child and family, so that informed decisions can be made. Issues of age and development will impact on the types of information given to children. Creative use of drawings, play, puppets and dolls can aid in the information process (DoH 2001a). Communication with children will require very different techniques depending on age and developmental needs. Once again it is not good enough to say, 'this is the way to communicate with a child' because infants will require very different methods to preschoolers or teenagers. The ability to judge a situation and intervene appropriately with individual children cannot be overestimated.

WWW

Visit the UNICEF website at:
• http://www.unicef.org
The full document The United Nations Convention on the Rights of the Child can be found at:
• http://www.unicef.org/crc/fulltext.htm

Child Protection Issues

Children participating in research have the same rights to protection offered all research volunteers by the declaration of Helsinki (World Medical Association (WMA) 2000). These issues will be discussed later in this chapter. In addition there is further protection from the Children Act (DoH 1989) and the NSF for Children (DoH 2003a), which stipulate requirements regarding the specific needs of children. This includes a Draft Standard on Child Protection stating:

Children have the right to be protected, and adults a responsibility to protect them from harm (DoH 2003a)

Families have a right to expect separate facilities, properly staffed by paediatricians, sick children's nurses and play therapists. Television, well-equipped playrooms and age-appropriate food are just some of the requirements. Collaboration between agencies is necessary, with multi-disciplinary development of child protection guidelines, policies and involvement in Serious Case Reviews. All staff must have child protection training and those who have direct contact with children require pre-employment police checks (DoH 2003a). For further information on child protection, see Chapter 19.

Activity

Look at the Child Protection policies when on different placements.
- How do they compare?
- How do they ensure that staff are properly trained in child protection?
- Have you had a police check?

Vulnerability and Autonomy

The lack of autonomy allowed children by society increases the vulnerability of young research volunteers. The amount of independence afforded to children is a matter of choice for society. It has been argued that children are unable to exercise choice due to cultural constraints rather than biological necessity. When children are not given the opportunity or permission to exercise their autonomy, it is often mistakenly assumed that they do not have the capacity to do so (Alderson & Montgomery 1996).

Activity

Discuss the following questions with your colleagues.
- How does the lack of autonomy increase the vulnerability of children?
- Have you seen examples of highly capable youngsters being prevented from participating fully in their healthcare?

The United Nations (UN) Convention on the Rights of the Child, Article 12 (UN General Assembly 1989) sets no minimum age for involvement in decisions and refers to children's 'evolving capacity', with adult members of society expected to foster participation.

Under UK law, children lack complete autonomy and are unable to make some decisions independently. Although they always have the right to assent or agree to participate, their parents usually make legal decisions and consent on their behalf (DoH 2001a). Issues of Gillick competency, consent and assent will be discussed later, as will involving children actively in the research process. The NSF for Children mandates the delivery of child-centred care and staff to support children 'to be active partners in decision making' (DoH 2003a). The child must come first and his or her needs are paramount within any research project.

At the basis of the research process is the trusting relationship between volunteer and researcher. It is critical that the research nurse prepares the child properly, taking into account the unique needs of each child with respect to age, development and social/family considerations. Research professionals must also put the needs and best interests of their volunteers first, ahead of research aspirations (DoH 2001b). Using age- and developmentally appropriate interactions and information, research nurses can be strong, dependable advocates for their young patients. Theories of growth and development, combined with an understanding of physical differences and needs of children, provide guidelines for researchers working with children and young people. However, assessing each child as a unique individual will increase the likelihood of successful interactions and research. Alderson & Montgomery (1996) warn there is a risk of holding on to outdated misconceptions that can result in the infantalisation of highly capable children and young people. Balancing the amount and types of support given to children can be difficult to judge and adults are often overcautious in assessing children's capabilities. Research nurses must ensure young volunteers are looked after in an appropriate and safe manner. Investing time to build a relationship will allow informed dialogue so that children are given the protection they need and the choices they deserve.

Issues of Informed Consent and Assent

Consent is a legal contract entered into by an adult or individual with parental responsibility; assent is the voluntary permission of an individual without legal status (Lamprill 2002).

HOW DO YOU OBTAIN CONSENT FROM CHILDREN?

In the document *Seeking consent: working with children* (DoH 2001a), the DoH stipulates that for consent to be considered valid, the person giving consent must be:

- competent: capable of making the decision
- acting voluntarily
- informed by the researcher to enable a decision to be made.

In the UK, children and young people acquire the right to give or withhold consent for treatment in stages. At 18 years of age, young people in England, Wales and Northern Ireland become legal adults with the absolute right to give or refuse consent (DoH 2001a). Under Scottish law, young people achieve this right at 16 (Age of Legal Capacity (Scotland) Act 1991). No one can consent on behalf of another competent adult. In the rest of the UK, 16–17 year olds are presumed competent to give consent for treatment. However, this becomes complicated when the child refuses consent, because the parents can override the wishes of their dissenting 16–17-year-old child. Under 16s are *not* legally competent unless they are deemed to be 'Gillick competent', i.e. if they have sufficient understanding and intelligence to enable them to understand fully what is proposed. Therefore, there is no specific age when a child becomes competent; it depends on the individual child and complexity of treatment (DoH 2001a).

For a young or non-Gillick competent child, consent must be given by a parent or person with 'parental responsibility', someone with legal responsibility for the child as stated in the Children Act (DoH 1989). It is important to note that unmarried fathers and stepfathers might not have this legal right unless afforded so by a court of law or by a Parental Responsibility Agreement with the mother. Therefore professionals must ensure that consent is obtained from an adult with this right of parental responsibility (DoH 2001a).

WHAT DOES THE NMC SAY REGARDING CONSENT?

The NMC in the Code of Professional Conduct (NMC 2002) clause 3.2 states that consent must be informed and given voluntarily by a competent person. It also recognises the patient's right to advocacy regardless of age in clause 2.2:

You are personally accountable for ensuring that you promote and protect the interests and dignity of patients and clients, irrespective of gender, age . . .

A clear guideline regarding competency is issued in clause 3.4:

You should presume that every patient and client is legally competent unless assessed by a suitable practitioner . . .

However, these statements are modified in relation to children and young people in clause 3.9:

No-one has the right to give consent on behalf of another competent adult. In relation to obtaining consent for a child, the involvement of those with parental responsibility in consent procedure is usually necessary, but will depend on the age and understanding of the child. If the child is under the age of 16 in England and Wales, 12 in Scotland and 17 in Northern Ireland, you must be aware of legislation and local protocols relating to consent.

 WWW

For more information on Gillick competency and the landmark court case go to:
- http://www.confidential.oxfordradcliffe.net/gillick

What is Competency?

The issue of competency can be complicated but the DoH (2001a) has given some guidelines. Someone is deemed competent if they:

Comprehend and retain information material to the decision, especially as to the consequences of having or not having the intervention in question . . .

Use and weigh this information in the decision-making process (DoH 2001a)

Children's competency is not an issue when they agree to treatment – it is when they refuse that questions of competency are raised (Alderson 1995). Until the youngster is 16 in Scotland, or 18 in the rest of the UK, parents have the legal authority to reverse the wishes of their child and give consent for treatment even if the youngster withholds consent (Age of Legal Capacity (Scotland) Act 1991, DoH 2001a). This creates a double standard for consent, with young people under the age of 18 free to agree and give consent but not able to disagree and withhold consent (Alderson 1995). The NSF for Children (DoH 2003a) states that:

Consent policies should include what to do when there is disagreement between a competent young person and their parent.

Therefore it is advisable to check local policies regarding consent. In extreme cases of disagreement, the courts can decide whether or not treatment is given (DoH 2001a).

 WWW

Visit the Department of Health website to review consent guidance:
- http://www.dh.gov/consent

The full Declaration of Helsinki document can be found at the World Medical Association website:
- http://www.wma.net/e/policy/b3.htm

Activity

Read the consent policies on your ward placement;
look at the consent forms:

- How often do you see 16-year-olds sign their own forms?
- Do you observe younger Gillick competent children signing consent for procedures?

What Makes Consent Informed?

The DoH Research Governance Framework (2001b) states that 'informed consent is at the heart of ethical research'. That is to say that information must be given so that consent is based on sufficient knowledge of what is planned and any possible risks involved. Extensive patient information sheets are required for each study and are ethically approved as part of formal research protocols. When children are involved in studies, special age-appropriate information sheets are needed (Robinson 2001). As stated in part 22 of The Declaration of Helsinki (WMA 2000), there is clear stipulation as to the type of information researchers are mandated to provide. This includes information regarding:

Aims, methods, sources of funding, any possible conflicts of interest, institutional affiliations of the researcher, the anticipated benefits and potential risks of the study and the discomfort it may entail.

The DoH (2001a) clearly states that children should be involved in decision making and suggests the use of toys, pictures and play and to ensure that written information is given in age-appropriate language. Prospective volunteers should be given this information in advance of their participation, ideally at least 24 h prior to the signing of consent forms. This enables them to consult with their family, GP or any person with whom they choose to discuss the study and possible concerns. It also allows time to formulate questions for the researcher prior to participation (Alderson 1995). The person obtaining consent must also 'check the child's understanding' (DoH 2001a). This can be achieved by including a simple quiz, which can be kept as a record of comprehension with other study forms (Lamprill 2002).

What About Research?

Participation in research is not mandatory. Participants in research studies are called 'volunteers'. That word describes an individual who freely takes part in the research process. Protection and care of the research subject is enshrined in internationally accepted guidelines.

The first international standard was written in 1947 as a reaction to the atrocities of the Second World War, and later became known as the Nuremberg Code. The ten principles have become the basis for ethical research practice involving humans. These principles include freely given consent, capacity to consent, freedom from coercion, comprehension of the risks and benefits, minimisation of risk and harm with a favourable risk/benefit ratio, the presence of qualified investigators using appropriate research designs and freedom for the subject to withdraw at any time. Children were excluded from participating in research by the stipulation of informed, voluntary consent free of coercion (Burns 2003).

The WMA Declaration of Helsinki, adopted in 1964 and then regularly amended (WMA 2000), has since allowed the participation of children in research as long as there is consent from a parent or 'legally authorised individual in accordance with applicable law'. It also states that when the subject is a 'minor child' and 'able to give assent to decisions about participation in research, the investigator must obtain that assent in addition to the consent from a legally authorised representative'. This document distinguishes between therapeutic research, described as 'research combined with medical care', and non-therapeutic research involving 'healthy volunteers'.

The principles of the Declaration of Helsinki (WMA 2000) led to the creation of an international standard for clinical trials involving human subjects. The International Conference on Harmonisation guideline for good clinical practice (ICH GCP) came into effect in 1997 with the objective of providing a 'unified standard for the European Union, Japan and the United States to facilitate the mutual acceptance of clinical data by the regulatory authorities in these jurisdictions'. The principles established in ICH GCP guidelines 'may also be applied to other clinical investigations that may have an impact on the safety and well-being of human subjects', not just clinical trials (ICH 2002).

In the UK, the DoH has developed the Research Governance Framework for Health and Social Care (DoH 2001b) to set standards and improve research quality by promoting good practice. In section 1.1, it recognises the need for health and social research while ensuring public confidence through 'high scientific, ethical and financial standards, transparent decision-making processes, clear allocation of responsibilities and robust monitoring arrangements' (DoH 2001b).

WWW

The Department of Health Research Governance Framework can be found at the DoH research and development website:
- http://www.dh.gov.uk/research

Risk Versus Benefit

The DoH (2001a) states that children may participate in therapeutic research based on new treatment that may be as effective or more effective than standard treatment. Participation in non-therapeutic research is possible if doing so is 'not against the interests of the child and imposes only a minimal burden'. In both cases it is stipulated that sufficient information must be given prior to participation. Minimal burden is not clearly defined and it is left to the researcher to assess each child and gives the examples of bone marrow donations and more simple injections. The bone marrow would require a therapeutic benefit to the child but an injection would not. However, as there is considerable variation in response to injections researchers must bear in mind the individual reaction of young volunteers. Some children might not consider an injection a 'minimal burden'.

The risk/benefit ratio first mentioned in the Nuremberg Code remains a source of debate. Alderson (1995) argues that 'risk' is vague and refers to both possible and definite harms, whereas 'benefits' implies there will be definite good. She states that 'risk and hoped-for benefits' is a more balanced phrase. These terms can be misleading depending on their context, with clarity needed regarding who is at risk and who will benefit. There is potential for great benefit to society at the great expense of a few volunteers. However, the Declaration of Helsinki (WMA 2000) states 'the considerations related to the well-being of the human subject should take precedence over the interests of society'. This ethical stance is reaffirmed in the DoH Research Governance Framework, which mandates 'The dignity, rights, safety and well being of participants must be the primary consideration in any research study' (DoH 2001b).

Is your Volunteer Acting Voluntarily?

ASSENT, GILLICK AND THE RIGHT TO REFUSE

Wherever possible assent or agreement to participate should be obtained from all children and young people. Researchers must take time to prepare parents to provide consent and pre-Gillick competent children to provide assent. Importantly, the DoH (2001a) states that even when the parent has given consent for participation in 'non-therapeutic research', if a child of any age disagrees then the research should not go ahead. It is interesting to note that this does not include 'therapeutic' research. So it would seem that the child once again has the right to consent but not the complete right to dissent. In the case of participation in a research study, it

would be foolish to include a child in a study against his or her parents' wishes (Lamprill 2002). Whereas a competent child may consent for participation without parental approval, this would be highly unrealistic and impractical (Robinson 2001). Best practice would dictate that with proper preparation a trusting relationship between the child, family and research team would prevent the occurrence of such extreme situations. The research nurse must be an advocate for the young volunteer and support them to have a voice in the research process.

Assessing Gillick competency for research consent requires determining the youngsters' understanding of research protocols. This includes complicated concepts such as placebos and their use in randomised controlled trials. Montgomery (2001) suggests that all projects need Gillick assessment and that a child may have sufficient understanding of one study but not of another. This creates a situation where a child is Gillick competent for one research project but not necessarily for all studies. Therefore it is imperative that children and young people are properly assessed for each study in which they participate.

Another fundamental component of consent for research is the right for the volunteer or parent to change their minds. This was first stated in the Nuremberg Code, and reaffirmed in the Declaration of Helsinki (WMA 2000):

The subject should be informed of the right to abstain from participation in the study or to withdraw consent to participate at any time without reprisal.

Consent forms and patient information sheets must state that participation is optional (Lamprill 2002). Children and young people need to understand this right and researchers must be certain that young volunteers and their parents feel able to stop at any time during the study without it affecting their care.

> ### Scenario
>
> Ten-year-old Aidan and Leo, his 16-year-old brother attend a CRF as part of a research study investigating the genetics of phenylketonuria (PKU) Jane, a second year Child Branch student nurse is assisting Research Nurse Sylvia. Ross, the boys father is very abrupt with the nurses as Sylvia goes over the Patient information Sheets and consent forms with him and the boys. "This isn't necessary just give them to me and I'll sign them. I must get back to work." Sylvia tries to explain she must be certain the boys understand and agree and she also asks Leo for his consent. "Don't be ridiculous, he's just a boy and of course they agree" What should Sylvia say? What would you do?

Advocacy and Best Interest

International Conference on Harmonisation (ICH) Document E11 (ICH 2000) gives clear guidelines regarding the need to balance the protection of young, potentially very vulnerable research volunteers with the benefits to be gained from participation in research. Research nurses must be the advocates for their young volunteers and empower them to make decisions free of any coercion. Recruitment must be free from inappropriate inducements to the parent or child and while reimbursement for expenses is allowed, it must be included in the protocol and approved by the ethics committee (ICH 2000).

The UN Convention on the Rights of The Child, Article 12 (United Nations General Assembly 1989) states that children have a right to participate in the decision-making process that may be relevant to their lives. Adults are also expected to promote and empower children so that they may express their views and influence decisions. Standards for healthcare professionals in the NSF for Children (DoH 2003a) include the need to provide a child-centred service, with the needs of the child put first. Choices should be offered to all children and young people regarding aspects of treatment. Young people must 'never feel that decisions are being made over their heads' (DoH 2001a). This should be the ethos of the multidisciplinary research team. In *Advocating for children*, the Royal College of Paediatrics and Child Health (RCPCH) (2000) has adopted as an overall aim 'To advocate the rights of children and young people in society and to promote their health needs and services'. It refers to the concept of 'best interest' enshrined in the UN Convention on the Rights of The Child, and expects 'all members to act within the framework'. This clear guidance for all professionals working with children, combined with the mandate of the NMC (2002), requires the research nurse to advocate for the best interests of young volunteers. This includes working with the research team and family to facilitate the child's participation as a partner in the research process. Providing information, choices and support for young volunteers will allow the continued development of safe, accurate and successful research.

Professional Conversation

Jane is a student nurse on placement with her mentor Sylvia, a research nurse.

Issues regarding children's assent and parental consent for participation in research

I have been on placement in the clinical research facility for 3 weeks. My mentor Sylvia and I had a difficult morning with a family participating in a genetic study. During lunch we chatted about the issues of consent and assent and how to include competent children in the con-senting process. I understand that young people must be involved and sometimes nurses must be advocates for youngsters – even if that means disagreeing with their parents.

How Research is Conducted with Children

Involving children in research requires the same child-centred approach as caring for sick children in a ward setting (DoH 2003a). Successful completion of any research project involving children demands careful planning, organisation, implementation and evaluation.

Researchers have to find ways of engaging children using negotiation rather than imposition (Barker & Weller 2003). To be successful, researchers need to think about how children will perceive them (Balen et al 2001). Children like to meet a person they can trust and someone who is fun to be around, therefore researchers need to make an effort to ensure they are creative (Curtin 2000) and provide an age-appropriate approach. Instead of employing existing adult methodologies, child-led methodologies have been developed to enable children to communicate using qualitative methods, e.g. drawing, dairies and photography (Avery 2003, Balen et al 2001). Such methods aim to build a rapport, trust and confidence, allowing children to clearly articulate their views and opinions. Hence by giving information in a child-centred way the researcher can empower young people, gain their trust and cooperation and obtain their assent to be active participants in research.

When designing information sheets, consent forms and constructing quantitative research tools such as questionnaires, child-centred researchers should be aware of the significance children and young people place on language. It is also important to consult with children about the development of appropriate research methods. Researchers should not impose their own interpretations, made up of adult feelings and presumptions, which can suppress or misrepresent the voices of children (Barker & Weller 2003).

 www

Visit this website for access to programmes that help to ensure the language used is reading age appropriate:
• http://www.sharedlearning.org.uk/
and follow FOG link

 Activity

When conducting a study with many components, consider how best to facilitate the young child's coping ability. For example, the use of star charts enables a child to plot their progress and at the same time provide a simple reward.

Construct a star chart for use in your working environment that would help children in your care cope with procedures.

Research Methodology and Design that is Suitable for Use with Children

Research methods can be divided into two main approaches, quantitative and qualitative:

- Quantitative research is structured, usually experimental and employs standard methods, e.g. randomised controlled trials. It produces data amenable to statistical analysis.

- Qualitative research methods are holistic, observational, unstructured or semi-structured, and the data are presented in the form of quotations or descriptions, though some basic statistics may be presented. Increasingly the two approaches (triangulation) are combined within one research project (Scanlon 2003).

Before deciding on which method to use the researcher needs to be satisfied that they have chosen the most appropriate design, which provides suitable answers to the following questions (Edwards & Talbot 1994):

- Is this method going to provide the kind of information required?

- Is this method going to build up as accurate a picture of the events as possible?

- Is this the most suitable design for the children concerned and can it be done in the time available?

By combining a range of research methods within one study, known as triangulation, a picture can be built up of the phenomenon under investigation from a range of perspectives (Morrow 2001). For example, in their pilot study, Avery et al (2003) used a quality of life questionnaire and the children took photographs of how their lives were affected by their illness and then wrote about their feelings when they took their photographs.

A pilot study can be described as a 'dummy-run' and enables the researcher to see whether the methods chosen do indeed collect the data needed to answer the chosen research question. This also provides an opportunity to get feedback from children themselves on the chosen methodology and their experience of participation (Balen et al 2001).

Research with children is carried out for many different reasons, and therefore different child-centred methods are required to elicit information.

Activity

- Is there an aspect of nursing care for children you are involved in that you would like to investigate further?

- Discuss with your colleagues what approach you might use for conducting this investigation.

Health-related Quality of Life Studies

WHAT IS QUALITY OF LIFE?

The World Health Organization (1996) has defined quality of life as:

An individual's perception of their position in life in the context of the culture and value systems in which they live and in relation to their goals, expectations, standards and concerns. It is a broad ranging concept affected in a complex way by the person's physical health, psychological state, level of independence, social relationships and their relationship to salient features of the environment.

 WWW

Read the article by Camilleri-Brennan 1999:
- http://www.rcsed.ac.uk/journal/vol44_4/4440010.htm

Children can be reliable informants, presenting accurate accounts of their experiences. However, engaging children in research and ensuring their voices are heard requires a specific non-adult approach (Curtin 2000). By involving children in research, we can learn about children's perspectives on their worlds, and the personal meanings children attribute to events and actions. By actively participating in research children can be given a voice and children can have practice in making life decisions.

Quality of life can be determined by the extent to which hopes and ambitions are matched by experience. Participating in a study can clarify a child's perceptions of their position in life, in relation to their goals, expectations, standards and concerns within the surroundings of their culture and value systems. Such quality of life studies can be used both to establish things children regard as important in their lives and to evaluate a child's current state against some ideal. The use of quality of life measures in clinical practice can help to ensure that treatment and evaluation focus on the child rather than the disease (Higginson & Carr 2001).

Other ways of assessing the quality of life from the perspective of children and adolescents include self-reporting questionnaires, interviews and computer-assisted forms. The researcher may want to obtain a complete family-centred analysis and should consider the quality of life of the children's families. By asking the parents and – if possible – siblings for their perception of a sick child's quality of life as well as their rating of their own quality of life, a fuller picture can be obtained (Bullinger et al 2002).

Illness, especially chronic illness and its consequences, affects the lives of children but little is known about the effects of ill health or medical interventions on children's development and how they adjust or compensate for the negative effects of hospitalisation, intrusive medical procedures and the uncertainty of survival. To understand these effects it is important to fully assess children's quality of life. There have been various definitions of health related quality of life, however researchers agree that quality of life is a multidimensional, subjective and dynamic concept (Camilleri-Brennan 1999).

Activity

Go to your local nursing library, access and read Avery et al (2003) and discuss with colleagues what aspects of your nursing care given to a cohort of children could similarly be investigated.

Discuss what insight this would give you into the quality of life of the children and their families, and how could you then change your practice to improve the children's quality of life?

When adults wish to communicate with children it is important that they develop strategies that recognise children's age specific cognitive development, attention span and language. Like adults, children make sense of their worlds and define meanings using previous experience. Unlike adults they have limited past experiences to make sense of new events (Fleitas 1998). Children are continually developing and changing with age so assessing quality of life in children differs from quality of life in adults.

Children's quality of life should be looked at within four categories:

1. Children's physical development.

2. Children's developing concepts of quality of life.

3. Children's cognitive development: the researcher should be aware that children's understanding of various spheres, including health, appear to be more related to experience than age or level of cognitive development.

4. Content of the questionnaire: as quality of life is usually measured by a questionnaire, the content of questionnaires should be suitably child-centred for the group being investigated (Bradding & Horstman 1999, Vincent & Higginson 2003).

Such quality of life questionnaires can be used to gather relatively straightforward information and can be employed to study groups or children with a particular problem. This allows comparisons with other groups. When developing or

using a validated questionnaire it is important to ensure it will produce the type of information sought (Hinds 2000). However, using questionnaires with children can produce misleading information. A child may not be able to recall the necessary information, have sufficient language skills to understand the meaning of the question or may lack the written skills to produce a comprehensible response. The resourceful researcher can be creative in the production of questionnaires, placing importance on both the visual presentation and the order in which the questions are presented. Questions should gradually shift from least to most sensitive, general to detailed, concrete to abstract. Children find it easier to answer questions about the present and events they have just experienced than about the past. It is important to use appropriate vocabulary to suit the age and literary ability of the children concerned (Curtin 2000, Oppenheim 2002). To produce valid responses clear instructions should be given for the use of scaled responses to questions, e.g. with a rating of 1 'not at all' to 6 'very much'. Or the researcher may consider the use of pictures instead of words: six simply drawn faces numbered 0 to 5 with various degrees from smiling through neutral to misery (iconic Likert scale). The child is asked to indicate how much he or she likes or dislikes a statement. Alternatively the researcher can use linear scales (visual analogue scale) based on a horizontal line with a mark at one end indicating the most positive aspect and a mark at the other end indicating the worst aspect (Dockerell 2000).

PowerPoint

Access the companion PowerPoint presentation to view an iconic likert scale and a visual analogue scale.

www

Visit the 'Wong on web' website for examples of rating scales:
• http://www3.us.elsevierhealth.com/WOW/faces.html

www

For an interactive online version of the Quality of Life Research Unit, University of Toronto Adult Quality of Life Profile, and descriptions of a variety of studies involving children, adolescents and families, visit:
• www.utoronto.ca/qol

Conducting Research Interviews with Children and Young People

When seeking children's views and opinions, researchers act as facilitators. An alternative technique they can employ is the interview. Interviews should be conducted in child-friendly surroundings, where the child is made to feel safe and comfortable; this might be in their home, or school or suitable playroom within the hospital setting. The researcher should be constantly aware of the children's perspective, develop innovative approaches and ensure the environment is child-centred. Before asking questions in an interview, the researcher should inform children that there are no right or wrong answers and that it is all right if they do not have an answer. The interviewer should use open-ended questions when asking children to report directly on their beliefs or knowledge as such questions allow children themselves to structure the type and extent of their responses (Curtin 2000, Dockerell 2000).

Williamson & Butler (1995) suggest children and young people can attempt to conceal the problems of their worlds from adults to avoid 'being humiliated by misunderstanding, misrepresentation and misplaced responses'. This concealment can be a considerable barrier to adults involved in gathering data from children. The answers given may not reflect the child's true opinion but be what they think the adult wants to hear. Rather than impose a series of questions, the creative researcher can encourage children to talk more by using activities that most children enjoy:

- Brainstorming: spider diagrams, mind maps.
- Sentence completion: e.g. 'Having a peanut allergy affects my life at school because . . .
- Prompt cards: single cards with pictures or words.
- Pictorial vignettes: a series of pictures.
- Ranking exercises: pictures or sentences on cards which children are asked to put in order of importance.
- Play: encouraging the child to describe his or her ideas, thoughts or emotions through a third person, e.g. teddy.
- Role-play: generating ideas, thoughts and emotions about a scenario the child acts out.

These methods can give children their own voice and ensure their ideas and explanations are heard and understood. Sorensen (1989) suggests the use of children's diaries or journals for data collection in research. The researcher must ensure the child understands what is required, by giving clear instructions, yet keeping the layout as open as possible. They may then discover the child's viewpoints of daily life, unhampered by observer presence or other formal data collection methods. Diaries give children freedom of thought and expression, by the use of their own language and drawings.

Activity

Go to your local nursing library, access and read Kennedy et al 2003 on the use of interactive data collection (IDC) software for collecting research data with school age children.

- Discuss this approach with your colleagues.

The Write and Draw Method

Young children and those with lesser abilities are under-represented in research studies. These groups can find the non-verbal approach an easier way to express themselves because they can find it hard to convey feelings verbally, especially with adults they do not know well. The use of play, painting or drawing can enable children to express themselves clearly. Practically all school-aged children are familiar with producing drawings and writing about them. The write and draw method involves children being invited to draw pictures related to aspects of health or ill health and to write about what is happening in their pictures (Backett-Milburn & McKie 1999). This is considered to be child-friendly, non-threatening and facilitating the expression of views by children. It does not necessitate the adult being continually involved in the process, so the children are free to concentrate and think about their own ideas but they are able to ask for adult help to communicate their thoughts in writing when they wish (Bradding & Horstman 1999).

When a child asks the researcher to scribe draw-and-talk, the researcher should do so verbatim, without prompting or influencing the child's thoughts and emotions. Different approaches can be used: draw and write, as previously described, and draw and label, when children choose to draw pictures and label them to show aspects of the theme, e.g. health or ill-health. The write only method, which Pridmore & Lansdown (1997) suggest, is a quick way of identifying major categories of information. The researcher can expand on the issues identified by using more enjoyable activities such as drawing and dialogue. These methods have been used successfully with individuals as well as in larger groups of children.

www

Visit the web site:
- http://her.oupjournals.org/cgi/content/ful/14/3/387
Read the full text of Backett-Milburn & McKie (1999) for a critique of the write and draw method.

Using Focus Groups

Focus group research involves a planned conversation with a selected group of children or young people to gain information about their views and experiences about a subject. Children participating in research need to feel safe. Children generally find safety in numbers so focus groups can provide a comfortable way of interaction between children; a well-chosen group of five or six children provide social support to each other. This methodology can be used to gain information relating to how children think, what their views are and capture their experiences by obtaining several perspectives about the same topic and the ways in which others influence individuals in a group situation (Gibbs 1997). This approach allows children to explain their perceptions of an event, an idea or an experience. Such groups are useful when there is a need for more insight and understanding of the child's experience and when seeking the perspective of children (Hinds 2000). In such a forum children need to fully understand what is expected of them. It is therefore essential that the questions be posed clearly, concisely and unambiguously in child-led language (Balen et al 2001). The moderator or facilitator needs to help the children feel at ease and facilitate interaction between all the children in the group by asking open questions, at times probing for more detail, keeping the session focused by steering the conversation back on course and ensuring everyone participates and has a chance to speak (Gibbs 1997).

Activity

Ask children about the quality of care they receive and in what ways they think the nursing care they receive could be improved:
- How best could you do this?
- Discuss this with your colleagues.

Randomised Controlled Trials

A randomised controlled trial (RCT) is the gold standard of research (Glasper & Ireland 2000). This method is the favoured design used to find out the effectiveness and safety of new clinical treatments including drug trials and explore different approaches to disease management. Patients are randomly assigned to a treatment (intervention) group or control (comparison) groups, sometimes blindly (i.e. the patient and family do not know which group they are in). Additionally, many studies use double blinding (neither the patient nor researcher know who is in which group). Only during analysis is the blinding removed.

Randomisation helps to minimise bias and ensures that children are allocated to either arm of the trial in the fairest way possible, taking into account all the risks and benefits. The active group receives the new treatment under investigation and the control group receives a placebo, or the best historically known treatment to date (Forman & Ladd 1995). At the end of the trial the results are collected and unblinded when necessary. Everyone then knows who was on which arm of the trial and the outcomes of the treatment from the children in both groups. Both groups are followed up over a period of time to see if there are any differences in the outcome.

RCTs are often run by commercial companies and are conducted over a period of time, from different sites (hospitals), and in different countries. This ensures that the findings are not unique to one setting and gives extra validity to the results (Swage 2000).

Conducting such a clinical trial with adults is one thing but to do so with children is even more challenging (Robinson 2002). It is only feasible with the cooperation and collaboration of all those involved. This includes groups of people, i.e. children, parents, investigators, research nurses, pharmaceutical sponsors and ethics committees, all of whom have varying roles to play, with different perceptions. This can lead to conflicting priorities. Lamprill (2003) calls for pharmaceutical sponsors to adopt a more child-friendly approach to their studies, taking child and family needs into account when planning protocols. Although parents do have altruistic motives for consenting to their children taking part in research studies, Rothmier et al (2003) suggest that most parents give consent to learn more about their child's disease. Similarly, Lamprill (2003) suggests that parents will not allow their children to be exposed to more than minimal risk or suffering. However, they may accept higher risk if there is a chance the child could benefit significantly from taking part in the study.

Pharmaceutical sponsors should remember that families live in the 'real world', so when the unexpected occurs – as it often does – this can hinder the smooth running of a paediatric trial. Lamprill (2003) describes a child who dropped his inhaler down the lavatory, a dog who ate a large pot of study medication, and a courier who arrived before the blood sample was prepared! Paediatric adverse events can be non-specific; children are often described as 'off food' or 'off colour'. As children's nurses are aware, there may be no specific symptoms but children can feel generally unwell and cannot express themselves, this is difficult to record in the formality of a drug trial.

Whatever the problems that arise during paediatric clinical trials, researchers should never lose sight of their purpose. In many instances this is to ensure that medication used to treat children is properly adapted for use in the growing child, and to establish appropriate safe doses that achieve maximum effect with minimal side effects.

This section has provided a brief overview of how research is conducted with children; other research methods can equally well be employed. Whatever methodology is used, the thoughtful, sensitive, and responsible child researcher must be mindful of adapting the method to the age and capacity of the children concerned, and to leave the child, of whatever age, enriched for having participated in the research process and feeling good about her or his contribution (Brown & Hayler 1989).

PowerPoint

Access the companion PowerPoint presentation for examples of other research methods.
For further information on research methods suitable for use in research with children see
Greig A, Taylor J 1999 Doing Research with Children Sage Publications London
Lewis A Lindsay G 2000 Researching children's perspectives Open University Press.

Why is it Necessary to Undertake Research With Children?

Children have a right to benefit from relevant research. Historically, health professionals have been reluctant to include children in research studies and clinical trials due to their vulnerability and their inability to give informed consent (Rosato 2000). It can no doubt be argued that they have been doing the childhood population a great disservice by denying them the most appropriate medicines and treatments. Children have a right to be given medication and treatments that are safe and effective whatever the age of the child. The Children's National Service Framework (NSF) (DoH 2003a) states that the use of medicines in children should be guided by the best available evidence of clinical effectiveness, cost effectiveness and safety, ideally derived from clinical trials conducted with children. When including this vulnerable population in clinical trials it is vital that the research nurse is familiar with issues surrounding informed consent and children's assent. There should be a proper balance between the need to recruit children to clinical trials and research studies and the need to protect their rights as human subjects (Meaux & Bell 2001).

As mentioned earlier, children are not simply small adults: their bodies are constantly growing and developing and metabolic rates change with age. In many cases data based on studies performed on adults cannot be directly applied to children. This is because on a pharmacological and pharmacokinetic level a child does not behave in the same way as an adult, yet many medicines prescribed for children have never been studied in children (Vasmant 2003). Children require treatments that are disease specific to them. A medicine may not be metabolised at the same speed in a child as in an adult, a child may not absorb a cream applied to the skin in the same way as an adult and an aerosol inhaler may not be dispersed in the lungs of a child as in an adult (ICH 2000). Therefore it is necessary to study these differences and to improve our knowledge of medicines used to treat children. This will enable professionals to make informed decisions when prescribing drugs for children.

Unlicensed and 'Off-label' Medicines and Therapies

Children need to be protected from use of unlicensed and 'off-label' medicines and therapies:

- Unlicensed medicine: has no product licence for use in the UK.
- 'Off-label' use of medicines: a drug has a UK licence but is being used outside the licence for a purpose or with a population for which it has not been approved, e.g. dose, suitable formulation, route of administration or age group (RCPCH 1999).

Too few drugs are licensed for use with children and hence some children are denied treatment (Wilson 1996). Good practice also includes using medicines for which there is a sound theoretical basis for believing they are effective in children. Therefore, many medicines prescribed for children in the UK are prescribed outside of licensed indications, i.e. 'off-label' or unlicensed. The use of such medicines is necessary in paediatric practice when there is no suitable alternative. The RCPCH and The Neonatal and Paediatric Pharmacists Group statement (1999) clearly states that 'such uses are informed and guided by a respectable and responsible body of professional opinion'.

It can be argued that the use of unlicensed and 'off-label' drugs to treat children has resulted in children being used as research subjects but without the controlled supervision of a clinical trial or systematic commitment to learn how to use the drug (Rosato 2000). When a child becomes sick, the paediatrician or GP must decide whether to prescribe a drug, considering the risk versus benefit. If a drug is not licensed for children in the UK, a doctor prescribing it for a child needs to extrapolate from the adult dose a suitable dose for that child, which may lead to inaccuracies. However, failing to prescribe the drug 'off-label' may deny the child the most effective intervention available.

The Children's NSF (DoH 2003a) acknowledges that the use of 'off-label' and unlicensed medicine has particular implications for clinical governance and in 2003 an NSF Working Group was set up to work towards improving medication safety particularly in babies and young children.

American and European Perspectives

Over the past decade in the USA, research into medicines for children has been encouraged (Meaux & Bell 2001). The National Institutes for Health (NIH) maintain a policy that children (i.e. individuals under the age of 21) must be included in all human subjects research conducted or supported by the NIH unless there are scientific and ethical reasons not to include them (NIH 1998). The European

Commission (EC) has introduced a similar approach to the USA (Vasmant 2003). The European Health Council's Resolution on Paediatric Medicinal Products in December 2000 stated that children have their own varying characteristics and cannot be treated like adults, and called on the EC to make appropriate proposals to develop clinical research and development into medicines for children.

Activity

Access the American NIH Policy and Guidelines on the Inclusion of Children as Participants in Research Involving Human Subjects:
- http://grants.nih.gov/grants/guide/notice-files/not 98-024.html

Discuss with your colleagues the importance of conducting clinical trials in medicines used with children. Is this in the best interest of the individual child or children as a population?

How Research Provides a Foundation for Evidence-based Practice

Children's nurses strive for excellence in planning the care of individual children and their families. The UK government's framework of clinical governance makes clinical nurses, doctors and managers accountable for the care they deliver. Child health nursing practice is required to develop clinical nursing protocols and interventions based on sound evidence-based research, rather than a nursing practice based on 'custom and practice', 'myths and rituals' (Glasper & Ireland 2000). The Children's NSF (DoH 2003a) expects clinical practice to follow the best available research evidence. By using evidence-based protocols and guidelines, professionals can achieve high standards of care for children and young people in all areas in which they are cared for.

Evidence-based nursing care is on the basis of partnership and multidisciplinary collaboration. Nurses are able to learn from the work and experience of nursing, medical and allied professional colleagues who undertake child health research, which can then be applied to clinical practice (Glasper & Ireland 2000). The evidence showing the effectiveness of interventions is reported, i.e. published, in research papers and is known as primary research, which is either quantitative or qualitative and directly focuses on patients. An increasing, enormous, base of primary research is available (Swage 2000). To view the broad picture, systematic reviews are used to search and filter out the good quality from the lesser quality primary research, to gather reliable evidence that is scientifically robust enough for

decisions to be made on what care to provide for children and their families (Casey 2000).

To carry out a systematic review, a researcher needs to perform a literature search, i.e. collect and review primary papers on the chosen subject, then to critically appraise the research articles and summarize the evidence presented according to standard criteria (Swage 2000). Finally, by using professional judgement, the researcher can interpret and evaluate the evidence and make an informed decision about using the findings in their evidenced-based clinical practice.

Activity

From your nursing library access this well documented example of a systematic review, which has led to a change in practice:
- Creery D, Mikrogianakis A 2003 Sudden infant death syndrome: what are the effects of intervention to reduce the risk of sudden infant death syndrome? Clinical evidence. BMJ Publishing Group, London

This is available online at:
- http://www.clinicalevidence.com

How to Critique a Research Paper

Nurses do not have to be researchers to practise evidence-based nursing, however they do need to be able first to assess research outcomes in a critical way, and second to separate insignificant and unsound research findings from significant studies that are worthy of interest. The critiquing process is about systematically reviewing and questioning each stage of the research process (Crombie 1996).

When reading a research paper it is useful to use a formal approach using a framework of questions that deal with all the aspects of the research process; the following is adapted from Bayea & Nicoll (1997):

1. What is the research question?
2. What is the basis for the research question?
3. Why is the research question important?
4. How was the research question studied?
5. Does the study method make sense?
6. Were the correct subjects selected for the study?
7. Was the research question answered?
8. Does the answer make sense?
9. What is the implication for practice?
10. What is next?

WWW

Visit the Critical Appraisal Skill Programme (CASP) and Evidence-based Practice website for further guidance on how to critique qualitative and quantitative research papers:

* http://www.phru.nhs.uk/~casp/casp.htm

You will need to use your judgement and experience to evaluate the appropriateness of the research study. Consider the strengths and weaknesses of the study design, methodology, data analysis and interpretation of the findings. You should indicate reasons for your judgements and the findings should be as objective as possible.

Activity

Before critiquing a research paper, read: Chapter 25 (Evaluating research reports) in Polit DF, Hungler BP (1995) Nursing research: principles and methods, 6th edn. Lippincott, Philadelphia

* Select a topic of interest to you and find a research article, which you can critique.

HOW TO CONDUCT A LITERATURE REVIEW/SEARCH

Visit your local nursing/medical library where you can access nursing and medical journals

Conduct on line searches using MEDLINE, EMBASE, CINAHL, NICE

Access search engines on the internet

www.cochrane.org

www.infotrieve.com

www.pubmed.com

How Research Studies are Beginning to Identify the Origins of Disease and Contribute to its Prevention in Later Life

Adults are grown up children and carry the legacy of their childhood with them throughout their lives (DoH 2003a). Research aiming to help prevent disease throughout life is focusing more on the search for the inborn determinants of disease. Parents and their children are being studied as both genes and the environment influence a child's development during fetal and early life. Research has shown this to have a long-term impact on an individual's health throughout life. The 'fetal origins' hypothesis proposed that alterations in fetal nutrition and endocrine status result in developmental adaptations that permanently change structure, physiology and metabolism, thereby predisposing to disease in adult life (Godfrey & Barker 2001).

Activity

Visit your local nursing library, access and read: Godfrey KM, Barker DJP 2001 Fetal programming and adult health. Public Health and Nutrition 4(2B):611–624

* Discuss this article with your colleagues.

In fetal life, the tissues and organs of the body go through critical periods of development. Humans are 'plastic' in their early life and are moulded by the environment. The growth of a fetus is influenced by its genes; this can be influenced by the environment, in particular the nutrients and oxygen received by the mother. 'Programming' describes the process that occurs during pregnancy whereby a stimulus or insult during a critical period of development has lasting or lifelong effects (Godfrey & Barker 2001). Research suggests that alterations in maternal nutrition can have long-term effects on the offspring in later life. It has been shown that coronary heart disease, hypertension and type 2 diabetes originate in impaired intrauterine growth and development (Godfrey & Barker 2000).

Paediatric research groups in various countries throughout the world are searching for reasons and answers to the increased prevalence of allergic disorders, such as eczema, asthma, hay fever and food allergy. Studies have been following children from the fetal period or from birth onwards. It has been found that allergic disease results from an extremely complex interaction of genetic traits and environmental influences (programming), such as the exposure to allergens, infections and variations in nutrient intake (Warner et al 2000a,b). A more comprehensive understanding of these events is required before researchers are able to prevent the onset of such diseases. Until such time, they require the help of children and their parents with research studies. Research into allergy and coronary heart disease are two examples of how research with children can show genetic and early environmental factors that influence the development of both paediatric and adult disease.

What about Children and Young People as Researchers?

With support, children and young people are able to organize and conduct research studies. Engaging with children and young people directly results in services better able to meet their needs (DoH 2003a). The DoH document *Strengthening accountability, involving patients and the public: practice guidance of the Health and Social Care Act* (DoH 2001c) states that 'the single most important piece of advice is to talk to the target group about the best way to consult and involve them'. However, children and young people are included in Section 9 of this document, 'Involving specific groups that the NHS has traditionally found hard to reach' and states that additional support may be required for such groups (DoH 2001c).

Attitudes that continue to marginalize children highlight the need for those who work with this 'hard to reach' group to make the investment of time and resources, to engage them so they are given a voice. It is this marginalisation of children that increases the need for their involvement. From a very early age children are able to express their views and they must be listened to (DoH2001c). This is mandated by Article 13 of The United Convention on the Rights of the Child (UN General Assembly 1989): 'the child shall have the right to freedom of expression; this right shall include freedom to seek, receive and impart information and ideas of all kinds'.

As is detailed elsewhere in this chapter, research can result in life-changing, life-prolonging results for the individual and others, and research will be more relevant if young people are involved in identifying the topics studied. Reaching the target group, in this case children and young people, can prove difficult for adults; young researchers are better able to access their peers. Youngsters often create a less formal, relaxed environment conducive to open and honest dialogue. In addition, their involvement can have an impact on professionals by exposure to young people's lives and concerns while providing valuable personal development for the young researchers (Kirby 1999).

 www

Visit the following website to see how The Children's Trust is involved in head injury and disability research:
- http://www.thechildrenstrust.org.uk

How Can Young Patients and Volunteers be Involved?

Guidance for involving the public as active partners in research is given in the Research Governance Framework (DoH 2001b). It states that participants should be involved in the design, conduct, analysis and reporting of research.

The NSF for Children (DoH 2003a) states that children and young people should be 'involved in the planning and improvement of services'. Methods for involvement might include:

- compliment and complaint boxes
- surveys and questionnaires
- consultation exercises: large or small groups
- creative consultations using drama, music, games
- facilitate young people to provide a service: take part in staff development and recruitment, provide mentor advice
- establish advisory groups (DoH 2001d).

Patient and volunteer involvement can encompass a variety of methods. Within Hospital Trusts, corporate and directorate leads work to meet national and local clinical governance key performance standards (KPS). The new confusingly named patient and public involvement forums (PPIFs) are statutory, independent bodies, different from the existing groups, also known as patient and public involvement (PPI) or user's groups, set up to meet clinical governance KPS (DoH 2003b). One important KPS requires active PPI groups in each directorate, including child health and other areas that treat children such as outpatients and emergency departments. Members of PPI groups are patients or carers who meet and address areas of concern they have, giving a voice to patients and volunteers, including children (DoH 2001c). Activities should be group led, but might include a review of patient information leaflets using a DoH toolkit. This allows direct input into the design and content of patient information and helps to ensure they are clear, attractive and understood by the people who use them, with children reviewing child-oriented information (DoH 2000b).

 www

Search for the complete DoH toolkit at
- http://www.dh.gov.uk

 Activity

Go to Chapter 37 for more on patient information leaflets:
- Read information leaflets on your ward placements.
- Are there separate ones for children and teenagers?

Models of Involvement

INVOLVE (formerly Consumers in NHS Research) is an organization that promotes NHS, public health and social care research. It has clearly identified three levels of public participation in the research process:

- The first level has been defined as consultation: information is given to the public by a group of healthcare providers or researchers.
- The next step is collaboration: there is a partnership between the two groups and a sharing of ideas.
- The highest level of participation would be user control: when the public takes charge and manages the research study (Hanley et al 2000).

 www

Visit the following website to see how a small group of children and parents have set up and run a foundation to fund research into familial dysautonomia, a rare (less than 600

patients worldwide) genetic disease. Their participation has led to improved treatments and discovery of the gene:

• http://www.familialdysautonomia.org

Another model is the public involvement continuum, which ranges from minimum to maximum involvement and is described in *Strengthening accountability, involving patients and the public: practice guidance of the Health and Social Care Act* (DoH 2001c). This document offers advice and practical ideas to put PPI into practice. It gives the following categories with many examples of activities:

● Giving information: exhibitions, leaflets, the press.

● Getting information: public panels, radio phone-ins, questionnaires, interviews.

● Forums for debate: focus groups, patient/carer groups, seminars.

● Participation: expert patients, health panels, shadowing, story telling.

● Partnership: community development, large group processes.

All the above methods can be used with children. Specific advice includes:

● Develop links with schools and youth groups.

● Ensure information is in appropriate language, style and format.

● Speak directly with and involve children and young people – not just their parents.

● Consider using video, interactive material and the internet (DoH 2001c).

Facilitating Involvement of Young Researchers

Participation early in the research process is recommended, ideally at the first step of deciding what topic should be researched, as greater influence can be achieved with early involvement (Joseph Rowntree Foundation 2000). Ideally, topics for research would be determined by children and young people, and not imposed by medical or scientific researchers (Kirby 1999). This requires support for the young people, who probably will not have experience of research or engaging with others in this way. As with older 'non-professional' researchers, training in research methods such as interviewing skills, questionnaire completion and data recording, will be necessary, as will clear guidelines for confidentiality and data protection issues (Kirby 1999). *Young people as researchers* – a learning resource pack (Worrall 2000) – includes exercises and handouts for use with novice researchers. Its aim is to 'provide materials for workers train-

ing young people in participatory research' and gives practical advice for engaging young researchers in projects.

INVOLVE also provides in depth briefing notes for researchers through the NHS Research Support Unit (Hanley et al 2000). These notes illustrate various aspects of involvement and practical guidelines that can be utilised. By breaking down the research process into stages it is possible to see how each step leads to the next. With support, young researchers can participate at any stage.

WWW

Visit the INVOLVE website for more information on involving your patients as active partners in research, and the full text of their briefing notes for researchers:

• http://www.invo.org.uk

Activity

• How might you involve youngsters in hospital?
• How could you determine which topics are important to them?
• What techniques might work best with children who can't read?

Difficulties Involving Children and Young People as Researchers

Young researchers can experience many of the same difficulties that adult or professionals encounter. These youngsters have reported a shift in perception during interviews from being a peer to authoritative figure, with the subjects becoming defensive. Young researchers might also be reluctant to probe for details. In addition, recruiting volunteers through a peer group might be successful but will not yield a suitably diverse group. It might be difficult for some young people to approach others whom they do not know. They can also face problems accessing youngsters through recruitment routes such as schools (Kirby 1999).

Young people researching adults rather than peers will face other issues. Young researchers might intimidate some adults, or adults might use jargon or words the youngster does not understand, which could lead to intimidation of the young person. Young people will require support, especially if interviews reveal sensitive or upsetting information. Child protection issues must be considered so that young researchers and subjects are safe. Working in pairs, interviewing in public areas such as schools or cafes, providing mobile phones, ID cards, and submitting daily plans of activity are possible strategies to safeguard involved children (Kirby 1999).

WWW

Visit the Department of Education and Skills website for the full texts of the *Learning to listen plan and report.*
- http://www.dfes.gov.uk/listening to learn

Scenario

David and Jonathan are 15 years old and have volunteered for training as young researchers on a study being set up at a local youth group. They will be interviewing children and their parents about the ways they travel to and from school.

What kind of training and support might they need? What are some of the problems they might encounter in the community?

How is the Governmenment Supporting Public Involvement in Healthcare and Research?

A framework for quality improvement was outlined in *A first class service: quality in the new NHS* (DoH 1998). This included the development of national service frameworks underpinned by clinical governance frameworks that assure the quality of clinical services. Hospital Trust directorates are mandated to meet the agendas of clinical governance frameworks in seven key areas. The patient and public involvement (PPI) section ensures patient and public participation at all levels of healthcare delivery. At the same time, the independent Commission for Health Improvement (CHI, which has since become the Commission for Health Audit and Inspection [CHAI]) was developed to monitor quality and progress and initiate a continuing programme of national patient surveys, addressing various issues that impact on patient care and satisfaction (DoH 1998).

This commitment to provide a patient-centred health care service was reaffirmed in the NHS Plan (DoH 2000a). The Commission for Patient and Public Involvement in Health (CPPIH) was founded in January 2003 to fund, establish and manage Patient and Public Forums (PPIFs) in every trust and PCT. These forums are a resource for the public, promoting their involvement and monitor Patient Advice and Liaison Service (PALS). PALS provide information about health services and about independent complaints advocacy services (ICAS). PPIFs will have legal powers to inspect, report and make recommendations based on patient views and experiences, with the aim to have a PPIF member on every NHS Trust Board (DoH 2003b). INVOLVE promotes public involvement in the NHS, public health and social care research, and recommends the principle of public representatives in NHS research and development programmes (DoH 2001b). A commitment to public involvement is now firmly in practice and extends to healthy research volunteers, including child volunteers and their families.

How Involved are Children and Young People?

In the *Learning to listen* action plan published by the Children's and Young People's Unit (DoH 2001d), the DoH set out the following core principles regarding the participation of youngsters:

- a visible commitment to involving children and young people
- that their involvement be valued
- equal opportunity to get involved
- that standards for participation are provided, evaluated and improved.

Therefore, the onus is on the health professionals to ensure that these principles are met. The subsequent *Learning to listen report* (DoH 2003c) describes many examples of good involvement by children and young people. It mentions the CPPIH and its role to ensure 'children's and young people's views are represented on patient forums' and also states that children should be supported as forum members, with the use of child-friendly information.

In addition, it gives details of the 'Building a culture of participation' research project to illustrate the benefits of involvement. This project aimed to give an indication of participation, provide information and advice on involvement, and report on the creation of a 'participatory culture'. This research project found:

- There is no single way to involve children, but depends on many factors.
- Listening must lead to change to ensure all the current activity actually makes a difference.
- There are real benefits from listening and acting on children's views, including improved service development as well as support for children and personal development.
- However, too little attention is given to studying outcomes of participation and support is needed at all levels of management to create participatory organisations.

The report concludes that challenges remain and more resources are needed. Monitoring methods, sharing information and widening involvement into more government work will help to develop necessary standards that can be applied to a range of organisations. Providing a forum for expression and participation will help children and young people play an active part in society (DoH 2003c).

> ● Seminar discussion topic
>
> Select an area of clinical practice from your current clinical placement. Conduct a full review of the research literature. Is there a strong enough evidence base to warrant its continued application?

Summary

The unique and specific qualities of children make child-oriented research an absolute necessity. Child-friendly methodologies allow youngsters to freely give their assent for participation as research volunteers. With proper training and support it is also possible to actively involve them as researchers. Regardless of how, or why, they are involved, the interests of each individual child are paramount. It is essential that professionals involving children in healthcare research follow the broad principles of good clinical practice with the highest scientific and ethical standards. Children's nurses are the guardians of good research practice.

Acknowledgements

The authors would like to thank the Wellcome Trust Clinical Research Facility (WTCRF) at Southampton University Hospitals Trust for permission for use of printed materials and photographs for the PowerPoint presentation, and colleagues there for their support. They would also like to acknowledge the initial contribution of Julie Mitton, former Education and Development Coordinator at the WTCRF.

References

Age of Legal Capacity (Scotland) Act 1991 HMSO, London

Alderson P 1995 Listening to children. Barnardo's, Ilford, pp 21, 23, 55, 56

Alderson P, Montgomery J 1996 Health care choices: making decisions with children. Institute for Public Policy and Research, London, pp 6, 10–12, 18

Avery NJ, King RM, Knight S, Hourihane J O'B 2003 Assessment of quality of life in children with peanut allergy. Pediatric Allergy and Immunology 14:378–382

Backett-Milburn K & McKie L 1999 A critical appraisal of the draw and write technique. Health Education Research 14(3):387–398

Balen R, Holroyd C, Mountain G, Wood B 2001 Giving children a voice: methodological and practical implications of research involving children. Paediatric Nursing 12:10

Barker J, Weller S. 2003 'Is it fun?' Developing children centred research methods. International Journal of Sociology and Social Policy 23:1–2

Bayea SC, Nicoll LH 1997 Ten questions that will get you through any research report. AORN Online 65(5):978–979

Behrman R, Kleigman R eds 1998 Nelson's essentials of paediatrics, 3rd edn. WB Saunders, Philadelphia, pp 4–9, 192, 213 482, 483

Bradding A, Horstman M 1999 Using the write and draw technique with children. European Journal of Oncology Nursing 3(3):170–175

Broome ME, Richards DJ 2003 The influence of relationships on children's and adolescent's participation in research. Nursing Research 52(3):191–197

Brown MS, Haylor M. 1989 Nursing research with preoperational age children: the use of standardized tests. Journal of Paediatric Nursing 4:1

Bullinger M, Schmidt S, Petersen C, Disabkids Group 2002 Assessing quality of life of children with chronic health conditions and disabilities: a European approach. International Journal of Rehabilitation Research 25:197–205

Burns J 2003 Research in children. Critical Care Medicine 31(suppl 3):S131–S136

Camilleri-Brennan J, Steele RJC 1999 Measurement of quality of life in surgery. Journal of the Royal College of Surgeons Edinburgh 44:252–259.

Casey A 2000 The role of professional journals in promoting evidence-based care. In: Glasper EA, Ireland L (eds) Evidence-based child health care challenges for practice. Palgrave, Basingstoke

Creery D, Mikrogianakis A 2003 Sudden infant death syndrome: what are the effects of intervention to reduce the risk of sudden infant death syndrome? Clinical evidence. BMJ Publishing Group, London

Crombie IK 1996 The pocket guide to critical appraisal. BMJ Publishing Group, London

Curtin C 2000 Eliciting children's voices in qualitative research. The American Journal of Occupational Therapy 55:3

Department of Health (DoH) 1989 The Children Act. HMSO, London

Department of Health (DoH) 1998 A first class service: quality in the new NHS. HMSO, London

Department of Health (DoH) 2000a NHS plan. HMSO, London

Department of Health (DoH) 2000b Toolkit for producing patient information. HMSO, London

Department of Health (DoH) 2001a Seeking consent: working with children. HMSO, London

Department of Health (DoH) 2001b Research governance framework for health and social care. HMSO, London

Department of Health (DoH) 2001c Strengthening accountability, involving patients and the public: practice guidance of the Health and Social Care Act. HMSO, London

Department of Health (DoH) 2001d Learning to listen – core principles for the involvement of children and young people. HMSO, London

Department of Health (DoH) 2003a Getting the right start: National Service Framework for Children Standard for Hospital Services. HMSO, London

Department of Health (DoH) 2003b Advice note, patient and public forums, 4 December 2003. DoH, London

Department of Health (DoH) 2003c The learning to listen report. HMSO, London

Dockerell J 2000 Researching children's perspectives: a psychological dimension. In: Lewis A, Lindsay G (eds) Researching children's perspectives. Open University Press, Buckingham

Edwards A, Talbot R 1994 The hard-pressed researcher. A research handbook for the caring professions. Longman, London

Fleitas J 1998 Spinning tales from the world wide web: qualitative research in an electronic environment. Qualitative Health Research 8(2):283–292

Forman EN, Ladd RE 1995 Ethical dilemmas in pediatrics, a case study approach. University Press of America, London

Hanley B, Bradburn J, Gorin S et al 2000 Involving consumers in research and development in the NHS: briefing notes for researchers. Consumers in NHS Research Support Unit, Eastleigh

Higginson J, Carr AJ 2001 Measuring quality of life: using quality of life measures in the clinical setting. British Medical Journal 322(7297):1297–1300

Hinds D 2000 Research instruments. In: Wilkinson D (ed.) The researcher's toolkit. The complete guide to practitioner research. Routlege Farmer, London

Gibbs A 1997 Focus groups. Social research update. Online. Available at: http://www.soc.surrey.ac.uk/sru/SRU19html

Glasper EA, Ireland L 2000 Evidence-based child health care. Palgrave, Basingstoke

Godfrey KM, Barker DJP 2000 Fetal nutrition and adult disease. American Journal of Clinical Nutrition 71(5 Suppl):1344S–1352S

Godfrey KM, Barker DJP 2001 Fetal programming and adult health. Public Health and Nutrition 4(2B):611–624

International Conference on Harmonisation (ICH) 2000 Topic E11 Clinical investigation of medicinal products in the paediatric population. EMEA, London

International Conference on Harmonisation (ICH) 2002 Guideline for good clinical practice. EMEA, London

Joseph Rowntree Foundation 2000 Involving young people in research projects. Joseph Rowntree Foundation, York

Kennedy C, Charlesworth A, Chen J 2003 Interactive data collection benefits of integrating new media into pediatric research. Computers, Informatics, Nursing 21(3):120–127

Kirby P 1999 Involving young researchers. Joseph Rowntree Foundation, York, pp 14, 16–19, 21, 26, 39, 64, 125

Lamprill J 2002 Asking for children's assent to take part in clinical research. Good Clinical Practice Journal 9(8):9–12

Lamprill J 2003 Prioritise and plan for children's needs. Good Clinical Practice Journal 10(8):17–19

MacGregor J 2001 Introduction to the anatomy and physiology of children. Routledge, London, pp 21, 30, 42, 113

Meaux JB, Bell PL 2001 Balancing recruitment and protection: children as research subjects. Comprehensive Pediatric Nursing 24:241–251

Montgomery J 2001 Informed consent and clinical research with children. In: Doyal L, Tobias S (eds) Informed consent in medical research. BMJ Publishing Group, London, p 178

Morland B 2003 Why children with cancer benefit from phase 1 studies. Good Clinical Practice Journal 10(8):11–14

Morrow V 2001 Using qualitative methods to elicit young people's perspectives on their environments: some ideas for community health initiatives. Health Education Research 16(3):255–268

National Institutes of Health (NIH) 1998 Policy and guidelines on the inclusion of children as participants in research involving human subjects. Online. Available at: http://grants.nih.gov/grants/guide/notice-files/not98-024.html

The Nursing and Midwifery Council (NMC) 2002 Code of professional conduct. NMC, London

Oppenheim AN 2002 Questionnaire design, interviewing and attitude measurement. Continuum International Publishing Group – Academi, London

Polit DF, Hungler BP 1995 Nursing research: principles and methods, 6th edn. Lippincott, Philadelphia

Pridmore PJ, Lansdown RG 1997 Exploring children's perceptions of health: does drawing really break down barriers? Health Education Journal 56:219–230

Robinson S 2001 Informed consent in children. Good Clinical Practice Journal 8(8):5–6

Robinson S 2002 Child-friendly concerns. Good Clinical Practice Journal 9(8):15

Rosato J 2000 The ethics of clinical trials: a child's view. The Journal of Law, Medicine and Ethics 28(4):362–378

Rothmier JD, Lasley MV, Shapiro GC 2003 Factors influencing parental consent in pediatric clinical research. Pediatrics 111(5):1037–1041

Royal College of Paediatrics and Child Health (RCPCH) 2000 Advocating for children. RCPCH, London

Royal College of Paediatrics and Child Health (RCPCH) and The Neonatal and Paediatric Pharmacists Group 1999 The use of unlicensed medicines or licensed medicines for unlicensed application in paediatric practice. Policy statement. RCPCH, London

Scanlon M. 2003 Issues in research. In: Wilkinson D (ed.) The researcher's toolkit the complete guide to practitioner research. Routlege Farmer, London

Sorensen ES 1989 Using children's diaries as a research instrument. Journal of Pediatric Nursing 4:6

Swage T 2000 Clinical governance in health care practice. Butterworth Heinemann, Oxford

United Nations General Assembly 1989 Convention on the rights of the child. UNICEF, Geneva

Vasmant D 2003 Europe grows impatient over delays in paediatric initiatives (guest editorial). Good Clinical Practice Journal August:1–3

Vincent KA, Higginson IJ 2003 Assessing quality of life in children. In: Carr AJ, Higginson J, Robinson S (eds) Quality of life. BMJ Publishing, London

Warner JA, Jones CA, Jones AC, Warner JO 2000a Prenatal origins of allergic disease. Journal of Allergy and Clinical Immunology 105(2):493–496

Warner JO, Jones CA, Kilburn AS, Vance GHS 2000b Prenatal sensitization in humans. Pediatric Allergy and Immunology Suppl 13:6 8

Williamson H, Butler I 1995 Children speak: perspectives on their social worlds. In: Brannon J, O'Brien M (eds) Children and parenthood. Proceedings of the International Sociological Association Committee for Family Research Practice 1994, London. Institute of Education, University of London, London, pp 294–330

Wilson JT 1996 Strategies for pediatric drug evaluation: a view from the trenches. Drug Information Journal 30:1149–1162

Wong DL, Baker CM 1988 Pain in children: comparison of assessment scales. Pediatric Nursing 14:9–17

World Medical Association (WMA) 2000 52nd General Assembly: Declaration of Helsinki. WMA, Edinburgh

Worrall S 2000 Young people as researchers, a learning resource pack. Joseph Rowntree Foundation and Save the Children, London, pp 2–7

Chapter Sixteen

16

Ensuring Quality and the Role of Clinical Audit

Janice Watson

ABSTRACT

The aim of this chapter and the companion PowerPoint presentation is to introduce key quality issues that arise during the provision of services and care to children and their families. Current government initiatives and key policy documents are identified and their impact on the provision of quality services explored. In particular, the central importance of clinical audit is discussed and the key stages of the audit cycle described.

Learning Outcomes

- Discuss clinical governance, with reference to the key elements, activities and processes associated with the clinical governance framework.

- Consider what quality means in a healthcare context.

- Explore recent government policy on quality in the NHS.

- Review key quality tools and their use in providing quality services.

- Demonstrate a sound understanding of the audit process and its importance to the quality agenda.

- Examine the role of key agencies in assuring quality improvements in health care.

Introduction

In 1983, the World Health Organization (WHO) stated that by 1990 all member states should have built effective mechanisms for ensuring the quality of patient care within their healthcare system, thus clearly identifying the global, central importance of quality in health care.

Arguably, quality in health care was first recognised by Florence Nightingale, who was a pioneer of systematic observation, standard setting and improvement of care and who clearly advocated the importance of quality in healthcare as early as the 19th century. During the Crimean War, Nightingale realised that admission to a battle hospital actually increased a soldier's chances of death, so she set standards against which she measured practice. This process led to a drastic reduction in the rates of hospital-acquired infection and dramatically cut the mortality rate. Furthermore, Nightingale (1863) reiterated the need to collect data and measure outcomes in healthcare:

> *In attempting to arrive at the truth, I have applied everywhere for information, but in scarcely an instance have I been able to obtain hospital records fit for any purpose of comparison . . . They would show subscribers how their money was being spent, what amount of good was really being done with it or whether the money was doing mischief rather than good.*

In 1959, the publication of the Platt Report, entitled *Welfare of Children in Hospital Report* (Ministry of Health 1959), was an early attempt to raise standards in the care of sick children in hospital, although the aspirations of this report went largely unfulfilled. For several decades the wise words of Nightingale and the key features of the Platt Report went relatively unheeded, although voluntary organisations maintained an impetus for the need to improve quality of care. In particular, the work of Action for Sick Children, previously known as the National Association for the Welfare of Children in Hospital (NAWCH) made important contributions to the quality of care afforded children in hospital and introduced a Charter for Children in Hospital in 1984. This charter encouraged nurse managers to monitor standards of care in children's departments.

In general, the nursing profession had an interest in quality care, which grew with the development of the Royal College of Nursing and the RCN Standards of Care Project (Parsley & Corrigan 1999a). From this work, nursing embraced the dynamic standards-setting system based on the Donabedian (1966) structure–process–outcome framework, but three main factors have resulted in an upsurge of interest in quality in recent years:

- Public expectations.
- The sheer complexity of healthcare organisations and interventions.
- Recognition of the opportunities for improvement through good practice, but also following the rising rate of litigation and high-profile cases of major failures in the NHS, such as the Bristol Royal Infirmary heart surgery tradegy.

In response to these factors, the UK government introduced a significant set of reforms in the NHS, which shifted the focus towards quality of care and formed one of the main principles underpinning the incoming Labour government's agenda for the NHS. In the White Paper *The New NHS: Modern Dependable* (Department of Health (DoH) 1997), the government declared that the new NHS would have quality at its heart; quality was to be the driving force for decision making at every level of the service and the agenda for quality was set in the White Paper *A First Class Service* (DoH, 1998). This paper identified three main components for ensuring high-quality care.

- The setting of clear standards and the introduction of the National Institute for Clinical Excellence (NICE) and the National Service Frameworks (NSFs).
- Delivering these standards at local level: clinical governance.
- Monitoring of standards: to be done by the Commission for Audit and Inspection (CHAI; previously the Commission for Health Improvement (CHI)), the NHS Performance Assessment Framework and the National Patient and User Surveys (Brocklehurst & Walshe 1999).

Figure 16.1 shows the relationship between these components; clinical governance being pivotal to this model.

Defining quality in health care has been fraught with difficulties, with many examples of attempts to describe in detail what good quality is in any service. The work of Donabedian (1966) highlights the inherent dangers in this, stating that the criteria of quality are nothing more than value judgements. Basically, quality can be almost anything to anyone, based on their own values, beliefs and goals within both health care and society in general.

Quality as a concept is important in so far as we want to be able to measure it to improve it, and the identification of components of quality are one way in which this has been attempted. One such example is Maxwell's six dimensions of quality (1984), which are:

- access to service
- relevance to need
- effectiveness
- equity
- social acceptability
- efficiency and economy.

Activity

Jot down what you believe constitutes a quality service or experience within a healthcare setting:
- How do these relate to your own values and beliefs?

Fig. 16.1 • The NHS quality framework.

Student nurse Kelly Jones has read in her local paper that her local hospital has been awarded only two stars. She asks her assessor how these ratings are awarded.

Maxwell's (1984) six dimensions of quality are reflected in the NHS Performance Assessment Framework, a set of performance indicators, or measures, that allow the performance of health authorities and NHS Trusts to be compared; some have been published in the form of league tables (Swage 2000). Individual trusts are assessed against these indicators and, depending on their score, a star rating is awarded, with five stars being the highest any Trust can achieve. These dimensions are:

- *Health improvement and reducing health inequalities.*
- *Fair access irrespective of geography, socio-economic group, ethnicity, age or gender.*
- *Effective delivery of appropriate health care that complies with agreed standards.*
- *Efficiency and the achievement of value for money.*
- *Patient/carer experience by assessing the way in which patients/carers view the quality of care they receive to ensure the NHS is sensitive to individual needs.*
- *Health outcomes of NHS care to assess the direct contribution of NHS care to improvement in overall health closing the loop back to the goal of health improvement (Pickering & Thompson 2003, Scally & Donaldson 1998, Swage 2000).*

Activity

The value of hospital league tables has been hotly debated in the media. Go to:

- http://www.chi.nhs.uk/ratings

and choose the England ratings and Acute Trust indicators in the left hand menu. In particular, review the ratings for Great Ormond Street Children's Hospital and Birmingham Children's Hospital:

- What were their star ratings and do you think these are a fair way to represent the performance of any Trust?
- Do you feel the indicators give a snapshot of the true activity of the hospital and the quality of the services they provide?
- Do you feel these ratings help families make an informed choice about the quality of care they can expect to receive from any given Trust?

Importantly, the information gained from such performance measures is only meaningful if it is used to bring about improvement. It is therefore more useful to consider quality as a cycle of improvement (Fig. 16.2).

Quality is therefore represented as being a continuous process, which is an organisation-wide endeavour. Two such

Fig. 16.2 • The quality improvement cycle.

organisational approaches, which have been adopted within the NHS, are total quality management (TQM) and continuous quality improvement (CQI). CQI aims at embedding continuous quality improvement at all levels and across all services with the goal of achieving changes in practice that improve patient outcomes. Within the NHS, TQM and CQI are often used synonymously and interchangeably.

Total Quality Management

TQM is a business philosophy that was first introduced by Deming and Juran in the USA. It is a method of managing quality issues throughout every aspect of an organisation. Deming – one of the proponents of TQM – advocated a systematic approach to problem solving and promoted the PDCA cycle: Plan, Do, Check and Act. Juran, who is considered the father of quality, established a theory of quality management which evolved during the 1940s, 1950s and 1960s (Parsley & Corrigan 1999) and involves everyone and everything that happens in an organisation. Quality is therefore a continuous process expanding across departments and professional boundaries; it is:

. . . an integrated, corporately led programme of organisational change designed to engender and sustain a culture of continuous improvement based on customer orientated definitions of quality (Joss & Kogan 1995 p 13)

KEY TQM PROCESSES

- Focus on the needs and expectations of the market and consumers (i.e. healthcare and its patients).
- Achieve top quality performance in all areas of activity.
- Install whatever operating procedures – simple or complex – are necessary to achieve top quality performance.

- Critically and continuously examine the processes to reduce and remove non-productive activities, inefficiencies and waste.
- Develop and monitor measures of performance, set standards against which this performance is measured and identify required improvements.
- Understand the need for, and develop, an effective communication strategy.
- Develop a non-hierarchical team approach to problem solving and delegate responsibility for change.
- Develop good procedures for communication and feedback to staff at any level of good work.
- Continuously review the above processes to develop a culture for never-ending improvement.

The aim is to 'get it right first time every time'.

Professional Conversation

Student nurse Jones has been reading an article in a nursing magazine, which has referred to TQM. She asks her assessor how TQM works in the NHS

Clinical governance is an example within the NHS which reflects the TQM philosophy of managing quality issues. The key processes identified with TQM can be directly related to systems and processes associated with clinical governance. These include quality improvement activities like audit, data collection, and record keeping; clear lines of responsibility and accountability, risk management policies, procedures for identifying poor performance, and public and user involvement. So, you see, TQM is very relevant to the NMS.

Activity

Spend 20 minutes reflecting on your clinical experience and see if you can identify any quality processes that are or were evident in your day-to-day practice.

The Rise of Clinical Governance

For healthcare to become more patient focused, and if quality improvements are to be made, then healthcare professionals need to embrace the wider aspects of care, which include:

- recognising the contribution of other colleagues from other disciplines
- organisational behaviour and change
- clinical audit
- working in teams.

A substantial shift in the culture of the NHS was required so that quality improvement became central to the work of the NHS, with an emphasis on collaboration rather than competition. To achieve this cultural shift the government determined that clinical governance would be used as a framework, with the patient–professional partnership at the pinnacle of a temple model supported by seven pillars (Scally & Donaldson 1998) (Fig. 16.3).

Each pillar represents professional and managerial processes integral to quality improvement. Clinical governance acts like an umbrella under which all aspects of quality can be gathered and monitored and the WHO's description of quality as being composed of four elements forms the basis for the development of clinical governance. These four elements are:

1. professional performance: technical quality
2. resource use: economic efficiency
3. risk management
4. patient satisfaction (Buetow & Roland 1999).

Clinical governance is defined as:

A framework through which NHS organisations are accountable for continuously improving the quality of their services and safeguarding high standards of care by creating an environment in which clinical care will flourish (DoH 1998)

Clinical governance is to be the framework used to bring about a new culture, which places quality as central to the work of all in the NHS. It covers the organisations' systems and processes for monitoring and improving services. This culture will be manifest in the ten C's of clinical governance (Heard et al 2001):

- clinical performance
- clinical leadership

Fig. 16.3 • The temple model of clinical governance.

- clinical audit
- clinical risk management
- complaints
- continuing health needs assessments
- changing practice though evidence
- continuing education
- culture of excellence
- clear accountability.

Importantly, clinical governance encourages healthcare professionals to take control and demonstrate their ability to self-regulate and maintain public service accountability. Healthcare professionals are to take the lead in quality improvement strategies within a structure of increased external accountability. Clinical governance is part of a strategy for quality improvement in the context of a nationally coordinated programme of clinical guideline development with a nominated individual in each organisation responsible for clinical governance. Clinical governance is quality at a local level and focuses on processes of care, which include clinical decision making, appropriateness, clinical effectiveness and evidence-based practice (Pickering & Thompson 2003, Swage

2000). The key features of clinical governance (Scally & Donaldson 1998) are:

- clear lines of responsibility and accountability for quality
- programme of quality improvement activities
- clear risk reduction policies
- procedures for identifying and addressing poor performance
- public and user involvement.

Figure 16.4 is a mind map of the key activities associated with clinical governance.

Activity

Put yourself at the centre of a mind map like the one in Fig. 16.4 and then identify how you can contribute to the clinical governance agenda. You might want to include things like:
- clinical supervision
- reflection
- education and training
- involvement in ward meetings.

Fig. 16.4 • Mind map of the key activities associated with clinical governance.

USER INVOLVEMENT

The involvement of service users is an important tenet to the implementation of clinical governance. This presents a challenge to those who are involved in the provision of healthcare services to children. Although children can be reliable informants who are able to accurately reflect their own lived experiences of being a patient in hospital, it is often assumed that they are not competent to offer a legitimate viewpoint on their experience of healthcare services (Glasper 2004, Woodfield 2001).

Since the publication of the Bristol Inquiry and the Children's National Service Framework, government recommendations have been quite strident in their call for greater patient and public involvement. The Commission for Patient and Public Involvement in Health (PPI) is tasked with giving the public a voice in decisions that affect their health and is operationalised through the Patient Advisory Liaison Service (PALS) at individual Trust level. Importantly, an innovative audit tool is being developed for CHAI to access Trusts against the Children's NSF based on a model already in use by *Essence of care* (NHS Modernisation Agency 2003), which will allow individual organisations to benchmark themselves against the NSF standards. It is hoped that this will help to raise the voice of children and truly involve them in their own healthcare services.

BENCHMARKING

Benchmarking is not new in paediatrics. The North West Paediatric Benchmarking Project was established in 1994 and today includes in its membership a large number of NHS and academic staff, although the origins of benchmarks are in fact in industry. Benchmarking provides a structured approach to the sharing of best practice utilising all levels of evidence in identifying standards of excellence (Ellis 2000).

Clinical practice benchmarking focuses on practice in which practitioners identify the structures and processes that contribute to good practice, provides a scoring system to measure the structures and processes and comments on the actual practice. Furthermore, an external review panel reviews the benchmarking statements. The comparison of scores enables sharing, which leads to development and innovation. The scoring system aims to be as objective as possible to maximise reliability and validity, although it is recognised that, due to the nature of the evidence on which the scores are based, there will always be some element of subjectivity. The comments made in relation to the scores are therefore very important and are used to support the development of action plans (Ellis 2000).

Clinical practice benchmarking is identified as being a valuable quality improvement initiative with several groups established in a variety of specialities throughout the UK. Repetition of effort is eliminated and vital time and resources saved, making it a cost-effective system for ensuring quality care. By involving practitioners in the process motivation is increased and an environment for change established with practice development an ongoing activity (Stark et al 2002).

ESSENCE OF CARE

The NHS Plan (DoH 2000) reinforced the need to get back to basics and get them right. It provides a tool to help practitioners take a patient-focused approach and a structure to sharing and comparing practice. Furthermore it is an across the age continuum tool. *Essence of care* (NHS Modernisation Agency 2003) has resulted in the identification of benchmarks covering nine fundamental aspects of care, which are:

- communication
- food and nutrition
- privacy and dignity
- continence and bladder and bowel care
- personal and oral hygiene
- pressure ulcers
- record keeping
- safety of clients with mental health needs in acute mental health and general hospital settings
- principles of self-care.

Of particular relevance are the benchmarks for communication between patients, carers and healthcare personnel, and in particular coordination of care, which requires that the wishes of patients and/or carers are listened to, considered and acted on appropriately, and that patients and/or carers are involved in person-centred planning, the single assessment process and discharge planning (NHS Modernisation Agency 2003). If benchmarking is used in the spirit for which it is intended then the voices of the children should be heard as we strive to improve the quality of care afforded to this client group. The benefits of *Essence of care* are that it:

- improves quality of care
- involves patients, users and carers
- has a structured approach to sharing and comparing practice
- requires the development of action plans to remedy poor practice
- is integral to the clinical governance agenda.

National Service Frameworks

The National Service Frameworks (NSFs) were set up as a rolling programme in 1998 to improve the quality of statutory services (NHS and the Social and Education services). They were established to tackle variations in care by setting national guidelines. The aim of an NSF is to:

- set national standards for a defined service or care group
- put in place strategies to support the implementation of these standards
- establish milestones against which progress will be measured.

Each NSF concentrates on a different area, with one having been specifically set up for children. The Children's NSF was established in February 2001 and is focused on developing new national standards for children across the NHS and in Social Services and the Education system. Most importantly, the Children's NSF is about putting children and young people, and their families, at the centre of their care and building services around all their needs. The Children's NSF has three main aims:

- improving services
- tackling inequalities
- enhancing partnerships (DoH 2003).

Within the Children's NSF there are individual external working groups (EWGs). These groups work together to ensure all children are receiving high quality services; they concentrate on:

- the health of all children
- maternity services
- child and adolescent mental health services
- children in special circumstances
- hospital and acute services
- use of medicines in children
- disabled children.

Source: CHI, 2004

Clinical Audit

The primary principle of clinical audit has always been to develop healthcare practice, something that practitioners have been attempting to do for generations. Clinical audit is a key quality improvement activity and NHS Trusts are now mandated through government legislation (DoH 2000) to have a comprehensive programme of quality improvement activity that includes clinicians participating fully in clinical audit. Clinical audit is taking a leading role in ensuring qual-

ity improvement activity is done collaboratively and systematically, influenced by the publication of numerous NHS policy statements (DoH 1997, 1998, 1999, 2000).

Healthcare systems need to find ways to ensure healthcare professionals are able to provide patients with the highest possible, and affordable, standards of care. Rawlins (1999) states that there is an abundance of evidence that the clinical care given to patients too often departs from best practice.

As a result of the 1998 public inquiry into paediatric cardiac surgical services at Bristol Royal Infirmary (DoH 2001), subsequent recommendations regarding audit were fully accepted by the government. In particular, the inquiry recommended that audit should be at the core of a system of local monitoring of performance and be fully supported by Trusts, to ensure that healthcare professionals have access to the necessary time, facilities and advice. All Trusts should have a central audit office to coordinate audit activity, provide advice and support and bring together the results of audit. Finally, clinical audit should be compulsory for all professionals providing clinical care and the requirement to participate should be included as part of the contract of employment.

In 1993 the NHS Executive (Mann 1996) set out the fundamental principles associated with clinical audit. These state that clinical audit should:

- be professionally led
- be seen as an educational process
- form a part of routine clinical practice
- be based on the setting of standards
- generate results that can be used to improve outcome of quality care
- involve management in both process and outcome of audit
- be confidential at the individual patient/clinician level
- be informed by the views of patients/clients.

The developing role of evidence-based medicine and clinical effectiveness has led to more recent policy statements by the NHS Executive, which have focused on the role that clinical audit has to play in clinical effectiveness by getting research into practice (Thomas 1999). Mann (1996) reported that clinical audit is, and should remain, a clinically led initiative that seeks to improve the quality and outcome of patient care through clinicians examining and modifying their practices according to standards of what could be achieved, based on the best evidence available.

The need for high-quality audit has been driven forward over recent years, within the NHS, primarily through the introduction of clinical governance. This was introduced into the NHS to indicate integration of clinical quality improvement with organisational and service performance at all levels. Scally & Donaldson (1998) highlighted that clinical quality, through clinical governance, would enable it to be integrated with financial control and service performance, at all levels of organisations, providing health care that will be managed well.

Clinical audit therefore plays a central role in this process. It is firmly placed in professional practice and is an essential pillar of clinical governance. This was confirmed by Johnson et al (2000), who state that well-planned audit is in a good position to be applied effectively to improve both clinical decisions and organisational efficiency. However, they stressed, to ensure clinicians play a pivotal role in this, greater attention needs to be made on the factors that have been shown to allow audit to flourish and those that have been shown to impede its progress.

An important point to note is that much of the local clinical audit activity that takes place in the UK is not published and therefore important and valuable information is not being shared.

Scenario

Student nurse Kelly Jones has been asked to participate in an audit of family satisfaction by giving families a discharge questionnaire. She asks her assessor 'What is a clinical audit?' and 'How is it undertaken?'.

WHAT IS CLINICAL AUDIT?

Clinical audit is a systematic review of care against explicit criteria, which seeks to improve patient care and outcomes through the implementation of change. For audit to succeed there needs to be a supportive organisational environment, with staff who are well prepared and fully understand the methods to be used (NICE 2002). The environment refers to both the structure and culture, and it is structure that provides the link back to the business of clinical governance, professional regulation and life-long learning. Culture, on the other hand, refers to an environment that encourages openness and creativity, and where errors and failures can be reported and investigated with no fear of blame (Morrell & Harvey 1999, NICE 2002).

Clinical audit can be described as having five principal stages (NICE 2002):

1. preparing for audit
2. selecting criteria
3. measuring performance
4. making improvements
5. sustaining improvements.

A variety of methods may be used at each of these stages requiring the use of a broad range of methods from a number of disciplines. These include organisational development, statistics and information management. Individual healthcare staff or groups of professionals in single or multi-disciplinary teams, usually supported by clinical audit staff, undertake clinical audit, which may be a project involving all services in a region or country. Effective systems for managing audit and implementing change are important and this might mean that more time is spent on creating the right environment than on the method itself (Dixon 1996).

CONDUCTING A CLINICAL AUDIT

Stage One: Preparing for Audit (NICE 2002)

Good preparation is essential to ensure a successful audit project and requires:

- Project management: consisting of topic selection, planning and resources, communication.
- Project methodology: project design, data issues, how the project will be implemented, stakeholders to be involved and the level of support for local improvement.

There are five key elements to address when preparing for audit:

1. **Involvement of users and sources of user information**: The involvement of users in decisions about their care and healthcare services is central to government strategy. Their voice can be heard through, for example:
   - the Patient Advisory Liaison Service (PALS)
   - patient stories or focus groups.

2. **Topic selection**: This will be based on an organisation's individual local priority, reflecting national targets, NICE guidelines and the implementation of National Service Frameworks. Or it might be as a result of:
   - letters of comment or complaint
   - critical incident reports
   - direct observation of care
   - direct conversations
   - following a clinical governance review
   - through benchmarking
   - appraisal of new or existing evidence.

3. **Purpose of the audit**: The need for clear objectives is fundamental to successful audit and enables the identification of suitable audit methods (Morrell & Harvey 1999). The aims of an audit may be couched in some of the following terms:
   - to improve . . .
   - to change . . .
   - to enhance . . .
   - to ensure . . .

4. **Provision of necessary structures for the conduct of a successful audit:** Such as:
   - time
   - funding
   - meetings.

5. **A skilled audit team:** This is needed to ensure that the audit is valid and robustly conducted. These skills include:
   - project leadership, organisation management
   - clinical, managerial leadership
   - audit method skills
   - change management skills
   - facilitation and negotiation skills.

Stage Two: Selecting Criteria (NICE 2002)

Criteria are used to access the quality of care provided by an individual, team or organisation; they are also commonly stated as standards. Criteria refer to a level of performance and can be classified into three groups:

1. Structure: staffing, skill mix, equipment.

2. Process: actions and decisions taken, e.g. communication, assessment, documentation, discharge planning.

3. Outcomes of care: physical or behavioural responses to an intervention, e.g. drug therapies.

The selection of valid criteria is essential if improvements are to be made in care. Valid criteria are measurable and based on the best available evidence (Parsley & Corrigan 1999b).

External Sources of Valid Criteria
- NICE: National Institute for Clinical Effectiveness.
- SIGN: Scottish Intercollegiate Guidelines Network.
- Systematic reviews: Cochrane Library.
- Benchmarking: *Essence of care* (NHS Modernisation Agency 2003).

Internal Sources of Valid Criteria
Following the systematic review of relevant literature:
- patient care pathways
- local protocols
- local guidelines.

Importantly, there needs to be an external peer review process of internally developed criteria with service user involvement through, for example, focused groups. The process used to obtain criteria for audit from evidence should be methodical, relate to important aspects of care and it should be measurable. Also, if the standards are incomplete or based on views of professionals or groups, formal consensus methods are preferred.

Stage Three: Measuring Performance (NICE 2002)

Methods of data collection should be carefully considered and, where possible, the use of existing data should be used. The audit group needs to consider who will collect data, and must ensure that they are capable, acceptable and non-threatening to patients and staff. Morrell & Harvey (1999) highlight the need to consider the consent of patients and staff before data collection begins and stress that guidance (e.g. the General Medical Council's 2004 *Confidentiality: protecting and providing information*) needs to be followed to address issues of confidentiality.

Four key areas should be addressed when measuring levels of performance:

 Activity

Access the guidance on *Confidentiality: protecting and providing information* at:
- http://www.gmc_uk.org/standards

Write down the key points from this guidance and why this is important to our practice.

1. Planning data collection:
   - User groups need to be identified (e.g. all premature infants between 32 weeks and 36 weeks gestation receiving care within the neonatal intensive care unit) and exceptions noted.
   - Which healthcare professionals are involved in the users care.
   - The time period over which the criteria apply.

2. Selecting the sample:
   - How big a sample do you need to be confident in the findings?
   - Resource constraints: time, access, costs.

3. Data collection: this is generally done retrospectively, after the care has been provided, although it can be collected concurrently to provide almost immediate feedback. As information technology becomes more advanced, concurrent audit becomes a more viable option. A tool is developed; this is usually a form, which identifies the precise information that is to be obtained. Any data collection tool should be piloted before use to ensure it captures the information required and to check that there is no ambiguity in the interpretation of the form by those who will collect the data. The form needs to be user friendly to ensure full data collection. Data can be collected using computerised programmes specifically designed for audit.

4. Data analysis:
   - How the data is analysed influences what and how the information is collected and should be identified at an early stage.

● Data can be qualitative, qualitative or a combination of both. Findings from an audit can be a simple percentage representation of the data, tables and graphs through to full qualitative description

Stage Four: Making Improvements (NICE 2002)

This is vital for effecting change. Practitioners frequently recognise the need to complete the audit cycle but may not have the skills, time, patience, authority or resources needed to improve the quality of care. Changes in practice may be achieved more effectively if a strategy involving several different types of action is used (Malby 1995).

Related factors that may also influence the likelihood of change include what the implication of the change is to service users, the effectiveness of teamwork, and the organisational environment. All these may therefore need to be considered when implementing change (Fig. 16.5).

Stage Five: Sustaining Improvement (NICE 2002)

Although improving performance is the primary goal of audit, sustaining that improvement is also essential. Any systematic approach to changing professional practice should include plans to monitor and evaluate change and ways to maintain and reinforce that change (NHS Centre for Review and Dissemination 1999). Leadership plays a vital role in this, with quality improvement embedded in all aspects of an organisation's work, sustained through monitoring and re-audit (NICE 2002).

New health technologies are sometimes adopted into everyday clinical practice without adequate evidence of their clinical effectiveness and cost effectiveness. Conversely, clinicians can be too slow to introduce new methods of practice even when they have been shown to be effective and give value for money. Clinicians do not have the time and expertise to evaluate each

and every possible new intervention but, when this is done for them, the resulting guidelines or guidance are too often of an inadequate or indeterminate quality, and are indigestible or inaccessible. It was for these reasons that the National Institute for Clinical Excellence (NICE) was established.

Examples of Improving Care through Audit

Evidence-based Practice

Implementing a children's day assessment unit in a district general hospital (from Beverley et al 1997)

The implementation of a paediatric day assessment unit to a district general hospital was as a result of increasing numbers of children being referred for admission over the previous decade and questioning of the appropriateness of the referral and admission of these children. The implementation of short-stay assessment facilities has been used in Australia and found to be an effective patient management strategy. Within this district hospital, issues were identified that required a review of the paediatric service. These issues included large peaks and troughs in patient activity exacerbated by uncoordinated admission procedures, with 20 different consultant surgeons from five different surgical specialities admitting children for elective surgery, which occasionally resulted in cancellations due to a lack of beds. Furthermore, there was the desire to meet the Audit Commission's recommendation for there to be two children's trained nurses on duty at all times on the children's wards.

Fig. 16.5 ● The clinical audit cycle (NICE 2002).

In planning for the introduction of a day assessment unit, representatives from the surgical and primary care teams were included in the project team and analysis of historic paediatric patient activity undertaken. Operational protocols were developed and key facilities secured for the assessment unit, e.g. a play-room, treatment areas. Furthermore, families discharged home from the assessment unit were given a contact telephone number in case they required further advice or support once at home.

An audit of the first year's activity demonstrated a fall in the number of children admitted overnight as an emergency, 658 children were assessed as an emergency but did not require admission to the inpatient ward, and a fall in staff nurse costs.

Evidence-based Practice

Telephone follow-up after paediatric day surgery (from Higson & Bolland 2000)

Following a review of the literature it was clearly identified that telephone follow-up calls are an effective tool in providing support and advice to families following discharge from hospital. Together with geographical, financial and staff resource considerations, day surgical units within a children's teaching hospital worked together to produce standards of care for telephone follow-up. To measure the effectiveness of the introduction of telephone call follow-up an audit tool was developed so the process of the telephone call follow-up could be evaluated. This was completed every 6 months. Concerns identified were with regard to pain management following certain surgical procedures, which resulted in children being prescribed stronger analgesia to take home with them following surgery. Patient information was also addressed and evidence-based information leaflets were developed using the information gained from the follow-up telephone calls, which were given to the children and their families during their admission.

Evidence-based Practice

Integrated care pathway for infants with bronchiolitis (Peter & Fazakerley 2004)

Integrated care pathways are structured multi-disciplinary care plans detailing essential steps in the care of a patient with a specified condition. They are regarded as a means by which local protocols and evidenced-based clinical guidelines can be combined, incorporating the means by which to evaluate the outcomes through the utilisation of variance analysis. There is, however, a recognised lack of empirical evidence of their effectiveness in clinical care therefore the audit process was used to evaluate the effectiveness of the introduction of a clinical pathway for infants with bronchiolitis.

A retrospective review of a number of case notes was undertaken over a 3-year period, 70 prior to implementation of the pathway, 70 following introduction of the pathway and a further 70 following revision of the pathway. Aspects audited included hospital admission criteria, oxygen therapy, hydration, investigations and drug therapy. Staff knowledge of bronchiolitis and satisfaction was also assessed before and after implementation. Improvements identified were increased staff knowledge and satisfaction, less inappropriate chest radiographs, less unnecessary antibiotic administration and improved A&E triage assessment.

Activity

To familiarise yourself with the audit process, contact your local clinical audit office and ask if you can see a completed audit relevant to your area of speciality. Ask yourself the following questions:

- Why was the topic chosen?
- Who were involved and was there user involvement?
- What was the purpose of the audit?
- What criteria did they use and what was the evidence base for these criteria – were they internal or external?
- How was the data collected and was any tool used? If so, was the tool user friendly?
- Was the data collected retrospectively or prospectively?
- How was confidentiality addressed?
- Who was the user group for the audit and was it specific?
- How was the sample size chosen?
- Was the data collected over a specified time period?
- How was the data analysed and was it easy to understand?
- What was the outcome of this audit – did it result in a change in practice?
- Was there an action plan for the implementation of any change?
- What have you gained by completing this activity?

The Role of the National Institute for Clinical Effectiveness

NICE has been charged with providing NHS staff with robust, authoritative and reliable guidance on current 'best practice'. Guidance from NICE covers individual technologies as well as the management of a wide range of conditions. NICE will also advise on appropriate methods of clinical audit in those areas where it has provided guidance. It has been established as a Special Health Authority with its own corporate and legal identity and has direct responsibility to the Secretary of State for Health (NICE 2002). NICE currently provides three kinds of guidance:

1. Appraisal and guidance on new and existing health technologies, e.g. newer drugs for epilepsy in children, juvenile idiopathic arthritis (Etanercept).

2. To develop clinical guidelines for practice through a variety of national collaborating centres, e.g. National Collaboration Centre for Women's and Child Health. Developing clinical guidelines on the diagnosis and management of type 1 diabetes in children and young people.

3. Interventional procedures: makes recommendations about whether interventional procedures used for diagnosis or treatment are safe enough and work well enough for routine use.

Activity

Go to http://www.nice.org.uk/cms/ipsearch.aspx, insert paediatrics in the relevant speciality and identify interventional procedures that are specific to paediatrics – one example is Coblation tonsillectomy:
- Do you think this kind of guidance is helpful?
- How do you think this might improve the quality of care children might receive from healthcare services?

NICE has developed guidance for the NHS on clinical audit and coordinates the results from the National Confidential Enquiries. Although the guidance it provides to health authorities, NHS Trusts, primary care groups and health professionals is in the form of advice and, as a whole, is not mandatory, there is an expectation that its recommendations will be universally accepted. Although it is widely acknowledged that strict adherence to clinical guidelines is not in the best interests of some patients, health professionals are wise to record their reasons for non-compliance in patients' medical records.

The four National Confidential Enquiries are also encompassed within NICE to ensure greater clarity and coherence to their findings, and to inform the Institute on areas for which guidance is needed. The Confidential Enquiry into Maternal and Child Health (CEMACH) was launched in April 2003. CEMACH incorporates the Confidential Enquiry into Maternal Deaths (CEMD) and the Confidential Enquiry into Stillbirths and Deaths in Infancy (CESDI) covering the period from 22 weeks' gestation to 28 days, but will also be extending its remit to encompass morbidity and a new national enquiry into child

health (NICE 2002). This, however, is due to change and responsibility for the National Confidential Enquiries will be transferring from NICE to the National Patient Safety Authority (NPSA).

To ensure transparent public and user involvement in the work of NICE, a citizens' council has been established. This is a 30-member group involving representatives from all sections of society who are able to have their say on the wider issues and have their judgements considered by NICE when they are issuing guidance to the healthcare sector (NICE 2002).

Ensuring Trusts have robust audit programmes in place to monitor the implementation of these guidelines is now the role of the Health Commission, whose legal name is the Commission for Healthcare, Audit and Inspection (CHAI; it was previously known as the Commission for Healthcare Improvement (CHI)).

The Role of the Health Commission – The Commission for Healthcare Audit and Inspection

The Health Commission was formed on 1 April 2004 under the Health and Social Care (Community Health & Standards) Act 2003. It replaces:

- the Commission for Health Improvement (CHI)
- the National Care Standards Commission
- the Audit Commission.

The Healthcare Commission has a wide range of functions, the main ones being to:

- Independently assess the performance of the health service from patients' perspectives.
- Coordinate NHS inspections with a range of other healthcare organisations: clinical governance reviews.
- Identify how effectively public funds are used within healthcare.
- Develop an independent second stage for complaints about the NHS that cannot be resolved locally.
- Investigate serious failures.
- Publish regular ratings of NHS hospitals and Trusts and provide an annual report on healthcare in England and Wales.
- Report on key issues, such as coronary heart disease.
- Publish data on staff and patient surveys.
- Manage the clinical audit programme.
- Report to the Secretary of State any serious concerns about the quality of public services or how they are run.

Activity

To familiarise yourself with clinical governance reviews, go to:

- http://www.chi.nhs.uk/eng/organisations/west_mid/brm_childrens/2002/brm_childrens.pdf
- What are the key areas of action the trust needs to address?
- What were CHI's conclusions at Birmingham Children's Hospital?

The Healthcare Commission will use core standards to establish the quality of care patients can currently expect and develop standards, which represent the aspirations for the future.

Seven domains are identified for the proposed standards, which take account of the NSFs and guidance issued by NICE, these are:

1. safety
2. clinical and cost effectiveness
3. governance
4. patient focus
5. accessible and responsible care
6. care environment and amenities
7. public health.

Activity

Having appraised yourself of a clinical governance review go to:

- http://www.chi.nhs.uk/eng/organisations/london/gosh/2003/gosh.pdf.

Identify the key issues evident in this review.

Now go to:

- www.chi.nhs.uk/eng/organisations/london/gosh/2003/gosh_action_plan.pdf

You should have found the action plan to address the issues raised from this review.

- Do you think this action plan demonstrates clearly what is to be achieved, by whom and within what time frame?
- What do you think could affect the implementation of this action plan?

By visiting http://www.heatlthcarecommission.org.uk healthcare professionals and the public can gain access to the work undertaken by the Healthcare Commission. In particular, information for service providers falls into seven key areas:

1. reviews and inspections
2. performance ratings
3. standards and criteria

4. NHS surveys
5. self-assessment
6. guidance for the NHS: an example being ward staffing guidance
7. national clinical audit: new/current and proposed.

By publicly identifying where improvement is required and sharing good practice within the service, the Healthcare Commission aims to help the NHS raise standards of patient care.

In due course, the Healthcare Commission is expected to take over the functions of the Mental Health Act Commission.

Summary

The importance of providing high-quality healthcare services is key to current government policy, with several important national directives and policy documents promoting a culture of quality in health care. Several support agencies and national bodies have been appointed to help embed quality in the NHS, with clinical governance being a central framework to drive the required changes at local Trust level. Importantly, quality is promoted as an individual enterprise, which is to be encouraged across all healthcare professionals and the central role of clinical audit is widely acknowledged as a key tool in providing quality services. All healthcare professionals, at whatever level, need to be familiar with key quality activities and recognise the centrality of providing quality care, thereby ensuring a quality service to children and their families.

References

Beverley DW, Ball RJ, Smith RA et al 1997 Planning for the future: the experience of implementing a children's day assessment unit in a district general hospital. Archives of Disease in Childhood 77:287–293

Brocklehurst N, Walshe K 1999 Quality in the new NHS. Nursing Standard 13(51):46–53

Buetow SA, Roland M 1999 Clinical governance: bridging the gap between managerial and clinical approaches to quality of care. Quality in Health Care 8:184–190

Commission for Health Improvement (CHI) 2004 Getting the right start: national service framework for children, young people and maternity services, published part 1: standards for hospital services

Department of Health (DoH) 1997 The new NHS: modern dependable. HMSO, London

Department of Health (DoH) 1998 A first class service: quality in the new NHS. HMSO, London

Department of Health (DoH) 1999 Making a difference. HMSO, London

Department of Health (DoH) 2000 The NHS plan. HMSO, London

Department of Health (DoH) 2001 Learning from Bristol: the report of the public inquiry into children's heart surgery at the Bristol Royal Infirmary 1984–1985. Cmd 5363. HMSO, London

Department of Health (DoH) 2003 Children's National Service Framework. HMSO, London

Dixon N 1996 Good practice in clincal audit. A summary of selected literature to support criteria for clinical audit. National Centre for Clinical Audit, London

Donabedian A 1966 Evaluating the quality of medical care. Milbank Memorial Fund Quarterly 44(3):166–206

Ellis J 2000 Sharing the evidence: clinical practice benchmarking to improve continuously the quality of care. Journal of Advanced Nursing 32(1):215–225

Glasper EA 2004 Preserving and enhancing standards of care in the NHS. British Medical Journal 13(6):293

Harvey G 1996 Relating quality assessment and audit to the research process in nursing. Nurse Researcher 3:3 35–46

Heard SR, Schiller C, Aitken M et al 2001 Continuous quality improvement: educating towards a culture of clinical governance. Quality in Health Care 10(Suppl II):ii70–ii80

Higson J, Bolland R 2000 Telephone follow-up after paediatric day surgery. Paediatric Nursing 12:30–32

Johnson G, Crombie IK, Davies HTO et al 2000 Reviewing audit: barriers and facilitating factors for effective clinical audit. Quality in Health Care 9:23–36

Joss R, Kogan M 1995 Advancing quality: total quality management in the National Health Service. Open University, Buckingham

Malby B 1995 Clinical audit for nurses and therapists. Scutari Press, Middlesex

Mann T 1996 Clinical audit in the NHS. Using clinical audit in the NHS: a position statement. NHS Executive, Leeds, p 36

Maxwell RJ 1984 Quality assessment in health. British Medical Journal 288:1470–1472

Ministry of Health 1959 Committee of the Central Health Services Council. Report of the Committee on the Welfare of Children in Hospital. Ministry of Health, London

Morrell C, Harvey G 1999 The clinical audit handbook. Ballière Tindall, London

National Institute for Clinical Effectiveness (NICE) 2002 Principles for best practice in clinical audit. Radcliffe Medical Press, Oxford

NHS Centre for Review and Dissemination 1999 Getting evidence into practice. Effective Health Care 5, University of York, York

NHS Modernisation Agency 2003 Essence of care. NHS Modernisation Agency, London

Nightingale F 1863 Notes on hospitals, 3rd edn. Longmans, Roberts and Green, London

Parsley K, Corrigan P 1994a Quality improvement in nursing and healthcare. Chapman and Hall, London

Parsley K, Corrigan P 1999b Quality improvement in healthcare: putting evidence into practice, 2nd edn. Stanley Thornes, Cheltenham

Peter S, Fazakerley M 2004 Clinical effectiveness of an ICP for infants with bronchiolitis. Paediatric Nursing 16(1):30–35

Pickering S, Thompson J 2003 Clinical governance and best value. Churchill Livingstone, London

Rawlins M 1999 NHS: in pursuit of quality: the NICE. Lancet 353(9158):1079–1082

Scally G, Donaldson L 1998 Clinical governance and the drive for quality improvement in the NHS in England. British Medical Journal 317:297–298

Stark S, MacHale A, Lennon E, Shaw L 2002 Benchmarking: implementing the process in practice. Nursing Standard 16(35):39–42

Swage T 2000 Clinical governance in healthcare practice. Butterworth Heinmann, Oxford

Thomas B 1999 Research and audit in effective health services. Nursing Standard 13(33):40–42

Woodfield T 2001 Involving children in clinical audit. Paediatric Nursing 13(30):12–16

World Health Organization (WHO) 1983 The principles of quality assurance: report on a WHO meeting. WHO, Geneva

Useful Websites

http://www.nice.org.uk

http://www.chi.org.uk

http://www.york.ac.uk

http://www.healthcarecommision.org.uk

http://www.gmc-uk.org/standards

Chapter Seventeen

17

The Management of Acute Pain in Children

Alison Twycross, Joanna Smith

ABSTRACT

The aim of this chapter and its companion PowerPoint presentation is to outline current best practice in relation to managing pain in children. Although focusing on the management of acute pain in children, the principles can be applied to other types of pain. Effective assessment is an integral part of pain management, and is treated as the first step of pain management and therefore explored in more depth. General pain management strategies are discussed.

Learning Outcomes

- Recognise the importance of managing children's pain effectively.

- Understand the current best practice guidelines relating to managing pain in children and the steps needed to manage pain effectively.

- Identify appropriate pain assessment tools for different ages of children.

- Be aware of the different types of analgesic drugs that can be used to relieve pain in children.

- Identify non-drug methods of pain-relief.

Introduction

Clinical guidelines developed for the management of pain in children in both the USA and the UK (Agency for Health Care Policy and Research (AHCPR) 1992, Royal College of Nursing (RCN) 1999), ensure that information about best practice is readily available. This chapter starts by defining pain management and summarising the gate control theory of pain. The evidence indicating that children feel as much pain as adults is summarised and the reasons for effective pain management are identified. Children's perceptions of their postoperative pain management are discussed and an outline of how children's perception of pain develops as they mature cognitively is provided. Recommendations from clinical guidelines relating to pain in children will be used to outline the steps nurses need to take to manage children's pain effectively.

What is Pain?

Pain is a complex multifaceted phenomenon. The definition of pain given by the International Association for the Study of Pain (IASP) acknowledges this and explains how the many facets of pain interrelate and affect pain perception:

Pain is an unpleasant sensory and emotional experience associated with actual or potential tissue damage, or described in terms of such damage (IASP 1979 p 249)

However, although supporting the concept of pain as a subjective phenomenon, this definition falls short in relation to those unable to communicate verbally, including neonates and young children. Pain perception is an inherent quality of life present in the early stages of development and serves as a signalling system for tissue damage. The IASP definition has recently been amended to incorporate this aspect:

The inability to communicate in no way negates the possibility that an individual is experiencing pain and

is in need of appropriate pain relieving treatment
(IASP 2001 p 2)

WWW

Find out more information about the IASP definition of pain at:
- http://www.iasp-pain.org/terms-p.html

Various theories have been postulated to explain the physiological and psychological processes involved in the pain experience and the modulation of pain pathways (Hawthorn & Redmond 1998). Wall & Melzack (1989) proposed the 'gate control' theory of pain, which proposes that there is a 'gating' mechanism in the dorsal horn of the spinal cord through which peripheral information passes (Fig. 17.1). The degree to which the 'gate' is opened or closed determines the degree of the pain perception. The theory attempts to explain the three interrelated components that result in the uniqueness of the pain experience: sensory/perceptual, emotional and cognitive (Weisenberg 1980).

Two interactive systems influence the 'gating' mechanism. The first is competitive peripheral input, where in certain situations the 'gate' can remain closed despite stimulation by a nerve impulse originating from a noiceceptor (Wall & Melzack 1989). The classic example of this competitive nerve input explains the pain inhibition that occurs when 'mummy rubs it better'. A kick on the knee would activate noiceceptors and if the stimulus was large enough a nerve impulse would be initiated, the 'gate' would open and allow interconnections to be made via the spinal cord to the brain. The brain would interpret the sensation as pain. However, if the knee is rubbed vigorously, non-painful sensory fibres would also be activated, competing with the nociceptor stimulation. The stronger impulse would dominate.

The second type of modulation at the dorsal horn relates to the influence of the descending nerves from the brain, which again influence whether the gate opens or closes (Wall & Melzack 1989).

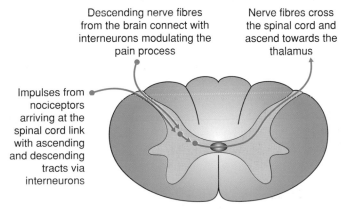

Descending nerve fibres from the brain connect with interneurons modulating the pain process

Nerve fibres cross the spinal cord and ascend towards the thalamus

Impulses from nociceptors arriving at the spinal cord link with ascending and descending tracts via interneurons

Fig. 17.1 • Spinal cord pathways.

Does Pain in Children Differ from Pain in Adults?

The neurophysiological mechanisms that produce pain sensation appear to work in the same way in children as in adults. Despite this, some healthcare professionals still believe that, in a similar situation, children do not feel as much pain as adults. Such beliefs possibly stem from the fact that children in pain behave differently from adults (McCaffery & Pasero 1999, Royal College of Surgeons and College of Anaesthetists 1990). Evidence shows that children experience as much pain as adults (Table 17.1).

Professional Conversation

Ian is 11 years old and has had repeated orthopaedic surgery throughout his life. He is extremely anxious about experiencing pain postoperatively. He had been involved in planning postoperative pain methods with the staff and it has been decided to use a patient-controlled analgesia (PCA) system postoperatively. Ian has been reviewing the pain assessment tool and familiarising himself with the equipment.

Ian's dad is his main carer. He has approached James, a mature student, and expressed anxieties about 'Ian injecting himself' with morphine and feels that Ian is at a vulnerable age and needs to be 'warned about the danger of drugs not encouraged to use them'.

Issues affecting the relationship between James, Ian and his dad

James is undertaking his first placement within child branch and has built up a good working relationship with Ian. He is concerned about Ian's dad's attitude and feels Ian is able to make his own choices.

What issues do you think are important for James to discuss with his mentor in relation to Ian and his family?

Why do We Need to Manage Pain Effectively?

Activity

Why do you think it is important to manage children's pain effectively?

Painful experiences are part of life for every child (Perquin et al 2000, Van Cleve et al 1996). However, unrelieved pain has a number of undesirable physical and psychological consequences that may delay and complicate the recovery of children postoperatively and/or following an acute illness.

Table 17.1 Children Feel as Much Pain as Adults

Misconception	Evidence
Infants do not feel as much pain as adults	Pain pathways (although immature) are present at birth and pain impulses are able to travel to and from the pain centres in the brain (Coskun & Anand 2000, Fitzgerald 2000, Wolf 1999) Neonates exhibit behavioural, physiological and hormonal responses to pain (Abu-Saad et al 1998, Carter 1997, Franck 1986, Hogan & Choonara 1996, Stevens 1999)
Infants cannot feel pain because of an immature nervous system	Complete myelination is not necessary for pain to be felt (Volpe 1981) Painful stimuli are transmitted by both myelinated and unmyelinated fibres (Craig & Grunau 1993, Volpe 1981) Incomplete myelination implies only a slower conduction speed in the nerves, which is offset by the shorter distances the impulse has to travel (Anand & Hickey 1987, Volpe 1981)
Children cannot indicate where pain is located	Children as young as 4 years old can demonstrate on a body chart where they hurt without knowing the names of body parts (Van Cleve & Savedra 1993) Children are able to report the intensity of pain by the age of 3–4 years (Harbeck & Pederson 1992)
Active children are not in pain	Increased activity is often a sign of pain (Eland 1985a) Children use play as a diversion and as a coping mechanism (Eland 1985a, Mather & Mackie 1983, McCaffery 1972, McCaffery & Pasero 1999)
A child engaged in playing activities cannot be in pain	Children can use play as a diversion and coping mechanism (McCaffery 1972) Children are particularly gifted in the use of distraction (McCaffery & Beebe 1989)
Sleeping children cannot be in pain	Sleep may be the result of exhaustion because of persistent pain (Hawley 1984)

The potential consequences of unrelieved acute pain, include (Eland 1990; Fisher & Morton 1998):

- psychological consequences such as recurrent nightmares and increased anxiety
- consequences for decision making in future healthcare interventions
- bronchiectasis and atelectasis due to inadequate lung expansion
- alkalosis due to increased respiratory rate and shallow breathing
- chest infection due to increased sections accumulating from inadequate cough and lack of spontaneous movement
- rapid respirations, increased heart rate, increased perspiration and increased metabolic rate, which will increase fluid losses.

CHILDREN'S VIEWS ABOUT HOW WELL PAIN IS MANAGED IN PRACTICE

Activity

Consider how well you think children's pain is managed in your clinical area.

Children's perceptions of how well their postoperative pain is managed have been examined in several studies (Alex & Ritchie 1992, Doorbar & McClarey 1999, Polkki et al 2003, Woodgate & Kristjanson 1996). Children suggested that nurses need to take a more active role in pain management. More specifically, children indicated that:

- pain is managed poorly in hospital
- nurses need to communicate with them about their pain and to listen to what they were saying about their pain
- nurses should ask them about their pain on an hourly basis
- they wished nurses had given them more or stronger analgesic drugs when they asked for them.

Although some pain is likely to be experienced postoperatively, children should not experience unrelieved moderate to severe pain. Using a rating scale of 0–10 (with 0 equating to no pain and 10 representing the worst pain possible; see Fig. 17.4) nurses should aim to maintain children's postoperative pain intensity below 3. Recent studies have found that children continue to experience unrelieved moderate to severe pain postoperatively (Hamers et al 1999, Kotzer 2000, Polkki et al 2003, Swallow et al 2000), suggesting that current guidelines are not being implemented effectively into practice.

Seminar discussion topic

Children continue to experience moderate to severe unrelieved postoperative pain (Hamers et al 1999, Kotzer 2000, Polkki et al 2003, Swallow et al 2000). This is despite the evidence to guide practice (both clinical guidelines and research evidence) being readily available:
- Discuss what steps children's nurses can take to ensure that postoperative pain is managed effectively.

Cognitive Development and Perception of Pain

When managing pain in children it is important to understand how children develop concepts relating to pain. This will enhance the quality of care that nurses provide and enable nurses to:

- provide appropriate explanations of illness and hospitalisation
- provide sensitive reassurance for children
- gain greater understanding of what children are saying to them
- gain some insight into how children interpret all the strange occurrences that can accompany illnesses.

Activity

Think about your interactions with children of different ages:
- How do you think perception of pain changes as children mature cognitively?

Children's perceptions of pain at different ages are outlined in Table 17.2.

Activity

How do you think recurrent pain/painful procedures affect a child's perception of pain?

Children who have experienced pain may have a different perception of pain than their healthy counterparts (Blos 1978, Eiser 1985). The 1990s saw a shift away from the traditional Piagetian emphasis on children moving through a series of stages in their development in relation to understanding the cause and effect of illness. It is now thought that the content of knowledge changes (Rushforth 1996, Yoos 1994), which develops at different ages in each child

(Sternberg 1989) and is determined by a child's experiences (Bernstein et al 2000). In relation to pain, Carey (1985) suggests that children move from novice to expert as they experience pain. If a child has had a number of painful experiences this may affect his or her perception of pain.

How Should Pain in Children be Managed?

In the context of nursing, pain management equates well to the stages of the nursing process (Yura & Walsh 1988) – assessment, planning, implementation and evaluation – to the treatment of pain. The first stage in the process is the assessment of the child's pain. This is followed by planning which pain-relieving interventions (non-drug methods or analgesic drugs or both) are appropriate, implementing these interventions and then evaluating their effectiveness. Nurses should communicate with the child and parents at each stage, and ensure that appropriate documentation is completed.

Evidence-based Practice

A review of clinical guidelines relating to the management of pain in children indicates that effective management of pain requires nurses to:
- Take a pain experience history from child and parent on admission.
- Assess children's pain using a valid and reliable, age-appropriate pain assessment tool.
- Take into account children's behavioural cues and physiological indicators of pain when assessing pain.
- Administer appropriate analgesic drugs.
- Use non-drug methods of pain relief.
- Involve parents in their child's pain management.
- Adopt a multidisciplinary approach.
- Document pain scores and interventions.
- Reassess pain having given time for pain-relieving interventions to take affect and, if necessary, alter the plan of care.
- Communicate with children and their parents about all aspects of pain management.

Developed from AHCPR 1992, RCN 1999, 2000.

www

Further information about the RCN's clinical guideline relating to the recognition and assessment of pain in children can be found by logging onto:
- http://is.dal.ca/~painsrc/docs/pps68.html

The steps that need to be taken to manage acute pain effectively are outlined in Fig. 17.2.

Table 17.2 Age-Specific Perceptions of Pain in Children and Implications for Practice

Piaget's stage of development	Perception/presentation of pain	Implications for practice
Sensorimotor (0–2 years)	Pain is a physical experience primarily expressed by changes in behaviours such as restlessness, irritability, tense, abnormal crying/grizzling/screaming, abnormal posture/movements	Understanding the normal activities and behaviours for each child and comparing these to those presented during illness is paramount Excellent observational skills are necessary, particularly in relation to interpreting verbal sounds/words, facial expression and body language
Preoperational (2–7 years)	Pain is primarily perceived as a physical experience, with an inability to distinguish between the cause of pain and its effect Children often perceive pain to be a result of their own behaviour, e.g. as a punishment for a wrongdoing Pain may also be perceived as the responsibility of someone else and the child may believe magical acts can remove the pain Increased ability to verbalise needs will correlate to language skills developments	Carers must be aware that the child may be aggressive when offered help and will not understand the connection between treatment and pain relief Allowing the child to express his or her feelings is important; children should be encouraged to describe the pain in their own language Much reassurance is needed to explain pain is not a punishment Family input is vital, although parents may not have seen their child in pain before and may not understand change in behaviours Guidance relating to comforting their child and distraction techniques will be necessary
Concrete operational (7–12 years)	There is more understanding of the physical properties of pain and can relate pain to body parts Fear about the consequence of pain and damage to the body are great, vivid imagination can lead to fears of total body destruction Towards the end of this period some rational thinking develops Pain concepts beginning to form and can describe effects that influence pain, the 'if' and 'when' scenarios	The child needs clear explanations about cause of pain and treatments and opportunity to discuss fears and beliefs and reassurance relating to body destruction
Formal operational (12 years and older)	There is the beginnings of depth of understanding, but may not be consistent due to limited life experiences and therefore may imagine sinister consequences of the pain	Adolescents need clear explanations about cause of pain and treatments and opportunity to discuss fears and beliefs about the potential impact of the pain

Adapted from Gaffney et al 2003, Twycross 1998a

Reflect on your Practice

- Think about your pain management practices.
- Does your pain management practice always conform to this best practice checklist and/or to the postoperative pain management algorithm shown in Fig 17.2?

TAKING A PAIN HISTORY

A pain experience history has been identified as an important element of pain management (AHCPR 1992, Hestor & Barcus 1986, Hestor et al 1998, RCN 1999). A pain experience history provides information about the child's likely

Fig. 17.2 • A decision-making algorithm for postoperative pain management in children.

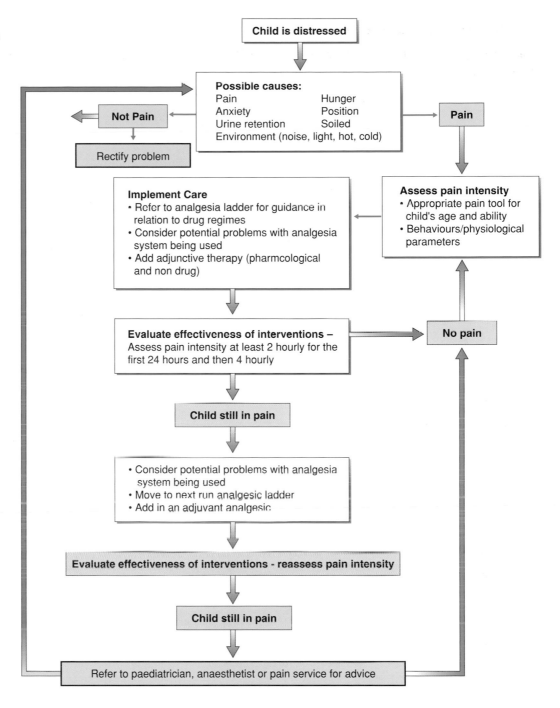

Child is distressed

Possible causes:
Pain   Hunger
Anxiety   Position
Urine retention   Soiled
Environment (noise, light, hot, cold)

Not Pain

Pain

Rectify problem

Assess pain intensity
• Appropriate pain tool for child's age and ability
• Behaviours/physiological parameters

Implement Care
• Refer to analgesia ladder for guidance in relation to drug regimes
• Consider potential problems with analgesia system being used
• Add adjunctive therapy (pharmcological and non drug)

Evaluate effectiveness of interventions – Assess pain intensity at least 2 hourly for the first 24 hours and then 4 hourly

No pain

Child still in pain

• Consider potential problems with analgesia system being used
• Move to next run analgesic ladder
• Add in an adjuvant analgesic

Evaluate effectiveness of interventions - reassess pain intensity

Child still in pain

Refer to paediatrician, anaesthetist or pain service for advice

response to pain and could be invaluable in deciding on effective treatments for pain. An outline of questions to include in a pain experience history is provided in Table 17.3.

Activity

• What do you think should be included in a pain history?
• How will this information help you manage a child's pain more effectively?

ASSESSING THE CHILD'S PAIN

Determining the level of pain a person is experiencing is difficult (Baker & Wong 1987, Bradshaw & Zeanah 1986, Franck et al 2000). Even with patients who can communicate about their pain, pain assessment is complex. However, even young children are able to indicate how much pain they have provided the right techniques are used (LaFleur & Raway 1999, Ross & Ross 1984). Knowing how

Table 17.3 Pain Experience History (Hestor & Barcus 1986, Hestor et al 1998)

Questions for child	Questions for parent
Tell me what pain is	What word(s) does your child use in regard to pain?
Tell me about the hurt you have had before	Describe the pain experiences your child has had before
Do you tell others when you hurt? If yes, who?	Does your child tell you or others when he or she is hurting?
What do you do for yourself when you are hurting?	How do you know when your child is in pain?
What do you want others to do for you when you hurt?	How does your child usually react to pain?
What don't you want others to do for you when you hurt?	What do you do for your child when he or she is hurting?
What helps the most to take your hurt away?	What does your child do for him- or herself when he or she is hurting?
Is there anything special that you want me to know about when you hurt? (If yes, have child describe)	What works best to decrease or take away your child's pain?
	Is there anything special that you would like me to know about your child and pain? (If yes, describe.)

much pain a child is experiencing is the first step to providing effective relief (McGrath & Unrah 2000, Price 1994). Pain assessment is therefore an essential component of pain management.

Reflect on your Practice

What methods do you use to assess pain in children?

Ask the Child

Children will not always speak about their pain unless they are specifically asked about it (Polkki et al 2003, Romsing et al 1996). Using a pain assessment tool allows children to indicate their pain intensity and facilitates a systematic assessment process (Franck et al 2000, RCN 1999, Taylor 1998). Indeed, nurses' assessments of children's pain correlate more closely with children's self-report when a validated pain assessment tool is used (Colwell et al 1996, Manne et al 1992).

The selection of a pain assessment tool should be based on the child's age and cognitive ability (Franck et al 2000, McGrath et al 1995, McGrath & Unrah 2000).

Pain Assessment Tools for the Verbal Child

Pain assessment tools used most commonly with verbal children are the visual analogue scale (VAS), the simple descriptive scale, the faces scale and the numerical scale.

The VAS is composed of a line with the words 'no pain' on the left and 'worst pain possible' on the right. The child marks the position on the line that he or she feels correlates with the pain intensity. The VAS is useful for children with limited language skills but the child needs to be able to translate experiences into an analogue format and to understand proportionality; the VAS can therefore be used only with older children.

The simple descriptive pain rating scale is composed of a horizontal or vertical 100mm line with descriptors written along the line starting at the left with 'no hurt' to 'worst possible hurt' on the right. This can be used with children from 9–15 years.

The faces pain scale and the numerical pain rating scale are described in Figs 17.3 and 17.4.

Several other pain assessment tools are available for use with children who can express their pain verbally. These are summarised in Table 17.4.

Pain Assessment Tools for Children Unable to Verbalise their Pain

An example of a tool used for preverbal children is the Face, Legs, Activity, Cry, Consolabilty (FLACC) (Merkel et al 1997) (Table 17.5). This has been validated for postoperative children aged 2 months to 7 years. The scores for each category are added together to give a rating of 0–10. Other pain assessment tools validated for use in this age group are listed in Tables 17.6 and 17.7.

This is one example of a faces pain scale initially developed by Beiri et al (1990) and later modified by Hicks et al (2001).

The use of neutral *no* pain face and the lack of tears on the *worst pain* possible face avoid the possibility of confusing pain severity with happiness/sadness.

Faces pain scales have been developed using cartoon faces. These are popular with children and parents but have been shown to be less accurate (Chambers et al 1999).

The nurse must explain to the child that the first face represents *no hurt at all* and that the last face represents *as much as they can possibly imagine.*

Fig. 17.3 • The faces pain scale. Reproduced with permission of the International Association for the study of pain (IASP) from Hicks CL,von Baeyer CL, Spafford P, von Korlaar I, Goodenough B. The faces pain Scale – Revised: Toward a common metric in paediatric pain measurement. Pain 2001; 93:173–183

Fig. 17.4 • A numerical pain-rating scale.

Table 17.4 Pain Assessment Tools for Use with Verbal Children

Tool and reference	Validated	Indicators	Comments
CHEOPS McGrath et al 1985, Barrier et al 1989	Yes	Alertness, calmness/agitation, respiratory response, physical movement, blood pressure, heart rate, muscle tone, facial tension	Complicated behavioural scale May not track pain well in 3- to 7-year-olds as pain behaviour is inhibited 10 categories, 4 of which are similar Confusing (high score = low pain) Cannot be used with intubated or paralysed patient
Colour scales Eland 1981, Beyer & Wells 1989	Yes	Child chooses pens or crayons and colours the outline of the child's body to indicate where their pain is and the intensity of that pain	Quickly engages the child's interest Fun Colour allows expression of other aspects of pain Child describes exact site of pain
COMFORT Ambuel et al 1992	Yes	Alertness, calmness/agitation, respiratory response, physical movement, blood pressure, heart rate, muscle tone, facial tension	Complicated: 8 categories and many subcategories Cannot be used with intubated or paralysed patients
Faces McGrath et al 1985a, Manukesla et al 1987, Whaley & Wong 1987, Bieri et al 1990	Yes	Set of faces in various stages of pain Number of faces ranges from 4 to 6	Simple and quick Younger children tend to choose extremes Some children confuse with happiness measure A neutral no pain face appears to produce more accurate pain ratings than a scale with a smiling no pain face

Table 17.4 Pain Assessment Tools for Use with Verbal Children

Tool and reference	Validated	Indicators	Comments

FLACC
Merkel et al 1997
  (see also Table 17.5)
	Yes	Face, legs, activity, cry, consolabilty	Behavioural scale
			Postoperative pain
			5 categories to score (0–2)
			Easy to use in practice
			Validated for postoperative children aged
			  2 months to 7 years

OPS
Hannallah et al 1987,
  Broadman et al 1988,
  Norden et al 1991
	Yes, against
	CHEOPS
	and faces
		Blood pressure, crying, movement, agitation,
		  verbal evaluation/body language
			Easy to use
			5 categories
			Reliable between observers
			Tracks pain and score decreases with
			  analgesia
			BP measurements may upset neonates
			Cannot use with intubated paralysed
			  babies

OUCHER
Beyer & Aradine 1987,
  Aradine et al 1988,
  Beyer & Wells 1989
	Yes	Photographs of children in 6 stages of distress
		  aligned to a vertical scale marked 0–100 rating
		  the degree of pain
			Can use either or both scales to fit
			  child's comprehension/ preference
			Self-report tool
			3 multi-ethnic versions available
			Validated for 3- to 12-year-old
			  postoperative children

Poker chip tool
  Hestor et al 1990,
  Beyer & Wells 1989
	Yes	4 red chips or 4 red and 1 white chip (no pain).
		Chips represent pieces of hurt
			Useful for children aged 4–13 years

TPPPS
Tarbell et al 1992
	Yes	Verbal pain, complaint/cry, groan/moan/grunt,
		  scream, open mouth, squint, brow bulge, restless
		  motor behaviour, rub/touch
			Validated for postoperative children
			  aged 1–5 years
			Tracks pain relief and effects of analgesia
			Correlates with nurse and parental
			  pain assessments
			7 categories to score

VAS
Scott & Huskisson 1979
	Yes	Vertical or horizontal 100 mm line with verbal anchors
		  representing a continuum of pain intensity
			Reliable and versatile
			Children must understand concept of
			  proportionality
			Intervals may not be equal from a
			  child's perspective

CHEOPS, Children's Hospital of Eastern Ontario Pain Scale; FLACC, Face, Legs, Activity, Cry, Consolabilty; OPS, Objective Pain Scale; TPPPS, The Toddler/Pre-Schooler Post-Operative Pain Scale. VAS, Visual Analogue Scale. Adapted from Royal College of Nursing 2000

www

Further information about pain assessment tools that are validated for use in children can be found in the RCN Clinical Guidelines relating to the recognition and assessment of pain in children, by logging on to:

- http://is. dal.ca/~painsrc/docs/pps68.html

Reflect on your Practice

- Which pain assessment tools are available in your clinical area?
- Are there pain assessment tools available for children across all age ranges?
- How often do you use these pain assessment tools?

Table 17.5 The FLACC (Face, Legs, Activity, Cry, Consolability) Pain Assessment Tool

Categories	Behaviours	Scoring
Face	No particular expression or smile	0
	Occasional grimace or frown, withdrawn, disinterested	1
	Frequent to constant quivering chin, clenched jaw	2
Legs	Normal position or relaxed	0
	Uneasy, restless, tense	1
	Kicking or legs drawn up	2
Activity	Lying quietly, normal position, moves easily	0
	Squirming, shifting back and forth, tense	1
	Arched, rigid or jerking	2
Cry	No cry (awake or asleep)	0
	Moans or whimpers, occasional complaints	1
	Crying steadily or sobs, frequent complaints	2
Consolability	Content. Relaxed	0
	Reassured by occasional touching, hugging to being talked to, distractable	1
	Difficult to console or comfort	2

Table 17.6 Pain Assessment Tools for Use with Neonates (0–1 Month)

Tool and reference	Validated	Indicators	Comments
CHEOPS See Table 17.4			
COMFORT See Table 17.4			
CRIES Krechel & Bildner 1995	Yes	Cries, oxygen saturation, heart rate/blood pressure, expression, sleeplessness	Easy to remember and use Valid and reliable down to 32 weeks gestational age Reliable between observers Tracks pain and the effect of analgesics Uses oxygenation as a measure; this can be affected by many other factors BP measurements may upset babies
LIDS Hogan & Choonara 1996	Yes	Spontaneous movements, spontaneous excitability, flexion of fingers and toes, facial expression, quantity of crying, sleep pattern and amount	Advantages Assesses postoperative pain 0–5-point scale
NFCS Grunau et al 1990	Yes	Bulging brows, eyes squeezed tightly shut, deepening of nasolabial furrow, open lips, mouth stretched, taut tongue	Anatomically based system for assessing facial expression
NIPS Lawrence et al 1993	Yes	Facial expression, cry, breathing patterns, arms, legs, state of arousal	Uses 6 categories, 2 of which are similar Hard to remember Cannot be used with intubated or paralysed patients

Table 17.6 Pain Assessment Tools for Use with Neonates (0–1 Month)—Cont'd

Tool and reference	Validated	Indicators	Comments
OPS See Table 17.4			
PIPP Stevens et al 1996	Yes	Gestational age, behavioural state, heart rate, oxygen saturation, brow bulge, eye squeeze, nasolabial furrow	Each indicator evaluated on a 4-point scale Total score dependent on infant's gestational age 7 indicator pain measures

CHEOPS, Children's Hospital of Eastern Ontario Pain Scale; CRIES, Crying, Requires O_2 for saturation above 95, Increased vital signs, Expression and Sleeplessness; LIDS, Liverpool Infant Distress Score; NFCS, Neonatal Facial Coding System; NIPS, Neonatal Infant Pain Scale; OPS, Objective Pain Scale; PIPP, Premature Infant Pain Profile. Adapted from RCN 2000

Table 17.7 Pain Assessment Tools for Use with Infants and Toddlers (1 Month to 3 Years)

Tool	Comment
CHEOPS	See Table 17.4
FLACC	See Tables 17.4 and 17.5
COMFORT	See Table 17.4
OPS	See Table 17.4
TPPPS	See Table 17.4

Adapted from RCN 2000

Table 17.8 Behavioural Indicators of Pain in Children

General behaviours	Specific behaviours
Changed behaviour	Banging head
Irritability	Pulling ear
Flat effect	Curling up on side
Unusual posture	Refusal to move limbs
Screaming	Constantly rubbing specific region
Reluctance to move	
Aggressiveness	
Increased clinging	
Unusual quietness	
Loss of appetite	
Restlessness	
Whimpering	
Sobbing	
Lying 'scared stiff'	
Lethargy	
Disturbed sleep pattern	

BEHAVIOURAL CUES

Activity

Consider when you think behavioural cues are a useful way of establishing whether a child is in pain?

Behaviour is a useful measure of pain in children (Chambers et al 1996, Reid et al 1995) (Table 17.8). There are no hard and fast rules about which behaviours indicate pain; a change from normal behaviour can indicate pain. Consulting parents about their child's normal behaviour is therefore essential. However, relying on pain behaviours can sometimes be misleading (Beyer et al 1990, Tesler et al 1998). Behavioural cues should be used in conjunction with other methods of pain assessment.

PHYSIOLOGICAL CUES

Activity

Consider whether you think physiological signs are a useful way of establishing whether a child is in pain?

Physiological signs can be used to establish whether children are in pain (Table 17.9) and are particularly useful when a child is unable to verbally communicate his or her pain. If pain persists over a period of time, adaptation occurs decreasing sympathetic responses (Gildea & Quirk 1977, McCaffery & Pasero 1999). Physiological cues also change as a result of anxiety, crying or handling, and should therefore be used in conjunction with other variables to assess pain (Bournaki 1997, RCN 1999).

Table 17.9 Physiological Signs Used to Assess Pain

Observation	Change in observation
Heart rate	Increases when in pain (after an initial decrease)
Respiratory rate	There is conflicting evidence about whether this increases or decreases, but there is a significant shift from baseline
Blood pressure	Increases when a child is in acute pain
Oxygen saturation	Decreases when a child is in acute pain

Adapted from Coffman et al 1997, Sweet & McGrath 1998, Tyler et al 1993

Professional Conversation

"

Joe is 6 months old and had a cleft lip and palate repaired 3 days ago. Claire, the student nurse looking after him, has noticed that he is not drinking much orally and that every time Joe smiles he bursts into tears. She overhears Joe's mother on the phone saying 'He doesn't seem himself today. I thought he might be in pain but the nurses say that he isn't.'

"

Claire begins to wonder whether Joe might be in pain and decides to speak to her mentor about this.

Issues affecting the relationship between Jane, Joe's mother and the staff

• What information might Claire want to find out before discussing the issue with her mentor?
• Is there anything Claire could do to establish whether Joe is in pain?
• What issues do you think are important for Claire to discuss with his mentor in relation to whether Joe is in pain or not?

Analgesic Drugs

Appropriate analgesic drugs should be administered based upon the pain assessment. Analgesic drugs should be given regularly to control pain and be appropriate for the severity of the pain (AHCPR 1992, McCaffery & Pasero 1999). A lower dose of analgesia can be effective if it is given before the pain becomes unbearable (McCaffery & Pasero 1999).

Three main types of drug are used to manage pain in children: non-opioids, weak opioids and strong opioids. An analgesic ladder simplifies and guides the prescription of analgesia but should be flexible and sensitive enough to meet a child's individual needs (Moriarty 1998, World Health Organization 1998). This can be achieved by having four drug choices that have a range of actions and potencies, such as paracetamol, diclofenac, codeine phosphate and morphine (Moriarty 1998). An example of an analgesic ladder is provided in Figure 17.5. The actions of the different types of analgesic drugs are outlined in Table 17.10.

ANALGESIC TECHNIQUES

Analgesic drugs can be administered using several routes: orally, rectally, epidurally, by patient-controlled analgesia (PCA), by nurse-controlled analgesia (NCA), intravenously and subcutaneously. The choice of route and method of administration will depend on many factors, including the:

● pain intensity score

● cause of pain and predicted duration of acute pain

● child's cognitive abilities: this is particularly important when considering PCA systems

● child's physical status: e.g. oral medication is not suitable if a child is vomiting or has impaired gut motility; subcutaneous administration may not be suitable if there is poor tissue perfusion and intravenous administration may not be appropriate if venous access is problematic

● ability to monitor the child

● time available to prepare the child and family: this is particularly important when using PCA

Fig. 17.5 ● An analgesic

Increasing pain intensity score

Prn paracetamol

Regular paracetamol
Prn codeine phosphate

Regular mild opiod:
codeine phosphate
Prn paracetamol

Regular strong opioid:
morphine
Regular paracetamol

Adjuvant analgesia such as diclofenac

Table 17.10 The Action of Analgesic Drugs

Drug type	Action
Paracetamol	The most commonly prescribed analgesic in children (Carter 1994) Appropriate for mild pain or as an adjunct to more potent analgesics Thought to act by inhibiting prostaglandin synthesis in the brain Probably impairs the perception of pain
Non-steroidal anti-inflammatory drugs (NSAIDs), e.g. ibuprofen, diclofenac	Used for mild to moderate pain Have an inflammatory, anti-pyretic and analgesic action and inhibit/block the action of cyclo-oxygenase, an enzyme necessary in the formation of prostaglandins (Day 1997, Russell 1992) This decreases pain as prostaglandins sensitise the pain receptors and thus make them more likely to become activated by other chemicals released during trauma (Walsh 1997) Contraindicated if there is a renal impairment, hypovolaemia, low platelets or tendency to bleed, liver disease, children under 6 months, gastric ulceration, immuno-compromised children and should be used with caution in children with asthma (may increase symptoms) (Moriarty 1998)
Opioids, e.g. codeine, morphine	Used for moderate to severe pain Act on the body's opioid receptors which are found throughout the central nervous system (Day 1997, Russell 1992) Opioid analgesics bind to these receptors and activate them, mimicking the effect of the endogenous encephalins (Atkinson et al 1987) Most opioid drugs are agonists, resulting in stimulation of the receptor Opioid 'partial agonists' (e.g. buprenorphine) bind to receptor sites but elicit only a partial response. They may antagonise the effects of more potent pure agonists by occupying the same binding sites. For this reason, drugs such as buprenorphine and morphine should not be given together (Russell 1992) Antagonists (e.g. naloxone) work by blocking the receptor sites and reversing the action of opioids (Day 1997)

- support available from anaesthetic and/or pain service
- local practice, policies and guidelines.

Advanced analgesia systems are an important part of acute pain management. Several of these will now be described.

Epidurals

Epidural analgesia is produced by injecting or infusing local anaesthetic and/or an opioid into the epidural space. The effect of epidurals is related to the types of drugs infused; local anaesthetics block the nerve function at the site of the catheter which usually corresponds to the wound site, and opioid analgesics block opioid receptor sites within the spiral horn (Ochsenreither 1997). Local anaesthetics may be given alone, and this is often effective in children (Howard 2003). However, a combination of local anaesthetics and opioids can produce a synergistic effect; this allows a reduction in drug dosages and concentrations while achieving a good level of analgesia with minimal side effects (Al-Shaikh

1997, Jacques 1994, Ochsenreither 1997). Table 17.11 outlines the observations required when caring for a child with an epidural.

An ice cube can be used to assess the level and extent of the motor block by detecting loss of cold sensation. The point at which the child perceives cold sensation is the level of the block.

Activity

Think about what other nursing care might be needed if a child has an epidural infusion?

Intravenous Infusion of Opioid Drugs

Continuous intravenous morphine infusions have been used in the management of postoperative pain following major surgery in children since the early 1980s (Bray 1983, Bray et al 1986) because of their ability to produce more consistent analgesia levels and the facility to add bolus doses as

Table 17.11 Observations Required When a Child Has an Epidural Infusion

Observation	Rationale
Pain intensity	To ensure effective pain relief is being provided
Pulse	May increase if child's pain is not adequately controlled
Respiratory rate and oxygen saturation levels	To detect respiratory depression (potential problem with opioids) To detect rostral spread of local anaesthetic which would cause respiratory failure
Temperature	Epidural catheters pose a potential infection risk
Blood pressure	Opioids and local anaesthetics can potentially cause vasodilatation and hypotension – this is uncommon in children younger than 8 years
Level of block	To ensure the block is not unilateral or too high
Sensation	Indicates the level of the block
Motor movement	Tested alongside the level of the block
Pressure areas	Indicates any problems with mobility Motor paralysis indicates excessive local anaesthetic
Site of epidural	To check for leakage and inflammation
Sedation	A possible side effect of opioids
Side effects of drugs	Nausea and vomiting Pruritus Urine retention Local anaesthetic toxicity – oral tingling followed by a rapid decrease in blood pressure, confusion and fitting
Volume infused used	To ensure that the epidural infusion is running as prescribed
Patency of intravenous cannula	To ensure intravenous access is available to give antidote if required

required. Hourly observations of pulse rate, respiratory rate, volume delivered, oxygen saturation, pain score, sedation score and nausea and vomiting should be recorded. It may be necessary to adjust the rate of the infusion to maintain the child in a pain free state and minimise side effects. This is best accomplished by the prescription being written as a sliding scale.

Patient-controlled Analgesia

Patient-controlled analgesia (PCA) was developed to enable analgesia requirements to be tailored to individual requirements and refers to the intravenous administration of small bolus doses of an opioid drug triggered by the child pressing a button (Lloyd-Thomas 1993). Most children aged 5 years and older can use PCA effectively and the analgesia provided compares favourably with continuous morphine infusions in the older child (Morton 1998). Some younger children are also able to use PCA; this depends on the ability of the individual child. Children require a detailed explanation on how the lockout system works (this is a built-in safety device that is designed to prevent children from receiving an overdose of opioid when using PCA). PCA is usually commenced intraoperatively and the most common opioid used is morphine. In children, PCA is often used in combination with a background infusion of the opioid. Children receiving PCA should be monitored closely and have hourly observations of pulse rate, respiratory rate, the volume delivered, oxygen saturation, pain score, sedation score and incidents of nausea and vomiting.

Parental education is important, because their support is essential to the child in the postoperative period. Parents need to be informed about how PCA works. Many children's wards and units provide written information for both the child and parent. It is important that parents understand that they must not press the button for the child.

Nurse-controlled Analgesia

The use of NCA has become popular for children under 5 years of age (Lloyd-Thomas & Howard 1994). This is essentially a morphine infusion with the ability to administer controlled boluses of the drug at times of increased pain. To prevent an overdose of morphine, a longer lockout time is employed than when using PCA. Nurses should consult the child and parents about the need for extra analgesia but it is the responsibility of the nurse to press the button (administer the drug). The same observations are carried out as when using PCA.

Subcutaneous Analgesia

When it is not possible to use PCA or epidurals, a catheter can be inserted subcutaneously at the time of the operation (Lloyd-Thomas 1993). This allows for intermittent boluses of opioid analgesia to be administered without having to give an intramuscular injection. It is important to check the needle site regularly for signs of infection or displacement.

When weaning a child from any of the above methods it is important to ensure that oral medication is prescribed and administered before the effective of the intravenous/subcutaneous medication has worn off. The aim of pain management is to maintain children in a pain-free state rather than waiting for them to be in pain before administering analgesia.

Seminar discussion topic

Heidi is a third year nursing student undertaking a specialist placement on a high-dependency surgical ward. She is enjoying her placement and has been learning to care for children with complex surgical needs, particularly enhancing her practical skills in relation to managing acute pain in children and the use of complex analgesia systems.

Heidi has been caring for Luke, 9 months old, who has undergone major bowel resection for Hirschsprung's disease. Luke had initial complications due to a delayed paralytic ileus and abdominal distension.

Heidi felt able to care for Luke in relation to ensuring all his physical needs were met and managing his IV infusion of analgesia. However, she found it difficult to assess Luke's pain and often felt that because he had had an epidural infusion of morphine that staff felt this was dealing adequately with any pain experienced.

What issues do you think are important to discuss in relation to this scenario within Heidi's learning set?

MISCONCEPTIONS RELATING TO ANALGESIC DRUGS

Despite successful use over the past two decades, with research supporting their efficacy and safety in older children (Berde & Sethna 2002), there are still misconceptions about the use of opioids in children (Broadbent 2000). Many nurses believe that the risk of a patient becoming addicted to opioid analgesics is high and use this as the reason for their reluctance to administer opioid analgesia (Bauwens et al 2001, McCaffery & Ferrell 1997, McCaffery & Robinson 2002, Van Niekerk & Martin 2001). This appears to be due to a lack of understanding of addiction. Addiction has been defined by the American Pain Society (2003 p 2) as:

. . . a primary, chronic neurobiological disease, with genetic, psychosocial and environmental factors influencing its development and manifestations. It is characterised by behaviours that include one or more of the following: impaired control over drug use, compulsive use, continued use despite harm, and craving.

 WWW

More information about the American Pain Society's definition of addiction can be found at:
- http://www. ampainsoc.org/advocacy/opioids2.htm

Very few patients become addicted to opioids; a review of the medical records of patients (both adults and children) who became addicted usually demonstrates a previous history of drug abuse or contributory socio-economic factors (Morrison 1991, Porter & Jick 1980). McCaffery & Wong (1993) note that fear of creating opioid addiction should never be a reason for withholding opioid analgesics from anyone who needs them for pain relief.

Nurses often confuse physical dependence (withdrawal symptoms) with addiction. Withdrawal symptoms will not occur if the opioid is decreased gradually and they are rarely a problem in clinical practice. If withdrawal symptoms *do* occur, this does not mean that the patient is addicted to the opioid; they occur because of the sudden withdrawal of a chemical (opioid) which the body has become used to (American Pain Society 2003, McCaffery et al 1990, McCaffery & Pasero 1999). Tolerance to both the analgesic effect and the toxicity of opioids occurs with sustained use (Miser 1993); as tolerance develops, increasing doses of opioids are required to produce effective analgesia (Yaster & Maxwell 1993). The use of opioids as analgesia is therefore extremely unlikely to cause addiction in children.

Several studies have examined the occurrence of respiratory depression in clinical settings and found that the risk in children is no greater than in adults provided that the dose is appropriate (Dilworth & MacKellar 1987, McCaffery & Wong 1993, Miller & Jick 1978). Severe consequences such as respiratory arrest can be prevented because respiratory slowing occurs well before severe respiratory depression. Appropriate interventions such as slowing or stopping the infusion can be implemented. The risk of using opioids in children is therefore no greater than using them in adults. Body clearance of morphine is reduced in neonates; therefore additional monitoring and facilities to allow rapid airway intervention are paramount for this group of children (Berde & Sethna 2002).

Non-drug Methods

Activity

- Which non-drug methods of pain relief do you use/have you seen used?
- With reference to the gate control theory explain how these pain relief methods work.

Several non-drug pain-relieving strategies are available and should be used in conjunction with analgesic drugs (AHCPR 1992, Chen et al 2000, Rusy & Weisman 2000). Many non-drug techniques can be taught or facilitated by nurses. This means that the child and his or her family can take over this part of pain management (Carter 1994, Twycross 1998b), thus giving the child and family some control. Feeling in control reduces the anxiety and stress associated with a hospital stay (Bernstein et al 2000). Other techniques such as aromatherapy and hypnosis require specific training (Carter 1994, Twycross 1998b). Table 17.12 summarises some of the non-drug methods used to manage pain in children.

The skills of the multidisciplinary team are important; play therapists and clinical psychologists, in particular, have an important role when using non-drug methods (Chen et al 2000, Twycross 1998b).

INVOLVING PARENTS IN THEIR CHILD'S PAIN MANAGEMENT

Parents can identify their children's pain behaviours (Chambers et al 1996, Finley et al 1996, Reid et al 1995, Watt-Watson et al 1990, Wilson & Doyle 1996). However, many parents believe that nurses will also know if their child is in pain and therefore leave pain management to them (Eland 1985b, Woodgate & Kristjanson 1996).

Children describe parental presence as being an excellent distracter from things that hurt, and they help to reduce the anxiety related to being in hospital and being in pain (Alex & Ritchie 1992, Polkki et al 2003, Woodgate & Kristjanson 1996). Recent studies have suggested that when parents are taught how to distract their child during a painful procedure, rather than simply being a reassuring presence, the child experiences less anxiety and pain (Greenberg et al 1999, Kleiber et al 2001, Manimala et al 2000). If parents are not prepared for their role in their child's pain management their presence can be counterproductive. Nurses therefore need to ensure that parents are adequately prepared to support their child through a painful procedure.

Parents also need information about managing their child's pain at home following discharge (Howard 2003, RCN 1999). This should include:

- the site and intensity of the pain
- the expected duration of the pain
- how much analgesia to give and when
- whether it is OK to give more than one analgesic drug
- possible side-effects
- how to obtain further advice or help.

Reflect on your Practice

- How often do you discuss children's pain management with their parents?
- Do you prepare parents for managing their child's pain after discharge?

INVOLVING THE MULTIDISCIPLINARY TEAM

Managing pain effectively involves the whole multidisciplinary team (Royal College of Paediatrics and Child Health (RCPCH) 1997, RCN 1999). However, nurses are the healthcare professionals who are with the child 24 hours a day (Broome & Slack 1990, RCPCH 1997). It is therefore nurses' responsibility to ensure that pain-relieving interventions are implemented and that they are effective.

Evaluation of Pain-relieving Interventions

Once pain has been assessed and a treatment plan implemented the success of interventions must be evaluated. Pain should be assessed frequently and if the child's pain has not been relieved the plan of care should be amended (AHCPR 1992, RCN 1999). In acute pain, pain assessment should be carried out every one to two hours, depending on the severity and type of analgesia system. If an advanced analgesia system is being used pain should be assessed every hour. More frequent assessments should be made if the pain is not relieved (AHCPR 1992).

Reflect on your Practice

- How often do you evaluate the effectiveness of the pain-relieving interventions you have used?
- How often do you assess a child's pain postoperatively?

Table 17.12 Non-drug Methods of Pain Relief

Method	Comments
Acupuncture	The Chinese explanation of how acupuncture works is based on the idea that life force flows round certain lines on the body known as meridians (Mayer et al 1976, Melzack & Wall 1996, Rusy & Weisman 2000)
	Needling points on these lines is thought to correct an abnormal flow of life forces (Mann 1971, Melzack & Wall 1996, Rusy & Weisman 2000)
	Another explanation is that acupuncture stimulates the production of natural endorphins (Mayer et al 1976, Melzack & Wall 1996)
	Often helpful in treating chronic pain (Kemper et al 2000, Sofaer 1998)
Aromatherapy	Uses essential oils extracted from aromatic plants as a means of relaxation and is often associated with a special form of massage (Carter 1995)
	Used as a means of reducing stress, relaxing, treating symptoms and providing relief from pain and other symptoms
	Promotes healing on different levels: physical, emotional and mental
	Should only be practised by a trained practitioner
Distraction	Best for relatively short duration pain such as procedural pain (Carter 1994)
	Makes pain more tolerable or bearable by putting pain at the periphery of awareness (Kleiber et al 2001, McCaffery and Pasero 1999)
	Attention is focused on the distracter rather than the pain (Carter 1994, Chen et al 2000)
	To determine an effective distraction strategy the nurse involves the child and parents in identifying what is particularly interesting to them (McCaffery & Wong 1993)
	Distraction has a positive effect on children's distress behaviour (Cohen et al 1999, Dahlquist et al 2002, Kleiber et al 2001)
Hypnosis	Defined as focused attention, an altered state of consciousness or a trance, often accompanied by relaxation (Valente 1991)
	Found to be of value in the care and management of children with both acute and chronic pain (Carter 1994, Chen et al 2000, Rusy & Weisman 2000)
	Children having bone marrow aspirations have found hypnosis reduced pain and anxiety (Liossi & Hatira 1999)
Imagery	The use of imagination to modify the response to pain (Doody et al 1991, McCaffery & Pasero 1999, Rusy & Weisman 2000)
	Can be used in a guided way so that the child imagines something about their pain which will help reduce it; for example, a child who has pain can picture the pain flowing out of their body (Carter 1994, Rusy & Weisman 2000)
	Has been shown to reduce children's postoperative pain
Massage	The systematic manual manipulation of the soft tissues of the body to produce relaxation of the muscles (Beck 1988)
	Promotes circulation of the blood, relief for pain, restoration of metabolic balance as well as other physical and emotional benefits (Beck 1988)
	An ancient method of maintaining and improving health (McCaffery & Pasero 1999)
	A review of research evidence over the past 20 years suggests that massage may be useful in the care of infants and children (Ireland & Olson 2000)
Relaxation	A patient cannot be relaxed and anxious concurrently. Pain tolerance should be increased if the patient is relaxed (Weisenberg 1980)
	An effective coping strategy for procedural, chronic or on-going pain (Chen et al 2000, McCaffery & Wong 1993)
	For pain that lasts most of the day a relaxation technique may be performed several times a day (McCaffery & Wong 1993)
	Presence of a parent is useful in helping to reduce distress associated with pain for all age groups (McCaffery & Wong 1993)
	Ideally taught prior to painful procedures
Touch	A two-way process involving sensation and cognition (Carter 1994)
	The need to be touched is present at birth and is a continuing and developing need
	Provides one of the strongest means of communicating care and empathy

Continued

Table 17.12 Non-drug Methods of Pain Relief—Cont'd

Method	Comments
Transcutaneous electric nerve stimulation (TENS)	Useful in localised pain; thought to increase endorphin levels and act as a counter-irritant (McCaffery & Pasero 1999) Little research in children (Eland 1993) Should be used in combination with other treatment methods (Eland 1993) Relieves pain by blocking the physiological gate in the dorsal horn; it is non-invasive and safe (Eland 1993) The TENS device delivers controlled low-voltage electricity to the body via electrodes (Eland 1993; Rusy & Weisman 2000) Recipients often describe a sensation of tingling when the device is working (McCaffery & Pasero 1999) Useful for both acute and chronic pain (Rusy & Weisman 2000, Sofaer 1998)

COMMUNICATION

Communicating with the child and their parent is an essential part of pain management (Carr & Mann 2000, Francke & Theeuwen 1994, RCN 1999). Ineffective communication results in children's pain not being managed effectively and affects the quality of the child's pain relief. A child's self-report of pain must be considered the gold standard. Nurses should therefore communicate with children about their pain whenever possible.

Reflect on your Practice

How often do you communicate with children about their pain and how it can/will be managed?

DOCUMENTATION

Good documentation improves communication about the child's pain management and subsequently results in better continuity of care (Salantera et al 1999). Systematic documentation results in patients (both children and adults) reporting a decrease in pain intensity (Faries et al 1991, Scott 1994, Stevens 1990). Nurses should therefore document children's pain scores and the pain-relieving interventions used for each child in the nursing kardex. Pain intensity scores should also be re-evaluated and recorded frequently.

Pain Management: An Ethical Imperative

In its Declaration of the Rights of the Child, the United Nations General Assembly states that children should in all circumstances be among the first to receive protection and relief, and should be protected from all forms of neglect, cruelty and exploitation (United Nations General Assembly 1989). This can be applied to the management of pain, particularly as good practice guidelines are available. The UNICEF Child Friendly Hospital Initiative (UNICEF 1999 p 8) states that:

A team will be established in the hospital whose remit is to establish standards and guidance in the control of pain and discomfort (psychological as well as physical) in children.

Not providing children with satisfactory pain relief can be considered a violation of their human rights. Indeed, when the consequences of unrelieved pain are taken into account, managing children's acute pain effectively is an ethical imperative (Franck 1998, Kachoyeanos & Zollo 1995, Rich 2000).

Reflect on your Practice

Think about the documentation about pain management you have seen in the clinical area:
- How thorough is it?
- What is included?

www

The following website contains protocols, policies and procedures relating to pain in children from across the world:
- http://is.dal.ca/~painsrc/

References

Abu-Saad HH, Bours GJ, Stevens B, Hamers JP 1998 Assessment of pain in the neonate. Seminars in Perinatology 22(5):402–416

Agency for Health Care Policy and Research 1992 Acute pain management in infants, children and adolescents: operative and medical procedures. Department of Health and Human Sciences, Rockville, MD

Alex JA, Ritchie MR 1992 School-aged children's interpretation of their experience with acute surgical pain. Journal of Pediatric Nursing 7(3):171–180

Al-Shaikh B 1997 Epidural analgesia in ICU. Care of the Critically Ill 13(3):20–24

Ambuel B, Hamlett KW, Marx CM, Blumer JL 1992 Assessing distress in pediatric intensive care environments: the COMFORT scale. Journal of Pediatric Psychology 3:11–23

American Pain Society 2003 Definitions related to the use of opioids for the treatment of pain. Online. Available at: www.ampainsoc.org/advocacy/opioids2.htm [accessed 26 June 2003]

Anand KJS, Hickey PR 1987 Pain and its effects in the human neonate and fetus. New England Journal of Medicine 317:1321–1329

Aradine CR, Beyer JE, Tompkins JM 1988 Children's pain perception before and after analgesia: a study of instrument construct validity. Journal of Pediatric Nursing 3:11–23

Atkinson R, Atkinson C, Smith EE, Hilgard ER 1987 Introduction to psychology, 8th edn. Harcourt Brace, London

Baker C, Wong D 1987 QUESTT: a process of pain assessment in children. Orthopaedic Nursing 6(1):11–21

Barrier G, Attia J, Mayer MN et al 1989 Measurement of post-operative pain and narcotic administration in infants using a new clinical scoring system. Intensive Care Medicine 15:S37–S39

Bauwens S, Distelmans W, Storme G, Kaufman L 2001 Attitudes and knowledge about cancer pain in Flanders. The educational effect of workshops regarding pain and symptom control. Palliative Medicine 15:181–190

Beck M 1988 The theory and practice of therapeutic massage. Milady, New York

Berde CB, Sethna NF 2002 Drug therapy: analgesics for the treatment of pain in children. New England Journal of Medicine 347(14):1094–1103

Bernstein DA, Clarke-Stewart A, Penner LA et al 2000 Psychology, 5th edn. Houghton Mifflin, Boston

Beyer J, Aradine CR 1987 Patterns of pediatric pain intensity: a methodological investigation of a self-report scale. Clinical Journal of Pain 3:130–141

Beyer J, Wells N 1989 The assessment of pain in children. Pediatric Clinics of North America 36(4):837–854

Beyer J, McGrath PJ, Berde CB 1990 Discordance between self report and behavior measures in children aged 3–7 years after surgery. Journal of Pain and Symptom Management 5(6):350–356

Bieri D, Reeve RA, Champion GD et al 1990 The faces pain scale for the self assessment of the severity of pain experienced by children: development, initial validation and preliminary investigation for ratio scale properties. Pain 41:139–150

Blos P 1978 Children think about illness: their concepts and beliefs. In Gellert E (ed.) Psychosocial aspects of pediatric care. Grune and Stratton, New York

Bournaki MC 1997 Correlates of pain-related responses to venepuncture in school-age children. Nursing Research 46(3):147–154

Bradshaw C, Zeanah P 1986 Pediatric nurses' assessments of pain in children. Journal of Pediatric Nursing 1(5):314–321

Bray RJ 1983 Post-operative analgesia provided by morphine infusion in children. Anaesthesia 38:1075–1078

Bray RJ, Woodhams AM, Vallis CJ et al 1996 A double blind comparison of morphine infusion and patient controlled analgesia in children. Paediatric Anaesthesiology 6:121–127

Broadbent C 2000 The pharmacology of acute pain. Nursing Times 96(26):39–41

Broadman LM, Rice LH, Hannallah RS 1988 Comparison of a physiological and a visual analogue pain scale in children. Canadian Journal of Anaesthesia 35:S317–S318

Broome ME, Slack JF 1990 Influences on nurses' management of pain in children. American Journal of Maternal Child Nursing 15(3):158–162

Carey S 1985 Conceptual changes in childhood. MIT Press, Boston

Carr ECJ, Mann EM 2000 Pain: creative approaches to effective pain management. Macmillan Press, Basingstoke

Carter B 1994 Child and infant pain: principles of nursing care and management. Chapman and Hall, London

Carter B 1995 Complementary therapies and the management of chronic pain. Paediatric Nursing 7(3):18–22

Carter B 1997 Pantomimes of pain, distress, repose and lability: the world of the preterm baby. Journal of Child Health Care 1(1):17–23

Chambers CT, Reid GJ, McGrath PJ, Finley GA 1996 Development and preliminary validation of a postoperative pain measure for parents. Pain 68:307–313

Chambers CT, Giesbredit K, Craig KD et al 1999 A comparison of faces scales for the measurement of pediatric pain: children's and parents' ratings. Pain 83:25–35.

Chen E, Joseph M, Zeltzer LK 2000 Behavorial and cognitive interventions in the treatment of pain in children. Pediatric Clinics of North America 47(3):513–525

Coffman S, Alvarez Y, Pyngolil M et al 1997 Nursing assessment and management of pain in critically ill children. Heart and Lung 26(3):221–228

Cohen LL, Blount RL, Cohen RJ et al 1999 Comparative study of distraction versus topical anesthesia for pediatric pain during immunizations. Health Psychology 18(6):591–598

Colwell C, Clark L, Perkins R 1996 Postoperative use of pediatric pain scales: children's self-report versus nurse assessment of pain intensity and affect. Journal of Pediatric Nursing 1(6):375–381

Coskun V, Anand KJS 2000 Development of supraspinal pain processing. In: Anand KJS, Stevens BJ, McGrath PJ (eds) Pain in neonates, 2nd edn. Elsevier, Amsterdam, pp 23–54

Craig KD, Grunau RVE 1993 Neonatal pain perception and behavioural measurement. In: Anand KJS, Stevens BJ, McGrath PJ (eds) Pain in neonates. Elsevier, Amsterdam, pp 67–105

Dahlquist LM, Busby SM, Slifer KJ et al 2002 Distraction for children of different ages who undergo repeated needle sticks. Journal of Pediatric Oncology Nursing 19(1):22–34

Day R 1997 A pharmacological approach to acute pain. Professional Nurse 13(1):S9–S12

Dilworth N, MacKellar A 1987 Pain relief for the pediatric surgical patient. Journal of Pediatric Surgery 22(3):264–268

Doody SB, Smith C, Webb J 1991 Non-pharmacological interventions for pain management. Critical Care Nursing Clinics of North America 3(1):69–75

Doorbar P, McClarey M 1999 Ouch! Sort it out: children's experiences of pain. RCN Publishing, London

Eiser C 1985 The psychology of childhood illness. Springer-Verlag, New York

Eland J 1981 Minimising pain associated with pre-kindergarten intra-muscular injections. Issues in Comprehensive Pediatric Nursing 5:361–372

Eland J 1985a Myths about pain in children. The Candlelighters Childhood Cancer Foundation, V(1)

Eland J 1985b The child who is hurting. Seminars in Oncology Nursing 1(2):116–122

Eland J 1990 Pain in children. Nursing Clinics of North America 25(4):871–884

Eland J 1993 The use of TENS with children. In: Schechter NL, Berde CB, Yaster M (eds) Pain in infants, children and adolescents. Williams and Wilkins, Baltimore, pp 331–339

Faries J, Mills D, Goldsmith KW et al 1991 Systematic pain records and their impact on pain control. Cancer Nursing 14:306–313

Finley GA, McGrath PJ, Forward SP et al 1996 Parents' management of children's pain following 'minor' surgery. Pain 64:83–87

Fisher S, Morton N 1998 Pain prevention and management in children. In Morton N (ed.) Acute paediatric pain management: a practical guide. WB Saunders, London, pp 1–11

Fitzgerald M 2000 Development of the peripheral and spinal pain system. In: Anand KJS, Stevens BJ, McGrath PJ (eds) Pain in neonates, 2nd edn. Elsevier, Amsterdam, pp 9–22

Franck L 1986 A new method to quantitatively describe pain behavior in infants. Nursing Research 35(1):28–31

Franck LS 1998 The ethical imperative to treat pain in infants: are we doing the best we can? Neonatal Intensive Care 11(5):28–34

Franck LS, Greenberg CS, Stevens B 2000 Pain assessment in infants and young children. Pediatric Clinics of North America 43(3):487–512

Francke A, Theeuwen I 1994 Inhibition in expressing pain: a qualitative study among Dutch surgical breast cancer patients. Cancer Nursing 17(3):193–199

Gaffney A, McGrath PJ, Dick B 2003 Measuring pain in children: developmental and instrument issues. In: Schechter NL, Berde CB, Yaster M (eds) Pain in infants, children and adolescents, 2nd edn. Lippincott Williams and Wilkins, Philadelphia

Gildea J, Quirk T 1977 Assessing the pain experience in children. Nursing Clinics of North America 1:631–637

Greenberg RS, Billett C, Zahurak M, Yaster M 1999 Videotape increase parental knowledge about paediatric pain. Pediatric Anaesthesia 89:899–903

Grunau RVE, Johnston CC, Craig KD 1990 Pain expression in neonates: facial action and cry responses to invasive and non-invasive procedures. Pain 42:295–305

Hamers JPH, Abu-Saad HH, Geisler FEA et al 1999 The effect of paracetamol, fentanyl and systematic assessments on children's pain after tonsillectomy and adenoidectomy. Journal of Perianesthesia Nursing 14(6):357–366

Hannallah RS, Broadman LM, Belman AS, Abramowitz MD 1987 Comparison of caudal and ilioingual/iliohypogastric nerve blocks for control of post orchiopexy pain in pediatric ambulatory surgery. Anaesthesiology 66:832–834

Harbeck C, Pederson L 1992 Elephants dancing in my head: a developmental approach to children's concepts of specific pains. Child Development 63:138–149

Hawley D 1984 Postoperative pain in children: misconceptions, descriptions and interventions. Pediatric Nursing 10(1):20–23

Hawthorn J, Redmond K 1998 Pain causes and management. Blackwell Science, Oxford

Hestor NO, Barcus CS 1986 Assessment and management of pain in children. Pediatrics: Nursing Update 1(14):1–8

Hestor NO, Foster R, Kristensen K 1990 Measurement of pain in children: generalizability and validity of the pain ladder and the poker chip tool. In: Tyler DC, Krane EJ (eds) Pediatric pain. Advances in pain research and therapy, vol 15. Raven Press, New York, pp 79–84

Hestor NO, Foster RL, Jordan-Marsh M et al 1998 Putting pain measurement into clinical practice. In: Finley GA, McGrath PJ (eds) Measurement of pain in infants and children. IASP Press, Seattle, pp 179–198

Hicks CL, von Baeyer CL, Spafford PA et al 2001 The faces pain scale revised: toward a common metric in pediatric pain measurement. Pain 93(2): 173–183

Hogan M, Choonara I 1996 Measuring pain in neonates: an objective score. Paediatric Nursing 8(10):24–27

Howard R 2003 Acute pain management in children. In: Rowbotham DJ, MacIntyre PE (eds) Clinical pain management: acute pain. Arnold, London, pp 437–462

International Association for the Study of Pain (IASP) 1979 Pain terms: a list with definitions and notes on usage. Pain 6:249–252

International Association for the Study of Pain (IASP) 2001 IASP definition of pain. IASP Newsletter 2:2

Ireland M, Olson M 2000 Massage therapy and therapeutic touch in children: state of the science. Alternative Therapies in Health and Medicine 6(5):54–63

Jacques A 1994 Epidural analgesia. British Journal of Nursing 3(14):734–738

Kachoyeanos M, Zollo M 1995 Ethics in pain management of infants and children. American Journal of Maternal/Child Nursing 20:142–147

Kemper KJ, Sarah R, Silver-Highfield E et al 2000 On pins and needles? Pediatric pain patients' experience with acupuncture. Pediatrics 105(4):941–947

Kleiber C, Croft-Rosenberg M, Harper DC 2001 Parents as distraction coaches during IV insertion: a randomised study. Journal of Pain and Symptom Management 22(4):851–861

Kotzer AM 2000 Factors predicting postoperative pain in children and adolescents following spine fusion. Issues in Comprehensive Pediatric Nursing 23:83–102

Krechel SW, Bildner J 1995 CRIES: a new neonatal postoperative pain measurement score. Paediatric Anaesthesia 5:53–61

LaFleur C, Raway B 1999 School-age child and adolescent perception of the pain intensity associated with three word descriptors. Pediatric Nursing 25(1):45–55

Lawrence J, Alcock D, McGrath PJ et al 1993 The development of a tool to assess neonatal pain. Neonatal Network 12:59–65

Liossi C, Hatira P 1999 Clinical hypnosis versus cognitive behavioral training for pain management with pediatric cancer patients undergoing bone marrow aspirations. International Journal of Clinical and Experimental Hypnosis 47(2):104–116

Lloyd-Thomas AR 1993 Postoperative pain control in children. Current Paediatrics 3:234–237

Lloyd-Thomas AR, Howard RF 1994 A pain service for children. Paediatric Anaesthesia 4:3–15

Manimala MR, Blount RL, Cohen LL 2000 The effects of parental reassurance versus distraction on child distress and coping during immunizations. Children's Health Care 29(3):161–177

Mann F 1971 Acupuncture: the ancient Chinese act of healing. Heinemann, Oxford

Manne S, Jacobsen P, Redd WH 1992 Assessment of acute paediatric pain: do child self-report, parent ratings and nurse ratings measure the same phenomenon? Pain 48:45–52

Manukesla EL, Olkkala KT, Korpela R 1987 Measurement of pain in children with self-reporting and behavioural assessment. Clinical Pharmacology and Therapeutics 42:137–141

Mather L, Mackie J 1983 The incidence of postoperative pain in children. Pain 15:271–282

Mayer DJ, Price DD, Rafii A 1976 Antagonism of acupuncture analgesia in man by the narcotic antagonist naloxone. Brain Research 121(2):368–372

McCaffery M 1972 Nursing management of the patient in pain. Lippincott, Philadelphia

McCaffery M, Beebe AB 1989 Pain: clinical manual for nursing practice. CV Mosby, St Louis

McCaffery M, Ferrell B 1997 Nurses' knowledge of pain assessment and management: how much progress have we made? Journal of Pain and Symptom Management 14(3):175–187

McCaffery M, Pasero C 1999 Pain: clinical manual, 2nd edn. Mosby, St Louis

McCaffery M, Robinson ES 2002 Your patient is in pain – here's how you respond. Nursing 32(10):36–45

McCaffery M, Wong D 1993 Nursing interventions for pain control in children. In: Schechter NL, Yaster M, Berde C 2003 Pain in infants, children and adolescents, 2nd edn. Lippincott Williams and Wilkins, Philadelphia

McCaffery M, Ferrell B, O'Neill-Page E et al 1990 Nurses' knowledge of opioid analgesic drugs and psychological dependence. Cancer Nursing 13(1):21–27

McGrath PJ, Unrah A 2000 Measurement and assessment of paediatric pain. In: Wall RD, Melzack R (eds) Textbook of pain, 4th edn. Churchill Livingstone, Edinburgh, pp 371–384

McGrath PA, Deveber LL, Hearn MT 1985 Multidimensional pain assessment in children. Advances in Pain Research and Therapy 9:387–393

McGrath PJ, Unrah AM, Finley GA 1995 Pain measurement in children. Pain: Clinical Updates 3(2):1–4

Melzack R, Wall P 1996 The challenge of pain, updated 2nd edn. Penguin, London

Merkel S, Voepel-Lewis T, Shayevitz JR, Malviya S 1997 The FLACC: a behavioral scale for scoring post-operative pain in young children. Pediatric Nursing 23(3):293–297

Miller WR, Jick H 1978 Clinical effects of meperidine in hospitalized medical patients. Journal of Clinical Pharmacology 18(4):180–189

Miser A 1993 Management of pain associated with childhood cancer. In: Schechter NL, Berde CB, Yaster M (eds) Pain in infants, children and adolescents. Williams and Wilkins, Baltimore, pp 411–424

Moriarty A 1998 The pharmacological management of acute pain. In: Twycross A, Moriarty A, Betts T (eds) Paediatric pain management: a multi-disciplinary approach. Oxford, Radcliffe Medical Press

Morrison R 1991 Update of sickle cell disease: incidence of addiction and choice of opioid in pain management. Pediatric Nursing 17(5):503

Morton NS 1998 Prevention and control of pain in children. Pain Reviews 5:1–15

Norden J, Hannallah RS, Getson P et al 1991 Concurrent validation of an objective pain scale for infants and children. Anesthesiology 75:A934

Ochsenreither JM 1997 Analgesia in infants. Neonatal Network 16(6):79–83

Perquin CW, Hazebroek-Kampschreur AAJM, Hunfield JAM et al 2000 Pain in children and adolescents: a common experience. Pain 87:51–58

Polkki T, Pietila A-M, Vehvilamen-Julkunen K 2003 Hospitalized children's descriptions of their experiences with postsurgical pain relieving methods. International Journal of Nursing Studies 40:33–44

Porter J, Jick H 1980 Addiction rare in patients treated with narcotics. New England Journal of Medicine 302(2):123

Price S 1994 Assessing children's pain. British Journal of Nursing 3(20):1046–1048

Reid GJ, Hebb JPO, McGrath PJ, Forward SP 1995 Cues parents use to assess postoperative pain in children. Clinical Journal of Pain 11(3):229–235

Rich BA 2000 An ethical analysis of the barriers to effective pain management. Cambridge Quarterly of Healthcare Ethics 9:54–70

Romsing J, Moller-Sonnergaard J, Hertel S, Rasmussen M 1996 Postoperative pain in children: comparison between ratings of children and nurses. Journal of Pain and Symptom Management 11(1):42–46

Ross D, Ross S 1984 Childhood pain: the school-aged child's viewpoint. Pain 20(2):179–191

Royal College of Nursing (RCN) 1999 Clinical guidelines for the recognition and assessment of acute pain in children: recommendations. RCN Publishing, London

Royal College of Nursing (RCN) 2000 The recognition and assessment of acute pain in children: technical report. RCN Publishing, London

Royal College of Paediatrics and Child Health (RCPCH) 1997 Prevention and control of pain in children: a manual for health care professionals. BMJ Publishing, London

Royal College of Surgeons and College of Anaesthetists 1990 Pain after surgery. Royal College of Surgeons, London

Rushforth H 1996 Nurses' knowledge of how children view health and illness. Paediatric Nursing 8(9):23–27

Russell K 1992 Pharmacology of pain. Surgical Nurse 5(6):18–22

Rusy L, Weisman J 2000 Complementary therapies for acute pediatric pain management. Pediatric Clinics of North America 47(3):589–599

Salantera S, Lauri S, Salmi TT, Aantaa R 1999 Nursing activities and outcomes of care in the assessment, management and documentation of children's pain. Journal of Pediatric Nursing 14(6):408–415

Scott IE 1994 Effectiveness of documented assessment of postoperative pain. British Journal of Nursing 3(10):494–501

Scott J, Huskisson EC 1979 Graphic representation of pain. Pain 2:175–184

Sofaer B 1998 Pain: principles, practice and patients, 3rd edn. Stanley Thornes, London

Sternberg RJ 1989 Domain generality versus domain specificity: the life and death of a false dichotomy. Merrill-Palmer Quarterly 35:115–130

Stevens B 1990 Development and testing of a pediatric pain management sheet. Pediatric Nursing 16(6):543–548, 556–557

Stevens B 1999 Pain in infants. In: McCaffery M, Pasero C (eds) Pain: clinical manual, 2nd edn. Mosby, St Louis

Stevens B, Johnston C, Petryshen P, Taddio A 1996 Premature infant pain profile: development and initial validation. Clinical Journal of Pain 12:13–22

Swallow J, Briggs M, Semple P 2000 Pain at home: children's experience of tonsillectomy. Journal of Child Health Care 4(3):93–98

Sweet SD, McGrath PJ 1998 Physiological measures of pain. In: Finley GA, McGrath PJ (eds) Measurements of pain in infants and children. IASP Press, Seattle, pp 59–81

Tarbell SE, Cohen IT, Marsh JL 1992 The toddler-preschooler postoperative pain scale: an observational scale for measuring postoperative pain in children aged 1–5. Preliminary report. Pain 50:273–280

Taylor A 1998 Pain assessment in children. In: Twycross A, Moriarty A, Betts T (eds) Paediatric pain: a multi-disciplinary approach. Radcliffe Medical Press, Oxford

Tesler MD, Holzemer WL, Savedra MC 1998 Pain behaviors: postsurgical responses of children and adolescents. Journal of Pediatric Nursing 13(1):41–47

Twycross A 1998a Children's cognitive level and their perception of pain. Paediatric Nursing 10(3):24–27

Twycross A 1998b Non-drug methods of pain control. Paediatric pain: a multi-disciplinary approach. In: Twycross A, Moriarty A, Betts T (eds) Paediatric pain: a multi-disciplinary approach. Radcliffe Medical Press, Oxford

Tyler DC, Tu A, Douthit J, Chapman CR 1993 Toward the validation of pain measurement tools for children: a pilot study. Pain 52:301–309

UNICEF 1999 Global millennium targets: UNICEF child-friendly hospital initiative. Paediatric Nursing 11(10):7–8

United Nations General Assembly 1989 Convention on the rights of the child. United Nations, New York

Valente SM 1991 Using hypnosis with children for pain management. Oncology Nurses Forum 18(4):699–704

Van Cleve L, Johnson L, Pothier P 1996 Pain responses of hospitalised infants and children to venipuncture and intravenous cannulation. Journal of Pediatric Nursing 11(3):161–168

Van Cleve LJ, Savedra MC 1993 Pain location: validity and reliability of body outline markings by 4 to 7 year old children who are hospitalized. Pediatric Nursing 19(3):217–220

Van Niekerk LM, Martin F 2001 Tasmanian nurses' knowledge of pain management. International Journal of Nursing Studies 38(2):141–152

Volpe J 1981 Neurology of the newborn. Saunders, Philadelphia

Wall PD, Melzack R 1989 Textbook of pain. Churchill Livingstone, London

Walsh D 1997. TENS: clinical applications and related theory. Churchill Livingstone, Edinburgh

Watt-Watson J, Evernden C, Lawson C 1990 Parents' perceptions of their child's acute pain experience. Journal of Pediatric Nursing 5(5):344–349

Weisenberg M 1980 Understanding pain phenomenon. Cited in: Carter B 1994 Child and infant pain: principles of nursing care and management. Chapman and Hall, London

Whaley L, Wong DL 1987 Nursing care of infants and children. Mosby, St Louis

Wilson GAM, Doyle E 1996 Validation of three paediatric pain scores for use by parents. Anaesthesia 51:1005–1007

Wolf AR 1999 Pain. Nociception and the developing infant. Paediatric Anaesthesia 9:7–17

Woodgate R, Kristjanson L 1996 A young child's pain: how parents and nurses 'take care'. International Journal of Nursing Studies 33(3):271–284

World Health Organization 1998 Cancer pain relief and palliative care in children. World Health Organization, Geneva

Yaster M, Maxwell L 1993 Opioid agonists and antagonists. In: Schechter NL, Berde C, Yaster M (eds) Pain in infants, children and adolescents. Williams and Williams, Baltimore, pp 145–172

Yoos H 1994 Children's illness concepts: old and new paradigms. Pediatric Nursing 20(2):134–140, 145

Yura H, Walsh MB 1988 The nursing process: assessing, planning and implementation, 5th edn. Appleton Lange, Norwalk, CT

Chapter Eighteen

Children and Surgery

Linda Shields, Ann Tanner

ABSTRACT

The striking difference in nursing children, as opposed to adults, through a surgical experience is that they do not come alone but are an integral part of a family group, with parents and/or caregivers as advocates for their treatment, and often siblings and other relatives in their extended family (Alsop-Shields 2000). As such, their care is more complicated and involved than it would be for a consenting adult patient. Parents of children admitted to hospital for surgery often have high levels of anxiety. If this anxiety is transmitted to the child, it can have a negative impact on the child's admission and surgery (Bellew et al 2002). Increased availability of preoperative information, in the form of written information sheets, coupled with the exchange of information by nursing and medical staff is likely to reduce parental anxiety. Children undergoing surgery are often anxious. This anxiety may initiate a stress response, which can delay wound healing and suppress the immune system (Koinig 2002). Reduction of anxiety for the child and their parent is an important role for the perioperative nurse.

Learning Outcomes

- Gain an overview of the nature of paediatric surgery.
- Understand the role of parents and family-centred care in paediatric surgery.
- Gain an overview of common paediatric procedures of different age groups and developmental stages.
- Understand the importance of education for parents and children throughout any surgical experience.
- Understand the ethical and legal ramifications of surgery on children.
- Recognise and understand common paediatric emergencies.
- Understand the flow through the operating theatres: preparation, admission, induction, procedure/surgery/anaesthetic, recovery, discharge, education.

Why Children Need Surgery

Paediatric surgery was not considered a specialised area separate to adult surgery until the first half of the 20th century (Mooney 1997). It encompasses a wide range of surgical procedures and differing ages, from premature infants weighing as little as 500–600 g to adolescents. There are many reasons why children need surgery. These can range from congenital malformations to accidental and non-accidental injuries, or a variety of disease processes (Shields & Werder 2002). A number of characteristic conditions and/or injuries for the varying age groups have been detailed in Table 18.1. These are representative of the general trends and are not indicative of all age groups or all types of surgery. Those highlighted have an accompanying photograph and a description of surgery.

HERNIA REPAIR (Fig. 18.1)

Hernias are one of the most common congenital abnormalities found in infants. There are several different types of hernia affecting both male and female children. The most frequently occurring hernias are indirect and direct inguinal

Table 18.1 A Sample of Paediatric Surgical Cases for Different Age Groups

Age	Type of surgery	Figures
0–2	Hernia repair (most common—inguinal)	18.1
	Repair of tracheo-oesphageal fistula	
	Diaphragmatic hernia repair	
	Repair of gastroschisis and exomphalos	18.2, 18.3, 18.4
	Insertion of ventricular-peritoneal shunts for hydrocephalus	
	Circumcision (medical and cultural)	18.5
	Correction of congenital abnormalities (removal of extra digits, cleft palate repair, repair of imperforate anus)	
	Craniofacial surgery for congenital abnormalities such as fusion of cranial sutures	18.6
	Hypospadias repair	18.8
	Eye surgery such as probing of tear ducts and examination under anaesthetic for tumours	
2–5	Common ENT procedures such as:	
	• insertion of grommets	
	• adenoidectomy	18.9
	• tonsillectomy	18.10, 18.11
	Urological surgery such as cystoscopy and ureteric reimplantation	
	Lacerations, dog bites	
	Repair of fractured limbs	
	Dental restorations and extractions for multiple dental caries	
	Eye surgery for squint repair	
	Burns grafts for scald burns	
	Brain tumours	
5–10	ENT: adenoidectomy, tonsillectomy	10.10, 10.11
	Repair of fractured limbs	
	Accidental injuries	
	Appendicectomy	18.12
	Orthopaedic surgery for congenital skeletal deformities	
	Brain tumours	
10–15	Accidental injuries	
	Lacerations	
	Repair of fractured limbs	
	Torsion of testes	
	Laparoscopic appendicectomy	18.12
	Bone tumours	
	Burns, grafts for flame burns	

hernias and hydroceles. Hernias occur when the processus vaginalis (a peritoneal diverticulum that extends through the inguinal ring) remains as a patent conduit with the peritoneal cavity instead of closing off and disappearing. During fetal development, the processus vaginalis attaches itself to the testes and is pulled down into the scrotum as the testes descend. If the processus vaginalis remains patent it is a potential hernia. Twenty per cent of individuals have a patent processus but remain asymptomatic. If bowel or other contents from the abdomen enter the processus it becomes an actual hernia. If only peritoneal fluid enters the processus it becomes a communicating hydrocele (Weber & Tracy 2000).

GASTROSCHISIS

Gastroschisis and omphalocele are two varieties of congenital abdominal wall defects resulting in a herniation of the abdominal contents in the developing fetus (Fig. 18.2). In

Fig. 18.1 • Inguinal hernia in a child.

gastroschisis the defect usually lies laterally to the umbilicus; the small and large bowel and often the stomach herniate through the defect and are not protected by a peritoneal membrane, but float freely within the amniotic fluid (Holcomb & Wallace 2000). The amniotic fluid acts as an irritant to the surface of the bowel, which forms a thick skin on the bowel surface. In an omphalocele, the umbilical ring is defective and can include a herniation of the entire small and large bowel, the stomach and the liver. Omphaloceles are protected by a layer of the peritoneal membrane. Atresia of the bowel can occur if the opening of the defect is narrow and the blood supply to the bowel has been compromised due to the subsequent stricture. For atresia, the affected bowel is resected. If the infant loses excess intestinal length 'short gut syndrome', which impairs reabsorption of sufficient fluids and nutrients, the child may be dependent on total parenteral nutrition for life. Treatment of gastroschisis depends on the size of the defect and the degree of herniation that has occurred. Infants born with gastroschisis and omphalocele usually have surgery within the first day of life. Smaller defects may be manually reduced and the defect sutured as a primary closure. Larger defects may have a silo bag applied (Fig. 18.3), which contains all the abdominal contents. The bag hangs suspended above the infant and gravity and time aid in

reducing the inflammation of the bowel, making it easier to manually reduce the hernia in a series of stages. If the abdominal wall defect is large, a prolene mesh graft may be used to assist in the closure of the defect. The defect can take years to close completely (Fig. 18.4).

CIRCUMCISION

Circumcision was once routinely performed at birth in many countries, although this custom has now mostly disappeared. However, it remains a reasonably common procedure although it is now performed for cultural/religious and medical reasons. A great deal of controversy surrounds circumcision for cultural and religious reasons. Medical circumcisions are required for two main conditions: phimosis, which is an inability to retract the foreskin, indicated by a ballooning of the foreskin on urination (Raynor 2000) and paraphimosis, which occurs when the foreskin which has retracted cannot be pulled back down, leaving it forming a stricture around the head of the penis.

Circumcision is usually performed under general anaesthetic and a penile nerve block. The surgeon makes a blunt dissection between the glans and the foreskin, the collar of the foreskin that has been isolated is then excised usually

Fig. 18.2 • Gastroschisis.

using diathermy, and the shaft skin is then sutured to the subcoronal skin using interrupted absorbable sutures (Fig. 18.5).

CRANIOFACIAL SURGERY

One of the more frequent types of craniofacial surgery is cranial vault remodelling for the correction of fused cranial sutures (Herron et al 2002). These children require surgery at around 6 months of age. It is preferable to operate this young because the bones are relatively malleable and the fusion of cranial sutures has not yet caused any brain damage. The child is positioned either prone or supine, depending on the skull shape and the region of deformity.

Cranial vault remodelling involves a neurosurgeon and a plastic surgeon. A large hemicircular incision is made, within the hairline, from ear to ear. The scalp is retracted back and periosteal elevators are used to scrape tissue off the periosteum (Fig. 18.6) in preparation for the craniotomy. The neurosurgeon performs the craniotomy (removal of the top half of the skull) and sutures any parts of the dura mater that might have been damaged during the removal. The plastic surgeon refashions the removed skull using bone cutters to make vertical cuts 3–5 cm in length into the skull around its circumference to widen and enlarge the skull. The refashioned skull is either wired or plated back onto the child's head, and the scalp sutured back into place. A head bundle dressing is applied and drains are occasionally required to prevent a build up of old blood and subsequent wound infection and break down.

HYPOSPADIAS AND REPAIR

Hypospadias (Fig. 18.7) is a developmental abnormality in which the urethra opens onto the ventral surface of the penis. The opening can occur anywhere from glans to the scrotum (Murphy 2000b) (Fig. 18.8). Surgical repair of hypospadias is often two staged. The repair involves the formation of a flap using the meatus to create a neourethra that opens at the tip of the glans. An indwelling catheter is left in situ for 7–10 days postoperatively, or until the dressing is removed.

ADENOIDECTOMY

Adenoidectomy is a common ENT procedure on children, particularly 2–5 year olds. General anaesthetic is given and the child lies supine, with a gel roll under the shoulders to tilt the head back (Herron et al 2002). The surgeon inserts

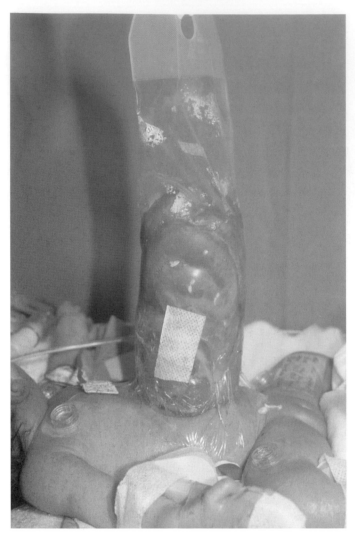

Fig. 18.3 • Repair of gastroschisis.

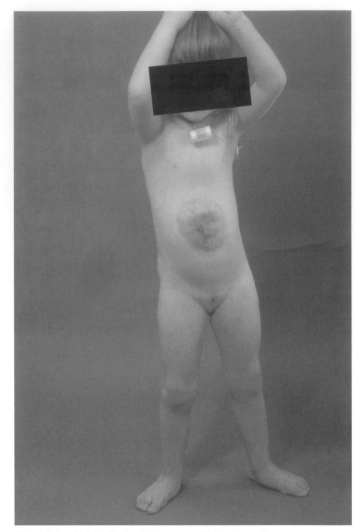

Fig. 18.4 • Child with healed gastroschisis at age 3.

a mouth gag, which both depresses the tongue and holds the jaw open. Two rods are used to support the gag in place and to keep the head in position (Fig. 18.9). An adenotome is used to scrape the adenoidal tissue from the adenoidal bed. Diathermy is not routinely used for adenoidectomy, rather haemostasis is obtained by firmly packing a swab into the adenoidal bed. This is removed after about 5 min and may be replaced with a fresh swab if bleeding persists. Adenoidal bleeding usually occurs if the adenoidal tissue has not been sufficiently scraped away, in this instance the surgeon may re-curette the tissue with the adenotome. Occasionally, suction diathermy is needed to cauterise any vessels that continue to bleed. Because Raytec® swabs are routinely packed into the adenoidal space for haemostasis, the scrub nurse's count is very important, as a bloody Raytec® is difficult to see and may cause a serious airway obstruction if left undetected.

TONSILLITIS (Figs 18.10 and 18.11)

Tonsillitis is a common illness of childhood, an infection which produces a purulent discharge which covers the inflamed tonsils and is accompanied by fever and often extreme discomfort. There is some controversy over the need for tonsillectomy and adenoidectomy and there is some suggestion that the operations are performed unnecessarily in some instances (Montgomery 1996). In children, adenotonsillectomy or adenoidectomy are performed to treat recurrent tonsillitis, obstruction of the naso-pharynx, and obstructive sleep apnoea (Nieminen et al 2000). Traditionally, there have been two methods for tonsillectomy – using a tonsil snare (guillotine) which loops over the tonsil and cuts it off at its base (Homer et al 2000), and more recently, by sharp or blunt dissection (Meether and Rothrock 1999).

Fig. 18.5 • Circumcision.

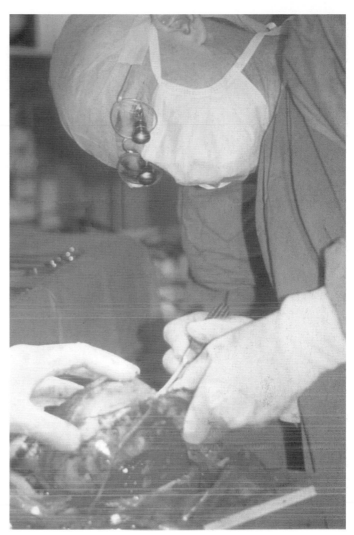

Fig. 18.6 • Craniofacial surgery.

LAPAROSCOPIC APPENDICECTOMY

Children presenting with acute appendicitis usually have a number of tell-tale signs and symptoms. The onset of acute appendicitis is usually over a period of 6–36 h. The child complains of abdominal pain, which commences around the umbilical area but moves to the right upper quadrant of the abdomen. If the appendix is inflamed the child may be febrile. In appendicitis, vomiting usually begins after the onset of pain; if the child begins vomiting before the onset of pain then the prognosis is more likely to be gastritis (Ein 2000). Diarrhoea does not usually commence unless the appendix has perforated, in which the case the sigmoid colon becomes involved and peritonitis may ensue.

Ultrasound is often performed to confirm a suspected appendicitis; laprascopic appendicectomy (Fig. 18.12) is now the preferred method, as opposed to an open laparotomy. It involves the insertion of a large port or trocar for the camera at the umbilicus, and one to two other ports (usually 5 mm wide) for the grasping instruments. The appendix is ligated away from the appendiceal mesentery using diathermy. Once freed, the appendix is tied off, dissected from the bowel and removed via a 10-mm port (which is inserted to replace one of the 5-mm ports) and routinely sent for pathology.

The Role of the Family

In times past, parents (the child's natural parent, stepparent, legal guardian or carer) were excluded from the hospital during a child's admission (Glasper & Charles-Edwards 2002). Such attitudes are now not widespread and parents are encouraged, and often expected, to stay for the duration of the child's admission. However, parental presence in the operating room is a more contentious issue.

Forty years ago, admission to hospital was portrayed as a positive, growth-promoting experience for children (Jessner et al 1952, Oremland & Oremland 1973) and the

Fig. 18.7 • Hypospadias.

experience of overcoming the emotional trauma associated with surgery was extolled as character-forming (Blom 1958); as late as 1992, Lansdown suggested that children could gain psychologically from a hospital admission. However, studies of the psychological trauma encountered by children and their parents before admission have highlighted the importance of adequate preparation of children for hospital admission and surgery (Strachan 1993).

Children have needs different to adults (Price 1994). The most important factor differentiating the needs of children from those of adults is their level of physical and psychological development.

A Child's Eye View of the Operating Room

Children are smaller and less developed physically and emotionally than adults, so have different visual and psy-

chological perspectives to adults. Consequently, the environment of the operating room looks different to a child (Figs 18.13 and 18.14). Also, children lack the rationalization skills that would allow them to integrate the environment perceptually, and so may become frightened.

The paediatric operating room environment must be planned with this in mind and should be as 'child-friendly' as possible, with pictures and cartoons on the walls, bright curtains and hangings, and colourful mobiles. Children are small, so pictures on walls need to be at relevant heights, for example, the bottom of walls for children who walk into the operating room, and higher for children who arrive on a trolley. Toys, books, television and videotapes are needed, as the children often are not premedicated and play until taken into the theatre. If possible, and if the parent is adequately prepared, parents should stay with the child until the child is anaesthetised, either in an induction room or in the operating theatre itself. Toy cars are fun for children to ride in from the ward to the operating room, or trolleys dressed up as boats or other 'fun' vehicles. Operating room dress is often redundant for children and they can be admitted to the operating room in their own pyjamas or clothes (Fig. 18.15).

Ethics and the Law in Paediatric Perioperative Settings

INFORMED CONSENT

Most hospitals have rigid, mandatory policies for obtaining consent for operation from a parent before their child's surgery. It is imperative that the parents are fully informed as to the reason for the operation, what is going to happen to their child, and the risks involved (Kerridge

Fig. 18.8 • Hypospadias repair.

Fig. 18.9 • Adenoidectomy.

Fig. 18.10 • Tonsillitis.

et al 1998). By law in many countries, it is the duty of the surgeon to explain the procedure and accompanying risks (Breen et al 1997), and the anaesthetist has responsibility for explaining the anaesthetic and its implications to the patient before the operation (Australia, New Zealand College of Anaesthetists 1996). It is the nurses' responsibility to ensure that the child (if able), and the parents have been told and that they understand what has been said (Murphy 2000a). This confirmation is done preoperatively by nurses on the ward, and by the nurse who receives the patient in the operating suite. In some hospitals, it is the admitting nurse in the operating suite who must check that the consent form has been signed; in others, the child cannot leave the ward for the operating room until the consent form is signed. Except in the most extreme emergency situations, no operation can begin without a signed consent form.

In some hospitals, older children have the right to sign their own consent forms, although usually, by law, it must be countersigned by the parent. The child must understand what he or she is signing, must understand what the operative procedure is and what it is for, and must be informed of the risks involved. Any communication with a child has to be age appropriate; tools such as puppets and calico dolls are useful explanation tools.

Parents and children need to know what to expect. Even for the most informed, intelligent and knowledgeable per-

son of any age, operating theatres and procedures are frightening, anxiety-causing events. The role of the paediatric perioperative nurse is to alleviate as much anxiety as possible for both children and parents (Shields & Waterman 2002).

PRIVACY

Children's privacy can be greatly compromised within the operating theatre. Some children are far more 'body-aware' and modest than many adults and to expose them unnecessarily is to affront their personal dignity, more so if they are anaesthetised. The anaesthetised child has no control over what is happening, his or her body may be exposed for the operation and there are numbers of people within the operating theatre at any one time. Theatre suites often have little provision for private conversations and procedure boards with patients' names and details are often on view to anyone who enters the suite. Perioperative nurses must ensure that children's privacy is respected at all times. Keep the patient covered as much as possible, restrict visitors to the operating theatres, and conduct conversations about private information away from heavy traffic areas. If a surgeon briefs the family on completion of a procedure, this should be done in a separate room away from other people.

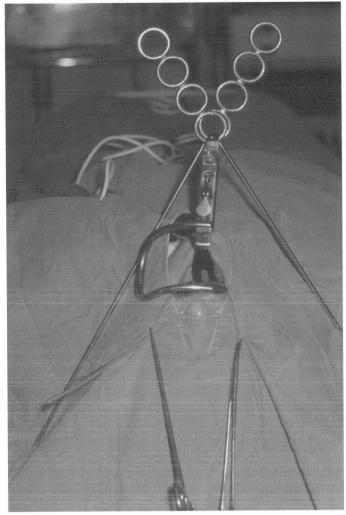

Fig. 18.11 • Patient prepared for tonsillectomy.

PATIENTS' RIGHTS

Every child, regardless of sex, race, religion or class, has the right to be cared for with dignity and respect. This is as true in the perioperative area as in any other part of a healthcare facility (Anonymous 1999). Extraordinary procedures, an alien environment, odd smells and sounds, people in bizarre clothes and strange surroundings make up the milieu of the operating room suite. Many children and parents' perceptions of an operating theatre are gained from the media, and often these are unrealistic. Some are terrified at the thought of entering such a foreign place, and anyone who comes to the operating room area requires support. Nurses have the communication skills to make children and their families less frightened by touch, reassurance, talking and explaining what is happening.

Parents and children have the right to know that their safety and spiritual, emotional and physical well-being are assured while in the care of perioperative nurses. Children often have operations for life-threatening illnesses, possibly for palliative care or to improve quality of life. Parents often accept the risks of a new procedure in the hope that their life will be improved. Nurses are most often those who recognise the fear and foreboding felt by the children and parents and are most able to support them effectively.

Children and parents from a culture different to the prevailing culture of the hospital have a right to have their religious and spiritual needs met. For example, Muslim parents will feel much more comfortable about their child having an operation for removal of a body part if they know they have the choice to decide if that body part will be given to them to dispose of according to their religious laws (Ebrahim 1995). Nurses are best situated to find out the wishes of people and to afford them the opportunity of having their wishes respected.

Children and parents always have choice and it is an important part of operating room procedure to ensure these choices are open to the patient. If, at the last minute, a patient decides that he or she cannot go through with a procedure, then those wishes must be respected. Nurses require good counselling skills to talk with the family, help address any queries and issues, and allow them to discuss the issues with the appropriate person, be it the surgeon, the anaesthetist or both. The nurse assumes the role of patient advocate and coordinates communication for the child and family so their best interests are assured.

Preadmission Programmes

Many paediatric hospitals use preadmission programmes as a means of educating the children and their caregivers about what to expect for their admission into theatre. Because this occurs before admission, it is generally in a more relaxed environment, which in turn is more conducive for child and parental education. The child may have a visit to the theatre admission area and, if possible, the recovery room, and receive an explanation as to what to expect during his or her own admission to theatre. Preadmission clinics save time on the day of surgery, particularly for day-surgery procedures, and are a means of obtaining an informed surgical consent in advance, gaining a familiarity in the theatre environment and allaying anxieties. Information sheets, particularly for day-surgery, can be given to children and parents at this stage, or posted to those unable to attend the clinic.

Activity

Search the Cochrane Library for a copy of the protocol for the review about the use of topical anaesthetics for needle insertion in children (Lander & Weltman 2003).

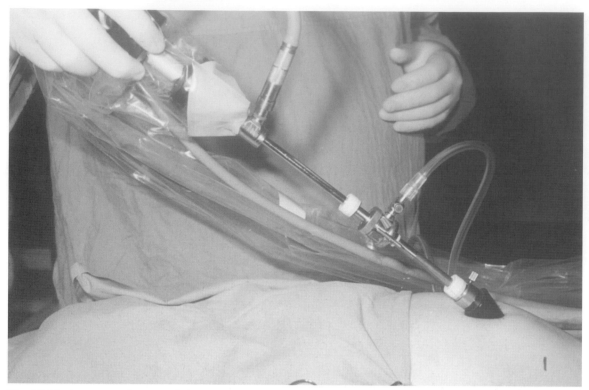

Fig. 18.12 • Laparoscopic appendicectomy.

www

Visit the Association for the Welfare of Child Health website to order their publications about parents in the operating theatre: *Parental involvement in their child's anaesthetic* (video) and *Policy relating to the provision of care for children undergoing anaesthesia*:

- http://www.awch.org.au/publications.html

www

Visit the Action for Sick Children website and see what information can be given to parents and children about going to the operating theatre:

- http://www.actionforsickchildren.org/vid-jane.html

Flow Through the Operating Rooms

1. ADMISSION: THEATRE RECEPTION

The first port of call in the operating rooms is the theatre reception area. Sometimes termed the 'holding bay', it is the public face of theatre. Unlike adults having surgery, the children, who are most often not premedicated, often walk in with their parents, may ride in on a toy vehicle, or babies may be carried in by their parents. The role of the nurse in this area is to check the incoming child to ensure the name band is labelled correctly with the correct spelling, date of birth, weight and possible allergies. The child's identification band must be checked with the accompanying notes and X-rays, scans or pathology results to ensure they match the patient. The consent is confirmed by checking both written and verbal consent and confirming the type and location of surgery that the child and family believe they are about to undergo. A preoperative checklist is completed to ensure that fasting times have been adhered to, that the presence of allergies and their reactions are documented, and that the child and their parent understands the procedure. During this admission, the nurse can ask the child and parent if they need to speak to the surgeon or anaesthetist once again before surgery. To alleviate anxieties, a relaxed, friendly, professional demeanour works best. This is the last stage for the child and their family before undergoing their anaesthetic, and can be a time of heightened emotions for both parties. Distraction works well at this time. Children's television and children's videos are often used as a distraction tool. Some operating rooms make use of volunteers, who help in play activities. Toys, books and ride-on cars and bikes can be effective. Some operating room staff encourage smaller children to ride a toy motor bike or car directly into the induction room, which keeps them distracted right up to anaesthetic induction. Of course, a quick assessment

Fig. 18.13 • A child's view from the operating table.

of the child's compliance needs to be done to ensure they can be coaxed off the bike or out of the car when it is time to do so.

2. INDUCTION

Paediatric anaesthetic induction is the process where an anaesthetist administers an anaesthetic agent either as a gas via a mask or intravenously. The child is usually cannulated to provide intravenous access essential for the anaesthetic and for the administration of emergency drugs should the child suffer laryngospasm and require emergency intubation to maintain an airway. Both processes (gas or intravenous or a combination of the two) anaesthetise the child, who is then ventilated by means of an endotracheal tube, a laryngeal mask airway or a Guedel's airway with a ventilator bag and mask. Physiological signs

Fig. 18.14 • A child's view of an anaesthetic mask.

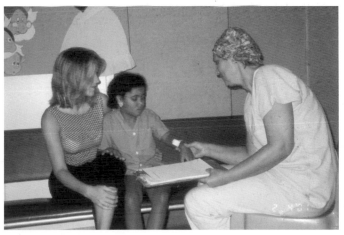

Fig. 18.15 • A child coming into the operating room in his own pyjamas.

are monitored. Electrocardiograph adhesive pads are placed on either side of the chest and one on the left flank. An oxygen saturation monitor is placed on the finger or toe so that the child can be safely monitored during surgery, and a blood pressure cuff is applied for further monitoring. The type of intubation and cannulation required depends on the type of surgery being performed. Once cannulated and intubated, the child is ready to be transferred onto the operating table and positioned appropriately for surgery.

The use of an induction room for paediatric anaesthesia is increasing. It provides a number of functions. First, based around the principles of family-centred care, it allows a parent or caregiver to accompany the child until he or she is anaesthetised, which in turn reduces the separation anxiety that may be felt by the child and parent. The presence of parents during the induction process arises from assessment of the child's developmental needs and the separation anxiety he or she might experience during traumatic events such as going to theatre. Unfamiliar faces and an unfamiliar environment impair the coping strategies in young children, and can cause feelings of vulnerability (LaRosa Nash & Murphy 1997). Adequate numbers of anaesthetic and paediatric nursing staff present facilitate case turnover, which vastly

SUMMARY RECOMMENDATIONS of THE CARLILE REVIEW
Information for parents about anaesthetic induction.
Educating parents before they accompany their child for an anaesthetic.

1. Tell the parents what is going to happen once the child arrives in the OR reception room.
2. Explain that the child will be checked for name, operation, surgeon, side of operation if relevant, allergies, any loose teeth, when the child last ate and drank, and that the consent form has been legally signed.
3. Explain that while the parent does not have to, they are allowed to accompany their child into the induction room or theatre itself until the child is fully asleep.
4. Tell the parent and child that the parent will have to don an overgown, theatre cap and overshoes before going into the theatre.
5. Explain that if the anaesthetic induction is going to be intravenous it will not hurt because the child will have had topical anaesthetic cream applied ready for the needle insertion, or it may be by use of a mask held over the child's face.
6. Allow the child and parent to hold an anaesthetic mask, to smell it and to feel what it is like on the face. Explain how the gases flow through it and that it smells 'funny'.
7. Describe the process of anaesthetic induction:
   - They will be taken into the room, the child may be placed on the operating table itself.
   - Large lights will be overhead.
   - People in the room will all have theatre gowns, hats and masks on.
   - There will be a lot of activity going on around them.
   - The anaesthetist and nurse will stay with the child and parent all the time.
   - The anaesthetist will insert the needle into the child's hand, or will place the mask over his/her face and tell them to breathe deeply, when the child is ready.
   - Describe to the parent the quick action of the induction – the child will be awake one minute and within five seconds will have gone to sleep and be limp and may appear to be not breathing. Explain that this is completely normal and everything is under complete control. THIS IS MOST IMPORTANT, as parents may become frightened to see their child go limp so rapidly.
   - Tell the parent that they will be escorted out of the theatre by a nurse and that any questions they may have will be answered.
8. Ask the child and parent if they understand what you have told them, ask them questions so you can gauge that they have understood and answer any queries they may have.

Links to Websites

Read about parent-present induction as described to parents at the Children's Hospital Boston:

http://web1.tch.harvard.edu/visiting/preparing/poparent.html

improves the turnaround time for longer lists. It also means that the instrument nurse can set up for the case in the theatre separate to the induction room. The anaesthetist is ultimately the one who decides if and when the parents can accompany their child during induction. Generally, for emergency anaesthetics when the standard fasting time is not possible, a rapid sequence induction is required and it is not common routine to have parents present.

Parental education is an effective means of reducing parental anxiety (Fig. 18.17). The provision of information during the preoperative admission process may reduce anxiety and improve understanding of the anaesthetic and surgical process (Bellew et al 2002). It is important that the accompanying adult is forewarned as to what to expect when the child is anaesthetised because, once induced, the child does not look to be merely asleep but looks lifeless. This can be extremely distressing for the parents and some will become upset and have to be escorted from the induction room. Obviously this is not the positive scenario sought during parent-present inductions.

Studies have found that it can be counterproductive to bring an anxious parent into the operating room without adequate preparation (Chan & Molassiotis 2002). Given sufficient education and reassurance before the day, and escorted immediately from the induction room once the child has received the anaesthetic agent, the process should successfully alleviate anxieties of the child by having the parent present until he or she is unconscious, and the parent is comforted by remaining with their child instead of leaving him or her among strangers (Fig. 18.16).

3. THE OPERATION

Once anaesthetised, the child is transferred from the induction room onto the operating table and is positioned as required. For example, the child may lie supine (which is the case for the majority of procedures) but could be placed prone or in a lateral position. Patient monitoring systems, such as oxygen saturation and an exhaled carbon dioxide monitor, are connected. These two non-invasive monitors provide the most valuable information to the anaesthetist regarding the child's condition during surgery (Binda & Mestad 2000). Blood pressure is monitored at regular intervals. If the surgery is major, arterial lines and central venous lines are inserted and taped securely so as not to dislodge once the child is positioned, prepared and draped. Most importantly, the airway is taped and secured and the child is not repositioned until the anaesthetist has control over the airway.

It is the instrument nurse's responsibility to check the patient's identification band with the chart, and to check the consent form. Usually, the scout nurse shows these to the instrument nurse, who is already 'scrubbed' and has set up for the case. The instrument nurse checks patient posi-

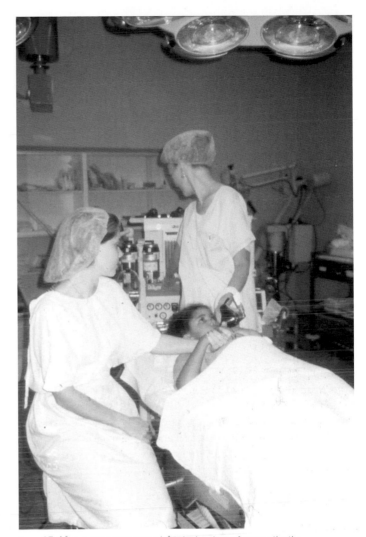

Fig. 18.16 • A parent present for induction of anaesthetic.

tioning and placement of the diathermy plate (Fig 18.17). The presence of allergies is rechecked. The child is then 'prepped' (using an antiseptic skin preparation such as aqueous betadine or chlorhexidine) and draped. Mayo tables and instrument trolleys are moved into position, suction and diathermy are connected before the surgeon puts knife to skin. The surgeon generally checks with the instrument nurse and the anaesthetist if they are ready to begin.

The instrument nurse's legal responsibility is to maintain a correct count of any instruments or swabs that have been placed in or around the wound, and to ensure that all are removed from the wound before it is closed. There are a standard three counts completed by the instrument nurse and the scout nurse together: the first before the commencement of surgery, and after all accountable items have been taken onto the sterile field. The second is completed at the initial stages of wound closure and the third when the surgeon commences closing the skin. Dressings are applied, drapes and diathermy removed and, when the anaesthetist is satisfied that the child's condition is stable, the child is extubated (unless transferring directly to intensive care intubated) and transferred to the postanaesthetic care unit (PACU).

4. POSTANAESTHETIC CARE UNIT

When the child arrives in the PACU the immediate tasks of the registered nurse are to secure the intravenous line, check that the child is breathing, ensure the airway is clear, reposition the airway (e.g. by supporting the jaw) if necessary, apply the oxygen saturation monitor, and place an oxygen mask on or next to the child's face, depending on the level of alertness and tolerance of the mask. Airway obstructions can occur in paediatric patients, particularly in those arriving deeply anaesthetised without mechanical airway support such as jaw support or a Guedel airway. Once these tasks have been done, the registered nurse checks the wound site for bleeding, assesses the pain level and documents vital signs. This process of checking, assessing and documenting is repeated at 5-min intervals for the duration of the child's stay in PACU, or less frequently if the child's condition is stable and the stay in PACU is extended. This is at the discretion of the registered nurse caring for the child. Because children's metabolism is rapid, they wake from anaesthetic much more rapidly than adults and can become quite active. For this reason, the nurse to patient ratio for paediatric recovery units is routinely 1:1.

The child remains in the PACU until he or she is awake and responsive to stimuli (such as calling his or her name), maintaining his or her own airway, oxygen saturation is satisfactory on room air, pain is fully controlled and the wound dressing remains dry and intact. If any bleeding has occurred, the wound is reinforced and if significant, reassessed by the surgeon in case the child needs to return to theatre.

Pain Management

Approximately 75% of children will say that they have considerable pain on the first day after surgery (Binda & Mestad 2000). Neonates are at risk of respiratory depression following the use of narcotics. For this reason, neonates require close monitoring if narcotics are required, preferably in an intensive care unit, and may need to remain intubated for their initial postoperative recovery. There is a greater risk of respiratory depression in any paediatric patient than in adults following narcotic use. An emergency scenario in the PACU is more likely to involve a respiratory arrest than a cardiac arrest. Close monitoring by experienced paediatric anaesthetic nursing staff is required. When the child has undergone a major or significantly painful procedure, narcotic analgesia is administered by means of a metered

dose system, which releases the prescribed amount. This can be patient-controlled analgesia (PCA) if the child is able to understand and use the device, or parent- or nurse-controlled analgesia (NCA) if the child is too young or not capable of administering a dose. Initially, these infusions may have a continuous background infusion and the parent, nurse or child can administer a bolus dose as prescribed according to a milligram per kilogram ratio. The pump is set with limits as to the number of bolus doses per hour. The child's level of pain and vital signs are closely monitored.

The role of the registered nurse in pain management is primarily one of acute assessment of the degree and severity of pain, and liaison with the anaesthetist to administer analgesics to bring the child's pain under control. Experienced paediatric nurses are essential for this assessment because children may withdraw from those around them in a response to their pain. In inexperienced hands this could be interpreted as an absence of pain. An increased understanding of the effectiveness of analgesia given as a premedication has markedly reduced the initial postoperative pain experienced by many children, particularly in the case of day-procedure surgery. In fact, pain is one of the factors inhibiting discharge following surgery and can significantly add to the health costs of day-case admissions if the child requires overnight stay for pain management.

 WWW

Examine pain management information on the internet:
- http://www.us.elsevierhealth.com/WOW/ PainAssessmentInfantsChildren.ppt
- http://www.oucher.org/the_scales.html

5. DISCHARGE FROM THE POSTANAESTHETIC CARE UNIT

Once the child has satisfied the PACU discharge requirements, including maintaining his or her own airway, satisfactory oxygen saturation on room air, controlled pain and a dry and intact wound dressing, he or she is ready to be transferred back to the wards. As with the admission of parents into the induction room, it is now becoming standard practice in many PACUs to admit the parents once their child is stable and awake. However, the same principles apply in terms of educating and preparing the parent prior to their admission to PACU and reassuring them when they see their child (Schulman et al 1967). If the parent is ill informed and not prepared for their visit to PACU they may become overcome with emotion. The role of the registered nurse is to support and explain procedural details and to outline the pain relief provided, and the location and type of dressings their child may have. Reassurance is the key word, and remaining calm, professional and friendly helps to comfort both the parent and child. The ward staff can be contacted to collect the child at the same time as the parents are invited into PACU. In this manner the parents and staff can benefit form the handover of the child's care.

Parents in the Anaesthetic Room and Postoperative Recovery

To ameliorate anxiety of both parent and child (Landers 1994, LaRosa Nash & Murphy 1996, Smerling et al 1988), many hospitals and anaesthetists encourage parental presence during anaesthetic induction (PPI). Empirical evidence confirms benefits to both child and parent (Cameron et al 1996) but it is important that parents are well prepared with thorough explanations of how their child will look as he or she becomes unconscious, that they are informed of everything that may occur, and that they are escorted from the theatre with

positive assurances (Fig. 18.18). Although research about PPI has been extensive, little research exists about the presence of parents in the PACU, but it can be assumed that similar benefits to the family accrue. Anaesthetic induction can be very rapid [Please access Fig. 18.19 at the Evolve website (http://evolve.elsevier.com/Glasper/childrensnursing)] so parents need to know what to expect, and how quickly their child can become unconscious.

PowerPoint

Access the companion PowerPoint presentation: *Ben's admission to PACU.*

STANDING ORDERS

Standing orders (Shields & Waterman 2002), i.e. orders written by a team within a unit (usually, in this case, comprised of the head anaesthetist, nurse in charge of the PACU and, if different, the nurse in charge of the operating room) are often used in situations such as PACU where the nurses work autonomously. They save time while providing safe practice guidelines for care while a child is in the unit. A sample of standing orders for the postoperative recovery of children who have had adenotonsillectomy are shown in the box titled "Sample of standing orders for child with tonsillectomy/adenoidectomy/obstructive sleep apnoea" at the end of this chapter.

DISCHARGE

Children of various ages require different strategies for discharge planning but an important factor is to ensure

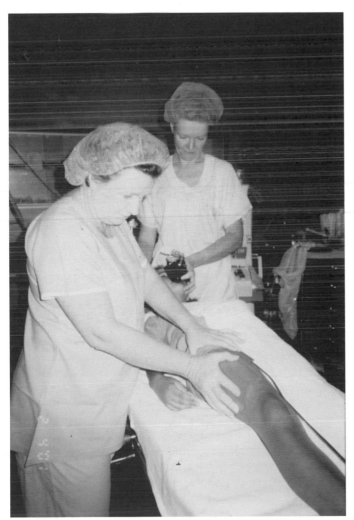

Fig. 18.17 • Positioning an anaesthetised child and applying the diathermy plate.

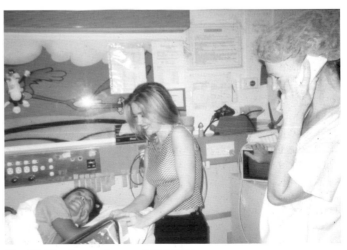

Fig. 18.18 • A parent present in PACU.

the parents are comfortable about taking the child home and that they are fully prepared to do so. Similarly, the child, if he or she is old enough, must feel secure about going home. Children of appropriate ages should be involved in all stages of planning for their care, as should their parents.

WWW

Examine the discharge planning in the paediatric clinical pathway used at Massachusetts General Hospital:

- http://www.mgh.harvard.edu/children/prof/Inpatient/Pedi%20General%20Pathway.pdf

In practical terms, discharge can be routine: when the child is awake, there is no bleeding from the wound site, the child has eaten and drunk and there is no vomiting or fever. The parents must be educated about:

- the child's care
- potential later complications
- when to call the hospital if something is wrong
- what the ward and A&E telephone numbers are
- what drugs to give and when and how
- when the child can return to a normal diet
- when the child can return to school, preschool, kindergarten or childcare
- how to identify infection
- when it is safe for the child to resume normal activity
- dressing and wound care
- potential changes in the child's behaviour relating to the hospital admission, how to recognise them and what to do about them
- appointment for the follow-up visit to the doctor or clinic.

However, with the best care in the world, things can sometimes go wrong.

PowerPoint

Access the companian PowerPoint presentation to find out what happened to Ellie during her tonsillectomy.

Issues affecting discharge planning and parental anxiety during the child's discharge from the PACU/recovery unit
I like to invite the parents into the PACU once I have established that their child's condition is stable, that the child can maintain its own airway, and that any pain has been assessed and the child has been given appropriate analgesics.

One of the most important ways for me to alleviate parental anxiety is to welcome the parents into the unit and let them know that their help in settling or comforting their child is appreciated. I like to immediately reassure them that their child is fine. I give the parents an informal handover of care, any details of the surgery will be explained to them by the surgeons, but many parents like to hear how their child was in their absence. If the child has any intravenous lines, or indwelling catheters or other drainage tubes, I point these out to the parents and, if needs be, explain what they are for. This is also the time to explain any patient-controlled analgesia, and to educate the parents as to how long the child will require the intravenous access. For example, day-surgery patients will usually return to the ward with an intravenous bung only, which the ward staff will remove before discharge.

I show the parents the dressings covering the wound site. There is often a small amount of blood or serous ooze on a freshly applied dressing after surgery, particularly if the local analgesia was given after the wound was sutured, and this initial inspection for the parents' benefit provides a timely education session as well, which includes the do's and don'ts of care of the dressing, what signs to look for (i.e. bleeding or wound infection) and the number of days they need to keep the dressing dry and intact before their follow-up surgical review. It has been my experience that the better informed about the care of their child the parents are, the less anxious they tend to be.

The PACU provides the first point of contact for the parents as to what to expect after their child's surgery and provides the initial education of care and discharge planning advice. This education needs to be reiterated by the ward staff, and the child's condition reassessed before discharge.

Discuss the paediatric nurses' role when children return to hospital for complications following surgery.

SAMPLE OF STANDING ORDERS FOR CHILD WITH TONSILLECTOMY AND ADENOIDECTOMY AND OBSTRUCTIVE SLEEP APNOEA

A sample of 'standing orders' used in PACU for children post-tonsillectomy (reproduced with the permission of Ms Lee-Anne Waterman and Greenwich Medical Media).

In the post-operative phase, a child with obstructive sleep apnoea (OSA) that has also had an ENT procedure is at risk due to post-op swelling and oedema. They should be closely monitored for signs of respiratory failure in addition to routine post-op observation.

Post-op oxygen standing orders

If a child's oxygen saturations drop below 90%:

1. Rouse the child.

2. Give oxygen if required.

3. If the child is unrousable commence resuscitation as per code procedure.

4. Call the consultant or registrar concerned.

5. 'Special' the child until review by medical staff.

N.B.   The child must not be left unattended with oxygen in situ while awaiting medical review.

Post-op pain relief orders for 'not for narcotic' children

It may be necessary for a child to be ordered narcotic pain relief and very close observation must then be undertaken for a minimum of two hours post administration. The child should be on pulse oximetry, and visual obs should include rousability and respiratory rate.

If a 'not for narcotic' child is in pain and requires stronger pain relief than ordered:

1. Call the ENT consultant or registrar concerned for a review of respiratory status and pain relief order.

2. Give pain relief as ordered.

3. Monitor oxygen saturations, respiratory rate and depth and rousability:
   - 5 minutely for 15 min
   - 15 minutely for 2 hours.

4. If oxygen saturations drop below 90%:
   - Rouse the child.
   - Give oxygen as required.
   - If unrousable commence resuscitation as per code procedure.
   - Call ENT registrar or consultant concerned.
   - 'Special' the child until medical review.

References

Alsop-Shields L 2000 Peri-operative care of children in a transcultural context. AORN Journal 71:1004–1020

Australia, New Zealand College of Anaesthetists 1996 P22 statement on patients' rights and responsibilities. Australia, New Zealand College of Anaesthetists, Melbourne. Online. Available at: http://www.anzca.edu.au/publications/profdocs/professional/p22_1996.htm

Bellew M, Atkinson K, Dixon G, Yates A 2002 The introduction of a paediatric anaesthesia information leaflet: an audit of its impact on parental anxiety and satisfaction. Paediatric Anaesthesia 12:124–130

Binda R, Mestad P 2000 Anaesthetic considerations. In: Ashcraft KW, Murphy JP, Sharp RJ et al (eds) Pediatric surgery, 3rd edn. WB Saunders, Philadelphia, pp 38–46

Blom GE 1958 The reactions of hospitalized children to illness. Pediatrics 22:590–600

Breen K, Plueckhahn V, Cordner S 1997 Ethics, law and medical practice. Allen & Unwin, St Leonards.

Cameron JA, Bond MJ, Pointer SC 1996. Reducing the anxiety of children undergoing surgery: parental presence during anaesthetic induction. Journal of Paediatric and Child Health 32:51–56

Chan C, Molassiotis A 2002 The effects of an educational programme on the anxiety and satisfaction levels of parents having parent present induction and visitation in a post anaesthesia care unit. Paediatric Anaesthesia 12:131–139

Ebrahim AF 1995 Organ transplantation: contemporary Sunni Muslim legal and ethical perspectives. Bioethics 9:291–302

Ein S 2000 Appendicectomy. In: Ashcraft KW, Murphy JP, Sharp RJ et al (eds) Pediatric surgery, 3rd edn. WB Saunders, Philadelphia

Glasper EA, Charles-Edwards I 2002 The child first and always: the registered children's nurse over 150 years. Part one. Paediatric Nursing 14:38–42

Herron A, Shields L, Tanner A, Waterman LA 2002 In: Shields L, Werder H (eds) Perioperative nursing. Greenwich Medical Media, London

Holcomb G, Wallace N 2000 Gastroschisis and omphalocele. In: Ashcraft KW, Murphy JP, Sharp RJ et al (eds) Pediatric surgery, 3rd edn. WB Saunders, Philadelphia

Homer JJ, Williams BT, Semple P et al 2000. Tonsillectomy by guillotine is less painful than by dissection. International Journal of Pediatric Otorhinolaryngology 52:25–29

Jessner L, Blom GE, Waldfogel S 1952 Emotional implications of tonsillectomy and adenoidectomy on children. Psychoanalytical Study of Children 7:126–169

Kerridge I, Lowe M, McPhee J 1998 Ethics and law for the health professions. Social Science Press, Katoomba

Koinig H 2002 Preparing parents for their child's surgery: preoperative parental information and education. Paediatric Anaesthesia 12:107–109

Lander JA, Weltman BJ 2003 Topical anaesthetics (EMLA and AMETOP creams) for reduction of pain during needle insertion in children (protocol for a Cochrane review). The Cochrane Library, Issue 3. Update Software, Oxford

Landers H 1994 Anaesthesia induction: should parents be present? Information for Nursing 25(4):10–12

Lansdown R 1992 The psychological health status of children in hospital. Journal of the Royal Society of Medicine 85:125–126

LaRosa Nash P, Murphy J 1996 A clinical case study: parent-present induction of anesthesia in children. Paediatric Nursing 22(2):109–111

LaRosa Nash P, Murphy J 1997 An approach to paediatric perioperative care; parent-present induction. Nursing Clinics of North America 32:183–198

Meeker RH, Rothrock JC 1999 Alexander's care of the patient in surgery, 11 edn. Mosby, St Louis

Montgomery WW 1996 Surgery of the nasopharynx. In: Surgery of the upper respiratory system, 3rd edn. Williams and Wilkins, Baltimore

Mooney K 1997 Perioperative management of the pediatric patient. Plastic Surgical Nursing 17:69–73

Murphy EK 2000a Preparation of the patient for the procedure: legal and ethical considerations. In: Phippen ML, Wells MP (eds) Patient care during operative and invasive procedures. WB Saunders, Philadelphia

Murphy J 2000b Hypospadius. In: Ashcraft KW, Murphy JP, Sharp RJ et al (eds) Pediatric surgery, 3rd edn. WB Saunders, Philadelphia

Nieminen P, Tolonen U, Copponen H 2000 Snoring and obstructive sleep apnea in children: a 6-month follow-up study. Archives of Otolaryngological Head and Neck Surgery 126:481–486

Oremland EK, Oremland JD 1973 The effects of hospitalization on children: models for their care. Charles C. Thomas, Springfield, MA

Price S 1994 The special needs of children. Journal of Advanced Nursing 20:227–232

Raynor S 2000 Circumcision. In: Ashcraft KW, Murphy JP, Sharp RJ et al (eds) Pediatric surgery, 3rd edn. WB Saunders, Philadelphia

Schulman JL, Foley JM, Vernon MA, Allan D 1967 A study of the effect of the mother's presence during anaesthesia induction. Pediatrics 39:111–114

Shields L, Waterman LA 2002 Psychosocial care of children in the perioperative area. In: Shields L, Werder H (eds) Perioperative nursing. Greenwich Medical Media, London

Shields L, Werder H 2002. Perioperative nursing. Greenwich Medical Media, London

Smerling AJ, Lieberman I, Rothstein P 1988 Parents' presence during the induction of anesthesia in children: parents' viewpoint. Anesthesiology 69(3A):A743

Strachan RG 1993 Emotional responses to paediatric hospitalization. Nursing Times 89(46):45–49

Weber T, Tracy T 2000 Groin hernias and hydroceles. In: Ashcraft KW, Murphy JP, Sharp RJ et al (eds) Pediatric surgery, 3rd edn. WB Saunders, Philadelphia, pp 654–662

Whaley LF, Wong DL 1995 Whaley and Wong's nursing care of infants and children 5th edn. Mosby, St Louis

Chapter Nineteen

19

Protecting Children: the Role of the Children's Nurse

Catherine Powell, Lorraine Ireland

ABSTRACT

This chapter explores the role of the children's nurse in protecting children from maltreatment. The chapter aims to equip students of children's nursing with the knowledge and understanding that will enable them to identify, and respond appropriately to, children who may be at risk of, or are actually suffering from, harm.

The chapter opens with an overview of child maltreatment that includes a definition of key terms, a discussion of the scale of the problem and a brief review of some of the theories and perspectives that seek to explain why some children and families are especially vulnerable to abuse. The chapter considers contemporary and emergent UK policy and guidance, and the way in which this impacts on nursing practice and professional responsibilities.

In taking a children's rights perspective, particular emphasis is given to the nurse's role in the prevention of maltreatment and the promotion of positive parenting skills. Child protection is a difficult and sensitive topic that touches the lives of many individuals and their families. Suggestions for accessing help and support are provided.

Learning Outcomes

- Define the major concepts associated with child protection.
- Understand the challenges of measuring the problem of child maltreatment.
- Critically review the theories that seek to explain child maltreatment.

- Assume professional responsibility in the prevention, identification and reporting of child maltreatment.
- Access help and support for child protection practice.

Introduction

> *The way in which a society treats its children is perhaps the best measure of its humanity (Lord Laming 2003)*

Child maltreatment is a major health and social problem that has recently been suggested to be the single biggest cause of morbidity in children (Hobbs 2003). For many abused children, the adverse effects on health and well-being will be life long. Furthermore, each week in the UK at least one child will die as a result of maltreatment (National Society for the Prevention of Cruelty to Children (NSPCC) 2004). There is little doubt that caring for a child who has been maltreated is one of the most difficult challenges that those working with children and families will face. It is work that is fraught with uncertainties and complexities, yet it can also be rewarding (Hall 2003).

At the time of writing this chapter, new child protection legislation is emerging following the death from maltreatment of Victoria Climbié. Victoria suffered immeasurable abuse at the hands of her great-aunt and her great-aunt's partner. In the foreword to the Inquiry Report that followed, Alan Milburn, the then Secretary of State for Health, commented that what made Victoria's death so appalling was the fact that she was in contact with many of the agencies that should have protected her. These agencies included not only social services and child protection police officers, but also two different hospitals. Health professionals, including children's nurses, who gave evidence at the inquiry, recalled serious child protection concerns (including bite marks and bruises) that at the time were neither recorded nor dealt with.

www

The Victoria Climbié Inquiry Report can be read online at:
• http://www.victoria-climbie-inquiry.org.uk/finreport/finreport.htm

This chapter aims to equip students of children's nursing with the knowledge and understanding that will enable them to identify, and respond appropriately to, children who may be at risk of, or suffering from, harm.

The chapter's underpinning philosophy reflects the words of the UK's best-known voluntary child welfare organisation, the NSPCC. This organisation acknowledges that the problem of child abuse and neglect will only be overcome when children's rights to physical and emotional integrity are respected (NSPCC 1996). We share this sentiment and hope that our readers will join with us in promoting and securing the best interests of children at individual, community and societal levels.

Definition of Key Concepts

Working at all levels to protect children requires a critical understanding of the notion of childhood, children's rights, child maltreatment and child protection. This section considers these key concepts and encourages students of children's nursing to challenge some mainstream ideas as to how children should be treated.

CHILDHOOD

Child protection activity is based on a tacit belief that children are a distinct group of vulnerable individuals who have not yet reached a certain chronological age. However, the notion of childhood (and therefore child maltreatment) is largely socially constructed and influenced by historical, social and cultural change. Although Qvortrup (1994 p 3) simply states that childhood is 'the life-space which our culture limits it to be', an analysis of contemporary childhood is an important precursor to an understanding of child maltreatment.

Activity

Discuss the nature and meaning of contemporary childhood in the UK. It may help to consider the following trigger questions:

• When does childhood start and end?
• Is childhood the 'golden age' it is often said to be?
• Are public places such as shops, pubs and restaurants 'child friendly'?
• Are school days really the 'best days of your life'?

Child protection policy in the UK rests on the legal definition of childhood that is reflected in the various Children Acts: The Children Act 1989 (England and Wales), The Children (Scotland) Act 1995 and The Children (Northern Ireland) Order 1995. Although this definition states that childhood lasts from birth to 18 years, recognition is given to the fact that action may need to be taken where there are concerns about an unborn child. Furthermore, the emerging legislation laid out in the Children Bill (House of Lords 2004) recognises that in certain circumstances (i.e. for people with learning difficulties) children's services may incorporate provision for those aged up to 25 years.

Although attainment of a chronological age is a useful parameter for defining childhood, there is clearly much more to consider. Perhaps one of the most important aspects of contemporary childhood is that it is often circumscribed in negative terms (Archard 1993). A good illustration of this is the use of the term 'childish' in our society. The following quote, although being written nearly 30 years ago, continues to reflect the subordinate and potentially damaging position of many children in the UK today:

The fact of being a 'child', of being wholly subservient and dependent on being seen by older people as a mixture of expensive nuisance, slave and super-pet, does young people more harm than good (Holt 1975 p 15)

CHILDREN'S RIGHTS

Children's rights theorists recognise the oppression of children as well as the lack of the constitutional rights that are accorded to others. Such oppression may be compared with the historical oppression of women, ethnic minorities and the proletariat. Franklin (1995) suggests that because children are politically disenfranchised they are frequently subjected to the sort of treatment that, if meted out to any other group in society, would be considered a moral outrage. Alderson (1993) illustrates this point by reflecting on the distressing circumstances that led to the death of 8-year-old Lester Chapman (Berkshire County Council 1979). Lester repeatedly ran away from home to escape daily beatings. Despite his protests, and the fact that the Police Surgeon compared his injuries with those of grievous body harm on an adult, Lester was always returned home.

The ongoing acceptance and use of corporal punishment in childhood, together with the readiness of the majority of adults to defend this practice, has been noted to be an 'obvious sign' of the low status of children (Newell 1995 p 215). Furthermore, as Alderson (1993) suggests, child maltreatment may be encouraged by beliefs about adult's rights over children's rights and the biblical notions of original sin and not sparing the rod. Powell (2002) recognises that nurses' views on the issue of corporal punishment reflect prevailing social and cultural practices. However, she also argues that the loss of extended family, community networks and increasing social isolation of young families, mean that nurses should be actively seeking opportunities to offer support, information and guidance to promote positive parenting practices.

Seminar discussion topic

At the current time, 'reasonable chastisement' remains legally acceptable in the UK. However, there is an increasing body of opinion among children's organisations that supports the view that hitting children is wrong. It is notable that all forms of physical punishment of children have been outlawed in Austria, Croatia, Cyprus, Denmark, Finland, Germany, Iceland, Israel, Latvia, Norway and Sweden. While recognising the effects of the prevailing social expectations, debate the case for a change in UK policy.

The children's rights movement is receiving support and global recognition in the inception of the United Nations (UN) Convention on the Rights of the Child, adopted by the General Assembly of the UN on 20 November 1989 (UN General Assembly 1989). The Convention, ratified by the UK in 1991, establishes a series of fundamental rights for children and young people and outlines the responsibilities of governments in ensuring that all services for children are offered in a child-centred, rights-based framework.

It is thus pleasing to see that current policy developments that influence the provision of children's services (including child protection services) are increasingly seeking to represent the views of children themselves. The recent Green Paper *Every child matters* (Department for Education and Skills (DfES) 2003) outlines proposals for the future provision of integrated services to help to support parents and carers and safeguard children from harm. Children who were consulted in the process of drawing up the paper wanted the provision of services and support that would help every child reach his or her potential, rather than a narrow set of services that intervened at times of crisis or failure. The key outcomes in childhood that are said to 'really matter' to children include: 'being healthy; staying safe; enjoying and achieving; making a positive contribution and economic well-being' (DfES 2003 p 14). Clearly, there is much to do to achieve these ideals, and children's nurses have a crucial role to play in helping to meet these important outcomes.

 www

Visit the United Nations Children's Fund (UNICEF) website to learn more about how this organisation advocates for children world-wide through facilitating the full implementation of the UN Convention of the Rights of the Child:
- http://www.unicef.org

Keep up to date with developments in the UK National Service Framework on:
- http://www.doh.gov/nsf/children

Progress on the Green Paper *Every child matters* and subsequent policy can be found on:
- http://www.dfes.gov.uk

Article 19 of the Convention provides a clear message in relation to child protection activity:

State parties shall take all appropriate legislative, administrative, social and educational measures to protect the child from all forms of physical or mental violence, injury or abuse, neglect or negligent treatment, maltreatment or exploitation, including sexual abuse, while in the care of parent(s), legal guardian(s) or any other person who has care of the child (UN General Assembly 1989)

Such protective measures should, as appropriate, include effective procedures for the establishment of social programmes to provide necessary support for the child and those who have care of the child, as well as for other forms of prevention and for identification, reporting, referral, investigation, treatment and follow-up of instances of child maltreatment.

Although 'coal-face' activity may sometimes seem far removed from the corridors of power, the child protection activities of children's nurses do reflect the essence of the above. Having considered how an understanding of the nature of childhood and children's rights thinking underpins child protection activity, the following section attempts to define child maltreatment.

CHILD MALTREATMENT: DEFINING THE PROBLEM

Defining child maltreatment is challenging and rests on historical, cultural and social contexts and beliefs, as well as the interests and concerns of the definers. As a result there are said to be 'thousands of different and conflicting definitions' (Corby 2000 p 68). The consequence of this state of affairs is that differences of opinions are a key feature of child protection work. Differences of opinion can arise amongst health professionals, between health professionals and workers from other agencies (such as Social Services or the Police Service) and, perhaps more importantly, they can arise between professionals and families and within families themselves.

Professional Conversation

Katy White is a qualified children's nurse who has been working on an acute paediatric medical ward for a number of years.

Over the years that I have been staffing on this ward we have admitted a number of children who have raised concerns about possible child maltreatment. Sometimes the issues are difficult to disentangle. For instance, we had a baby in recently whose weight was a cause for concern. I think things had not been going well for a while.

The health visitor had had difficulty finding the family at home and they did not attend the Well Baby Clinic. I believe that grandma had called the clinic to say that she was worried that her daughter was not looking after the baby properly, but that she didn't want her daughter to know about the call. In the end the Health Visitor got the baby seen by the GP, who referred him to us.

The paediatrician wanted to run some tests to see if there was an underlying cause for the poor weight gain, but we could see that the baby was simply underfed. It turned out that the mother was spending a lot of time out with her friends and leaving her baby son with a variety of babysitters, which in my mind is neglect. He also had a terrible nappy rash, which proves that he wasn't being well cared for.

However, the younger staff on the ward felt sorry for the mother, who was their sort of age and had not wanted to be tied down by a child. She was also very reluctant to come into hospital with her son and I reckoned that she was grateful for some free babysitting. A number of us felt that a child protection referral should be made, but the Social Worker thought a family support route would be better. I think we'll see that baby again.

One of the ways of approaching the difficulties in definition is to spend some time reflecting on what child maltreatment is *not*. 'Good enough parenting' is a term that can be used to describe the provision of child care that will help to ensure that the health, safety and developmental needs of children are met. Good enough parenting can be discussed in terms of the provision of care and control. Care involves anticipating children's age-appropriate needs through pre-natal care, adequate feeding, warmth and protection from harm. Control encompasses action to meet the child's safety requirements, as well as the setting of consistent limits to behaviour. Although the notion of 'control' might seem antithetical to the notion of children's rights, children

must be treated as people in their own right and the parents able to put the child's needs above their own.

Reflect on your Practice

- Is your interpretation of 'good enough parenting' congruent with that of your colleagues?
- Do you sometimes find yourself (or notice others) making negative judgements about parents' ability to parent their child?
- How can you ensure that the 'welfare of the child is paramount' when parents have a multiplicity of needs (e.g. they are trying to cope with financial difficulties, substance misuse, mental or physical health problems, domestic violence)?

Although it is helpful to consider the notion of 'good enough parenting' it is perhaps important to remember that, like child maltreatment, it is a concept that is heavily influenced by the prevailing social and cultural norms. Corby (2000) reminds us that professionals can become so accustomed to poor standards of parenting that they begin to accept them as normal, with potentially catastrophic consequences for children. Thus, although children's nurses clearly have a remit to provide culturally sensitive care and support to families, the focus on deciding whether or not a child has been maltreated should remain on the daily lived experience of the child.

The contextual nature of child maltreatment suggests that a broad sociological definition is a good starting point for determining what child maltreatment may be. The following definition, taken from a research report on prevention of maltreatment, remains one of our favourites:

Child abuse consists of anything which individuals, institutions, or processes do or fail to do which indirectly harms children or damages their prospects of safe and healthy development into adulthood (National Commission of Inquiry into the Prevention of Child Abuse (NCIPCA) 1996 p 2)

Activity

- Try and think of examples of how individuals, institutions and processes may cause significant harm in children.
- Was it difficult to reach agreement on some of the examples you raised?

Section 31-10 of the Children Act 1989 similarly recognises the importance of children's health and development in ascribing a concept of 'significant harm' to denote the threshold that justifies compulsory intervention in family life (i.e. the initiation of statutory child protection procedures). Nevertheless, no detailed definition of what constitutes 'significant harm' is given. Indeed, it has recently been suggested that:

Decisions about significant harm are complex and should be informed by a careful assessment of the child's circumstances, and discussion between the statutory agencies and with the child and family (DoH et al 2003 p 3)

The NCIPCA (1996) definition of child maltreatment and the legal concept of significant harm offer excellent vehicles with which to challenge the infringements of children's rights to physical and emotional integrity. However, their scope may be too broad for everyday practice. A more practical definition of child maltreatment, which is broadly applicable throughout the UK, is provided by government guidance in the document *Working together to safeguard children* (DoH et al 1999). Such guidance describes four 'categories' of maltreatment: physical abuse, emotional abuse, sexual abuse and neglect (*note*: there is significant comorbidity of the different types of abuse).

The document *What to do if you're worried a child is being abused* (DoH et al 2003) is a practitioner-friendly interpretation of the guidance that gives the following definitions of each of the categories:

Physical abuse may involve hitting, shaking, throwing, poisoning, burning or scalding, drowning, suffocating, or otherwise causing physical harm to a child, including by fabricating the symptoms of, or deliberately causing, ill health to a child.

Emotional abuse is the persistent emotional ill-treatment of a child such as to cause severe and persistent adverse effects on the child's emotional development. It may involve conveying to children that they are worthless or unloved, inadequate, or valued only insofar as they meet the needs of another person, age or developmentally inappropriate expectations being imposed on children, causing children frequently to feel frightened, or the exploitation or corruption of children.

Sexual abuse involves forcing or enticing a child or young person to take part in sexual activities, whether or not the child is aware of what is happening. The activities may involve physical contact, including penetrative (e.g. rape or buggery) or non-penetrative acts. They may include involving children in looking at, or in the production of, pornographic material, or encouraging children to behave in sexually inappropriate ways.

Neglect is the persistent failure to meet a child's basic physical and/or psychological needs, likely to result in the serious impairment of the child's health or development, such as failing to provide adequate food, shelter and clothing, or neglect of, or unresponsiveness to, a child's basic emotional needs (DoH et al 2003 pp 3–4)

Although the term 'diagnosis' is often used in relation to one or more of the types of maltreatment highlighted above, child maltreatment is perhaps more accurately described as a form of behaviour (Newman et al 1998) that will impact on a child's health and development. Children who are 'suffering from maltreatment' may present with overt signs of abuse that are immediately recognised (such as severe bruising in a non-mobile child) or abuse may be identified over a longer period of time (e.g. persistent failure to attend to health needs).

Identification of maltreatment will almost always depend on someone other than the child or parent recognising the problem. But this work is not easy, even for the most skilled and knowledgeable practitioner and it should never be undertaken in isolation. Thus we conclude this part of the chapter by returning to the work of Corby who notes that:

The only safe definition of child abuse is that it is a judgement reached by a group of professionals on the examination of the circumstances of the child, normally (in Britain) at a child protection conference (Corby 2000 p 70)

Activity

Are any of the following child maltreatment?*
Complete this activity alone and then discuss your responses with a partner.

	Yes	No	Not sure
A mother-to-be is using small amounts of heroin during her pregnancy			
An angry father lashes out at his child and causes minor bruising			
A teacher often tells a child that she is hopeless			
A 14-year-old girl is having sex with her 19-year-old boyfriend			
Parents with learning difficulties are feeding their small baby infrequently			
A 5-year-old frequently arrives at school without having had breakfast			
A 10-year-old is often left to care for her frail and demented grandmother			

	Yes	No	Not sure
A 14-month-old is found to have traces of cannabis resin in his urine			
A child with epilepsy has lower than expected levels of medication in his blood			
A stepfather insists on tucking his 10-year-old stepdaughter into bed – he says its their 'special time'			
A 3-year-old presents at the Emergency Department with a fractured femur – there is no clear history			
A 9-year-old with a squint has missed three appointments with an ophthalmologist			

THE SCALE OF THE PROBLEM

There is no doubt that in the UK and elsewhere child maltreatment is a major health and social problem. However, as the above section indicates, accurate measurement of the scale of the problem is hindered by complex difficulties in defining and reporting maltreatment. A balanced perspective may be that whereas fatal or grievous abuse is extremely uncommon (but newsworthy), a very large number of children have their health and development compromised by less severe, but ongoing, abusive and neglectful situations. This section considers some of the statistical evidence.

Fatal Maltreatment

Drawing on criminal statistics, the NSPCC reports that at least one child in the UK is killed every week as a result of maltreatment (NSPCC 2004). The risk of death from maltreatment is about three times greater for under-1s than for those aged between 1 and 4 years of age, with those aged 5 to 14 years facing half the risk of the 1 to 4 years age group (UNICEF 2003). With improvements to many areas of child health, deaths from maltreatment are becoming increasingly significant amongst the leading causes of death in childhood.

Some childhood deaths from maltreatment will be subject to a public inquiry, and thus become familiar to many of us through resultant press coverage (e.g. Victoria Climbié

and Lauren Wright). However, most fatal abuse cases are not made public, although in all cases where a child dies or is very seriously injured, and maltreatment is thought to have contributed to the death, a Serious Case Review will be undertaken in line with government guidance (DoH et al 1999). Here, all agencies that cared for the child will be asked to review their records of contacts and services provided to the child and their family. Because of the universal nature of health services, this process will inevitably involve health professionals and underlines the importance of good record keeping at all times. The purpose of a Serious Case Review is to establish whether there are lessons to be learnt about the way in which local professionals and agencies work together to protect children, to outline action plans as to how any lessons will be responded to and to improve local inter-agency working in the future. Serious Case Reviews are not enquiries into how a child died, or who was responsible for their death; these processes are determined by the Coroner and Criminal Courts.

Many of those working in child protection are concerned that the fatal abuse statistics underestimate the true picture. Certainly, the use of criminal statistics may not accurately identify all deaths that result from maltreatment, particularly as neglect is the leading cause of childhood deaths from maltreatment (UNICEF 2003). Current proposals to set up local 'screening groups' to review all unexpected childhood deaths (DfES et al 2003) may mean that, in the future, deaths from accidents, suicides and potentially treatable conditions such as pneumonia and gastroenteritis would be examined to ascertain whether maltreatment had played a part. Deaths resulting from diagnosed cancers or congenital abnormalities would clearly be excluded from such screening.

 Scenario

Jordan, aged 15 years, was being bullied at school for being overweight. Because of alcohol misuse and relationship difficulties, his parents were unable to provide adequate emotional support and guidance to their son. Deeply unhappy, Jordan took his own life. How should this death be classified?

Non-fatal Maltreatment

The NCIPCA (1996) report into the prevention of child maltreatment suggests a 'conservative estimate' of 1:10 of children in the UK experiencing abuse during the course of their childhood. Importantly (and at odds with a common misconception of 'stranger danger'), the NCIPCA report also recognises that most children who suffer maltreatment do so at the hands of someone that they know and trust. Although the figure of 1:10 was put forward as an estimate, a research study into the prevalence of child maltreatment has provided some evidence to substantiate this figure (Cawson et al 2000). This important and influential study is outlined in the box below.

Evidence-based Practice

Cawson et al (2000) report on the results of computer-assisted interviews on childhood experiences carried out with a random probability sample of 2869 young people, aged between 18 and 24 years and drawn from the general population. The age group was selected to overcome the problems of interviewing children, yet include those individuals close enough to childhood to be able to recall experiences of growing up. The use of computers allowed the participants to enter sensitive data and protect their confidentiality.

Some of the findings are illustrated by the analogy of a double-decker bus taking children home from school. On the bus, at least seven children would be going home to families who were not perceived as loving or close, ten children would be going home to do housework and care for parents who were incapacitated by health or social problems (including substance misuse), two or three children would be going home to face domestic violence between their parents and two or three children would be returning to a threat of physical violence and/or emotional abuse. A number of the children on the bus would be returning to several or all of these conditions.

The authors note that the study may (in common with other retrospective prevalence studies) underestimate maltreatment because events in early childhood might not be remembered.

As well as raising concerns about the prevalence of abuse, the NCIPCA (1996) report also notes that in many cases maltreatment is neither reported nor identified. The failure to recognise and report maltreatment has been a recurring feature of studies that have interviewed adult 'survivors' of abuse. The following quotes illustrate the difficulties that children may face:

I went to my doctor when I was 15 . . . and said there is something wrong with me down below . . . he just took it as needing to reassure me . . . later on I thought he might have said 'why is something troubling you?' or anything like that . . . it would have helped me say.

Somebody almost picked it up at [famous children's hospital] but they interviewed me in a room like a toilet with a gap under the door and my mother was outside and so I couldn't say; because afterwards I would have had to deal with her and why I hadn't told her (Walker 1992 pp 97–98)

The prevalence of child maltreatment and the evidence of the 'hidden nature' of the problem provide a number of important challenges to those working in the field. The Professional conversation box below gives insight into this work.

Professional Conversation

Sarah Greene is a Child Protection Nurse Specialist at a Children's Trust. Sarah has a background in health visiting and children's nursing and is the local 'Named Nurse' for child protection. Her role includes supporting and advising professionals who have child protection concerns, the development of local guidelines and policy and the provision of training to a wide variety of health care staff. Sarah has been involved in three Serious Case Reviews.

The evidence base for child maltreatment is important in underpinning good practice. I try and encourage a broad awareness of the prevalence of the problem and ensure that practitioners explicitly 'rule out' possible abuse as part of their decision-making, particularly when children present with unusual or vague histories. I promote the value and importance of listening to children and advocate for the provision of opportunities for children to speak to us alone.

I am particularly conscious of the prevalence of maltreatment when I am facilitating a training session. Out of the 20 or so staff in attendance you have to remember the possibility that two people could have suffered an abusive or neglectful childhood – sometimes the sessions bring up issues that may have been hidden or never disclosed at the time. I always try and ensure that support is available for those who need it.

One of the difficulties for people who have experienced maltreatment is that such individuals may find themselves unwilling/unable to become involved in cases they might meet in the course of their work. If this is the case, it is an issue that other staff may need to recognise and respect. However, it is vitally important that no children who use our services fall through the safety net. Above all we encourage an open and supportive way of working that means that concerns can be identified and shared and measures put in place to safeguard the child.

OFFICIAL STATISTICS

A further source of statistics that may underpin our knowledge of child protection is the number of children who are on Local Authority Child Protection Registers (see below). These figures are published each year as a point prevalence statistic (i.e. how many children are on the register on a particular date). Although the figures may indicate some useful trends, we urge our readers to remember that the Child Protection Register is dynamic (with names being added and removed on a daily basis) and that the names held represent only those children who have identified, current and unresolved child protection concerns. Such concerns may include the notion of being 'at risk' rather than suffering from 'actual harm', hence the register is sometimes referred to as the 'At Risk' Register.

The DfES website recorded a total of 26,600 children whose names were on Child Protection Registers as of 31 March 2003. This figure represents a rate of 24 children per 10,000 of the population and is for England only. Although the figure showed a small increase from the previous year, it is lower than the rate 5 years previously. If the figures are broken down by category of maltreatment (see the section on definitions above) these are as follows:

- neglect: 39%
- physical abuse: 19%
- sexual abuse: 10%
- emotional abuse: 18%
- mixed categories: 15%.

This section has attempted to portray the scale of the problem of child maltreatment. We have noted the impact of the difficulties of definition and the hidden nature of childhood abuse as fundamental to the challenge of portraying the scale of the problem with any great accuracy. However, we have seen that neglect (i.e. where there are acts of omission by parents and carers) features highly both in terms of its links with fatal maltreatment and as the leading reason for children to have their names on the Child Protection Registers.

Theories of Maltreatment

Children's nurses pride themselves on being able to work openly and in partnership with children and their families. Clearly, when children require healthcare services and maltreatment (perpetrated by a parent or someone acting in that role) is suspected, the dynamics of this relationship will be compromised.

Two important points need stressing here: first, that the majority of children who suffer maltreatment will be returned to their families (albeit with the provision of services to monitor and safeguard their future well-being); second, that in many instances there will be a non-abusive parent who will be both witnessing the unnecessary suffering of their child and coming to terms with the fact that a much-loved spouse or partner may have perpetrated this event. An understanding of the aetiology of maltreatment may help the nurse to provide sensitive and supportive care to all the family.

Corby (2000) suggests that three main groups of theories seek to explain the causation of child abuse: psychological; social psychological and sociological. Within these groupings, a variety of ideas are proposed. These include such disparate theories as the survival instinct of the sociobiological school, the acceptance of intrafamilial violence of the social-cultural theorists and the institutionalisation of male power proposed by the radical feminists. However, as Corby recognises, there is an inherent danger to adopting single-cause explanations of the problem. What seems to be becoming more widely accepted is the notion of an integrated approach to understanding child maltreatment. Such an approach was postulated by Belsky (1993), whose ecological model recognises the dynamic and mutually dependent nature of individual characteristics, interactions within families, the social environment and the broader structural factors (such as societal attitudes to violence). Hence, the way in which these different levels interact with each other at specific moments in time will affect the likelihood of maltreatment (or not). An understanding of the ecological model of abuse may be useful in helping practitioners overcome prejudices and lessen the likelihood of apportion of blame to the vulnerable and needy individuals who find themselves unwontedly harming their children.

Scenario

Jade, a preterm baby now aged 6 weeks, has been admitted to the Paediatric Intensive Care Unit after suffering a subdural bleed. Her condition is giving cause for concern and it is feared that she has suffered irreversible brain damage. Gemma, Jade's mother, has reported that Jade cried a great deal and that she was often anxious about upsetting the neighbours in the bed-sit where she has been living since being thrown out of her childhood home by her mother and stepfather. Jade's father is a known drug user who has a number of other children. He is not allowed to visit the Children's Unit because he has been violent towards staff on another occasion. Gemma reports that she is depressed and lonely and that life with Jade has been a 'struggle'. She denies harming her. The health visitor has only managed to visit once because she is covering the caseload of a sick colleague.

Risk Factors for Child Maltreatment

In an effort to apply theory to practice, a number of researchers have attempted to draw up checklists of risk factors (or vulnerability) for child maltreatment (e.g. see Browne et al 1988). However, as the researchers themselves acknowledge, this work is beset with difficulties that include high rates of false positives and the dangers of 'labelling' families. There is always a need to recognise that information gathering and assessment should balance the positive aspects of children's lived experiences against any possible concerns. However, some risk factors are worthy of special consideration here.

The particular vulnerability of children with disabilities to abuse and neglect is being increasingly recognised. A report by the National Working Group on Child Protection and Disability (2003) suggested that this vulnerability may be a result of a number of factors. These include societal attitudes and assumptions (e.g. disabled children are not abused), inadequacies in service provision (e.g. communication systems that lack the language necessary to disclose abuse) and factors associated with impairment (e.g. the need for intimate care that may increase the risk of exposure to abusive behaviour).

Reflect on your Practice

- Children with disabilities are frequent users of community and hospital health services.
- How well are their special needs met?

Although children with disabilities represent an important group of vulnerable children, other groups have been identified. *Safeguarding children* (DoH et al 1999) outlines four key 'sources of stress for children and families' that impact on the health and development of children and lead to situations where children may suffer significant harm:

- Social exclusion: caused by factors such as poverty, poor housing and racism.
- Domestic violence: including the threat to an unborn child where kicks and punches may be directed to the mother's abdomen.
- Mental illness in the parent or carer: including the effects of postnatal depression.
- Drug and alcohol misuse: including harm caused by maternal transmission of substances during pregnancy and the diminished parenting capacity of those under the influence of drugs and/or alcohol.

Children's nurses and others may be in a position to recognise these factors and offer early intervention and support to help to ensure the best outcomes for the child.

Research has tended to show a social class bias towards higher rates of child maltreatment in social classes D and E. However, it is important to remember that abuse and neglect feature across the social spectrum. Indeed, the authors of this chapter know of cases of overt child maltreatment, where there has been reluctance amongst health professionals to refer the case to Statutory Agencies simply because of the social standing of the parents. Likewise, although recognising that child maltreatment is more common amongst families on low incomes, Cawson et al (2000) suggest that the highest rates of *undetected* child maltreatment may rest in the professional classes.

In conclusion, this section has aimed to provide a brief overview of the factors that may cause a child to be maltreated. However, best practice rests on being open to a possibility of maltreatment in all contacts with children and, where age and developmental status allow it, listening to what the child has to say.

Professional Responsibilities

This section considers the professional responsibilities of the nurse in safeguarding children and promoting their welfare. Before moving on to discuss the recognition and referral of child maltreatment, we will consider ways in which children's nurses may support vulnerable children and their parents and thus potentially help to prevent maltreatment.

CHILDREN IN NEED

Children who are defined as 'children in need' under the Children Act 1989 (Section 17) are those who need extra support and services to help them reach or maintain a satisfactory level of health and development. Such children will include those with chronic health conditions, physical disabilities and learning differences, as well as those living in poor socio-economic circumstances.

Students of children's nursing will gain valuable experience of family life and the provision of health and social services when undertaking their community placement. It is important that children's nurses seek and maintain links with health visitors, school nursing services and hospital social workers, and know how to refer children and families in need of extra health, social or financial support. For children with complex needs, discharge planning should take into account the need to coordinate a range of services.

In recent times there has been greater investment in the provision of services for children in need. New services include early years' education and child care through the Sure Start programme, the setting up of a range of local projects for 5- to 13-year-olds supported by Children's Fund moneys and the creation of Connexions to provide advice, guidance and personal development opportunities for young people aged 13–19 years.

Activity

Find the details of any local Sure Start, Children's Fund and Connexions in your area. If possible, arrange to visit these projects and find out how children, young people and their families can access these services.

SUPPORT IN THE PARENTING ROLE

Children's nurses may also be in a position whereby they can help to advise and support parents on aspects of child care, thus reducing stress and possibly helping to reduce the likelihood of maltreatment. The falling birth-rate and increasing social isolation of young families, combined with geographical mobility, mean that many adults have extremely limited experience of child care before embarking upon parenthood. Children's nurses are well-placed to advise parents on normal development (e.g. when it is reasonable to expect a child to be clean and dry), positive parenting techniques (i.e. rewarding good behaviour and ignoring bad behaviour) and the benefits of play. Sometimes, however, it is just a sympathetic ear that is needed. As Wilczynski (1997 p 103) succinctly comments:

Parenting can be a very exhausting and stressful task even for the most ideal of candidates.

RECOGNITION OF CHILD MALTREATMENT

Children who have been maltreated may present for health care following a single traumatic event (such as a shake injury) or as a result of the compilation of a number of significant events, which may include neglect of healthcare needs. Child maltreatment may also be suspected during the course of a hospital admission or other encounters with health professionals for unrelated problems. Physical indicators of possible child maltreatment include bruising, bite marks, burns, scalds and fractures. Behavioural indicators include age-inappropriate behaviour, self-harm, wariness of certain individuals and 'frozen watchfulness'. A full review of physical and behavioural indicators of maltreatment is provided by Hobbs et al (1999).

Although there are no indicators that are 100% 'diagnostic' of maltreatment, it is important to carefully evaluate each child's history and presentation, taking into account their developmental needs and abilities.

Scenario

Scott, a 10-week-old baby, was seen in the Emergency Department with a cut above his left eye. He was accompanied by his mother, who explained that he had been out with his father that morning and managed to fall out of the buggy. On examination, bruising was noticed on Scott's abdomen.

Delays in presentation and inconsistencies in history giving are suspicious for maltreatment. Injuries of differing ages and repeated presentation to healthcare professionals are also of concern. Wherever possible, the child should be asked to give his or her own history. In some cases, children will spontaneously disclose abuse and, if this happens, it is vitally important that the child is allowed to talk freely, not openly questioned (this may affect criminal procedures), and that detailed, contemporaneous records are kept.

Fabricated or induced illness (FII) is a relatively rare, but important, form of child maltreatment that sometimes leads to the death of a child. Here, carers (usually the mother) repeatedly present the child to healthcare professionals with falsified accounts of various signs and symptoms. The child may then undergo multiple investigations (which in themselves may be harmful) without a firm diagnosis being reached. In more severe cases, symptoms are induced through the misuse of medication or other substances (e.g. table salt) or hospital equipment, such as infusion lines, might be tampered with. FII is a form of abuse that can be very difficult to detect but concerns relating to a possibility of this type of maltreatment should be managed within interagency child protection procedures (DoH 2002). Health professionals who have unwittingly colluded with perpetrators of this type of harm will themselves need support through activities such as 'debriefing' (Terry 2004).

Recognition of maltreatment often relies on a professional's 'gut feeling' that all is not well. In all cases it is important to check concerns with a senior colleague and to keep accurate records. Reviewing past records and history may also be helpful, as will informal discussions with other professionals who have contact with the child and family.

RESPONDING AND REFERRAL

Although it may well be a nurse who identifies possible indicators of child maltreatment, the decision to make a child protection referral to Social Services will normally be made by a senior paediatrician following careful evaluation of the child's presentation and history. Because nurses spend more time with patients there may be situations in which interprofessional disagreements arise. In these instances it is wise to seek the help of local child protection specialists (such as Named Professionals) to help to resolve differences in opinion and to ensure the child's welfare.

Social Services will undertake an initial assessment and make a decision as to whether they believe that the child is at risk of, or suffering, actual significant harm. If this is the case they will call a Strategy Discussion, which will involve the Police and other relevant agencies. This process can take up to 7 working days but may be more immediate if there are urgent concerns about a child's welfare and a need for urgent protective measures. Should the Strategy Discussion lead to a decision that there are concerns about a child's safety then a full inquiry (under Section 47 of the Children Act 1989) will be undertaken. A social work manager will be responsible for convening a Child Protection Conference within 15 working days of the Strategy Discussion, if the enquiries substantiate the concerns. The purpose of a Child Protection Conference is to decide whether the child is at continuing risk of harm and if so, to place his or her name on the Child Protection Register and draw up plans to safeguard him or her from the risk of further harm. Alongside the child protection procedures, the Police may undertake a criminal investigation. This may involve undertaking a joint interview with the child.

Children's nurses and other health professionals will be invited to contribute to the above proceedings. In doing so they may be required to share confidential information without the consent of the patient or client. Although the Nursing and Midwifery Council's (NMC) Code of Professional Conduct (2002) requires nurses to protect confidential information, provision is made for nurses to act in the public interest and in accordance with national and local child protection policies (NMC 2002 Section 5.3 pp 7–8).

Child protection procedures involve detailed interagency working and rest on the principles of openness and partnership with children and their families. The document *What to do if you're worried a child is being abused* (DoH et al 2003) provides more detailed guidance on procedures, although imminent legislation in the wake of the Victoria Climbié Inquiry may lead to new guidance.

Summary

The chapter has aimed to equip students of children's nursing with the knowledge and understanding that will enable them to identify, and respond appropriately to, children who may be at risk of, or suffering from, harm. We hope that this work will give future children's nurses confidence in their abilities to be part of this important area of child health. The emphasis on the rights of the child has been deliberate – children's nurses will work with many vulnerable and needy families in the course of their practice. To lose the focus on the daily lived experience of the child is

to court the possibility of another child maltreatment tragedy. We wish you well.

Child Protection Helplines and Websites

Childline (24 hours): 0800 1111; http://www.childline.org.uk/

Contact-A-Family (9 a.m. to 5 p.m. Monday to Friday): support for parents of children with disabilities: 020 7222 2695; http://www.cafamily.org.uk/

Cry-sis (9 a.m. to 5 p.m. Monday to Friday): persistently crying and/or sleepless babies: 020 7404 5011; http://www.cry-sis.com/

Family Rights Group (1.30 p.m. to 3.30 p.m. Monday to Friday): support with child protection procedures: 020 7249 0008; http://www.frg.org.uk/index.asp

Kidscape (9.30 a.m. to 5 p.m. Monday and Wednesday): deals with bullying, stranger danger, threats of abuse: 020 7730 3300; http://www.kidscape.org.uk/

NCH Action for Children: 01772 25492; http://www.nchafc.org.uk/

NSPCC Child Protection Line (24 hours): acts in cases of neglect and abuse of children: 0808 800 500; help@nspcc.org.uk

National Association for People Abused in Childhood (NAPAC): for adult survivors of abuse: 0800 085 3330; http://www.napac.org.uk/

Respond: sexual abuse and people with learning disabilities: 0845 606 1503; http://www.respond.org.uk/

Survivors (Incest): 020 7833 3737; http://www.survivors.org.uk/

Women's Aid: emergency accommodation for abused women and children: 0117 963 3542; http://www.womensaid.org.uk/

References

Alderson P 1993 Children's consent to surgery. Open University Press, Buckingham

Archard D 1993 Children: rights and childhood. Routledge, London

Belsky J 1993 Etiology of child maltreatment: a developmental-ecological analysis. Psychological Bulletin 114(3):413–434

Berkshire County Council 1979 Lester Chapman inquiry report. Berkshire County Council, Reading

Browne K, Davies C, Stratton P (eds) 1988 Early prediction and prevention of child abuse. John Wiley, Chichester

Cawson P, Wattam C, Brooker S, Kelly G 2000 Child maltreatment in the United Kingdom: a study of the prevalence of child abuse and neglect. NSPCC, London

Corby B 2000 Child abuse: towards a knowledge base, 2nd edn. Open University Press, Buckingham

Department for Education and Skills (DfES) 2003 Every child matters. The Stationery Office, London. Online. Available at: http://www.dfes.gov.uk/everychildmatters/pdfs/EveryChildMatters.pdf

Department for Education and Skills (DfES), Department of Health (DoH), Home Office (2003) Keeping children safe: the government's response to the Victoria Climbié inquiry report and joint chief inspectors' report safeguarding children. The Stationery Office, London

Department of Health (DoH) 2002 Safeguarding children in whom illness is fabricated or induced. DoH, London

Department of Health (DoH), Home Office, Department for Education and Employment (DfEE) 1999 Working together to safeguard children: a guide to inter-agency working to safeguard and promote the welfare of children. DoH, London

Department of Health (DoH), Home Office, Department for Education and Skills (DfES) 2003 What to do if you're worried a child is being abused. DoH, London

Franklin B (ed.) 1995 The handbook of children's rights. Routledge, London

Hall D 2003 Protecting children, supporting professionals. Archives of Disease in Childhood 88:557–559

Hobbs C 2003 In: Department for Education and Skills (DfES), Department of Health (DoH), Home Office (2003) Keeping children safe: the government's response to the Victoria Climbié inquiry report and joint chief inspectors' report safeguarding children. The Stationery Office, London

Hobbs C, Hanks H, Wynne J 1999 Child abuse and neglect: a clinician's handbook, 2nd edn. Churchill Livingstone, London

Holt J 1975 Escape from childhood: the needs and rights of children. Penguin, Harmondsworth

House of Lords 2004 Children Bill. The Stationery Office, London

Lord Laming 2003 The Victoria Climbié inquiry: report of an inquiry by Lord Laming. The Victoria Climbié Inquiry. Online. Available at: http://www.victoria-climbie-inquiry.org.uk/finreport/finreport.htm

National Commission of Inquiry into the Prevention of Child Abuse (NCIPCA) 1996 Childhood matters, vol I and II. Stationery Office, London.

National Society for the Prevention of Cruelty to Children (NSPCC) 1996 A cry for children campaign: child protection agenda. NSPCC, London

National Society for the Prevention of Cruelty to Children (NSPCC) 2004 Online. Available at: http://www.nspcc.org.uk/

National Working Group on Child Protection and Disability 2003 It doesn't happen to disabled children. Child protection and disabled children. NSPCC, London

Newell P 1995 Respecting children's rights to physical integrity. In: Franklin B (ed.) 1995 The handbook of children's rights. Routledge, London, pp 215–226

Newman M, Otvos B, Harris-Hendriks J 1998 Evaluating the risks to children. In: Dent RJ (ed.) Dangerous care: working to protect children. The Bridge Child Care Development Service, London, pp 22–27

Nursing and Midwifery Council (NMC) 2002 Code of professional conduct. NMC, London

Powell C 2002 There is no such thing as a child receiving 'a good smack'. British Journal of Nursing 11(22):1425

Qvortrup J 1994 Introduction. In: Qvortrup J, Bardy M, Sgritta G, Wintersberger H (eds) Childhood matters: social theory, practice and politics. Avebury, Aldershot, pp 1–23

Terry L 2004 Fabricated or induced illness of children. Paediatric Nursing 16(1):14–18

United Nations General Assembly 1989 Convention on the rights of the child. UNICEF, Geneva

United Nations Children's Fund (UNICEF) 2003 A league table of child maltreatment deaths in rich nations. Innocenti Report Card No. 5. UNICEF Innocenti Research Centre, Florence. Online. Available at: http:// www.unicef-icdc.org

Walker M 1992 Surviving secrets. Open University Press, Buckingham

Wilczynski A 1997 Child homicide. Greenwich Medical Media, London

Chapter Twenty

20

Ethics in Children's Nursing

E Alan Glasper, Jim Richardson

ABSTRACT

The primary aim of this chapter is to examine, within the context of recent developments in child health practice and research, some underlying ethical demands and dilemmas facing children's nurses. A description of the Nuremberg Code, the Helsinki Declaration, The UN Convention on the Rights of the Child and the Human Rights Act will form the backdrop to this chapter and a range of contemporary examples will be used to illuminate these issues. Within this arena, the four major principles that underpin healthcare ethics will be investigated and past examples of historical unethical practice and research acknowledged. The vulnerability of children and their families to potential coercion and the role of research ethics committees will be discussed.

Learning Outcomes

- Achieve an overview of the major ethical principles in child health care.

- Recognise how these principles can be applied in everyday child health nursing.

- Appreciate dimensions surrounding some ethical controversies in relation to research involving children.

Introduction

It might appear to the newly qualified children's nurse that the recent history of the profession is tarnished with examples of unethical healthcare practice and violation of basic human rights. With no less than four major official investigations related to ethical aspects of childcare published since the start of the 21st century (NHS Executive 2000, DoH 2001a,b, National Assembly for Wales 2002) it can be appreciated that urgent action is necessary to restore public confidence in the NHS. However, before examining contemporary issues related to child health care it is worth remembering that it was the activities of German healthcare professionals during the years of the Second World War that finally galvanised an exhausted post-war world to do something about unethical healthcare practice and research. When the full scale of the dreadful experiments carried out on human beings, including children, against their will became fully known, perpetrators were prosecuted at the trials in Nuremberg, although not all were severely punished. In the wake of the Nuremberg trials, a code of practice was developed that became subsequently known as the Nuremberg Code (Eby 1995).

 WWW

Read the Nuremberg Code online at:
- http://www.ohsr.od.nih.gov/nuremberg.php3

The Nuremberg Code particularly related to the ethical conduct of research. Although the elements that make up valid consent are the same in consent to research as in consent to treatment (information, capacity and freedom from coercion), research carries two extra dimensions that increase the potential vulnerability of research subjects to exploitation: (i) research may be risky and the potential benefit to the subject might be slight, unknown or absent; and (ii) the aims of the research may conflict with the therapeutic aims of treatment.

The Nuremberg Code and Past Unethical Practice

Ten key directives are highlighted, which pertain to the conduct of human experimentation. These include:

- That the voluntary consent of the human subject is absolutely essential.

- That the experiment should be designed to yield fruitful results for the benefit of society. The experiment should avoid all unnecessary physical and mental suffering and injury.

- No experiment should be conducted where there is reason to believe that death or disabling injury will occur except perhaps where the experimenters themselves serve as subjects.

- The degree of risk should never exceed the humanitarian importance of the problem to be solved through the research. Adequate facilities should be provided to protect the experimental subject from injury, disability or death.

- Experiments should be carried out only by appropriately qualified persons.

- Human subjects should be able to terminate the experiment whenever they wish.

- During the experiment, the principal investigator must be prepared to terminate the experiment at any stage if there is reason to believe that continuation is likely to result in injury, disability or death of a subject.

Despite the universal condemnation of the German atrocities committed in the name of scientific progress, unethical research on human beings has, unfortunately, continued. Perhaps the most flagrant abuse of human rights during a longitudinal government-sponsored medical investigation occurred in the USA between the years 1932 and 1972 during the Tuskegee syphilis study.

 WWW

You can find out more about this infamous research at:
- http://www.med.virginia.edu/hs-library/historical/apology/index.html

In the study, 399 African-American men were denied treatment for syphilis; they were deceived by public health officials who were fully aware that effective treatment was available. Such has been the damage to the US government's reputation that it was necessary, in 1997, for the then President to issue a formal apology on behalf of the nation. Although the presidential words may have closed one chapter in the catalogue of human rights abuses, it would be naïve to believe that unethical research is currently not being conducted. A report in the *Lancet* (1997)

revealed that the US Centre for Disease Control had supported unethical trials of new drugs for the treatment of human immunodeficiency virus (HIV), in which a placebo group of women were allowed to infect their children perinatally. These examples demonstrate the particular vulnerability of certain groups to exploitation. Children are a classic example of such a group.

The Helsinki Declaration

Although the Nuremberg Code is explicit in its recommendations for healthcare researchers, the Tuskegee scandal demonstrated that harm was still being done in the name of good. The World Medical Association therefore adopted the recommendations contained in the document *Guiding physicians in biomedical research involving human subjects* at the 18th World Medical Assembly in Helsinki, Finland, in June 1964. This 'Helsinki Declaration' was subsequently amended several times, the last being at the World Medical Association General Assembly in Edinburgh in October 2000. Importantly, the Helsinki Declaration highlights the necessity of obtaining informed consent. Additionally, it advises caution if the research subject is in a dependent relationship with the researcher or if the individual might consent under duress. This is particularly pertinent for children's nurses, who purport to act as advocates for the family while also contributing to the research process.

The Declaration uses the term 'legal incompetence', whereby physical or mental incapacity makes it impossible to obtain informed consent or when the subject is a minor. In these cases the Helsinki protocol recommends the gaining of permission from a responsible relative. Although this is advocated, importantly the gaining of consent from the child is stressed in addition to that of the minor's legal guardian.

The UN Convention on the Rights of the Child and the Human Rights Act

The General Assembly of the United Nations adopted the convention on the Rights of the Child in November 1989; this came into force in the UK in January 1992.

 WWW

You can access the UN Convention at:
- http://www.unhcr.ch/html/menu3/b/k2crc.htm

 Activity

Read through the summary of the Convention on the Rights of the Child. Make notes against each article on its relevance to:

- research involving children
- clinical children's nursing practice.

When you have done this, consider to what extent the requirements of these two fields of practice differ from each other in their ethical requirements.

The UK's second report to The UN Committee on the Rights of the Child (DoH 1999) demonstrated that considerable effort was being made to meet the UN targets. However, UNICEF suggests that the government's 1999 report is 'little more than an uncritical review of aspects of government policy related to children' (UNICEF 2000).

The Human Rights Act of 1998, which came into effect on 2 October 2000 highlighted the potential of some areas of health and social care practice to affect the rights and freedoms promised under the Act. Power (2002) discusses Article 3, among others, of the Act, which relates to torture and degrading treatment or punishment and highlights the implications for child health nurses, especially when restraining children for healthcare interventions.

www

You can find the text of the Human Rights Act at:
- http://www.doh.gov.uk/humanrights/qa.htm

The implementation of these policies is beginning to impact on the way in which children are cared for in hospital and the Child Friendly Hospital Initiative spearheaded by UNICEF has been embraced by a number of children's hospitals in the UK such as The Royal Hospital For Sick Children Glasgow.

www

You can details of the Child Friendly Hospital initiative at:
- http://www.childfriendlyhealthcare.org

The Four Principles of Healthcare Ethics

Although the NMC Code of Professional Conduct (NMC 2002) provides explicit guidance on consent for all nurses, Section 3.9 discusses children in particular. Additionally the Royal College of Nursing (RCN) has issued guidelines for nurses involved with research (RCN 1977). These and other guidelines implicitly or explicitly use the four principles of healthcare ethics first proposed by Beauchamp & Childress in 1979.

1. AUTONOMY

The primary interpretation of this word is self-determination. The complexity of this concept is increased by its link with liberty. Personal liberty, although a common value of Western life, may have different value in other countries and other social groups, where decisions may be made by a group, such as a family, rather than espousing individual rights. Autonomy and childhood have in the past been perceived as mutually exclusive but there is now a growing awareness that children are able to make their own decisions if given information in an age-appropriate manner (Alderson 2000, British Medical Association (BMA) 2001).

When the term 'autonomy' is applied to contemporary healthcare practice and research the focus is on the right to informed consent (Behi 1995). Although every individual has this right, it must be appreciated that some, but especially children, may not be able to articulate this or may be prevented from doing so. The Gillick case (*Gillick v West Norfolk and Wisbech AHA* [1986]), in which a mother unsuccessfully challenged the legal right of doctors to withhold information about their advice and treatment of a minor from parents when it was thought to be in the young person's best interest, was a high-water mark in the enfranchisement of children (Alderson & Montgomery 1996). Since then, children who are deemed competent in line with 'Fraser guidelines' are, in the eyes of the law, able to make informed choices. When this conveniently matches the decision of the healthcare professional or guardian, this inclusion in decision making is seen as an example of good practice. When it does not, the rights of the child may be diluted on the basis that adults know best. Although this paternalistic approach within both treatment and research is in decline, competent children remain a group whose rights to consent or refuse consent are easy to overlook.

In the case of younger, pre-autonomous children, respect for autonomy is shown by ensuring that parents agree to give proxy consent to treatment and research. The cases detailed below demonstrate the loving commitment of parents to the well-being of their child and their deep sense of betrayal if their child is harmed by health professionals.

Scenario

14-year-old Sam has been suffering from lethargy, unusual tiredness and a tendency to bruise easily. Bloods drawn by his GP have yielded a very pathological result. Sam needs further investigation for a potentially serious illness. He absolutely refuses to tell his parents about this situation or to allow his parents to be told by a member of the care team.

Activity

Consider the factors to be taken into account in judging whether Sam is mature enough to make this decision alone. What are the ethical requirements of this situation, e.g. what are the rights and responsibilities of all the players in this scenario?

2. BENEFICENCE

Beneficence means the duty to do good to others, to act in their best interests. However, if this principle was universal and we were required always to do good to everyone, the duty would be too onerous. Beneficence is a constituent part of a special duty of care such as that which exists between a nurse and patient or between a parent and child (Charles-Edwards 1995). Cases such as that of the GP Harold Shipman are particularly horrifying because of the breach of this duty of care.

One of the ambiguities at the heart of health care is the duty to act in the patient's best interests while avoiding the danger of following only the principle of beneficence and ignoring that of autonomy; 'the doctor knows best' phenomenon. The contemporary insistence that patient (and parent) must be given an informed choice attests to this and to the anachronism of paternalistic attitudes: 'Partnership between patient and healthcare professional is the way forward' (Kennedy 2001 p 13).

3. NON-MALEFICENCE

Florence Nightingale is reported to have said 'first do the patient no harm' and non-maleficence simply means to do no harm. However, this has to be tempered with the reality that inadvertent harm may befall a child during a caring intervention, which may not have been foreseen. Iatrogenic illness or illness precipitated by medical treatment is now a common cause of death and was first highlighted 25 years ago by Ivan Illich (1977). It is the duty of every nurse to avoid harming others, and this is reflected in the use of policies, procedures and protocols that are designed to minimise this. Some hospitals include this philosophy in their mission statements, e.g. The Great Ormond Street Hospital for Children has as its motto 'The child first and always'.

4. JUSTICE

When applied to health care, justice is used in the context of an equitable use of healthcare resources. There is consequently a dichotomy between wanting to give the best for each patient (beneficence) and the recognition of competition for scarce resources among the whole of the client group. In the 1995 court case of Child B or Jaymee Bowen (*R v Cambridge Health Authority, ex parte B* [1995]) the principle of justice was at the heart of the controversy as

portrayed by the media (Ham & Pickard 1998). Jaymee was aged 10 at the time and had suffered from acute lymphoblastic leukaemia, which she had developed at the age of 5 and for which she had a successful bone marrow transplant. She was admitted to hospital with acute myeloid leukaemia. Senior childhood cancer consultants advised against treatment believing it not to be in the child's best interests. Her father refused to accept this decision and sought other opinions. A London-based consultant offered to treat the child in the private sector at a cost of £75,000. The local health authority refused to underwrite the cost and the father started legal action, which was not successful. The case attracted much publicity and an anonymous benefactor eventually paid for the treatment. Sadly, the treatment did not have the lasting effects hoped for and Jaymee died just 17 months later. The case was cited as an example of healthcare rationing, now widely referred to as 'postcode health care', although the high-risk, low-benefit outcome of the proposed treatment was central to the medical decision that further treatment would be futile. The ethical dilemmas presented by participation in experimental treatment, such as that proposed in Jaymee's case, and not underpinned by peer-reviewed published evidence will always be problematical.

 Activity

Consider the rights and responsibilities of each of the individuals/agencies involved in the above situation. Think about the ethical implications and consequences of the available courses of action, e.g. treating or not treating.

Advocacy

For the sake of completeness, it will be useful to consider the role advocacy might have in such ethically demanding situations. Advocacy is an idea that is widely discussed in nursing circles (Wheeler 2000). The concept is based on the fact that there will always be some who will need someone else to speak out on their behalf to protect their best interests. Although all of us are likely to require such assistance at some point in our lives, there are certain groups in society who have been identified as potentially in need of such help. Children who have not yet achieved the developmental skills for autonomous decision making are an obvious example of this (Mallik 1997).

Although advocacy is usually assumed to be benign in character and well-intentioned (Willard 1996), it must be recognised that the basis of advocacy is that the advocate has the power to speak with effect whereas the person advocated for does not. This power gradient must be recognised and acknowledged for what it is if advocacy is to be constructive. Checks and balances must be in place to ensure that paternalism, at best, and abuse, at worst, is avoided. With a realistic view of its potential advantages and disadvantages, advocacy can be a strong contributor to child well-being. Parents have long been advocates!

Contemporary Examples of Child Healthcare Practice and Research Where the Rights of the Child or Family have Been Breached

Despite the existence of charters and declarations that purport to protect the public from the potential hazards of healthcare practice and research, pockets of questionable practice related to children and their families have undermined the otherwise good reputations of healthcare researchers.

CONSENT FOR ORGAN RETENTION AT THE ROYAL LIVERPOOL CHILDREN'S HOSPITAL (ALDER HEY)

As the news relating to the wholesale removal of organs from the bodies of dead children without parental consent at the Alder Hey Children's Hospital was breaking, it quickly become apparent that many other hospitals throughout the UK also had collections of children's organs. An audit conducted by the Chief Medical Officer Professor Liam Donaldson (DoH 2000) revealed that hospitals collectively had stored anywhere between 40,000 and 50,000 organs from deceased individuals. The scandal that emanated from the Alder Hey Children's Hospital covered the period 1988–1996, when organs were removed from the bodies of dead babies for research purposes without adequate consent.

The primary lesson of the Royal Liverpool Children's Inquiry (DoH 2001a; the Redfern Report, which represents the official report of events at the Alder Hey Children's Hospital) is that there was a gross mismatch between the understanding of the parents, who thought giving consent for tissue removal meant only small specimens, and the doctors, who believed such consent implied they could take what they wanted, including whole body systems.

It is perhaps timely to examine the origins of the Human Tissue Act, introduced in 1961. The law was originally introduced because of a shortage of eyes for corneal grafting. The Act made it lawful for doctors to authorise the removal of body parts for medical education and research purposes 'if having made such reasonable inquiry as may be practicable, he [sic] has no reasons to believe that any rela-

tive objects.' Hence a law introduced for medical expediency at a particular time in history opened the floodgates for abuse. It was the way in which some doctors interpreted and implemented this law that is the cause of this recent controversy (Glasper & Powell 2001).

Few people doubt the benefits to patients that are derived from human tissue research but the flagrant abuse of rudimentary consent procedures linked to the existing Human Tissue Act 1961 has resulted in a level of public scepticism that, if not rectified, will have a negative impact on future research and organ donation in particular. Indeed, in the days following the publication of the Redfern Report, world transplant pioneer Professor Magdi Yacoub was warning the public about a backlash against giving consent for organ donation and revealed an acute shortage of donors (Editorial 2001).

The media reports also reveal the strength of public disquiet at the events at Alder Hey (Bentham 2001). A key finding of the report was the abundant evidence of failure on the part of clinicians to obtain appropriate consent. During the inquiry, doctors who gave evidence acknowledged that it was difficult to reconcile their traditional benign paternalistic attitudes, which made them seek to protect families from distressing events, to the wording of the Human Tissue Act in which the details of the procedure were supposed to be fully and frankly discussed. However, the inquiry concluded that, on the evidence, the medical profession did not properly consider the Act in the first place. This resulted in doctors believing they could have access to any part of a child's body that they wished. However, this only partially explains why the pathology department at Alder Hey systematically collected body organs from children in numbers that could not be reconciled with the research programmes being conducted at the hospital.

Nurses must acknowledge that existing consent procedures will have to be strengthened to avoid a repetition of the events at Alder Hey (Glasper & Powell 2000) and the other centres that retained organs. Although the DoH (2001c) has now produced a new reference guide to consent for examination and treatment, which includes a guide for children and young people, it must be acknowledged that families will continue to rely on nurses to be their advocates. This is particularly poignant in the light of the second scandal to encroach on the otherwise flawless reputation of Alder Hey. Only a year after the publication of The Redfern Report, the hospital was again accused of retaining the organs of children without parental consent, with managers being accused by the family solicitors of 'learning nothing' (Editorial 2002).

Children's nurses are in a unique position to support the appropriate implementation of the enquiry's recommendations for consent. Alan Milburn, who was then the Secretary of State for Health, stated on the day of the report publication:

For trust to thrive there has to be informed consent, not a tick-in-the-box regime – consent that is based on constructive dialogue and where consent is actually sought and positively given (Bosley 2001)

These recommendations emphasise that fully informed consent means that a person must have all the information required to make a final decision. Although many clinicians will find it difficult to provide the details recommended by the enquiry, e.g. about the post-mortem examination and what this entails, nevertheless it is now incumbent for this to become accepted and standard practice. The Chief Medical Officer (DoH 2000) stated:

When a child dies that child is still the parent's child – not a specimen, not a cause, not an unfortunate casualty of a failed procedure, but someone's baby, someone's child. In life the parent is responsible for every aspect of a child's well being. In death that responsibility should not be taken away.

To help parents fully understand the need to retain some organs for histological analysis, and that such examinations cannot take place for several weeks because of the scientific process, the information sharing that now must take place should also encompass parental wishes regarding the subsequent respectful disposal of the organ. Only if this process is strictly adhered to will relatives be able to begin, experience and complete the necessary process of human grieving.

CONSENT FOR MAJOR HEART SURGERY AT THE BRISTOL ROYAL INFIRMARY

The situation of Bristol Royal Infirmary is linked to that of Alder Hey in that both concern children but also have ramifications for nursing as a whole. Alison Norman, the President of the UKCC said of the events 'it is a tragedy that it took the death of more than 30 children to act as a catalyst for cultural change within the NHS' (UKCC 2001). However, long before the 3-year public inquiry into children's heart surgery at the Bristol Royal Infirmary, chaired by Professor Ian Kennedy, was finally published, healthcare professionals were acknowledging that the old health service needed reform (Glasper 2001). The inquiry was initiated after it was revealed that mortality figures at Bristol for children undergoing heart surgery were higher than in comparable units in other parts of the country. The Bristol inquiry (DoH 2001b) showed that some healthcare professionals had not treated families with the proper respect due to them and had failed to obtain fully informed consent from parents before surgery. The lessons of Bristol emphasise the necessity for all children's nurses to accept the benefits of clinical governance, in which the family holds centre-stage in

a continuous cycle of quality improvement. Furthermore, the recommendation that calls for children to be cared for only by professionals who have been specifically educated in the care of children reinforces the message of previous reports and has helped inform the ongoing development of the National Service Framework for Children.

The report had ramifications for the NHS in general, and in particular the need for openness in the giving of information. If information-giving is indeed the key to empowerment (Robertson 1995) then families must be given all the information they need to make critical decisions about their children. In the wake of Bristol a new regulatory body for NHS managers was being established whose maxim is a re-emphasis on patients first. The DoH's response to the public inquiry ratifies the findings and reaffirms the commitment of the government to transform the health service. Importantly, consent is highlighted as a continuous process, not a one-off event. This has important ramifications for children's nurses, as children, because of their developmental parameters, will require innovative methods of obtaining informed consent.

Conducting Research and Protecting the Rights of Children and their Families

The BMA has been prompted to publish explicit guidelines for those who wish to conduct research with children (BMA 2001). Furthermore, the Royal College of Paediatrics and Child Health (RCPCH) have published guidelines on the involvement of children in research (RCPCH 2000 p 177) in which it states:

Many children are vulnerable, easily bewildered and frightened, and unable to express their needs or defend their interests. Potentially with many decades ahead of them, they are likely to experience, in their development and education, the most lasting benefits or harms from research.

 Activity

Obtain and read in detail the Royal College of Paediatrics and Child Health's useful set of guidelines (RCPCH 2000).

A number of questions related to research with children and young people have been raised and discussed by Alderson (1995):

- Are children likely to suffer any harm as a result of the research, in the form of emotional distress or intrusion?
- Do the benefits of the research clearly outweigh these possible risks?

- Who will benefit from the research—children or just the researchers?
- Are children given the proper information about the research?
- Are children offered the opportunity to refuse to participate or answer particular questions?

Despite the large volume of recommendations related to consent available to children's nurses from a variety of auspicious bodies, there is little evidence that children are actively involved with their own healthcare decision making in a meaningful way (Feasy 2001). Children are not used to being listened to and adults have difficulties about listening to children (O'Quigley 2000), and these inherent communication difficulties place children in a vulnerable position during healthcare interventions.

THE ROLE OF LOCAL RESEARCH ETHICS COMMITTEES (LREC)

All NHS areas host research ethics committees, whose role it is to maintain high ethical standards in the conduct of all clinical research undertaken on patients and healthy volunteers and to safeguard the rights of human research subjects as defined by the Declaration of Helsinki, the reputation of the health professions and their institutions. It should be clarified that the LRECs are independent of the Trusts and are answerable to the National Health Service Executive outposts. The lines of accountability are changing with the introduction of a Research Governance Framework to ensure that any research carried out in health and social care has full ethical approval (for more information, see http://www.doh.gov.uk/research/rd3/nhsrandd/ research-governance.htm).

- This includes all types of studies whether therapeutic or non-therapeutic on patients and normal subjects.
- The committees are accountable to a Health Authority and membership includes a lay chairperson and members in addition to doctors, nurses and other healthcare professionals. These committees meet monthly and consider all LREC applications.
- Applications can be approved fully, given conditional approval where amendments are necessary or approval can be withheld where there are concerns. It remains to be seen if newly organised LRECs will be able to safeguard children better than they did in the past.

Summary

The world of healthcare practice and research remains a moral minefield. Child health nurses, working within their philosophy of family care, are often at the forefront of activity and therefore open to criticism. It is incumbent upon all nurses to make themselves aware of the ethical dimensions of any research or clinical care they might be involved with no matter how peripherally. It will not be possible to protect the rights of the child unless they do so. If we do not learn the lessons of the past then we are destined to repeat them.

References

Alderson A 2000 Young children's rights: exploring beliefs, principle and practice. Jessica Kingsley, London

Alderson P 1995 Listening to children; children, ethics and social research. Barnardos, Ilford

Alderson P, Montgomery J 1996 Health care choices: making decisions with children. Institute of Public Policy Research, London

Beauchamp T, Childress J 1979 Principles of biomedical ethics. Oxford University Press, New York

Behi R 1995 The individual's right to informed consent. Nurse Researcher 3(1):14–23

Bentham M 2001 Report shows half of hospitals involved in body parts scandal. Headline News January 28 2001, p 26

British Medical Association (BMA) 2001 Consent, rights and choices in health care for children and young people. BMJ Books, London

Bosley S 2001 Grotesque breach of trust at Alder Hey. The Guardian January 29 2001, p 6

Charles-Edwards I 1995 Moral, ethical, and legal perspectives. In: Carter B, Dearmun AK (eds) Child health care nursing. Blackwell Scientific, London, pp 61–74

Department of Health (DoH) 1999 Convention on the Rights of the Child. DoH, London

Department of Health (DoH) 2000 The removal, retention and use of human organs and tissue from post mortem examination (Advice from the Chief Medical Officer). DoH, London

Department of Health (DoH) 2001a The Royal Liverpool children's inquiry: summary and recommendations. The Stationery Office, London

Department of Health (DoH) 2001b The report of the public inquiry into children's heart surgery at the Bristol Royal Infirmary 1984–1995. Learning from Bristol. DoH London

Department of Health (DoH) 2001c Reference guide to consent for examination or treatment. DoH, London

Eby M 1995 Ethical issues in nursing research: the wider picture. Nurse Researcher 3(1):5–13

Editorial 2001 Heartless, mindless, living children should not pay the price for the dead. The Times February 3 2001

Editorial 2002 New organ retention row hits Alder Hey. The Guardian May 13 2002

Feasy S 2001 Children' participation in decision making (research and commentary). Paediatric Nursing 13(10):12

Gillick v West Norfolk and Wisbech AHA [1986] AC 112, 1985 3WLR 830, 3 All ER 402 HL

Glasper EA 2001 Nurses must enhance care in the wake of Bristol. British Journal of Nursing 10(15):966

Glasper EA, Powell C 2000 Children need protecting in death as well as life. British Journal of Nursing 9(1):5

Glasper EA, Powell C 2001 Lessons of Alder Hey; consent must be informed. British Journal of Nursing 10(4):213

Ham C, Pickard S 1998 Tragic choices in health care: the case of Child B. Kings Fund, London

Illich I 1977 Limits to medicine; medical nemesis, the expropriation of health. Penguin, Harmondsworth

Kennedy I 2001 Learning from Bristol: the report of the inquiry into children's heart surgery at Bristol Royal Infirmary 1984–1995. The Stationery Office, London

Lancet 1997 The ethics industry (editorial). Lancet 350:297

National Assembly for Wales 2002 Too serious a thing/Peth rhy Ddifrif: the review of safeguards for children and young people treated and cared for by the NHS in Wales. National Assembly for Wales, Cardiff

NHS Executive West Midlands Regional Office 2000 Report of a review of the research framework in North Staffordshire Hospital NHS Trust (Griffiths Report). NHS Executive, Leeds

Nursing and Midwifery Council (NMC) 2002 Code of professional conduct. NMC, London

Mallik M 1997 Advocacy in nursing: a review of the literature. Journal of Advanced Nursing 25(1):130–138

O'Quigley A 2000 Listening to children's views: the findings and recommendations of recent research. Joseph Rowntree Foundation, York

Power K 2002 Implications of the Human Rights Act 1998. Paediatric Nursing 14(4):14–19

R v Cambridge Health Authority, ex parte B [1995] 22 All ER 129(CA)

Robertson R 1995 The giving of information is the key to family empowerment. British Journal of Nursing 4(12):692

Royal College of Nursing (RCN) 1977 Ethics related to research in nursing. RCN, London

Royal College of Paediatrics and Child Health (RCPCH) 2000 Guidelines for the ethical conduct of medical research involving children. Archives of Diseases in Childhood 82:177–182

UKCC 2001 UKCC response to Bristol public inquiry says that children should be nursed by properly-qualified children's nurses. Register Number 37, Autumn p 5

UNICEF 2000 The UN Convention on the Rights of the Child. UNICEF, London

Wheeler P 2000 Is advocacy at the heart of professional practice? Nursing Standard 14(36):39–41

Willard C 1996 The nurse's role as patient advocate: obligation or imposition. Journal of Advanced Nursing 24(1):60–66

Chapter Twenty One

21

Legal Aspects of Child Health Care

Louise M Terry, Anne Campbell

ABSTRACT

This chapter summarises the judicial system and identifies the meaning of 'child' and 'parent' in law. It explores issues around consent to treatment. The concepts of 'duty of care' and 'negligence' are examined.

Learning Outcomes

- To appreciate significant aspects of child and family law and their impact on the well-being of children and their families.

- To understand and correctly apply key legal terms in a child health setting.

- To reflect on the relevance and impact of key cases on the present and future management of child health/illness situations.

- To understand consent issues.

- To appreciate what a 'duty of care' entails and to reflect on the impact and consequences of negligence.

The Legal System

The legal system of England and Wales differs from that of Scotland and Northern Ireland. All share a common law tradition in which both judge-made law (case law) and parliament-made law (statutes) play a part. Judges interpret statutes (Acts of Parliament) and use previous case law (precedents) to guide their decisions. If no statute exists, judges rely on legal principles and precedent to reach a decision. The Civil courts are separate from the Criminal courts.

The Family Division of the High Court hears cases involving medical treatment decisions. Appeals against the decision can go to the Court of Appeal (Civil Division) and then to the House of Lords. In cases involving disputes over the treatment of children, the child will be represented by a guardian ad litem, usually from the Child and Family Court Advisory and Support Service (CAFCASS) the Official Solicitor may act as guardian ad litem. The guardian ad litem will try to ascertain the views of the child, if he or she is able to express them. Claims for compensation for negligently caused harm are heard in the Civil courts unless the negligence was criminally culpable. The Magistrates courts, which have a 'bench' of three lay Justices of the Peace hear many criminal cases and some family cases, e.g. contact disputes.

Activity

Attend a session at your local Magistrates court to see justice in action.

Cases involving breaches of the 1950 European Convention for the Protection of Human Rights and Fundamental Freedoms can be heard in all British courts now since the Human Rights Act 1998 came into force in 2000. Appeals from the House of Lords can go to the European Court of Human Rights. However, although the UK has ratified the 1989 United Nations Convention on the Rights of the Child, this is not yet part of domestic law.

Activity

Visit the Houses of Parliament or listen to/watch a House of Lords debate on radio or television.

www

Look at the European Court of Human Rights website on:
- http://www.echr.coe.int

WHO IS A CHILD?

The Family Law Reform Act 1969 confirms that a child or 'minor' is any person who has been born but is under the age of eighteen.

● Seminar discussion topic

Should unborn children have rights? If so, what rights would you give them? Does the journey down the vaginal tract into the outside world change their moral status?

WHO HAS PARENTAL RESPONSIBILITY?

1. The gestational mother (who may or may not be the biological mother).

2. The biological father if he:
   - was married to the gestational mother when the child was born.
   - has since married the gestational mother.
   - has, with the child's mother, jointly registered or re-registered the child's birth if the child was born after 1 December 2003, when relevant parts of the Adoption and Children Act 2002 came into force.
   - has a residence order.
   - has a court order that gives him parental responsibility.
   - has a formal 'parental responsibility agreement' with the mother.

3. The husband of the gestational mother is presumed to be the legal father of the child but this can be rebutted by evidence, e.g. DNA samples. If the child was conceived using in vitro fertilisation treatment in a licensed clinic and the husband of the gestational mother consented to the use of another man's sperm, he will be the legal father.

4. A guardian of the child.

5. Someone who holds a custody or residence order in respect of the child.

6. A local authority that has a care order in respect of the child.

7. Someone who has an emergency protection order in respect of the child.

8. Any man or woman who has adopted the child.

There is a presumption by the courts that it is in the child's best interests to know his/her biological parentage: *Re H and A (paternity: blood tests)* [2002] 1 FLR 1145.

● Seminar discussion topic

In the case of *The Leeds Teaching Hospitals NHS Trust v Mr and Mrs A and others* [2003] EWCA 259 (QB), Mrs A – the gestational mother – was found to be the biological mother of twins born using in vitro fertilisation but, because of a mix-up, Mr B's sperm was used instead of Mrs A's husband's. The presumption that Mr A was the legal father was rebutted and the court decided Mr B was the legal father. Mr and Mrs A may apply to adopt the twins to regain Mr A's legal status as father; Mr B can oppose the adoption order.
- Do you have concerns about this?
- What if the mix-up had occurred the other way around and Mr A was the biological father, Mrs A the gestational mother but Mrs B the biological mother?

DECISION-MAKING REGARDING CHILDREN

The Children Act 1989 reflects the following principles:

1. The welfare of the child is paramount.

2. The child's views, in the light of his or her age and understanding, are to be taken into account.

3. There should be partnership with parents and other family members and support for the child within the family whenever possible.

CONSENT TO TREATMENT

Respect for autonomy is one of the principles underpinning the need to obtain consent before performing any healthcare intervention. Another is the right to bodily integrity. Lord Donaldson in *Re W (a minor) (medical treatment)* [1993] Fam 64 explains that consent has a clinical purpose of ensuring patient cooperation with treatment, and a legal purpose of providing a 'flak jacket' against criminal charges of assault or battery (e.g. Offences Against the Person Act 1869 s47 – liability for causing actual bodily harm), or civil claims for damages for trespass to the person. Failure to adequately inform or advise may give rise to negligence claims. In *Schloendorff v Society of New York Hospital* (1914), Cardozo said 'Every human being of adult years and sound mind has a right to determine what shall be done with his own body.' Increasingly, children's rights to determine what is done to them are being recognised in both law and ethics (Brazier & Bridge 1996, Hendrick 2000 pp 36–38, Terry & Campbell 2001).

Activity

Does your ward have information leaflets telling children what to expect from their stay? If not, why not design one? If you have got information leaflets, are they available in the languages your patients speak?

There are three forms of consent:

1. Orally, e.g. the patient says 'I need my dressing changed'.
2. Implied, e.g. the patient holds out his or her arm for a cannula to be inserted.
3. In writing, e.g. a signed consent form.

Each form is equally valid unless statute law expressly says otherwise, as in the Human Fertilisation and Embryology Act 1990, which requires written consent. The law also prohibits certain procedures regardless of patient or family wishes. For example, the Prohibition of Female Circumcision Act 1985 s1(1) makes it a criminal offence for any person (whether a healthcare professional or not) to 'to excise, infibulate or otherwise mutilate the whole or any part of the labia majora or labia minora or clitoris of another person' or 'to aid, abet, counsel or procure' such mutilation. The Female Genital Mutilation Act 2003 made it a criminal offence to take a child abroad for such mutilation.

 WWW

Look up 'female circumcision' on the internet to find information about this practice. Try:
* http://www.google.co.uk
The following is one of the sites you might have found. How far should the law interfere with cultural norms?
* http://www. religioustolerance.org/fem_cirm.htm

OBTAINING VALID CONSENT

Consent to medical or surgical treatment is usually obtained by a clinician but this duty can be delegated to a nurse who is suitably knowledgeable and competent to do this task. For consent to be valid, it must be:

* given by a competent person
* freely given
* informed.

 Activity

Observe how different doctors inform patients and help children make decisions.

THE GIVING OF CONSENT BY A COMPETENT PERSON

The competent person may be the child or someone with parental responsibility. The law treats the giving of consent to treatment differently depending on the age of the child.

For instance, consent for very young children is very different from that for mature adolescents. Each situation will be considered in turn.

The Infant or Very Young Child

The obvious decisional incapacity of the child means that decisions will be made on its behalf usually by one or both parents. Usually, the consent of only one person with parental responsibility is required. Parental decisions should be made in the child's best interests and the welfare of the child is paramount. The ethical principles of beneficence (doing good) and non-maleficence (avoiding harm) underpin the decision (Beauchamp & Childress 2001). Doctors have dual obligations: to act in accordance with a responsible body of medical opinion when identifying treatment options and to act in the best interests of the incompetent patient (*Re S (Sterilisation: Patient's Best Interests)* [2000] 2 FLR 389).

 Activity

Read the article by Bridgeman (2003). What can you learn for your practice?

When there is doubt or conflict over what constitutes a child's best interests, the court may be asked to decide. Education and communication are preferable to litigation, which can polarise views because of the adversarial nature of legal decision making in this country. The child might even be lost to medical scrutiny.

 Reflect on your Practice

How can you show respect for a person's religious or cultural beliefs while ensuring that you practice within legal and professional boundaries?

The School-age Child

Normal childhood development leads to increasing ability to act autonomously (British Medical Association (BMA) 2001 pp 92–104). Alderson & Montgomery (1996) suggest that children as young as 5 years should be deemed as autonomous unless the evidence or the complexity of the decision suggests otherwise. Thus, a young child might be able to consent to a grazed knee being cleaned but not consent to X-rays and surgical resetting of a broken limb.

Nurses can help educate even very young children about medical treatment in a variety of ways. The child's views can be obtained, even though decisions will ultimately be taken in the child's best interests.

Scenario

Jake, a 6-year-old boy, is admitted for a tonsillectomy. His parents insist he is not told any details of his surgery, so he is not able to be fully informed and prepared by the health professionals.

- Identify the difficulties this could cause and evaluate possible interventions by healthcare professionals.

The Mature Minor Under 16 Years Old

Maturity and insight into medical treatment has to be measured on an individual basis. A 10-year-old child who has undergone years of treatment for leukaemia might be sufficiently competent to make his or her own decisions regarding further chemotherapy. In *Gillick v West Norfolk and Wisbech AHA* [1986] AC112 at p114, the House of Lords held that a child under the age of sixteen can consent to medical treatment if she had 'sufficient understanding and intelligence to enable her to understand fully what was proposed'. It is for the doctors to decide whether the child has a 'full understanding and appreciation of the consequences both of the treatment in terms of intended and possible side-effects and equally important, the anticipated consequences of a failure to treat' (*Re R (a minor)(wardship: consent to treatment)* [1992] Fam 11 at p26 per Lord Donaldson MR). In this case, the girl who suffered from psychosis was deemed incompetent due to her fluctuating understanding.

'Gillick competent' children can consent to medical treatment even if their parents are opposed to it: 'parental right yields to the child's right to make his own decision' (per Lord Scarman) although their rights to refuse treatment are more limited. Their confidentiality should be upheld so their parents have no right to know that they have sought treatment. In *Re B (wardship: abortion)* [1991] 2 FLR 426, a 12-year-old girl was held to be 'Gillick competent' and could consent to a termination of pregnancy, although the court also said that had she not been competent the termination would be allowable in her best interests. Nurses should encourage children to involve their parents, particularly when surgery is proposed.

Professional Conversation

Anne, a registered children's nurse on Part 15 of the professional Nursing and Midwifery Council (NMC) register works in Accident and Emergency.

Gillick competency, confidentiality and partnerships in care

I was on duty when a 13-year-old girl Muslim girl was brought in with abdominal pains. The doctor found she was 4 months pregnant and bleeding per vagina. She was very frightened and upset. Her parents were waiting outside asking what was wrong with her. I didn't know how to do my best for her. The doctor said she was Gillick competent but she seemed very immature to me so I wasn't sure. But I thought, 'If her parents are told what is wrong, what might happen to her?' All I could think of was reading in a newspaper about a Muslim girl who got pregnant and her family killed her for dishonouring it.

The 16–17-Year-Old Child

The Family Law Reform Act 1969 s8(1) States that:

The consent of a minor who has attained the age of sixteen years to any surgical, medical or dental treatment which, in the absence of consent, would constitute a trespass to his person, shall be as effective as it would be if he were of full age; and where a person has by virtue of this section given an effective consent to any treatment, it shall not be necessary to obtain any consent from his parent or guardian.

'Treatment' includes diagnosis, anaesthesia and ancillary procedures.

Activity

Compare and contrast examples of completed consent forms. Can you identify weaknesses?

The Parent of Questionable Competency

Competency can be affected by learning disabilities, mental illness or other conditions. Where the parent is obviously incompetent, consent must be obtained from another person with parental responsibility or the court. In the case of adults and children over 16 years, competency requires being able to comprehend and retain the information given and weigh it in the balance to reach a decision: *Re C (adult: refusal of treatment)* [1994] 1 FLR 31 approved in *Re MB (medical treatment: consent)* [1997] 2 FLR 1097. Although Anglo-Welsh law does not fully recognise the concept of the emancipated minor, marriage or fighting for one's country have been deemed to free minors from parental control. Regardless of her age, the girl who becomes a mother has parental responsibility for her child. Her parents will not automatically have parental responsibility for the grandchild. In cases where the child-parent's ability to consent for her own child is doubtful, it may be necessary to apply to the court.

Freely Given Consent

Duress can invalidate consent, even if it has been applied in the best interests of the patient. Persuasion is acceptable, coercion is not and is likely to cause a breakdown in the relationship between the various parties. Even adults can be placed under duress to accept or reject treatment as in the case of *Re T (adult: refusal of treatment)* [1993] Fam 95, whose Jehovah Witness mother persuaded her to reject blood transfusions. A court later allowed transfusion on the grounds that T was incompetent due to pain and pethidine at the time of her decision and was placed under duress. Children may be less able than adults to withstand emotional pressure. Regarding *Re E (a minor)(wardship: medical treatment)* [1993] 1 FLR 386, a 15-year-old Jehovah's Witness boy with leukaemia who was refusing blood transfusions, Brazier & Bridge (1996) question whether his refusal was 'free choice'.

Duress of circumstances is inadequately recognised within medicine. A 14-year-old may appear 'Gillick competent' but her fear of 'what my parents will say if they find out' might mean she does not fully consider the risks of abortion.

Scenario

A 15-year-old girl underwent a termination of pregnancy without her parents' knowledge. Complications arose and she underwent an emergency hysterectomy. On arrival in intensive care, a decision had to be made about notifying her parents but a senior manager was strongly opposed to this on confidentiality grounds. Discuss and justify your reasoning.

www

Look at the recommendations regarding the principles underpinning the use of patient information given to Caldicott guardians on:

- http://www. doh.gov.uk/confiden/cgmintro.htm

Informed Consent

The World Medical Association's Declaration of Helsinki 1964 states:

> *If it is at all possible, consistent with patient psychology, the doctor should obtain the patient's freely given consent after the patient has been given a full explanation.*

Difficulties arise over provision of information. A balancing act is often performed, which can leave the patient or parent underinformed. The House of Lords decision in *Sidaway v Board of Governors of the Bethlem Royal Hospital and the Maudsley Hospital* [1985] AC 871 meant that for years the 'Bolam test' for negligence governed the provision of information about benefits, risks and side-effects of treatment (*Bolam v Friern Hospital Management Committee* [1957] 1 WLR 582; see later). The standard was how much information would the 'reasonable' doctor disclose. In the Bristol Royal Infirmary inquiry, Professor Ian Kennedy was critical of the failure by surgeons to provide adequate information about the risks to children undergoing complex heart surgery (Kennedy 2001). The Department of Health (DoH) now issues guidance and the standard of 'what would the reasonable patient want to know?' is appearing.

www

Read the DoH guidance on consent on:

- http://dh.gov.uk/(search for consent)

www

Read the recommendations made by Professor Ian Kennedy in the Bristol Inquiry report at:

- http://www.bristol-inquiry.org.uk

In *Chester v Afshar* [2005] 1 AC 134, the House of Lords held that patients are entitled to be given proper warnings about risks of surgery. They can recover damages for non-negligent complications if they can show they would not have had the operation at that particular time if warned, even if they might have had it later. Patients and parents are increasingly likely to actively seek medical information, particularly via the internet (Ham & Pickard 1998). The difficulty lies in understanding and interpreting it but patients, and families, are no longer silent partners in medicine.

Refusal of Treatment

REFUSAL BY PARENTS

Decisions should be made in the best interests of the child. Cases may arise in which it is obvious that the parents' decision is coloured by personal preferences or beliefs and seems clearly contrary to the child's best interests. In the case of a life-threatening emergency, treatment can be given in the child's best interests to save 'life and limb' under the common law doctrine of necessity. In other cases, if doctors believe treatment is appropriate and persuasion has failed, they can refer the decision to the courts. A Specific Issue Order can be given under the Children Act 1989 or the court can exercise its inherent jurisdiction and make a declaration as to lawfulness of treatment.

Activity

When a child's treatment is the subject of dispute, a guardian ad litem will want to meet the child:

- What arrangements exist in your hospital regarding such meetings?
- How can you ensure that your professional responsibilities under the NMC Code of Professional Conduct, in particular, Clause 2, are fulfilled?

In *Re B (a minor) (wardship: medical treatment)* [1981] 1 WLR 1421, where the child had Down syndrome and needed life-saving emergency surgery but the parents refused consent, the Court of Appeal concluded 'it is not for this court to say that life of that description ought to be extinguished'. The lack of peer/judicial review contributes to the 'haphazard and often arbitrary nature of the practice' of interpreting best interests according to Robertson (1986). Caring for the disabled presents 'substantial burdens to parents, family, and even taxpayers', which not all are prepared to take on (Robertson 1986 p 217). The burdens on others are irrelevant under the Children Act 1989 according to Lord Justice Ward (*Re A (conjoined twins: medical treatment)* [2001] 1 FLR 1 at p52). In this case, the Catholic parents opposed the separation of conjoined twins, which would result in the inevitable death of the weaker twin. BMA (2001 p 4) advice that 'the implications for the family of treatment or non-treatment' should be considered when establishing a child's best interests now seems out-dated.

Activity

Next time the media discloses a contentious medical treatment case, read reports in different newspapers. Does your opinion change as you read the different versions?

Re J (a minor) (wardship: medical treatment) [1991] Fam 33 at p55, which involved a severely brain-damaged baby, held that 'the correct approach is for the court to judge the quality of life the child would have to endure if given the treatment'. *Re A (conjoined twins)* shows how difficult it is to determine 'best interests'. Sanctity of life, quality of life, the parents' views and the lawfulness of the operation were all considered. Lord Justices Ward and Brooke held the separation was not in Mary's best interests, although it was allowable. Lord Justice Walker was, according to Foster (2000), '...scarily clear [that] a short, terribly disabled and possibly painful life was a life not worth living' consequently, separation (and death) was in Mary's best interests. It was suggested that refusing to give one twin the chance of life could constitute abuse contrary to the Children and Young Persons Act 1933, which makes it a criminal offence to ill-treat, neglect or abandon a child under 16 years. In *Re S (a minor)(medical treatment)* [1993] 1 FLR 376, the court authorised blood transfusions for a 4-year-old child with T-cell leukaemia against her parents' religious objections.

In other cases, it is much less certain which viewpoint is the correct one. As Ham & Pickard (1998 p 22) point out, differences of opinion:

. . . reflect the individualistic values to which medicine has always subscribed, particularly in the case of clinicians who have reached the top of the hierarchy and feel they possess sufficient expertise to act on the basis of their own judgement.

Re ZM and OS (sterilisation: patient's best interests) [2000] 1 FLR 523 at p533, a case involving incompetent adults, the judge held that expert opinion is not conclusive and should be 'weighed and judged by the court'. The seeking of independent medical advice by the Court of Appeal in *Re A (conjoined twins)* is new and to be encouraged but judges may struggle when critiquing medical information.

Only rarely is the refusal of treatment for minors allowed. In *Re T (wardship: medical treatment)* [1997] 1 FLR 502, involving a child in need of a liver transplant whose parents removed him from the UK, it was unclear that treatment was ethically appropriate and unlikely that the child would survive into adulthood even if the transplant went ahead. Freeman (2000 p 258) believes that the court was 'taken in' by the knowledge of the parents, who were healthcare professionals.

The emphasis placed on parental opinion in *Re T* cannot be seen as decisive following *Re MM (medical treatment)* [2000] 1 FLR 224. The child, MM, was a temporary resident in the UK while his Russian parents studied here. There was no definite diagnosis of his immunological condition and the parents seemed as knowledgeable as the doctors. The parents wanted to continue his existing treatment because, if started on immunoglobulins as English doctors wished, he would have to continue with them but they would be difficult to obtain in Russia. Using telephone conferencing, the judge was able to help the parents and doctors reach a compromise position.

REFUSAL BY CHILDREN

Young children lacking understanding may struggle and fight against those delivering necessary care. In such circumstances, when explanations or reassurances have failed to help, minimal restraint in the child's best interests is allowable. Guidance is available from the DoH (1993) and the Royal College of Nursing (1999).

Activity

Read the article by Jeffrey (2002).

Reflect on your Practice

How would you give a 2-year-old child an intramuscular injection when she is fighting, crying and her mother can't stand injections either?

The Children Act 1989 (s38, 43, 44) gives the court powers to order medical or psychiatric examination and treatment but, if the child is of sufficient understanding to make an informed decision, the child has the right to refuse medical/psychiatric examination. If a competent child refuses examination, the doctor will be unable to make a diagnosis and recommend treatment. A competent child is unlikely to refuse examination because he or she will recognise the need for diagnosis. Consequently, a refusal of examination could be evidence of incompetence. The child's welfare is the paramount consideration although the court should take into account the factors in s1(3) of the Children Act 1989. The child's wishes are only one factor to be considered.

Scenario

Jenny is 12 years old. She has achondroplasia. Her mother wishes her to have leg-lengthening operations but she refuses. Discuss.

The courts have held that a child's refusal of treatment can be overriden by anyone with parental responsibility or by the court. In *Re W (a minor) (medical treatment)* [1993] Fam 64, a 16-year-old girl with anorexia refused force feeding. As the Family Law Reform Act 1969 s8 does not use the word 'refuse' her powers to refuse treatment were not absolute – others could give permission. In *Re R (a minor)(wardship: consent to treatment)* [1992] Fam 11, the court held that even if the 15-year-old were 'Gillick competent', her refusal of antipsychotic medication could be overridden.

A Metropolitan Borough Council v *DB* [1997] 1 FLR 767 concerned a 16-year-old pregnant crack cocaine addict suffering from eclamptic fits who was admitted to hospital but discharged herself. Two days later she underwent a Caesarian section. The hospital wanted to monitor her so the local authority asked the court to place her in secure accommodation – the maternity ward. The court agreed she was incompetent to make her own decisions and granted the order.

The more sheltered an upbringing, the less likely a child is to be found competent, as in *Re L (medical treatment: Gillick competency)* [1998] 2 FLR 810. This involved a 14-year-old with epilepsy who had suffered serious scalding. She, and her parents, refused life-saving blood transfusions because of their Jehovah's Witness faith. Doctors preferred not to upset the child with details of how painful her death without treatment would be and asked the court for permission. Had she been told, she may have consented (Terry & Campbell 2001). The judge granted permission while acknowledging this could condemn her to 'life in the wings'. Judges, and doctors, must recognise that some patients may legitimately prefer death.

In *Re M (child: refusal of medical treatment)* [1999] 2 FLR 1097, a 15½-year-old girl refused consent to a heart transplant. Although her mother had consented, doctors wanted judicial backing and obtained it when the judge held M to be incompetent. Mason et al (2002 p 330) suggest this represents 'the outermost reaches of acceptable paternalistic practices'. In a case involving an adult refusing consent to a life-saving Caesarian section (*R* v *St Georges NHS ex parte S* [1998] 2 FLR 728, the Court of Appeal held that even if the patient is not told of alternative procedures, the court should be if its permission is sought. In *Re M* (at p 1099) the court was told 'no other medical option was available', although life-saving alternatives such as mechanical hearts, which may have been medically better as well as more acceptable to the patient did, at the time, exist (Rogers 2000a). When treatment is refused, particularly if it involves physical maim, alternatives should be sought and considered before resorting to enforcement of the doctor's preference against the wishes of the mature minor.

A risk in *Re M* is non-compliance with antirejection medication once she reaches adulthood. The boy in *Re E* exercised his right to refuse further blood transfusions once he reached 18 and died. Bailey-Harris (2000 p 137) believes 'teenagers with deeply held convictions' should be regarded as mature and 'entitled to their full autonomy rights'. Douglas (1992) argues that the courts have rejected the right of a competent person to make mistakes and 'entrenched not welfare, but paternalism, as its guiding principle'. Bridgeman (1993) criticises the harsh treatment of *W*, who had already been dealt with harshly by fate. Huxtable (2000) questions the existence of the doctor's 'flak jacket' regarding mature minors.

THE MENTALLY ILL CHILD

If the child has mental illness, statutory powers under the Mental Health Act 1983 allow enforced treatment, although there is marked reluctance to use them because of the stigmatising nature of mental illness and being sectioned. Reluctance to use these powers left one child barricaded in her room, manipulating her family and not receiving the psychiatric help she needed before the court was eventually asked to exercise its jurisdiction (*South Glamorgan CC v W and B* [1993] 1 FLR 574). In *Re C (a minor) (detention for medical treatment)* [1997] 2 FLR 180, an order was made under s100 of the Children Act 1989 so that a 16-year-old with anorexia could be returned to a clinic for treatment. She had a history of absconding and was at risk of significant harm.

End-of-life Issues

Lord Justice Hoffman, in *Airedale NHS Trust v Bland* [1993] AC 789 at p 834, felt that whether 'it would be lawful to provide or withhold the treatment or care is a matter for the law' not doctors. This reflects public opinion that doctors are accountable and patients have protectable rights. Imminent, unavoidable death constitutes well-established grounds for ending treatment (*Re C (a baby)* [1996] 2 FLR 43, concerning a baby left brain-damaged following meningitis). Establishing brainstem death is difficult in very young children but in *Re A* (1992) 3 Med LR 303, it was accepted that the 2-year-old was brainstem dead and that it was appropriate to disconnect the ventilator. In *Re C (a minor) (wardship: medical treatment)* [1989] 3 WLR 240, it was appropriate to withhold treatment enabling a baby with severe hydrocephalus to 'die peacefully with the greatest dignity and the least of pain, suffering and distress'. *Re J (a minor) (wardship: medical treatment)* [1991] Fam 33 (at p 53) held that 'it is settled law that the court's prime and paramount consideration must be the best interests of the child'. There is a 'strong presumption' in favour of preserving life except in 'exceptional circumstances', with Lord Justice Taylor stating 'it can not be too strongly emphasised that the court never sanctions steps to terminate life' (p 53). In *Re C (medical treatment)* [1998] 1 FLR 384, concerning a terminally ill child with spinal muscular atrophy type 1, the court held that 'whilst the sanctity of life is vitally important, it is not the paramount consideration. The paramount consideration here is the best interests of little C' (at p 393). The Orthodox Jewish parents wanted reventilation to remain an option because of their vitalist approach to sanctity of life.

Among other factors, the court will consider 'whether the life of this child is demonstrably going to be so awful that in effect the child must be condemned to die' (*Re B (a minor) (wardship: medical treatment)* 1981 1 WLR 1421, at p 1424). However, pain alone is no defence for ending life unlawfully, as Dr Cox found after gave his patient potassium chloride to end her intolerable pain (*R v Cox* [1992] 12 BMLR 38).

In *A National Health Service Trust v D & Ors* [2000] FLR 677, the resuscitation status of a severely disabled child was considered. The court listed the four principles to be applied:

1. The paramount consideration is the best interests of the child.
2. The court has a clear duty to respect the sanctity of life, which imposes a strong presumption in favour of taking all steps to preserve it.
3. Actions to accelerate death or terminate life cannot be approved by the court.
4. The court cannot order a doctor to give treatment that the doctor is unwilling to give and which is contrary to the doctor's clinical judgement.

In *Re A (conjoined twins)*, Lord Justice Ward held that 'Mary may have a right to life, but she has little right to be alive' (p 54); in effect, Mary's twin, Jodie, had a stronger right to life than Mary. The impact of the Human Rights Act 1998, which came into force in October 2000 just after the conjoined twins case, has been considered in several end-of-life cases. In *NHS Trust A v Mrs M and NHS Trust B v Mrs H* [2000] it was held that Article 2 (the right to life), Article 3 (the right not to be subjected to degrading or inhuman treatment) and Article 8 (the right to respect for private life) did not bar the withdrawal of treatment that was not in the patient's best interests.

CONFLICT BETWEEN PARENTS AND DOCTORS

In *R v Cambridge District HA, ex parte B* [1995] 1 FLR 1055, the father of 'Child B' obtained a judicial review of the Health Authority's decision not to fund further treatment for his daughter, a 10-year-old suffering from leukaemia. His refusal to accept the doctor's non-treatment decision represented a 'direct challenge' to the doctors involved in her care (Ham &Pickard 1998). The court held that further treatment would not be in her best interests. If the court decides the doctor's stance is contrary to the patient's best interests, it can order the transfer of the patient to another doctor. This option was considered in *Re T* (the child needing a liver transplant). Doctors at Great Ormond Street Hospital requested the transfer of the conjoined twins in *Re A* on the grounds that they had the necessary expertise to do the separation, although they also said they might accede to the parental wishes not to operate (Rogers 2000b).

Parents may be concerned that their child is being used as a teaching tool and not receiving appropriate care, as in the case of a baby with Goldenhaar syndrome. When the parents sought to remove the child from the hospital, a child protection order banning this was obtained (Mahendra 2002).

Parents and doctors may conflict over when the child's condition should be considered terminal. In *Royal Wolverhampton Hospitals NHS Trust v B* [2000] 1 FLR 953, Bodley J concluded that the breakdown in trust between the parties required that the doctors were given permission to not treat the child dying from chronic lung disease due to prematurity if they thought fit, not just because this was in the patient's best interests but as 'a kindness to the parents' (p 957). The cases of babies Charlotte Wyatt ([2005] EWHC 693) and Luke Winston Jones ([2004] EWHC 2713) involved parents challenging medical decisions not to provide life-prolonging treatment and resuscitation.

GOOD CARE AND COMMUNICATION SEEM VITAL TO PREVENT CONFLICTS

In the David Glass case, doctors gave David, a severely disabled boy with respiratory failure, the respiratory depressant diamorphine against his mother's clearly expressed objections (*R v Portsmouth NHS Trust ex parte Glass* [1999] 2 FLR 905). The family was outraged and, *en masse*, invaded the ward and resuscitated David amid scenes of violent disorder during which two doctors and the mother of another child were injured. Three of them were later jailed for assault (*R v (1) Davies (2) Wild (3) Hodgson* (2000) CA 28 July 2000 unreported). In March 2004, the European Court of Human Rights ruled that 'the decision to impose treatment on the first applicant (David) in defiance of the second applicant's (his mother's) objections gave rise to an interference with the first applicant's right to respect for his private life, and in particular his right to physical integrity' (*Glass v The United Kingdom* Application No 61827/00 ECHR 9 March 2004 paragraph 70). The Court concluded that the situation was not one of such urgency that treatment could proceed without the mother's consent because it was clear that the hospital had had sufficient time to secure a police presence on the ward and 'the doctors and officials used the limited time available to them in order to try to impose their views on [the mother]' (paragraph 81). In regard to the fact that the doctors' notes indicated the mother had consented at one point to the therapeutic use of diamorphine, even though a solicitor's letter the next day made her opposition clear, the Court held 'it cannot be stated with certainty that any consent given was free, express and informed' (paragraph 82).

The UK government was ordered to pay compensation to David and his mother jointly, because the Court recognised 'the stress and anxiety' she suffered in her own right as well as 'feelings of powerlessness and frustration in trying to defend her own perception of what was in the best interests of her child' (paragraph 87). David was discharged into the care of his GP a few hours after the violent incident and was still alive at the time of writing. The final word perhaps belongs to Judge Casadevall:

In the particular circumstances of [this case] maternal instinct has had more weight than medical opinion.

WWW

Find the *Glass v United Kingdom* judgement on the European Court of Human Rights website:
* http://www.echr.coe.int/Eng/Judgments.htm

CONFLICT BETWEEN PARENTS

An exception to the rule that only one person with parental responsibility need consent arose in *Re J (child's religious upbringing and circumcision)* [2000] 1 FLR 571, when the non-practising Muslim father of a child wanted him to be circumcised against the non-practising Christian mother's wishes. The court ordered that circumcision required the consent of both parents or, when old enough to decide for himself, the child's consent.

In *Re C (welfare of child: immunisation)* [2003] EWHC 1376 (Fam), the fathers of two girls aged 4 and 10, both of whom lived with their mothers who were opposed to vaccination, asked the court to order that the children be vaccinated against tetanus, poliomyelitis and other diseases. The court held that immunisation was in the children's best interests. Article 8 of the European Convention on Human Rights did not mean that the right to privacy and family life meant the court could not protect the health of the child.

Consent to Non-therapeutic, Controversial or Experimental Treatment

Although the incompetent patient has a right not to be subjected to non-consensual touching, which is waived only if inhumane not to, children have been allowed to donate bone marrow to siblings or other relatives, with minimal, or no, interference by the courts. Child B's sister was the donor for the failed bone marrow transplant (*R v Cambridge District HA, ex parte B* [1995] 1 FLR 1055). In most such cases, providing the parents, doctors and child (if old enough to be involved) agree, the courts are not involved. In the Australian case of *Re GWW and CMW* (1997) 21 Fam LR 612, a 12-year-old boy was allowed to donate bone marrow to his aunt. It was clear that this was his own, voluntary decision. Although Month (1996) argues that preventing children from donating bone marrow may not be in their best interests, it is important for nurses to be alert for signs of duress or distress. In the American case of *Hart v Brown* (Super 1972) 29 Conn Supp 368, permission was given by the courts for a kidney donation from a healthy 7-year-old to his seriously ill, identical twin brother.

An example of controversial treatment is the use of plastic surgery to alter the facial features of Down syndrome children. One retired consultant paediatrician has called for such surgery to be outlawed like female circumcision (Jones 2000).

Where conventional medicine holds no hope, and death is certain, experimental treatment might be allowed. In *DS v (1) JS (2) An NHS Trust* and *PA v JA (2) An NHS Trust and Secretary of State for Health* [2002] EWHC 2734 (Fam) the court allowed two sufferers of variant Creuzfeldt–Jakob disease (JS, an 18-year-old and JA, a 16-year-old, neither of whom had capacity any more to make their own decisions) to be given an untested treatment – pentosan polysulphate – directly into their brains, even though the procedure itself might kill them.

Negligence

Healthcare interventions are not always successful. Where consent to risks has been sought and given, if those risks come about, the 'flak jacket' protects against being sued. When harm is caused through negligence, either by an omission to act appropriately or by errors in the actions performed, the injured child, or his or her family, might make a claim for compensation in the Civil Courts under the Tort of Negligence. To win compensation, the claimant must prove the following:

- The patient was owed a duty of care by the defendant.
- The defendant (doctor, nurse, hospital) breached the duty of care by failing to reach the standard required of them by law.
- The breach caused harm of a type that was foreseeable.

A request for patient records may indicate that a negligence action is being considered.

WWW

Read the DoH information on accessing patient information on:
- http://www.doh.gov.uk/ipu/confiden/faq.htm

DUTY OF CARE

A duty of care is owed once the hospital, doctor, surgeon, nurse or other person undertakes to perform certain tasks for the child. It is owed once the patient presents for treatment (*Barnett v Chelsea and Kensington HMC* [1968] 1 All ER 1068) and may continue after the patient has been transferred from one professional to another, has left the GP's surgery or hospital, or the nurse has left the patient's house.

BREACH OF THE STANDARD OF CARE

Many nurses act in an extended role. The court will decide whether the healthcare professionals, or other carers, have met the standard that the law expects them to meet. The standard of care is found in *Bolam v Friern Hospital Management Committee* [1957] 1 WLR 582 (the 'Bolam test'):

The test is the standard of the ordinary skilled man exercising and professing to have that special skill. A man need not possess the highest expert skill, . . . It is a well-established law that it is sufficient if he exercises the ordinary skill of an ordinary competent man exercising that particular art.

The key words are 'exercising' and 'professing'.

- Professing is what you say you are, e.g. children's nurse, doctor.
- Exercising is what you do: what task were you actually doing?

Reflect on your Practice

What are the legal and professional responsibilities of the Named Nurse? Can conflict exist between the two?

The court will hear expert witness evidence to determine what standard was acceptable. In *Bolitho v City and Hackney HA* [1998] AC 232, a child was left brain-damaged following a respiratory arrest. The ward sister had asked the doctor to attend with a view to preventively intubating him but the doctor failed to arrive. The House of Lords held that not only should a responsible body of opinion uphold the act or omission but there must be a logical basis to the opinion given. This reflects the trend for evidence-based healthcare.

Learners and their instructor must together meet the standard of the qualified person; inexperience is no excuse – the standard goes with the post. In *Wilsher v Essex AHA* [1986] 3 All ER 801, a junior doctor misplaced a catheter and miscalculated the oxygen for a premature baby who then suffered retrolental fibroplasia.

Written standards, guidelines, protocols, and Do Not Attempt Resuscitation (DNAR) policies are useful for providing consistent care. They need updating regularly and can be used as evidence in a court of law – failure to comply with standard guidance may be seen as proof of a failure to meet the relevant standard of care.

Activity

Attend a hearing of the NMC Professional Conduct Committee. Places are limited so book in advance.

CAUSATION OF FORESEEABLE HARM

Experts for the claimant will provide evidence to persuade the court 'on the balance of probabilities' that the breach of the standard of care caused the harm complained of. The defence will produce its own experts. The question the court asks is 'But for the negligent act or omission, would the harm complained of have occurred?' In *Barnett v Chelsea and Kensington HMC* [1968] 1 All ER 1068, a doctor who failed to examine three men who fell ill after night duty was found to have breached his duty of care. However, this breach did not cause the death of one of the men, which was held to be inevitable due to arsenic poisoning.

Where there are multiple possible causes of the harm, as in *Wilsher v Essex AHA* [1986] 3 All ER 801, unless the claimant can prove on the 'balance of probabilities' that one was the cause, the claim will fail. In *Wilsher*, the blindness could have been caused by several factors, not just the excess oxygen, so the child's claim failed. Likewise, in *Temple v South Manchester Health Authority* [2002] EWCA Civ 1406, negligent treatment of a 9-year-old's diabetic ketoacidosis had not, on the balance of probability, caused his irreversible brain damage. Where there are two equal acts of negligence, either of which could have resulted in the harm complained of, but science cannot provide the necessary proof, *Fairchild* [2002] 3 WLR 79 now holds that the court can decide that both were 'material causes'.

Compensation may sometimes be recovered for psychiatric damage. In *North Glamorgan NHS Trust v Walters* [2002] EWCA Civ 1792, a mother was compensated for suffering psychiatric injury caused by the shock of seeing the distressing final 36 h of her son's life following a negligent failure to diagnose his acute hepatitis.

The doctrine of *Res Ipsa Loquitur* (the thing speaks for itself) simplifies the proof of negligence and causation. If forceps are left inside a patient after an operation, there was obvious negligence and the subsequent peritonitis will be attributed to this.

Unforeseeable harms cannot be protected or insured against so claimants will not be able to recover compensation for harms no one knew existed. If the professional should have known, liability can be established; continuing professional development is important.

WWW

Read the NHS Litigation Authority advice on how to reduce negligence in the NHS:
* http://www.nhsla.com

Accurate record keeping is vital. This is your defence when asked to justify your actions or inactions months or years later. In *Juliff v (1) Dr Hillard (2) Dr Trigg (3) Dr Lukaszewicz* (2001) QBD 24 June unreported, the medical notes were 'conscientiously, properly and accurately recorded' and demonstrated that the defendants had 'discharged their duties with conspicuous care and conscientiousness'. They were not to blame for the child's stroke, which followed a difficult-to-diagnose case of meningitis.

Reflect on your Practice

Look at a nursing record you made a week ago. How clearly can you recall the patient's care? How well could you do this if asked in 8 years time when a solicitor's letter arrives?

WWW

Read the DoH (2001) guidance in *The essence of care: patient-focused benchmarking for healthcare practitioners* on:
* http://www.publications. doh.gov.uk/essenceofcare/index.htm

Read the NMC's (2002) *Guidelines for records and record keeping* on:
* http://www.nmc-uk.org

Activity

* How can record keeping in your practice area be improved?

VICARIOUS LIABILITY

Under the doctrine of vicarious liability, the employer will be held liable for the employee's negligence providing the employee was working within the course and scope of his employment. In *Townsend v Worcester and District HA* [1995] 23 BMLR 31, the defendants were vicariously liable for brain damage caused by the excessive force applied to the baby's head during a forceps delivery.

LIMITATIONS FOR LEGAL ACTIONS

In the case of negligent harm occurring during pregnancy, delivery or any time in childhood, the child retains a right to sue for 3 years after becoming an adult or becoming aware of the negligent act if no legal action has commenced before then.

Criminal Liability

GROSS NEGLIGENCE MANSLAUGHTER

Where negligence causes death, criminal charges of gross negligence manslaughter might follow, as in *R v Adomako*

[1993] 3 WLR 927 in which an anaesthetist's negligence led to his patient's death.

Activity

Visit your local Coroner's court, particularly if there is a paediatric case being heard.

MURDER

Intentional neglect resulting in death may constitute murder or attempted murder. In *R v Arthur* (1981) 12 BMLR 1, Dr Arthur prescribed sedation and nursing care only for a Down syndrome baby rejected by his parents. Initial charges of murder were reduced to attempted murder when a post-mortem revealed the baby would have died anyhow because of his medical condition.

DELIBERATE HARM BY PARENTS, CARERS OR OTHERS

Child protection issues are covered in a separate chapter of this book. However, it is worth noting here that following Lord Laming's 2003 report into the death of Victoria Climbié, which identified failings on the part of health and other professionals in contact with Victoria, a new Children's Commissioner will be introduced, along with new duties of cooperation between all the different agencies in contact with children to minimise risk for all children as part of the Children Act 2004.

www

Look at the Children Act 2004 on:
- http://www.hmso.gov.uk/acts/acts2004/20040031.htm

and the explanatory notes on:
- http://www.parliament.the-stationery-office.co. uk/pa/ld200304/ldbills/035/en/04035x—.htm

Look at the Climbié report, in particular, the sections on the health services:
- http://www.victoria-climbie-inquiry.org.uk/finreport/finreport.htm

Summary

This chapter summarises legal issues relating to child health care as they stand at the time of writing. It is important for all health care professionals to remember that the law is not static. Changes to legislation and new cases testing out the boundaries of care occur regularly. It is your duty to keep yourself up to date to ensure that you continue to practice safely and within the law.

References

Adoption and Children Act 2002 The Stationery Office, London

Alderson P, Montgomery J 1996 Health care choices: making decisions with children. Institute for Public Policy Research, London

Bailey-Harris R 2000 Patient autonomy – a turn in the tide? In: Freeman M, Lewis A (eds) Law and medicine: current legal issues, vol 3. Oxford University Press, Oxford, pp 127–140

Beauchamp TL, Childress JF 2001 Principles of biomedical ethics, 5th edn. Oxford University Press, Oxford

Brazier M, Bridge C 1996 Coercion or caring: analysing adolescent autonomy. Legal Studies 16:84–109

Bridgeman J 2003 After Bristol: the healthcare of young children and the law. Legal Studies 23(2):229–250

Bridgeman J 1993 Old enough to know best? Legal Studies 13:69–80

British Medical Association (BMA) 2001 Consent, rights and choices in health care for children and young people. BMA, London

Children Act 1989 HMSO, London

Children Bill 2004 The Stationery Office, London

Department of Health (DoH) 1993 Guidance on permissible forms of control in children's residential care. HMSO, London

Department of Health (DoH) 2001 Essence of care: patient-focused benchmarking for health care professionals. The Stationery Office, London

Douglas G 1992 The retreat from Gillick. Modern Law Review 55:569–576

Family Law Reform Act 1969 HMSO, London

Foster C 2000 Rocks and hard places. Solicitors Journal 13 October:922–923

Freeman M 2000 Can we leave the best interests of very sick children to their parents? In: Freeman M, Lewis A (eds) Law and medicine: current legal issues, vol 3. Oxford University Press, Oxford, pp 257–268

Ham C, Pickard S 1998 Tragic choices in health care: the case of Child B. King's Fund, London

Hendrick J 2000 Law and ethics in nursing and health care. Stanley Thornes, Cheltenham

Human Rights Act 1998 The Stationery Office, London

Huxtable R 2000 Re M (medical treatment: consent) Time to remove the 'flak jacket'? Child and Family Law Quarterly 12(1):83–88

Jeffrey K 2002 Therapeutic restraint of children. Paediatric Nursing 14(9):20–22

Jones RB 2000 Parental consent to cosmetic facial surgery in Down's syndrome. Journal of Medical Ethics 26:101–102

Kennedy I (Chair) 2001 Learning From Bristol: the report of the public inquiry into children's heart surgery at Bristol Royal Infirmary Inquiry 1984–1995. Final Report. Cmd 5207. The Stationery Office, London. Online. Available on http://www.bristol-inquiry.org.uk

Laming, Lord (Chair) 2003 The Victoria Climbié inquiry. The Stationery Office, London. Online. Available at: http://www.victoria-climbie-inquiry.org.uk/finreport/finreport.htm

Mahendra B 2002 Facing up to a child's dilemma. New Law Journal 152(7024):426

Mason JK, McCall Smith RA, Laurie GT 1999 Law and medical ethics, 5th edn. Butterworths, London

Mental Health Act 1983 HMSO, London

Month S 1996 Preventing children from donating may not be in their best interests. British Medical Journal 312:241–242

Nursing and Midwifery Council (NMC) 2002 Guidelines for records and record keeping. NMC, London

Robertson JA 1986 Legal aspects of withholding treatment from handicapped newborns: substantive issues. Journal of Health Politics, Policy and Law 11(2):215–230

Rogers L 2000a Mini heart pump to end transplants. The Times 9 April 2000

Rogers L 2000b Doctors may not operate on twins. The Sunday Times 1 October 2000

Royal College of Nursing (RCN) 1999 Restraining, holding still and containing children: guide for good practice. RCN, London

Terry LM, Campbell A 2001 Are we listening to children's views about their treatment? British Journal of Nursing 10(6):384–390

Chapter Twenty Two

22

Assessing Children's Health Care Needs over the Telephone: Using NHS Direct as an Exemplar

Felicity Thompson, Rosalyn Moore, Susan Bourner

ABSTRACT

The primary aim of this chapter and its companion PowerPoint presentation is to explore the development of NHS Direct and outline the key elements of the service that provides 24-hour access to healthcare advice and information. The processes of care undertaken when consulting over the telephone are discussed and applied to the specific needs of children and their carers. Examples of practice are illustrated and put into context with the description of a child's journey through the call made to NHS Direct.

Learning Outcomes

- Understand the aims of NHS Direct as an integral part of NHS service provision.

- Describe the roles of NHS Direct staff and the interaction with children and their parents or carers.

- Comprehend the stages and key processes of the care undertaken in telephone consultation.

- Follow a parents or carers journey through the call made to NHS Direct.

- Understand the case mix of calls that are received about children to NHS Direct.

Glossary

Algorithm:
A sequence of questions that are arranged in order of importance or priority and work on a yes/no principle to provide a structured framework for decision making and documentation.

Call handler:
A trained member of staff working for NHS Direct who answers the telephone call, takes patient information and details, establishes the reason for the call and assigns a level of priority for the assessment of needs.

Clinical decision support system (CDSS):
Tools that incorporate clinical questions and information with patient information to provide a structured framework to aid decision making in clinical practice.

GP out-of-hours services:
Provided to give 24-hour access for the public to primary care outside normal working hours. Some out-of-hours services have links to NHS Direct to provide an integrated approach to access to health advice and information.

Health information advisers:
Trained health professionals working within NHS Direct who provide specialist advice and information on a wide range of simple and complex health information enquiries from the general public.

NHS clinical assessment system (NHS CAS):
The computerised clinical decision support system procured and developed for use within the NHS. At present it is used mainly within NHS Direct and Walk-in centres.

NHS Direct:
The 24-hour nurse-led telephone assessment service available in England and Wales that provides access to healthcare advice and information for people to enable them to better care for themselves and their families.

NHS 24:
The 24-hour telephone assessment service, similar to NHS Direct, that is provided in Scotland.

NHS Direct Online:
The internet-based advice and information service that is an integral part of the NHS Direct to provide easy to

access, consistent and high-quality health advice and information. The web address is: http://www.nhsdirect.nhs.uk

Nurse adviser:

An experienced nurse working within NHS Direct who sorts, assesses and manages the healthcare needs of the person who has made the telephone call.

Telephone consultation:

The process of care that occurs when assessing the needs of patients on the telephone. Initial triage of the healthcare problem, combined with the assessment of symptoms, a management decision and the provision of advice and information combine to form a complete episode of care.

INTRODUCTION

Ambulatory care is one of the fastest growing branches of child health care in Western societies. The transition from tertiary inpatient care – which began for children in 1852 with the opening of The Hospital for Sick Children, Great Ormond Street, London, and culminated in the building of large district General Hospitals – to an essentially primary health care led health service has created the conditions necessary for the development of ambulatory care services.

Ambulatory care encompasses a range of services that share one element: providing care that does not involve an overnight stay and bridges service provision gaps that may inhibit a seamless web of care being delivered to children and their families. The term 'ambulatory care' is defined as 'health services provided on an outpatient basis to those who visit a hospital or clinic and depart after treatment on the same day' (Mosby 1995). This section of the book is not exhaustive and readers who wish to explore the full parameters of ambulatory care provision should consult Glasper and Lowson (1998). There is no doubt that children's nurses have led the way in the design, implementation and evaluation of ambulatory care services for families.

The renewed energies of children's nurses within this area are also indicative of the growth in specialisation linked to the clinical nurse specialist movement, which has concentrated on the area of ambulatory care. The technical sophistication of tertiary medicine, coupled with the changing roles of junior doctors, has also been a causative factor in placing ambulatory care in the spotlight of change. Nurses have been quick to grasp and exploit these new opportunities to promote their expertise. Their commitment to partnership with families has influenced the strategic development of many ambulatory care services, including those discussed in this section of the book.

The process of ambulatory care is constant for the patient, requiring flexibility and careful management. It is essential in all practice that the patient and family's journey is escorted by healthcare professionals constantly reviewing their practice and evaluating care.

It is worth reflecting that the father of paediatric ambulatory care, an eighteenth century physician named Dr George Armstrong, was conscious of the role of parents and carers in the successful management of sick children. It was for this reason that he was opposed to inpatient care, believing that economic pressures would prohibit parents' ability to care for their children in hospital. It is however important to stress that in contemporary healthcare ambulatory provision might be more economically debilitating for parents and carers than inpatient care. This is because a parent may have to make special provision to take time off work, thus losing salary, especially important among low-income families. Despite this, Armstrong's legacy to modern child health, the assertion that 'to take a sick child away from its parents breaks its heart immediately' (Palmer 1993), does not reflect the reality of the slums of London in the eighteenth century and the appalling conditions in which children lived. It was the very failure of ambulatory care during this era which led to the opening of the UK's first children's hospital (see Chapter 1 for a full review of the historical aspect of the development of children's nursing).

For ambulatory care to flourish, it is necessary to have an established and sophisticated primary healthcare system that is able to work in a seamless manner with the other arms of the healthcare service. With up to one child in four attending an emergency department in any one year in the UK (Audit Commission 1993), it is not surprising that ambulatory care provision and its relationship with primary care trusts is now under the spotlight. The way in which children presenting with emergencies are managed is the primary focus of this section of the textbook.

The following aspects of ambulatory care for sick children will be addressed:

- Assessing children's health care needs over the telephone
- Using NHS Direct as an exemplar The role of Paediatric Emergency Assessment Units (PEAU)
- Emergency department management of sick children

The Development of NHS Direct

NHS Direct was developed in response to the Labour government's vision for a modern and dependable National Health Service (Department of Health (DoH) 1997). The service was established to provide 'easier and faster advice and information for people about health, illness and the NHS so they are better able to care for themselves and their families' and also to direct people to the most appropriate level of care (DoH 2001, 2003a, NHS Direct 2003) It was first established as a pilot in 1998 to test the feasibility and modelling of such a service as an integral part of healthcare provision and the service was rapidly expanded to cover all of England and Wales by 2000. Scotland has also set up a similar service provision called NHS 24, which started in 2002.

Clear objectives were set for the service, which aims to be patient-centred, enabling people to make decisions about their own health or their family's health:

- Provide a confidential, reliable and consistent source of professional advice on health care 24 hours a day so that people can manage many of their problems at home or know where to turn to for appropriate care.

- Provide simple and speedy access to a comprehensive and up-to-date range of health and health-related information.

- Improve quality, increase cost effectiveness and reduce unnecessary demand on other NHS services by providing more appropriate response to the needs of the public.

- Allow professionals to develop their role in enabling patients to be partners in self-care and help them focus on those patients for whom skills are most needed.

PowerPoint

Acess the companion PowerPoint presentation.

The core service of NHS Direct has rapidly grown since its development and by 2003 it had dealt with more than 18 million calls. It is now seen as the largest and most successful healthcare provider of its kind in the world (NHS Direct 2003).

PowerPoint

Access the companion PowerPoint presentation.

Working alongside the 24-hour telephone health advice and information line is the internet-based service NHS Direct Online. This was launched in 1999 and is one of the most successful health websites in the UK. It seeks to provide high-quality health information in a format that is readily accessible, consistent and easy to use; it recently launched a new access point through digital television.

Activity

Log onto the NHS Direct website and explore its components, then search for advice on managing cold and flu symptoms in a child:
- http://www.nhsdirect.nhs.uk

The rapid growth of the service from a modest project to an extensive national service has highlighted the need to evaluate and study the service and its ability to meet the objectives that were set at its inception. Evaluation studies and

observational reports by the University of Sheffield (Munro et al 2000, 2003), the National Audit Office (2002) and the House of Commons (2002) have provided feedback of how NHS Direct is performing as a service.

Activity

- What conclusions do you think might have been drawn about the strengths and challenges for NHS Direct?
- Make some brief notes about your ideas and then compare them with Table 22.1, which sets out perceived strengths and challenges of NHS Direct.

PERCEIVED STRENGTHS AND CHALLENGES OF NHS DIRECT

Research and study findings (Munro et al 2000, 2003, National Audit Office 2002) evaluating NHS Direct are shown in Table 22.1.

The main findings of the studies provide a detailed guide as to how the service is perceived by its users and other NHS healthcare professionals and its position in health service provision. The Consumers Association has undertaken two investigations (Ratcliffe 2003, Williams 2000) to investigate how it perceives NHS Direct is performing as a service. In both reports (published in the *Which?* magazine) it provided examples of good and poor practice, and identified areas where it feels the service needs to improve.

Activity

Find the relevant copies of *Which?* (August 2000 and July 2003) and read the Consumers Association's perspective of NHS Direct as a service:
- What does the association think of NHS Direct as a service?
- What things does the service do well?
- How well does the service assess the needs of children?
- What improvements does the association suggest for the service?

Research, audit and feedback are key to the governance processes of NHS Direct and play an integral part of the services commitment to the provision of high-quality healthcare advice and information as demonstrated in the recent strategy document outlining the development of NHS Direct over the next three years (NHS Direct 2003).

The aims of NHS Direct have changed now that it is becoming part of the NHS infrastructure. The main aim now is to provide patient-centred care that in turn

Table 22.1 Strengths of and Challenges Facing NHS Direct

Strengths of NHS Direct as a service	Challenges for NHS Direct
60% of the population are aware of NHS Direct as a service	Raising awareness of the service and its objectives
The service has made large advances in tackling inequity of access	Scope to improve the access to and use of NHS Direct in some social groups – younger people, older people, ethnic minority groups, less advantaged social groups and those with disabilities
Public satisfaction with the service is consistently high, with over 90% of callers being satisfied with the advice and information given	Continue to maintain and improve the service for callers and their families or friends
Good safety record	Rising call volumes and increased need for capacity will increase the risk of serious adverse events. Measures such as performance frameworks and governance processes will ensure that quality issues are addressed
Education, training and development are competency based and underpin the service provision	Provide an environment for life-long learning that meets the needs of all staff groups and prepares them to provide high quality care
Improved access to other NHS providers (pharmacists and dentists) and generating more appropriate use of other NHS services	Increased call volumes necessitate the need to plan strategically to manage capacity and referral to other NHS agencies
Development of performance framework	Continually measure and monitor outcomes and demands of the service
Quality assurance of health information available	Provide consistent high quality information for both service users and health professionals
Providing 'added value' to service users by reassuring callers and reducing unnecessary anxiety	Provide high quality care that is safe, effective and appropriate to callers' health care needs

Activity

Read the National Audit Office report (2002) and think about:
- How successful was the development and implementation of NHS Direct as a service?
- What does the public think about NHS Direct?
- How does the public use NHS Direct as a service?
- What impact has NHS Direct had on the rest of the NHS?
- What are the major challenges to NHS Direct as a service?

empowers members of the public to make safe and appropriate decisions about their health and well-being. It also aims to aid the modernisation of the health service by re-engineering attitudes to health care and maximising the advent of information technology and telephony to deliver care by new methods. A further aim is to support change in other areas, particularly GP out-of-hours services.

NHS Direct also strives for reliability and has clear national clinical and performance standards to manage

PowerPoint

Access the companion PowerPoint presentation.

capacity to meet the increased demand on the service. It also works to clear governance standards on clinical effectiveness and uses evidence-based advice and information to aid consistency of approach. The service aims to provide a generalist service that sorts, manages and refers appropriately to a varied and complex caseload of callers with approximately a third of all calls being made about children.

NHS Direct and Caring for Children

PowerPoint

Access the companion PowerPoint presentation.

NHS Direct sets out to try and put children and their families or carers at the centre of the care given over the telephone. By means of a computerised record of care, and making use of the ability to electronically transfer to other healthcare providers, the service seeks to provide a seamless and integrated journey for the child and family. It also tries to take a holistic view of the care of children and, with the aid of the decision support tool, to provide high-quality care to a child or their carer regardless of their sex, age, race faith or disability. A decision support tool provides the supportive framework for the nurse to structure the assessment of the child's physical, social and psychological needs and offers a source of evidence-based information and advice. The system also provides a means of contemporaneously capturing a record of the assessment and advice given and supplies an aid for reflection and learning.

PowerPoint

Access the companion PowerPoint presentation.

Caring over the telephone involves one of the key nursing skills: communication. Specialist workshops in both induction courses and ongoing learning programmes provide theoretical elements of communication and customer care skills. These are applied to working on the telephone by the use of role play and in experiential sessions in the call centre where interpersonal skills are reviewed and reflected on to provide a focus for practice. Key elements of communication within the call, such as questioning and listening, are all regularly reviewed as part of the NHS Direct quality improvement framework (DoH 2003a).

By listening to the child's parent or carer, and by using skilled information gathering, a whole picture of the emotional, psychological, physical and social needs of the child and family is built and then assessed to provide a way forward to manage the problem. However, as a gateway rather than a treatment service, NHS Direct will refer parents or carers to the right service to meet those needs.

All sources of evidence point to a high level of demand from parent and carers ringing about children. Call volumes to NHS Direct relate directly to the number of children in the population. Lattimer et al (1998), when evaluating the safety and effectiveness of nurse telephone consultation, found that calls about children under 4 years exceeded the proportion of this age group of children in the population. The numbers of calls therefore reflect the fact that nothing matters more to parents than the health, well-being and safety of their children (DoH 2003b).

Activity

What social factors do you think might account for the high levels of demand for NHS Direct by parents and carers?

The social profile in the UK changed significantly during the 20th century. We have witnessed a rise in family breakdown and a proportional increase in the number of households containing only one adult (The Stationery Office 2004). This has been accompanied by greater social and geographic mobility and ever-increasing numbers of women going out to work, which have contributed to a shift in the traditional structure of families and nature of family relationships. Consequently, parents and carers may well turn to NHS Direct for the sort of advice and reassurance they would have previously obtained from family members. Alongside this, we have seen the advent of the '24-hour society' and rising expectations as a result of technology (including the use of mobile telephones) and improvements in the availability of information. Parents and carers now expect more convenient and more accessible health care for their children – when they need it.

These trends are reflected in the National Service Framework for Children (DoH 2003b), which provides some key areas for the improvement of patient experience these sit well with the key aims of service provision within NHS Direct:

- improving access and waiting
- more information and choice
- building closer relationships
- safe, high-quality, coordinated care.

NHS Direct is a confidential service and callers are asked for their consent to transfer information whenever necessary or during out-of-hours periods. A core service is provided on the 0845 4647 number 24 hours a day and a gateway triage service is provided for GPs in out-of-hours periods. It is anticipated that, by 2005, all out-of-hours calls will be dealt with by NHS Direct in conjunction with Primary Care Trusts.

NHS Direct provides other services that are agreed as part of local health care provision, such as mental health crisis lines, prison support, telehealth and social alarms.

PowerPoint

Access the companion PowerPoint presentation.

The entire call transaction is recorded in a computer database, which supplies the nurse with a decision support tool (NHS CAS) and a record of the consultation. The computerised decision support system provides a structured format for the collection of patient information and details, such as the child's name, date of birth, address, the name of the person calling, and the address if different from where they normally live. The details of their GP are also collected, when appropriate, in case of onward referral for a face-to-face consultation. Information is given at the beginning of the call about the confidentiality aspects of the service and every effort is made to make the parent or carer feel comfortable about imparting personal details and information.

Negotiating skills form a key part of the training programmes to ensure that staff remain sensitive to parents or carers needs and wishes. A record of the questions and advice given asked by the nurse in the consultation is also captured in the structured sequence in which they appear. This provides a unique record of the episode of care that can be accessed to provide extra information should the parent or caller phone again. All call records are stored and accessed according to the principles of the Data Protection Act. Extra advice and information might be given at the time of the call by a health information adviser, who obtains quality-assured local and national information from databases that link with the computerised record. All information and data are captured.

As the main gateway and referral service for health and social care in England and Wales, NHS Direct makes possible the more integrated approach to health care that has long been the goal of government. One area where this is most prominent is in the care of children and particularly child protection.

Working with Other Services to Improve Child Health and Safeguard Children

The 2003 enquiry into the death of Victoria Climbié, and the subsequent report, highlighted a woeful lack of collaboration and information sharing between the various services charged with her welfare. There is a stark lesson in the report for all services in contact with children and NHS Direct, following a unique partnership with the NSPCC, has invested significantly in staff training and provision in this area.

In a multi-sited, geographically dispersed organisation such as NHS Direct, it is essential to have a consistent and integrated approach to child protection that ensures the rapid and proactive identification, and appropriate referral, of children at risk or in need, wherever they live. Therefore child protection is deemed a universal responsibility – not the province of experts, nursing or medical staff, as was sometimes the case in the past. All staff having direct or indirect contact with children and families or having access to information about them in the course of their everyday work have a responsibility to safeguard and promote the welfare of children (DoH 2003c). This means that, regardless of where the caller is located geographically, the child protection concerns are handled by the site receiving the call and the person who identifies the concern.

During the course of their work staff may also encounter children and families who are not deemed as being 'in need or at risk' but who, in the judgement of the individual nurse or other staff member, would benefit from additional health and/or social care support.

Activity

Consider for a moment how this fits in with the claim to provide a confidential service.

Liaison and family support is seen as a core role for NHS Direct staff and, in the case of a child or family who might benefit from additional support, the person dealing with the call will seek consent to contact the appropriate service by telephone, logging the contact on the patient record.

In situations where the child is deemed at risk of harm or in need, the case is less clear cut. It is always best practice to obtain consent from the caller for a referral, unless it is judged that to do so would be detrimental to the child's welfare or where seeking consent might prejudice a police investigation. All staff recognise that information about patients and colleagues should be treated as confidential. However, the Laming Report (2003) is clear that better information sharing between services and individuals is crucial to child protection and must take place with or without consent. Therefore child protection presents nurses and other staff with a situation where the safety of the child takes precedence over the caller's legal rights to confidentiality and data protection. To facilitate this, clear guidelines are in place for sharing information with other services on a 'need to know' principle and staff must comply with those requirements. To ensure information sharing within the service, all children known by other services or child protection agencies are flagged in accordance with proposed government policy (Department of Education and Skills (DfES) 2003) by a 'special note' attached to the patient record, with access allowed only on a need-to-know basis.

How NHS Direct Provides Care for Sick Children

PowerPoint

Access the companion PowerPoint presentation.

Three groups of staff work within the call centre environment; other staff work behind the scenes to ensure that service provision is underpinned by a safe and effective infrastructure.

The three groups are:

- call handlers
- health information advisers
- nurse advisers.

All staff groups at NHS Direct are recruited using a competency-based assessment and then undertake a preparation programme and period of preceptorship to prepare them for their new role. The nature of the service is such that these staff groups for the most part work in generalist rather than specialist roles and must be equipped to deal with any call that presents. The decision to adopt a model of call taking whereby calls are answered according to their clinical need rather than by specialist area was taken early in the service development when it became clear that, whereas call volumes could be predicted, there was no way of predicting call type (Thompson 2001). Therefore new ways of working, involving all branches of nurse training and those with specialist paediatric knowledge and skills, are essential to provide staff who are competent to assess the needs of children and to maximise opportunities for development and flexibility of the service.

However, this approach has been challenged by several studies and observational reports (McClellan 1999, 2004, Monaghan 2003), which proposed that all calls relating to children should be undertaken by registered sick children's nurses.

Activity

What do you think?
- Read the paper by Monaghan et al (2003).
- When you have read this paper, think about your own opinion on whether a registered sick children's nurse should assess all calls about children to NHS Direct?
- If you think they should, how could you ensure that there were enough competently trained nurses to deal with all calls relating to children 24 hours a day?

However sound an idea this may be, the lack of nurses in general, and the small number of registered sick children's nurses in particular, makes this an impossibility and lateral solutions need to be created to provide care that is fit for this purpose for the needs of children. Elston & Thomas (2002) report on the shortage of children's nurses in their report to the Royal College of Nursing and the Royal College of Paediatrics and Child Health and provide evidence that this will increase unless solutions are found to improve the care given to sick children. NHS Direct is doing this through educational activity focusing on the role of staff in telephone consultation and the competencies needed to safely and effectively assess and manage the healthcare needs of all patients.

Communication and interpersonal skills form the basis of the programme, with other sessions providing background to local health needs, how to use the computerised decision support tool and how past knowledge, experience and skills are meshed into the complex multi-tasking activities of working on the telephone. Specialist input is given to provide the generalist nurses with strategies and knowledge to safely and effectively manage the needs of children, callers with mental health needs, those calling out of hours and those with special individualised needs.

TELEPHONE CONSULTATION

Telephone consultation is characterised by several key elements, which form a total episode of care that uses a sequence or framework for practice. An early model of care that highlighted the areas of practice was devised by a working party convened by the Royal College of Nursing (RCN 1998) and this has been further built on by Lattimer & Crouch (1999). A competency framework developed by Moore (2001) outlines and defines the role of nurse advisors in NHS Direct and describes the key processes of telephone consultation. These have since been extended to other staff groups.

Early work outlining the use of the telephone in health care describes the process as 'telephone triage'. This term was initially used to describe the process of sorting to determine the urgency of the intervention and then prioritising the action and providing advice as appropriate. Further observation has provided the newer definition of care provided over the telephone.

The processes of information gathering, internalisation of knowledge, decision making in conjunction with the caller, and the provision of advice and information forms a complete episode of care. This complex method of care therefore becomes a total consultation and is performed by an autonomous practitioner who is competent to perform the whole process.

Telephone triage services featured prominently in healthcare provision across the world before the planned development of the national NHS Direct service. A service established in the Sick Children's Hospital in Toronto was established in the 1970s to provide advice and reassurance for worried parents. Call centres developed rapidly in North America in response to insurance companies managing health care and these provided a triaging and advice and routing service to patients with healthcare needs (Dundas & Casler 1998).

Telephone advice has been utilised by staff working in Accident and Emergency departments and acknowledged by studies reporting the activities and outcomes of using this method (Buckles & Carew-McColl 1991, Edmonds 1997, Eggleston 1994).

Telephone triage has become well established as part of the primary care provision in Sweden (Marklund & Bengtsson 1989, Timpka & Arborelius 1994) and the experiences of these services have been mirrored in the setting up of out-of-hours nurse triage in England and Wales. Lattimer et al (1998) undertook a randomised controlled trial to study the safety and effectiveness of nurse telephone consultation in out-of-hours primary care. The study concluded that the model tested was safe and effective; these findings enabled the set-up of NHS Direct.

Early telephone consultation relied on the nurse's ability to structure and assess the caller's needs using their own knowledge, skills and past experience. Early work in North America by Quilter & Wheeler (1993) outlined the need for a structured framework and the use of evidence to aid decision making in the assessment process. Glasper (1993) describes working over the telephone as being 'analogous to nursing with yours eyes closed and your hands tied behind your back'.

It was also acknowledged that nurses undertaking this new kind of role need training and support to enable them to work in this new complex way. Early guidance on protocols that could be used to help nurses to make decisions were postulated by Quilter & Wheeler (1993) and Briggs (2002), who developed a series of paper-based protocols to use when working on the telephone. Further research has been undertaken to study how nurses make decisions when consulting on the telephone. Edwards (1994, 1998) and Lyneham (1998) found that nurses use different skills that link to help them make a decision using analytical reasoning skills.

Pettonari & Jessop (2001) discuss how the nurse determines a mental image of the patient or in other words 'builds a picture' of the caller and their healthcare needs as part of the assessment process. These examples provide an illustration the multifaceted nature of assessing and caring on the telephone. Work undertaken by Lattimer et al (1998) highlighted the use of computerised decision support in telephone consultation. Computerised guidelines and protocols aid the nurse to structure and competently assess the needs of a caller over the telephone. They are designed to supplement the nurse's clinical knowledge and judgement and enhance the lateral and critical thinking used in decision making. Crouch (2002) describes the different approaches to decision support and how they underpin nursing practice. NHS Direct strives to maintain high-quality care and perceives that computerised decision support provides structure and consistency to each care episode. The decision support tool relies on the clinical judgement and skills of the nurse and how they apply the information gathered from the caller.

Experience shows that effective teleconsultation is built on the interaction between three key variables described first by Valanis et al (2003) and adapted since by the authors to reflect the particular needs of children at NHS Direct (Fig. 22.1).

Activity

Conduct a literature search to determine the evidence base of telephone consultation using the following key terms:

- telephone triage
- telephone consultation
- nurse triage
- clinical decision support software
- NHS Direct
- children.

Variables

The System

Different structures, whether they are paper guidelines or computerised protocols or algorithms, will affect the outcome. The interface of how these support tools are used operationally to guide practice will also affect the outcome and consistency of approach. Different items of clinical content and the evidence on which they are based may also vary how the consultation progresses (Fig. 22.2).

Fig. 22.1 • NHS Direct.

Variables

Decision support
- The responsiveness of the algorithms to symptoms in infants and children
- The functionality of the system
- The quality and relevance of the clinical content to the needs of children
- The interface with other algorithms and with other patients services

The parent or carer calling
- The demographics profile of the caller and child
- The ability to communicate or accurately articulate their concerns and the child's symptoms
- Health status of the child and the parent/carer
- Health beliefs of the caller
- Previous experience of healthcare and the NHS (recent and general)

The consultation process
- Parent or carer satisfaction with access and management to date
- Level of trust and rapport built
- The power process between caller and nurse
- Day and time call
- Call volumes and capacity
- The length of the call
- The clinical judgement being exercised
- Expectations of desired outcome of the consultation
- Barriers to following advice
- Local variations in the health economy

Nurse advisor
- Education and experience
- Critical thinking abilities
- Perception of autonomy
- Risk assessment skills
- Critical thinking
- Health beliefs
- Cultural competency

Fig. 22.2 • Factors affecting the progress of a consultation.

The Nurse

Nurses undertaking these new roles will have different nursing backgrounds and skill sets and will therefore have different perceptions and values when assessing callers on the telephone as previously outlined. The educational preparation is fundamentally important to provide a solid base from which to practice. Caring for individual health needs in a complete episode of care inevitably means the nurse is working autonomously in conjunction with the caller. Past knowledge, beliefs and experience used 'critically' to reason and laterally think might also provide different outcomes for the call. High levels of self-awareness and critical reflexivity are crucial.

PowerPoint

Access the companion PowerPoint presentation.

The Parent or Carer Calling

Callers to NHS Direct bring their own individuality and needs that contribute to the consultation process. Social and emotional factors play a key role in determining the appropriate endpoint for the call. This is particularly evident in parents or carers calling about a child, who often identify specific reasons for calling, a need for reassurance and also confirmation of their own ideas. Past experience of using other healthcare services often influences the outcome and decision made about the care of their child (Thompson 2001).

Scenario

A call was received by a nurse adviser at 17.30 on a Wednesday evening from an anxious mother. She had been preparing tea for her three children aged 8½ years, 6 years, and 12 months. The two eldest children had been fighting over toys and she had gone to sort out the argument, forgetting that the youngest was playing on the kitchen floor. On returning to the kitchen she found the baby eating cat litter from the tray on the floor. She called NHS Direct to find out if the cat litter could be harmful to the baby.

She expressed anxiety around her child and what would happen if the cat litter was poisonous but also talked about her feelings of guilt about not thinking about lifting the cat litter tray from the floor to prevent the accident occurring.

The nurse using the decision support system elicited the reason for the call and asked the mother a series of questions to assess the nature of the symptoms and to ensure the child was not seriously ill following the incident and that the all three children were happy and safe. Having established the main focus of the call and the type of cat litter, the nurse reassured the mother, allowed her to talk and explain the incident and then talked her through the next steps. The nurse then telephoned the poisons helpline to access the appropriate information for the mother. Three minutes later the nurse phoned the mother back to tell her that the cat litter would not harm her baby. She provided some further advice and some 'watch out fors' and the possibility that he may be sick and asked if there was anything else she was worried about. The mother was greatly relieved by the news, reassured that her son was all right and felt comforted by the fact that she had been able to talk to somebody about the event. The call ended by the nurse reiterating that if anything changed, new symptoms appeared or if the mother was worried to call back the service.

CONSULTATION

Strong interpersonal skills are essential to building a good relationship, which enables a positive outcome for both caller and nurse. The influence of personal bias, values and beliefs may provide a barrier to communication. Callers often telephone with an outcome in mind and dissatisfaction may occur because the assessment does fulfil their expectations. This may be due to the denial of the seriousness of the symptoms or purely acknowledging what has happened, or the symptom may be less serious than perceived by the caller. This is perhaps more evident when dealing with parents or carers who are anxious, feel out of control or isolated (Thompson 2001). These feelings may be exaggerated by the time of call; children often have worrying symptoms late at night when other support networks are not available. Other influences on the outcome of a call can include the ability of the caller to understand and follow the advice given by the nurse. This may be due to social, cultural or economic reasons. One of the challenges facing the nurse in the consultation process is to negotiate, reflect and check the caller's understanding.

Scenario

A call was received from Karen Hall at 23.00 about her 6-year-old son Ian, who had woken up and was crying and seemed hot. On questioning, Ian was responding normally to her and had no symptoms that would need an emergency response. Further questioning aided by the decision support tool and taking in to account Ian's past medical history (past ear infections, insertion of grommets) established that Ian felt hot and that he had a very painful left ear.

Having completed a full assessment of Ian's needs and enquired what Karen has already done, the nurse explains to Karen that the symptoms she is describing (hot to touch, pain in the left ear, crying but responding normally) could be dealt with by some advice on how to reduce the temperature and relieve the pain. Karen is

not happy with this action because whenever this has happened in the past the doctor has been to visit them at home and prescribed antibiotics. She tells the nurse that she is also alone at home with her three children as her husband is working away.

The nurse reflects about how she came to make the decision and discusses this with Karen using the decision support tool to provide evidence-based information to support the conversation. A joint decision is made by Karen and the nurse that Karen, although she is feeling vulnerable, will try and use the advice given about reducing Ian's temperature and relieving his pain and that she will call back if his symptoms change or worsen or if she is still worried.

The use of the clinical information captured by the system questions enables clinical risk to be confirmed or eliminated. Answering the clinical question determines the direction of the assessment ending in referral to another healthcare provider or self-care. At the end of the assessment a disposition is offered and at this point the nurse can select an alternative that takes into account the psychological, social and emotional issues of the situation. A national decision support tool has been procured and has been developed acknowledging the experience and theoretical underpinning of decision making and the importance of assimilating information gathered from a caller. The system provides a systematic and reliable framework in which a record of care is documented. A robust evidence base underpins the clinical content to provide clinically effective information at the point of care. Data can be retrieved from all phases of the consultation to aid quality programmes service analysis.

Activity

Imagine you have just undertaken a call from a father of a 5-year-old girl, who rang because he thought he had given his daughter too much Calpol for her high temperature. After assessing the child's needs and symptoms you decide that you can give the father some advice to help him manage the problem:
- What type of advice would you give to the father?
- What resources would you use to obtain appropriate advice?

An extensive IT infrastructure supports the delivery of the system to the nurse. Other electronic resources are available for the nurse to use to aid decision making such as links to Toxbase and eBNF.

Specific telephone consultation or triage services for paediatrics have been developed in North America. These are mainly hospital-based paediatric department services, many of whom demonstrate successful effective outcomes. Studies of these services provide observational evidence around the use of protocols, effective training to aid consistency of approach (Barber 2000, Belman 2002, Wachter 1999).

The journey through NHS Direct is outlined in Fig. 22.3.

Parents make a decision to call NHS Direct on 0845 46 47 because of a health need or problem. The reasons they make the decision to call NHS Direct are outlined below:

- no access to GP
- used the service before
- recommended to use the service
- long wait to see their GP
- want health information
- redirected from other services: GP out-of-hours services and A&E
- not wanting to bother the doctor
- for a second opinion.

Scenario

Mrs Morris is worried about her 3-year-old son. He has a temperature and is having problems with his breathing. She has just separated from her husband and is waiting to move back up north to where her family lives so feels very alone. She has just rung the number for her GP's surgery but has got a voice-mail message directing her to NHS Direct.

Scenario

Heather Payne has just been diagnosed with multiple sclerosis after several months of tests and trips to the doctor and the hospital. She has been told that NHS Direct keeps information about the disease and also can give her some addresses and telephone numbers of groups that can help people with multiple sclerosis.

Fig. 22.3 • The journey through NHS Direct.

Scenario

John Boyle has rung his GP practice because he is aching all over and feels unwell. The receptionist has told him that there are no appointments for the next 3 days and that he should ring later to see if there any cancellations. His friend at work tells him about NHS Direct and gives him the number to ring.

Activity

Ask friends and relatives if they have called NHS Direct. Explore that experience with them. Why did they ring, what was the outcome and were they satisfied with the service they received?

PowerPoint

Access the companion PowerPoint presentation.

Before speaking to anyone at NHS Direct, the caller is presented with a statement about the nature of confidential information and how it is handled by the service. Callers are then directed to the first available operator at NHS Direct by the telephone network.

All interactions that occur within the call are recorded in the computerised system known as the NHS Clinical Assessment System (NHS CAS). The call handlers log patient details and information, and further interactions are documented as the call progresses. Following the documentation of the demographic details, the clinical aspects of the call are recorded with the use of the algorithms to aid decision making and information aspects are recorded along with notes of what information and advice was given.

Specialist services are employed by the call handler if is there is a communication barrier such as hearing impairment or English not being the first language of the caller. These translation services are employed throughout the service to aid and support effective communication.

The calls to the service fit into two categories: health information and symptomatic advice calls. A description of the progress of each call type follows.

A call handler takes essential demographic information and ascertains the reason for the call and rapidly performs a first-level assessment to exclude a life-threatening situation. These callers are immediately transferred to the ambulance service. Other callers are assigned a priority level. These include direct transfer to a nurse or being placed in a queue to be called back.

PowerPoint

Access the companion PowerPoint presentation.

A health information advisor telephones callers requiring health information. This group of staff comes from a diverse range of backgrounds and many will have worked in other health or customer care services. The nature of health information calls is split into two groups, those callers needing access to local health services, such as dentists and pharmacies, and those who want to know more information about health related issues. Informational databases (Fig. 22.4) provide a very extensive range of information that can be given over the telephone or with the caller's consent through the post. These databases can tailor the results to account for the caller's location restricting responses to those available to the caller locally if needed. Specialist information can be provided on medicines and the use of alternative therapies, and on conditions rare syndromes. More complex issues are sent to a specialist researcher, who searches for further evidence to answer the enquiry. A specialist pilot is being undertaken to test the effectiveness of providing health information by e-mail, which is proving to be very popular.

Those callers who require advice about their symptoms are either transferred directly to a nurse or called back from a queue. The dialogue begins with confirmation of the details given earlier. Then a call progresses through four phases. In the introduction phase the nurse establishes a relationship with the caller and uses his or her interpersonal skills to elicit information from the caller to explore and validate the call reason given during the first-level assessment by the call handler. The call then moves onto the exploration phase, in which the nurse undertakes a second-level assessment. During this, information around lifestyle, past medical history, current treatments, allergies and medications are obtained and documented within the NHS CAS system. This information is synthesised and is used throughout the call to link information about the patient with the symptom.

PowerPoint

Access the companion PowerPoint presentation.

The nurse selects the most suitable algorithm to further assess the presenting symptom. If there is a set of complex problems, the nurse identifies the most significant symptom to the caller to select the algorithm. The algorithm provides the nurse with a series of structured questions to establish the most appropriate venue for the management of the presenting symptom. This may range from sending an

Fig. 22.4 • A screen from an NHS Direct informational database.

ambulance, attending an Accident and Emergency Department, speaking to a GP, attending a walk-in centre or managing the symptom at home with advice from the nurse. The algorithm is not the only source of information used during this process. Background noise and other non-verbal cues also provide the nurse with important supporting information.

Scenario

Sarah Clarke, a child minder, phones about David, one of the children she looks after. She has just been to collect him from school and he has been playing in the garden. He has jumped off the garden wall and fallen over awkwardly on his leg. He got up and tried to walk but found it difficult. David is 9 years old and has no past medical history of note. He is now complaining that his leg hurts.

The nurse undertakes an assessment of David's needs by asking a structured set of questions about David's injury and any other factors, such as past medical history, that need to be taken into account. She has established that there are no life-threatening symptoms as a consequence of his injury and that he is safe but ascertains that he is now unable to weight bear and is in a lot of pain.

The nurse then recommends that David needs to attend the Accident and Emergency department because of his symptoms and the need for further investigations and treatment. She discusses this with Sarah and between them they organise a solution for David's parents to come and take him to the Accident and Emergency department.

Closure of the call is the final phase in the process and involves the nurse providing the individual with advice that supports the outcome reached during the assessment. Using his or her clinical judgement, the nurse may decide that the system recommendation is not be suitable for the child's situation and may recommend an alternative outcome. Checking the parent's or carer's understanding and providing them with instructions on how to manage should the symptoms deteriorate are essential components of this process.

Key elements of all the phases in the call are involvement of the parent or carer in the decision-making process and ensuring their confidence in the recommendations of the nurse. The call ends by the parent or carer confirming their acceptance of these recommendations and the nurse ensures that the documentation represents a true and contemporaneous record of the call.

Some calls may present difficult ethical and moral dilemmas and prove challenging to the nurses. The record of the consultation collected by the NHS CAS system provides an excellent tool to promote reflection. Nurses are encouraged to debrief and provide support to one another alongside programmes of formal supervision.

Child Health-related Calls to NHS Direct

Parents calling on behalf of their children form part of the largest group of users of the service. Recent figures from NHS Direct suggest around 34% of all calls are by or on behalf of children, with two-thirds of those being about the under 5's (NHS Direct 2003).

Children are classified into three groups for reporting purposes. These groups are reflected in the algorithms available: under 1 year, 1 year to 4 years and 11 months, and 5 to 16 years. Data are routinely collected and analysed to provide the service and its stakeholders with an accurate picture of the service usage and referrals made to other healthcare providers. The most commonly used algorithms by nurses for the management of presenting symptoms in NHS Direct are shown in Table 22.2.

The top ten lists consistently contain the same symptoms and are subject to very little seasonal variation. The three lists contain many commonalities and any variations are consistent with the ability of children to articulate the source of their distress or discomfort.

An algorithm is based on a clinical symptom and is a series of questions that are placed in order of priority or urgency. The nurse uses the questions as prompts to sort and assess bearing in mind the lack of visual cues and to structure the decisions that are taking place. It is a complex task for the nurse to undertake because of the multidimensional sources of information that are used and the application of clinical reasoning and judgement. The algorithms are therefore structured to aid the clinical knowledge and skills of the nurse to undertake a safe and effective consultation. Figure 22.5 demonstrates how algorithms provide a structure for the user.

In children under the age of 1 year, it is difficult to assess the specific nature and location of symptoms. A default algorithm entitled *Crying or unwell* is therefore provided, which provides a thorough and systematic approach to assess the needs of very young unwell children. Where appropriate, all other algorithms have newborn, infant and toddler versions.

PowerPoint

Access the PowerPoint presentation.

Activity

Jean Foster calls NHS Direct on a Sunday morning about her 2-year-old granddaughter Leanne, who she is caring for while her daughter is at work. She thinks Leanne has earache. She tells the nurse that Leanne is normally fit and well and thinks she has had all her immunisations. She has been miserable and crying at times which 'is not like her', she also seems to be pulling at her ear and appears flushed and looks pink. She wants 'lots of cuddles' and has not eaten any breakfast but still is drinking cola:

- What questions would you want to ask the caller?
- Devise a template to help you document the answers to the questions.

A national package of training has been devised to ensure that nurses who come from a background that was not child-health focused are prepared to competently assess the needs of children and their carers over the telephone. In addition, a CD ROM provides scenarios with which the nurse can

Table 22.2 The Most Commonly Used Algorithms

Top ten algorithms for patients aged < 1 year	Top ten algorithms for patients aged 1 year to 4 years 11 months	Top ten algorithms for patients aged 5 to 16 years
Vomiting	Fever	Rash
Fever	Rash	Abdominal pain
Rash	Vomiting	Fever
Cough	Cough	Vomiting
Diarrhoea	Ingestion of toxic material	Sore throat
Unwell/crying newborn	Diarrhoea	Head injury
Unwell/crying infant	Head injury	Headache
Head injury	Unwell/crying toddler	Cough
Constipation	Abdominal pain	Ingestion of toxic material
Skin problems	Sore throat	Ear pain

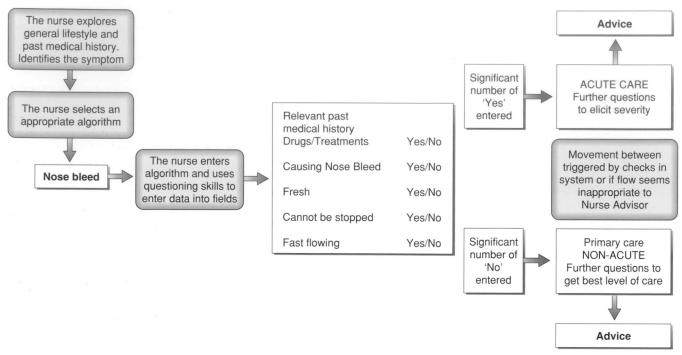

Fig. 22.5 • An NHS Direct algorithm.

explore debate and reflect on some of the more challenging issues they may encounter working for NHS Direct.

As highlighted previously, one of the challenges to working on the telephone is in identifying potential child protection issues. Specific questions in the algorithms provide prompts to the nurse to think laterally around the possibility of abuse and neglect. A national educational package has been devised in conjunction with NSPCC and will shortly be implemented across the service. Strategic planning for future service provision will include recommendations from the National Service Framework for Children to ensure that children have equitable access to quality care. Clear lines of communication with local child protection services at every site are in place to safeguard and protect children. Dilemmas will occur when dealing with phone calls about children and this will usually result in the nurse expressing his or her concerns. The following scenario illustrates the type of issues that may arise.

Professional Conversation

> A nurse advisor took a call from a female caller aged 24 at 22:00 on a Tuesday night. The original presenting reason for call was that the caller was feeling depressed. After a long consultation, the call outcome resulted in an emergency referral to the out-of-hours social work team to review the safety of the caller's four young children and a referral to the out-of-hours GP service for the caller.

The nurse advisor asked her supervisor to review the outcome of the call with her the next day. She wanted to review the progression of the consultation and the outcomes because, although she had previous experience with patients with mental health problems, she had limited child health experience. Because of the nature of the request from the nurse advisor, the supervisor asked another nurse advisor from a health visiting background to join the review.

Very early on, listening to the call, the health visitor stopped the tape and asked the nurse advisor what she had just heard that might cause an alarm bell to ring. The nurse advisor did not see anything at this point to ring alarm bells. The health visitor pointed out the time of the call and the fact that four very young children can be heard in the background still up and about. The nurse advisor, who had no children of her own, had not considered that it was inappropriate that small children should still be up at that time of night.

References

Audit Commission 1993 Children first. A study of hospital services. HMSO, London

Barber JW, King WD, Monroe KW, Nichols MH 2000 Evaluation of emergency department referrals by telephone triage. Pediatrics 105(4):819–821

Belman S, Murphy J, Steiner JF, Kempe A 2002 Consistency of triage decisions by call center nurses. Ambulatory Pediatrics 2:396–400

Briggs JK 2002 Telephone triage protocols for nurses, 2nd edn. Lippincott, New York

Buckles E, Carew-McColl M 1991 Triage by telephone. Nursing Times 87:26–28

Crouch R 2002 Computerised decision support. In: Thompson F, Dowding D (eds) Clincial decision making and judgement in nursing. Churchill Livingstone, Edinburgh

Department of Education and Skills (DfES) 2003 Every child matters. Cmd 0240. The Stationery Office, London

Department of Health (DoH) 1997 The new NHS: modern and dependable. The Stationery Office, London

Department of Health (DoH) 2001 NHS Direct: a new gateway to health care. Directorate of Access and Choice, DoH, London

Department of Health (DoH) 2003a Developing NHS Direct: a strategy for the next three years. Directorate of Access and Choice, DoH, London

Department of Health (DoH) 2003b Getting the right start: National Service Framework for Children. Emerging findings. Department of Health, London

Department of Health (DoH) 2003c What to do if you are worried a child is being abused. Health Services Circular 2003/007. DoH, London.

Dundas J, Casler C 1998 Can I talk to a nurse? Nursing Management 29(12):37–40

Edmonds E 1997 Telephone triage: 5 years experience. Accident and Emergency Nursing 5:8–13

Edwards B 1994 Telephone triage: how experienced nurses make decisions. Journal of Advanced Nursing 19:717–724

Edwards B 1998 Seeing is believing—picture building: a key component of telephone triage. Journal of Clinical Nursing 7:51–57

Eggleston CV, Kelly HC, Cope AR 1994 Use of telephone advice line in an accident and emergency department. British Medical Journal 308:31

Elston S, Thomas R 2002 Children nursing workforce. A report to the Royal College of Nursing and The Royal College of Paediatrics and Child Health. RCN, London

Glasper A 1993 Telephone triage: a step forward for nursing practice? British Journal of Nursing 2(2):108–109

House of Commons Committee of Public Accounts 2002 NHS Direct In England. Fortieth report of session 2001–2002, together with Proceedings of the Committee and Minutes of Evidence, HC610. The Stationery Office, London

Laming WH 2003 The Victoria Climbié inquiry/report of an inquiry by Lord Laming. The Stationery Office, London

Lattimer V, Crouch R 1999 Nurse telephone consultation. In: Salisbury C, Dale J, Hallam L (eds) 24 hour primary care. Radcliffe Medical Press, Oxford

Lattimer V, George S, Thompson F et al 1998 Safety and effectiveness of nurse telephone consultation in out of hours primary care: randomised control trial. British Medical Journal 317:1054–1059

Lyneham J 1998 The process of decision making by emergency nurses. Australian Journal of Advanced Nursing 16:2

Marklund B, Bengtsson C 1989 Medical advice by telephone at Swedish health centres: who calls and what are the problems. Family Practice 6(1):42–46

McClellan NJ 1999 NHS Direct: here and now. Archives of Disease in Childhood 81:376–379

McClellan NJ 2004 NHS Direct: virtually engaged. Archives of Disease in Childhood 89(1):57–59

Monaghan R, Clifford C, McDonald P 2003 Seeking advice from NHS Direct on common childhood complaints: does it matter who answers the phone? Journal of Advanced Nursing 42(2):209–216

Moore R 2001 A framework for telephone nursing. Nursing Times 97:16

Mosby's Pocket Dictionary of Nursing, Medicine and Professions Allied to Medicine 1995 Mosby, London

Munro J, Clancy M, Knowles E 2003 Evaluation of NHS Direct, impact and appropriateness. Medical Care Research Unit, University of Sheffield. Report to the Department of Health, October 2003

Munro J, Nicholl J, O'Cathain A et al 2000 Evaluation of NHS Direct first-wave sites: final report of the phase 1 research. Medical Care Research Unit, University of Sheffield. Report to the Department of Health, July 2000

National Audit Office 2002 NHS Direct in England. Report by the comptroller and Auditor General. HC505, Session 2001–2002, 25 January 2002

NHS Direct 2003 Online. Available at: http://www.nhsdirect.nhs.uk

Palmer SJ 1993 Care of sick children by parents: a meaningful role. Journal of Advanced Nursing 18:185–191

Pettonari CJ, Jessop L 2001 'Your ears become your eyes' Managing the absence of visibility in NHS Direct. Journal of Advanced Nursing 36:668–675

Quilter Wheeler S 1993 Telephone triage. Theory, practice and protocol development. Delmar, Albany, NJ

Ratcliffe N 2003 NHS Direct help or hindrance. Health Which? August:12–16

Royal College of Nursing (RCN) 1998 Nurse telephone consultation services information and good practice. RCN Publications, London

The Stationery Office 2004 Social Trends 34: a portrait of British society. National statistics. The Stationary Office, London

Thompson F 2001 Telling the story; experiences of making a call to NHS Direct. Unpublished thesis, Southampton University

Timpka T, Arborelius E 1994 The primary care nurses' dilemmas: a study of knowledge and need during telephone consultations. In: Smith J (ed.) Research and its application. Blackwell Scientific Publications, London

Valanis B, Tanner C, Randles Moscato S, Shapiro S 2003 A model for examining predictors of outcomes of telephone nursing advice. Journal of Nursing Administration 33(2):91–95

Wachter DA, Brillman JC, Lewis J, Sapien RE 1999 Pediatric telephone triage protocols: Standardised decision-making or a false sense of security. Annals of Emergency Medicine 33(4):388–394

Williams S 2000 NHS Direct investigated. Health Which? July:10–13

Chapter Twenty Three

23

The Role of Paediatric Emergency Assessment Units

Penny Aitken, E Alan Glasper, Maureen Wiltshire

ABSTRACT

The primary aim of this chapter is to raise the understanding of the key issues surrounding the emergency assessment of the sick child and family. The specialist skills required by paediatric nurses and the importance of the environment in which the child is admitted and treated will be explored.

The introduction of NHS Direct, walk-in centres and the changing role of both the GP and community nurse require all nurses working within the NHS to explore new ways of working in line with recent government directives. These nurses work with the child and family to provide hospital acute care when appropriate and support for the child to be cared for at home whenever possible.

Learning Outcomes

- Recognise the nursing skills required in the assessment of the acutely ill child.

- Appreciate the development of nurse-led initiatives in the care of the child and family.

- Understand the importance of recent inquires and government policies in the development of evidence-based practice for emergency care.

- Recognise the importance of family-centred care in the emergency assessment setting.

- Appreciate that children should only be admitted as inpatients when other services are inappropriate.

Introduction

Children should be admitted to hospital only if the care they require cannot be as well provided at home or on a short stay basis in hospital (DoH 1991)

The Royal College of Paediatrics and Child Health (RCPCH) supports this view and has highlighted the acute assessment unit as an example of best practice in the management of acute paediatric illness, which can prevent inappropriate admissions (RCPCH 1988). Such units are often sited adjacent to inpatient wards or within emergency departments and rely on skilled children's nurses. Meates (1997) has outlined the crucial role that they play in helping parents to provide self-care, thus reducing the need for overnight admission. Perhaps the most important objectives in establishing a Paediatric Emergency Assessment Unit (PEAU) are to place the child at the centre of care and to recognise the importance of the family in contributing to the care of their child (DoH 2003).

Children admitted to hospital for assessment are often seen in inappropriate areas, such as Emergency Departments without designated paediatric areas or treatment areas on wards. Of great concern to nurses and paediatricians is the risk of premature discharge of children without the opportunity to evaluate treatment and monitor improvement at home for 24 hours. The key objectives in establishing a PEAU are to:

- Assess all GP and other referrals and reduce unnecessary admission to hospital.

- Improve the quality of short-stay care and reduce family disruption.

- Adopt different ways of working to provide more effective use of resources.
- Provide the family with support to care for their sick child at home.
- Bridge any boundaries that may exist between primary and acute paediatric care.

This chapter and the companion PowerPoint presentation will follow an ill child from the initial consultation with the GP, admission to a PEAU, observation, discharge planning for care at home, follow-up next day telephone call and communication with other healthcare professionals.

Referral and Admission to PEAU

Many PEAUs have been designed to enhance services to local GPs and a study by Aitken et al (2003) demonstrated that the majority of admissions were initiated from this source. The changing nature of initial contact between a family and the health service is ensuring that triage or the determination of urgency of healthcare intervention is taking place in a variety of geographical locations and mediums.

The use of the telephone by nurses has grown enormously in the UK since the inception of NHS Direct, and telephone nursing reflects the growth in the use of the telephone in contemporary British society (Glasper & Wilkins 1998). The safety and effectiveness of nurse telephone consultations was described by Lattimer et al (1998) who, in a seminal randomised controlled trial of equivalence between GPs and nurses, found that there were no adverse outcomes for patients.

In 2003, Aitken et al (unpublished data) reported a survey of GPs following a nurse-led initiative of accepting direct referrals. This clearly demonstrated that GPs are happy to refer sick children to a PEAU via a dedicated telephone referral system. Although not all acute assessment units provide this service, the advantage of the GP speaking to the nurse ultimately receiving the child provides a clearer picture of the nature of the condition. This saves time for both the family and GP and therefore enhances a seamless service through the healthcare system.

WWW

Read summaries of the three chapters of the National Service Framework for Children's hospital services document and then look up the Chief Nursing Officer's ten key roles for nursing. In particular, explore the nurse's role in direct referrals:

- http://www.doh.gov.uk/NSF/children.htm
- http://www.doh.gov.uk/newrolesfornurses

Scenario

Ann-Marie is a 4-year-old girl who lives at home with her parents, her two sisters aged 12 and 10 years old and her 8-year-old brother. Ann-Marie attends a local playgroup and has no previous admissions to hospital. Ann-Marie was taken to her GP with a 3-day history of cough, a temperature and reluctance to eat and drink. On arrival at the Paediatric Emergency Assessment Unit her respiratory rate = 40, pulse = 128, temperature = 38.2°C and oxygen saturations = 96% in air.

Activity

- What are the normal parameters for temperature, heart rate, respiratory rate, oxygen saturations and weight for a 4-year-old?
- What immediate nursing intervention would Ann-Marie require?
- In relation to the ten key roles of the nurse that you have previously explored, which patient group directives have been agreed in your clinical area?
- What training is required nationally to allow nurse prescribing?

WWW

Read the Paediatric Resuscitation guidelines online:

- http://www.resus.org.uk/pages/guide.htm

Explore a clinical decision support information system online:

- http://www.isabel.org.uk/

Children's nurses working with ill children and their families are required to develop a wide range of advanced skills that meet the expectations of paediatric emergency assessment (Box 23.1). It is important that the nurse establishes a good professional relationship on meeting the child and family. This will enable the nurse to carry out a full nursing assessment to include a physical, developmental and social history and negotiate a plan of care. The very nature of childhood illnesses can result in some children presenting with a life-threatening condition and it is therefore essential that all staff undertake a recognised paediatric advanced life support course.

As the role of the children's nurse develops, the skills become more enhanced and the paediatric nurse practitioner will be first-line assessing and managing ill children. Although the majority of paediatric episodic illnesses are relatively benign and resolve completely, the implications of a missed diagnosis could become life threatening. Therefore, regardless of the type of illness, the basic information and skills required in the acute assessment of an ill child are for the most part the same in all children. Before the history-taking process begins it is essential that the

Box 23.1

Types of conditions likely to be encountered in a PEAU

Although every assessment unit will offer slightly different services, the principles behind the units will be similar, in that they offer first-line emergency assessment of acute illness. Which specialities are seen within a unit will depend on the service requirements, however it is likely to include a vast variety of conditions and illness. Below are examples of the conditions that may be seen within a PEAU:

- abscesses
- appendicitis
- asthma
- bronchiolitis
- constipation
- convulsions
- croup
- diabetes mellitus/ketoacidosis
- failure to thrive
- gastroenteritis
- head injuries
- Henoch–Schönlein purpura
- hernias
- Hirschsprung's disease
- intussusceptions
- irritable hip
- jaundice
- Kawasaki disease
- meningitis
- pyrexia unknown origin
- rashes
- septic arthritis
- testicular problems
- urinary tract infection.

Child protection issues will also be encountered.

nurse who is looking after the child and family introduces him- or herself, puts them at their ease and makes them feel welcome. A child-friendly environment should be encouraged, with age-appropriate toys and distraction. Privacy should be ensured throughout.

A well-taken and documented medical and social history of an ill child is crucial for the diagnosis and management of care for both the child and family. Open-ended questions should be used to ensure a full response from the child and family. At all times children should be encouraged to participate and tell their 'own story'. During the history-taking process it is helpful to maintain as much eye contact as possible with the child and family.

Even before the nurse lays a single hand on the child, a major element of the physical examination should have taken place. While undertaking the history from the child and family, the nurse will have been observing both child and family members to answer the questions:

- How do the parents relate to the child, and the child to its parents?
- Do the parents appear anxious, upset or distressed?

- Does the child happily separate from his or her parents?
- Does the child play age appropriately?
- Is the child unusually distressed?

Nurses working in an emergency assessment environment are frequently practising at a nurse practitioner level, which includes physical assessment, history taking, venesection, cannulation and prescribing (Box 23.2) (Dearmun & Gordon 1999, Rushforth 2002, Rushforth & Glasper 1999). Additionally, such nurses – using established protocols – admit children as inpatients and discharge them home with support of follow-up services (this will be discussed later in the chapter).

Professional Conversation

Hayley Anderson is a second-year student nurse on clinical placement on a Paediatric Emergency Assessment Unit. Ellen Lancaster, her mentor, is a staff nurse within the unit.

Issues relating to physical and social history taking

While undertaking the assessment of Ann-Marie, Hayley asks her mentor to explain areas of the assessment and care that all children admitted to the unit are subjected to:

'I've been on the ward for three shifts and I just don't understand why whenever a child presents we have to take such a detailed physical and social history – why do we need to know the surname of who lives in the home, if all the siblings have the same parents, and if they have a social worker or not? And why do we need to undress Ann-Marie, she's experiencing shortness of breath – she has a chest problem, she doesn't have abdominal pain, she hasn't experienced any lower limb trauma?'

Ellen explains to Hayley how every child requires a full social and medical history to ensure nothing is missed:

'Bringing a child to hospital can be very stressful and therefore by ensuring we follow a structured assessment process we are reducing the risk of missing information that may be vital in the diagnoses and treatment of the child. By observing a child prior to a physical assessment, a relationship can be built and in taking this social and medical history, time is allowed for this.'

Reflect on your Practice

Could you explain to a parent why there is a need for a full physical examination of all children presenting to an emergency assessment unit, as well as documenting a full social and medical history?

Activity

- Review the admission paperwork for children in your own practice area; do they meet the recommendations following the Victoria Climbié inquiry.
- Draw your own family tree. Could a colleague easily identify the age, sex and occupation of your parents and siblings? Could they identify who lives in the family home?

Box 23.2

Types of skills likely to be developed when working on a PEAU

With the various learning opportunities offered within PEAU, both qualified and student nurses should have the opportunity to enhance their skills in many areas, not least in some of the examples below, whether by doing or assisting:

- cannulation
- collection of specimens
- distraction and play
- emergency procedures
- fluid management
- health promotion
- history taking
- inhaler techniques
- initial assessment of a sick child
- liaison with multidisciplinary team
- lumbar punctures
- managing pyrexia
- nasogastric tube management
- nebulisation
- negotiating with children
- negotiating with parents
- neurological observation
- ongoing assessment of a sick child
- pain management
- physical assessment
- pulse oximetry
- venesection.

www

Read the Victoria Climbié report online:

- http://www.victoria-climbie-inquiry.org.uk/finreport/inquiry.htm

Read the *Safeguarding children* document online:

- http://www.doh.gov.uk/safeguardingchildren/index.htm

Observation

The problems associated with short-stay admissions inappropriately admitted to acute children's wards are many but include time-consuming admission procedures and admissions to inappropriate wards where specialist nurses or equipment may not be at hand. Additionally, beds for elective admissions are effectively blocked. Consultant ward rounds are delays that impact on discharge and, importantly, an undermining of parental confidence in self-managing minor illnesses in the home. Furthermore, the economic costs in terms of bed occupancy and resource allocation should not be underestimated.

Although hospital inpatient care is undeniably expensive, in both fiscal and social domains, for the families of sick children and the admitting hospital, the reasons for admission to paediatric beds has only recently been investigated in the UK. Much of the literature is focused on the appropriateness of hospital admission and MacFaul (1997) has indicated that 50% of paediatric emergencies are discharged within 1 day and reports a significant reduction in overnight stays after the opening of a short-stay acute illness assessment facility.

Similarly, an Australian review of paediatric admissions (Numa & Oberklaid 1991) concluded that 65% of eligible admissions would have been fit for discharge within 12 hours had there been a short-stay unit available. A subsequent Australian study (Browne 2000) revealed considerable approval in terms of parental satisfaction with short-stay and cost savings when a 23-hour short-stay unit was attached to the emergency department.

The mean stay for children entering a PEAU in the study by Aitken et al (2003) was 2 hours 57 minutes. Although the NHS is inextricably focusing on waiting times, which are now linked to a wide range of Ministerial Directives, White Papers and Health Service Circulars (DoH 2000), the overall satisfaction of the family encounter with the healthcare facility must remain high. Accordingly, benchmark standards of care are a high priority for nurses and other healthcare professionals involved with service delivery. The publication of documents such as *The essence of care* (DoH 2001) encourages all healthcare professionals to 'think out of the box' when reconciling innovation with improved levels of family satisfaction.

In the absence of such units, unnecessary delays often prolong the admission. Beattie & Moir (1993), in reporting the first annual audit of a 24-hour short-stay ward attached to an emergency department, studied 829 children of whom 25% stayed less than 12 hours. The most common cause of admission reported in this audit was head injury, with 479 cases documented.

Professional Conversation

> Second-year student nurse Hayley Anderson is discussing Ann-Marie's case with staff nurse Ellen Lancaster, her mentor in the PEAU.

Nursing observation after medical treatment
Following a good response to paracetamol, when Ann-Marie's temperature has reduced and she appears much

more happy and content in herself, student nurse Hayley Anderson asks her mentor Ellen (who is sharing Ann-Marie's care with her) when the family will be discharged home. Staff nurse Ellen explains the need for a period of observation to ensure that Ann-Marie's parents are happy with fever management at home, that she tolerates good volumes of oral fluids and that her condition remains stable.

Ellen goes on to explain to Hayley that this period of observation also gives the opportunity for the nurse to address any educational or health promotion needs of the child and family.

Interestingly, the justification for a 24-hour PEAU service has been rejected in at least one large North American study (Bond & Weigand 1997), which concluded that a single observation bed would be inadequate 25% of the time and empty 37% of the time. In a retrospective study conducted by Rajaratnam (1991) of admission case notes of children, between 15% and 20% of the 620 randomly selected cases were considered by the assessors not to have required admission. Furthermore, between 3% and 9% of the admissions were judged to be for social and not medical reasons.

Medical and social factors associated with paediatric emergency admissions to hospital have been the subject of some scrutiny. Steward et al (1998) have linked self-referral by parents to an accident and emergency department as being associated with socio-economic deprivation. It is the appropriateness of childhood emergency admissions that continues to be linked to the evolution of services such as a PEAU. Although Esmail et al (2000) cite evidence of rises in paediatric admissions to UK hospitals, with these possibly being linked to poor social circumstances, in a retrospective review of 3324 paediatric admissions from 13 district general hospitals only 8% were found to be inappropriate. This perhaps reflects the discriminatory prowess of the robust UK primary healthcare services and, importantly, in this study inappropriate admissions were not linked to GP referrals.

Of interest is a report of a study on 18,057 children by Raffles et al (1999), which compared admission rates to a child health unit before and after the creation of a dedicated six-bedded PEAU situated within a busy emergency department. The reduction in overnight admission rates was calculated at 19% in the first year of operation of the PEAU.

Reductions in overnight stays in a climate of increased emergency admissions of children generally to hospital are clearly linked to the development of PEAUs and a French report (Lamireau et al 2000) concludes that a short-stay unit can provide cost-effective, comprehensive care linked to a reduction of fears among clinicians of inappropriate discharge.

Discharge and Follow-up Care

Hospital admission involving an overnight stay is always disruptive to the families concerned and Rajaratnam (1991) highlights these and the potential opportunity costs in discussing the reconfiguration that some hospitals have made to their paediatric inpatient facilities in the light of changes in the management of emergency admissions.

A quadrennial review of data during one calendar month by Aitken et al (2003) related to emergency patient length of stay revealed a substantial rise in the number of children admitted for less than 1 day and therefore avoiding an overnight stay since the opening of the unit in 1998. The rise in overall numbers of short-stay children was also accompanied by a corresponding fall in the number of children staying overnight in hospital during the same time period. Lamireau et al (2000) and Beverly et al (1997) have reported similar magnitudes of raises in short-stay patients.

Activity

Discharge planning is a key part of the admission process. Review your local discharge process and paperwork in relation to Ann-Marie.

Reflect on your Practice

What skills are needed to empower parents and children with both the knowledge and confidence to be cared for at home?

One of the increasing concerns expressed by some authors is that of inappropriate or premature discharge (MacFaul 1997). It is important to stress that during the study by Aitken et al (2003) only one child was readmitted to the PEAU within 24 hours of discharge; three children who had attended the PEAU within the previous week were readmitted, as were three who had been discharged within the previous month. A total of 20 children in the study had been inpatients within the previous month with 56 children attending the emergency department within the previous month.

In a study by Lal & Kibirige (1999), who investigated the relationship between paediatric assessment units, quality of care and unscheduled return visits, only 2% (n = 65) of children were identified. The primary identified reason stated for these returns was parental perceptions of the illness with only two re-referred by their family doctor. Such findings reinforce the crucial role of the PEAU nurse in the giving of discharge information, ensuring that in partnership parents are fully involved in the decision making process and that all concerns are fully addressed.

Proactively, the nursing staff in some PEAUs have introduced weekday 24-hour open access and an extended period to cover weekend and bank holiday read-mission to PEAU for just such eventualities. The establishment of an open access process for children, without the necessity of re-consulting a GP is thought to be reassuring for parents who might have residual worries after discharge. Additionally, some PEAUs offer a routine, morning-after-discharge nurse-led telephone consultation to all parents. A survey of parental satisfaction with paediatric emergency care revealed that parents found both the open access arrangement and follow-up telephone call reassuring (Aitken et al 2003, unpublished data).

Professional Conversation

> Hayley Anderson, a second-year student nurse on clinical placement on a PEAU, asks staff nurse Ellen Lancaster, her mentor, about follow-up procedures on the unit.

Follow-up after discharge from hospital

The morning after Ann-Marie's discharge, student nurse Hayley asks staff nurse Ellen why she is telephoning the family, as they have been discharged home and been given 24 hours open access if they are concerned. She expresses concerns about the amount of nursing time this takes up. She further discusses the view that NHS Direct gives advice over the telephone and that the NHS Direct nurses are supported by computerised decision support software. She asks 'Should nurses really be doing such telephone interaction without such tools?'

Ellen explains that although it is true that parents can contact the unit if they are concerned, the telephone follow-up allows nursing staff to reinforce any information given on discharge and provides an important link between the nursing staff and family. Parents/carers may well wish to clarify certain issues or concerns and feel reluctant to 'bother' busy health professionals. The follow-up telephone call allows parents to ask questions about the previous day's treatment and for nursing staff to address any concerns.

Activity

- Explore the cost of an overnight admission and the effect of an unnecessary admission to hospital on a child and their family.
- Examine the legalities of telephone advice and the introduction of NHS Direct.

Reflect on your Practice

- Consider the importance of team working in the assessment and planning of individual care for the acutely sick child and the consequences of a breakdown of communication in the multidisciplinary team.
- Reflect on a recent example of a breakdown in communication within your own working environment.

Summary

The study by Aitken et al (2003) reinforced the importance of service evaluation as part of a child health unit commitment to clinical governance. The development of the PEAU cited in this study was very much a nurse-led initiative and the success of the service is indicative of children's nurses' pledge to family-centred care. In avoiding an unnecessary hospital stay, potential emotional child and family upset may be avoided. In this way, seminal contemporary child health policy publications (DoH 1996) can be enacted and adhered to.

However, new opportunities for nurses to work in this expanding field of practice will require an appropriate educational preparation, which includes physical history taking and examination (Rushforth et al 1998).

KEY POINTS

- Emergency assessment short-stay units appear to be an effective way to manage some children not requiring overnight hospital stay.
- Although difficult to calculate, the economic benefits of short-stay units should not be underestimated.
- Fears of inappropriate premature discharge, although important, do not appear to be a cause for concern.

References

Aitken P, Birch S, Cogman G et al 2003 Quadrennial review of a paediatric emergency assessment unit. British Journal of Nursing 12(4):234–241

Beattie TF, Moir A 1993 Paediatric accident and emergency short-stay; a 1 year audit. Archives of Emergency Medicine 10:181–186

Beverly DW, Ball RJ, Smith RA et al 1997 Planning for the future; the experience of implementing a children's day assessment unit in a district general hospital. Archives of Disease in Childhood 77(4):287–292

Bond GR, Wiegand CB 1997 Estimated use of pediatric emergency department observation unit. Annal of Emergency Medicine 29:739–742

Browne GJ 2000 A short stay or 23 hour ward in a general and academic childrens hospital; are they effective? Paediatric Emergency Care 16(4):223–229

Dearmun A, Gordon K 1999 The nurse practitioner in children's ambulatory care. Paediatric Nursing 11(1):18–21

Department of Health (DoH) 1991 Welfare of children and young people in hospital. HMSO, London

Department of Health (DoH) 1996 The patients charter. Services for children and young people. HMSO, London

Department of Health (DoH) 2000 The NHS Plan. A plan for investment, a plan for reform. HMSO, London

Department of Health (DoH) 2001 The essence of care. Patient-focused benchmarking for health care practitioners. Online. Available at: hhtp://www.doh.gov.uk/essenceofcare

Department of Health (DoH) 2003 The children's national service framework. DoH, London

Esmail A, Quayle JA, Roberts C 2000 Assessing the appropriateness of paediatric hospital admissions in the United Kingdom. Journal of Public Health Medicine 22(92):231–238

Glasper EA, Wilkins V 1998 Telenursing – the provision of information by telephone: the implication for paediatric nursing. In: Glasper EA, Lowson S (eds) Innovations in paediatric ambulatory care – a nursing perspective. Macmillan, Basingstoke, pp 31–47

Lal MK, Kibirige MS 1999 Unscheduled return visits within 72 hours to an assessment unit. Archives of Disease in Childhood 80(5):455–458

Lamireau T, Llanas B, Fayon M 2000 A short stay observation unit improves care in the paediatric emergency care setting. Archives of Disease in Childhood 83(4):371

Lattimer V, George S, Thompson F et al 1998 Safety and effectiveness of nurse telephone consultation in out of hours primary care: randomised controlled trial. British Medical Journal 317:1054–1059

MacFaul R 1997 Commentary – planning for the future. The experience of implementing a children's day assessment unit in a district general hospital. Archives of Disease in Childhood 77(4):292–293

Meates M 1997 Ambulatory paediatrics – making a difference. Archives of Disease in Childhood 76:468–476

Numa A, Oberklaid F 1991 Can short hospital admissions be avoided? A review of admissions less than 24 hours duration in paediatric teaching hospital. Medical Journal of Australia 155(6):395–398

Raffles A, Foo WL, Chowdhurt T, Dustagheer L 1999 Does a paediaric acute assessment unit influence paediatric admissions? Proceeding of the Royal College of Paediatrics and Child Health Spring Meeting. Tuesday 13 April 1999. RCPCH, London

Rajaratnam G 1991 A study of admissions to paediatric beds. Postgraduate Medical Journal 67:50–54

Royal College of Paediatircs and Child Health (RCPCH) 1998 Ambulatory paediatric services in the UK. Report of a working party. RCPCH, London

Rushforth H 2002 Study of the factors influencing decisions by acute care nurses to undertake expanded roles traditionally associated with medical practice. Final study report for the UKCC. UKCC, London

Rushforth H, Glasper EA 1999 Implications of nursing role expansion for professional practice. British Journal of Nursing 8(22):1507–1513

Rushforth H, Warner J, Burge D, Glasper EA 1998 Nursing physical assessment skills: implications for UK practice. British Journal of Nursing 7(16):965–970

Steward M, Werneke U, MacFaul R et al 1998 Medical and social factors associated with admissions and discharge of acutely ill children. Archives of Disease in Childhood 79:219–224

Chapter Twenty Four

24

Emergency Department Management of Children

Julie Flaherty, E Alan Glasper

ABSTRACT

The primary aim of this chapter and its companion PowerPoint presentation is to review emergency care for children and the role of children's nurses in emergency departments. The role of the children's nurse in maintaining the integrity of the family unit during emergency interventions is highlighted. A case study scenario based around a child with epilepsy is utilised in this chapter.

Learning Outcomes

- Develop the specialist knowledge required to safely administer medicines to children.

- Understand how the triage process is operationalised in paediatric emergency departments.

- Explore how children presenting with fits are managed in emergency departments.

- Appreciate positive attributes of the environment of care in emergency departments in the overall care of children.

- Review pain management for children in emergency departments.

- Consider how the philosophy of family-centred care is promoted in emergency departments.

- Appreciate the role of paediatric emergency nurse practitioners.

The National Picture

A 1997 report of national trends in the UK between 1979 and 1997 identified that in one year alone 459 children died as a result of accidents. Approximately 3.5 million children attend local A&E departments for their injuries each year and 10,000 children become permanently disabled every year. The cost to the NHS has been estimated at £100 million per annum; the personal cost is unquantifiable.

Since the inception of the NHS, medical care has been comprehensively provided for all. In the early 1960s the term 'casualty' became synonymous with that part of the NHS receiving and stabilising acutely ill and injured patients. The portal of entry into the hospital setting for the ill and injured was through the 'casualty' department. At the same time as the acutely ill and injured attended, those members of the public who felt their physical and mental health need required urgent medical attention took advantage of the casualty department's ever open door.

In 1961, the Standing Medical Advisory Committee of Central Health Services undertook an investigation into NHS acute hospital arrangements for receiving and stabilisation of acutely ill and injured patients. The subsequent report for the first time formally recognised the concept of 'casual attendees' within the casualty department. Within the report, acknowledgement was given to the very skilful and important work undertaken in casualty departments. In recognition that this work should continue to develop, the concepts of 'casualty' and 'casual attendees' needed to be refocused and the term 'Accident and Emergency' A&E department was created.

Many subsequent reports, including the Court report *Fit for the future* (Department of Health and Social Services (DHSS) 1976), *Welfare of children and young people in hospital* (Department of Health (DoH) 1991), *Children first. A study of hospital services* (Audit

Commission 1993) and *The patient's charter – services for children and young people* (DoH 1996), all advocated and determined recommendations and standards for health services, with specific reference to A&E services for children. Furthermore, there is now evidence that some of the recommendations of the many working groups are now taking shape, although slowly. Within the current climate of the modernising NHS (DoH 2000, 2004) there is now greater emphasis than ever on recognising and meeting the needs of families and children requiring A&E services.

There are currently many avenues to emergency services for children and young people. Importantly there are nine active children's A&E departments in the UK. Alternatively, there are 259 other A&E departments accommodating health needs of all ages either in teaching or district general hospitals. The general A&E departments vary tremendously from integrated child and family services, audiovisual separation of adults and children to co-location of child and adult services.

In an average year, 50% of children under 1 year of age will attend an emergency department, and 25% of older children. Additionally, one in 11 children will be referred to a hospital outpatient department (NHS Confederation 2003). Additionally, an important change has occurred in the utilization of emergency departments in recent years, with increasing numbers of children seeking hospital assessment, largely via self-referrals, but not requiring hospital admission (Boyle et al 2000).

Given the high profile that children have within an emergency department and Watson (2000) indicates that this client group makes up 30% of all attendees to emergency departments every year, it is not surprising to note that the National Service Framework (NSF) for children, young people and maternity services (DoH 2003) includes specific recommendations for accident and emergency departments. These include physical separation between children and adult areas within emergency departments and environments that are accessible, safe and suitable for babies, children and families.

Partridge (2001) has highlighted that children attending emergency departments have not generally been either treated or seen in separate facilities by registered children's nurses. This situation will begin to change in light of the NSF recommendations, which will be audited by the Commission for Health Audit and Inspection (CHAI). Furthermore, Partridge argues that nurses who work in emergency departments must recognise that the treatment of children and adults within the same space is fraught with difficulties. This sharing of facilities such as waiting rooms ensures that at least some children will be exposed unnecessarily to hostile sights and hostile sounds. It is, however, to be hoped that the token obligatory box of broken toys in a dark corner of the waiting room of some emergency depart-

ments, as described by Glasper (1995), is a thing of the past. However, nurse managers within emergency departments recognise these important aspects of care and are increasingly requiring registered nurses not holding a recognised children's nursing qualification to undertake shortened child branch courses at local universities.

Scenario

Sheila Putman is 4 years and 6 months. She had a grand-mal convulsion in the school playground and sustained a laceration to the scalp, which bled profusely. She is dazed and confused after the convulsion, crying and asking for her mother. The teacher calls an ambulance and travels with Sheila to the local emergency department. Sheila's mother is eventually located at her work address on the outskirts of the city. She arrives at the emergency department 30 minutes after Sheila's arrival.

Transportation to the Emergency Department

By far the best way for critically ill and injured children to travel to hospital is by ambulance. However, parents and carers are often unaware of the severity of illness and injury that children suffer. Often because of their size, children are 'scooped up' and brought by people unaware of the risks they are taking escorting children in critical conditions by private car, public transport or taxi. Only 6% of children attend emergency departments by ambulance.

Taking this figure into account, it is important that A&E staff are aware that seriously ill and injured children often arrive in the emergency department 'in arms', and should receive early triage for this very reason. Conveying to the public the message about appropriate use of ambulances in urgent and emergency situations has been ongoing for years. There are, however, numerous accounts of situations when an ambulance has been called inappropriately by someone who has misjudged the situation. The nationally available NHS Direct telephone advice service is available for parents and carers (tel: 0845 46 47). The nurses can provide emergency advice about a child's health status and mobilise an ambulance if necessary.

Ninety per cent of all children attending A&E do so between 8.00 a.m. and midnight; the remaining 10% attend between midnight and 8.00 a.m. The busiest period for children in A&E is between mid-day and 4.00 p.m., when over 55% children attend for unscheduled care; 80% of children with traumatic injury arrive between 4.00 p.m. and midnight.

Macfaul & Werneke (2001) conducted a study in which presenting problems were recorded in 842 admissions. Fifty-six per cent of children presented with one of three problems: breathing difficulty (25%), fit (16%), or feverish illness (15%). Feeding problems and diarrhoea together accounted for a further 21%. Seizures as a high cause of emergency admissions have come under considerable scrutiny by healthcare professionals working in such environments. The introduction of clinical guidelines (or care pathways) for the management of children presenting with fits in emergency departments is linked to improvements in the effectiveness of care delivery (Arnon et al 2004).

Activity

Critically review the Arnon et al (2004) paper. Access this online at: http://www.archdischild.com
Read the article by Watts et al (2003) and look at the Joanna Briggs Institute, Adelaide website. Access this at: http://www.joannabriggs.edu.au

What are Fits, Convulsions or Seizures?

WWW

The following text is based on *About seizures*, a leaflet produced by the Royal Children's Hospital Melbourne. Access the original document at:
* http://www.rch.org.au/cep/epilepsy/

Many people in society suffer from fits, convulsions or seizures. One in 20 (5%) of all children will have a fit of some kind during childhood. About 1 in 200 (0.5%) children have epilepsy, i.e. a neurological condition in which the child has a predisposition to recurrent, unprovoked fits.

Epileptic fits occur when there is a transient disarrangement of the electrical and chemical neurotransmitters in the brain, which results in brain cells discharging impulses in an abnormal fashion. This may create a temporary disturbance in the way the brain controls awareness and responsiveness, which commonly causes unusual sensations or abnormal movements and postures. What happens during a fit reflects what parts of the brain are involved.

There are many different types of fit. The following describes the classification of seizure types from the International League Against Epilepsy (ILAE). A major distinction that healthcare professionals try to make is between partial (focal) fits, where the abnormal activity arises in a localised part of the brain (usually on one side), and generalised fits, where epileptic activity begins all over the brain simultaneously.

PARTIAL (FOCAL) FITS

Partial (focal) fits occur when the abnormal activity arises in a localised part of the brain, usually on one side, and consciousness may or may not be impaired. The manifestations of the seizure depend on the part of the brain involved with the abnormal electrical discharge. Partial fits are classified according to whether there is impairment of consciousness:

* **Simple partial fits**: arise in parts of the brain not responsible for maintaining consciousness, typically the movement or sensory areas. Consciousness is *not* impaired and the effects of the fit relate to the part of the brain involved. If the site of origin is the motor area of the brain, bodily movements may be abnormal (e.g. limp, stiff, jerking). If sensory areas of the brain are involved, the person may report experiences such as tingling or numbness, changes to what he or she sees, hears or smells, or very unusual feelings that may be hard to describe. Young children might have difficulty describing such sensations or may be frightened by these.

* **Complex partial seizures**: arise in parts of the brain responsible for maintaining awareness, responsiveness and memory – typically parts of the temporal and frontal lobes. Consciousness is lost and the person may appear dazed or unaware of his or her surroundings. Sometimes the person experiences a warning sensation, or aura, before losing awareness, essentially the simple partial phase of the fit. Behaviour during a complex partial fit relates to the site of origin and spread of the fit. Often, the person's actions are clumsy and the individual will not respond normally to questions and commands. Behaviour may be confused and the person might exhibit automatic movements and behaviours, e.g. picking at clothing, picking up objects, chewing and swallowing, trying to stand or run, appearing afraid and struggling with restraint. Colour change, wetting and vomiting can occur in complex partial fits. Following the fit, the person may remain confused for a prolonged period and may not be able to speak, see, or hear if these parts of the brain were involved. The person has no memory of what occurred during the complex partial phase of the fit and often needs to sleep.

* **Partial seizures becoming secondarily generalized**: fits that begin as simple or complex partial seizures may progress due to a spread of epileptic activity all over one or both sides of the brain, leading to a secondary generalised seizure. This part of the fit looks like a generalised tonic clonic seizure.

GENERALISED SEIZURES

Generalised fits occur when epileptic activity begins all over the brain simultaneously and consciousness is always impaired in generalised seizures:

- **Tonic clonic fit:** sometimes called a 'grand mal' fit: produces a sudden loss of consciousness, with the person commonly falling to the ground followed by stiffening (tonic) and then rhythmic jerking (clonic) of the muscles. Shallow or jerky breathing, bluish tinge of the skin and lips, drooling of saliva and often loss of bladder or bowel control generally occur. The seizures usually last a couple of minutes and normal breathing and consciousness then returns. The person is tired following the seizure and may be confused. There is no aura prior to a tonic clonic seizure.

- **Absence fit:** sometimes called a 'petit mal' fit: produces a brief cessation of activity and loss of consciousness, usually lasting 5–30 seconds. Often, the momentary blank stare is accompanied by subtle eye blinking and mouthing or chewing movements. Awareness returns quickly and the person continues with the previous activity. Falling and jerking do not occur in typical absences.

- **Myoclonic fit:** sudden and brief muscle contractions that may occur singly, repeatedly or continuously. They may involve the whole body in a massive jerk or spasm, or may only involve individual limbs or muscle groups. If they involve the arms, the person might drop or spill what he or she was holding. If they involve the legs or body, the person may fall.

- **Tonic fit:** characterised by generalised muscle stiffening, lasting 1–10 seconds. Associated features include increased pulse, brief cessation of breathing, flushed face, bluish skin discoloration and drooling. If a tonic seizure occurs suddenly while the person is awake, he or she may fall violently to the ground, causing injury. Tonic seizures often occur during sleep. Fortunately, tonic fits are rare and usually only occur in severe forms of epilepsy.

- **Atonic fit:** produces a sudden loss of muscle tone, which, if brief, may only involve the head dropping forward ('head nods'), but may cause sudden collapse and falling ('drop attacks').

From these descriptions, it can be appreciated that the exact type of fit may be difficult for a witness to determine. For example, a fit with stopping and staring could be a complex partial seizure or an absence seizure. A large, convulsive fit (grand mal) may be a generalised tonic clonic fit, a myoclonic fit, a tonic fit or a partial fit that became secondarily generalised. A sudden fall to the ground ('drop attack') can occur with a myoclonic, a tonic or a atonic fit or a partial fit involving the movement areas. Determination of the exact type of fit is important and is obtained from patient and observer descriptions, home video recordings, and EEG testing and sometimes video EEG monitoring.

It is also important to remember that many episodic behaviours and disorders in children can mimic epilepsy, including breath-holding spells, normal sleep jerks, daydreaming, fainting, migraine, heart and gastrointestinal problems and psychological problems.

MANAGING ACUTE SEIZURES AND STATUS EPILEPTICUS

Activity

Think about the management of a brief seizure by putting yourself into the position of witnessing a child, known to have epilepsy, who is having a seizure in school:
- What would you do?
- What would you not do?

www

Advice relating to seizure management can be readily found on the following websites:
- Epilepsy Action (British Epilepsy Association) search for seizure-first aid: http://www.epilepsy.org.uk
- National Society for Epilepsy search for first aid for epilepsy: http://www.epilepsynse.org.uk

Rapid treatment has the potential to minimise the morbidity and mortality associated with acute seizures and convulsive status epilepticus (Scott et al 1998, Scott & Neville 1999). Although status epilepticus is described as a disorder in which epileptic activity, a seizure or series of seizures persists for 30 minutes or more, clinically, most seizures that do not stop spontaneously within 5 minutes progress for 30 minutes or more (Appleton et al 2000, Scott et al 1998, Tasker 1998). Seizure activity dramatically increases the brain's demands for oxygen and glucose. After 30 minutes compensatory mechanisms fail, resulting in cerebral oedema, metabolic acidosis and circulatory collapse and an increasing risk of cerebral damage (Shovron 2001). Causes of acute seizures in children include (Shovron 2000):

- Acute cerebral dysfunction:
  - trauma
  - infection
  - tumours
  - metabolic disturbances
  - febrile seizures.

- Pre-existing epilepsy:
  - drug withdrawal
  - progression of underlying cause
  - acute illness.

The aim of management is to control the seizure before cerebral damage and life-threatening sequelae occur (Scott et al 1998, Tasker 1998). Clear protocols with structured interventions are necessary to ensure prompt and consistent management of seizures and status epilepticus (Appleton et al 2000, Scott & Neville 1999, Shovron 2001, Tasker 1998) (Table 24.1).

Children who have repeated episodes of convulsive epilepticus may need an adapted acute protocol to reflect their individual response to treatments and interactions with regular anticonvulsants (Scott & Neville 1999, Tasker 1998). Individual protocols will require the inclusion of parental home treatment regimes.

Emergency Care Teams

Given that accidents are the foremost cause of death in children over 1 year of age, response to the care of the most seriously ill and injured children must be delivered speedily and following a professionally competent model backed up by the right facilities. A team approach allows critically ill and traumatised patients optimal chances for survival.

The Royal College of Surgeons recommends that the emergency care team should include a team leader, usually the A&E consultant, a surgical consultant, a medical consultant, and an anaesthetic or intensivist consultant. Other team members will be registered nurses and allied health professionals (AHP); the numbers will vary but it has been suggested that the trauma team should include four senior doctors, five nurses and a radiographer. It was clearly stated in the National Confidential Enquiry into Perioperative Deaths (1989 p 7) that:

Consultants who take responsibility for the care of children . . . must be competent and must keep up to date in the management of children.

The Royal College of Paediatricians and Child Health stipulates that a nominated consultant anaesthetist, suitably

Table 24.1 Principles of Managing Acute Seizures and Status Epilepticus (Appleton et al 2000, Scott & Neville 1999, Shovron 2001, Tasker 1998)

Stage	Action	Rationale
Immediate assessment and stabilisation	• Rapid cardiopulmonary assessment • If necessary maintain and secure airway • Give oxygen • Monitor vital signs and pulse oximetry • Confirmation/history of seizure/child's past medical history	Recognise respiratory failure and shock Airway obstruction will compound hypoxia Ensure management is appropriate for the individual child
Immediate seizure control (5–10 minutes)	Administer first-line anticonvulsant: • If IV access available, administer IV lorazepam • If there is no venous access, administer either rectal diazepam or intramuscular midazolam or intramuscular paraldehyde. Obtain IV or intraosseous access • Obtain bloods for electrolytes and glucose • Commence intravenous fluids. Repeat further IV dose of lorazepam if no response after 10 minutes • Repeat cardiopulmonary assessment. Prepare for intensive support	Lorazepam has longer duration of action compared with diazepam and lower risk of drug accumulation. It may be less effective in children taking regular benzodiazepine anticonvulsants Paraldehyde may result in abscess formation at injection site
Second-stage treatment (15 minutes onwards) Intensive care management	If no response administer further anticonvulsants: • Phenytoin infusion • Intubate and ventilate, transfer to intensive care • Ventilate, monitor pulse/BP/temperature/ urine output, EEG • Phenobarbitone infusion If no response consider IV bolus of midazolam or thiopentone	Phenytoin is effective within 10–30 minutes and has a long duration of action and may prevent recurrent seizures Phenobarbitone is effective but may take time to reach therapeutic levels and may cause lowering of the blood pressure Midazolam is water soluble and easy to administer, less irritant to veins and appears to be effective in stopping seizures that have been unresponsive to other drugs

BP, blood pressure; EEG, electroencephalogram; IV, intravenous.

trained in paediatric anaesthesia, should be responsible for children's services. It is important to train the right team members, with the right skills and abilities; successful results in a trauma situation are determined by the training and abilities of the trauma team.

A paediatrician should be included in the emergency care team for seriously traumatised children. After initial resuscitation and stabilisation, children should be transferred to the care of paediatric surgeons in a specialist facility with paediatric intensive care back-up. More recently, a joint report from the Royal College of Surgeons and the British Orthopaedic Association (RCS/BOA 2000) recommended that:

> Any hospital receiving and caring for the severely injured child must have on-site support from paediatricians and paediatric anaesthetists.

The Audit Commission (1993 p 48) highlights the fact that A&E departments do not always have or receive timely back-up from other specialists or allied health professionals to support diagnostic investigations. Further, the Audit Commission (1993 p 49) appraises a list of favourable specialists that should work synergistically with A&E services. Some speciality back-up seems obvious, such as anaesthesia, orthopaedics, general surgery and medicine. Support services that need to co-locate at A&E include critical care facilities, radiology, ultrasound, online CT scanner and 24-hour pathology services.

Disappointingly, the report *Better care for the seriously injured* (RCS/BOA 2000) dedicates only one of fifty-five pages to the severely injured child. However, the report does acknowledge that there is a much higher frequency of serious head, chest and abdominal injuries in children than in adults. It berates less experienced doctors for their indecision and late intervention when managing a seriously injured child and is also the only report of all those mentioned above to relate and conclude that severely injured children present the greatest opportunity for organ salvage.

CHILDREN'S NURSES IN EMERGENCY DEPARTMENTS

The development of Accident and Emergency nursing has been at the forefront of role extension within the UK and the development of a faculty of emergency nursing within the Royal College of Nursing (RCN) has allowed nurses working within the domain to agree and establish levels of clinical competencies (Endacott et al 1999). Bentley (1996) has defined role categories for children's nurses who work in emergency departments, which include the development and use of protocols in the management of sick children. Despite this, Cleaver (2003) has highlighted the feelings of vulnerability experienced by children's nurses who work in emergency departments, who are perceived by their adult/general nurse colleagues as being experts in the care of sick children. Cleaver's study reveals that the children's nurses themselves, having acquired and mastered new roles, move from feeling vulnerable to feeling frustrated when they are not allowed to develop autonomous practice.

THE ENVIRONMENT IN THE A&E DEPARTMENT

Often, the first point of contact or portal of entry to hospital is through the A&E department. The A&E department can be a distressing place, full of unfamiliar sights and sounds and little opportunity to prepare children for this experience (DoH 2003). Depending on their particular stage of cognitive development, children will interpret the situations into terms they can conceptualise. In turn, the child's perceptions and experiences in the A&E or emergency room will affect future attendances; the right staff and the right environment can have a dramatic impact (Audit Commission 1993, DoH 1991, 2003).

The provision of services for children should be appropriate to their cognitive and developmental needs. Children should be cared for in an environment that is audiovisually separate from the main A&E department and they should be attended to by staff who have been suitably trained and educated to care for children. The value of children's nurses in A&E is enormous; children's nurses possess skills in assessing children's development stage, communicating with child and family and developing care plans that meet the individual child's needs.

Triage in Emergency Departments

Triage is an integral part of the modern emergency department. The use of a recognised triage system has many advantages for the emergency department, including reference to a recognised decision-making structure and support in the form of a professionally accepted and validated system. Many units use the Manchester triage system, which is a method of identifying high-priority patients. The word 'triage' comes from the French 'to sort' and has its origins in the management of battlefield casualties. Although there are a number of definitions and Scoble (2004), for example, describes triage as a process of nurse assessment of a patient on arrival in an emergency department, all the definitions are consistent in that they describe triage as the categorising of sick or injured patients according to severity in order to coordinate care and ensure the most efficient and efficient use of emergency department staff and facilities (Box 24.1).

The Manchester triage system uses 52 flow charts, which allocate patients to one of the five national triage categories described above. Although the Manchester system is widely used and works well for prioritisation, Willis (2001) believes that it fails to encourage nurses using it to query in the case of a child the reason for the emergency attendance. In particular, the possibility of non-accidental injury as the cause of admission has prompted Willis (2001) to describe an enhancement to the Manchester triage system known as CWILTED (Willis 2001):

C = Condition: area of pain, problem, child protection.

W = Witness: name, position and designation of person who actually saw the incident; if nobody saw the incident write 'none'.

I = Incident: mechanism that caused the injury.

L = location: home address, school, childminder (name and address), park or play area.

T = Time: time accident occurred and date, time first aid given (including medication), time of last meal.

E = Escort: it should not be automatically assumed that an accompanying adult is a parent. Does this person have parental responsibility? If he or she is not witness to the accident, how do they know what happened?

D = Disability: initially this had been 'description' but this tended to repeat 'condition' and triage staff have modified this to be disability caused by the incident or diagnosis if known at the time. Willis (2001) notes that the staff of the emergency department at St Peters Hospital in Surrey reverted to 'description', i.e. to mean what the child looks like, is behaving like, etc. because 'disability' did not always appear appropriate when the child had a medical presentation.

www

CWILTED was cited by the Commission for Health Inspection (CHI) in a report of interagency working as being commendable practice. Read this report online at:

- http://www.chi.nhs.uk/eng/about/publications/safeguards/surry.pdf

Willis (2001) is critical of the Manchester triage system because important child protection issues might be missed and recommends that CWILTED is used as an adjunct to this method of identifying and prioritising patient problems. The Manchester system has also been criticised by Woolwich (1999), who laments the mechanistic approach of applying a computer algorithm to the identification of prioritised patient symptoms, believing that this isempowers nurses conducting the triage by reducing their professional judgement, clinical expertise and intuitive acumen.

Box 24.1

Triage categories

Triage category 1
- People who need to have treatment immediately (in practice, within 2 minutes) are called immediately life-threatening patients.
- People in this group are critically ill and require immediate attention. Most would have arrived at the emergency department by ambulance. They would probably be suffering from something like a critical injury or cardiac arrest.

Triage category 2
- People who need to have treatment within 10 minutes are called imminently life-threatening patients.
- People in this group would probably be suffering from something like a critical illness or very severe pain. People with serious chest pains, difficulty in breathing and severe fractures are included in this group.

Triage category 3
- People who need to have treatment within 30 minutes are called potentially life-threatening patients.
- People in this group would probably be suffering from something like severe illnesses, major bleeding from cuts, major fractures or dehydration.

Triage category 4
- People who need to have treatment within 1 hour are called potentially serious patients.
- People in this group would probably have less severe symptoms or injuries with something like a foreign body in the eye, sprained ankle, migraine or earache.

Triage category 5
- People who need to have treatment within 2 hours are called less urgent patients.
- People in this group probably have minor illnesses or symptoms that may have been present for more than a week, like rashes or minor aches and pains.

Triage categories 1 to 5 were previously described as resuscitation, emergency, urgent, semi-urgent and non-urgent.

Triage using the National Triage Scale (Mackway-Jones 1997) has been widely adopted and is generally considered an efficient way of 'sorting' those very urgent needs from those with less urgent needs, and in managing emergency departments. Triage, however, can only be truly effective if the process takes place on arrival. Triage also needs to be a continual process, so that deterioration in children with initially lower priority can be recategorised (Mackway-Jones 1997 p 2). Immediate and continued triage requires nursing staff to be constantly available and assigned to triage duties. This is often difficult with a less than optimal nursing establishment. The emergency situation that can be visualised is more likely to take precedence than the potential one waiting for triage. One needs to be reminded of the 'duty care' to all patients and the emergency department shift coordinator holds the ultimate responsibility for deployment of nursing and medical colleagues.

Immediate triage is crucial for young children and babies. This can be a lengthy process because it can take some time taken to remove layers of clothing from small children. This will create a 'knock on' effect in delay for the next waiting child.

Less than 0.25% of all children attending emergency services require paediatric intensive care. However, it is widely known and accepted that half of this 0.25% will have been carried 'in arms' to the emergency department, with the consequent risks of further injury. Although only a small fraction of children attending emergency departments require paediatric intensive care services, level one dependency accounts for 61% of all PICU admissions.

Activity

Read the grey chapters in the Advanced Life Support Group (2003):
Chapter 1 Introduction
Chapter 2 Why treat children differently
Chapter 4 Basic life support
Chapter 5 Advanced support of the airway and ventilation
Chapter 6 Management of cardiac arrest
Chapter 8 The structured approach to the seriously ill child
Chapter 15 The structured approach to the seriously injured child

Scenario

What would really happen?
On arrival by ambulance, Sheila is taken into the paediatric emergency area, where the children nurse undertakes a quick visual assessment – **A**irway, **B**reathing, **C**irculation – to determine if there is any immediate life threat. Sheila is triaged and the nurse observes that she is in pain.

Sheila is a known epileptic who has anticonvulsant therapy. She is alert and conscious and is able to express that she is feeling sore on her head. The nurse recognises that Sheila needs some analgesia. Paracetamol is the drug of choice.

The cause of Sheila's fit could range from meningitis or encephalitis, metabolic causes such as diabetic ketoacidosis, hypoglycaemia, electrolyte disturbances or from head injury, drug or poison ingestion or intracranial haemorrhage – all of which have the potential for respiratory, circulatory failure and shock. It should take less than a minute to identify any potential respiratory, circulatory or neurological failure, with resuscitation given immediately as necessary. Prompt recognition and treatment are essential if the extreme situation of cardiopulmonary arrest and a poor outcome is to be avoided. Respiratory failure is a clinical state characterised by inadequate ventilation or oxygenation and by circulatory failure. Because children have lower pulmonary reserves than adults they compensate quickly and are therefore susceptible to both cardiorespiratory failure and shock.

Recognition and Assessment of Pain

Integral to the process of triage, children have their pain assessed. Triage priority is often determined by severity of pain. This allows for the child's pain to be managed at the earliest opportunity. Once pain management is determined and the child made more comfortable, it may be possible to recategorise to a lower priority.

Pain assessment in the emergency department is often difficult, particularly with children. Having sustained an injury or illness causes the child anxiety. Children will be frightened of being in a strange environment and not knowing what is going to happen next, and often think that what happened is their fault and fear punishment. Children often imagine the worst outcome of their pain, or they will deny their pain entirely. Many healthcare professionals hold unfounded beliefs that because children are not crying they cannot be in pain. By the same rule it is often said, 'that children who make the loudest noise usually experience the least pain'.

Pain assessment tools used in conjunction with triage protocols, fall into three main types (Mackway-Jones 1997): verbal descriptor scales, visual analogue scales and pain behaviour tools. The ideal pain assessment tool in the emergency department should be age appropriate, user friendly and simple, quick to use and incorporate the three main types.

Verbal descriptor scales when working with children are extremely helpful. Depending on their cognitive stage of development, children often are unable to express the intensity of their pain. By understanding the mechanism of injury and the effect the injury has on the child, it is not unreasonable to anticipate the level of pain when a child is unable to express the intensity. An example of pain management would be the child who has amputated the end of a finger but is for many reasons unable to express how much pain he or she is experiencing. By using verbal descriptors weighted within a pain ruler (Mackway-Jones 1997 p 25) it would not be unreasonable to assess the pain between 6 and 7. Verbal descriptors for level 6 suggests pain is described as very bad/severe.

PAIN RELIEF FOR CHILDREN IN EMERGENCY DEPARTMENTS

One of the elements of the Manchester triage scale is its insistence that a patient's pain must be assessed during the triage process. However, in reality, pain relief is often not managed to the patient's satisfaction. Maurice et al (2002) give a comprehensive review of emergency analgesia in childhood emergencies and counsel against using intramuscular injections because the rate of absorption of the drug is not predictable and, if the child is in shock, the drug will not be disseminated adequately around the body in the way that an intravenous injection would. Furthermore, the potential for the need for top-up injections coupled with the development of potential or actual needle phobia make this method of pain relief unacceptable. Maurice et al (2002) argue that the ideal analgesia in childhood emergencies is easily and painlessly administrated, has a rapid onset, and has predictable and effective pain reliving actions and importantly no unwarranted side effects (Box 24.2).

Activity

- What other methods of pain relief are available to emergency nurses?
- Discuss the role of distraction and complementary therapies.

Making Medicine Administration and Drug Calculations Safer

After working through this section of the chapter you should be able to calculate drug doses accurately and safely.

In the minds of most children, 'getting better' is associated with taking medicine. At a very early age children are introduced to paracetamol when they have a fever or feel unwell. At 3 months most children receive their first immunisation. If illness occurs then various drugs with a wide range of side effects will probably be required.

The treatment of an individual child or young person with medicine is a process that involves prescribing, dispensing, administering, receiving and recording. Thus treatment with medicines is a partnership between the doctor, the pharmacist, the nurse and the patient.

It is the trained nurses' responsibility to ensure safe and reliable medicine administration, to monitor the effects, to ensure patients understand their medication and to sign the prescription sheet.

As a student nurse you should be able to assist the trained nurse to:

- identify the correct patient
- select the correct, in-date medicines
- calculate and measure the dose required
- administer the dose by the correct route.

Box 24.2

Methods of relieving childhood pain in emergency departments (after Maurice et al 2002)

- Local anaesthesia infiltrated into the wound: simple and safe but potentially painful. This can be counteracted by using a small-bore needle or a warmed solution.
- Topical anaesthesia: ELA (not for infants under a year) or Ametop (not for infants under 1 month). Good for preparing for cannulation or venepuncture but not for use in open wounds or mucous membranes which makes them unsuitable for use in the cleaning or suturing of wounds.
- Field block: local anaesthesia is injected around the perimeter of a wound or abscess a centimetre away from the edge. Takes longer to work but prevents the reduction of the desired anaesthetic effect, which occurs when local is infiltrated into infected areas which have increased vascularity.
- Peripheral nerve block: this involves the injection of local into the area of a peripheral nerve to provide anaesthesia to the area of the body distal to the area being infiltrated. Commonly used to provide femoral (good for fractures of the shaft of femur before X-ray and application of traction) or digital nerve block (good for avulsed finger nails or draining of paronychia).
- Paracetamol: good for mild pain (can be given rectally).
- Non-steroidal anti-inflammatory drugs such as ibuprofen: not recommended for children younger than 1 year but useful for moderate pain, especially that caused by musculoskeletal trauma. Contraindicated in patients with a history of gastrointestinal bleeding or renal impairment. Can cause bronchospasm in asthmatic children.
- Nitrous oxide: in a mixture of 70% with 30% oxygen this gas is effective for venous cannulation. It is painless to administer and the children can control their own dispensation through a mouthpiece. In a 50:50 mixture, nitrous oxide has good analgesic effect.
- Opioids: codeine is a good drug for mild to moderate pain; its effect is enhanced when it is combined with paracetamol. Morphine is an excellent choice for severe pain such as that caused by burns or fractures; the intravenous route is preferred. Diamorphine administered intranasally has been shown to be effective in children with fractures of the long bones. Pethidine has shorter duration than morphine with less sedative effects. However, pethidine can cause nausea and sometimes convulsions. Fentanyl is a synthetic opioid that can be administered intravenously or intranasally. It has rapid onset and short duration but can cause respiratory depression. It should be used with caution in emergency departments. Ketamine has analgesic, anaesthetic and dissociative state properties but also has side effects such as increase in blood pressure, which makes it unsuitable for patients with raised intracranial pressure.

ACCURACY

When calculating drug doses for children, accuracy is of the utmost importance. Often, doses are very small, particularly for infants, and an overdose can have a catastrophic effect. In 1995 a junior doctor at Rotherham District General Hospital intended to give 150 micrograms of morphine to a premature baby. She miscalculated the decimal point and gave 15 milligrams of morphine; the baby died. This is not meant to alarm you but to emphasise the importance of ensuring your ability to undertake calculations accurately. Please remember if you are unsure about a calculation *stop and get help*. Do not give medicines unless you are confident in your calculation. Practice calculations using the prescription charts on the wards and test your competence with your clinical assessor, clinical skills coordinator or academic tutor.

It is essential that you can undertake all medicine calculations without using a calculator. The reason for this is that it is too easy to press the wrong button and come out with an entirely wrong answer. Furthermore, you need to have a reasonable idea of the amount of drug you are expecting to give; in other words to understand what is a logical amount. If you work the dose out first by hand it is acceptable to then check it using a calculator.

UNITS USED IN MEDICINE

Many different units are used in medicine for drug strength and dosages. You need to understand the units in which drugs can be prescribed and how to convert from one unit to another.

The first step is to check out your knowledge of these units, which are based on the International Système of units (SI units) or metric system for weight, volume and amount of substances.

Activity

Complete the following:
- 1 kilogram (kg) = . . . grams (g)
- 1 gram (g) = . . . milligrams (mg)
- 1 milligram (mg) = . . . micrograms (mcg or µg)
- 1 microgram (mcg) = . . . nanograms (ng)
- 1 litre (L) = . . . millilitres (mL)
- 1 mole (mol) = . . . millimoles (mmol)
- 1 millimole (mmol) = . . . micromoles (mcmol or µmol)

Please ensure that you fully understand these units. If you have any difficulty you should consult one of the 'drug calculation for nurses' books (e.g. Lapham & Agar 1995).

Activity

Now try these unit conversions:
- 1 mol = . . . mcmol

- 1 kg = . . . mcg
- 1 mg = . . . mcg
- 1 g = . . . ng

You must be able to convert from one unit to another fluently, so practise until you can.

WEIGHT

Without doubt, the most rapid increase in height and weight occur in the first year of life. The average baby at birth weighs 3.2 kg and will treble its weight by its first birthday to 9.6 kg. By the second birthday the toddler will have quadrupled its birth weight to 12.8 kg.

In the emergency situation, it is important to ascertain the child's weight as a matter of urgency. Most drugs and therapies are given as the dose per kilogram. Given the impracticalities of weighing children in the emergency situation, a number of methods can be used to estimate a child's weight. The most widely known formula if age is known is:

Weight (kg) = 2 (age + 4)

IS THE DOSE CORRECT?

Before you give a medicine to the child you must be sure that the dose is correct. Drug dosages are commonly calculated on the child's weight. Every time you give medicines you must find out the child's weight and check in a paediatric formulary to find out the recommended dose per kilogram of body weight (the Royal College of Paediatrics and Child Health book *Medicines for children* is a good reference source). If there is a discrepancy it must be checked with the prescriber.

Activity

Check these calculations:
- Jennifer is 18 months old and weighs 14 kg. She has an abscess on her index finger and has been prescribed 200 mg of paracetamol 4–6 hourly for pain. The recommended dose is 15 mg/kg.
- Robert, aged 13, has had an accident. He chopped off the top of his finger with a skateboard. Following a course of intravenous antibiotics he has now changed to oral. He is prescribed oral cephalexin 500 mg at 06.00 hours and 18.00 hours. He weighs 43.3 kg. The *Medicines for children* formulary recommends 25 mg/kg daily in divided doses. What do you notice about this prescription?
- Paracetamol is the drug of choice for mild to moderate pain. A loading dose of paracetamol would be given at 20 mg/kg for children between 2 and 12 years of age

(RCPCH 2003). Paracetamol oral solution/suspension is available in 120 mg in 5 mL and 250 mg in 5 mL. Calculate the dose of paracetamol for Sheila.

- 1% lidocaine is most commonly used for local anaesthetic infiltration prior to suturing children's wounds. This drug comes as 10 mg/mL and maximum dosages to achieve local anaesthesia are 3 mg/kg. Sheila weighs:

(Age 4½ years + 4) × 2 = 17 kg.

Please remember that someone could have made a mistake when writing the child's weight on the drug chart. You *must* assess whether the weight shown makes sense in relation to the child's age. Until you are familiar with children's weights you should check using growth charts.

IS THE ROUTE CORRECT?

Check in the formulary that the prescribed route is correct. Some drugs have different doses for different routes, so check correct dose for correct route. Also, check on the bottle or vial that you are using the correct formulation of the drug for the route you are using.

SIDE EFFECTS

It is also your responsibility to know the side effects and interactions of all the medicines that you give. Some of the side effects are pivotal to nursing care. For example, one of the side effects of morphine is respiratory depression. Thus it is vital that sedation level and respiratory function are rigorously monitored. Please ensure that you know and monitor the possible side effects for all the medicines commonly used in each of your clinical placements.

Activity

List ten medicines, with their side effects, which you have seen administered in your clinical placements. Include morphine whether you have seen it administered or not.

CALCULATIONS

If the prescribed dose is straightforward, calculation is simple. However, if the prescribed dose is a small fraction of the available medicine then this simple formula can be used:

(Strength required [what you want] ÷ Strength available [what you have got]) × stock solution (volume the drug is in)

The 'what you want' and 'what you have got' should be in the same unit.

Box 24.3

Example

The prescription is for oral ampicillin 80 mg. The bottle contains 125 mg in 5mL. How many millilitres should you give?

$$(80 \div 125) \times 5 = 3.2 \ mL$$

There are various ways of denoting the concentration of drug in a liquid medicine. The most usual way is in mg of drug in mL of liquid, i.e. mg/mL. For example, paracetamol comes in oral suspensions of either 120 mg in 5 mL or 250 mg in 5 mL.

Activity

How many mL of paracetamol 120 mg in 5 mL will you give if the prescription is for:
- 50 mg?
- 75 mg?

How many mL of paracetamol 250 in 5mL will you give if the prescription is for?
- 100 mg?
- 150 mg?

Prescriptions must be:

- legible and not altered
- written in block capitals
- signed using a full name
- give the drug generic name, not the trade name.

www

Visit the Association of Chief Children's Nurses website and access the Paediatric Nursing Journal information on drug calculations
http:\\www.accnuk.org

Additionally, prescriptions for controlled drugs must:

- give maximum number of doses that may be administered
- give minimum dose interval
- have a separate prescription for each route of administration
- be administered and signed for by two people.

Any allergies must be recorded on the patient's prescription sheet. You must check for these.

Do not try to guess if you cannot read the prescription. A child was written up for 350 mg of an antibiotic. The prescription was illegible so the nurse guessed and gave 850 mg. The potential consequences of this guesswork are dangerous. There could be toxicity leading to permanent disability, severe reactions and litigation.

Activity

Try the following calculations:

Drug	Dose prescribed	Drug comes as:
Tegretol	70 mg	100 mg/5 mL
Paracetamol	60 mg, 240 mg	120 mg/5 mL
Erythromycin	100 mg	125 mg/5 mL
Flucloxacillin	62.5 mg	125 mg/5 mL
Atropine	150 micrograms	600 micrograms/1 mL
	240 micrograms	600 micrograms/1 mL
Digoxin	15 micrograms	50 micrograms/1 mL
	12 micrograms	0.05 mg/mL
Phenytoin	10 mg	30 mg/5 mL
Diazepam	3 mg	2 mg/5 mL
Morphine	3 mg	10 mg/1 mL

Answers can be found in the companion PowerPoint presentation.

Family-centred Care in the Emergency Department

Traditionally, families have not been allowed to participate in or be present at certain invasive procedures involving children in emergency departments. There has been a growth in family-centred care in the UK and elsewhere, with writers such as Darbyshire (1994) and Smith et al (2002) articulating the role nurses can play in not only acting as family advocates but, importantly, in helping remove the barriers that impede the implementation of family-friendly protocols and procedures. The admission of parents/guardians to areas of the hospital that have traditionally excluded them has been slow and emergency departments have only recently acknowledged that the presence of parents during invasive procedures is actually helpful not only for the practising nurse but also for the child and family as a whole. Eppich & Arnold (2003) describe how family members can contribute to the overall care of the child during such procedures and, furthermore, can be present during cardiopulmonary resuscitation (CPR). A large body of evidence suggests that parental presence during hospital procedures is helpful to a child during a stressful procedure (Coyne 1995, Glasper & Powell 2000).

There are not always sufficient children's nurses on duty to ensure that all children are appropriately managed. Sue is working an early shift with her mentor Sally and they are reflecting on an event the previous day, when a mother was refused entry to the resuscitation room. The 18-month-old child was not successfully resuscitated and the mother later complained that she regretted not being present during this last period of her child's life.

PAEDIATRIC RESUSITATION

Although paediatric events that require resuscitation are rare, it is important that all nurses understand the principles of successful resuscitation. Castle (2002) suggests that most district general hospitals will have less than one paediatric cardiac arrest per week. It is the rarity of this event that makes it emotionally difficult for those in emergency departments. Seminal work by Ellison (1998) in Manchester showed that relatives want to be present during their child's resuscitation. It is, however, important to recognise that there are both positive and negative aspects of family presence during this stressful event. Although family presence during a resuscitation procedure is becoming more usual in emergency departments, many members of the interprofessional team still have concerns and doubts about it. Kidby (2003) believes that nurses should take into account the views of relatives, although resuscitation procedures should never be compromised by the presence of family members. Evidence suggests that it can improve the grieving process for families and be helpful to patients who survive (Rattrie 1999).

PAEDIATRIC INTENSIVE CARE

A study of trauma victims by the Royal College of Surgeons concluded that as many as one-third of those who died could have been saved. As discussed earlier, the starting point in caring for acutely ill and injured patients is an appropriate skilled workforce that is competent in assessment and management of such patients (Mackway-Jones 1997 p 35). The team approach allows critically ill or traumatised patients optimal chances for survival. The distribution of trauma deaths has been described as being 'trimodal'. Fifty percent of all trauma deaths occur before medical attention can be provided. The first peak in mortality occurs at the time of injury or shortly after. The second peak of the trimodal experience occurs within the first hours of injury. It is in this phase that the emergency care team response can make a difference in provision of care to prevent death as a result of 'airway, breathing and circulatory problems'. The term the 'golden hour' is often used to describe this second phase of the trimodal theory. Having survived the initial trauma, resuscitation and stabilisation patients who die in the third trimodal stage commonly die in intensive care from multisystem failure.

The paediatric intensive care report *Framework for the future* (NHS Executive 1997 p 7) describes three levels of care for the critically ill or injured child. Level one, often referred to as high-dependency care, is greater than that care provided on an acute paediatric ward or department. Children requiring level-one care require close observation, continuous heart monitoring, non-invasive blood pressure monitoring or single organ support not including respiratory support. Children who fall into level one may be experiencing severe breathing difficulties like croup, suspected intestinal obstruction or poisoning (NHS Executive 1997 p 9). Level two is defined as the level of care for children requiring assisted ventilation either due to respiratory absence or single system failure requiring respiratory support. Level three is defined as children with multisystem failure requiring advanced respiratory support.

CHILD PROTECTION

Activity

Obtain the following references:
- Castle N 1999 Paediatric resuscitation. Emergency Nurse 7(1):31–39
- Castle N 2002 Paediatric resuscitation: advanced life support. Nursing Standard 17(11):47–52.

Discuss paediatric resuscitation in your clinical skills groups.

If you are a subscriber to any journal published by the RCN, you can obtain these papers from *The Nursing Standard* website searchable archive.

Children's nurses must be able to recognise potential problems in relation to children and their interaction with their immediate family or carers. Child protection issues are often identified when observing the dynamics between the child and family. While undertaking assessment of any child it is important to identify non-verbal information as much as the verbal information gathered. The non-verbal clues might indicate lack of eye contact, withdrawn body posture, facial expression and tone of voice. These are all factors that can encourage or discourage the flow of information between the nurse and the parents.

Nurses who use verbal cues such as open-ended questions, active listening and empathy, can demonstrate to the parents that what they are saying is important and is helping in the care of their ill child. This is a continual process and should be two-way between the parent and nurse to facilitate the development of trust and confidence in the nursing and medical staff. This can begin the development of a partnership with the parents in care.

Social interaction manifest in numerous forms of non-verbal communication; children's nurses use non-verbal cues to eliminate, amplify or expand on what is expressed in words. The use of eye contact during conversations is a process by which each individual demonstrates attention and involvement in the conversation by regularly looking into the eyes of the other, staring intently can indicate evasiveness. Facial expressions, gestures and body posture can convey what is really meant even when nothing is actually said.

Parental involvement and partnership have been advocated since the publication of the Platt report (Ministry of Health 1959). Since this time, government policy has reaffirmed that the care of children should be provided in part by partnerships with parents and their families (DoH 1991). Most recently, *Getting the right start: national service framework for children* (DoH 2003, 2004) advocates that children, young people and parents are partners in care and that partnership and parental involvement are recognised as important issues in services for children.

When children are unwell, parents often seek help because they do not have the knowledge or skills to care for their children at home; there is an implicit and explicit dependence on professional knowledge and expertise. However, this dependence is not one-sided. The professionals are dependent on the parents sharing information to enable appropriate care. This sharing of information can empower the family and reduce the vulnerability felt by the parents.

Partnership in care can have difficulties in the emergency situations as distress and anxiety can interfere with the parent's ability to formulate and rationalise decisions.

Scenario

In line with the NICE guidelines (available online at: http://www.NICE.org.uk) for head injuries, Sheila does not require a skull X-ray or computer tomography. However, her scalp wound does require closure. The wound to Sheila's head is no more than 3 cm in length and is deep dermal. The wound does not require to be sutured and can be closed by simple application of wound glue (of which there are many on the therapeutics market at the present time). Two of the most popular are Liquiband and Histoacryl.

WOUND MANAGEMENT IN EMERGENCY DEPARTMENTS

The wound on Sheila's head needs to be cleansed and closed. For a young child this is a very frightening procedure and Sheila will require a lot of psychological preparation for this to be accomplished. The hospital play therapist and Sheila's mother will try to distract her attention as much as possible. This may be by blowing bubbles or by playing a game or reading a storybook. Depending on the presentation of the wound there are different methods for closure. Sutures are still very common but will not be undertaken unless the child is able to understand what suturing entails. No child should ever be held down or wrapped in a blanket so that painful procedures can be undertaken. Children who have wounds and are non-compliant with therapies should either undergo conscious sedation or referral to surgeons. Often, wounds are 'steristripped' (previously known as butterfly stitches) and then kept dry for 5 days.

THE ROLE OF PLAY

The provision of therapeutic play facilities within emergency departments is of crucial importance in the management of children attending. The obligatory box of broken toys cited by Glasper (1995) is no longer acceptable and Smith (1998) believes that a play specialist in emergency departments can help reduce the fear and anxiety experienced by children attending. A good hospital play therapist will be aware of a child's developmental needs and can often determine the toys and therapeutics that each child needs for distraction from painful procedures.

PAEDIATRIC NURSE PRACTITIONERS

The expansion of roles within the emergency departments has been described by Jones & Smith (1998), who articulate the challenge of assessing and treating children in the emergency department for independent practitioners. To date, there is no national recognised course for the training and development of registered children's nurses to become ENPs. However, there has been an area of growth around clinical assessment of children although again this has yet to gain national recognition.

OBSERVATIONS

Observation of all Sheila's vital signs remains stable throughout her treatment and stay in the emergency department. Her scalp wound has been cleansed and closed using wound glue. Sheila's immunisation status is checked and she is up to date with all her immunisation and does not require a tetanus booster. Having been given instructions and advice on how to care for Sheila at home, both Sheila and her mum are ready for discharge. Sheila is given an out-patient appointment for follow-up care for her epilepsy and her mum feels confident that she can manage Sheila's fits at home.

Summary

First contact emergency care for children and young people is a growing area of nursing. A number of national initiatives including the National Service Framework highlight the pivotal role of emergency departments in the care of sick children and their families. Children and young people nurses will continue to play a big role in ensuring that emergency care for their client group is commensurate with the age group continuum of growth and development.

References

Advanced Paediatric Life Group 2003 Advanced paediatric life support: the practical approach, 3rd edn. BMJ Books, London

Appleton R, Choonara I, Martland T et al 2000 The treatment of convulsive status epilepticus in children. Archives of Disease in Childhood 83(5):415–419

Arnon K, MacFaul R, Hemmingway P et al 2004 The impact of presenting problem-based guidelines for children with medical problems in an accident and emergency department. Archives of Disease in Childhood 89:159–164

Bentley J 1996 Child-related services in general accident and emergency departments. Journal of Advanced Nursing 24:1184–1193

Boyle R, Smith C, McIntyre J 2000 The changing utilization of a children's emergency department. Ambulatory Child Health 6(1):39

Castle N 2002 Paediatric resuscitation: advanced life support. Nursing Standard 17(11):47–52

Cleaver K 2003 Developing expertise – the contribution of paediatric accident and emergency nurses to the care of children and the implications for their continuing professional development. Accident and Emergency Nursing 11:96–102

Coyne I 1995 Partnership in care: parents views of participation in their hospitalised child's care. Journal of Clinical Nursing 4:71–79

Darbyshire P 1994 Living with a sick child in hospital: the experiences of parents and nurses. Chapman and Hall, London

Department of Health (DoH) 1991 Welfare of children and young people in hospital. HMSO, London

Department of Health (DoH) 1996 The patient's charter – services for children and young people. HMSO, London

Department of Health (DoH) 2000 The NHS plan: a plan for investment, a plan for reform. The Stationery Office, London

Department of Health (DOH) (2003) Online. Available at: http://www.doh.gov.gov.uk/nsf/children/gettingtherightstart.htm

Department of Health (DoH) 2004 The national service framework for children, young people and maternity services. Online. Available at: http://www.dh.gov.uk

Department of Health and Social Security (DHSS) 1976 Fit for the future (the Court Report). The Report of the Committee on Child Health Services. HMSO, London

Ellison G 1998 Witnessed resuscitation; the relatives' experience. Emergency Nurse 5(8):27–29

Endacott R, Edwards B, Crouch R et al 1999 Towards a faculty of emergency nursing. Emergency Nurse 7(5):10–15

Eppich WJ, Arnold L 2003 Family member presence in the paediatric emergency department. Current Opinion in Paediatrics 15(3):294–298

Glasper EA 1995 Paediatric ambulatory care: shop window or back door. British Journal of Nursing 4(7):384

Glasper EA, Powell C 2000 First do no harm: parental exclusion from anaesthetic rooms. Paediatric Nursing 12(4):14–17

Jones SJ, Smith JM 1998 Expanding roles and practice within paediatric A and E departments – The children's nurse practitioner. In: Glasper EA, Lowson S (eds) Innovations in paediatric ambulatory care: a nursing perspective. Macmillan, Basingstoke

Kidby J 2003 Family witnessed cardiopulmonary resuscitation. Nursing Standard 17(51):33–36

Lapham R, Agar H 1995 Drug calculations for nurses, a step by step approach. Arnold, London

MacFaul R, Werneke U 2001 Recent trends in hospital use by children in England. Archive of Disease in Childhood 85:203–207

Mackway-Jones K (ed) 1997 Emergency triage. Manchester triage group. BMJ Publishing, London

Maurice SC, O'Donnell JJ, Beatie TF 2002 Emergency analgesia in the paediatric population. Part II: pharmacological methods of pain relief. Emergency Medicine Journal 19:101–105

Ministry of Health 1959 Committee of the Central Health Services Council. Report of the Committee on the Welfare of Children in Hospital. Ministry of Health, London

NHS Confederation 2003 Getting the right start: standard for hospital services. Briefing June 2003 N87.

NHS Executive 1997 Paediatric intensive care: a framework for the future. Report of the National Co-ordinating Group on Intensive Care to the Chief Executive of the NHS Executive. NHSE, London

Partridge T 2001 Children in accident and emergency: seen but not heard? Journal of Child Health Care 5(2):49–53

Rattrie E 1999 Witnessed resuscitation: good practice or not? Nursing Standard 14(24):32–35

Royal College of Paediatrics and Child Health (RCPCH) 2003 Medicines for children. RCPCH, London

Royal College of Surgeons (RCS) and the British Orthopaedic Association (BOA) 2000 Better care for the seriously injured. RCS, London

Scoble M 2004 Implementing triage in a children's assessment unit. Nursing Standard 18(34):41–44

Scott RC, Neville BRG 1999 Pharmacological management of convulsive status epilepticus in children. Developmental Medicine and Child Neurology 41:207–210

Scott RC, Surtees RAH, Neville BRG 1998 Status epilepticus: pathophysiology, epidemiology, and outcomes. Archive of Diseases in Childhood 79(1):73–77

Shovron S 2001 Management of status epilepticus in children. Journal Neurology, Neurosurgery, Psychiatry 70 (suppl II):ii22–ii27

Smith F 1998 Caring for children. Emergency Nurse 6(6):20–24

Smith L, Coleman V, Bradshaw M (eds) 2002 Family centred care: concept, theory, and practice. Palgrave, Basingstoke

Tasker RC 1998 Emergency treatment of acute seizures and status epilepticus. Archive of Diseases in Childhood 79(1):78–83

United Kingdom Central Council for Nursing, Midwifery and Health Visiting (UKCC) 2000 Guidelines for the administration of medicines. UKCC, London

Watson S 2000 Children's nurses in accident and emergency department: literature review. Accident and Emergency Nursing 8:92–97

Watts R, Robertson J, Thomas G 2003 Nursing management of fever in children: a systematic review. International Journal of Nursing Practice 9:S1–S8

Willis MA 2001 CWILTED Emergency Nurse 8(9):18–22

Woolwich C 1999 Putting the nurse back into triage. Emergency Nurse 7(5):8–9

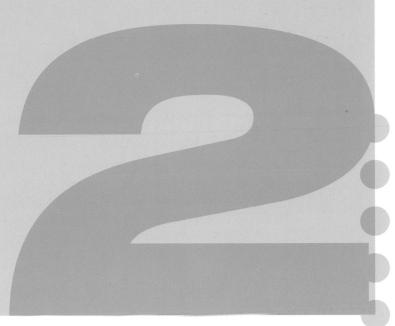

25 Children with complex motor disability 371

26 Caring for children with body fluid and electrolyte imbalance 389

27 Caring for children with genitourinary problems 405

28 Respiratory illness in children 423

29 Caring for children with gastrointestinal problems 445

30 Caring for children with cardiovascular problems 460

31 Caring for children: the role of the immune system in protecting against disease 476

32 Caring for children and adolescents with malignant disease 490

33 Caring for a child with neurological dysfunction 507

34 Caring for children with diabetes and other endocrine disorders 535

35 Caring for children with orthopaedic disorders 558

Children with Complex Motor Disability

Jackie Parkes, Sonya Clarke

ABSTRACT

The aim of this chapter is to describe the needs and nursing care of children with complex motor disabilities, and to consider the support that the families of such children require. Complex motor disability has been defined as those conditions resulting in a significant motor impairment in association with other impairments affecting the senses, learning, communication and/or problems with active seizures. Particular reference is made to the condition cerebral palsy as an 'indicator' condition for complex motor disability.

This chapter is divided into two broad parts. The first part describes the wider context related to children with complex motor disability – the numbers of children with severe disability, sources of information, the impact of having a child with a complex disability, the aims of services and parents' expectations and need for those services. Reference is made to where the children's nurse 'fits in' to the wider service context. The second part of the chapter deals with a small number of care needs that are commonly present in children with complex motor disability, and includes a description of a nursing assessment and possible interventions related to these problems.

Learning Outcomes

- Appreciate the perspectives of individual level and population-based approaches to assessment and planning care for children with complex motor disability.

- Describe the leading causes of complex motor disability in childhood.

- Recognise the relative contribution to be made by the medical and social models of disability.

- Be able to locate and interpret information (routine and other) on children with complex motor disability in the UK.

- Recognise the central role of parents as experts in the management of children with complex disability.

- Understand the role of the children's nurse in identifying unmet need through competent nursing assessment of the child with complex motor disability and their family.

- Be able to critically apply proposed outlines for nursing assessment in the care of the child with complex motor disability and their families.

Introduction

The aim of this chapter is to focus on the care of the child with complex motor disability, and on the issues faced by their families, in the context of community and hospital. The chapter uses both an individual-level and a population-based perspective to explore both the needs of children with complex motor disability and the needs of their families. An individual level approach focuses on the needs and unique experiences of an individual – a child, his or her parents and siblings. This perspective is important in developing an individualised assessment of need and tailored plan of nursing care. It contrasts with a population-based approach, which considers the needs and experiences of groups of children and their families with similar conditions and usually living in the same geographic area (for example in a Health and Social Services Trust or one region of the UK). This perspective is important for prevention of disease, health promotion and planning and targeting services to those in greatest need. The children's nurse has a role to play at both levels of assessment and intervention in relation to child health and more specifically with regard to children with complex motor disability.

Definitions, Numbers, Needs and Services

DEFINITION OF COMPLEX MOTOR DISABILITY

The term 'complex motor disability' is interpreted here to mean children whose primary problem is a significant disorder of movement and whose condition is affected and complicated by the presence of other associated impairments such as sensory deficits, problems with learning, communication or active seizures. Cerebral palsy is a good example of such a condition and most children with cerebral palsy have at least one additional, associated impairment in conjunction with problems related to movement. Cerebral palsy can be severe: approximately one in three children are unable to walk and one in four have no useful arm or hand function (Parkes et al 2001a). The impact of disability experienced is further increased by the presence of other severe associated impairments: one in four children with cerebral palsy have severe learning disability (IQ < 50) and one in ten have no useful vision (Parkes et al 2001a).

In addition, some children with complex motor disability will depend on technology to sustain their lives, for example requiring assisted ventilation, artificial feeding or care associated with having a colostomy, ileostomy, urostomy or catheterisation (Glendinning et al 2001). It should be noted that the terms 'complex motor disability', 'complex healthcare needs' and 'technology-dependent children' are not interchangeable, although many of the same children are common to all three groups.

LEADING CAUSES OF MOTOR DISABILITY

The numbers of children with disabilities and conditions requiring medical intervention has increased in the last 30 years (Gordon et al 2000, Kirk 1999). Advances in medical care have helped to improve and prolong the life expectancy of some babies and children who would have previously died (Pharoah et al 1996). For example, neonatal intensive care has helped to improve the survival of extremely premature or low birthweight babies, who are at particularly high risk of developing problems like cerebral palsy (Johnson & King 1998, O'Shea et al 1998, Pharoah et al 1996). Also, interventions like chemotherapy and ventilation, now available in the community, have improved the life span of children with degenerative conditions.

Although it is important for the children's nurse to appreciate the underlying medical diagnoses and pathology

of complex motor disabilities, medical diagnosis alone does not predict service needs (Gordon et al 2000, World Health Organization (WHO) 2001). For this reason, only a short overview of medical causes is presented here.

Activity

For a comprehensive overview of causes, complications and resulting conditions leading to complex physical disability, see McCarthy et al (1992) pp 18–21.

The leading causes of complex motor disability that may give rise to complex needs in children include cerebral palsy, spina bifida, Duchenne muscular dystrophy and other degenerative and neuromuscular conditions like spinal muscular atrophy. Cerebral palsy is the leading cause of physical disability in childhood (Parkes et al 2001a, Surveillance of Cerebral Palsy in Europe (SCPE) 2000) and has been defined as 'an umbrella term covering a group of non-progressive but often changing motor impairment syndromes secondary to lesions or anomalies of the brain arising in the early stages of its development' (Mutch et al 1992 p 549). A number of rare metabolic disorders (e.g. Lesch–Nyhan syndrome) and genetic syndromes (e.g. Turner syndrome) can also result in neuromotor impairments and disability. For some children, the underlying medical diagnoses remain uncertain.

Some of these conditions will invariably lead to premature death (e.g. Duchenne muscular dystrophy), whereas others are likely to mean the child and family will have a life-time of disability requiring specialist help and support (e.g. cerebral palsy). Although conditions like cerebral palsy and spina bifida are not fatal *per se*, premature death is associated with more severe forms (Crichton et al 1995, Hutton et al 1994). It has been estimated that of those with the most severe disabling cerebral palsy (unable to walk, no useful arm or hand function and with intellectual impairment) 70% will survive to age 10; 50% to age 20; and 40% to 30 years (Hutton & Pharoah 1998).

MEDICAL AND SOCIAL MODELS OF DISABILITY

As children's nurses we need to be aware and appreciate the 'larger' issues around disability as a political, social and emerging academic discipline in its own right. Generally speaking, we are taught and tend to assume the 'medical model' in assessing and intervening in the care of children with disability and their families. The medical model supposes that disability is the result of pathology and impairment, resulting in deficit of function and rendering the person disabled and unable to participate fully in 'normal' life. Our interventions are aimed at the level of the individual and include pre- and postoperative surgical care, medication, rehabilitation and the provision of aids and appliances to help the individual adapt and 'fit into' mainstream society. Although it could be argued that this perspective is at least partially appropriate, the contrasting social model of disability has gained increasing validity and recognition.

The social model of disability conceives that impairments do not make a person disabled but rather that it is society who disables people by failing to accommodate their differences (Priestley 2003). The manifestation of this 'failure to accommodate' means that people with disabilities are excluded from mainstream life through segregated education, few and poorly paid employment opportunities problems, and difficulty gaining access to buildings and using public transport, among other things (Priestley 2003). In the social model of disability the level of intervention is aimed at changing societal attitudes and societal behaviour towards people with disability.

The distinction between these models is not merely an academic one because how we think about disability will influence our nursing practice. The children's nurse has a clear responsibility to provide nursing care and meet the immediate physical and psychological needs of the child and family. We also have a wider role to play.

Seminar discussion topic

Can children's nurses act as advocates at the societal level, raising awareness about inclusion for children with disability in 'mainstream' society and helping to change attitudes?

THE WORLD HEALTH ORGANIZATION AND DISABILITY

In 1980, the World Health Organization (WHO) published the much cited International Classification of Impairments, Disabilities and Handicaps (ICIDH). This defined **impairment** as 'any loss or abnormality of psychological, physiological or anatomical structure or function'; **disability** as 'any restriction or lack (resulting from impairment) of ability to perform an activity in the manner within the range considered normal for a human being'; and **handicap** as 'a disadvantage for a given individual, resulting from an impairment or a disability, that limits or prevents fulfilment of a role that is normal'.

This framework has now been revised to form a more positive 'components of health' classification called the International Classification of Functioning, Disability and Health (or ICF; WHO 2002). Previously, the ICIDH was a 'consequences of disease' classification that focused on the impact of disease on the individual (WHO 1980). By contrast, the ICF focuses on health and measuring function regardless of the reason for the impairment (WHO 2002). The terms and concepts of 'disability' and 'handicap' have now been replaced by the terms 'activity limitations' and 'participation restrictions', respectively.

 WWW

Read a beginner's guide to the ICF called *Towards a common language for functioning, disability and health* online at:
- http://www3.who.int/icf/icftemplate.cfm?
  myurl=homepage.html&mytitle=Home%20Page

Click on 'Beginner's Guide'. In particular, see p 6 regarding ICF applications in service provision. Alternatively, for a more detailed account click on 'Introduction'.

The ICF provides a conceptual framework for the 'definition, measurement and policy formulations for health and disability' (WHO 2002 p 2) for use in health care and at the levels of individual, institution and population. Finally, one of the additional unique features of the ICF is recognition and classification of the environmental factors (such as social attitudes and social structures), which are derived from the social model of disability. Assessment of these features is necessary to complete the 'picture' of health and disability.

In the context of children's nursing it is important to appreciate the ICF because it is relevant and could be used in nursing practice in the following ways (adapted from WHO 2002):

- To provide standardised descriptions and a conceptual framework of health and health-related states for individual children and their families. For example, it could be used in relation to assessing and planning care for children with complex motor disability.

- Use of standardised language to promote interdisciplinary communication (with physiotherapists, occupational therapists, paediatricians for example) and make comparisons about health, health care and health outcomes in children with complex needs within geographic areas and between geographic areas.

- More generally, to provide reliable summary measures of population health for surveillance purposes and monitoring health outcomes.

- The ICF promotes assessment of the 'contextual factors' or barriers that limit the participation of individual children with complex motor disability or populations of children with complex motor disability and their families.

- It provides a systematic coding scheme for health care information systems.

Reflect on your Practice

What would be the advantages and disadvantages of including the ICF as part of routine nursing assessment in the care of children with complex motor disability?

SOURCES OF INFORMATION ON CHILDREN WITH COMPLEX MOTOR DISABILITY

Information about the numbers of children with complex motor disability or other forms of disability have been described as 'invisible' from the routine statistics published by government (Gordon et al 2000). Most regions within the UK have a formal, computer-based system for monitoring child health – a child health surveillance system. The sorts of information recorded on child health surveillance systems include birth notifications, immunisations, preschool health checks and the identification of any special needs. These systems tend to be orientated towards provision of services and have limited use as complete sources of information on specific conditions like cerebral palsy (Parkes et al 1998). Furthermore, these routine information systems could, but generally do not, publish information on children with complex needs as part of routine statistics.

Some of the gaps in the routine information about children with special and complex needs have been filled by *ad hoc* ('one-off') surveys carried out in Great Britain and Northern Ireland. In Great Britain, the Office of Population Censuses and Surveys conducted surveys of childhood disability in 1985 and 1988 (Bone & Meltzer 1989), which were subsequently reanalysed by Gordon et al (2000). Glendinning et al (1999, 2001) also reported on the numbers of technology-dependent children living in the UK; Beresford (1995) on the numbers of parents caring for a severely disabled child at home (in England) and Roberts & Lawton (2001) on severely disabled children whose families have accessed the Family Fund.

WWW

The Family Fund Trust is an independent organisation that provides financial support and information services to families caring for a severely disabled or ill child (under 16 years of age). The Family Fund Trust is government funded. Read more about the Family Fund at:
• http://www.familyfundtrust.org.uk

In Northern Ireland, sister OPCS surveys were conducted by the Policy, Planning and Research Unit in 1989 and 1990 (Duffy 1995, Smith et al 1992). A survey was undertaken in Scotland to identify the numbers and service needs of children with motor impairment and their families (Gough et al 1993). The results of these surveys are summarised in Table 25.1.

Some caution must be used in the interpretation of Table 25.1 because differences between surveys will be partly due to differences in the way 'disability' and 'severe disability' have been defined. It should be noted that the impact of disability may increase with age and studies of disability need to take this into account.

Some longitudinal studies of childhood motor disability do exist in the form of dedicated case registers of children with cerebral palsy. Currently, five such registers are actively recording cases in Northern Ireland, parts of England and Scotland. These registers fulfil an important function in providing unique information about the prevalence, severity and survival of children and young adults with cerebral palsy in the UK. The registers are also used to monitor trends over time and between areas and act as a sampling frame for research into causation and services.

Table 25.2 summarises some of the literature on the numbers and prevalence of children with cerebral palsy in different parts of the UK, including information from the five registers referred to above.

WWW

The five registers of children with cerebral palsy in the UK are part of a working collaboration. Read about the UK Collaboration of Cerebral Palsy Registers online at:
• http:///www.liv.ac.uk/PublicHealth/UKCP.htm

Although it could be argued that disability and complex motor disability remains relatively rare, the following extract written by a parent clearly highlights the impact on the child and family and their need for ongoing, intensive support to cope.

THE IMPACT OF HAVING A CHILD WITH COMPLEX MOTOR DISABILITY

The following 'real life scenario' written by a parent provides a unique and special insight into the parent's feelings and experiences of having a child with complex needs. It is strikingly similar to other accounts by parents who have reiterated many of the same messages (see Beresford 1994, Kingdom & Mayfield 2001).

In the account presented here, the parent does not elaborate on the precise 'medical equipment' she uses. However Beresford (1995) identified the following equipment being used by 1100 families for a severely disabled child at home:

Table 25.1 Summary of Surveys of Childhood Disability and Technology-dependent Children in the UK

Author and year	Geographical area	Definition used	Numbers and proportions of children with a disability (including children with severe/ multiple problems where known)
OPCS Bone & Meltzer 1989	England, Wales, Scotland	'Disabled' as defined by the ICDIH (WHO); aged 0–15 years	360,000 disabled children (3.2% of the child population in the UK) 327,000 disabled children in England & Wales
OPCS Gordon et al 2000	As above	Re-analysed OPCS data and redefined disability and identified clusters of disability	45,000 children with the most severe and multiple disabilities
PPRU Smith et al 1992, Duffy et al 1995	Northern Ireland	'Disabled' as defined by the ICDIH (WHO); aged 0–15 years	14,600 disabled children (3.5% of the child population in NI) 2,600 'severely disabled'
Gough et al 1993	Scotland	Motor impairment of central origin born 1985–86 and resident in Scotland 1991–92	244 children with a motor impairment of central origin (0.3% of child population in Scotland) Two thirds had moderate–severe disability in relation to personal care; more than half had severe learning disability
Beresford 1995	UK (using the Family Fund database)	Been helped by the Family Fund and been in recent contact with the Family Fund; children < 16 years	Collected data on 1100 families caring for a severely disabled child Estimate 150,000 families are caring for a severely disabled child
Glendinning et al 2001	UK	Technology-dependent children	Estimates 6000 technology-dependent children in the UK (although some double counting may have occurred) 2800 children receiving artificial feeding (British Artificial Nutrition Survey cited by Glendinning et al)

nasal feeding tubes (18%), suction equipment (16%), nebulisers and inhalers (10%), gastric feeding tubes (12%), a feeding pump (12%), catheters (7%), oxygen (9%), ventilators (7%), other things (14%). Clearly, parents have to develop advanced clinical skills to look after their child at home. The children's nurse has a clear role to play in teaching families these skills, sourcing and providing equipment, anticipating and preventing potential problems and supporting parents at home to provide the highest quality care.

Scenario

Real-life scenario by a parent of a child with complex motor disability

'My son Daniel [a pseudonym] was born in 1998 and what should have been a wonderful event became a tragedy. Daniel has athetoid cerebral palsy. He is now four and a half years old and is a 24-hour job.

Apart from physical exhaustion looking after a handicapped child, the mental torment is nearly worse. Watching your child day to day and wondering if he will see another one or if the next illness will be the last and you have to say 'goodbye'.

The needs of the child are great and this can be where health services mainly focus. However, the needs of the parent often fall by the wayside. Practical help is required from the start in the form of advice, supplies and respite care. I 'fell' through the net and did not receive any real help until my son was two and a half years old. Daniel was then assigned a community nurse who realised our plight and set out to help. She organised all supplies, including nappies and medical equipment. Something as simple as this eased the load and was something less to worry about. She was excellent for advice on Disability Living Allowance and Motability transport. She also

Table 25.2 Studies of Children and Young People with Cerebral Palsy

Reference (alphabetical)	Geographical area	Method	Birth years	Number of children	Rate per 1000 live births
Colver and Mackie 1998	North East of England	Case register	1991–93	287	2.4
Edmond et al 1989	Great Britain	British Perinatal Mortality & Birth Survey	1958, 1970	40, 41	2.5
Ingram 1955	Edinburgh	Ad hoc survey	1938–52	208	1.9
Jarvis et al 1985	North East of England	Case register	1960–75	421	1.6
Johnson & King 1998	Oxford	Case register	1984–91	697	2.5
MacGillvary & Campbell 1995	Avon	Taken from a handicap register	1969–88	489	2.1
Parkes et al 2001b	Northern Ireland	Case register	1981–93	784	2.2
Pharoah et al 1990	Mersey	Case register	1980–84	309	1.9
Pharoah et al 1998	Mersey, Oxford & Scotland	Case registers	1984–89	1649	2.1
Williams et al 1996	North East Thames	Case register	1980–86	672	1.6

arranged hospice and respite care, which are wonderful, and tried to make life that little bit easier.

Too many parents are struggling on their own with limited information and resources as all too often one parent has to give up work to be the carer. This is what happened to me. There are few day-care facilities who can deal with a child with a nasogastric tube, a tracheostomy and epilepsy.

Emotional support is rare. It does not have to be an expensive organisation. Someone to talk to, have a coffee with and who does not mind if you have a good cry to get things off your chest, is often all that is required, but it is not out there. If it does exist, many parents are not told.

This might all sound like 'me, me, me', however to give Daniel a good life, I have to be strong mentally as well as physically. To put Daniel in care if I have a breakdown would cost approximately £700 per week. Me caring for my son is free.

I cannot describe the mental torture of knowing my son will die. Only a mother who walks a day in my shoes could possibly understand the constant struggle for help and advice. The situation has not improved a great deal in the last twenty years.'

AIM OF SERVICES

In 1991 the UK government ratified the United Nations Convention on the Rights of the Child (United Nations General Assembly 1989) and by doing so undertook to commit to the principles laid out by the Convention. Several articles within the Convention are relevant to children with disabilities (Articles 2, 3 and 12). More specifically, Article 23 states:

. . . a mentally or physically disabled child should enjoy a full and decent life, in conditions which ensure dignity, promote self-reliance, and facilitate the child's active participation in the community.

Article 23 should form the basis for providing services and interventions to the child with complex motor disability and his or her family. The overall aim of services to children with complex motor disability must also include early detection (and prevention where possible), early intervention and family support. The ultimate aim for all children with health or special needs must be to help them achieve the maximum potential and the best quality of life as possible:

Children with profound and multiple disabilities and/or complex and continuing health care needs should enjoy the highest quality of life possible, receiving quality health, social and educational services which meet their needs and the needs of those who care for them, and respect their lifestyle and culture (Ward et al 2003)

● Seminar discussion topic

Use the real-life scenario presented above and the account provided by Kingdom & Mayfield (2001):

- What issues or 'patient' problems can you identify? Distinguish between child-centred problems and parent-centred problems.
- To what extent do the parents' experiences and perceptions match the aims of services for children with disability specified above?
- Discuss the role of the children's nurse in addressing each of the issues or problems identified.
- What other professionals might the children's nurse interact with to help ensure the needs of this child and family are met?

FAMILIES' EXPERIENCES OF SERVICES

As we have already heard from parents, help and support is available from a wide range of services and professionals, some of whom focus directly on helping the child, whereas others concentrate on assisting the parents and family. Sloper & Turner (1992) found that parents of severely disabled children were in contact with a large number of professionals, as many as ten in any one year, with a range of 5–17. Similarly, in a study of children with moderate to severe cerebral palsy, Parkes et al (2002) also found that families were in contact with an average of seven service providers in a 6-month interval, range 1–13. Not surprisingly, parents of children with disability have reported problems related to coordination of services and fragmentation of care. Bamford et al (1997) described this as 'deficiencies in the total care concept'.

Sloper & Turner (1992) found that many parents reported that they had encountered problems in finding and coordinating services, particularly in the early days after diagnosis, as reported elsewhere (Bamford et al 1991, Haylock et al 1993, Watson et al 2002). In particular, parents have reported that professionals often duplicate work and seem unable to detect where the gaps in services are (Rees 1983). Haylock et al (1993) found school (i.e. special education) offered families a form of integration of care that they very much appreciated; again, this has been reported elsewhere (McConachie et al 1999).

The inadequacies of respite care for families with a child with special needs, both in terms of quantity and quality of services available, have been repeatedly identified in the literature (Beresford 1994, 1995, McConkey & Adams 2000, Stalker 1990). The children's nurse has a particular role to play here in terms of finding respite facilities, giving families good information and helping and preparing them psychologically to avail of services (Miller 2002, Ross & Parkes 2004). Families with a child with complex problems that require nursing care (e.g. problems with active seizures requiring medication) may find it more difficult to find respite from both the formal and informal sector because of their child's specialist requirements and the level of responsibility required of carers (Beale 2002, Parkes 1998). Families of children with severe and complex needs are at higher risk of stress and feelings of being unable to cope (Sloper & Turner 1993).

WWW

Read about a model of good practice in relation to providing holistic care for children with complex healthcare needs and their families. See the Children's Trust, Tadworth, Surrey, a charitable organisation providing specialist care, therapies and education for children with severe disabilities, at:

- http://www. thechildrenstrust.org.uk/

There are many examples of good practice in the care of children with complex motor disability both in the literature and in our local communities. Ross & Parkes (2004) outlined a model of good practice for the children's community nurse in relation to the care of a child with complex motor disability and the child's family. This paper highlights the unique role that the children's nurse can play in coordinating a multidisciplinary response that helps to 'cut down' excessive visits by numerous professionals while at the same time tailoring services to meet with the child and family's individual needs.

A number of 'care interfaces' and transitional phases may exist for the child with complex motor disability and their family, which the children's nurse must be aware of and anticipate. These interfaces exist where the child and family 'move' from one service arrangement to another, for example from community to hospital or from child to adult services, as a result of changing need or developmental stage. These interfaces and transitional phases are times when the child and family may need extra help and support to cope and where service providers are 'at risk' of failing due to inadequate planning, poor cooperation or coordination between multiagencies.

The children's nurse in collaboration with the child's paediatrician, the family and other members of the multidisciplinary team, can act as coordinator of health and social care services and ensure that adequate advance planning takes place before discharge from hospital or transfer to another setting. Children with complex needs often receive hospital services at a number of hospital locations (McConachie 1997) and this highlights the importance of children's nurses communicating with one another across institutional boundaries.

WHAT FAMILIES WANT FROM SERVICES

Based on research involving families with a disabled child, Baldwin & Carlisle (1994) identified the attributes of a quality service for children with disability. A number of their findings have been supported from research conducted by others. The results have implications for children's nursing practice and are summarised below.

Evidence-based Practice

The following has been taken from Baldwin & Carlisle (1994), whose findings are supported by other research (the references of which are included here). Families with a disabled child want:

- An individual, comprehensive assessment of the needs of each child and family. Sloper & Turner (1992) also found that services that focus purely on the child's needs may put the family under more pressure.
- Regular review and assessment of need, particularly at times of transition. Hirose & Ueda (1990) identified the time of diagnosis, starting school, changing school and leaving school as times of stress for families with a child with disability.
- An opportunity to make informed choices about services.
- Involvement in the design and delivery of a package of services.
- A 'key worker' for each child and family, who maintains close contact, acts as a link person between the different agencies involved in their child's care, acts as an advocate and represents their views (Audit Commission 1994, Beresford 1994, Sloper 1999).

Research evidence additional to Baldwin & Carlisle's recommendations suggests that families need regular breaks that are tailored to their individual requirements (Beresford 1994, McConkey & Adams 2000).

For a more detailed account of the evidence regarding service models to support parents of disabled children, see Sloper (1999).

SETTING STANDARDS: THE CHILDREN'S NATIONAL SERVICE FRAMEWORK

In 1998, the government launched a programme of National Service Frameworks (NSFs) for a number of key patient groups with the aim of 'driving the modernisation agenda' within the NHS. The aims of the NSFs are to set national standards for key interventions, develop strategies to support the implementation of interventions and to increase quality and decrease variation in service provision. An outline of the development of the Children's NSF is provided by Smith (2003). The Standards for Hospital Services is the first part of the Children's NSF and is available online.

www

Find the latest information on the development of the Children's National Service Framework, including a downloadable copy of the Standards for Hospital Services, at:
- http://www.doh.gov.uk/nsf/children/index.htm
There is also a Children's NSF Bulletin *Getting the right start*, which is available at the same website address.

An external working group on disabled children was set up to specifically address the unique and particular needs of children with disability and/or complex and life-limiting illness. This group comprises parents, professionals, voluntary workers and researchers. It also has a series of seven task groups set up to address specific issues related to early diagnosis task group, family support, equipment, therapy services, transition services, children's and family participation and children with severe disability and long-term conditions. Many of these priorities are reflected in the evidence-based work by Baldwin & Carlisle (1994) and from the accounts given by parents, including the real-life scenario described above. A number of key areas under consideration for the proposed standards and interventions for children with complex and continuing health needs have been specified in a draft 'work in progress' document.

www

Access the draft document at:
- http://www.doh.gov.uk/nsf/children/externalwgdisabled.htm

For earlier work on the development of a charter for children with disabilities and their families, see Milner et al (1996).

Nursing Assessment and Interventions

This section addresses a small number of activities of living that should be assessed by the children's nurse involved in the care of a child with complex motor disability – at home in the community, or on admission to hospital. Reasons for hospitalisation can include orthopaedic surgery, nutritional management including surgery, and other medical reasons such as management of a chest infection or pneumonia and respite care. The issues discussed here include mobility, eating and drinking and communication. These areas have been identified as the subject of specialist referrals in the literature (Cass et al 1999) and as relevant on the basis of our own clinical and research experience. Other problems not mentioned here, but addressed elsewhere in this book, include the management of the child with seizures, sensory impairments and pain management.

Many of the problems encountered by children with complex motor disability are interrelated and require complex analyses by the children's nurse to understand the relationship between patient problems and their underlying causes. Cass et al (1999) identified a useful hierarchy of assessment involving consideration of six levels. This model proposes that problem solving 'high'-level functions, like communication, depends on the resolution of lower-level functions affecting communication (e.g. head control). Sensory impairments can affect the ability to communicate; the presence of active seizures may impact on the child's general alertness and motivation and can affect eating and drinking. These examples underline the importance of taking a holistic approach to assessing and planning care for children with complex motor disability and listening carefully to parents and carers. They also highlight the importance of undertaking an assessment in a multidisciplinary environment where joint planning can be undertaken (Cass et al 1999).

In the context of children's nursing, the Roy adaptation model (1976) has much to offer the assessment of children with complex problems. This model focuses on the responses of the 'adaptive' person to a constantly changing environment (Fawcett 1995). Roy's nursing assessment comprises two stages:

1. Stage one: identification of 'adaptive' and 'maladaptive' behaviours in relation to four domains:
   - physiological mode
   - self-concept mode
   - role function mode
   - interdependence.
2. Stage two: identification of the stimuli that are thought to be responsible for the maladaptive behaviours. These stimuli are grouped into:
   - focal stimulus: the one most directly and immediately confronting the patient (as defined by nurse, child (where possible) and family)
   - contextual stimuli: all other stimuli present that influence the behaviour being observed
   - residual stimuli: the wider influences the patient may experience related to parent and family knowledge, beliefs, motivations, confidence and abilities.

The principles of competent nursing assessment include use of an appropriate model in which to frame: the assessment; the involvement of the parents and the child, where possible; use of positive language about what the child is able to do, as well as what he or she is unable to do, and regular review of the assessment undertaken. The emphasis within assessment will change according to the child's age and developmental stage and the family's needs (Cogher et al 1992). However, we propose core elements for consideration under the problems 'mobility', 'eating and drinking' and 'communication'.

Parents are increasingly being recognised for the experts that they are in the care and the management of their child

with disability (Beresford 1994, 1995, de Geeter et al 2002, Taanila et al 2002, NSF 2003). It is vital that nursing assessment takes place in meaningful dialogue with the parent. Assessment will involve observation of the parent–child interaction and of the child alone and against developmental milestones, as well as through nursing interventions (e.g. taking vital signs).

The principles of competent nursing intervention with the child with complex motor disability include establishing a meaningful, working partnership with the child and family; meeting the child's prioritised needs for nursing care; identifying and meeting the child and family's information needs and promoting their adaptation to the environment in which they are being cared for. Communicating with and coordinating other service providers is vital to avoid duplication or the opposite – opening a new gap in the family's support network. In the case of hospitalisation, preparation for discharge should be begin on the day of admission.

Reflect on your Practice

Read about an initiative to develop individualised, continuous documentation for children with special needs by Tippett (2001):
- What are the strengths of this approach?
- Are there any disadvantages to this approach?

MOBILITY

Complex motor impairment involves dysfunction of postural control, especially in children with cerebral palsy (Brogan et al 1998, Westcott et al 1997). Posture will be significantly affected in children with other conditions affecting truncal control and muscle strength (e.g. spina bifida, spinal muscular atrophy). Posture has been defined as the ability to maintain or control the centre of mass in relation to the base support (Westcott et al 1997). A sitting position is defined as a static balance, in comparison to a dynamic balance, which relates to walking. Attaining static balance is a prerequisite of dynamic balance.

In the long-term management of the child with complex motor disability, specialist physiotherapists and occupational therapists jointly oversee the assessment and planning of mobility (Fig. 25.1) and seating arrangements. This service is usually run in conjunction with the skill and expertise of specialist technicians in seating, aids and appliances. These professionals aim to optimise the child's posture and comfort, which will then enhance the child's respiration, eating, drinking, digestion, ability to communicate and help with moving and handling by the child's parents and carers. Physiotherapy services tend to be arranged, as might be expected, to provide the most intense levels of treatment to those most severely affected (Gough et al 1993, Haylock et al 1993, Parkes 2002). The aims of the

Fig. 25.1 • Postural control walker. This walker or rollator can be pushed or pulled (in reverse). It encourages the child to adopt a good posture, with the shoulders back, upright posture and leg extension.

Fig. 25.2 • Powered wheelchair. This chair has a child-operated control panel to give the child more independence. This example is suitable for a child with head control, although a head rest can also be added, and should be for all children during transport. Note the seat belt and foot plates to ensure good positioning and safety. An electric battery sits under the seat and must be charged regularly.

physiotherapy for the child with complex motor disability are likely to be conservative and directed towards preventing further complications, as well as advising and supporting families to continue with 'good practice' at home. The physiotherapist is the most common professional seen by the population of children with cerebral palsy (Parkes et al 2002), but is likely to be only one of the many key providers for children with complex problems. The children's nurse has a responsibility to liaise closely with the child's physiotherapist and occupational therapist to ensure good practice in relation to mobility, seating and positioning; and to adopt strategies aimed at preventing contractures or pressure areas and ensure these are incorporated in the plan of nursing care. Also any new developing problems, for example hip pain or dislocation, need to be identified and appropriate nursing interventions taken as early as possible. In the absence of independent walking, useful arm and hand function becomes particularly important to achieve independent mobility as a wheelchair user.

Bottos et al (2001) found that the introduction of powered wheelchairs (Fig. 25.2) for children with severe motor disability, including those with coexisting severe learning disability, enabled 21 of 27 children to move around independently and led to improved socialisation, but interestingly not to overall quality of life. The majority of parents in this study were not in favour of the introduction of powered wheelchairs at the beginning of the study but 23 of 25 expressed positive feelings at the end of the study.

There is evidence that the mobility of children with cerebral palsy is also affected by the environment or setting (Palisano et al 2003), which should be taken into consideration by the children's nurse when undertaking assessment of the child and family. Palisano et al (2003) found there was increased independence at school or in the community with wheelchair use, although few children self-propelled or used powered wheelchairs. However, this independence diminished at home for the most severely affected children, 39% of whom were carried about by a parent. Capturing information about the child's functional abilities in different settings (Figs 25.3 and 25.4) is therefore very important and should include a description of abilities at home, in school and in the community.

Orthopaedic surgery can lead to improvements in the day-to-day management of children in relation to personal hygiene, dressing and mobility. More specifically, the aims of orthopaedic surgery for the child with complex motor disability includes improving function, preventing pain, improving hygiene and appearance (Cogher et al 1992). Innovative treatments such as botulinum toxin also have a role in assisting management of limbs and joints affected by spasticity. Botulinum toxin is injected in minute amounts into targeted muscles and creates a temporary paralysis (see Korman et al (2003) for recent guidelines on the use of botulinum toxin injections for spasticity associated with cerebral palsy children).

Nursing Assessment of Mobility

In relation to assessment of the child's mobility and seating, we suggest the criteria in Box 25.1 are considered as part of

Fig. 25.3 • Prone stander. A prone stander offers an alternative position to help prevent deformities. It offers optimum hip symmetry and ensures a prolonged, passive stretch at the hips, knees and feet and ankles. This stander can also promote alertness and has an adjustable work surface to help prevent the child drooping forward.

good practice to ensure a complete and accurate assessment of need is conducted. Some of these suggestions are derived from an assessment form developed by Evans et al (1989), aimed at standardising the description of children with motor impairment of central origin. We have adapted the content of the box to reflect an assessment form using the Roper, Logan, Tierney model for nursing practice (1990 p 56) and this template is used throughout.

Fig. 25.4 • Adapted tricycle. This tricycle comes with a seat belt and foot plates with straps. Riding the tricycle encourages good positioning, postural control and muscle strength. It is suitable for children who are non-ambulant. It promotes reciprocal movement by breaking total body synergy associated with involuntary movements.

Box 25.1

Proposed nursing assessment of mobility for children with complex motor problems

Therapy history
- Take a brief physiotherapy history.
- Who usually treats the child? Where? How often?
- Do the parents conduct any regimes at home?
- Describe usual parental practice.
- Discuss any preventive strategies with the parents, e.g. does the child wear splints at night?
- Check when and how these are applied.

Type of motor impairment
- Describe the nature of the motor impairment.
- Is there altered tone? If yes, is it increased or decreased?
- Are there abnormal or involuntary movements?

Extent of motor impairment
- Describe the distribution of the impairment.
- How many limbs are affected?
- Is one side of the body more affected than the other?
- Are the legs more affected than the arms?
- Are the arms more affected than the legs?

Head, neck and trunk control
- Describe the distribution of the impairment.
- Is the child able to hold his or her head up? For how long?
- If not, what is the most comfortable way to support the child's head?
- Can the child sit unsupported? For how long?
- If not, what is the best way to support the child in a sitting position?
- Is there any evidence of curvature of the spine?

Leg function
- Assess the level of motor independence.
- Is the child able to walk 15 steps unaided?
- How far can the child walk (give approximate distance)?
- Comment on the use of aids for walking (e.g. crutches, sticks, rollator).
- If the child uses a wheelchair, can he or she mobilise independently? How far?

Arm function
- Assess the level of motor independence.
- Does the child have any self-care or self-mobilising skills?
- Does the child require assistance with dressing? If yes, how much assistance?
- Does the child require any help with eating or drinking? If yes, how much?

Aids and appliances
- Assess and describe good handling and posture regimes for the child: include seating, standing and mobility.
- Describe any other appliances used, e.g. night splints.

Complications
- Assess if any complications exist.

Continued

Proposed nursing assessment of mobility for children with complex motor problems—cont'd

- Describe any contractures that are present and describe position, severity and impact on child's ability. Check ankles, knees, hips, elbows and wrists.
- Describe the child's feet and footwear noting any abnormalities of posture (e.g. valgus) or problems related to comfort.
- Note the presence of scoliosis or kyphosis because this may have important implications for positioning and comfort.

Nursing Interventions in Mobility

The children's nurse, and particularly those with specialist orthopaedic training, has much to offer the child with complex motor disability and their family in terms of skill and knowledge in relation to mobility.

Adaptive seating can prevent or delay musculoskeletal deformities, enhanced postural control, upper limb control and oral motor control (Roxborough 1995). The treatment can also increase comfort, improve physiological function, enhance function abilities and increase the child's social interaction. Cogher et al (1992 pp 152–166) provide a detailed description of the types of seating available. A wheelchair can offer independent mobility and transport but also a position for eating and drinking, as well as a place to play with toys. Arranging suitable seating should include consideration of body posture, head control, and feet and limb positioning. Restraining straps, cushion requirements and material type are also vital in assuring the safe transport, tissue viability and hygiene needs of the child.

Providing equipment for mobility and positioning, especially if spinal curvature is present or has undergone correction, will often involve a dedicated orthotic team. Specialist technicians whose purpose is to maximise function, comfort and social acceptability will individually craft orthotic equipment (Fig. 25.5). Standard equipment will be adjusted to meet the needs of the individual. The parent will also require easy storage of equipment at home and during transportation, with ease of assembly and disassembly a high priority. If the equipment is static, consideration of space within the home is an important factor.

A main intervention in relation to seating and mobility is teaching parents about safe lifting and handling of the child; about continuing therapy routines at home and about safe use and storage of the equipment. The equipment can then be used for a trial period to review its effectiveness for both parent and child. Adjustments are often required, especially if the child's medical or physical status has changed. The developing child implies a limited life span for such equipment, for this reason, frequent check-ups and adjustments

Fig. 25.5 • Adaptable chair. This chair can be raised or lowered, enabling the child to participate in different activities that take place at different heights – eating, playing or working at a desk. Note the knee blocks to help maintain hip position. The chair also has trunk and lateral supports with adjustable foot plates.

by technicians are essential for optimum use. Care must be taken not to 'overburden' the family with too high expectations about what they can manage at home, given that they may have other children or family commitments, and may also work.

EATING AND DRINKING

An association between severe neurodevelopmental conditions like cerebral palsy and impaired oromotor function leading to eating problems has been identified (Gisel & Alphonce 1995). Samson-Fang et al (2003) cited that 27% of children with moderate to severe cerebral palsy included in a North American follow-up study were found to be malnourished (as measured by skin-fold thickness). Problems with eating and drinking vary from mild problems related to control of salvia or chewing ability to severe problems with disturbances of gut motility, reflux and vomiting.

One of the most important assessment indicators of health in children is growth and a primary reason for intervening in eating and drinking is concern about the adequacy of nutrition as evidenced by poor growth. Children with severe oromotor impairment can take from 2–12 times longer to manipulate and swallow a standard amount of pureed food and 1–15 times longer to chew and swallow solid food (Gisel & Patrick 1988). These children are at higher risk of experiencing poor growth and weight gain, although artificial feeding techniques have been found to be effective in helping to establish weight gain. Furthermore, persistent feeding problems in young children with cerebral palsy have been identified as a marker for poor feeding, growth and developmental outcome later in childhood and could be used to identify those children with cerebral palsy who might benefit from gastrostomy feeding (Motion et al 2002). Given the complexity of the problems, a team approach to assessment is most effective and usually consists of parents, teacher, speech and language specialist, occupational therapist, physiotherapist, dietician, paediatrician and children's nurse.

Nursing Assessment in Eating and Drinking

The severely affected child is assessed for his or her ability to coordinate sucking and breathing during feeds, with evidence of problems recognised during weaning. An inability to gain weight and the deterioration to low-weight-for-age-specific percentiles within the first year of life are characteristic. The assessment of eating and drinking impairment is based on measures of growth and eating skills: eating efficiency and oral motor skills (Gisel & Alphonce 1995). To make a detailed eating and drinking assessment, knowledge of what happens at meal times along with aspects of proposed change by the parent/carer is necessary. A profile of contributing factors is also required as part of the assessment and planning prior to professional intervention.

A second component that relates to the assessment and planning of eating and drinking is drooling. This problem is again often associated with cerebral palsy children with poor oromotor function. Intensive drooling leads to negative social interactions, schooling issues and physical effects: chapped and sore lips and chin, sodden clothes and often an unpleasant smell (Lloyd Faulconbridge et al 2001). The multidisciplinary team assesses such drooling along with individual planning and intervention.

In relation to assessment of the child's eating and drinking, the criteria in Box 25.2 are considered part of good practice to ensure that a complete and accurate assessment of need is conducted. Some of the suggestions in the box are derived from Evans et al (1989) and Cogher et al (1992).

Nursing Interventions in Eating and Drinking

If it is apparent that adequate nutrition is being achieved, parents may just need reassurance, especially if eating is very messy. Simple alterations to posture and seating can prove very effective in enhancing dietary intake. Oral fluid intake may be altered through a thickening agent; a thicker consistency prevents reflux, choking and aspiration. This approach can also encourage a higher fluid intake and prevent dehydration. Food consistency may also be changed, for example from mashed to puréed textures. A change in

---

Box 25.2

Proposed nursing assessment of eating and drinking for children with complex motor problems

Adequacy of nutrition
- Assess growth: height, weight.
- Assess rate of growth.
- Compare parent and professional assessment of growth and nutritional status.
- Take feeding history: length of time to complete a meal; assess daily intake and daily loss (vomiting).
- Describe amount and type of food intake.

History
- Find out about early feeding habits.
- Seek and include histories of dietetic and speech and language therapy input.
- Assess if any referrals might be necessary.

Oral skills
- Note dentition, any structural problems that might make eating or breathing while eating difficult.
- Observe and comment on ability to chew, swallow, clear palate, control saliva.
- Look for drooling.

Tolerance
- Assess if the child is prone to choking, coughing, spluttering, vomiting. Record frequency.
- Cogher et al (1992) emphasise the importance of assessing tolerance through behaviours – turning away, refusing to eat, crying, grimacing, gagging or vomiting.

Food preferences
- Describe the child's food preferences.
- Also describe the preferred texture (lumpy, solid, puréed); preferred feeding utensils.

Feeding technique
- Describe breathing pattern while eating and assess the risk of aspiration as far as possible.
- Describe the parents' technique.
- How do the parents position the child for eating and drinking?
- What special utensils do they have, or are preferred?

Digestion and elimination
- Is there any evidence of pain and discomfort on eating and drinking?
- Is there any history of constipation or other gastrointestinal problems: reflux, obstruction, rupture?

Parents' attitudes
- Find out about parents' feelings towards their child's nutrition and eating and drinking: are these associated with stress?

---

equipment – spoons (Fig. 25.6) and cups (Fig 25.7) – often works in harmony with feeding techniques, which again reduce the risk of choking and aspiration. Cogher et al (1992) also suggest desensitising the child's face and mouth

Fig. 25.6 • Spoons. Flexi-spoons are available to help children feed more easily and independently.

before eating by the use of touch if behaviour intolerance or an excess of involuntary movements are present.

Alternatively, a period of hospitalisation may be necessary often for the insertion and parental education of nasogastric tube feeding. Failure of such a system due to either non-compliance or tube insertion issues may lead to a long-term option, that of a gastrostomy feeding system. Gastrostomy is not without risk, although the benefits of adequate nutrition usually outweigh the risks of complications. Gastrostomy feeding has been associated with improved growth and quality of life in children with cere-

Fig. 25.7 • Cups and straws. A cup with an angled rim means that the child does not have to throw the head back if self-feeding. If being fed from these cups, the feeder has extra control in the amount of liquid the child receives. The straw has non-return valve that helps children with poor sucking ability. Note the non-slip mat to prevent spillages.

bral palsy (Smith et al 1999). This system, established by insertion of a tube through the abdominal wall into the stomach, is for long-term use. Regardless of the feeding method utilised, oral hygiene of the mouth is essential to reduce tooth decay and other related medical problems. Support and trouble-shooting for all feeding interventions can be sought within the community from a variety of healthcare professionals and at relevant hospital clinics.

Evidence-based Practice

The American Academy for Cerebral Palsy and Developmental Medicine (AACPDM) undertook a systematic review of the outcomes of gastrostomy feeding in children with cerebral palsy (Samson-Fang et al 2003). The findings of the systematic review are summarised below:

- 10 studies met all the inclusion criteria and were included in the review. The 10 studies contain results on a total of 281 individuals.
- All the studies were described by Samson-Fang et al (2003) as comprising 'very low levels of evidence' when evaluated against the AACPDM quality rating scheme.
- Overall, however, there was consistency in the results, which favoured gastrostomy feeding.

This systematic review provides an excellent example of how to investigate the evidence base for practice in a rigorous way and could be used as 'gold standard' in assessing the evidence for children's nursing.

Feeding and language-related problems often go together in children with severe cerebral palsy, even though speech production does not inevitably correlate with earlier oral-motor patterns (Dormans & Pellegrino 1998). The next section considers the related area of communication.

COMMUNICATION

Speech and language facilitate learning and regulate behaviour, they are also critical developmental tasks that form the basis for all social interactions. The ability to communicate is fundamental to expressing personal need or opinion. Children will often use their natural modes of communication, such as vocalisation, eye-pointing, gesture and body movements. Play can also enhance communication through motivation, imagination and the development of social skills. Several examples of good practice exist in the literature (Brodin 1999, Crawford & Raven 2002) and make useful suggestions to strengthen play opportunities for this group. Children restricted by physical and cognitive limitations who are not given adequate opportunities for free play are being further disadvantaged.

Children with significant neuromotor impairments may experience problems related to articulation of speech and language and/or problems related to intellectual ability and the ability to communicate and express themselves. Pennington & McConachie (1999) studied the interaction between non-verbal children with severe motor impairment and their carers. The findings indicated that the adults took control of conversations, instigated topics, asked questions and issued commands. The children provided the required responses, using a restricted range of communicative functions. This highlights the importance of children's nurses understanding how to communicate with non-verbal children. However, work conducted by Beail (1985) found that nurses had low-level and poor-quality interactions with children with multiple disabilities; it is to be hoped that awareness and practice have changed since then.

Nursing Assessment in Communication

In relation to the assessment of a child's communication abilities, the criteria in Box 25.3 are considered part of good practice to ensure a complete and accurate assessment of need is conducted. Some of the suggestions are derived from Evans et al (1989) and Cogher et al (1992).

Nursing Interventions in Communication

Effective assessment is imperative to optimise a child's communication and development potential. Impairments, including hearing, visual, cognitive (learning disability), attention deficits, respiratory problems, orthopaedic anomalies and other medical conditions (e.g. seizures, respiratory problems, gastroesophageal reflux), may all affect the child's ability to communicate (Cass et al 1999). The key interventions to facilitate communication in the child with complex motor problems as described by Cogher et al (1992) should focus on good positioning – to maximise eye contact and minimise involuntary movements and facilitated expression through constructive play and augmented communication systems (Figs 25.8 and 25.9).

To maximise the successful use of augmentative communication systems, the child should be introduced to the system as early as possible, professionals and parents need to be trained to facilitate the child and there needs to be planning and cooperation between the professional multi-agencies (Ko et al 1998). During a period of hospitalisation it is essential that the children's nurse supports the child to continue to use and develop his or her skills in augmentative communication systems as far as possible.

Ineffective communication can lead to frustration, which is sometimes interpreted as 'bad behaviour' in the child. Frustration can be expressed through non-compliance to care with rigid or thrashing torso and high vocalisation. The child may be expressing a need to change position or to

Box 25.3

Proposed nursing assessment of communication for children with complex motor problems

Oromotor abilities
- Are problems related to articulation of speech apparent (dysarthria)?
- Record history of speech and language therapy.

Social interaction
- What motivates the child to communicate: happy? sad? hunger? pain? Assess in conjunction with parents.
- Describe child's experiences and knowledge of play?
- Is the child able to participate in symbolic play?

Means of expression
- Describe means of expression: verbal or non-verbal.
- Alternative methods of communication: eye pointing? sounds?
- Formalised systems such as Makaton?
- Describe if any involuntary facial expressions are apparent – these can sometimes be misleading.

Non-verbal skills
- Describe non-verbal skills, especially if the child is unable to speak.
- Describe eye contact, vocalisation, body movements (head control, unwanted movements, facial grimacing).
- Describe if the child is able to 'take turns' in any interaction, assess attention span.

Comprehension
- Is there a reliable yes/no response: to nurse, to parents, to others?
- Ask parents level of understanding.
- Also record type of school attended; psychologist's reports.

Use of expressive language
- Describe use of expressive language: range and depth of vocabulary. Age appropriate?

Phonology
- Describe how the words sound: accurate?

Family communication
- Describe any child and family communication strategies that might exist, in particular the role of play, particular games.
- Describe how the parents and siblings communicate with the child.

resolve hunger, toiletry needs or pain. Free play can help alleviate such communication difficulties through development of the whole child. Behavioural cues may be misleading so parents and health professionals must be cautious in their assessment and planning. Facial impressions can be misunderstood due to low muscle tone and vocalisations can be misinterpretated due to increased laryngeal spasticity.

Promoting function requires the building of skills as well as developing compensatory mechanisms to help the child

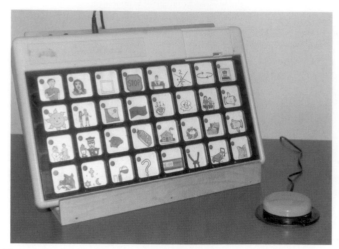

Fig. 25.8 • Symbols for communication. Picture symbols can be used to communicate. This communications board is activated by a switch. The child practises controlling the switch through work and play.

best function within the limits of his or her motor and cognitive abilities. Once a child's communication deficits and potential have been established, the specialist team of speech therapist and medical consultant must implement a phase of planning. Such planning will be shared within a larger team, to include paediatric nurse, health visitor, teacher, physiotherapist and occupational therapist. The aim is to develop all areas that will facilitate optimum communication for the child. If speech is not an available option, alternative skills such as pointing, picture boards, and non-verbal cues will be developed to ensure the child's needs are met. If the child is visually and hearing impaired, non-verbal responses such as body language along with the positive communication of a familiar parent/carer is vital for effective child communication.

Fig. 25.9 • More symbols. This Makaton system is another example of symbols for communication. It is based on picture symbols. The child points at the words and, with practice, can build up relatively sophisticated communication. A booklet can be customised for each individual child.

Summary

This chapter has brought together a number of perspectives in the consideration of children with complex motor disability. Although complex motor disability is relatively rare, as are the conditions that give rise to it, the level of need and support required by children and their families is high and life long. Multiple agencies are involved in the provision of care and services to these children and care must be taken not to overburden families with too many professionals but at the same time ensure their needs are met. Parents caring for a child with complex motor disability are experts in their own right and a valued partner for the children's nurse. This chapter considered a small number of predominant problems experienced by children with complex needs. In particular, detailed consideration was given to what the children's nurse should assess and how they should intervene in the areas of mobility, eating and drinking and communication.

Acknowledgements

We would like to thank Daniel's Mum for her frank and honest account of her experiences caring for her son. We would also like to thank Mrs Sheila McNeill, Paediatric Physiotherapist, and Mrs Julia Maskery, Paediatric Occupational Therapist, for advice on the use of aids and adaptations as featured in the photographs and accompanying text; and Mrs Doris Corkin, Nurse Lecturer, for reading and commenting on an earlier draft.

References

Audit Commission 1994 Seen but not heard: coordinating community child health and social services for children in need. HMSO, London

Baldwin S, Carlisle J 1994 Social support for disabled children and their families. A review of the literature. Social Work Services Inspectorate, HMSO, London

Bamford D, Griffith H, Kernohan G 1991 I felt like running away: the social and emotional implications of cerebral palsy. Boys' and Girls' Welfare Society, London

Bamford D, Griffith H, Kernohan G 1997 Analysis of consumer satisfaction with cerebral palsy care. British Journal of Social Work 27:605–614

Beail N 1985 The nature of interactions between nursing staff and profoundly multiply handicapped children. Child: Care, Health and Development 11:113–129

Beale H 2002 Respite care for technology-dependent children and their families. Paediatric Nursing 14:18–19

Beresford B 1994 Positively parents. Caring for a severely disabled child. Social Policy Research Unit, HMSO, London

Beresford B 1995 Expert opinions. A national survey of families caring for a severely disabled child. Policy Press, Bristol

Bone M, Meltzer H 1989 The prevalence of disability among children. HMSO, London

Bottos M, Bolcati C, Sciuto L et al 2001 Powered wheelchairs and independence in young children with tetraplegia. Developmental Medicine and Child Neurology 43:769–777

Brodin J 1999 Play in children with severe multiple disabilities: play with toys – a review. International Journal of Disability, Development and Education 46:25–34

Brogan E, Hadders-Algra M, Forssberg H 1998 Postural control in sitting children with cerebral palsy. Neuroscience and Behavioural Reviews 22:591–596

Cass H, Price K, Reilly S et al 1999 A model for the assessment and management of children with multiple disabilities. Child: Care, Health and Development 25:191–211

Cogher L, Savage E, Smith MF 1992 Cerebral palsy. The child and young person. Chapman & Hall Medical, London

Colver AF, Mackie P 1998 North of England collaborative cerebral palsy survey. Annual Report

Crawford C, Raven K 2002 Play preparation for children with special needs. Paediatric Nursing 14:27–29

Critchton JU, MacKinnon M, White C P 1995 The life expectancy of person with cerebral palsy. Developmental Medicine and Child Neurology 37:567–576

de Geeter KI, Poppes P, Vlaskamp C 2002 Parents as experts: the position of parents of children with profound multiple disabilities. Child: Care, Health and Development 28:443–453

Dormans JP, Pellegrino L 1998 Caring for children with cerebral palsy: a team approach. Brooks Publishing, London

Duffy B 1995 PPRU surveys of disability report 5: disabled children in Northern Ireland: services, transport and education. Policy Planning and Research Unit, Belfast

Edmond A, Golding J, Peckham C 1989 Cerebral palsy in two national cohort studies. Archives of Disease in Childhood 60:1113–1121

Evans PM, Evans SJW, Alberman E 1989 A standard form for recording clinical findings in children with a motor deficit of central origin (letter). Developmental Medicine and Child Neurology 31:121–127

Fawcett J 1995 Analysis and evaluation of conceptual models of nursing, 3rd edn. FA Davis, Philadelphia

Gisel EG, Alphonce E 1995 Classification of eating impairments based on eating efficiency in children with cerebral palsy. Dysphagia 10:268–274

Gisel EG, Patrick J 1988 Identification of children with cerebral palsy unable to maintain a normal nutritional state. Lancet 1:283–286

Glendinning C, Kirk S, Guiffridda A, Lawton D 1999 The community based care of technology dependent children in the UK: definitions, numbers and costs. National Primary Care Research and Development Centre, University of Manchester, Manchester

Glendinning C, Kirk S, Guiffridda A, Lawton D 2001 Technology-dependent children in the community: definitions, numbers and costs. Child: Care, Health and Development 27:321–334

Gordon D, Parker R, Loughran F, Heslop P 2000 Disabled children in Britian. A re-analysis of the OPCS disability survey. The Stationery Office, London

Gough D, Li L, Wroblewska A 1993 Services for children with a motor impairment and their families in Scotland. Public Health Research Unit, University of Glasgow

Haylock C, Johnson AM, Harpin VA 1993 Parents' views of community care for children with motor disabilities. Child: Care, Health and Development 19:209–220

Hirose T, Ueda R 1990 Long-term follow up study of cerebral palsy children and coping behaviour of parents. Journal of Advanced Nursing 15:762–770

Hutton J, Cook T, Pharoah POD 1994 Life expectancy in children with cerebral palsy. British Medical Journal 309:431–435

Hutton J, Pharoah POD 1998 Life expectancy in people with cerebral palsy. Abstract from an annual meeting. In: Colver A, Mackie P North of England collaborative cerebral palsy survey. Annual report, November:19–25

Ingram TTS 1955 A study of cerebral palsy in the childhood population of Edinburgh. Archives of Disease in Childhood 60:1113–1121

Johnson A, King R 1998 Oxford register of early childhood impairments. Annual Report 1997. National Perinatal Epidemiology Unit, Oxford

Kingdom S, Mayfield C 2001 Complex disabilities: parents preparing professionals. Paediatric Nursing 13:34–38

Kirk S 1999 Caring for children with specialised health care needs in the community. Health & Social Care in the Community 7:350–357

Ko MLB, McConachie H, Jolieff N 1998 Outcome of recommendations for augmentative communication in children. Child: Care, Health and Development 24:195–205

Korman LA, Paterson Smith B, Ballrishnan R 2003 Spasticity associated with cerebral palsy in children. Pediatric Drugs 5:11–23

Lloyd Faulconbridge RV, Tranter RM, Moffat V, Green E 2001 Review of management of drooling problems in neurologically impaired children: a review of methods and results over 6 years at Chailey Heritage Clinical Services. Clinical Otolaryngology 26:76–81

MacGillivray I, Campbell D 1995 The changing pattern of cerebral palsy in Avon. Paediatric and Perinatal Epidemiology, 9:146–155

McCarthy GT, Cork M, Crone S et al 1992 The baby and young child. In: McCarthy GT (ed.) Physical disability in childhood. An interdisciplinary approach to management. Churchill Livingstone, Edinburgh, pp 13–52

McConachie H 1997 Organization of child disability services. Guest editorial. Child: Care, Health and Development 23:3–9

McConachie H, Salt A, Chadury Y et al 1999 How do child development teams work? Findings from a UK national survey. Child: Care, Health and Development 25:157–168

McConkey R, Adams L 2000 Matching short break services for children with learning disabilities to family needs and preferences. Child: Care, Health and Development 26:429–443

Miller S 2002 Respite care for children who have complex healthcare needs. Paediatric Nursing 14:33–37

Milner J, Bungay C, Jellinek D, Hall DMB 1996 Needs of disabled children and their families. Archives of Disease in Childhood 75:399–404

Motion S, Northstone K, Emond A et al 2002 Early feeding problems in children with cerebral palsy: weight and neuro-developmental outcomes. Developmental Medicine and Child Neurology 44:40–43

Mutch L, Alberman E, Hagberg G et al 1992 Cerebral palsy epidemiology: Where have we been and where are we going? (Annotation) Developmental Medicine and Child Neurology 34:547–551

National Service Framework (NSF) 2003 Online. Available at: http://www.doh.gov.uk/nsf

O'Shea TM, Preisser JS, Klinepeter KL, Dillard RG 1998 Trends in mortality and cerebral palsy in a geographically based cohort of very low birthweight neonates born between 1984 to 1994. Pediatrics 101:642–647

Palisano RJ, Tieman BL, Walter SD et al 2003 Effect of environmental setting on mobility methods of children with cerebral palsy. Developmental Medicine and Child Neurology 45:113–120

Parkes J 1998 Children with cerebral palsy in Northern Ireland: needs and services. Unpublished PhD Thesis. Queen's University, Belfast

Parkes J, Dolk H, Hill AE 1998 Does the child health computing system adequately identify children with cerebral palsy? Journal of Public Health Medicine 20(1):102–104

Parkes J, Dolk H, Hill N, Pattenden S 2001b Epidemiology of cerebral palsy in Northern Ireland: 1981–1993. Paediatric and Perinatal Epidemiology 15:278–286

Parkes J, Donnelly M, Dolk H, Hill N 2002 Use of physiotherapy and alternatives by children with cerebral palsy: a population study. Child: Care, Health and Development 28(6):469–477

Parkes J, Donnelly M, Hill N 2001a Focusing on cerebral palsy: reviewing and communicating needs for services. Scope, London

Pennington L, McConachie H 1999 Mother–child interaction revisited: communication with non-speaking physically disabled children. International Journal of Language and Communication Disorders 345:391–416

Pharoah POD, Cooke T, Cooke RWI, Rosenbloom L 1990 Birthweight-specific trends in cerebral palsy. Archives of Disease in Childhood 65:602–606

Pharoah POD, Platt M, Cooke T 1996 The changing epidemiology of cerebral palsy. Archives of Disease in Childhood 75:F169–F173

Pharoah POD, Cooke T, Johnson A et al 1998 Epidemiology of cerebral palsy in England and Scotland 1984–1990. Archives of Disease in Childhood F21–F25

Priestley M 2003 Disability. A life course approach. Polity Press, Cambridge

Rees SJ 1983 Families' perceptions of services for handicapped children. International Journal of Rehabilitation Research 6:475–476

Roberts K, Lawton D 2001 Acknowledging the extra care parents give their disabled children. Child: Care, Health and Development 27:307–319

Roper N, Logan WW, Tierney AJ 1990 The elements of nursing. Churchill Livingstone, Edinburgh

Ross A, Parkes J 2004 Making doors open: the role of the children's community nurse in caring for a child with severe cerebral palsy. Paediatric Nursing, in press

Roxborough L 1995 Review of the efficacy and effectiveness of adaptive seating for children with cerebral palsy. Assistive Technology 7:17–25

Roy C 1976 Introduction to nursing: an adaptation model. Prentice-Hall, Englewood Cliffs, NJ

Samson-Fang L, ButlerC, O'Donnell M 2003 Effects of gastrostomy feeding in children with cerebral palsy: an AACPDM evidence report. Developmental Medicine & Child Neurology 45:415–426

Sloper P 1999 Models of service support for parents of disabled children. What do we know? What do we need to know? Child: Care, Health and Development 25:85–99

Sloper P, Turner S 1992 Service needs of families of children with severe physical disability. Child: Care, Health and Development 18:259–282

Sloper P, Turner S 1993 Risk and resistance factors in the adaptation of parents of children with severe physical disability. Journal of Child Psychology and Psychiatry 34:167–188

Smith F 2003 'Getting the right start': the children's national service framework. Paediatric Nursing 15:20–21

Smith M, Robinson P, Duffy P 1992 PPRU surveys of disability report 2: the prevalence of disability among children in Northern Ireland. Policy, Planning and Research Unit, Belfast

Smith SW, Camfield C, Camfield P 1999 Living with cerebral palsy and tube feeding: a population-based follow-up study. Journal of Pediatrics 135:307–310

Stalker K 1990 Share the care: an evaluation of family-based respite care. Jessica Kingsley, London

Surveillance of Cerebral Palsy in Europe (SCPE) 2000 Surveillance of cerebral palsy in Europe: a collaboration of cerebral palsy surveys and registers. Developmental Medicine and Child Neurology 42:816–824

Taanila A, Syrjala L, Kokkonen J, Jarvelin MR 2002 Coping of parents with physically and/or intellectually disabled children. Child: Care, Health and Development 28:73–86

Tippett A 2001 All about me: documentation for children with special needs. Paediatric Nursing 13:34–35

United Nations General Assembly 1989 Convention on the Rights of the Child. UNICEF, Geneva

Ward T, Worswikc J, Inglis A et al 2003 Children with complex, continuing health needs and/or life-limiting conditions. Report of the task group. Children's national service framework: disabled children external working group. Online. Available at: http://www.doh.gov.uk/nsf/children

Watson D, Townsley R, Abbot D 2002 Exploring multi-agency working in services to disabled children with complex healthcare needs and their families. Journal of Clinical Nursing 11:367–375

Westcott SL, Lowes LP, Richardson PK 1997 Evaluation of postural stability in children: current theories and assessment tools. Physical Therapy 77:629–645

Williams K, Hennessey E, Alberman E 1996 Cerebral palsy: effects of twinning birthweight and gestational age. Archives of Disease in Childhood 75:F178–182

World Health Organization (WHO) 1980 International classification of impairments, disability and handicap (ICIDH). World Health Organization, Geneva

World Health Organization (WHO) 2001 Beginner's guide. Towards a common language for functioning, disability and health (ICF). World Health Organization, Geneva

World Health Organization (WHO) 2002 International classification of functioning, disability and health. World Health Organization, Geneva

Chapter Twenty Six

26

Caring for Children with Body Fluid and Electrolyte Imbalance

Agnes B Kanneh

ABSTRACT

Body fluids are the biochemical environments in which chemical reactions take place, thus the biological and clinical relevance of adequate hydration and electrolyte balance. It is essential that positively charged particles balance negatively charged particles. Balance in volume and solute composition is ensured by the well-coordinated and integrated action of the homeostatic organs, carefully matching intake with output. Scientific explanations offered on the structure and biological functions of water affirm the notion that water is the chemical of life, second only to oxygen (Martini 2004).

The availability of and access to safe drinking water is a basic human right. Body fluid and electrolyte balance relates to equilibrium between water intake and output, or between gain and loss, to maintain homeostasis. Therefore, imbalances occur when the body contains more or less of the required amounts.

In any human environment, water intake in the form of drinking is necessary to ensure a balance that maintains effective organ system function. Indeed food, nutrition, bladder and bowel control feature as essential elements of care in the government document *Essence of care* (DoH 2001). Here, children – and especially the very young – are dependent on their parents and carers, including healthcare professionals, to meet these fundamental human needs because of limited self-care ability. Maintenance of an adequate fluid and electrolyte balance in children is therefore pivotal in both child health care and paediatrics, and the area plays a major role in childhood morbidity and mortality on both national and global scale. Sadly, 3–5 billion children under 5 years of age worldwide experience acute gastroenteritis annually, causing 4 million childhood deaths in children 0–5 years of age. In the UK, 204 of every 1000 GP consultations and 7 of every 1000 hospital admissions of children under 5 years are due to acute diarrhoea. Although death is uncommon in developed countries, acute diarrhoea causes considerable morbidity due to body fluid and electrolyte imbalance (Dalby-Payne & Elliott 2004). Acute diarrhoea is the leading cause of body fluid and electrolyte imbalance in children worldwide.

Learning Outcomes

- Specify the main functions of water and electrolytes in the growing and developing child.

- Identify and examine possible causes of body fluid and electrolyte imbalance in children.

- Explain the clinical manifestations in the child with dehydration and electrolyte imbalance.

- Detail the principles of nursing care in the child who presents with body fluid and electrolyte imbalance caused by acute diarrhoea and vomiting.

Water Composition of the Body

BODY FLUIDS

From birth to the end of adolescence, the child is a biological, psychological and sociological human being, whose body is made up of trillions of cells. The cell is the fundamental unit of life and metabolism and an adequate intake of water is essential to the survival and everyday activities of the growing and developing child in both health and disease. Body fluids constitute total body water (TBW), with its dissolved chemical particles. Throughout life a large proportion of the body is water (these proportions change as age progresses, in accordance to the sex and body fat composition) (Fig 26.1).

Life on earth is a water-based phenomenon, postulated to have originated in water. Water is essential to the existence of all living organisms and water is the most abundant molecule of their cell mass (Horton et al 2002). Two-thirds of the total body weight is water and it is the body's single most important constituent (Martini 2004). Table 26.1 shows the water composition of various tissues in the average individual. In the absence of water, chemical reactions, metabolic processes and regulatory systems will become severely compromised and eventually cease to occur. A healthy adult can survive for around 10 days without water; a healthy child will survive only 3–4 days without water. To appreciate the value of water to the growing and developing child, and hence the deleterious effects of uncorrected body fluid and electrolyte imbalance, an understanding of the chemical and physical properties of water is essential (see Martini 2004, Chapter 27).

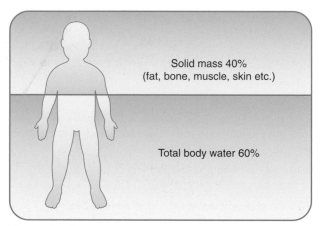

Fig. 26.1 • The percentage of total body water from age 1 year (Ichikawa 1990).

Table 26.1 Water Composition of Body Tissues in the Average 75-kg Male

Tissue	Percentage of water	Litres of water	Percentage of total body water
Skin	72	9.72	22
Skeleton	22	2.47	5
Blood	83	3.11	7
Adipose	10	0.90	2
Muscle	76	24.51	55

BODY FLUID COMPARTMENTS

Children are multicellular human organisms and their body fluid is functionally divided into compartments. These are specific enclosures in which the fluid exists in relation to cell anatomy, with the cell membrane forming the interface between the compartments. Body fluid compartments differ in both their volume and solute composition. The solute composition, because of the osmotic movement of water, is in equilibrium between the extracellular fluid and intracellular fluid. The specific composition of each compartment establishes the optimal environment for the biochemical reactions that occur within them. The absolute and relative size and volume of each compartment varies with the age and sex of the individual. In relation to tissue cells, total body water exists in two main compartments and a third minor compartment:

- Intracellular fluid (ICF) compartment: constitutes the fluid existing inside tissue cells.
- Extracellular fluid (EFC) compartment: constitutes body fluid existing outside and between tissue cells.
- Transcellular fluid: an extra small compartment.

The body of the average adult contains approximately 42 litres of water (Fig. 26.2), which is divided into the various body fluid compartments (Guyton & Hall 2000). Figure 26.2 and Table 26.2 illustrate the distribution of body water within the compartments and Figures 26.3 and 26.4 apply specifically in the various imbalances in the child, where fluid shifts can occur, thereby changing the osmolality of fluids within the three compartments.

Intracellular Fluid

Intracellular fluid constitutes the body water that exists inside the trillions of cells that make up the child's body, and accounts for 35–40% of the total body water. The intracellular fluid is contained within a closed space (the cell) so it is not easy to estimate and there is a limit to which it can expand without causing stress to the cell membrane. For this reason, pure water is not administered intravenously because pure water is hypotonic.

In a theoretic intravenous administration, plasma water in the blood vessels is diluted, which causes the cells (e.g. erythrocytes) to exist in a hypotonic environment relative to their intracellular space. Water will then move by the process of osmosis into the erythrocytes, causing them to swell until the cell membrane is unable to accommodate the increase in the cell volume and the erythrocyte bursts (cell lysis). A similar situation will occur in water intoxication or overhydration with acute hyponatraemia. Here, the cells most vulnerable to osmotic fluid shift into their intracellular compartment are brain cells. Ultimately, cytotoxic cerebral

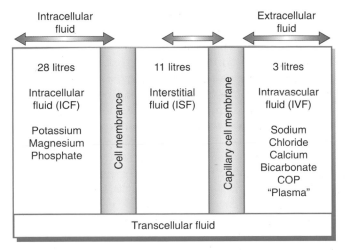

Fig. 26.2 • Distribution of total body water within compartments in the average adult; showing all the body fluid compartments and their corresponding constituents. The intravascular fluid (IVS) is the effective circulating blood volume (CBV), maintained largely with the help of the plasma proteins, with albumin maintaining 70–80% of the colloid oncotic pressure (COP). Colloid solutions with the same COP as plasma will stay in the IVS and thus are most efficient in restoring the CBV in hypovolaemia. Alternatively, crystalloid solutions administered intravenously are isotonic to plasma and thus distributed to the extracellular fluid (ECF), with the majority of it to the interstitial space (ISS). The sodium/potassium (Na+/K+) ATPase pump actively pumps sodium into the extracellular space (ECS) and potassium into the intercellular space (ICS) although glucose-containing fluids are evenly distributed in the ICS to rehydrate cells (Hillman et al 1997).

Table 26.2 The Body Fluid Composition During the Lifespan (Ichikawa 1990)

Age	TBW (%)	ECF (%)	ICF (%)
Preterm neonate	80	45	35
Full-term neonate	75	40	35
1–12 months	65	30	35
1–12 years	60	20	40
Adult			
male	55	25	30
female	50	20	30

ECF, extracellular fluid; ICF, intracellular fluid; TBW, total body water.

oedema, with its attendant raised intracranial pressure (ICP), occurs. Cerebral function is altered, and this is reflected in an abnormal score on the Glasgow Coma Scale (GCS). Unrelieved, cerebral neuropathy resulting from the raised intracranial pressure can cause seizures, coma and death.

Extracellular Fluid (Ichikawa 1990, Martini 2004)

The extracellular fluid exists outside and between tissue cells, and therefore cells are supported and nourished by – and bathe in – extracellular fluid. It accounts for 20–45% of the total body weight in children and is further subdivided into two subcompartments:

- intravascular fluid compartment
- interstitial fluid.

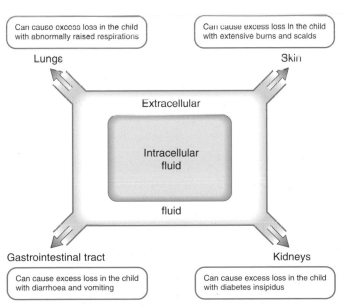

Fig. 26.3 • The relationship between intracellular fluid, extracellular fluid and exchange with the external environment within the body.

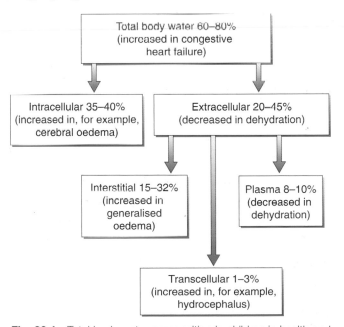

Fig. 26.4 • Total body water composition in children in health and disease.

Extracellular fluid is fundamental to the regulation and balance of body fluids and electrolytes because it is the changes in this compartment that the regulatory systems are in contact with and which therefore trigger regulatory actions.

Intravascular Fluid Compartment

The components in the intravascular fluid compartment enable the cardiovascular system to meet the metabolic needs of the body by ensuring:

- thermoregulation
- body defences
- maintenance of homeostasis
- delivery of oxygen and nutrients to cells
- removal of carbon dioxide and other toxic metabolic waste products
- distribution of synthesised and administered molecules within the body, facilitated by the intravascular fluid volume.

The cardiovascular system is a continuous, closed, blood-filled circuit equipped with a double pump (the heart) that maintains the pulmonary and systemic circulation. The cardiovascular system consists of:

- the heart: an electrical muscular pump that establishes the pressure gradient that ensures effective blood flow to tissue cells
- blood vessels: the channels or passageways through which blood flows within the body
- blood: the biological load and transport medium, which contains plasma water, suspended blood cells and dissolved particles.

By causing a deficit in plasma water, hypovolaemia increases blood viscosity and the packed cell volume, which can increase the propensity for thromboembolic episodes in a child with nephrotic syndrome, for example.

The intravascular fluid constitutes plasma water and makes up 8–10% of the total body water. It includes the entire amount of fluid inside the blood vessels (excluding the fluid inside the blood cells). The intravascular space is bounded by the capillary endothelial cell membrane. Plasma water, the suspended blood cells and dissolved particles constitute the circulating blood volume (CBV). This is the actual fluid volume perfusing the tissue cells and is in contact with – and the stimulating factor of – the volume receptors and baroreceptors in the vena cavae and aorta, respectively. Plasma is the fluid component of blood and contains salts, organic and inorganic compounds and hormones. Serum is plasma minus the clotting factors, in particular fibrinogen.

Interstitial Fluid

The interstitial fluid (ISF) constitutes the fluid interposed between the intravascular space and intracellular space. The interstitial fluid is the fluid between the cells, i.e. it bathes the cells. Nutrients and respiratory gases, plus enzymes, hormones and other substances, reach tissue cells via the arterial ends of the capillaries. Cells need to be cleared of their metabolic waste products and this is a function of the venous end of capillary; the process enables the waste products to reach their designated depots such as the kidneys and lungs for disposal.

Interstitial fluid is tissue fluid and the interstitial space can be viewed as a 'biological bureau de change'. Effective distribution of fluid between the intravascular and interstitial compartments is determined by the difference between the hydrostatic pressure, which is generated by myocardial contractility and arteriolar vasoconstriction, and the opposing plasma oncotic pressure, which is generated by plasma proteins. This partially explains oedema in the child with nephrotic syndrome who becomes hypoproteinaemic or one who develops pleural effusion in congestive heart failure. In children, the majority of the extracellular fluid is interstitial fluid.

Lymph, the fluid that circulates in the lymphatic vessels, is part of the interstitial fluid. It is an important fluid because it reclaims the small amounts of fluid or protein that remain in the interstitial space back into the intravascular space, thus preventing fluid backlog leading to oedema. Although body fluids are compartmentalised, they are all in communication with one another. Therefore fluid shifts occur in dehydration because fluid will tend to move into the compartment with the deficit.

Activity

Critical reflection on theory

With reference to the descriptions above, explain why a dehydrated child might manifest abnormal physical features of the skin and mucous membranes.

Transcellular Fluid

Transcellular fluid is a minor part of the total body water, forming 1–3%. Its function is to lubricate and provide smooth movement between two closely related layers or membranes, e.g. the pleural membranes. In terms of the circulating blood volume, transcellular fluid is non-functional or vestigial. This is because it is not readily available to support the circulating blood volume in time of need, as in hypovolaemia for example. Transcellular fluid can, however, act as a third-space fluid in pathological conditions that cause accumulation of fluid in this space. Transcellular fluid constitutes:

- cerebrospinal fluid (CSF) (excess = hydrocephalus)
- pericardial fluid (excess = pericardial effusion)
- pleural fluid (excess = pleural effusion)
- synovial fluid (excess = swollen joints)
- intraocular fluid (excess = glaucoma).

Biological Functions of Water

The descriptions and explanations above highlight the critical role adequate hydration plays in the effective functioning of the growing and developing child's body at any age, particularly infancy. It also supports Eastwood's (1997) notion of water being the chemical of life. Table 26.3, explains why children, especially the very young, are at increased risk of body fluid and electrolyte imbalance. Also, the organ systems that maintain water balance are imma-

ture in children, so young children in particular are at risk of fluid and electrolyte imbalance. The well-hydrated child should therefore feel warm, have pink and moist mucous membranes, vital signs that are normal for their respective age band, and pass a minimum of 1 mL of urine per kilogram of body weight per hour (Table 26.4).

Table 26.4 Maintenance Fluid Requirement (Ryan & Molyneux 1996)

Weight (kg)	Fluid requirement
2.5–6 kg	150 mL/kg/24 hours
6–10 kg	120 mL/kg/24 hours
10–20 kg	100 mL/kg/24 hours
20 kg and over	75 mL/kg/24 hours

Table 26.3 Why Children Need More Water than Adults

Concept	Rationale(s)
Higher ratio of extracellular fluid volume to that of intracellular fluid volume	Blood plasma forms part of the ECF and it is this body fluid that is in direct contact with the environment, e.g. that perfusing the subcutaneous capillaries underneath the skin The close encounter of ECF with the environment thus means a higher turnover rate of ECF in the child than the adult
Children have a large surface area to volume ratio meaning a higher insensible fluid loss from the skin and airways	The surface area-to-volume ratio of a small child is greater than that of an adult. This increases water loss from the child through the skin in heat loss by radiation to the environment The concept thus adds to the child's increased biological need for water
Children have a higher metabolic rate	Children are highly metabolic individuals because of their ongoing growth and development, as well as their other life activities. Children therefore have a higher metabolic rate than adults, which in turn require water for both intercellular and intracellular synthesis and excretion of metabolic wastes
Children have a high rate of heat exchange	The high metabolic rate in the child means an increased energy expenditure, one of which is thermal energy, thus a high rate of heat exchange. Water is required to facilitate this heat exchange, which increases the day-to-day water requirement for the child as compared with the adult
Children are not miniature adults	The homeostatic organs of children, especially infants, are immature and the control centre/brain (and their interconnecting pathways) require time to attain functional competence. Even the interaction between hormones and their target organ receptors takes time to mature in children Therefore, the respective gains of control are less effective and at times exaggerated as in the case of peripheral vasoconstriction in hypovolaemia. Children's homeostatic systems are thus not very well able to respond and make the necessary adjustments in sudden and extreme changes in set-points. Finally, the self-care abilities in particular in infants are limited with the total dependence on parents/carers

ECF, extracellular fluid.

THE MAIN ELECTROLYTES, THEIR FUNCTIONS AND REGULATORY SYSTEMS

Ions and Electrolytes

An ion is an electrically charged atom or groups of atoms. Electrolytes are inorganic molecules that, when dissolved in water or an aqueous solution, separate into their ionic components and dissolve into positive (cations) and negative (anions) to carry their respective electrical charges. They are chemical substances that exist as charged or ionised molecules (Horton et al 2002). Cations are electrolytes that migrate towards the negative pole of an electrical field. Anions alternatively migrate towards the positive pole, hence the adage 'opposites attract'. The physical and chemical properties of electrolytes enable them to carry out their respective biological roles in the body of the growing and developing child: maintaining total body water, acid–base balance and energy balance. Also, electrolyte composition of plasma is crucial for effective functioning of tissue cells, in particular those of excitable form, i.e. neurons and myocytes. The key electrolytes in the body and their chemical symbols are shown in Table 26.5.

It is essential that the positively charged ions are in balance with the negatively charged ions, otherwise fluid and electrolyte imbalance results, which can be detrimental to the child. For this reason, most of the essential biological processes are dependent and affected by electrolyte imbalance, which cannot be tolerated for a long time. Sodium and potassium are the chief positively charged ions. Sodium, potassium, chloride and bicarbonate are most likely to show in electrolyte imbalance. Changes in the concentration of one ion usually cause changes in the others.

The high metabolic, growth and developmental needs of the child in health and disease make both electrolytes and water critical to the child's biological being. Table 26.6 shows the daily electrolyte requirements in children and Table 26.7 shows the normal reference values for electrolytes in children. These figures are biologically determined reference values but can vary in different clinical conditions on an individual basis (Ichikawa 1990, Somers & Harmon 1999).

Table 26.6 Daily Electrolyte Requirements in Children (Green, 2004)

Electrolytes	
Sodium	1–3 mmol/kg/day
Potassium	1–3 mmol/kg/day
Chloride	2–3 mmol/kg/day
Calcium	0.7–1.5 mmol/kg/day
Phosphorus	0.9–1.5 mmol/kg/day

Table 26.7 Plasma Reference Values for Electrolytes in Children and Neonates (from Ichikawa 1990, Clayton & Round 1994)

Electrolyte	Childhood reference value	Neonatal reference value
Sodium	135–145 mmol/L	132–145 mmol/L
Chloride	100–106 mmol/L	90–110 mmol/L
Potassium	3.5–5.5 mmol/L	3.6–5.9 mmol/L
Calcium	2.2–2.6 mmol/L	1.9–2.85 mmol/L
Magnesium	0.75–1.0 mmol/L	0.71–1.1 mmol/L
Phosphorus	1.45–2.1 mmol/L	1.4–3.0 mmol/L
Bicarbonate	24–30 mmol/L	
Urea	3–7 mmol/L	1–5 mmol/L
Creatinine	18–70 micromol/L	<20–150 micromol/L
Glucose	3.9–6.9 mmol/L	
Osmolality	275–295 mOsm/kg H_2O	280–300 mOsmol/L
Anion gap	7–16 mmol/L	

Table 26.5 Major Metabolic Cations and Anions

Cations	Anions
Sodium (Na^+)	Chloride (Cl^-)
Potassium (K^+)	Bicarbonate (HCO_3^-)
Calcium (Ca^{2+})	Phosphate (HPO_4^{2-})
Magnesium (Mg^{2+})	'Proteins/amino acids' (A^-) Organic acids

Electrolytes

Electrolytes are obtained from the child's diet in health (Martini 2004):

- Water is absorbed mostly by the process of osmosis, with sodium playing a major role.
- Sodium diffuses into the villi of the enteroctyes and is then actively pumped into the bloodstream by the sodium/potassium (Na^+/K^+) pump.
- Glucose is co-transported with sodium and used by the cells, with the help of insulin, to make energy.
- Amino acids also use a co-transport system together with sodium.
- Calcium, phosphate and sulphate absorption require active transport accelerated by calcitonin and parathyroid hormone.

- Magnesium absorption requires carrier proteins.
- Chloride and bicarbonate are absorbed by diffusion or carrier-mediated transport.
- Potassium absorption in the small intestine is mainly by passive diffusion, influenced by net water movement and in response to the electrochemical gradient.

Urea

Urea is a waste product of protein metabolism and is removed from the blood via the kidneys. Neonatal and childhood plasma urea concentration levels are lower than in adulthood, reflecting the heightened amino acid utilisation for protein synthesis in childhood. Adult values are reached between 10 and 12 years of age.

Creatinine

Creatinine in the blood is the product of muscle energy metabolism and thus has a direct relationship with muscle mass. Plasma creatinine levels therefore vary with the age and sex of the individual. Creatinine is cleared/excreted from the blood via the kidneys (Linné & Ringsrud 1999, Walmsley & White 1994).

Glucose

Glucose is the simple sugar that is the immediate energy source for cell metabolism. It is the preferred source of energy for brain cells, which rely on an adequate blood sugar because the brain has very limited glycogen stores. Glucose is derived from carbohydrates, which are digested in the gut to produce glucose as the end product. Together with oxygen, glucose is used by cells to synthesise adenosine triphosphate (ATP), a high-energy molecule that provides the chemical energy for effective cellular function.

The Anion Gap

The anion gap is the calculation of the mathematical difference between the anions chloride (Cl^-) and bicarbonate (HCO_3^-) and the cations sodium (Na^+) and potassium (K^+):

- $[Cl^- + HCO_3^-] - [Na^+ + K^+] =$ anion gap
- Normal value in children is 7–16 mmol/L
- Raised levels [>14 or more] suggests metabolic acidosis as in diabetic ketoacidosis.

Blood urea and electrolyte (U&E) assay, although invasive and therefore unpleasant for the child and family, is a valuable biological and clinical assessment tool whenever the integrity of blood biochemistry is in question, e.g. there is a possible body fluid and electrolyte imbalance. The test estimates essential elements and the chemical components in the blood and urine. Depending on the child's clinical state and technological facilities, the test result can be known within minutes, hours or days. Although reference values are offered here, individual units tend to operate on their laboratory-validated reference ranges that are calibrated to take into account the sources samples are obtained from and the machines used to carry out the assays. It is therefore the responsibility of all nurses to familiarise themselves with the accepted reference values in their own unit and to act promptly when results are outside these ranges.

Homeostasis

Understanding of the various regulatory mechanisms in balance – or homeostasis – has been helped by the application of control theory (Taylor et al 1997). Guyton & Hall (2000) suggest that thousands of control systems exist in the body, with genetic control systems the most fundamental and intricate. The systems, mainly the hypothalamus, adrenal glands, and kidneys carry out their delicate activities to maintain intracellular and extracellular functions in the process of keeping the individual organism alive and healthy. Martini (2004) offers two general mechanisms of control in homeostatic regulation. A third is added here because it is important when caring for children:

- Autoregulation, also called intrinsic control: the process that occurs when a mechanism within the biological system detects a change and adjusts automatically in response to that change.
- Extrinsic regulation: change is made possible by the activities of the nervous system or the endocrine system.
- Behavioural responses (Fig. 26.5): the child at birth has an internal drive/motivation to prevent fluid loss. So, for example, a toddler left 'home alone' will quench their thirst by drinking the most accessible water (e.g. from

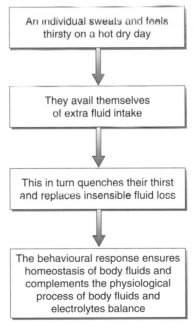

Fig. 26.5 • A behavioural response to increased insensible fluid loss on a hot day.

the toilet), whereas older children will express their thirst and have an inner drive to obtain food and drink. However, the limited self-care abilities of young children make them depend on their carers for self-preservation of homeostatic actions.

Dehydration in Children

Children, and especially infants, are at risk of body fluid and electrolyte imbalances (Rao et al 2001, Marie-Cardine et al 2002). The reasons why children require an increased intake of water than adults were explained in Table 26.3. As the extracellular fluid is in direct contact with the outside world, and given that, the younger the child, the higher the proportion of extracellular fluid volume, any illness or situation in which fluid intake in the child is reduced or fluid is lost (e.g. acute diarrhoea and vomiting) creates potential or actual imbalances.

For example, a fever above 38°C requires an increase in the child's fluid intake of 10–12% because of the increased radiant, and thus water, loss. Tachypnoea similarly increases the child's fluid requirement two- to three-fold. Children undergoing surgery (because of the period of fasting involved and anaesthesia-related vasodilation), on cancer chemotherapy, who have sustained moderate to severe burns and scalds, or presenting with vasco-occlusive sickle-cell painful crisis are all at risk of body fluid and electrolyte imbalance. Finally, any major systemic disease or trauma, and limited paediatric knowledge and expertise in both nursing and medical practice, can increase the risk of body fluids and electrolyte imbalance in children. It is important that when a child enters into a healthcare setting, the people who care for that child know and care about what they are doing, highlighting possible inadvertent care deficits and attendant risks in managing the child's fluid and electrolytes requirement.

DEFINITION AND CAUSES OF DEHYDRATION IN CHILDREN

Dehydration means an excessive loss of body water. The phenomenon is usually accompanied by electrolyte imbalance, which causes fluid shifts to occur between the intracellular, interstitial and extracellular fluid compartments. It results in a low fluid volume in all three compartments, with the child being in a negative fluid balance. Children, and especially infants, have an increased propensity to dehydration because their total body water exceeds solid body mass.

Water forms a significant proportion of the child's body weight and therefore weight loss, except in circumstances such as malnutrition, is a reliable method of ascertaining body fluid deficit in children. Any recent weight loss in excess of 3% of previous weight is indicative of body fluid deficit. In circumstances where a previous or current weight cannot be ascertained, the physical appearance and cardiovascular parameters of the child are useful alternatives.

Acute diarrhoea and vomiting from gastroenteritis is the most common cause of dehydration in children (see the scenario later in this chapter). Dehydration in the child can occur for any of the reasons below:

- Reduced fluid intake:
  - frank neglect or water inavailability
  - inadvertent fluid restriction that underestimates maintenance requirement
  - poor swallowing as in severe cerebral palsy or undiagnosed oesophageal atresia
  - uncompensated intake in excessive renal loss as the infant/toddler with diabetes insipidus
  - anorexia due to psychiatric illness or adverse effects of drugs
  - the unconscious child or one in a coma especially if they are alone/undiscovered.

- Increased body fluid loss:
  - excessive gastrointestinal loss
  - vomiting/emesis due to systemic disease or adverse effects of drugs, e.g. chemotherapy
  - acute or chronic diarrhoea, such as viral or bacterial infection of the gastrointestinal tract or malabsorption syndromes causing osmotic diarrhoea
  - excessive loss from stomas or fistulae.

- Excessive renal loss:
  - adverse effects of osmotic or other forms of diuretics
  - adrenal insufficiency
  - salt-losing nephropathy
  - chronic renal failure
  - diabetes insipidus, especially in young children unable to compensate their renal loss by thirst satiety.

- From skin and respiratory tract:
  - hyperpyrexia
  - heat exposure
  - cystic fibrosis
  - severe burns.

TYPES OF DEHDRATION IN CHILDREN

Biochemical classification of childhood dehydration considers sodium as the principal extracellular cation and, as such, embodies the contextual classification. Symptoms usually appear in the child when the plasma sodium is less than 120 mmol/L or more than 150 mmol/L (Awazu et al 1990, Weinstein 1997).

Isonatraemic Dehydration

- plasma sodium 130–145 mmol/L
- plasma osmolality 275–295 mOsm/kg H_2O.

Isonatraemic dehydration is the most common form of dehydration, affecting approximately 70% of children who present with body fluid and electrolyte imbalance. Here, the solute loss equals water loss in the relatively healthy child with effective renal compensation. No change occurs in the tonicity or osmolality of fluids within the three compartments, thus there are no transmembrane fluid shifts. The extracellular compartment, being the most accessible to the external environment, bears the brunt of the fluid loss and contracts, reducing the circulating blood volume, with the attendant hypovolaemia. Losses from the gastrointestinal tract, such as diarrhoea and vomiting, are the most common cause of isotonic dehydration in children.

Hyponatraemic Dehydration

- plasma sodium <130 mmol/L
- plasma osmolality <275 mOsm/kg H_2O.

Hyponatraemic dehydration may be seen in about 10% of children. Causes include excessive solute loss in urine (as in diuretic therapy), severe burns, vomiting and acute/chronic diarrhoea. In this condition the net fluid loss contains more salt than water. Children may be inadvertently managed with hypotonic intravenous fluids or encouraged to drink large volumes of sugary drinks to counterbalance the fluid loss. The cells will take up the glucose and leave the extra water in the extracellular compartment. As a result, a transmembrane fluid shift will occur from the extracellular to the intracellular compartment. So, the predominant water loss is once more from the extracellular compartment, resulting in reduced circulatory blood volume and hypo volaemia. Here, the symptoms of dehydration can be more severe and should be considered in the child who presents with circulatory shock even in the absence of an apparent significant history of fluid loss.

Hyponatraemic dehydration should be distinguished from hyponatraemic water intoxication or hypervolaemia in the child with SIADH.

Hypernatraemic Dehydration

- plasma sodium >145 mmol/L
- plasma osmolality >295 mOsm/kg H_2O.

This form of dehydration affects about 20% of the children seen. Here, water loss occurs without the corresponding salt loss, i.e. a proportionally greater loss of water than salt. Examples include diabetes insipidus in the child with limited self-care, increased insensible loss of hyperpyrexia and hyperventilation or an inadvertent excess hypertonic intravenous fluid administration. As the extracellular fluid compartment is hypertonic, fluid moves across the membrane from the intracellular to the extracellular compartment to dilute the more concentrated plasma. It includes hyperglycaemia and hypocalcaemia also; the exact reason for the latter unknown. In the end, both the intracellular and extracellular compartments are fluid depleted but the clinical manifestations may not be very obvious in the early stages. It is difficult to predict the degree of dehydration in young children (Duggan et al 1996).

Scenario

Nicola is a 12-week-old infant who presented with 10% dehydration caused by acute diarrhoea. She was born at term weighing 3.3 kg. She is admitted to the ward with her mother, and has a 2-day history of vomiting and passing frequent loose watery stools. She appears irritable, her cry is weak and she has poor muscle tone. Her recorded weight 1 week ago was 5.0 kg.
Conclusion from investigations and clinical assessment indicates a state of 10% dehydration caused by her acute diarrhoea.

Nicola's clinical assessment and investigations
- Present body weight: 4.500 kg
- Blood urea: 8.0 mmol/L (normal range: 3–7)
- Axilla temperature: 38°C (normal range: 36–37°C)
- Plasma sodium: 146 mmol/L (normal range: 135–145)
- Plasma potassium: 5.4 mmol/L (normal range: 3.5–5.5)
- plasma osmolality: 300 mOsm/kg/kg H_2O (normal range: 275–295)
- At rest:
  - heart rate per minute: 180 (normal range: 110–160)
  - packed cell volume: 48% (normal range: 28–42)
  - respiratory rate per minute: 52 (normal range: 30–40)
  - systolic blood pressure: 68 mmHg (normal range: 70–90)
- Extremities = cold and mottled
- Eyes contour = sunken
- Mucous membranes = dry lips and tongue
- Skin = hot, dry and lax
- Urine = small quantity; very concentrated
- Stools = loose and watery
- 10% dehydration from acute diarrhoea

PRINCIPLES OF ASSESSING AND CARING FOR THE CHILD PRESENTING WITH DEHYDRATION

Nursing assessment is the first and principal step in the care of the child presenting with dehydration, as in the case of Nicola. The assessment process should be holistic, comprehensive, child-focused and family-centred, regardless of the conceptual framework or nursing model around which it is based. Assessment is the process of gathering, validating and communicating accurate and reliable data about a child (Kozier et al 2000, Smith et al 2004). To assist with Nicola's assessment, the following questions will be asked:

1. What Evidence – from the Most Reliable Clinical Manifestations in this Child – Predicts the Degree of Dehydration?

This question is fundamental in the effective management of the child with suspected body fluid and electrolyte imbalance. The data derived during the process of assessment must be the most reliable possible if effective decision making for the subsequent management of the child is to be made. There are differing opinions as to which clinical features suggest an accurate degree of dehydration. Categories such as 'mild', 'moderate' and 'severe' have been, and continue to be used in the clinical setting. Current evidence suggests that there is a fine divide between mild and moderate dehydration and consequently the categories 'none', 'some' and 'severe' have been adopted. A comprehensive work by Duggan et al (1996) on the validity of the clinical signs of dehydration in young children identifies the following as the most reliable data for estimating the degree of dehydration in infants aged 3–18 months with acute diarrhoea:

- integrity of skin fold
- neurological status
- quality of pulse
- nature of oral mucous membranes
- quality and nature of breathing
- warmth of extremities.

Mackenzie et al (1989), in a study involving 0–4-year-old children, identified the following as reliable signs of dehydration:

- decreased skin turgor
- decreased peripheral perfusion
- deep (acidotic) breathing
- blood urea >6.5 mmol/L
- blood pH <7.35.

The nature of the fontanelle was found to be the least reliable sign, which correlated poorly with the degree of dehydration in the children in Mackenzie et al's study. Weight loss is the 'gold standard' for estimating fluid deficit, and weight gain is used as the criterion from which to estimate progress or recovery from the state of dehydration. This is because recent weight loss in the otherwise well child usually means some loss of total body water, and not loss of mean mass.

2. What Information is Needed about Nicola?

- Medical examination and outcomes.
- Blood investigations and results.
- Urine investigations and results.
- Her:
  - illness history present and past
  - physical appearance
  - physiological parameters
  - behaviour, activity, alertness.

Objective data are obtained by the nurse assessing the child; subjective data are information obtained from the child, as age permits, or his or her parent.

Why is this Information about Nicola Required?

- Baseline observation of her vital signs provide a reference point for future care and management.
- Changes and/or trends in her baseline observations suggest improvement or further deterioration, and thus guide practice.
- Helps establish actual and potential problems to be used in planning, implementing and evaluating care.

3. How are Data about Nicola Ascertained?

- Prerequisite knowledge-base:
  - common sense: assessment process
  - intellectual sense: child development.
- Age-related parameters.
- Effects of hospitalisation on the child (Nicola) and family.
- Effective communication skills: with Nicola, with her mother and with colleagues participating in her care.
- Accurate measurement:
  - technical skills and competence
  - use of equipment.
- Analysis and synthesis of data collected from which biological or clinical relevance should emerge.
- Accurate documentation of data.
- Clinical reasoning to guide prompt appropriate and safe action in Nicola's care, e.g. nursing care, fluid and electrolytes therapy, communication/liaison with colleagues.

4. What Happens to the Data When they have been Collected?

- Categorised and used to structure care.
- Accurate, timely and complete documentation of care, i.e. not haphazard or on bits of paper.
- Clinical analysis and reasoning.
- What the data mean.
- The significance of the data:
  - how ill she is
  - is she getting better?
  - is she getting worse?

- Whether the findings from the data require immediate action.
- Who to communicate with within the multiprofessional team.
- Nursing care following observations in Nicola's best interest.
- Identification of Nicola's:
  - actual problems
  - potential problems
  - healthcare needs
  - parents' needs.
- Planning Nicola's nursing care by setting child- and family-centred goals or suggesting child-focus expected outcomes of care
- Prioritising and implementing Nicola's care.
- Evaluating her care.
- Adapting/making changes in her care accordingly.

Nursing Assessment and Biochemical Investigations

The scenario suggests that Nicola is very ill, with 10% dehydration, which is a life-threatening condition meaning that her vital organs (brain, heart, lungs, kidneys) require effective support. For this reason, the Roper–Logan–Tierney (1990) nursing model is applied for Nicola's care delivery and management. Data collection would start in the accident and emergency department (A&E) and be completed in the admission or ambulatory unit. It would include the following:

BREATHING

This relates to Nicola's heart and lung function. Baseline observations will be made on admission onto ward:

- Readings at rest:
  - respiratory rate per minute

- respiratory quality: effort, rhythm, depth
- heart rate per minute
- quality of heart rate: regularity; volume
- capillary refill less or over 2–3 seconds
- blood pressure: mean arterial pressure; systolic value.
- Colour and warmth of her limbs/extremities.
- Comparison with age group as young infant.

The scenario indicates tachycardia and tachypnoea because the 10% dehydration is tasking her heart and lungs.

EATING AND DRINKING

Nicola's physical appearance, cardiopulmonary parameters and biochemical assays indicate that she is severely dehydrated, which is a life-threatening condition. Her clinical features are congruent with the contents of Table 26.8. Her ongoing assessment should include:

- Body weight: degree of weight loss. A cloth or towel would be put on a clean scale, zeroed then used to record Nicola's weight without her nappies on.
- Whether she is bottle- or breast-fed.
- Amount of feeds for that day, if any.
- Whether she is retaining or vomiting the feeds.
- Consistency and amount of vomitus.
- Onset and history of diarrhoea.
- Volume, consistency and frequency of diarrhoea.
- Integrity of Nicola's skin and mucous membranes.
- Integrity and contour of her eyes.
- Fullness of her anterior fontanelle.

There is evidence to suggest that the skin turgor and neurological status of the child who is dehydrated are the best reliable clinical data to show the degree of dehydration in children (Duggan et al 1996).

Table 26.8 Reasons for Abnormal Blood Chemistry in Diarrhoea

Nicola's blood chemistry	Possible reasons
Elevated plasma urea	Reduced CBV thus reduced GFR and excretory capacity of the kidneys as less water is delivered to them
Raised plasma sodium and potassium	Reduced ECF and ICF volume/water content means a higher solute concentration
Raised plasma osmolality	Reduced ECF means less water in blood vessels and thus a concentrated plasma
Raised packed cell volume	Reduced CBV means a reduction in the usual 55% plasma content of blood, thus a raised cellular component of the blood

CBV, circulating blood volume; ECF, extracellular fluid; GFR, glomerular filtration rate; ICF, intracellular fluid.

PERSONAL CLEANSING AND DRESSING

This aspect of assessment will focus on Nicola's general state, and will ascertain the following:

- Nicola's skin:
  - cleanliness
  - any rash
  - redness
  - integrity of her nappy area.
- Clothing: not necessarily new/expensive but clean.
- How her mother usually meets her hygiene needs, i.e. baby soap/cream/lotion, etc.
- General status of her scalp, eyes and face in general to note, e.g. cradle cap or sticky eyes.
- Nicola's state of physical comfort.
- The healthy state of her mouth, e.g. presence or absence of oral thrush.

Microbiological studies to rule out any other forms of infection, e.g. urinary tract infection. Stool specimens may be requested to rule out any bacterial infection but, as the scenario shows, the conclusion is that she has acute diarrhoea of viral origin.

MAINTAINING A SAFE ENVIRONMENT

Here, both the physical safety and psychological safety will be assessed:

- How restless or irritable Nicola is, in view of what is indicated in the scenario.
- How settled she is between handling.
- Whether she appears to be in pain or not.
- Physical environment of her room and cot area:
  - suction equipment, oxygen and emergency bell in working order
  - basic equipment for basic life support
  - safety of her cot in terms of contents/breaks
  - safety of all other equipment required for her care, e.g. intravenous volumetric pumps, cardiac monitors, apnoea alarm
  - basic equipment to facilitate effective infection control, e.g. hand washing utensils, disposable units, gloves and aprons.
- Nurse call alarm in her room in working order.
- Necessary documents, e.g. fluid balance charts, observation charts, treatment chart, intravenous prescription chart.
- Awareness of the nurse for their areas of accountability and responsibility.
- Ensuring that Nicola's mother knows and understands the safety aspects of her care, in particular infection control.

- How anxious Nicola's mother is.
- Ascertaining main areas of anxiety for Nicola's mother, e.g. contact with her husband/partner about Nicola's admission.
- Contacting Nicola's father – by her mother or ward if appropriate.

ELIMINATING

This will build on what was presented in the scenario, covering Nicola's:

- Urine output:
  - volume
  - specific gravity
  - frequency.
- Stools:
  - characteristics
  - consistency
  - amount
  - colour
  - frequency
  - odour.
- Changes in urine output and bowel habit as noted by her mother.
- Whether tears are present when she cries.
- Vomitus:
  - amount
  - frequency
  - colour
  - consistency.
- An estimate of 10 mL/kg/stool or vomitus.

A urine bag or pad may be applied on Nicola to obtain and carry out a clinitest on her urine. A concentrated urine with a raised specific gravity (SG) and osmolality that shows nothing else abnormal is indicative of dehydration.

Nicola's nappies may be weighed to assess urine output. The dry nappies are weighed before being applied on Nicola. The wet nappies are then weighed after removal and the gram-by-gram difference assumed as the amount of urine passed as 1 g dry weight is equivalent to 1 mL water.

COMMUNICATING

Communication with Nicola will be three-fold, i.e. that with Nicola even as an infant; with her parents, in particular her mother, on admission; and interprofessional and multidisciplinary communication:

- With Nicola: communication involves mainly obtaining data from her physical, behavioural biochemical and physiological assessment:

- making use of observation skills
- concrete data
- elusive/indirect data
- individual hunches.

- With Nicola's parents:
  - history of the onset and progress of Nicola's diarrhoea and vomiting
  - changes observed in their child
  - their main worries and anxieties
  - specific information they wanted to know about Nicola, her care/treatment.

- With colleagues:
  - accurate documentation
  - who the key members of the team are
  - their key areas of responsibility
  - nursing areas of accountability and responsibility: who is to be informed about her admission and assessment data.

MOBILISING

As well as the presentation in the scenario (p 397), the following areas will be assessed:

- Nicola's:
  - general activity
  - muscle tone: twitching; excessive tone
  - crying pattern
  - restful state or irritability
  - muscle weakness: potassium deficit
  - abdominal distension: potassium deficit
  - sleep state/alert state
  - quality of chest movement on respiration.

- Nicola's physical care: how often she will be cared for physically.

- Anticipatory information on future:
  - home environment
  - health education/health promotion.
  - discharge home: any socio-economic issues to be addressed, e.g. home environment and parenting skills.

WORKING AND PLAYING

As Nicola is acutely ill at present, this relates mainly to her environment and the interaction with her:

- How much humanizing and distressing her room/cot area is.
- What type of toys are safe and appropriate in the area.

CONTROLLING BODY TEMPERATURE

This area of assessment will similarly build on what was presented in the scenario on p 397.

- Ambient temperature: room temperature noted: too hot/too cold.
- Nicola's body temperature:
  - safest route of measurement 'axilla' abdominal
  - whether pyrexia is resolving
  - how hot her skin/cheeks appear and feel
  - warmth of her extremities.

EXPRESSING SEXUALITY

Nicola's assessment in this area will relate mainly to the manner in which her parents present her:

- clothes she wears
- any preferred favourite clothing by her mother
- which toys to be displayed in her cot.

DYING

Nicola's parents will be very anxious because their daughter is acutely ill. Many questions will be going through their minds about their daughter's illness, prognosis and future. Assessment thus includes:

- Nicola's parents' main areas of worry
- their understanding of her illness
- their understanding about her treatment
- their conception of the reasons and use of machinery in her room
- areas they would like to discuss with medical staff
- specific close family members they would like to know and have for support during their daughter's hospitalisation.

From the assessment and scenario content, the actual and potential problems are identified and care prioritised, planned and implemented and evaluated.

BIOCHEMICAL INVESTIGATIONS

Medical investigations of the child with body fluid and electrolyte imbalance include physical examination to establish the degree of dehydration. Routine urea and electrolytes tests are no longer thought necessary for all children but are essential in the child who requires intravenous hydration or suspected of hypernatraemia (Armon et al 2001). Many of the important metabolic functions of the body depend on the maintenance of normal electrolytes concentration. Biochemical assays should include plasma or serum electrolytes, osmolality, urea, pH, bicarbonate, glucose, calcium and also urine osmolality. Deviations from the norm or reference values shown in Table 26.7 usually means that the child's body is unable to maintain normal control or balance either by excretion or conservation of body water or electrolytes (Linné & Ringrud 1999). Because an accurate chemical analysis of body fluids depends on their appropriate collection, handling and care, each specimen must be obtained, stored and transported to the laboratory in the correct manner. Hyperkalaemia can be misdiagnosed in the child who has had a traumatic specimen collection or a blood specimen stored or transported wrongly to cause haemolysis and thus release intracellular potassium from the red blood cells.

It is essential that nurses know the age-related reference 'normal' values and understand the clinical significance of any changes the tests show. This way, they can become aware of what the change means for the child's biological function (see Table 26.8) and take timely and appropriate nursing action, e.g. alerting or summoning the medical staff to prescribe the necessary adjustment in the child's fluid and electrolyte therapy.

Personal experience shows that failure to take a timely and appropriate action on receiving a child's blood results may end with a gravely ill and prostrated/collapsed child by the end of a shift, so knowing the normal reference values and being aware what they mean for the child are fundamental aspects of care in the child with body fluid and electrolyte imbalance.

There is current evidence to suggest that simple urine tests for specific gravity and ketonuria are appropriate in assessing the child with moderate (some) degree of dehydration (Nager & Wang 2002).

Therapeutic Strategies in Caring for the Child with Body Fluid and Electrolyte Imbalance

Severe dehydration and electrolyte imbalance such as that depicted in Nicola is a life-threatening situation. Indeed, body fluid loss (e.g. blood loss or acute diarrhoea) or fluid maldistribution (e.g. oedema in heart failure or nephrotic syndrome) are major causes of cardiac arrest in children. As such, the ABCD principles of paediatric resuscitation apply (BMJ 1999). The scenario shows that Nicola's respiratory status, although overworking to compensate for her dehydrated state, is not in any immediate danger. However, her cardiovascular status is very compromised because of the 10% dehydration state. The ultimate goal of any therapeutic strategy is thus to restore her circulating blood volume and improve her tissue cell perfusion, especially her vital organs such as the brain, heart and kidneys. A rational fluid and electrolyte regime must therefore be commenced with the following therapeutic goals (Arfors & Buckley 1997, Armon et al 2001, Johnson & Sullivan 2003):

- Carry out a comprehensive and holistic assessment to accurately estimate Nicola's degree of dehydration and fluid deficit.
- Restore her circulating blood volume or intravascular fluid volume to establish an effective cardiac output, colloidal osmotic pressure and tissue perfusion.
- Maintain Nicola's interstitial and intracellular fluid and electrolytes by administering the most appropriate colloidal plasma substitute or physiologically balanced crystalloid solutions.
- Establish and treat the cause of her dehydration through the most appropriate differential diagnosis.
- Prioritise and carry out her nursing care safely, effectively and humanely.
- Evaluate care and adapt management accordingly.

WWW

- http://www.archdischild.com
- http://www.WHO.org
- http://www.ESPGAN.org

Fluid Therapy in Acute Diarrhoea in Children

The fundamental role of an accurate assessment is crucial because it informs the decision-making process in managing Nicola's much-needed fluid and electrolyte therapy safely and effectively. There is now ample evidence to assure clinicians and practitioners that oral hydration solution (ORS) is efficient and effective in the management of children with some degree of dehydration. However, many myths and doubts still exist among healthcare professionals, as well as parents, about the usefulness of oral hydration solution. Parents, in particular, might doubt its effectiveness because they cannot see the instantaneous improvement that is sometimes evident in intravenous therapy. Healthcare professionals similarly think that oral hydration solution is more time-consuming and costly in terms of hospital stay.

Evidence-based Practice

Oral hydration therapy

Conners et al 2000, Atherley-John et al 2002, Nager & Wang 2002, Sandhu 2002 suggest:
- Oral hydration solution is effective and safe in the management of children with moderate (i.e. some) dehydration caused by uncomplicated diarrhoea.
- Therapy with oral hydration solution reduces hospital stay from 2.8 days to 1.8 days.
- Oral hydration therapy is cost effective in terms of staff time and period of treatment.

- Oral hydration therapy has elicited good parent satisfaction.
- There is no increase in iatrogenesis from hypernatraemia.
- Children show a reduction of treatment-related complications.
- There is a low rate of failure warranting intravenous therapy.

In severe dehydration, an isotonic solution is administered rapidly to restore the intravascular fluid volume. In so doing, venous return to the heart is enhanced, which in turn improves the cardiac output and thus an effective circulating blood volume. Once this is achieved, tissue perfusion has to be re-established, which is achieved in the child with some dehydration using oral hydration solution by oral or nasagastric route, or by half-strength dextrose saline intravenously. This helps to re-establish the interstitial fluid volume, which subsequently ensures tissue perfusion and effective cellular–blood exchange. Deficit replacement is achieved over 4–8 hours. Not to be omitted here is the child's usual maintenance fluid requirement, usually administered in the form of oral hydration solution or intravenous dextrose 4.0% saline 0.18% intravenous solution. The child with hypernatraemic dehydration is rehydrated slowly to avoid rebound cerebral oedema.

CALCULATION OF PERCENTAGE DEHYDRATION

Nicola's pre-illness weight = 5.0 kg
Nicola's present weight = 4.5 kg [1 kg = 1000 g]

NICOLA'S FLUID DEFICIT

Pre-illness weight (kg) – Present weight (kg)

$$5000 - 4500 = 500 \text{ g} = 500 \text{ mL fluid deficit}$$

$$1 \text{ g} = 1 \text{ mL}.$$

Calculating Nicola's fluid requirement will determine her fluid deficit plus her maintenance requirement.

Summary

Helmstadler (1998) contends that applied clinical knowledge, on which assessment skills and professional judgement depends, has always been the defining characteristic of an effective nurse. Nursing, as any other practice-based discipline, requires a body of professional knowledge, and this is critical to effective clinical reasoning and decision making (Higgs & Tichen 2000). On this note, research evidence continues to highlight the knowledge deficits and practices of caregivers (Bachrach & Gardner 2002) and parents (Datta et al 2001), as well as conflicts between the beliefs and knowledge of doctors about the nutritional management of children with acute diarrhoea (Carral-Terrazas et al 2002). Such evidence has implications for the management and health promotion education role of health professionals. It is also proposed that logical thinking and common sense should prevail, as this promotes safe use of knowledge that guides the clinical judgement, clinical reasoning and the decision-making process.

Ask any parent what they wish for most for their child's imminent hospitalisation and the answer will probably be that their child comes home intact in mind and body. This natural aspiration is unlikely to be realised if the healthcare professionals managing that child's care do not have an adequate and appropriate knowledge to inform their practice.

The chapter has provided the evidence and knowledge base that can be applied to the holistic, comprehensive, child-focused and family-centred care of the child with body fluid and electrolyte imbalance.

References

Arfors EK, Buckley PB 1997 Pharmacological characterists of colloids. Ballières Clinical Anaesthesiology 11(1):15–41

Armon K, Stephenson T, MacFaul R et al 2001 An evidence and consensus based guideline for acute diarrhoea management. Archives of Diseases in Childhood 85:132–142

Atherley-John YC, Cunningham SJ, Crain EF 2002 Randomised trail of oral vs intravenous rehydration in a pediatric emergency department. Archives of Pediatric and Adolescent Medicine 156:1240–1243

Awazu M, Kon V, Barakat AY 1990 Volume disorders. In: Ichikawa I (ed.) Pediatric textbook of fluids and electrolytes. Williams and Wilkins, Baltimore

Bachrach LR, Gardner JM 2002 Caregiver knowledge, attitudes and practices regarding childhood diarrhoea and dehydration in Kingston, Jamaica. Revista panamericana de salud publica [Pan American Journal of Public Health] July(1):37–44

Carral-Terazas M, Martinez H, Flores-Huerta S et al 2002 Beliefs and knowledge of a group of doctors about the nutritional management of the child with acute diarrhoea. Salud publica de Mexico 44(4):303–314

Clayton BE, Round JM 1994 Clinical biochemistry and the sick child. Blackwell Scientific, Oxford

Coffee JC 1998 Metabolism. Fence Creek Publishing, Madison, WI

Conners GP, Barker WH, Mushlin AI et al 2000 Oral versus intravenous: rehydration preferences of pediatrics emergency fellowship directors. Pediatric Emergency Care 16(5):335–338

Dalby-Payne J, Elliot E 2004 Gastroenteritis in children. Clinical Evidence 11:1–3

Datta V, John R, Singh VP et al 2001 Maternal knowledge, attitude and practices towards diarrhoea and oral rehydration therapy in rural Maharashtra. Indian Journal of Pediatrics 68(11):1035–1037

Department of Health (DoH) 2001 Essence of care. Department of Health, London

Duggan C, Refat M, Hashem M et al 1996 How valid are clinical signs of dehydration in children? Journal of Pediatric Gastoenterology and Nutrition 22:56–61

Eastwood M 1997 The principles of nutrition. Chapman and Hall, London

Green M 2004 Nutrition. In: O'Callaghan C, Stephenson T (eds) Pocket Paediatrics, 2nd edn. Churchill Livingstone, Edinburgh

Guyton AC, Hall JE 2000 Textbook of medical physiology, 10th edn. WB Saunders, Philadelphia

Helmstadler C 1998 RCN annual conference paper. RCN, London

Higgs J, Tichen A 2000 Knowledge and clinical reasoning, In: Higgs J, Jones M (eds) Clinical reasoning in the health professions. Butterworth-Heinemann, Oxford

Hillman K, Bishop G, Bristow P 1997 The crystalloid versus colloid controversy: present status. Ballières Clinical Anaesthesiology 11(1):1–11

Horton HR, Moran LA, Ochs RS et al 2002 Principles of biochemistry, 3rd edn. Prentice Hall, Upper Saddler River, NJ

Ichikawa I (ed) 1990 Pediatric textbook of fluids and electrolytes. Williams and Wilkins, Baltimore

Johnson JE, Sullivan PB 2003 The management of acute diarrhoea. Current Paediatrics 13:95–100

Kozier B, Erb G, Berman AJ et al 2000 Fundamentals of nursing. Prentice Hall, Upper Saddler River, NJ

Linné JJ, Ringrud KM 1999 Clinical laboratory science: the basics and routine techniques, 4th edn. Mosby, St Louis

MacKenzie A, Barnes G, Shann F 1989 Clinical signs of dehydration in children. Lancet 2:605–607

Marie-Cardine A, Gourlain K, Mouterde O et al 2002 Epidemiology of acute viral gastroenteritis in children hospitalised in Rouen, France. Clinical Infectious Disease 34(9):1170–1178

Martini F 2004 Fundamentals of anatomy and physiology 6th edn. Prentice Hall, New Jersey

Nager AL, Wang VJ 2002 Comparison of nasogastric and intravenous methods of rehydration in pediatric patients with acute dehydration. Pediatrics 109(4):566–572

Parsons KC 2003 Human thermal environments. Taylor & Francis, London

Rao MR, Naficy AB, Savarino SJ et al 2001 Pathogenicity and convalescent excretion of campylobacter in rural Egyptian children. American Journal of Epidemiology 154(2):166–173

Roper N, Logan WW, Tierney AJ 1990 The elements of nursing. Churchill Livingstone, Edinburgh

Ryan S, Molyneux E 1996 Acute paediatrics. Blackwell Science, Oxford

Sandhu BK 2001 Rationale for early feeding in childhood. Gastroenteritis 33:513–516

Smith SF, Duell DJ, Martin BC 2004 Clinical nursing skills: basic to advanced skills. Pearson Prentice Hall, Upper Saddle River, NJ

Somers MJG, Harmon WE 1999 Clinical electrolyte and fluid management. In: Barrat TM, Avner ED, Harmon WE (eds) Pediatric nephrology, 4th edn. Lippincott Williams and Wilkins, Baltimore

Taylor DJ, Green NPO, Stout GP 1997 Biological sciences 2: systems maintenance and change. Cambridge University Press, Cambridge

Walmsley RN, White GH 1994 A guide to diagnosis in clinical chemistry, 3rd edn. Blackwell Science, Oxford

Weinstein SM 1997 Plummer's principles and practice of intravenous fluids, 6th edn. Lippincott, Philadelphia

Caring for Children with Genitourinary Problems

Kevin McFarlane

ABSTRACT

The kidneys play a major role in maintaining homeostasis. They eliminate waste and maintain the balance of water, pH and electrolytes in the body. Disorders of the genitourinary system may impact on kidney function and present a severe threat to health. The aim of this chapter and the companion PowerPoint presentation is to provide the reader with an insight into common genitourinary tract problems. The chapter focuses on urinary tract infection, nephrotic syndrome, poststreptococcal glomerulonephritis, vesicoureteric reflux, Wilms' tumour, hypospadias, cryptorchidism, circumcision, acute renal failure, and chronic renal failure.

Learning Outcomes

- Discuss common genitourinary tract conditions with reference to:
  - pathology
  - presenting symptoms
  - diagnosis
  - nursing management
  - medical management
  - potential complications
  - education and prevention.

Introduction

Urinary tract infections (UTI) occur in 1% of boys and 3% of girls before they are 11 years old (Stull & Lipuma 1991). Overall, urinary tract infection is more common in girls but in the first 3 months after birth it is more common in boys.

The term 'urinary tract infection' refers to an infection anywhere in the renal tract. It is convenient to categorise urinary tract infections into two groups:

- Lower urinary tract infection: involves the bladder and urethra and tends not to be associated with long-term sequelae.
- Upper urinary tract: involves the ureters and kidneys. Acute pylonephritis (APN) is the most serious upper urinary tract infection. It is associated with arterial hypertension and chronic renal failure (Jodal 1987).

Escherichia coli

The most common causative organism associated with urinary tract infection is *Escherichia coli* (*E. coli*). This organism is responsible for 80% of infections. *E. coli* is normally found in the large bowel, where it is involved in vitamin K production. The bacteria enter the urethra via the perineum. The cell membrane of the *E. coli* bacterium contains protein structures called adhesions, which facilitate bacterial adhesion to the surface of urogenital cells. This adhesion prevents the bacteria from being washed away during micturition. The infection ascends the urethra and enters the bladder, where the bacteria adhere to the cells that line the internal surface.

Susceptibility to Urinary Tract Infection

Some children are more susceptible than others are to urinary tract infection. Uncircumcised boys under 1 year old are more prone than circumcised boys; the short female urethra increases susceptibility in girls. Constipation is linked to repeated urinary tract infection. Constipation impairs voiding by compressing the urethra or the bladder neck. It leads to a high urine residual. This creates the conditions in which bacteria can flourish. Treatment of constipation may result in the resolution of urinary tract infection (Loening-Baucke 1997). Finally, congenital abnormalities of the renal tract place the child at risk. Vescoureteric reflux is the most common congenital abnormality of the genitourinary tract. Obstructive uropathies are also significant causes of urinary tract infection (Roth et al 2002b).

PowerPoint

Access the companion PowerPoint presentation, where you will find information on the common obstructive uropathies.

Diagnostic Problems

Urinary tract infection in children is problematic because it is not always obvious. In addition, when it is identified it may be difficult to distinguish between a lower urinary tract infection and upper urinary tract infection. The younger the child, the more likely these problems are to occur.

Diagnosis in an older child tends to be a little more obvious. An older child with a lower urinary tract infection may present with specific symptoms such as frequency, urgency, dysuria and secondary enuresis. If the infection is in the upper urinary tract, e.g. pylonephritis, the child may present with fever, flank pain and is obviously ill.

Babies and infants are more difficult to diagnose. This is because presenting symptoms are often non-specific and may not particularly point to genitourinary origins. Possible non-specific symptoms are irritability, vomiting, diarrhoea, poor feeding and failure to thrive. These signs do not generally allow medical staff to predict whether the infection is in the upper or lower genitourinary tract. Fever is the only factor that may point to an upper urinary tract infection but its absence does not negate the possibility.

Collecting Urine

In children older than 3 years, a midstream specimen of urine is the method of choice. The logic underpinning the collection of a midstream specimen is that the initial passage of urine flushes bacteria from the urethral orifice and thus reduces the likelihood of contamination. For those younger than 3 years who cannot or are unable to cooperate, an alternative approach is to obtain a clean-catch specimen. The procedure can be time consuming so it is helpful

if a parent can be the person collecting the urine. The baby or infant is positioned over a sterile container until voiding takes place.

The use of U-bags is controversial. Collections made by this method are notorious for becoming contaminated; as many as one-third of specimens taken in this way yield false-positive results (Li et al 2002). Uncircumcised boys are particularly at risk. U-bags are commonly used for non-toilet trained children but should not be used in high-risk cases (Al-Orifi 2000).

Urine can also be gathered from absorbent collection pads placed inside nappies. The pads are checked every 10 minutes until the child is found wet. A syringe is then used to aspirate urine from the pad. Although pad specimens are still prone to contamination, there is some evidence that they are more effective than bag specimens (Feasey 1999). There is also evidence that parents prefer to use the pad method when home collection is required (Liaw et al 2000).

The most effective means of attaining an uncontaminated specimen of urine from a child is by suprapubic stab or by catheterisation. Because of pain and the invasive nature of these procedures, they are reserved for high-risk cases. Febrile babies less than 3 months old should have specimens taken by these means. Older non-toilet trained children with features of upper urinary tract infection or a history of urinary tract infection or with known abnormalities should be catheterised to obtain a specimen.

Irrespective of the method of obtaining urine for culture, the specimen should be transferred to a specimen bottle within 30 minutes of collection. It can then be stored in a fridge at 4°C until processing.

Reflect on your Practice

- What methods of urine collection are you familiar with?
- Are you totally familiar with the manufacturer's recommendations concerning applying a U-bag?
- Are there times when you use U-bags when a more effective method could be used?

Urine Testing

Urine should be screened at ward level. The nurse should be alert to the amount of urine that is produced; it may be diminished in urinary tract infection. The colour is also significant. Healthy urine will lie somewhere between clear and straw coloured. Infected urine is commonly cloudy. The smell of urine is traditionally thought to be a significant factor but it appears not to be a reliable indication of urinary tract infection in children (Struthers et al 2003).

Dipstick testing may prove positive for blood and/or protein. These substances are not particularly predictive of a urinary tract infection; they may be present but equally they may not. Much more predictive is the presence of nitrite and leucocyte esterase. Nitrate is a substance that is normally found in urine. Most bacteria convert nitrate to nitrite; it takes them around 4 hours to do this. This is why morning testing for nitrite is a good idea. A dipstick can also be used to detect the presence of leucocyte esterase. This is an enzyme produced by white blood cells; its presence indicates infection. A urine sample that is positive for leucocyte esterase and nitrites strongly suggests urinary tract infection. Definitive diagnosis is on urine culture.

Antibiotic Therapy

Neonates (0–2 months) have immature immune systems. There is a likelihood that an infection could spread beyond the urinary tract. These babies are managed as if they have systemic sepsis and are prescribed parental antibiotics that are given for 2–3 weeks.

Children between 2 months and 2 years may also be hospitalised to receive intravenous antibiotics. A child who is unwell, with features such as fever, rigors, vomiting or dehydration, should be admitted. Rapid treatment is required because delay increases the risk of renal damage (Smellie et al 1994). Parental antibiotics are administered for a period of 24–48 hours. This should be followed by a 7–10-day course of oral antibiotics.

Children who are considered to have a lower urinary tract infection and do not appear ill can be managed at home. They are prescribed oral antibiotics. There is a debate about how long the course should be. Some physicians prefer to prescribe a 7–10-day course whereas others prescribe a short course of 2–4 days. There is conflicting evidence in the literature (Keren & Chan 2002, Michael et al 2003) and the debate remains unresolved. Amoxicillin, trimethoprim–sulfamethoxazole and cephalosporin are the drugs of choice (Riccabona 2003).

Nursing Considerations

Assessment must include pain, hydration stasis and temperature. The type of pain and the location varies. Pain may occur only on micturition. Bladder spasms may occur. Loin pain may be present. Non-pharmacological methods such as distraction and heat pads should be considered. Analgesia should be prescribed and administered as required. The child may be dehydrated because of reduced intake and increased insensible loss. It is necessary to observe for signs of dehydration and record input and output. The child's weight should also be recorded. Older children can be encouraged to consume adequate fluids but younger children might require intravenous support. Temperature con-

trol may be necessary. Children with lower urinary tract infections may have a mild temperature rise. Those with upper urinary tract infections may have more substantial temperature rises. Cooling measures should be implemented and antipyretics administered.

Investigations

Imaging is used during the acute illness and later to identify any damage to the kidneys and any predisposing causes of urinary tract infection. Babies and infants are most likely to be in danger of renal damage associated with genitourinary abnormalities (American Academy of Pediatrics (AAP) 1999). This age group is more likely to be investigated intensively. The diagnostic imaging methods that are usually considered include ultrasonography, dimercaptosuccinic acid scanning and voiding cystourethrogram.

Ultrasonography is a non-invasive test that provides information about the structure of the renal tract and dilation of the collecting system. It can identify dilated or duplicated ureters, ureteroceles and horseshoe kidneys. The test is limited because it cannot identify acute pyelonephritis or subsequent renal scarring. It may also fail to detect hydronephrosis.

Dimercaptosuccinic acid (DMSA) scanning is used during an acute urinary tract infection when an upper urinary tract infection is suspected. It can detect inflammation of the kidney substance and confirms the diagnosis of acute pyelonephritis. Later DMSA scanning can be used to determine the presence of any scarring. It is estimated that between 60 and 65% of children will have a renal scar following an initial insult of acute pyelonephritis (Jakobsson & Soderlundh 1992).

Micturating cystourethrogram (MCU) provides information about the bladder and flow of urine. It identifies the presence of vesicoureteric reflux and the grade of reflux. An MCU can be carried out before or after the child has completed their initial antibiotic course (Mahant et al 2001). The procedure involves catheterisation and instillation of contrast media. Preparing the child and family before investigation can reduce the distress associated with the procedure. Story-telling and play have both been found to be effective (Phillips et al 1998).

Education and Prevention

Children who have had one urinary tract infection are at risk of further infections. There are means of limiting the likelihood of a second infection. Detailed discussion concerning these means must take place. Information given to parents (and children) should be verbal and reinforced on paper.

Parents and children should be taught the gross anatomy of the urinary tract and the nature of ascending infection. From this point they can then appreciate the recommended hygiene habits that must be practised. If a child is in nappies, these should be changed as soon as possible after soiling. Perineal hygiene is important in girls, stroking away from the urethra is recommended. Cotton underwear is advisable because synthetic materials may increase heat and sweating and encourage bacterial growth. Bubble baths should not be added to bath water and perfumed soaps are inadvisable. Using bubble baths and perfumed soaps may disturb the urethral flora and encourage bacteria to ascend.

Stasis of urine should be avoided so the child should drink frequently and also be given the opportunity to void every hour or two. Cranberry juice has been recommended as a suitable fluid because of its ability to acidify the urine, this is said to prevent binding of *E. coli*. Some authors find in its favour (Kontiokari et al 2001) whereas others debate its efficacy (Schlager 1999).

It is also necessary to teach parents to look for the features of a urinary tract infection. They may also have to learn how to obtain specimens and test them for nitrite and leucocyte esterase. Finally, the importance of complying with antibiotic therapy should be discussed and the necessity to attend follow-up clinic appointments and investigations should be stressed.

The Nephrotic Syndrome

The most common form of the nephrotic syndrome (NS) is idiopathic, which accounts for over 85% of presentations (International Study of Kidney Disease in Children 1978) and is the subject of this section. However, there are other causes: in a small number of cases the disorder is congenital, the most common congenital presentation being Finnish-type, an autosomal recessively inherited disease (Holmberg et al 1996). The nephritic syndrome may also be a consequence of another disease; glomerulonephritis is most commonly implicated.

PATHOLOGY

Substances filter from the glomerulus into the nephron through a selective barrier called the basement membrane. Substances move through the barrier on the basis of size and electrical charge. In the nephritic syndrome the selectivity of this membrane is impaired and the glomerulus allows albumin to escape from the blood into the filtrate. Urine therefore tests positive for protein; the amount of protein lost is often described as massive. The loss of albumin interferes with the body's ability to balance fluids between the various body compartments. Normally, albumin levels provide oncotic pressure that counterbalances the effect of hydrostatic pressure at capillary level. In effect, normal levels of albumin are necessary to maintain fluid within the vascular space. When albumin is lost in the filtrate, hypoalbuminaemia occurs and oncotic pressure falls. The effect is that hydrostatic pressure acts with minimum opposition, fluid shifts into the interstitial space and oedema results.

Sodium levels also play a role in oedema formation. Sodium retention occurs. Traditionally, it was thought that fluid shifts cause hypovolaemia, which triggers the renin–angiotensin mechanism, which, in turn, promotes sodium retention. An alternative view is that nephrotic syndrome causes a primary defect at the tubular level, and that this causes sodium retention (Orth & Ritz 1998).

Hypoalbuminaemia is one consequence of the nephrotic syndrome; hyperlipidaemia is another. The levels of cholesterol and triglycerides in the blood rise as a result of increased synthesis by the liver and decreased clearance by the kidneys. Although the exact mechanisms for this are unknown, the potential consequences are a cause for concern. High cholesterol levels have a known association with atherosclerosis and high triglyceride levels may also have atherogenic properties and can cause further renal injury (O'Donnell 2001).

DIAGNOSIS

Nephrotic syndrome should be suspected when a child presents with oedema and proteinuria. In the paediatric age group, urinary protein loss of 50 mg/kg per 24 hours or greater is a firm diagnostic criterion (Roth et al 2002a); other markers are hypoalbuminaemia and hyperlipidaemia. Diagnosis is usually made without resorting to biopsy during the initial illness. This approach is taken because the majority of children have idiopathic nephrotic syndrome and their biopsies reveal the same results: they demonstrate damage to the glomerular epithelial foot processes. This is called minimal change nephrotic syndrome. A biopsy is reserved for children who do not respond to treatment. Although biopsy in these cases is still likely to reveal minimal change nephrotic syndrome (International Study of Kidney Disease in Children 1978), a few will identify other microscopic changes that might signify a different approach to treatment and different long-term outlook.

MEDICAL TREATMENT

Corticosteroids are used to treat nephrotic syndrome, prednisolone being the drug of choice. The standard course is 8 weeks. A typical protocol might be 2 mg/kg daily for 4 weeks, then 1.5 mg/kg on alternate days for 4 weeks. Some children will relapse and require long-term maintenance. The earliest predictor that suggests a relapsing course is the time it takes the child to enter remission after prednisolone treatment is initiated (Constantinescu et al 2000). The child on long-term maintenance may receive prednisolone daily or every second day. There is evidence that alternate day regimes may be more beneficial and produce fewer side effects (Hiraoka et al 2003). If the child is commenced on long-term maintenance then the parents must be aware of possible side effects, such as increased appetite, weight gain and cushingoid symptoms. Parents also have to know about possible psychological side effects. Anxiety, depression and difficult behaviour are all possibilities (Soliday et al 1999).

Some children may be resistant to steroid therapy and others may suffer unacceptable side effects because of prolonged use. These children are likely to be prescribed immunosuppressive or immunomodulator drugs such as cyclosporine A, cyclophosphamide or levamisole. All these agents are associated with significant potential adverse effects and there is no consensus as to which is the most appropriate (Durkan et al 2001).

Diuretics are reserved for treating substantial oedema. Furosemide (Lasix) a loop diuretic is commonly prescribed. It is used judiciously because it may result in hypovolaemia, which in turn might increase the likelihood of thrombosis. Albumin may be used in conjunction with furosemide if severe oedema and complications such as pleural effusion or ascites are present.

COMPLICATIONS

Distribution of hydrostatic and oncotic pressure across the pleural and peritoneal membranes is altered. Fluid may shift into the pleural space and cause a pleural effusion. It may also shift into the peritoneal space and cause ascites. Both conditions impair lung expansion and respiratory distress may result. Treatment involves administration of diuretics and albumin.

Children with the nephrotic syndrome are prone to infection; chickenpox is a particular threat. Chickenpox is caused by the varicella-zoster virus and can have devastating effects on an immune-suppressed child. The child's immune status should be checked and, if not immune to varicella-zoster and exposed to chickenpox, then varicella-zoster immune globulin should be administered. Acyclovir prophylaxis may also be administered as an adjunctive (Goldstein et al 2000).

Peritonitis is also a potential threat. Any abdominal pain must be carefully assessed with this complication in mind. The causative organism is usually a pneumococcus and pneumococcal immunisation is recommended for all children. Penicillin prophylaxis may be given to some subgroups (McIntyre & Craig 1998).

The final complication is thromboembolism. Children are prone to both arterial and venous thrombosis. Disturbances in clotting and fibrinolytic systems occur; Antithrombin III levels may be depleted and fibrinogen levels raised. High cholesterol and triglyceride levels and low levels of albumin are other risk factors. The presence of dehydration and the use of diuretic also increase susceptibility. Nurses should be cognisant of the features of deep venous thrombosis and pulmonary embolism. With regard to the latter, the development of tachypnoea should raise concern because this might be a sign of pulmonary embolism (van Ommen et al 1998). Thromboembolism requires immediate anticoagulant treatment.

NURSING MANAGEMENT

Activity

A ten-year-old boy is admitted with significant oedema. His face, abdomen, legs and feet are particularly swollen. He reveals that his scrotum is also oedematous:
- What nursing interventions would you consider appropriate?

Check your answer with the companion PowerPoint presentation.

As the activity above suggests, caring for a child with oedema is a major focus when caring for a child with nephrotic syndrome. Fluid balance is also important. Fluid intake is normally controlled, the child's previous day's input and output being two of the factors that influence the amount prescribed. Diets high in protein (to increase albumin) or low in protein (to rest the kidneys) have been used in the treatment of this condition but they tend to be ineffective. The current approach is to determine the child's normal dietary protein requirements and ensure that these are met. Carbohydrate intake has to be sufficient to ensure that protein intake can be utilised appropriately and not used for energy purposes. Hyperlipidaemia is not generally a cause for concern during the initial illness. If the child does not respond to treatment and hyperlipidaemia becomes a chronic state, dietary measures such as reduced saturated fat and cholesterol intake are advisable. Medications to reduce cholesterol and triglycerides may also be recommended. Finally, because sodium levels may be elevated in the nephrotic syndrome, dietary sodium has to be controlled. Foods high in sodium should not be consumed and salt should not be added to foods during cooking or at meal times.

Measures must be taken to protect the child from infection and identify it if it occurs. To this end, visitors should be infection free and the number of visitors must be controlled. The child should also be observed for signs of infection such as cough, runny nose and sore ears. Temperature, pulse and respiration should also be recorded regularly.

PROGNOSIS

Deaths due to the nephrotic syndrome are rare but do occur. These deaths are normally attributed to peritonitis and thrombus. Most children with idiopathic nephrotic syndrome respond within 10–14 days of treatment; of these, two-thirds will relapse. The parents need to know about this possibility and be in the position to recognise it. They should monitor the child's weight and test urine for protein. These children will require repeated courses of steroids, often for a prolonged period of time. Most will return to normal, although it may take many years.

WWW

Obtain a fact sheet on the nephrotic syndrome at the Great Ormond Street Hospital website:
- http://www.ich.ucl.ac.uk/factsheets/diseases_conditions/congenital_nephrotic_syndrome/

Poststreptococcal Glomerulonephritis (PSGN)

Glomerulonephritis is an inflammation of the glomeruli of the kidneys. Poststreptococcal glomerulonephritis (PSGN) is the most common cause of acute glomerulonephritis in children and, as its name suggests, develops after a streptococcal infection. The site of infection is usually the pharynx or the skin. There is a latent period between the original infection and the presentation of poststreptococcal glomerulonephritis. If the source of infection is the pharynx the period is 1–2 weeks, whereas if the source is the skin it is 2–4 weeks. The condition is most often seen in boys and the age of onset is between 3 and 15 years (Simckes & Spitzer 1995).

PATHOPHYSIOLOGY

The pathogenesis of poststreptococcal glomerulonephritis is not fully elucidated. There is evidence that a streptococcal component becomes lodged in the glomerular basement membrane (Cu et al 1998); this is the 'planted antigen' theory. Antibodies then fix to the component/antigen, forming an immune complex. The immune complex triggers a second phase, which involves activation of complement. Complement triggers a cascade of events that result in glomerular inflammation. Glomerular capillaries become blocked and impairment of glomerular filtering function occurs. Protein and blood are lost in the urine. The glomerular filtration rate (GFR) falls and urine output diminishes. In some patients, the reduction in the glomerular filtration rate may be significant and the child may develop acute renal failure. The fall in the glomerular filtration rate results in sodium and water retention and the expansion of the blood volume. Body fluid is redistributed and oedema results. Hypertension also occurs. This is partially due to sodium and water retention but other factors are thought to be involved.

PowerPoint

Access the companion PowerPoint presentation for a full explanation of glomerular filtration rate.

SIGNS AND SYMPTOMS

The clinical severity of poststreptococcal glomerulonephritis is variable, with some children having mild disease and being asymptomatic (Tasic & Polenakovic 2003). When children have symptoms the onset is usually abrupt. The child suffers from haematuria, mild to moderate proteinurea and oedema. The degree of oedema varies. Mild periorbital oedema may occur or it may be more extensive. In some cases it may be severe with accompanying ascites or pleural effusion. Urine assumes a dark colour because of the presence of blood and protein. Urine output is diminished, some children are oliguric and, as mentioned above, may present with acute renal failure. Hypertension is common; this might be mild but can be severe. If severe, associated symptoms such as headache and visual disturbance occur. The child is usually fatigued. Anaemia, uraemia and hypervolaemia contribute to feelings of tiredness.

DIAGNOSIS

Diagnosis is made on history, examination and a number of investigations. Urinalysis reveals blood, protein and high specific gravity. Throat swabs (or skin swabs) may be positive for streptococcal infection. Blood samples are taken and examined for antibody to streptococci and their extracellular products (Lang & Towers 2001). Antistreptolysin O (ASO) is one example. The normal ASO is < 166 Todd units, in poststreptococcal glomerulonephritis this is raised. Blood is also examined for evidence of complement activity. A reduction in complement elements C3 and C4 are suggestive of poststreptococcal glomerulonephritis.

MANAGEMENT

Antibiotics are administered to eliminate any persistent streptococcal infection; penicillin is the drug of choice. Hospitalisation is not always required but when hypervolaemia, oedema or hypertension are concerns the child is admitted.

Hypervolaemia and the resultant oedema make fluid balance an important focus. All input and output should be accurately documented. The child's weight should also be recorded. Hypervolaemia and oedema can be addressed by restricting fluids and sodium intake. The child's diet should not contain salty foods and salt should not be added. Dietary manipulation alone may be insufficient to deal with more severe problems and diuretics may be required. Loop diuretics such as furosemide act quickly and effectively.

Hypertension may be mild, moderate or severe. The frequency of recording will differ depending on the circumstance. The dietary measures and administration of diuretics taken to relieve oedema and hypervolaemia may be all that is required to reduce the blood pressure. If hypertension is not alleviated by these means then antihypertensive agents are employed. Severe rises in blood pressure require intravenous antihypertensive agents.

PROGNOSIS

The prognosis of poststreptococcal glomerulonephritis is excellent (Kasahara et al 2001). Most children who develop the condition will recover, with blood pressure and renal function returning to normal. However, a small number of children do not recover and go on and develop renal failure (Baldwin et al 1974).

Vesicoureteric Reflux

Vesicoureteric reflux (VUR) is the abnormal back flow of urine from the bladder into the ureter or into the ureter and kidneys. The condition may be unilateral or bilateral. Vesicoureteric reflux is usually a primary disorder caused by an anatomical defect at the junction between the ureter and the bladder. There is solid evidence that vesicoureteric reflux has a familial basis (Noe et al 1992). Primary vesicoureteric reflux is thought to be an autosomal dominant disorder with incomplete penetrance and variable expression.

PATHOLOGY

The ureters enter the bladder at an oblique angle on the posterior right and left lateral surface. The oblique course is continued through the bladder wall. Each ureter terminates in a ureteral orifice found at both sides of the upper level of the trigone. When the intravesical pressure is increased during micturition the detrusor muscle contracts and the intravesical section of the ureters are passively compressed. This valvular mechanism normally prevents reflux. The effectiveness of this mechanism is dependent on an adequate length of intravesical ureter (Belman 1997).

REFLUX, URINARY TRACT INFECTION AND SCARRING

Vesicoureteric reflux predisposes to urinary tract infection because urine that is refluxed into the ureter(s) trickles back into the bladder, producing an increased urine residual, which provides the conditions for an infection to take place. Reflux then provides a route by which the infection can reach the kidney. Urinary tract infection with vesicoureteric reflux is associated with renal scarring and is an important cause of hypertension and chronic renal failure in later life.

INVESTIGATIONS

Children with urinary tract infection must be investigated promptly to determine vesicoureteric reflux. Young children are particularly at risk and are usually prescribed prophylactic antibiotics until imaging is complete. One of the mainstays in the diagnosis of vesicoureteric reflux is micturating cystourography (MSU). This is an invasive procedure involving the trauma of catheterisation, the potential for infection and exposure to radioactivity. There is controversy concerning when it should be used and protocols vary. Because children under 3 years are more prone to vesicoureteric reflux, they tend to routinely undergo the procedure. Abdominal X-ray and ultrasound are also usually carried out. Older children, who are not as at risk, may be spared MCU, although this is not always the case. Primary investigation of these children may include abdominal X-ray, ultrasound and DMSA scanning. If these tests suggest reflux then MCU may be required. A positive MCU allows reflux to be graded. Grading influences management.

MANAGEMENT

The objective of medical management is to keep the urine infection free while waiting for spontaneous resolution. This is an effective treatment and can work in all grades of reflux, but the higher the grade the less likely spontaneous resolution is. Medical management involves the prescription of continuous low-dose antibacterial prophylaxis. The drugs are usually given in a single nightly dose.

Prophylaxis is usually discontinued when reflux disappears. This can be expected between 6 and 10 years (Huang & Tsai 1995). Management also emphasises the importance of measures designed to minimise the likelihood of urinary tract infection. The parent/child is taught the importance of adequate fluid intake, appropriate wiping action, regular toileting, double voiding to expel refluxed urine, and avoidance of constipation.

Surgery is considered for patients with grade IV and V reflux. It is considered as an option because spontaneous resolution is less likely. Surgery is also considered when prophylaxis fails to prevent urinary tract infection or further renal damage. Open surgery involves re-implantation of the offending ureter or ureters. The aim of re-implantation is to create an adequate intravesical tunnel, to allow compression of the ureter against the detrusor muscle. The success rate of reimplanation is 95% (Birmingham Reflux Study Group 1984).

An alternative surgical technique avoids open surgery. Endoscopic injection therapy involves using a standard operating cystoscope to visualise the ureteric orifice. A substance is then injected below the epithelial layer, just inside the edge of the orifice. This narrows the lumen. The technique takes about 15 minutes and can be done on a day-patient basis. Teflon was the original injected substance but concerns arose concerning particle migration to lymph, liver and lungs. Bovine collagen was then used but was also considered unsatisfactory because it was reabsorbed. Other products are on the market but it seems that the ideal material has yet to be developed (Leonard 2002). The operation is available in some centres but it is not as successful as open surgery and reoccurrence is a problem.

FOLLOW-UP

Children who are being treated prophylactically have to attend clinics on a regular basis, usually 3-monthly. They have their urine checked for infection, and undergo blood pressure and growth monitoring. Clinic appointments also provide the opportunity to reinforce the importance of compliance with medication. Further radiological studies are always necessary to ensure that reflux has not worsened or, more hopefully, that it has actually resolved. If the child has been treated surgically, follow-up continues to be important but the nature of the surveillance changes with fewer specimens required and fewer radiological studies.

Wilms' Tumour (Nephroblastoma)

Wilms' tumour is the most common abdominal tumour in childhood, affecting 1 in 10,000 children (Birch & Breslow 1995). It most commonly presents between the ages of 1 and 3 years and is seen equally in boys and girls. The condition may be bilateral or unilateral and it may occur as an isolated problem or may be associated with other syndromes or abnormalities.

Wilms' tumour is a malignancy associated with the embryonic cells that form the kidney. Renal stem cells differentiate and are responsible for forming the nephrons and connective tissue. In Wilms' tumour, some of these stem cells are thought to persist and are referred to as 'nephrogenic rests'. These are present at birth and retain their embryonic differentiation potential; they are the precursors of Wilms' tumour. The cells that constitute the rests begin to multiply and differentiate. Wilms' tumours are found to contain normal kidney tissue but they may also contain squamous epithelium, skeletal muscle and cartilage tissue (Coppes et al 1999); sometimes the tumours do not contain any of these recognisable cell types. Anaplasia is the presence of uncharacteristic cell types. These tumours tend to be more aggressive and difficult to treat. Wilms' tumour invades local structures and spreads via the lymphatic system. The most common sites of metastasis are the lungs, liver and brain.

GENETIC ALTERATIONS

The genetic mechanism responsible for Wilms' tumour is complex. Approximately 1% of presentations occur in families in which susceptibility appears to be inherited. The pattern of inheritance is autosomal dominant with incomplete penetrance. There is strong evidence that the gene that predisposes to this is to be found on chromosome 17 (Rahman et al 1996). A similar percentage of presentations occur as part of recognised syndromes such as aniridia and Beckwith–Weidemann. The majority of cases of Wilms' tumour present sporadically. A number of genes that are implicated in sporadic cases have been identified. One such gene is found on chromosome 11 (11p13). It is known as the Wilms' tumour suppressor gene. Only 5–10% of sporadic Wilms' tumour cases are characterised by this defect. Circumstantial evidence suggests that other genes are involved but the location and identification of these genes are unknown. The involvement of different genes helps to explain why different areas of the kidney are affected and different cell changes take place. It may also explain why the condition is unilateral or bilateral. It is possible that increasing knowledge about the genetic origins of the disorder may lead to earlier diagnosis or even prevention of the condition.

PRESENTATION AND DIAGNOSIS

The most common initial indication of an isolated Wilms' tumour is an abdominal mass (McLorie 2001). These, often massive tumours, may be identified by a parent or by the GP. Alternative presenting features are malaise, hypertension, abdominal pain, and haematuria. Following identification of the mass, an ultrasound is carried out. The ultrasound can detect the solid nature of the tumour and distinguish it from other conditions such as hydronephrosis. Abdominal computerised tomography is then performed, followed by magnetic resonance imaging.

GRADING AND STAGING

Therapy involves chemotherapy and surgery for all patients. Radiotherapy is not usually used but may be required when metastasis is present or following surgery when remnants of the tumour are still present. The International Society of Paediatric Oncology (SIOP) has developed protocols that determine management. Staging and grading determine the duration of chemotherapy, and the specific chemotherapeutic agents. Staging involves determining the position and extent of the tumour. Staging is determined by visualising techniques such as computerised tomography and magnetic resonance imaging. Grading is concerned with histology; it involves determining the nature of the tumour cells. A needle biopsy of the renal mass prior to initiation of chemotherapy is recommended (Vujanic et al 2003). The histology is described as 'favourable' or 'unfavourable'. A favourable histology demonstrates a tumour composed of recognisable cell types; an unfavourable histology demonstrates anaplasia.

CHEMOTHERAPY AND SURGERY

When grading and staging are complete, the child commences on prenephrectomy therapy. The grading and staging determine the protocol the child embarks on. Cytotoxic therapy involves using at least two chemotheraputic agents. The first-line chemotherapy agents used to treat Wilms' tumour include vincristine, actinomycin D, and doxorubicin. Pre-nephrectomy chemotherapy induces a dramatic reduction in the size of the tumour (McLorie 2001). Following chemotherapy surgery is conducted. In the case of a unilateral tumour surgery is aimed at complete removal of the affected kidney. Bilateral tumours require a different approach. Surgery is carried out to remove the tumour while conserving functional kidney tissue.

NURSING CONSIDERATIONS

The child may present with an abdominal mass but might not feel ill. The focus of care at this point will be on the parents, who will be devastated when the diagnosis is made. One concern in terms of the child is related to the possibility of metastasis. Unnecessary palpitation of the abdomen should be avoided. The child should be handled carefully. There is a danger that malignant cells could be liberated from the tumour if these measures are not taken. Later nursing interventions will focus on problems associated with chemotherapy. Following chemotherapy, interventions are concerned with the preoperative and postoperative care of the child with a nephrectomy.

PROGNOSIS

There is an overall survival rate of 80% (Wilms' tumour: status report 1990). As SIOP continues to fine-tune drug therapy protocols and new drugs become available, even better results may be achieved. There is a low risk of developing secondary cancers related to treatment. Renal malignant neoplasms are more common in children who have been treated for Wilms' tumour than the general population (Cherullo et al 2001).

 WWW

For information about cancers see the Cancer UK Research website. Information on Wilms' tumour can be found at:
* http://www.cancerhelp.org.uk/help/default.asp?page=6521

Hypospadias

Hypospadias is a congenital anomaly of the male genitalia in which the urethral meatus is abnormally located on the ventral side of the penis anywhere from the glans to the perineum. In Europe, hypospadias has an estimated prevalence of 4.1 per 1000 male births (Calzolari et al 1986). Hypospadias may be proximal or distal; most are distal. In these situations the meatus is positioned in the glans.

The proximal form of hypospadias is more serious. Hypospadias here may be penoscrotal, scrotal or perineal. The condition may also be associated with other congenital malformations, such as undescended testes, inguinal hernias, upper urinary tract anomalies, and cardiac and gastrointestinal malformations (Albers et al 1997). Chordee may accompany both types of hypospadias; this term refers to curvature of the penis. It occurs in 15% of distal and at least 85% of proximal hypospadias (Snodgrass 1999).

CAUSES

There are a number of known causes of hypospadias. It is a feature of several chromosomal abnormalities. It is seen in XX male syndrome, Wolf–Hirschhorn syndrome and Drash syndrome. It is also a feature of a number of endocrine anomalies. Urethral development takes place between 8 and 20 weeks gestation. Before 8 weeks, male and female external genitalia appear identical. The action of androgens (e.g. testosterone, androsterone) trigger the development of the male genitalia. Partial androgen receptor insensitivity is a recognised cause of hypospadias. Another related cause is 5-alpha-reductase deficiency. Testosterone has to be transformed by 5-alpha-reductase so that it can activate androgen receptors. A deficiency of 5-alpha-reductase impairs testosterone action; hypospadias is one of a number of possible consequences.

SURGERY

Surgery is carried out between 6 and 18 months. Most hypospadias require a one-stage repair (because most are distal). A one-stage repair may also be sufficient to reverse proximal hypospadias but a two-stage repair may be necessary. Irrespective of the number of stages required, the objective is the same: to bring the urethral meatus to the tip of the penis, correct any chordee, and create a cosmetically acceptable glans and penile shaft. Numerous procedures have been developed to achieve this. Commonly documented examples are the Thiersch–Duplay, Mathieu, Mustardé, meatal advancement and glanuloplasty and tubularised incised plate (TIP) urethroplasty.

POSTOPERATIVE CARE

Pain is one of the major problems in the immediate postoperative period. Penile block, caudal or epidural analgesia are employed to minimise this. Postoperative pain assessment and regular analgesia are required. Following surgery, a dressing is wrapped round the penis to provide support and protection and to minimise discomfort. Because different techniques are used, there are variations in the use of catheters and stents; some techniques employ them and others do not (Bernie & Alagiri 2003). Irrespective of whether these adjuncts are used, assessment of adequate urinary output is essential. The nurse should attempt to ensure that the child does not tamper with the dressing, stents or catheters. Doing so is associated with negative postoperative outcomes such as fistula development (Grobbelaar et al 1996). The dressing stays on for 4–7 days.

Removal of the dressing is a source of anxiety for parents and is painful and upsetting for the child. Before removal of the dressing, the child is given analgesia. It is common practice to then place the child in a bath to soften the dressing material. Despite this, the dressing is often still difficult to remove without upsetting the child. Distraction techniques can be employed and parent participation encouraged as a means of reducing distress. This procedure is a focus of attention in the literature. Sanders (2003) suggests that a barrier film can be applied before a dressing is attached to ease removal. Alternative modes of dressings that promote ease of removal have been suggested. Other authors question the efficacy of using dressings, as there is evidence to suggest that dressings might not be necessary in routine hypospadias repair (McLorie et al 2001, van Savage et al 2000).

Immediate Postoperative Concerns

Postoperative complications include infection, retention and fistula formation. Antibiotics are prescribed to minimise the likelihood of infection. The nurse must still be alert for signs of infection such as elevated temperature, discharge from the wound and foul-smelling urine. Retention may be anatomical or drug induced. All children, irrespective of the surgical technique employed, should be observed for this complication. A fistula may occur in the week following surgery. Urine leaks from a point along the reconstructed tract. Spontaneous closure is rare and a second operation is required.

OUTCOME AND LONG-TERM PROBLEMS

Studies have identified a high level of satisfaction with the outcome of hypospadias surgery. Long-term problems concern micturition difficulties and problems with sexual function. Micturition difficulties are generally caused by stricture. Urethral dilation may be necessary and in some cases open urothroplasty may be required. Sexual function problems, such as erection and ejaculation difficulties, have been reported following repair of severe hypospadias.

WWW

For further information see the links on the Hypospadias and Epispadias Association (HEA) web page:

- http://www.hypospadias.net/

Cryptorchidism

Cryptorchidism (undescended testis) is categorised as congenital or acquired. The incidence of congenital cryptorchidism in full-term males at birth is 2–4% (Barthold & González 2003). In early fetal development the testes are located within the abdominal cavity. Mediated by hormonal and mechanical factors, the testes descend into the scrotum. Migration begins at 17 weeks' gestation and is usually complete by 33 weeks (Malas et al 1999). Sometimes one or both testes fail to descend; the former is more common. If one or both fail to descend they may still fall within the first year; this is particularly true in the case of premature babies. If by 1 year testes are still undescended then orchidopexy is normally required. Cryptorchidism may also be acquired. In this situation the testes are in a normal scrotal position initially but one or both become undescended later. The pathogenesis of acquired cryptorchidism is unknown although possible causal factors such as failure of the spermatic cord to elongate have been proposed. Because cryptorchidism can be diagnosed during infancy (congenital) and later childhood (acquired) boys undergo the operation at different ages.

UNDESIRABLE CONSEQUENCES

Children with cryptorchidism are at risk from a number of undesirable consequences. Compared with other males they have a greater risk of testicular torsion. This occurs when the testicle twists on the spermatic cord and results in disturbance of blood flow, ischaemia and infarction of the testicle. Emergency surgery is required to save the testicle.

INFERTILITY

The condition is also associated with infertility. If bilateral cryptorchidism remains untreated the adult male will be infertile. However, surgery does not ensure fertility. The treated male may be fertile, subfertile (Coughlin et al 1997) or infertile. A successful outcome appears to be related to the position of the testes before operation, the age at operation and an adequate blood supply to the testes following surgery.

TESTICULAR CANCER

Cryptorchidism is an established risk factor for testicular cancer. It is possible that hormonal conditions cause both cryptorchidism and testicular cancer. Another possibility is that the higher temperature, to which the undescended testicle is exposed, promotes tumour formation. There appears to be a relationship between the age at which the male undergoes orchidopexy and the likelihood of testicular cancer (Herrinton et al 2003). Early orchidopexy appears to be associated with a more positive outcome.

SURGERY

Trends in orchidopexy have fallen in recent years. This may be due to better diagnosis or a simple decrease in frequency (Mireille et al 2003). The operation is often carried out as a day-case procedure and involves mobilising the testes, spermatic cord and blood supply. The testes or testicle is then brought down into the scrotum and secured by suture.

On return from theatre a dry dressing may be in place. It is removed prior to, or during, a shower the following day. The stitches dissolve a week later. Initially there is considerable swelling and bruising of the scrotum. This will cause discomfort and moderate pain relief will be required. Quiet play should be encouraged. Energetic play/exercise should be avoided for 10–14 days. There are complications associated with the procedure. There may be damage to the blood supply or spermatic cord during the operation, testicular function may be lost, wound infection may occur but is rare.

The risk of testicular cancer is still present even though orchidopexy has been carried out. All males should carry out testicular examination at regular periods. Those who have had cryptorchidism have added reason to do so.

WWW

For information about self-examination for testicular cancer, see:

- http://tcrc.acor.org/tcexam.html

Circumcision

Circumcision refers to excision of the prepuce, the outer portion of the foreskin covering the penis. The prepuce normally covers the glans. In infancy the inner surface of the prepuce, the mucosa, adheres to the glans and over the next 2 years retraction normally becomes possible. The foreskin protects the glans and keeps it soft and moist. Circumcision may be carried out for religious reasons, prophylactic reasons or for Phimosis.

RELIGIOUS REASONS

The most common reason for circumcision is religious. Circumcision is a sacred ritual for Muslims and Jews. The timing differs for each religion. Jewish babies are circumcised on the eighth day of life. Muslim children are circumcised between the seventh day following birth and up to puberty.

PROPHYLAXIS

Arguments in favour of routine circumcision for prophylactic reasons focus on a number of conditions. Urinary tract infection is one. The literature suggests that there is an increased risk of urinary tract infection in the uncircumcised child in the first year of life (Schoen et al 2000). Human papillomavirus (HPV) is another condition in which circumcision may be beneficial. HPV is a sexually transmitted disease and strains of the virus are linked to cancer of the cervix. Castellsague et al (2002) present evidence that male circumcision is associated with reduced risks of penile HPV infection and cervical cancer in female partners. Circumcision may also have a positive impact on the transmission of human immunodeficiency virus (HIV). Szabo & Short (2000) explain that the inner lining of the foreskin, the mucosal layer, contains Langerhans' cells. These cells are targets for HIV. The authors suggest that during heterosexual intercourse the foreskin is pulled back leaving the vagina exposed to an area rich in virus. Circumcision, it is thus argued, would reduce the likelihood of HIV transmission. In sub-Saharan Africa, where HIV is rampant, circumcision as a means of prevention of HIV is being advocated as an additional HIV prevention strategy (Rain-Taljaard et al 2003). This position is not without its critics. Others argue that it is not acceptable citing medical, ethical and legal reasons (Hill & Denniston 2003).

Phimosis

Phimosis refers to a non-retractable foreskin. It is the most common medical indication for circumcision (Rickwood 1999). Balanitis xerotica obliterans (BXO) is an inflammatory disorder that affects the prepuce and glans; it causes phimosis. Balanitis xerotica obliterans is rare before 5 years and it peaks before puberty. Features include phimosis, which may be accompanied by bleeding, dysuria and acute retention. Phimosis caused by balanitis xerotica obliterans necessitates circumcision. Phimosis can be diagnosed in the absence of balanitis xerotica obliterans and circumcision is carried out in these cases too. Circumcision in these situations is contentious. It is argued that it may not be necessary because the foreskin will retract in time without surgical intervention (Farshi & Atkinson 2000).

MANAGEMENT

No matter what the reason for circumcision, there are risks attached. Bleeding, infection and retention are all possible complications. On return from theatre the wound may be exposed or a dressing such as Vaseline gauze may be in place. The penis will look swollen and child and parents should be prepared for this. The wound can be cleaned with moistened cotton balls. It should be observed for infection and bleeding. If bleeding does occur it is usually minor and self-limiting, severe bleeding is uncommon. A white/yellowish exudate forms after 48 hours; this should not be confused with pus. It is granulation tissue and part of the healing process. Pus has a thicker consistency and smells malodorous. Infection is a rare occurrence but if it does occur the wound is cleansed regularly and antibiotic therapy commenced.

 WWW

For further information read the circumcision information and resource pages at:
- http://www.cirp.org/

Acute Renal Failure

Acute renal failure (ARF) is the sudden loss of renal function. Failure occurs over a period of hours or days. The kidneys play a major role in maintaining homeostasis. They maintain the body's water, electrolyte and acid–base balance, as well as eliminating waste from the body. In acute renal failure this homeostatic balance is lost and waste is not eliminated effectively. The causes of acute renal failure are traditionally divided into three categories: pre-renal, post-renal and intrinsic.

 Activity
- Make a list of the functions of the kidneys.
- Compose a brief statement explaining each of the functions.
- Access the companion PowerPoint presentation and compare your answers.

Pre-renal causes of acute renal failure are associated with impaired renal blood flow. The kidneys are structurally normal. All types of shock possess the capability to cause acute renal failure. Shock results in inadequate perfusion pressure and reduction in glomerular filtration rate. Oliguria occurs and the kidneys can no longer maintain their homeostatic functions. If the initiating condition is reversed promptly, kidney damage is prevented. If the initiating condition is not reversed, sympathetic and hormonal activity cause intense renal vasoconstriction and ischaemic renal injury and cell death occurs.

Intrinsic renal failure is concerned with pathology within the kidney. Glomerulonephritis and nephrotic syndrome are both possible causes but the most common cause, across all age groups, is haemolytic uraemic syndrome (Moghal et al 1998). This condition is caused by verotoxin-producing *E. coli*, a strain that is carried by cattle. It is thought that meat becomes contaminated during the slaughter process. The organism is destroyed if food is cooked properly. When the child consumes infected meat, colitis occurs. The verotoxin is then absorbed from the intestinal tract and enters the circulation, where it fixes to receptor sites on renal epithelium. Damage to the glomeruli result in a significant reduction in glomerular filtration thus impairing the kidneys regulatory functions.

Post-renal causes of acute renal failure are associated with obstruction. Common conditions that cause obstruction are posterior urethral valves, ureteropelvic obstruction, and neurogenic bladder. These conditions impair the flow of urine and back pressure results. The pressure in the renal tubules rises. As filtration depends on the pressure in the glomerulus being higher than that in the tubules, the gradient diminishes and the glomerular filtration rate falls. The kidneys fail.

DIAGNOSIS

The predisposing causes of acute renal failure will alert those caring for the child to the possibility of the development of acute renal failure. The signs and symptoms are varied and may include oliguria (less than 0.5 mL/kg/h in children) or anuria, oedema, nausea, vomiting, hypertension, confusion or seizures. Blood chemistry reveals increasing blood urea nitrogen (BUN) and creatinine. Abnormalities in electrolyte and acid balance are also evident. Imaging studies such as ultrasound may be ordered to determine whether obstruction is a cause. Renal biopsy is not routine but may be carried out if diagnosis is unexplained (Kersnik et al 2001).

NURSING MANAGEMENT

This is a life-threatening condition and enormous sensitivity is required when dealing with the parents. They should be encouraged to verbalise their feelings. Issues should be discussed with honesty and information provided should be accurate. The parents should be encouraged to participate in care but only to the degree that they are comfortable with.

Physical management is aimed at eliminating the underlying cause, balancing fluid and electrolytes, controlling acidosis, sustaining nutrition and protecting the child from infection. There may be fluid depletion or overload, thus fluid may have to be replaced or removed. This makes accurate recording of the child's input and output critical. The child's weight is also significant and should be documented twice daily. If fluid has to be replaced, the choice is between crystalloid, colloids and blood. The cause of the renal failure influences the choice of fluid. In the case of fluid retention dietary measure can be taken. Sodium and fluid intake can be restricted. Diuretics such as mannitol and furosemide may be prescribed; dopamine is an alternative.

Electrolyte balance focuses on sodium and potassium. High sodium levels may occur and are associated with fluid retention and oedema formation and are thus undesirable. In the event of hypernatraemia, sodium restriction is necessary. High potassium levels are also cause for concern. They may approach dangerous levels due to increased production and decreased elimination.

Hyperkalaemia is life threatening because it disturbs the conductive mechanism of the heart. This may result in dysrhythmia. Cardiac monitoring may be ordered in anticipation of such an event. Initial management involves restricting potassium intake, administration of potassium binding agents, control of acidosis and diuretic therapy aimed at increasing urinary output. Glucose metabolism causes potassium to move into cells. Glucose and insulin may be administered to induce these events (Kemper et al 1996). Severe hyperkalaemia is one of the reasons for commencing renal replacement therapy.

Acidosis is undesirable for a number of reasons. Prominent among these is its impact on potassium levels. It promotes the movement of potassium from the intercellular fluid into the extracellular compartment, and thus promotes hyperkalaemia. Acidosis also impacts on cerebral function. Neurological observations are implemented if there is any evidence of confusion or mental impairment. Acidosis may be treated with sodium bicarbonate.

Acute renal failure is highly catabolic. Parental nutrition or enteral feeding may be ordered to meet the child's nutritional requirements. The nutritional components are tailored to the child's needs. The amount of energy provided is usually high so that the body does not metabolise body tissues. If body tissue is metabolised for energy, potassium is liberated into an environment where hyperkalaemia may already exist.

The child has to be protected from infection because the immune system is compromised when homeostasis is impaired. Sepsis is a frequent cause of death. Great care has to be taken to protect the child from nosocomial infections. Hand-washing and implementation protocols designed to eliminate the possibility of cross-infection should be strictly applied. The child should be observed for signs of infection and antibiotic therapy should be implemented promptly if infection is discovered.

The interventions described above, plus treatment of predisposing causes, may produce the desired response. In the event of continued fluid overload, hyperkalaemia, acidosis or severe uraemia renal replacement therapy will be required until renal function returns. Common modalities include peritoneal dialysis, intermittent haemodialysis and continuous haemofiltration or haemodiafiltration (Flynn 2002). The choice of modality depends on the child's age, clinical condition and local experience with the particular modalities.

PROGNOSIS

Prognosis depends on the underlying cause. The outcome for those suffering from haemolytic–uraemic syndrome is excellent. The mortality rate for other illnesses that cause acute renal failure is much higher. Wong et al (1996) recorded a mortality rate of 27%.

Chronic Renal Failure

There are numerous causes of chronic renal failure in children. The most common cause is vesicoureteric reflux. Other significant causes are the obstructive uropathies such as posterior urethral valves, ureterocele and ureteropelvic junction obstruction (Roth et al 2002b). Medical conditions that may result in chronic renal failure are nephrotic syndrome and glomerulonephritis.

Chronic renal failure is categorised according to changes in glomerular filtration rate. This is the amount of filtrate that flows into all nephrons in one minute. The normal rate in a child is 110–120 mL/min.

Creatinine is a waste product of protein metabolism. Serum levels of creatinine can be measured. Creatinine is eliminated from the body by the kidneys. A 24-hour collection of urine is obtained to determine the amount cleared. By comparing serum creatinine to levels cleared in the 24-hour collection, the glomerular filtration rate can be calculated.

Chronic renal failure is regarded as mild, moderate or severe. The criteria are as follows:

- mild: glomerular filtration rate 50–75 mL/min
- moderate: glomerular filtration rate 25 mL–50 mL/min
- severe: glomerular filtration rate less than 25 mL/min.

CLINICAL FEATURES

The kidneys are multifunctional. Impairment of these functions produces a variety of clinical features. Common features are poor appetite, stunted growth, anaemia (with associated features), increased or decreased urine output, oedema, hypertension, skin discoloration and pruritus.

DIAGNOSIS

Chronic renal failure diagnosis is based on history, clinical examination, altered laboratory values, various scanning techniques and biopsy. Laboratory values reveal elevated blood urea nitrogen, elevated creatinine, altered calcium:phosphorus ratio, acidosis and electrolyte imbalance. The diagnosis is confirmed by kidney biopsy.

MANAGEMENT

There are a number of causes of chronic renal failure and these affect the management. There are also different stages of severity and variable progression. Thus the management described here is generalised.

The child's dietary protein intake should be based on the recommended dietary allowances (RDA) for his or her chronological age. Additional increments may be desirable to ensure growth. Increasing dietary protein intake above the RDA has to be balanced against the kidneys' ability to rid the body of waste products of protein metabolism. The energy portion of the diet has to be high; it is given in the form of fat and carbohydrates. If energy intake is insufficient then protein will be utilised for energy purposes. This will impair the child's growth. Maintaining strict records of intake and output are necessary. Height and weight are also documented.

High sodium levels encourage fluid retention, oedema and also contribute to hypertension. In chronic renal failure, sodium and fluids are usually restricted. Sodium should not be added to cooked food and foods high in salt should be avoided. These measures may not suffice and sodium intake may have to be restricted to a specific amount. Elevated potassium levels due to decreased excretion are associated with arrhythmias and cardiac arrest. Foods high in potassium should thus be avoided.

Attempts to curb the onset of anaemia are initially made by encouraging the anorexic child to eat. The diet should be attractive and small portions offered. It should be rich in iron, folic and vitamin B12. These substances may also be given in supplement form. Anaemia is inevitable in chronic renal failure because of loss of erythropoietin production. As the degree of kidney failure progresses, erythropoietin production fails and anaemia breaks through. Treatment involves administration of erythropoietin. Elimination of anaemia with erythropoietin is very effective; it is known to enhance cardiac, muscular and immune functions (Vijayan et al 2000) and generally improve quality of life.

Hypertension has been linked to the progression of chronic renal failure. There are a number of mechanisms that may be responsible for hypertension in chronic renal failure. Sodium and fluid retention is one factor. Controlling sodium and fluid intake is therefore employed to control blood pressure. Another mechanism involves the triggering of the renin–angiotensin system (RAS). The mechanism is activated by a falling glomerular filtration rate. Angiotensin II (produced when the renin–angiotensin system is triggered) promotes sodium and water retention and causes widespread vasoconstriction. It also promotes inflammation, fibrosis and scarring of the kidneys (Soergel & Schaefer 2002). Diuretics and acetylcholinesterase inhibitors are used to counteract the activities of the renin–angiotensin system.

Activity

- Describe the renin–angiotensin system.

Compare your recall of the mechanism with the companion PowerPoint presentation.

A precursor of active vitamin D is manufactured in the skin. Another precursor is consumed in the diet and is absorbed from the bowel. Both liver and kidneys modify these precursors and produce biologically active forms. Active vitamin D stimulates the absorption of dietary calcium from the bowel. By doing so, it helps to maintain serum calcium levels. In chronic renal failure the damaged kidneys do not activate the precursors of vitamin D. The result is that calcium absorption from the bowel is impaired and hypocalcaemia results. The problem is compounded by abnormalities in serum phosphorous levels.

Serum phosphorous levels tend to be elevated in chronic renal failure. This is partly due to the damaged kidneys, which fail to eliminate the substance. High serum phosphate is undesirable. It binds to calcium and lowers blood levels and also impairs vitamin D action, which also adversely affects calcium levels. Hypocalcaemia stimulates the production of parathyroid hormone that promotes movement of calcium out of bones. Bone demineralisation takes place and the child develops osteodystrophy.

Efforts are made to maintain calcium levels. Because the damaged kidneys do not activate precursors of vitamin D, an active form has to be prescribed. Calcium supplementation may also be provided. Attempts are also made to control serum phosphorous levels. Food high in phosphorous should be avoided and binding agents, such as aluminium hydroxide or calcium carbonate, which prevent phosphorous absorption, are prescribed. These measures have a positive impact but as failure progresses bone demineralisation becomes inevitable.

Acidosis adversely affects protein metabolism and is strongly implicated in growth delay (Boirie et al 2000). As kidney disease progresses there is a failure to synthesis ammonia (a process necessary to ride the body of hydrogen ions). There is also a failure to effectively reabsorb bicarbonate. These two factors combine to cause acidosis. When serum bicarbonate falls to levels below 22 mmol/L it should be corrected (National Kidney Foundation 2000). Sodium citrate or sodium bicarbonate may be administered orally. When a child is on dialysis, the problem can be met by adapting the dialysate solution to include high sodium bicarbonate concentrations.

Dialysis

Continuous ambulatory peritoneal dialysis is the preferred form of dialysis. Its main advantage is that the child can pursue his or her normal activities. A catheter is inserted into the child's abdomen. Gravity is utilised to allow dialysate to flow into the abdominal cavity. It lies on one side of the peritoneal membrane. An exchange between dialysate fluid and body fluid on the opposite side of the membrane takes place. The process takes about 2 hours and then the now altered dialysate is removed by allowing it to drain into a bag attached to the catheter and placed below the abdomen. Peritonitis is a complication of peritoneal dialysis. If this occurs it may be necessary for the child to convert to haemodialysis. This is more efficient than peritoneal dialysis but is much more restrictive. The child has to attend a specialist unit for 3 or 4 hours two or three times a week.

www

For information about dialysis, refer to the National Kidney Federation website:

- http://www.kidney.org.uk/Medical-Info/pd.html

Transplant

The child is tissue-typed to ensure compatibility. The outcome has improved in recent years thanks to pharmacological innovations designed to prevent rejection. These pharmaceuticals suppress the child's immune system. T cell induction therapy, steroid therapy and chemotherapy are all utilised.

Summary

Paediatric nurses are required to care for children with compared and acquired anomalies of the genitourinary tract. This chapter has attempted to offer an insight into some of the more common anomalies. Nurses caring for children must have a well-developed knowledge about urinary tract infection (UTI) because it is very common and because of its association with impaired renal function, hypertension and end-stage renal disease. Vesicoureteric reflux was given prominence in this chapter because it is intrinsically linked to UTI and is the most common congenital abnormality of renal tract. The nephrotic syndrome and post-streptococcal glomerulonephritis warranted attention because they are the commonest disorders associated with glomerular pathology. Children are commonly subject to surgical procedures involving the genitourinary tract. To this end, circumcision, hypospadias, cryptorchidism and Wilms' tumour were included. Finally, acute and chronic renal failure were given prominence because they are complications associated with most of the previously mentioned anomalies.

References

Albers N, Ulrichs C, Gluer S et al 1997 Etiologic classification of severe hypospadias: implications for prognosis and management. Journal of Pediatrics 131(3):386–392

Al-Orifi F, McGillivray D, Tange S et al 2000 Urine culture from bag specimens in young children: are the risks too high? Canada Journal of Pediatrics 137:221–226

American Academy of Pediatrics (AAP) 1999 Practice parameter: the diagnosis, treatment, and evaluation of the initial urinary tract infection in febrile infants and young children. Pediatrics 103:843–852

Baldwin DS, Gluck MC, Schacht RG, Gallo GR 1974 The long-term course of poststreptococcal glomerulonephritis. Annals of Internal Medicine 80:342–358

Barthold J, González R 2003 The epidemiology of congenital cryptorchidism, testicular ascent and orchiopexy. Journal of Urology 170(6) Pt 1:2396–2401

Belman AB 1997 Vesicoureteral reflux. Pediatric Clinics of North America 44(5):1171–1190

Bernie J, Alagiri M 2003 Tubeless barcat: a patient-friendly hypospadias procedure. Urology 61(6):1230–1232

Birch J, Breslow N 1995 Epidemiological features of Wilms' tumor. Hematology/Oncology Clinics of North America 9:1157–1178

Birmingham Reflux Study Group 1984 A prospective trial of operative versus non-operative treatment of severe vesico-ureteric reflux: 2 years' observation in 96 children. Contributions to Nephrology 39:169–185

Boirie Y, Broyer M, Gagnadoux MF et al 2000 Alterations of protein metabolism by metabolic acidosis in children with chronic renal failure. Kidney International 58(1):236–241

Calzolari E, Contiero MR, Roncarati E et al 1986 Aetiological factors in hypospadias. Journal of Medical Genetics 23(4):333–337

Castellsague X, Bosch F, Munoz N et al 2002 Male circumcision, penile human papillomavirus infection, and cervical cancer in female partners. New England Journal of Medicine 346:1105–1112

Cherullo EE, Ross JH, Kay R et al 2001 Renal neoplasms in adult survivors of childhood Wilms' tumor. Journal of Urology 165(6) Pt 1:2013–2016

Constantinescu AR, Shah HB, Foote EF et al 2000 Predicting first-year relapses in children with nephrotic syndrome. Pediatrics 105(3) Pt 1:492–495

Coppes MJ, Wolff JE, Ritchey ML 1999 Wilms' tumour: diagnosis and treatment. Paediatric Drugs 1(4):251–262

Coughlin M, O'Leary L, Songer N et al 1997 Time to conception after orchidopexy: evidence for subfertility? Fertility and Sterility 67(4):742–746

Cu GA, Mezzano S, Bannan JD et al 1998 Immunohistochemical and serological evidence for the role of streptococcal proteinase in acute post-streptococcal glomerulonephritis. Kidney International 54(3):819–826

Denton MD, Chertow GM, Brady HR 1996 'Renal-dose' dopamine for the treatment of acute renal failure: scientific rationale, experimental studies and clinical trials. Kidney International 50(1):4–14

Durkan A, Hodson E, Willis N et al 2001 Non-corticosteroid treatment for nephrotic syndrome in children. Cochrane database of systematic reviews (4):CD002290

Farshi Z, Atkinson K 2000 A study of clinical opinion and practice regarding circumcision. Archives of Disease in Childhood 83(5):393–396

Feasey S 1999 Are Newcastle urine collection pads suitable as a means of collecting specimens from infants? Paediatric Nurse 11(9):17–21

Flynn JT 2002 Choice of dialysis modality for management of pediatric acute renal failure. Pediatric Nephrology 17(1):61–69

Goldstein SL, Somers MJ, Lande MB et al 2000 Acyclovir prophylaxis of varicella in children with renal disease receiving steroids. Pediatric Nephrology 14(4):305–308

Grobbelaar A, Laing J, Harrison D et al 1996 Hypospadias repair: the influence of postoperative care and a patient factor on surgical morbidity. Annals of Plastic Surgery 37(6):612–617

Herrinton L, Zhao W, Husson G 2003 Management of cryptorchidism and risk of testicular cancer. American Journal of Epidemiology 157(7):602–605

Hill G, Denniston G 2003 HIV and circumcision: new factors to consider. Sexually Transmitted Infections 79(6):495–496

Hiraoka M, Tsukahara H, Matsubara K et al 2003 A randomized study of two long-course prednisolone regimens for nephrotic syndrome in children. American Journal of Kidney Diseases 41(6):1155–1162

Holmberg C, Laine J, Rönnholm K et al 1996 Congenital nephrotic syndrome. Kidney International Supplement 53:S51–S56

Huang FY, Tsai TC 1995 Resolution of vesicoureteral reflux during medical management in children. Pediatric Nephrology 9 (6):715–717

International Study of Kidney Disease in Children 1978 Nephrotic syndrome in children: prediction of histology from clinical and laboratory characteristics. Kidney International 13:159–165

Jakobsson B, Soderlundh S, Berg U 1992 Diagnostic significance of 99mTc-dimercaptosuccinic acid (DMSA) scintigraphy in urinary tract infection. Archives of Disease in Childhood 67:1338–1342

Jodal U 1987 The natural history of bacteriuria in childhood. Infectious Disease Clinics of North America 1:713–729

Kasahara T, Hayakawa H, Okubo S et al 2001 Prognosis of acute poststreptococcal glomerulonephritis (APSGN) is excellent in children, when adequately diagnosed. Pediatrics International 43(4):364–367

Kemper MJ, Harps E, Müller-Wiefel DE 1996 Hyperkalemia: therapeutic options in acute and chronic renal failure. Clinical Nephrology 46(1):67–69

Keren R, Chan E 2002 A meta-analysis of randomized, controlled trials comparing short- and long-course antibiotic therapy for urinary tract infections in children. Pediatrics 109(5):E70–0

Kersnik Levart T, Kenig A, Buturovic Ponikvar J 2001 Real-time ultrasound-guided renal biopsy with a biopsy gun in children: safety and efficacy. Acta Paediatrica 90(12):1394–1397

Kontiokari T, Sundqvist K, Nuutinen M et al 2001 Randomised trial of cranberry-lingonberry juice and Lactobacillus GG drink for the prevention of urinary tract infections in women. British Medical Journal (Clinical research edition) 322(7302):1571

Lang MM, Towers C 2001 Identifying poststreptococcal glomerulonephritis. Nurse Practitioner: American Journal of Primary Health Care 26(8):34–42

Leonard M 2002 Endoscopic injection therapy for treatment of vesicoureteric reflux: a 20-year perspective. Paediatrics and Child Health 7(8):545–550

Li PS, Ma LC, Wong SN 2002 Is bag urine culture useful in monitoring urinary tract infection in infants? Journal of Paediatric and Child Health 38(4):377–381

Liaw LC, Nayar DM, Pedler SJ 2000 Home collection of urine for culture from infants by three methods: survey of parents' preferences and bacterial contamination rates. British Medical Journal 320(7245):1312–1313

Loening-Baucke V 1997 Urinary incontinence and urinary tract infection and their resolution with treatment of chronic constipation of childhood. Pediatrics 100:228–232

Mahant S, To T, Friedman J 2001 Timing of voiding cystourethrogram in the investigation of urinary tract infections in children. Journal of Pediatrics 139(4):568–571

Malas M, Sulak O, Öztürk A 1999 The growth of the testes during the fetal period. British Journal of Urology 84(6):689–692

McIntyre P, Craig JC 1998 Prevention of serious bacterial infection in children with nephrotic syndrome. Journal of Paediatrics and Child Health 34(4):314–317

McLorie G 2001 Wilms' tumor (nephroblastoma). Current Opinion in Urology 11(6):567–570

McLorie G, Joyner B, Herz D et al 2001 A prospective randomized clinical trial to evaluate methods of postoperative care of hypospadias. Journal of Urology 165(5):1669–1672

Michael M, Hodson EM, Craig JC et al 2003 Short versus standard duration oral antibiotic therapy for acute urinary tract infection in children. Cochrane database of systematic reviews 1:CD003966

Mireille B, Toledano L, Anna L et al 2003 Temporal trends in orchidopexy, Great Britain, 1992–1998. Environmental Health Perspectives 111:129–132

Moghal NE, Brocklebank JT, Meadow SR 1998 A review of acute renal failure in children: incidence, etiology and outcome. Clinical Nephrology 49(2):91–95

National Kidney Foundation 2000 Clinical practice guidelines for nutrition in chronic renal failure. American Journal of Kidney Disease 35(6 Suppl 2):S1–S140

Noe HN, Wyatt RJ, Peeden JN Jr et al 1992 The transmission of vesicoureteral reflux from parent to child. Journal of Urology 148(6):1869–1871

O'Donnell M 2001 Mechanisms and clinical importance of hypertriglyceridemia in the nephrotic syndrome. Kidney International 59(1):380–382

Orth SR, Ritz E 1998 Medical progress: the nephrotic syndrome. New England Journal of Medicine 338(17):1202–1211

Phillips DA, Watson AR, MacKinlay D 1998 Distress and the micturating cystourethrogram: does preparation help? Acta Paediatrica 87(2):175–179

Rahman N, Arbour L, Tonin P et al 1996 Evidence for a familial Wilms' tumour gene (FWT1) on chromosome 17q12-q21. Nature Genetics 13(4):461–463

Rain-Taljaard R, Lagarde E, Taljaard D et al 2003 Potential for an intervention based on male circumcision in a South African town with high levels of HIV infection. AIDS Care 15(3):315–327

Riccabona M 2003 Urinary tract infections in children. Current Opinion in Urology 13(1):59–62

Rickwood A 1999 Medical indications for circumcision. British Journal of Urology 83 Supplement 1:45–51

Roth K, Amaker BH, Chan JCM 2002a Nephrotic syndrome: pathogenesis and management. Pediatrics in Review 23(7):237–248

Roth K, Koo HP, Spottswood SE et al 2002b Obstructive uropathy: an important cause of chronic renal failure in children. Clinical Pediatrics 41(5):309–314

Sanders C 2003 Comparison of dressing removal following hypospadias repair. British Journal of Nursing 12(15) Supplement:S21–S28

Schlager TA, Anderson S, Trudell J et al 1999 Effect of cranberry juice on bacteriuria in children with neurogenic bladder receiving intermittent catheterization. Journal of Pediatrics 135(6):698–702

Schoen E, Colby C, Ray G 2000 Newborn circumcision decreases incidence and costs of urinary tract infections during the first year of life. Pediatrics 105:789–793

Simckes AM, Spitzer A 1995 Poststreptococcal acute glomerulonephritis Pediatrics in Review/American Academy of Pediatrics 16(7):278–279

Smellie JM, Poulton A, Prescod NP 1994 Retrospective study of children with renal scarring associated with reflux and urinary infection. British Medical Journal 308:1193–1196

Snodgrass W 1999 Changing concepts in hypospadias repair. Current Opinion in Urology 9(6):513–516

Soergel M, Schaefer F 2002 Effect of hypertension on the progression of chronic renal failure in children. American Journal of Hypertension 15(2) Pt 2:53S–56S

Soliday E, Grey S, Lande MB 1999 Behavioral effects of corticosteroids in steroid-sensitive nephrotic syndrome. Pediatrics 104(4):e51

Struthers S, Scanlon J, Parker K et al 2003 Parental reporting of smelly urine and urinary tract infection. Archives of Disease in Childhood 88(3):250–252

Stull TL, Lipuma JJ 1991 Epidemiology and natural history of urinary tract infections in children. Medical Clinics of North America 75:287–297

Szabo R, Short RV 2000 How does male circumcision protect against HIV infection? British Medical Journal 320:1592–1594

Tasic V, Polenakovic M 2003 Occurrence of subclinical post-streptococcal glomerulonephritis in family contacts. Journal of Paediatrics and Child Health 39(3):177–179

van Ommen CH, Heyboer H, Groothoff JW et al 1998 Persistent tachypnea in children: keep pulmonary embolism in mind. Journal of Pediatric Hematology and Oncology 20(6):570–573 *van Savage J, Palanca L, Slaughenhoupt B 2000* A prospective randomized trial of dressings versus no dressings for hypospadias repair. Journal of Urology 164(3) Pt 2:981–983

Vijayan A, Behrend T, Miller SB 2000 Clinical use of growth factors in chronic renal failure. Current Opinion in Nephrology and Hypertension 9(1):5–10

Vujanic GM, Kelsey A, Mitchell C et al 2003 The role of biopsy in the diagnosis of renal tumors of childhood: Results of the UKCCSG Wilms' tumor study 3. Medical and Pediatric Oncology 40(1):18–22

Wilms' tumour: status report 1990 National Wilms' tumour study committee. Journal of Clinical Oncology 9:877–887

Wong W, McCall E, Anderson B 1996 Acute renal failure in the paediatric intensive care unit. The New Zealand Medical Journal 109(1035):459–461

Respiratory Illness in Children

Janet Kelsey, Gill McEwing

ABSTRACT

The primary aim of this chapter is to give the reader a theoretical grounding from which to care for children and young people with respiratory illnesses. The anatomy of the respiratory tract and the mechanism of external respiration are described. The effects of incomplete development of the respiratory system in children, and its impact on nursing care, are discussed. A detailed account of respiratory assessment is given, outlining some of the skills and specialised equipment required. The common respiratory infections encountered in children are discussed with their nursing management.

Learning Outcomes

- Demonstrate an understanding of the anatomy and physiology of the respiratory tract.

- Gain an overview of the nature of respiratory illness in children.

- Appreciate the role of the nurse in caring for children with respiratory illness.

- Identify the signs of respiratory distress.

- Use relevant literature and research to inform the nursing care of children with respiratory illness.

Introduction

The most common illnesses in infants and children in the UK are disorders of the respiratory system. Respiratory tract infections in children, although common, are not usually serious. Frequent infections occur in children because the immune system has not been exposed to common pathogens and therefore infections tend to develop with each new exposure. The risk of infection is also increased in children because the respiratory tract is relatively short. Most of these infections do not cause a serious problem to the child; however children are particularly vulnerable to respiratory problems because of their relatively high oxygen requirements and the immaturity of their respiratory system (Carter 1995). Respiratory disease in early childhood can interfere with the development of the lungs and cause permanent lung damage. Acute respiratory failure can result from any airway, pulmonary or neuromuscular disease that impairs oxygen exchange or elimination of carbon dioxide (Mackway-Jones et al 1997).

Some respiratory problems are more common at specific ages. The same organism can cause different illnesses at different ages. For example, the respiratory syncytial virus (RSV) frequently causes bronchiolitis in infants but causes only a sore throat and cold symptoms in older children (Meadow & Newell 2002).

The majority of infections (80%) are restricted to the upper respiratory tract, approximately 20% of these will become severe and require medical intervention, these include conditions such as bronchiolitis, laryngotracheobronchitis, epiglottitus, pneumonia and acute asthma (Morton & Phillips 1992, Thompson 1990). These are major causes of morbidity in children and a common reason for admission to hospital (Meadow & Newell 2002).

Respiratory illness accounts for 30–40% of acute medical admissions to hospital of children and over 450 deaths in England and Wales each year. The Child Health Committee (1997) reported that the principal cause for admission to hospital (30.9%) of children aged 0–4 years in England between 1993 and 1994 was a respiratory problem.

Anatomy and Physiology of the Respiratory Tract

The human body requires a constant supply of oxygen. Children have a higher metabolic rate than adults, and thus an increased need for oxygen, which demands that their respiratory system functions effectively. The respiratory system consists of the lungs, the airways, the chest wall and the pulmonary circulation. The lungs (Fig. 28.1) are situated in the thorax, the sides of the thorax are bounded by the rib cage; linking the ribs are the intercostal muscles. At the base of the thorax is a flexible sheet of muscle known as the diaphragm.

The primary function of the respiratory system is the exchange of gases between the environmental air and the blood. There are three steps in this process: the movement of air in and out of the lungs, the movement of gases between air spaces in the lungs and the blood, and the movement of blood from the capillaries surrounding the lungs to the body's organs and tissues. The first two processes are functions of the respiratory system, the third is performed by the cardiovascular system (McChance & Heuther 2002).

The respiratory system can be divided into the upper and lower airways. The upper airways consist of the nasopharynx and the oropharynx. These structures are lined with highly vascular, ciliated epithelium. This warms and moistens the inspired air and removes foreign particles from it as it passes into the lungs. During quiet respiration, air passes through the nose, nasopharynx and oropharynx to the lower airways. During exercise or when the nose is obstructed the mouth and oropharynx are used for ventilation, however by this route the air is not filtered or humidified as efficiently as via the nasopharynx. The larynx connects the upper and lower airways; it is a cartilaginous structure that prevents collapse of the airways during inspiration. Air then flows into the trachea, which is supported by U-shaped cartilage. The trachea divides into the two main bronchi, which in turn divide into bronchioles; there are sixteen divisions in total, ending in the terminal bronchioles. This multiple subdivision causes a decrease in the velocity of the air flow into the lungs, which allows for maximum gaseous exchange to take place. The bronchioles have cartilage within their walls until the tenth division. The terminal bronchioles continue to divide into smaller respiratory bronchioles, and then into the alveolar ducts. These lead to the alveolar sacs, which are made up of numerous alveoli. The alveoli (Fig. 28.2) are the primary gas-exchange units of the lungs; it is here that oxygen enters the blood and carbon dioxide is removed (McChance & Heuther 2002).

There are 20 million alveoli at birth, increasing to 300 million alveoli in the fully formed lungs of the adult (Meadow & Newell 2002). This means that infants and young children have a relatively small alveolar surface area for gaseous exchange. Each alveolus has a network of capillaries wrapped around it. The walls of the alveoli and the capillaries are only one cell thick. A thin layer of liquid covers their surface, which aids gaseous exchange between the inhaled air and the circulating blood.

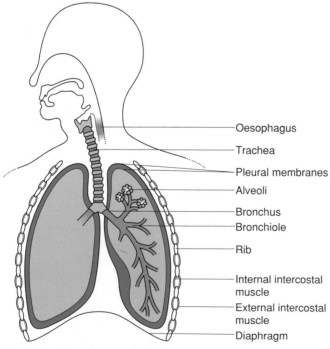

Fig. 28.1 • Basic structure of the lungs.

Oesophagus

Trachea

Pleural membranes

Alveoli

Bronchus

Bronchiole

Rib

Internal intercostal muscle

External intercostal muscle

Diaphragm

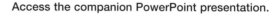

PowerPoint

Access the companion PowerPoint presentation.

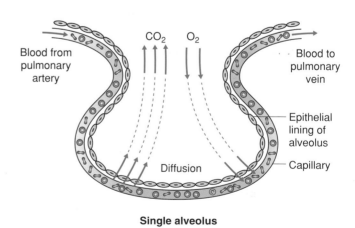

Single alveolus

Fig. 28.2 • A single alveolus.

Blood from pulmonary artery

CO_2 O_2

Blood to pulmonary vein

Epithelial lining of alveolus

Capillary

Diffusion

Inhalation involves the diaphragm contracting and flattening and the external intercostal muscles contracting, pulling the ribcage upwards and outwards. This increases the volume inside the thorax, decreases the pressure inside the lungs, and air is sucked in. When the diaphragm relaxes it domes up into the thorax and, as the external intercostal muscles relax, the rib cage drops down and moves inwards. This increases the pressure inside the lungs and forces air out. The internal intercostal muscles contract during strenuous breathing to pull the rib cage down to produce a forced expiration. There are two main considerations in infants and children. First, in the newborn, the diaphragm is not able to contract as effectively as in an older infant or child because it is attached higher at the front and is therefore longer. Second, infants and children have a relatively round thoracic cavity due to the horizontal position of the ribs, this places increased dependence on the diaphragm and abdomen as the primary means of ventilation.

PowerPoint

Access the companion PowerPoint presentation.

WWW

See respiratory movements online at:

- http://mywebpages.comcast.net/wnor/respiratory movements.htm

LUNG VOLUMES

The total capacity of a child's lungs increases from 1.4 litres in the 5-year-old child to 4.5 litres at the time of puberty (MacGregor 2000):

- At the end of quiet respiration, the air that remains in the lungs is termed the **functional residual capacity**.

- Following forced expiration, between 0.5 and 1.5 litres (depending on age) of air remains trapped in the alveoli, this minimal volume is called the **residual volume**.

- The additional volume of air forced out of the lungs during a forced expiration, between 0.5 and 1.5 litres is known as the **expiratory reserve volume**.

- During quiet respiration, the amount of air in the lungs increases from 0.7 litres at 5 years (or 2.25 litres at puberty) at the end of expiration to 0.8 litres at 5 years (or 2.55 litres at puberty) at the end of inspiration, this 0.1 litres (0.3 litres at puberty) of air moving in and out of the lungs is called the **tidal volume**.

- The **vital capacity** of the lungs is the amount of air moving when the patient is performing forced inspiration and forced expiration, which will be the sum of the inspiratory reserve volume, the expiratory reserve volume and the tidal volume. This volume is related to the size of the patient, at age 5 years it is approximately 1 litre; this increases to 3 litres at puberty (MacGregor 2000). The vital capacity can be increased if the patient stands up because the volume of blood in the lungs is reduced.

- The **peak flow** is the maximum velocity of air flow produced in a forced respiration. When this value is low it suggests that expiratory respiratory muscle activity is weak or that there is an obstruction to expiratory air flow due to some form of bronchoconstriction such as asthma.

NERVOUS CONTROL OF BREATHING

The respiratory centre is situated at the base of the brain and is made up of the medulla oblongata and the pons. The control of breathing has both automatic and voluntary components. Voluntary control allows for breathing to be integrated with voluntary actions such as blowing, singing and speaking. Automatic control involves input form two types of receptors, those that monitor the pH, carbon dioxide and oxygen levels in the blood and those that monitor breathing patterns and lung function.

Chemoreceptors assess the level of carbon dioxide and oxygen in the blood, messages are transmitted to the respiratory centre and ventilation is adjusted to maintain arterial blood gases within a normal range (Table 28.1). How much oxygen is in the blood depends on the:

- haemoglobin concentration in the blood (Hb g/dL)
- oxygen saturation of the haemoglobin (SaO_2)
- partial pressure of oxygen (PaO_2).

The central chemoreceptors located in the medulla oblongata monitor the carbon dioxide level in the blood by assessing the number of free hydrogen ions in the cerebrospinal fluid circulating around the medulla. This is important because the carbon dioxide level in the blood affects the pH level of the extracellular fluid of the brain. These receptors are extremely sensitive in the short term but long-term elevation of carbon dioxide levels, such as can occur in chronic respiratory disease, causes desensitisation of these receptors.

The carotid and aortic bodies are chemoreceptors that are sensitive to oxygen levels in the carotid artery and aorta, respectively. They are less responsive than the central

Table 28.1 Normal Arterial Blood Gas Values in Children

	Neonate at birth	Child
pH	7.32–7.42	7.35–7.45
$PaCO_2$	30–40 mm Hg	35–45 mmHg
HCO_3	20–26 mEq/L	22–28 mEq/L
PaO_2	60–80 mmHg	80–100 mmHg

chemoreceptors and are activated only when the oxygen level falls below 60 mmHg. Therefore hypoxia is the main stimulus for ventilation in persons with chronic hypercarbia (Porth 1994).

Reflect on your Practice

How would you explain to a junior nurse the importance of the correct level of oxygen administration when assisting a child with a chronic respiratory condition experiencing an acute respiratory illness?

The anatomy and physiology of the respiratory and cardio-vascular systems of children differs from that of adults. This influences the care given to children and hence must be considered when assessing and managing children with respiratory problems.

It is important to remember that anatomical differences influence the degree to which children respond to respiratory illness because of the smaller diameter of the airways (Fig. 28.3 and Table 28.2).

Poiseuille's law states that:

$$\text{Resistance } \alpha = \frac{1}{\text{Radius}^4}$$

Infant

1mm oedema=16 fold resistance increase

Adult

1mm oedema=2.4 fold resistance increase

Fig. 28.3 • Anatomical differences between the airways of an infant and of an adult.

That is, resistance to airflow is inversely proportional to the fourth power of the radius. In other words, a small amount of mucous or oedema in the airways will significantly increase resistance to airflow and therefore increase the work of breathing.

Powerpoint

Access the companion PowerPoint presentation.

Respiratory Assessment and Examination of the Chest

A calm manner should always be adopted when assessing any child with respiratory problems. The 'hands-off approach' can generate a lot of useful information gained through careful observation and this is particularly useful in very young children, who may resist physical examination. It is always important to leave the child with his or her carer in an upright position. Although observations focus on the respiratory status of the child, it is important to note the child's general appearance, level of engagement with carer, colour, hydration status and temperature. In addition, the ability of infants to feed should be noted. If at any time you feel the child needs immediate intervention, for example they are having difficulties breathing, then the assessment should be stopped and emergency care given to stabilise the child.

Assessment follows the ABC criteria for assessment in conjunction with neurological observations and provides a framework for rapid and effective nursing assessment of the child with respiratory problems. The survey should therefore include assessment of the following:

A. AIRWAY

Patency of the airway is assessed, observing for spontaneous ventilation and look, listen, feel. Note any presence of inspiratory noises. If the child is able to speak or is crying this indicates that the airway is patent. If there is no evidence of air movement then chin-lift or jaw-thrust should be carried out and the basic life support algorithm commenced.

B. BREATHING

To assess the adequacy of breathing the chest should be examined and the following assessed:

- The effort of breathing including respiratory rate, recession, grunting, use of accessory muscles and nasal flaring.
- The efficacy breathing including breath sounds and chest expansion/abdominal excursion.
- The effects of inadequate respiration including heart rate, oxygen saturation, skin colour and mental status.

Table 28.2 The Differences in the Anatomy and Physiology of the Respiratory and Cardiovascular Systems of Children (Cosby 1998 Cited by Dolan & Holt 2000, Hazinski 1992, Mackway-Jones et al 1997)

Factor	Nursing considerations
Airway	
Large head, short neck, inability to support head	Assistance required to maintain position of comfort
Large tongue	Airway is easily obstructed by tongue; proper positioning is often all that is necessary to open the airway
The floor of the mouth is easily compressible	Care is required when positioning of the fingers when holding the jaw
Infants less than 6 months old are obligate nose breathers	Obstruction of the nasal passages by mucus can compromise the infant's airway
Smaller diameter of all airways in a 1-year-old child. Tracheal diameter is less than the child's little finger	Small amounts of mucous or swelling easily obstruct the airways; child normally has increased airway resistance
The epiglottis is horseshoe shaped and projects posteriorly at 45%. The larynx is high and anterior	Tracheal intubation can be more difficult. A straight blade laryngoscope is used, cricoid pressure may be necessary to facilitate intubation
The trachea is short and soft. (The cricoid cartilage is the narrowest portion of neck)	Airway of infant can be compressed if neck is flexed or hyperextended. Tube displacement is more likely. Provides a natural seal for endotracheal tube
The cricoid ring is lined by pseudostratifed ciliated epithelium loosely bound to areolar tissue	Particularly susceptible to oedema. Uncuffed tubes are preferred in pre-pubertal children
Breathing	
Infants rely mainly on diaphragmatic breathing. The ribs lie more horizontally in infants and contribute less to chest expansion. Their muscles are more likely to fatigue compared with adults	Children are more prone to respiratory failure. Anything that impedes diaphragm contraction or movement, e.g. abdominal distension can contribute to the development of respiratory failure
Sternum and ribs are cartilaginous; chest wall is soft; intercostal muscles are poorly developed	Infant's chest wall may move inwards instead of outwards during inspiration (retractions) when lung compliance is decreased; greater intrathoracic pressure generated during inspiration. The compliant chest wall may allow serious parenchymal injuries to occur without rib fracture
Increased metabolic rate (about twice that of an adult); increased respiratory demand for oxygen consumption and carbon dioxide elimination	Respiratory distress increases oxygen demand, as does any condition that increases metabolic rate, e.g. fever
Lung compliance and high chest wall compliance in the neonate	Respiratory function inefficient during episodes of respiratory distress
Smaller amount of elastic and collagen tissue in the paediatric lung	May contribute to the increased incidence of pulmonary oedema, pneumomediastinum and pneumothorax in infants
Circulation	
Child's circulating blood volume is larger per unit of body weight (70–80 mL/kg) but absolute volume is relatively small; 70–80% of newborn's body weight is water, compared with 50–60% of an adult body weight; about half of this volume is extracellular	Blood loss considered minor in an adult may lead to shock in a child; decreased fluid intake or increased fluid loss quickly leads to dehydration. Acute blood loss produces symptoms when 20–25% of circulating volume has been lost. Dehydration will compromise peripheral perfusion when 7–10% of the infant or child's body weight and 5–7% of the adolescent or adult body weight is lost
Stroke volume is small and relatively fixed in infants. Cardiac output is directly related to heart rate	Stroke volume cannot increase to improve cardiac output. Response to volume therapy is therefore blunted
By the age of 2 years the myocardial function and response to fluid is similar to that of an adult	Tachycardia is the child's most efficient method of increasing cardiac output. However ventricular rates > 180–220 beats/min compromise diastolic filling time and coronary artery perfusion
Systemic vascular resistance rises after birth and continues to do so until adulthood	Children's normal values for blood pressure increase with age

Assessment of breathing therefore involves examination of the chest for the following:

- respiratory movements
- number rhythm, depth and quality of respirations
- character of breath sounds utilising the skills of palpation, auscultation and percussion.

Chest wall movement should be symmetric bilaterally and coordinated with breathing.

On inspiration, the chest rises and expands (Fig. 28.4A); on expiration, the chest descends and decreases in size (Fig. 28.4B). In children less than 6–7 years of age, respiratory movement will be mainly abdominal or diaphragmatic; in older children respirations are mainly thoracic.

To observe for chest expansion, stand at the child's head or feet and, looking down the midline, note any asymmetry of movement. Decreased movement on one side may be the result of foreign body obstruction, pneumonia, pneumothorax or atelactasis.

Respiratory movements can be felt by placing each hand flat against the chest or back with thumbs in the midline along the lower costal margin (Fig. 28.5). The hands move with the chest wall during respiration. The amount of respiratory excursion is evaluated and asymmetry is noted.

Palpation is carried out for voice conduction (vocal fremitus). Place the palmar surface of the hand on the child's chest and feel for vibrations as the child speaks. At the same time, move the hand symmetrically on either side of the sternum and vertebral column. Vocal fremitus is usually most prominent at the apex and least prominent at the base of the lungs. Absent or diminished vocal fremitus in the upper airway may indicate asthma or foreign body obstruction. Increased vocal fremitus may indicate pneumonia or atelectasis.

During palpation other abnormal vibrations that indicate pathological conditions are noted. These include pleural rub, which is felt as a grating sensation and is synchronous with respiration, and crepitation, which can be felt as a coarse crackly sensation and is the result of air escaping from the lungs to the subcutaneous tissue. This may be caused by injury or surgical intervention. Both crepitation and pleural rub can often be heard as well as felt.

The sinking-in of soft tissues relative to the cartilaginous and bony thorax may be noted in some respiratory disorders. This is recession, it is described as intercostal, subcostal, substernal, clavicular and suprasternal and it demonstrates increased work of breathing:

- Intercostal, subcostal or sternal recession show increased work of breathing.
- Recession is more easily seen in younger children whose chest wall is more compliant.

Fig. 28.5 • Respiratory movements.

A

B

Fig. 28.4 • Chest expansion.

- In children over 6 or 7 years, recession suggests severe respiratory problems.

- The degree of recession gives an indication of the severity of the breathing difficulty.

Powerpoint

Access the companion PowerPoint presentation.

Nasal flaring is also an indication of increased work of breathing. The enlargement of the nostrils helps to reduce nasal resistance and maintain airway patency; it is usually described as either minimal or marked. Head bobbing in the infant is a sign of dyspnoea.

Respiratory rates should be measured over a full minute (Table 28.3). It should be remembered that young children breathe diaphragmatically and therefore are observed by watching abdominal movement rather than the movement of the chest. A decreasing rate or rhythm may indicate deterioration rather than improvement in the child's condition (Mackway-Jones et al 1997). A resting rate of >60 breaths/minute is a sign of respiratory distress in a child irrespective of age (Cosby 1998 cited by Dolan & Holt 2000). Tachypnoea at rest indicates a need for increased ventilation.

Respiratory Rate

Further information about the severity of the child's illness may be gained by measurement of oxygen saturation (SaO_2) levels with a pulse oximeter (Fig. 28.6). A saturation of less than 92% while breathing air, or less than 95% when breathing oxygen, is low. Rajesh et al (2000) evaluated respiratory rate as an indicator of hypoxia in infants <2 months of age and concluded that a respiratory rate of >60/minute is a good predictor of hypoxia and that the infants should be treated with oxygen should the facility to measure SaO_2 not be available. It should be remembered that pulse oximetry is less accurate when the SaO_2 is less than 70%, when shock is present, and in the pres-

ence of carboxyhaemoglobin (Mackway-Jones et al 1997). If there is evidence of respiratory or circulatory failure then arterial blood gases are needed.

www

Learn about the oxyhaemoglobin dissociation curve at:
- http://www.ebme.co.uk

The effectiveness of breathing is also assessed by observing breath sounds. Auscultation allows assessment of breath sounds for pitch, intensity, quality, location and duration. Breath sounds are best heard if the child inspires deeply. Normal breath sounds are vesicular, soft and low pitched on inspiration followed by shorter sound on expiration; bronchial or tubular, similar to sounds heard upon auscultation over the larynx during respiration; and bronchovesicular, a mixture of bronchial and vesicular sounds. Vesicular are heard over most of the chest, except over the larynx and trachea, and, in infants, over the upper chest. Infants' breath sounds are bronchovesicular in the upper chest because of increased transmission (Thompson 1990). Fluid,

Fig. 28.6 • Measurement of oxygen saturation levels.

Age (years)	Breaths/min
<1	30–40
2–5	20–30
5–12	15–20
>12	12–16

Table 28.3 Normal Respiratory Rates (Mackway-Jones et al 1997)

air or solid masses in the pleural space all interfere with the conduction of breath sounds.

Consolidation or solidification of a portion of the lung caused by, for example, pneumonia will result in tubular or bronchial breathing being heard over the posterior chest due to increased transmission between the trachea and the periphery of the chest (Thompson 1990).

Alert, diminished or absent breath sounds are always abnormal.

Percussion or tapping of the lungs (Fig. 28.7) is carried out to determine the presence and location of air, liquid and solid material in the lung and to evaluate the densities, position and landmarks of the underlying organs. Normally, the percussion note in a lung full of air is resonant. When there is fluid in the chest, e.g. pleural effusion, the note becomes flat. With pneumonia where there is an increased amount of fluid but not in the chest the note becomes dull. With excess air, e.g. asthma, the note is hyperresonant. It is normal to find dullness over the liver and heart.

Activity

To help discriminate between hollow and flat sounds
Try tapping various parts of an internal wall, see if you can distinguish between the hollow sound of the unsupported plaster board and the flat sound of the solid wood or concrete support.

Voice sounds are also part of auscultation of the lung. Normally, vocal resonance or voice sounds are heard but the sounds are muffled and indistinct. Hearing clear distinct sounds is an abnormal finding and is caused by the same conditions causing abnormal vocal fremitus.

Various respiratory illnesses produce adventitious sounds that are not normally heard over the chest; these are not alterations in normal breath sounds but are additional abnormal sounds.

Fig. 28.7 • Percussion

The effects of inadequate respiration can be seen by examining heart rate, skin colour and mental status. These are linked to the examination of circulation and disability.

C. CIRCULATION

Adequacy of circulation is assessed by examining the cardiovascular status and looking for the effects of circulatory inadequacy on other organs (Mackway-Jones et al 1997).

Vital Signs

The child's vital signs should be appropriate for the child's age and clinical condition. A child normally has a faster heart rate (Table 28.4) and respiratory rate and a lower arterial pressure than an adult. The child's heart rate and pulse volume should be assessed by palpating both central and peripheral pulses. It is important to note that normal vital signs are not always appropriate when a child is seriously ill, indeed a normal heart rate and respiratory rate may indicate cardiopulmonary arrest is imminent (Hazinski 1992). Hypoxia produces tachycardia and is to be expected; bradycardia is a sign of respiratory failure and is a preterminal sign. Absent peripheral and weak central pulses are signs of advanced shock and hypotension in children (Mackway-Jones et al 1997).

An accurate pulse should be measured for a full minute and be consistent with the apex beat. If measuring the heart rate of children less than 2 years of age, a stethoscope should be placed over the apex of the heart and the beats counted for a full minute. Sinus tachycardia is common in the unwell anxious child and further assessment should be carried out to identify the cause.

Blood Pressure (Table 28.5)

Expected systolic blood pressure (BP) = 80 + (age in years × 2) The size of the child's limb must be taken into consideration when taking blood pressure. Make sure the width of the blood pressure (BP) cuff is about two-thirds the length of the child's upper arm (Fig. 28.8). A cuff that is too large may produce a reading that is too low; a cuff that is too small may give a false high reading (Thomas 1996).

Table 28.4 Normal Heart Rates (Mackway-Jones et al 1997)	
Age (years)	**Beats/min**
<1	110–160
2–5	95–140
5–12	80–120
<12	60–100

Table 28.5 Systolic Blood Pressure by Age (Mackway-Jones et al 1997)

Age (years)	Systolic blood pressure
<1	70–90
2–5	80–100
5–12	90–110
>12	100–120

Children in early shock may have a normal blood pressure reading initially, hypotension is often a late sign and preterminal sign of circulatory failure. Small quantitative changes in the child's blood pressure may indicate significant qualitative changes in the child's clinical condition (Hazinski 1992). It is therefore imperative that accurate and current observations are taken into account when assessing the child's circulatory status.

Skin Perfusion and Body Temperature

The skin colour and temperature should be consistent over the trunk and limbs. Clinical signs of poor perfusion include peripherally cool skin, pallor, mottling, peripheral cyanosis and capillary refill >2 seconds. By the time central cyanosis is visible in acute respiratory distress respiratory arrest is very

Fig. 28.8 • Observation of a child's blood pressure.

close (Mackway-Jones et al 1997). Capillary refill is a quick and easy method for determining the efficacy of respiratory function. A raised digit is pressed for 5 seconds and the time taken for blood to return to the area is estimated in seconds. A capillary refill time of greater than 2 seconds in a child and 3 seconds in a neonate is a sign of poor oxygenation. Ambient temperature should always be considered in the interpretation of capillary refill.

The normal circadian range of infant's temperatures over the 24-hour period has been described as ranging from 36°C at night to 37.8°C during active periods in the day (Table 28.6). In addition, there is now recognised to be a variable fluctuation between individuals of 0.5°C (Mackowiak et al 1992). Therefore we should accept individual variations in normal body temperature, recognising that time of day and age of child may affect expected normal values.

D. DISABILITY

Parents are usually the first to recognise any changes in their child's level of consciousness and it is therefore important to listen to what they say. A hypoxic child may be irritable or agitated early on but increasingly lethargic later. He or she might fail to recognise or interact, e.g. maintain eye contact, with the parents or might not respond to stimuli, e.g. unfamiliar nurses. A progressive drop in level of consciousness is a late sign of hypoxia and may be an indication of impending respiratory distress. Other factors that may lead to a decreasing level of consciousness are shock, sepsis, ingestion of depressants, metabolic abnormalities, hypothermia and head injuries (Thomas 1996). The level of consciousness should be assessed using the AVPU scale:

A = **a**lert

V = responds to **v**oice

P = responds to **p**ain

U = **u**nresponsive.

Any problem with ABC must be addressed before assuming that a decrease in conscious level is due to a primary neurological problem (Mackway-Jones et al 1997).

Table 28.6 Normal Variations in Temperature Related to Age

Age (years)	Temperature (°C)
<1	37.5–37.7
2–5	37.0–37.2
5–12	36.7–36.8
>12	36.6

The final but integral part of the child's assessment is their medical history. Factors to be taken into consideration include the following symptoms:

- Is the child breathless:
  - When? At rest, walking, talking, sleeping, feeding?
- Does the child have a cough?
  - What type?
  - How long has the child had this?
- When do the symptoms occur, daytime, night-time?
- Are the symptoms improving or worsening?
- Are there any aggravating or precipitating factors? Does anything relieve the symptoms?
- Are the symptoms associated with anything, e.g. feeding? Is the child able to take feeds?
- How long has the child been unwell, has this happened suddenly, did it occur over time?
- Does the child have a sore throat?
- Is there any nasal discharge, has the child a cough, is the cough productive, what colour is the sputum, how long have these been present?
- Has the child's sleep been affected?
- Is the child's breathing noisy, in what way? Ask the parents to describe any noises they have heard.
- What has the child's activity level been like?

Less specific symptoms to observe for include:

- pyrexia
- urinary output
- anorexia
- vomiting
- diarrhoea
- abdominal pain
- meningism.

In addition, the family will be asked about the child's previous medical history, family and social history, environmental factors and developmental history including immunisation status. It is of interest to note that Elphick et al (2001) found 'wheeze' to be a commonly chosen word used by parents to describe their child's noisy breathing. However, there was wide variation in what parents meant by this term, with many using the word inappropriately. The authors conclude that:

This highlights the need for accurate history taking, as parents' initial response may be to use words that they perceive as being a medical term. The responsibility lies with the doctor to ensure that interpretation of the language used by

Table 28.7 Terminology Used to Describe Different Patterns of Respiration

Term	Description
Tachypnoea	Increased rate
Bradypnoea	Decreased rate
Dyspnoea	Difficulty in breathing
Apnoea	Cessation or inability to breathe
Hypoventilation	Decreased and irregular depth of respirations
Hyperventilation	Increased rate and depth
Hypercapnia	Increased levels of carbon dioxide
Hypoxia	Low level of oxygenation
See-saw	Chest falls on inspiration and rises on expiration
Cheyne–Stokes	Altered rate and depth of respirations with periods of apnoea

parents reflects accurately the noise they mean to describe (Elphick et al 2001) (Table 28.7)

Summary

The diagnosis of acute respiratory disease in childhood is largely a clinical one. It rests on history and examination with the aid of chest radiograph when necessary. The clinical signs of respiratory failure include those demonstrating evidence of a significant increase in the work of breathing, e.g. severe retractions or grunting, inadequate ventilation rate, apnoea or gasping, reduced or absent inspiratory breath sounds and alterations in level of consciousness and evidence of compromise in systemic perfusion, e.g. significant tachycardia, bradycardia and extended capillary refill. Central cyanosis is a late sign of severe hypoxia and requires urgent treatment (Hazinski 1992, Morton & Phillips 1992).

Management of Respiratory Illness in Children

The aims of the management of respiratory disease are applicable to all respiratory illnesses in addition to the disease specific treatments. These aims of management include to:

- Monitor the child's vital signs, effort and efficacy of breathing and effect of inadequate respiration, i.e. oxygen saturations, colour and mental status.

- Facilitate respiratory effort and maximise oxygen delivery to maintain O_2 saturations above 92%:
  - position the child for maximum comfort and to facilitate respiratory movements
  - decrease oxygen demand by reducing stress, minimal handling and fever
  - provide humidified and monitored supplemental oxygen by age-appropriate means, i.e. head box for infants, mask for older children.
- Minimise intrusive examinations and treatments.
- Prevent complications such as hypoxia.
- Promote hydration and prevent dehydration by utilising nasogastric or intravenous fluids to maintain adequate fluid intake.
- Evaluate the effect of pyrexia on the child and administer antipyretics as appropriate.
- Provide nutrition.
- Instigate appropriate pharmacological interventions.
- Communicate effectively with the child and family.
- Provide psychological support for the child and family.
- Provide opportunistic health education.
- Prevent spread of infection.
- Provide clear and explicit discharge advice.

Respiratory Infection

Infections of the respiratory tract are described in a number of ways depending on the area of involvement (Fig. 28.9). However, the infections tend to spread from one area to another because of the continuous nature of the mucous membrane that lines the respiratory tract and the shorter distance between the anatomical structures in children. In addition, the short, open Eustachian tube allows easy access to the middle ear. Infections of the respiratory tract may therefore involve more than one structure.

The largest percentage of infections accounting for acute illness in children is caused by viruses. Infants under 3 months of age have a lower infection rate, which then rises between the ages of 3 and 6 months and remains high through the toddler years. However, by the age of 5 years viral infections are less frequent, although the incidence of *Mycoplasma pneumoniae* and group B streptococcal infections rises.

UPPER RESPIRATORY TRACT INFECTION

The average child has between four and twelve upper respiratory tract infections a year and 90% of these are viral, requiring symptomatic management only. Of the remaining 10%, group B haemolytic streptococcus is common and requires treatment with penicillin. However, we should

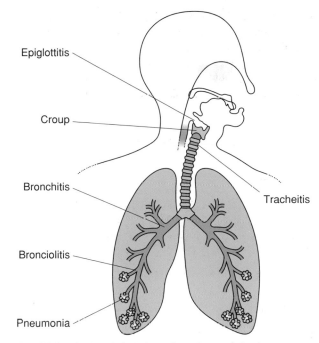

Fig. 28.9 • Anatomic location of respiratory infections.

always remain vigilant for the possibility that a child with a mild upper respiratory tract infection may have an accompanying illness such as meningitis.

Whooping Cough

Pertussis or whooping cough is an acute respiratory infection caused by *Bordetella pertussis*. It occurs mainly in non-immunised children and a single attack confers lifetime immunity.

Characteristics of Whooping Cough
Begins with the symptoms of an upper respiratory tract infection:

- Corzya.
- Sneezing.
- Low-grade temperature.
- Cough, which continues for some weeks and becomes more severe and paroxysmal. May consist of short rapid coughs followed by an inspiratory 'whoop' sound during which the child's face becomes flushed. This can continue until mucus is vomited.

Specific Treatment
The management of whooping cough includes administration of antimicrobial therapy, e.g. erythromycin, as this may reduce the period of infectivity. However, it does not alter the course of the illness. Household and other close contacts should also be treated.

Croup Syndromes

Croup is a general term that applies to any condition producing inspiratory stridor. Stridor is a harsh vibratory sound caused by partial obstruction of the upper airway. Croup syndromes include laryngotracheobronchitis (LTB), spasmodic croup, bacterial tracheitis and epiglottitis. LTB and croup are often used synonymously.

LTB is common cause of upper airway obstruction in children and is usually mild but sometimes can be serious (Geelhoed et al 1996). It is an acute inflammation of the upper and lower respiratory tract that occurs in children aged 6 months to 4 years, usually occurring in the winter months. The peak incidence is during the second year of life with boys more affected than girls.

Characteristics of Croup

Croup is usually preceded by an upper respiratory tract infection:

- rhinorrhea
- coryza
- low-grade fever
- sudden onset – often at night.

Presenting with:

- inspiratory stridor
- barking cough
- harsh cry/hoarseness.

If obstruction is severe:

- tachypnoea
- stridor
- intercostal, supraclavicular, substernal and suprasternal inspiratory retractions.

As condition worsens:

- cyanosis
- increased respiratory effort
- restlessness
- reduced stridulous sound (Rudolf & Levene 1999).

These symptoms are a result of oedema of the larynx and trachea. They are usually triggered by recent infection with the parainfluenza virus (Ausejo et al 1999), although other pathogens can be involved (respiratory syncytial virus, adenovirus, enterovirus and rhinovirus). The incidence of croup is 1.5–6 % of children less than 6 years of age, of these 1.5–31% are admitted to hospital (Marx et al 1997, cited in Ausejo et al 1999).

Activity

Review Poiseuille's law and consider the effect of a distressed child with a more turbulent airflow.

Specific Treatment

- Maintain airway, less than 5% require intubation and this is usually due to gradual deterioration rather than acute obstruction.

- Nebulised and/or oral glucocorticoids (Ausejo et al 1999, Geelhoed et al 1996) usually nebulised budesonide and oral dexamethasone (Rudolf & Levene 2003).

- Inhaled steroids reduce upper airway oedema (Rudolf & Levene 1999), which has a rapid and sustained effect (D'Amore & Campbell Hewson 2002).

- Nebulised adrenaline has been shown to provide temporary relief to patients with croup but is not thought to have long-term benefits (Waiisman et al 1992, cited by Ausejo et al 1999).

Evidence-based Practice

Cold humidified air (mist therapy) is not effective in improving clinical symptoms in children with moderate croup. Discuss.

Epiglottitis

This is mainly seen in children aged 2–5 years. The infection is usually caused by *Haemophilus influenzae* B and the condition is becoming rare as a result of the introduction of the HIB immunisation of infants (Tanner et al 2002).

WWW

Childhood immunization
Familiarise yourself with the guidance notes for professionals:
- http://www.doh.gov.uk/greenbook/greenbbookpdf/chapter-16-latout.pdf

Characteristics of Epiglottitis

- Short history.
- Fever.
- Stridor.
- Dyspnoea.
- Systemically unwell: pale, toxic, lethargic.
- May drool and unable to swallow but have minimal cough (Tanner et al 2002).
- Child often adopts the characteristic posture of sitting upright, mouth open and their chin thrust forward (Rudolf & Levene 1999).
- Extreme anxiety.

The infection causes inflammatory oedema of the supra-glottic area, which includes the epiglottis and the pharyngeal structures. If the condition is suspected, examination of the mouth must be avoided because acute or total airway obstruction could result. The child should be examined only with an experienced anaesthetist ready to intubate if required (Rudolf & Levene 1999). Do not lie the child down because this forces the epiglottis to fall backwards, leading to complete airway obstruction. Radiography of the neck is justified only if diagnosis is in doubt and should take place only if the child is stable; radiography in lateral position may also precipitate respiratory arrest due to complete airway obstruction (Tanner et al 2002). It is also not advisable to perform any procedure that may increase the child's anxiety (e.g. taking a blood specimen) as this could precipitate airway spasm and cause death (Porth 1994).

Specific Treatment

If epiglottitis is suspected then emergency intubation should be performed to protect the airway (Tanner et al 2002). Intravenous antibiotics are required immediately following intubation, usually chloramphenicol or ampicillin (Rudolf & Levene 1999). Recovery is usually rapid once the airway is established and antibiotic therapy given.

Apnoea

Temporary cessation of breathing can be the result of central respiratory depression or from mechanical obstruction. It can occur in the first 2 days of infections particularly respiratory syncytial virus and pertussis (Meadow & Newell 2002). When apnoea is associated with cyanosis or unconsciousness then possible causes that need to be considered are seizures, congenital heart disease or airway obstruction.

Aspirated Foreign Body

Usually occurs in toddlers who are mobile and put small objects in their mouths. Small beads, coins and foodstuffs are the most common objects aspirated. Peanuts are the most dangerous because they swell in the airway, becoming firmly embedded and difficult to remove because they fragment (Rudolf & Levene 1999). Initially, the child may suffer from acute choking but the aspiration of a foreign body may not be recognised. Obstruction may be complete or incomplete. Incomplete obstruction usually allows the passage of air either in both directions or one only. Complete obstruction prevents either inspiration or expiration.

Characteristics of Aspirated Foreign Body
- Acute onset.
- Respiratory distress.
- Wheeze often unilateral.
- Persistent cough.

- Asymmetry of chest.
- Mediastinal shift.
- Dull percussion if collapse has occurred (Rudolf & Levene 1999).

Specific Treatment

A bronchoscopy under general anaesthetic to remove the foreign body is required. It is important that this is performed as soon as possible to prevent coughing moving the object back up into the trachea, which may lead to more severe obstruction of the airway (Mackway-Jones et al 1997).

Activity

Look at your local health education literature to find the advice given to parents regarding suitable toys for toddlers and first aid in the event of aspiration of a foreign body.

WWW

Read the advice from the Child Accident Prevention Trust:
- http://www.capt.org.uk

Bronchiolitis

This condition is the most common cause of severe respiratory infection in infancy, usually occurring in the winter months. It is a viral infection with 75% of cases due to respiratory syncytial virus, other pathogens implicated include adenovirus, parainfluenza and rhinovirus. By the age of 2 years 90% of children are immune to respiratory syncytial virus (Meadow & Newell 2002). It usually occurs in children under the age of 18 months the most serious cases are infants under 6 months old. The mortality rate is 1 in 5000–20,000. The infection causes inflammatory obstruction of the small airways and necrosis of the cells lining the lower airways. The ciliary damage impairs the clearance of secretions and combined with increased mucosal secretion, submucosal oedema and desquamation of cells, there is obstruction at the bronchiolar level with atelactasis and hyperinflation. The child is often able to inhale but has difficulty exhaling. Air becomes trapped below the obstruction and interferes with gaseous exchange. Hypoxia and in severe cases hypercapnia may occur (Porth 1994).

Characteristics of Bronchiolitis (Meadow & Newell 2002, Mackway-Jones et al 1997)
- Initial coryza.
- Fever.
- Tachycardia.
- Tachypnoea.

435

- Irregular breathing, recurrent apnoea.
- Cough.
- Subcostal and intercostal recession.
- Irritability.
- Poor feeding.
- Widespread wheeze and crepitations.
- Hyperventilated chest.
- Cyanosis/pallor.

The typical appearance of a baby with acute bronchiolitis is therefore one with:

- marked breathlessness
- rapid respirations
- distressing cough
- retraction of lower ribs and sternum
- wheezing depending on degree of airway obstruction.

Many infants with bronchiolitis can be managed at home however careful assessment is required in deciding which infants need hospitalisation. The NHS Executive guidelines for the management of acute respiratory failure in normal infants and children recognise that a respiratory rate of > 50/minute, a heart rate of > 140/minute and O_2 saturation of < 92% in air, with the use of accessory muscles defines a moderately severe episode and requires hospitalisation (Table 28.8).

Respiratory failure may be preceded by cyanosis, pallor, listlessness and reduction or absence of breath sounds (Porth 1994) and hypoxia requires urgent intervention.

Specific Treatment
- Because of the risk of apnoea, small infants should be nursed using apnoea monitors or O_2 saturation monitors (Mackway-Jones et al 1997).
- Antibiotics, bronchodilators and steroids have no positive effect on this condition (Mackway-Jones et al 1997).
- Some infants (2%) suffer recurrent apnoea attacks, exhaustion or hypercapnia and hypoxia and require mechanical ventilation.

Reflect on your Practice

What advice have you witnessed being given to children's families regarding the spread of RSV?

Activity

Review the effect of a raised temperature on an infant's metabolic rate and oxygen requirements.
- Why is this important in infants with bronchiolitis?

Table 28.8 Assessment of Illness Severity

Clinical parameter	Severity	
	Mild	*Moderate to severe*
Activity level	Alert	Reduced level of consciousness, exhausted or fatigued
Heart rate	<140/min	>140/min
Respiratory rate	<50/min	>50/min
Oxygen saturation	>92%	<92%
Temperature	<380	>380
Recession	Mild	Marked
Nasal flaring	None	Some
Feeding	Taking three-quarters or more than half of normal feeds	Taking less than half of normal feeds
Colour	Pink	Pallor, mottling, cyanosed or grey
Level of hydration	Normal	Evidence of dehydration
Apnoea	None	History of
Capillary refill	<2 seconds	>2 seconds

Scenario

Emma is 3 months old, she is admitted to the assessment ward accompanied by her anxious parents. The GP visited her at home and organised for an emergency admission.

Emma has had a runny nose for 2 days and is off her feeds. She has felt hot since yesterday evening and over the past few hours she has become quite pale. However, her mother reports that Emma is not as irritable as last night and has at last stopped crying:
- What framework would you utilise to assess Emma's physiological status?
- What observations do you need to carry out?
- What would you expect these observations to be?
- Would you categorise Emma's present condition as mild, moderate or severe?
- Is there any information in the history given that would cause concern?
- What care would you expect to be initiated?
- What ongoing care would Emma require?

PowerPoint

Emma's scenario is repeated on the companion PowerPoint presentation. Work through it here or on the PowerPoint. Answers are provided at the end of the chapter or on the presentation.

LOWER RESPIRATORY TRACT INFECTION

Pneumonia

Pneumonia is an infection of the lower respiratory tract most commonly due to bacterial or viral pathogens. Pneumonia can be classified according to its anatomical distribution:

- Lobar pneumonia occurs when there is involvement of a large portion of or an entire lobe of a lung.
- In bronchopneumonia there is patchy consolidation involving several lobes of the lungs.
- Interstitial pneumonia involves the walls surrounding the alveoli and bronchioles; this type of pneumonia is usually caused by viral or mycoplasmal infections (Porth 1994).

Pneumonia is also classified by the infective pathogen e.g. streptococcus or mycoplasma. The incidence of bacterial pneumonia is highest amongst children < 2 years of age, with boys affected more than girls (2:1 ratio). Viral infections with RSV are also common in this age group; this is the most common cause of viral pneumonia. Death rates from pneumonia in England and Wales for children under one year are 111 per million population. Children aged 1–4 years 14 per million population and 5–14 years 3 per million population (Office of National Statistics 2003). Children who are chronically sick or have congenital abnormalities are at greater risk (Mackway-Jones et al 1997). Predisposing factors should always be considered in children who present with pneumonia such as congenital abnormality of the bronchi or inhaled foreign body (Rudolf & Levene 1999).

Bronchopneumonia

This condition occurs in young children and older children with chronic conditions that affect their respiratory function (Meadow & Newell 2002). A large number of different organisms can be responsible. Bronchopneumonia usually follows another respiratory illness such as bronchiolitis, whooping cough or viral infection.

Characteristics of Bronchopneumonia (Meadow & Newell 2002)
- Tachypnoea.
- Dry cough initially then productive with purulent sputum.

- Fever.
- Fretfulness.
- Intercostal/subcostal recession.
- Grunting in infants.
- Nasal flaring.
- Generalised crepitations.
- Cyanosis in severe cases.

Lobar Pneumonia

Around 90% of cases of lobar pneumonia are caused by *Streptococcus pneumoniae*.

Characteristics of Lobar Pneumonia (Meadow & Newell 2002)
- Sudden illness.
- High fever.
- Flushed.
- Tachypnoea.
- Cyanosis in severe cases.
- Respiratory distress.
- Intercostal/subcostal recession.
- Grunting in infants.
- Nasal flaring.
- Pleuritic pain – child leans forward towards affected side.
- May have referred pain in abdomen or shoulder tip.

Specific Treatment

Broad-spectrum antibiotics are usually administered, with choice of antibiotic being based on the most likely pathogen dictated by the child's age and clinical presentation. Physiotherapy is no longer considered beneficial in children with pneumonia.

 WWW

Read more about this condition online:
- http://kidshealth.org/parent/infections/index.html

Seminar discussion topic

There is an increased risk of pneumonia in the first year of life if parents smoke:
- What other potential health risks are there to children in a smoking household?
- Should smoking be banned completely?

TUBERCULOSIS

After years of decline in the incidence of this disease, the global incidence is now increasing. The World Health Organization (WHO) estimates that one-third of the world's population is infected with *Mycobacterium tuberculosis*. Infection rates are highest in South-east Asia, China, India, Africa and Latin America (Nelson 1996). Watson & Moss (2001) report that, in the year 2000 in England and Wales, 235 schoolchildren aged 5–14 were notified has having tuberculosis. Most of these will not have been infectious but some will have been smear positive and therefore potential sources of infection. Most children are infected by someone close to them but outbreaks also occur in other meeting places, e.g. schools. In 2001, the biggest ever school outbreak of tuberculosis recorded in the UK occurred in Leicester.

Common Presenting Symptoms

- Cough and respiratory symptoms.
- Mild dyspnoea.
- Weight loss and anorexia.
- Fever may occur.

These are gradual in onset and increase in severity as the disease progresses. Investigations include chest radiography, tuberculin test, gastric aspiration and sputum testing. Treatment is by antituberculosis drugs for between 3–6 months under the care of a clinician with experience in tuberculosis care.

Asthma

The changes in prevalence of asthma in children are difficult to determine because of changes in diagnostic practice (Magnus & Jaakkola et al 1997) but, however defined, asthma and wheezing in children has increased dramatically over the past few decades (Kaur et al 1998). Asthma is thought to affect approximately 10% of children and the incidence and severity of the disease appears to be increasing (Cross 1999). This increase is thought to be due to environmental factors (Caldwell 1998). It is difficult to diagnose asthma in the very young because it is hard to distinguish between asthma and other causes of wheezing. Epidemiological studies suggest that up to 30% of all children under the age of 3 years have had an acute episode of wheezing (Barnes 2003). This makes asthma the most common medical condition of childhood (Phelan 1994). There are approximately 2000 deaths (adult and children) each year in the UK due to asthma; 80% of these are thought to be preventable.

WWW

Read the most recent audits on the prevalence of asthma in the UK:

- http://www.asthma.org.uk/about/images/childrenaudit02.pdf

Asthma is a chronic inflammatory disorder of the airways. The National Heart, Lung and Blood Institute (1992, cited in Greyson 1993) describes asthma as 'airway obstruction that is reversible, airway inflammation, and increased airway responsiveness to a variety of stimuli'.

The aetiology of asthma is multifactorial (Barnes 2003). There is often a family history of atopy, asthma or allergies and, in addition to this, there are precipitating factors such as infection, allergic triggers, tobacco smoke or physical or emotional stress. Some of the possible reasons for an exacerbation of an asthma attack are:

- Predisposing factors such as:
  - a strong genetic factor (Smith 1995)
  - maternal smoking
  - not breast-fed for the first 4 months of life (Oddy et al 1999)
  - family atopy (Smith 1995).
- Indoor triggers such as:
  - allergy to house-dust mite (Smith 1995)
  - allergy to animal dander (Caldwell 1998)
  - tobacco smoke (Cook & Strachan 1997)
- Outdoor triggers:
  - allergy to pollen (Smith 1995)
  - cold weather (Caldwell 1998)
  - air pollutants
  - industrial chemicals (Smith 1995).
- Other possible triggers:
  - viral infection (Johnston et al 1995)
  - exercise (de Bisschop et al 1999)
  - food allergies (Valman 1993)
  - stress, emotion and laughing (Valman 1993)
  - high salt intake (Medici et al 1993).

Asthma is a hyperresponsiveness of the airways induced by a trigger (Barnes 2003). It commonly presents as a lower airway obstruction; the wheezing is generated by turbulent airflow causing oscillation of the bronchial wall.

Three factors are involved in the asthmatic response:

1. Bronchospasm:
   - narrowing of the bronchial walls due to contraction of the smooth muscle
   - more severe in the smaller bronchi and bronchioles, where there is no cartilage in the walls.

2. Inflammation:
   - causes the airways to become hyperresponsive and narrow easily in reaction to a wide range of stimuli

- further narrowing of the airways by the invasion of the mucosa, submucosa and muscle tissue by inflammatory cells.

3. Inflammatory cells:
   - mainly eosinophils but also contain neutrophils macrophages and mast cells
   - contain chemical mediators, including histamine, prostaglandins and leukotrienes, which cause vasodilation and increased capillary permeability
   - result in mucus production and oedema.

The lumen of the airways is therefore narrowed by contraction of the smooth muscle, mucosal oedema and the hypersecretion of mucus (Fig. 28.10) (Frakes 1997, Hunter 1995).

CHARACTERISTICS OF SEVERE ASTHMA (BARNES 2003, BARRY & O'CALLINGHAN 1997)

- Too breathless to talk.
- Chest recession/use of accessory muscles.
- Respiratory rate >50 breaths/minute (children under 5 years) or respiratory rate >30 breaths/min (children 5 years and over).

Normal

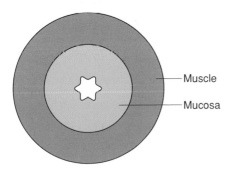

Inflamed airways

Fig. 28.10 • The asthma response.

- Heart rate >130 beats/minute (children under 5 years) or >120 beats/minute (children 5 years and over).
- Peak flow reduced to <50% of expected.
- Wheezing may or may not be a prominent feature.
- Use of accessory muscles of respiration.

CHARACTERISTICS OF LIFE-THREATENING ASTHMA (BARNES 2003, BARRY & O'CALLINGHAN 1997)

- Conscious level depression.
- Agitation.
- Exhaustion.
- Poor respiratory effort.
- Cyanosis.
- Oxygen saturation levels < 85% in air.
- Silent chest.
- Peak expiratory flow rate (PEF) < 30%.

There are two phases of the asthmatic response (Thompson & Gustafson 1996). The first phase occurs within minutes of the exposure to the stimuli, reaches a peak in about 30 minutes and subsides after approximately 2 hours. It includes oedema, mucus secretion and bronchospasm-induced wheezing (Frakes 1997). The second phase occurs about 4–12 hours after the exposure; it reaches a peak after about 4–8 hours but can last for more than 24 hours. This inflammatory reaction can lead to damage of lung tissue. The airways are hypersensitive to allergic stimulation in this phase, which can result in further inflammation and bronchoconstriction.

PRINCIPLES OF ASTHMA MANAGEMENT

In the event of an acute asthmatic attack the child should be given 2–4 puffs of a β2-agonist, via spacer and face-mask; alternatively, oral soluble prednisolone can be given (British Thoracic Society 2003).

If an acute attack fails to respond to the child's usual treatment then nebulised β2-agonists can be given driven by compressed oxygen (Brewin 1997, Mackway-Jones et al 1997). The dose required is 0.15 mg/kg (maximum dose of 5 mg) every 20 minutes for the first hour (Frakes 1997). In the case of life-threatening asthma, continuous nebulised β2-agonists may need to be used until the condition stabilises. Intravenous drugs may be necessary because inhaled drugs are not effective during severe asthmatic attacks because the airways are completely obstructed by inflammation and mucus (Jordan & White 2001). ECG monitoring should be used if frequent doses of nebulised salbutamol or intravenous salbutamol are given. In the event of a severe attack, a short course of oral steroids may be required. Prednisolone can be given for 3–4 days; this will not require tapering off and will not cause adrenal suppression or affect growth (Rudolf & Levene 1999).

In the event of a severe attack, a short course of oral steroids may be required.

In severe asthma, nebulised ipratropium bromide can be given in addition to maximal doses of bronchiodilators (Frakes 1997, Mackway-Jones et al 1997).

Humidified oxygen may be required to maintain the child's oxygen saturation. The method of oxygen administration chosen depends on the child's age and condition. Transcutaneous measurement of oxygen saturation is used for continuous oxygen assessment if the child is hypoxic, so that oxygen therapy can be titrated against the oxygen saturation levels. Arterial blood gas monitoring may be necessary if the child shows signs of severe respiratory distress this will help determine if the child is in respiratory failure and needs respiratory support. If necessary, assisted ventilation using endotracheal intubation may be used for a short period of time, usually 8–12 hours.

PowerPoint

Access the companion PowerPoint presentation.

The decision to admit the child to hospital or to discharge the child home is often difficult. Clear guidelines are available from The British Thoracic Society (2003). These are available on the Society's website (http://www.britthoracic.org.uk).

The step approach to drug management is advised by both national and international guidelines for the management of asthma in children (British Thoracic Society 2003). The National Institute of Clinical Excellence (NICE 2000) has also published a guide to the management of asthma and a useful review of the use of inhaler systems/devices in children.

WWW

Read the guide produced by NICE at:
* http://www.nice.org.uk

Look up the Kids Club for 7–14 year olds to help gain their compliance:
* http://www.asthmabusters.org

Scenario

It is 6 p.m. and Jason, a 12-year-old boy, is to be admitted to the children's ward. His mother is with him. Jason is a known asthmatic and he is prescribed regular medication. He was sent home from school earlier in the day with an acute exacerbation of his asthma. He is breathless and unable to carry out a conversation:

* What additional equipment would you get ready prior to Jason's arrival on the ward?
* When they arrive, what questions would you ask Jason and his mother?
* What observations would you carry out?
* What are the normal ranges for these observations for a child this age?
* What medications should have been administered during the day?
* What treatment should be given?
* What advice should be given to Jason and his mother before discharge from hospital?

Discussion of the Scenarios

BRONCHIOLITIS SCENARIO: EMMA

What Framework would You Utilise to Assess Emma's Physiological Status?

Assessment follows the ABC criteria for assessment in conjunction with neurological observations and provides a framework for rapid and effective nursing assessment of the child with respiratory problems. The survey should therefore include assessment of:

* airway
* breathing
* circulation
* disability.

What Observations do You Need to Carry Out?

* **Vital signs:** temperature, pulse and respiration. Remember that normal vital signs are not always appropriate when a child is seriously ill, indeed a normal heart rate and respiratory rate may indicate cardiopulmonary arrest is imminent.

* **Respiratory rates:** should be measured over a full minute.

* **Assessment of breathing:** involves examination of the chest including observation of respiratory movements, number, rhythm, depth and quality of respirations, and character of breath sounds utilising the skills of palpation, auscultation and percussion.

- Remember that the **degree of recession** gives an indication of the severity of the breathing difficulty and nasal flaring is a further sign of increased work of breathing. A resting rate of > 60 breaths/minute is a sign of respiratory distress in a child irrespective of age and an **oxygen saturation** of less than 92% while breathing air is low.

- The child's **heart rate and pulse volume** should be assessed by palpating both central and peripheral pulses for 1 minute. The **skin colour and temperature** should be consistent over the trunk and limbs. Clinical signs of poor perfusion include peripherally cool skin, pallor, mottling, peripheral cyanosis and **capillary refill** > 2 seconds. Remember that by the time central cyanosis is visible in acute respiratory distress respiratory arrest is very close.

What would You Expect These Observations to be?

- Mum reports Emma as struggling to get her breath and you count her respirations as 52 breaths/minute.

- Her peripheral temperature is 38°C.

- Her pulse is 155 beats/minute on an apex recording.

- Her oxygen saturations are 90% in air.

- She has marked recession and nasal flaring.

- She is pale and her capillary refill time is 3 seconds.

Would You Categorise Emma's Present Condition as Mild, Moderate or Severe?

Most likely she would be classed as severe because her pulse rate is above 140/minute, her oxygen saturations are below 92% in air, she has marked recession and nasal flaring. She has also become pale and stopped crying, which may be an indication of fatigue.

Is There Any Information in the History Given that would Cause Concern?

Emma has not been eating for 2 days. You need to ask exactly how much feed she has taken. You also need to ask when she last had a wet nappy and assess if her anterior fontanelle is sunken. You are assessing her state of hydration. She has had a reduced fluid intake, a raised temperature and fewer wet nappies, therefore you would expect her to be dehydrated. If you cannot remember how to classify dehydration, please review this now.

Emma has stopped crying, which may indicate that she is becoming fatigued and that her decreased oxygen saturation is altering her mental status. You would need to assess her against the AVPU scale.

What Care would You Expect to be Initiated?

- Regular **observations** of vital signs and capillary refill, continuous monitoring of oxygen saturations.

- Humidified and monitored **oxygen therapy** in a head box to maintain oxygen saturation > 92% (Fig. 28.11).

- Obtain a specimen of **nasopharyngeal aspirate** to determine cause of bronchiolitis.

- Nursing assessment of state of **hydration** to include amount of feed taken, urine output, temperature of peripheries, peripheral pulses, skin turgor, temperature gap, capillary refill time, state of mucous membranes and specific gravity of urine.

- Assessment of **ability to feed** orally and care planned accordingly to progress to either orogastric/nasogastric or intravenous fluids as condition determines.

- If oral feeding continues then reduce feed volume and increase frequency offered as condition determines returning to normal feeds and frequency as condition improves.

- If oral feeding discontinues then commence **mouth care**.

- If intravenous fluids are initiated then commence care of **intravenous infusion** and intravenous cannula site.

- Monitor **urine output**. Minimum required for an infant is 2 mL/kg/h. Weigh nappies before and after use; 1 g = 1 mL.

- Manage **fever** as appropriate. Remember that an increase in temperature raises basic metabolic rate and increases oxygen demand.

- Prevent spread of **infection**

What Ongoing Care would Emma Require?

Continuation of all above care and in addition·

- Minimal handling.

- Care of family to include all aspects of family-centred care.

Fig. 28.11 • Oxygen therapy.

- Education of family re ongoing care needs at home.

- Discharge planning including outpatient appointment, health visitor liaison and referral to community team as appropriate, discharge summary, completion of health visitor red book, medication, provision of written information/advice.

ASTHMA SCENARIO: JASON

What Additional Equipment would You Get Ready Prior to Jason's Arrival on the Ward?

- Oxygen.

- Nebuliser.

- Oxygen saturation monitor.

- Equipment for intravenous therapy.

- Extra pillows.

When They Arrive, What Questions would You Ask Jason and His Mother?

- What is his normal medication?

- What medication has he taken today, how frequently and when was it last given?

- What may have triggered this attack?

- Is his condition worsening or improving?

- How long has been breathless?

- Has he been in hospital recently for asthma?

- Response to treatment previously?

- How much has he had to drink today?

What Observations would You Carry Out?

- **Vital signs**: temperature, pulse and respirations. Remember that normal vital signs are not always appropriate when a child is seriously ill, indeed a normal heart rate and respiratory rate may indicate cardiopulmonary arrest is imminent.

- **Respiratory rates**: should be measured over a full minute.

- **Assessment of breathing** involves examination of the chest including observation of respiratory movements, number, rhythm, depth and quality of respirations, and character of breath sounds. The child's inability to speak is a relevant factor when assessing their respiratory distress.

- Remember that the **degree of recession** gives an indication of the severity of the breathing difficulty and nasal flaring is a further sign of increased work of breathing. A resting rate of >60 breaths/minute is a sign of respiratory distress in a child irrespective of age and an **oxygen saturation** of less than 92% while breathing air is low.

- The child's **heart rate and pulse volume** should be assessed by palpating both central and peripheral pulses for 1 minute. The **skin colour and temperature** should be consistent over the trunk and limbs. Clinical signs of poor perfusion include peripherally cool skin, pallor, mottling, peripheral cyanosis and **capillary refill** >2 seconds. Remember by the time central cyanosis is visible in acute respiratory distress respiratory arrest is very close.

- The child's **level of consciousness** should be noted. Is the child agitated or becoming lethargic?

What are the Normal Ranges for These Observations for a Child This Age?

- Normal respiratory rate 15–20 breaths per minute.

- Normal heart rate 80–120 beats per minute.

- Temperature 36.6–36.8°C.

- Oxygen saturation level 95–98%.

- Capillary refill < 2 seconds.

What Medications should have been Administered During the Day?

The following answers are based on British Thoracic Society (2003):

- Normal medications prior to acute exacerbation probably β2-agonist.

- When exacerbation occurred 2–4 puffs β2-agonist via spacer.

- β2-agonist increased to 2 puffs every 2 minutes up to total 10 puffs according to response. Do not exceed 10 puffs within each 4-hour period.

- Soluble oral prednisolone 30–40 mg may have been given under the direction of the GP.

- If seen in accident and emergency department then nebulised β2-agonist driven by oxygen may have been administered.

What Treatment should be Given?

- Depending on severity, continue treatment as above administering nebulised β2-agonist driven by oxygen until the attack is under control.

- Continue oxygen via face-mask or nasal prongs.

- If required give intravenous hydrocortisone 100 mg.

- Monitor Jason's vital signs.

- Position Jason for maximum comfort.

- Prepare for intravenous cannulation and infusion.

- Provide psychological support for Jason and his mother.

What Advice should be Given to Jason and His Mother before Discharge from Hospital?

The following answers are based on British Thoracic Society (2003):

- Continue with β2-agonist as prescribed.
- Continue with oral prednisolone for up to 3 days.
- Contact GP if asthma not controlled on prescribed treatment.
- Provided written asthma action plan.
- Check inhaler technique.
- Arrange GP follow-up.

References

Ausejo M, Saenz A, Pham B et al 1999 The effectiveness of glucocorticoids in treating croup: meta-analysis. British Medical Journal 319:595–600

Barnes K 2003 Paediatrics – a clinical guide for nurse practitioners. Butterworth Heinemann, London

Barry P, O'Callinghan C 1997 Nebuliser therapy in childhood. Thorax 52 (Suppl 2):77–88

Brewin A 1997 Comparing asthma and chronic obstructive pulmonary disease (COPD). Nursing Standard 12(4):49–55

British Thoracic Society 2003 The British guidelines on asthma management. Thorax 58:Supplement 1

Caldwell C 1998 Management of acute asthma in children. Nursing Standard 12(29):8–14, 49–54

Carter B 1995 Nursing support and care: meeting the needs of the child and family with altered respiratory function. In: Carter B, Dearman AK (eds) Child health care nursing. Blackwell, London, pp 275–305

Child Health Committee 1997 The specific health needs of children and young people, 2nd report. Child Health Committee, London

Cook D, Strachan D 1997 Parental smoking and prevalence of respiratory symptoms and asthma in school aged children. Thorax 52:1081–1094

Cross S 1999 Better care for people with asthma. Nursing Standard 13(46):4–10, 51–54

D'Amore A, Campbell Hewson G 2002 The management of acute upper airway obstruction in children. Current Paediatrics 12:17–21

de Bisschop C, Guenard H, Desnot P, Vergeret J 1999 Reduction of exercise-induced asthma in children by short, repeated warm ups. British Journal of Sports Medicine 33(2):100–104

Dolan B, Holt L 2000 Accident and emergency theory into practice. Ballière Tindall, London

Elphick HE, Sherlock P, Foxall G et al 2001 Survey of respiratory sounds in infants. Archives of Disease in Childhood 84:34–39

Frakes M 1997 Asthma in the emergency department. Journal of Emergency Nursing 23(5):429–438

Geelhoed G, Turner J, Macdonald W 1996 Efficacy of a small single dose of oral dexamethasone for outpatient croup: a double blind placebo controlled clinical trial. British Medical Journal 313:140–142

Greyson R 1993 Education for control management principles and inhaler techniques for childhood asthma. Child Health June–July

Hazinski M 1992 Nursing care of the critically ill child, 4th edn. Mosby, St Louis

Hunter S 1995 The use of steroids in asthma treatment. Nursing Standard 9(38):25–27

Johnston S, Pattemore P, Sanderson G et al 1995 Community study of role of viral infections in exacerbations of asthma in 9–11-year-old children. British Medical Journal 310:1225–1229

Jordan S, White J 2001 Bronchodilators: implications for nursing practice. Nursing Standard 15(27):45–55

Kaur B, Anderson HR, Austin J et al 1998 Prevalence of asthma symptoms, diagnosis, and treatment in 12–14-year-old children across Great Britain (International Study of Asthma and Allergies in Childhood; ISAAC UK). British Medical Journal 316:118–124

MacGregor J 2000 Introduction to the anatomy and physiology of children. Routledge, London

Mackowiak P, Wasserman SS, Levine MM 1992 A critical appraisal of 98.6°F the upper limit of the normal body temperature and other legacies of Carl Reinhold August Wunderlich. Journal of the American Medical Association 268:1578–1580

Mackway-Jones K, Molyneux E, Phillips B, Wieteska S 1997 Advanced paediatric life support. The practical approach, 2nd edn. BMJ Publishing, London

Magnus P, Jaakkola J 1997 Secular trend in the occurrence of asthma among children and young adults: critical appraisal of repeated cross sectional surveys. British Medical Journal 314:1795–1803

Maill L, Rudolf M, Levene M 2003 Paediatrics at a glance. Blackwell Science, Oxford

McChance K, Heuther S 2002 Pathophysiology – the biologic basis for disease in adults & children. Mosby, London

Meadow R, Newell S 2002 Lecture notes in paediatrics, 7th edn. Blackwell Science, Oxford

Medici TC, Schmid AZ, Hacki M, Vetter W 1993 Are asthmatics salt sensitive? A preliminary controlled study. Chest; the Cardiopulmonary Journal 104(4):1138–1143

Morton RJ, Phillips BM 1992 Accidents and emergencies in children. Oxford University Press, Oxford

The National Institute of Clinical Excellence 2000 Online. Available at: http://www.nice.org.uk

Nelson WE 1996 Textbook of pediatrics, 15th edn. WB Saunders, Philadelphia

Oddy WH, Holt PG, Sly P et al 1999 Association between breast-feeding and asthma in six year old children: findings of a prospective birth cohort study. British Medical Journal 319:815–819

Office of National Statistics 2003 Online. Available at: http://www.statistics.gov.uk

Phelan PD 1994 Asthma in children: epidemiology. British Medical Journal 308:1584–1585

Porth CM 1994 Pathophysiology – concepts of altered health states, 4th edn. Lippincott, London

Rajesh VT, Singh S, Kataria S 2000 Tachypnoea is a good predictor of hypoxia in acutely ill infants under 2 months. Archives of Disease in Childhood 82:46–49

Rudolf M, Levene M 1999 Paediatric and child health. Blackwell Science, Oxford

Smith E 1995 Guidelines for asthma treatment. Nursing Standard 9:23

Tanner K, Fitzsimmons G, Carrol D et al 2002 *Haemophilus influenzae* type b epiglottitis as a cause of acute upper airways obstruction in children. British Medical Journal 325:1099–1100

Thomas DO 1996 Assessing children – it's different. RN 59(4):33–44 (quiz 45)

Thompson R, Gustafson K 1996 Adaptation to chronic childhood illness. American Psychological Association, Washington DC

Thompson SW 1990 Emergency care of children. Jones & Bartlett, Boston

Valman H 1993 Bronchial asthma. British Medical Journal 306:1676–1681

Watson JM, Moss FM 2001 TB in Leicester: out of control, or just one of those things? British Medical Journal 322:1133–1134

Chapter Twenty Nine

29

Caring for Children with Gastrointestinal Problems

Julia M Winter

ABSTRACT

The aim of this chapter is to review the types, causes and management of both acute and chronic gastrointestinal disorders in infants and children. The chapter content will focus primarily on the most common causes of gastrointestinal disturbance, likely to be encountered by the children's nurse. Management will be considered both with reference to best evidence and also within the context of a family-centred approach to care. Additional information relevant to this chapter will be available on the Evolve website, with PowerPoint presentations on the chapter content.

Learning Outcomes

- Identify the causes and management of vomiting in infants and children.

- Identify the causes of acute and chronic diarrhoea in infants and children.

- Recognise and distinguish between presentation of acute and chronic disorders.

- Identify the causes of sudden acute gastrointestinal problems requiring surgery.

- Consider the management of both acute and chronic gastrointestinal disorders, adopting a family-centred approach to care.

- Review the changes in incidence in chronic gastrointestinal disorders, considering causes and implications for healthcare practice.

Glossary

Anal stenosis:
Narrowing or stricture of the anal canal and sphincter.

Atresia:
Absence or closure or a natural passage or channel, imperforation.

Bulimia:
An eating disorder, which is characterised by self-induced vomiting after eating.

Cell hyperplasia:
The abnormal multiplication or increase in the number of cells in normal arrangement in a tissue.

Cirrhosis
Liver disease characterised pathologically by loss of the normal microscopic structure.

Fundoplication:
Mobilisation of the lower end of the oesophagus and wrapping (plication) of the fundus of the stomach around it. Done as a treatment for reflux.

Haemolytic uraemic syndrome:
A pathological condition with involves the rupture (haemolysis) of red blood cells, subsequent anaemia, low platelet count and kidney failure.

Hirschsprung's disease:
Congenital aganglionosis of colon leading to loss of gut motility.

Imperforate anus:
A congenital obstruction of the anal opening.

Intussusception:
Telescoping of one portion of the intestine into another.

Jejunal biopsy:
Tissue sampling of the jejunum.

Malrotation:
Failure during normal embryonic development of normal rotation of all or part of an organ.

Meconium ileus:
Obstructed bowel due to impacted, tenacious meconium.

Myopathies:
Disease of muscles.

Neurofibromatosis:
Growth of neurofibromas (smooth soft or firm tumours) anywhere in the myelinated nervous system (autosomal inheritance).

Organic causes:
A disease that occurs as a result of anatomical or physiological abnormality.

Pyloric stenosis:
A congenital disorder in which the pylorus is thickened causing obstruction of the gastric outlet.

Scleroderma:
Hardening of skin.

Steatosis:
Fatty degeneration.

Systemic lupus erythematosus:
A chronic autoimmune disease.

Villous atrophy:
Wasting or flattening of the villi.

WWW

Use this site, or similar, to look up terms you are not sure of:
- http://www.nlm.nih.gov/medlineplus/mplusdictionary.html

Vomiting

Vomiting in infants and children is a common problem and therefore likely to be experienced by the majority of families and all children's nurses. Causes of vomiting are diverse and are summarised in Table 29.1. This table shows that causes of vomiting differ between infants and older children. Some are associated with anatomical dysfunction requiring surgery.

WWW

Go to:
- http://www.surgical-tutor.org.uk

and using the search facility identify:
- incidence
- pathophysiology
- diagnosis
- management

of pyloric stenosis, intussusception and Hirschsprung's disease. You can find images of most of the conditions mentioned at:
- http://images.google.co.uk

Table 29.1 Causes of Vomiting

Infant	Older child/adolescent
Overfeeding (> 200 mL/kg/day)	Gastroenteritis
Gastrointestinal obstruction	
Pyloric stenosis	
Duodenal or ileal atresia	
Congenital malrotation	
Hirschsprung's disease	
Meconium ileus (in cystic fibrosis)	
Intussusception	
Gastro-oesophageal reflux	Systemic infection
Whooping cough	Raised intracranial pressure
Systemic infection (e.g. urinary tract)	Migraine
	Bulimia
	Poisoning
	Pregnancy

Activity

Choose one of the problems requiring surgery:
- Using a systematic approach, plan the care the child would require before and after surgery.
- How could you make sure you adopted a family-centred approach?

You can check principles of pre- and postoperative care on the companion PowerPoint presentation.

Other causes of vomiting can be medically managed. One common problem, which lends itself in most cases to medical management, is gastro-oesophageal reflux.

GASTRO-OESOPHAGEAL REFLUX

Gastro-oesophageal reflux (refluxing of stomach contents into the oesophagus) is frequently seen, to varying degrees, in infants.

Aetiology

The most common cause is functional immaturity of the gastro-oesophageal sphincter. It is more frequently seen in children with a neurological condition, such as cerebral palsy, and also in children with Down syndrome. Whereas mild reflux (possetting) is generally harmless (although it increases the amount of laundry!) it becomes problematic when associated with failure to thrive or complications develop. These include oesophageal scarring, due to refluxing of gastric acid, which can lead to strictures. There is also the risk of aspiration and potentially apnoea. Diagnostic investigations aim to assess any aspiration risk, degree of severity and structural abnormality such as hiatus hernia.

 www

Look at the diagram showing relevant anatomy and position of affected sphincter at:
- http://www. mydr.com.au/default.asp?Article=3353

Diagnosis

Diagnostic investigations include:

- Contrast studies: show degree of reflux, strictures, altered anatomy of oesophageal junction.
- 24-h pH probe studies: detect presence of gastric acid in oesophagus.
- Ultrasound of gastro-oesophageal junction: can demonstrate reflux but no other anatomical defects.
- Radionuclide scan: aspiration.

Management

Management centres mainly on thickening feeds with products such as Carobel and nursing the infant in a more upright position. In more severe cases, drugs to increase gut motility and speed stomach emptying have been used. However, a recent Cochrane Review (Augood et al 2003) suggests that the benefits of cisapride are not proven and are outweighed by its side effects, which can be life threatening. Surgery (fundoplication) may be required for some children.

 www

Look at the information for parents offered online by Great Ormond Street Hospital:
- http://www.ich.ucl.ac.uk/factsheets/diseases_conditions/ gastro_oesphageal_reflux/

View the images of radiographic studies of reflux shown on:
- http://www.amershamhealth. com/medcyclopaedia/ Volume%20VII/GASTRO%20OESOPHAGEAL% 20REFLUX.asp

It is important that an accurate medical and nursing assessment is made of infants and children presenting with vomiting to identify and treat quickly any significant underlying medical problems. Key points to consider are (Miall et al 2003):

- The overall state of the child, including level of consciousness, circulatory and respiratory function. Does the child need urgent resuscitation?
- Feeding history: the child who is being overfed and vomiting the excess will seem happy and thriving, as will a child with some minor regurgitation. However, other more serious causes of vomiting will lead to weight loss, failure to thrive and in more severe cases potentially dehydration and death.
- Pattern of vomiting: e.g. projectile vomiting presenting from 3–6 weeks may indicate pyloric stenosis. Bile-stained vomiting is suggestive of obstruction and needs further investigation as a matter of urgency.
- Vomiting following paroxysms of coughing is suggestive of whooping cough: check immunisation status.
- Access to poisons such as medication, alcohol and other chemicals.
- Febrile: infection both within and outside of the gastrointestinal systems can cause vomiting. If diarrhoea is present, gastroenteritis is likely. If not it is useful to consider urinary tract infection, meningitis and middle ear infection.

Key investigations are summarised in Table 29.2.

Diarrhoea: Acute and Chronic

As with vomiting, diarrhoea is also a common childhood problem and may be experienced in conjunction with vomiting or on its own. Causes of diarrhoea can be broadly categorised as infectious, inflammatory/allergy mediated or due to malabsorption.

ACUTE INFECTIOUS DIARRHOEA

Acute infectious diarrhoea is a common medical problem of childhood accounting for significant numbers of hospital admissions. Although most cases are an unpleasant and debilitating experience, poor management – particularly in the vulnerable young child or in severe cases – can lead to life-threatening dehydration. It is a major cause of morbidity and mortality in developing countries.

Causative Organisms

These can be both viral and bacterial, with trends in seasonal causes seen and a correlation between age group and vulnerability to type of organisms. A summary is shown in Table 29.3.

 Activity

Other less common bacterial causes of diarrhoea include *Yersinia enterocolitica*, *Vibrio cholerae*, staphylococci and *Clostridium* spp:
- What can you find out about these organisms?

Table 29.2 Key Investigations for Vomiting (Miall et al 2003, Smart & Nolan 2000)

Investigation	Significance
Urea and electrolytes	Imbalance in gastroenteritis and pyloric stenosis
Chloride	Depleted in pyloric stenosis
pH and bicarbonate	Metabolic alkalosis common in pyloric stenosis
Toxicology	If poisoning suspected or to exclude
pH monitoring and barium swallow	To show gastro-oesophageal reflux
Presence of gastric peristalsis during feeding and presence of pyloric tumour on palpation	Indicate pyloric stenosis
Bile-stained vomit	Intestinal obstruction
Urine for culture	Presence of infection

As most acute episodes of gastroenteritis are self-limiting, management focuses primarily on assessment of the degree of dehydration and replacing fluid loss. This is successfully achieved in most cases with the use of oral rehydration solution (ORS). Other factors to consider from a nursing perspective include enabling family management of the child with an acute attack at home and education to minimise the risk of further episodes that might be caused, for example, by poor food handling and preparation techniques. If the child is admitted, minimising the risk of infection to other patients is also of considerable importance.

Reflect on your Practice

- What nursing interventions can you implement to reduce the risk of infection to others in the ward environment?
- How can you ensure that resident family is not posing an infection threat?

You will find additional guidance in the Royal College of Nursing (RCN) publication *Good practice in infection control* (RCN 2004).

Although acute gastroenteritis is the most common cause of diarrhoea, particularly in the preschool child, other causes of diarrhoea could be considered.

Malabsorption and Food Allergies

CYSTIC FIBROSIS

Aetiology

Cystic fibrosis (CF) is an autosomal recessive inherited disorder. It is more common in the Caucasian population, and currently affects 1:2500 live births in the UK. The gene responsible is located on the long arm of chromosome 7, with <F508 being the most common mutation, although 900 other variations were found between 1989 and 2001 (Cystic Fibrosis Trust 2001); 1 in 20 individuals is likely to be a carrier.

Activity

Check your understanding of autosomal recessive inheritance. Draw a diagram to illustrate this and check if you are correct by checking on the companion PowerPoint presentation.

The disease primarily affects the exocrine glands. Sufferers do not have normal life expectancy, although this is improving with treatment advances.

Exocrine glands regulate production of sweat and mucous. Affected individuals may present with varying symptoms, dependent on the degree of severity. Symptoms commonly include digestive and respiratory problems but overall can include:

- shortness of breath
- persistent cough
- hyperhydrosis (excessive sweating)
- limited lung capacity
- 'salty' skin
- wheezing
- abdominal pain
- pneumonia
- excessive appetite but little weight gain
- large, foul-smelling stools
- diarrhoea
- impaired fertility
- reduced bone mass.

Table 29.3 Summary of the Causative Organisms of Diarrhoea (McVerry 1999, Wong 1999)

Organism	Epidemiology/pathology	Symptoms
Rotavirus	Most common causative organism in UK, Particularly affecting the under 2s More common in cooler times of year Damages mucosa with severe inflammatory changes Incubation 1–3 days Transmission: faecal/oral	Fever >38°C for approx. 48 hours Vomiting, profuse watery diarrhoea, may last up to a week
Adenovirus	Second most common viral cause, most common in younger age groups More common in cooler months Mucosal damage (check if Norwalk group) Incubation within 24 hours Transmission: faecal/oral, person to person or droplet	May have associated respiratory infection Diarrhoea not usually vomiting
Giardia (protozoan)	Most common cause of non-bacterial diarrhoea in North America Favours cool moist conditions More common in children May be asymptomatic carriers Pathophysiology not proven – suspect either produces toxin or causes mechanical obstruction of the absorptive surface of intestine Incubation up to 1 week Transmission: contaminated food, water sources, person to person	Diarrhoea average 1 week May be longer and may be transient or persistent disaccharide intolerance
Escherichia coli	Common in newborns More common in summer Produces toxins, which bind to mucosal villi and cause profuse secretion of water and electrolytes. Can also invade and destroy epithelium Incubation variable Transmission: contaminated and undercooked food, person to person	Fever, green watery and explosive diarrhoea, abdominal distension Usually settles 3–10 days *Note: E. coli* 157 also causes abdominal cramps, haemorrhagic colitis and haemolytic uraemic syndrome
Salmonella spp	More common in toddler age groups More common in summer Invades connective tissue of small bowel and colon-local inflammation and secretion of fluids. Local oedema. Incubation period 6–72 hours Transmission: carried in poultry, eggs and other food sources; also by pets	Variable degrees of symptoms, including fever and chills, vomiting cramps and diarrhoea (may be bloody) Can have infection at other sites causing local symptoms or septicaemia *Note: S. typhi* causes fever, fatigue, cough, diarrhoea and weight loss
Shigella	More common in toddler age groups More common in late summer Causes enterotoxin production see above Incubation 1–7 days Transmission: person to person or fomites	Sudden high fever Abdominal cramps Watery diarrhoea with mucus and blood May also have headache, neck stiffness and potential for convulsions with fever
Campylobacter jejuni	More common in toddler age groups and young adults More common in late summer Enterotoxin production and loss of absorptive surface from villi Incubation 1–7 days Transmission: birds are most common host. Carried on foods and milk	Fever, watery or sticky diarrhoea may be blood and leucocytes Vomiting Usually self-limiting rarely leads to complications such as haemolytic uraemic syndrome, septicaemia Infectivity can be limited with erythromycin

Children affected by cystic fibrosis, regardless of symptom severity, have increased sodium and chloride levels in saliva and sweat. Children with cystic fibrosis are unable to effectively reabsorb sodium and chloride leading to increased losses, particularly in warmer conditions. This creates an increased risk of dehydration, hypochloraemia and hyponatraemia.

Symptoms are caused by production of viscous mucous, which accumulates, obstructing the mucous secreting glands in affected organs. There is also obstruction of small passages namely the bronchioles of the lungs, pancreatic and biliary ducts.

Respiratory Function

Failure to expectorate bronchial secretions by normal cilliary movement results in accumulation of secretions, which then create a medium for infection. Lung damage is progressive over time as continued obstruction causes atelectasis and emphysema. Colonisation with *Pseudomonas aeruginosa* is specific to cystic fibrosis sufferers. Eventually, there is destruction of bronchial epithelium and progressive fibrosis with impaired pulmonary function. Long-term treatment options include lung transplant.

Gastrointestinal Function

Gastrointestinal problems are due to occlusion of the pancreatic ducts with mucous concretions. Outflow of pancreatic enzymes is obstructed resulting in impaired digestion and absorption of nutrients, particularly fats and proteins. Over time, fibrosing of the pancreas occurs, which may account for the increased incidence of insulin-dependent diabetes in cystic fibrosis sufferers.

Diagnosis

Diagnosis is supported by presence of the symptoms described above but is confirmed by a 'sweat test'. This is achieved by collection of a minimum of 100 mg of sweat and measuring the quantity of sodium chloride contained within. Many parents of infants with cystic fibrosis will remark that their child 'tastes salty'. Normal sodium chloride levels are <40 mmol/L; sodium levels of >50 mmol/L and chloride levels of >60 mmol/L are abnormal (Smart & Nolan 2000).

Other diagnostic tests include (Cystic Fibrosis Trust 2001):

- prenatal chorionic villous sampling
- meconium ileus in neonatal period
- genotyping
- pancreatic function
- stool elastase.

Management

Gastrointestinal Symptoms

The aim of gastrointestinal management is to ensure the child achieves adequate nutrition for optimal growth with minimum gastrointestinal symptoms. The mainstay of treatment is pancreatic enzyme replacement (pancreatin), which contains the enzymes protease, lipase and amylase, which assist in the digestion of protein, fats and starch, respectively. Supplements are given orally. Pancreatin is inactivated by gastric acid and heat; therefore supplements are most effective in an enteric-coated form and given immediately prior to or with meals and snacks. If mixed with food and drink, care should be taken that it is not too hot. Pancreatin can cause perioral and buccal mucosa irritation, so children should be taught to swallow quickly and not retain it in the mouth. Large doses may cause perianal irritation. Pancreatin is currently available in both capsule and granular form. It is usually porcine in origin so this factor should be considered in relation to the child and family's religious beliefs. The dosage required is variable, influenced by the severity of the child's disease and the individual child's response to medication. However, it should be noted there is also an identified association between high-dosage pancreatin and fibrosing colonopathy, a condition that can lead to pain and intestinal obstruction (Dodge 2000).

Dietary Management

As absorption of nutrients from the small intestine is reduced in children with cystic fibrosis, their carbohydrate, fat and protein calorie requirements are in excess of the norms for their age, if optimal height and weight is to be maintained. It is recommended that their overall calorie requirements are between 120 and 140% of the RDA, with 40% of intake provided by fats. However, studies have found that within both preschool and school-age groups, a minimum of one-third of children did not meet the recommended calorie and fat intakes, demonstrated more meal-time negative behaviours and had lower measures of weight and height than children in the control groups (Powers et al 2002, Stark et al 1997).

Survival in cystic fibrosis is mostly mediated by the rate of deterioration in lung function, as the disease progresses. Deterioration in lung function is associated with worsening nutritional status. Although it is yet to be confirmed which of these factors is a precursor for the other, there is evidence that poor nutrition in childhood has a negative effect on lung growth, which may result in more rapid progression of lung disease. De Vizia et al (2003) found that omega-3 fatty acid supplements resulted in a decrease in inflammatory responses and antibiotic use in cystic fibrosis patients, so this may be a useful form of nutritional supplement. Optimal calorie intake may be supported by enteral and parenteral feeding in the community. However, the burden of responsibility and the resource implications for the child's family are significant and an assessment of benefits to the child and family and ongoing support is required (Puntis 2001). Achieving optimal nutritional management in a family-managed setting requires focused education in relation to the disease and nutritional needs. Although there is sometimes the belief among health professionals that the child and family with a chronic illness become 'experts', it has been shown that some children and care-givers are not fully aware of how to meet nutritional needs. Families showed a better understanding of the management of pancreatic enzyme supplements than of nutritional requirements overall (Stapleton et al 2000). Arguably, a key nursing management focus should be supporting optimal nutrition in the infant and growing child. Given the impact of chronic disease on the child and family as an integrated unit, adopting a family-focused approach, is good practice. The best outcomes are likely to be achieved by working with the multidisciplinary team members, including dieti-cians and community nurse specialists, where available. Clear communication and agreed care strategies should be developed between the acute and ambulatory care settings. Consideration should be given to the financial support the child and family might need.

As with all chronic health deficits, there is potential for emotional stress. There are indicators that children with cystic fibrosis have an altered perception of body image, which although negative, differs from the distortions shown by healthy children in control groups. It was shown that self-esteem in relation to body image was similar between groups of 7–12-year-olds with cystic fibrosis and a control group who were cystic fibrosis free. However, children with cystic fibrosis were significantly more likely to report their ideal body size as larger, differing from the control group, who were more likely to identify their ideal body size as smaller and thinner (Truby & Paxton 2001). This would seem to indicate the significance of the efforts children with cystic fibrosis must make to maintain their weight.

COELIAC DISEASE

Aetiology

Coeliac disease (gluten-sensitive enteropathy), although characterised by problems with absorption, is in origin a food allergy. Gastrointestinal food allergies include a range of disorders, which result from adverse responses to dietary antigens (Sicherer 2003). These are listed below:

- immediate gastrointestinal hypersensitivity (anaphylaxis)
- oral allergy syndrome
- allergic eosinophilic oesophagitis

- gastritis
- gastroenterocolitis
- dietary protein enterocolitis
- proctitis
- enteropathy
- coeliac disease.

Attributed, but not proven, are colic, gastro-oesophageal reflux and constipation.

Coeliac disease is still thought as of a relatively rare condi-tion, known to affect 1 in 1000 individuals in the UK. However, it is thought that this figure could be higher – up to 1 in 300 (Sullivan 1999) – and anecdotal evidence suggests that it may be under diagnosed. It has historically been thought of as a disease predominantly affecting the Caucasian population, with the classic phenotype described as blonde and blue eyed. However, there is an increasing incidence amongst Afro-Caribbean races, and suggestion that it may be a major cause of chronic diarrhoea in North Africa, India and the Middle East (Catassi 2002). Those affected have a per-manent intolerance to the α-gliadin protein that is found in wheat, barley and rye, and in hybrids of these. The mecha-nisms and origins of the abnormal allergic response to gluten are not fully understood, although some individuals have a genetic predisposition, which is dependent on specific alleles of the HLA system, the DQ2 and, less frequently, the DQ8.

On ingestion of gluten-containing cereals, first of all wheat and, secondly, barley and rye, traces of gluten-derived peptides come in contact with the antigen-presenting cells (APC) located in the lamina propria of the intestinal mucosa and activate, in DQ2- or DQ8-positive subjects, an abnormal immune response leading to the typical coeliac enteropathy – intestinal villous atrophy with crypt hyper-plasia (Catassi 2002). Essentially, there is an abnormal immune response, which is thought to be triggered by unknown factors such as an acute viral illness. As with many immune-mediated illnesses, the disease has familial ten-dencies and an increased risk of developing it if a close rel-ative is affected.

The villous atrophy decreases the absorptive surface of the gut wall and the amount of enzymes usually available on the villous surface. The result is passage of partly undi-gested food through the intestinal tract. This leads to diar-rhoea or, because of the large amounts of undigested fat, bulky, foul-smelling stools, which are pale in colour. These fatty stools are termed 'steatorrhoea'. As the disease pathology progresses, the ability to absorb proteins, carbo-hydrates, calcium, folic acid, iron and some vitamins also decreases and the child presents with diarrhoea/steator-rhoea and weight loss, including both fat and muscle. Symptoms may be noted from infancy as weaning intro-duces gluten-containing foods, but progresses until symp-toms become noticeable, usually in early toddler years

(Wong 1999). The classic 'coeliac toddler' presents with thin arms and legs, flat wasted buttocks, bloated abdomen, and with a miserable and lethargic appearance. Commonly, they are anaemic and may have rickets; slowing of bone growth may show on X-ray examination. However, it should be noted that coeliac disease is increasingly being identified in asymptomatic patients or with atypical presentation (Davison 2002). This is particularly relevant in children who have related or associated disorders, as discussed later.

Diagnosis

Diagnosis is made on history and presentation. Blood tests for the presence of α-gliadin antibodies (present in response to gluten) and anti-reticulin and anti-endomysial antibodies (which are present when the gut mucosa is damaged) may be made. Definitive diagnosis is made by jejunal biopsy and microscopic examination of the structure of the villi. Additionally, children with coeliac disease will demonstrate clinical remission of signs when given a gluten-free diet. Increasingly diagnosis is occurring later, including in adult years.

Management

The management is quite simple in that there is complete remission of gut changes if a gluten-free diet is followed. The diet is a permanent lifetime requirement. Oats are also usually excluded from the diet, as they are often contaminated with wheat (Sullivan 1999).

Managing the diet effectively and consistently can pose challenges for the child and family. Obvious gluten-containing foods such as bread, biscuits and cakes can be replaced but many of the products are less palatable, especially breads. In addition, gluten appears under many guises within foods. Examples include thickeners for commercially prepared meals and desserts, and flavourings in snack foods, such as crisps. Generally, food labelling is improving and many products now state whether they are gluten free, or use the symbol of two crossed heads of grain to show that the product is coeliac friendly. Support groups such as the Coeliac Society and the Coeliac Resource Centre, offer advice on gluten-free commercial products, recipes and special dietary products. Major supermarket chains are steadily increasing their range of specialist dietary products. Staple foods such as bread and flour are available on prescription. Referral to a paediatric dietician is useful.

Activity

Think of an average menu for a birthday tea party for a 4-year-old. How much of it is likely to contain gluten? How could you advise a parent to manage the normal social activity of party invitations?

Useful addresses:

- The Coeliac Society, PO Box 220 High Wycombe, Buckinghamshire. Website: http://www.coeliac.co.uk
- Coeliac Disease Resource Centre (Part of Nutricia Dietary Care), Newmarket Avenue, White Horse Business Park, Trowbridge, Wiltshire BA14 0XQ. Website: http://www.glutafin.co.uk

Complications/Related Problems

It is known that coeliac disease coexists in children with other conditions, and may be asymptomatic. As the potential complications of untreated coeliac disease include reduced fertility, reduced bone density and gastrointestinal malignancy, routine screening for coeliac disease may be considered for children with (Gale et al 1997, Holmes 2001):

- Down syndrome (prevalence of coeliac disease = 4–17%)
- Insulin-dependant diabetes (prevalence of coeliac disease = 1–17%)
- Ulcerative colitis and Crohns's disease.

The common factor with some of the above seems to be the existence of autoimmune problems. Coeliac disease is also associated with other complications or disorders, including:

- Arthritis: an association between coeliac disease and arthritis is suggested, with remission of arthritis symptoms with successful dietary treatment of coeliac symptoms.
- Dental defects such as defects in dental enamel: these are prevalent in children with coeliac disease. Children with enamel defects and a history of non-specific diarrhoea should be considered for further gastroenterology investigations.
- Infertility: has been shown to be a presenting factor in women with undiagnosed coeliac disease. Fertility improved with introduction of a coeliac diet.
- Liver dysfunction: is a noted complication in coeliac patients (Davison 2002) and the recognition of the autoimmune component to coeliac disease has led to the recognition of its association with other autoimmune disorders, including liver disease. Three types of liver disease are described:
  - Mild liver dysfunction: characterised by raised liver enzymes and some changes in histology, including Kupffer cell hyperplasia, mononuclear cell infiltration, mild fibrosis and steatosis. In most cases, liver enzymes revert to norm within 12 months of establishing a gluten-free diet.
  - Chronic liver disease: characterised by severe cirrhosis, fibrosis and hepatitis with associated biochemical changes. Despite the underlying damage, gluten free diets are shown to result in significant improvement.

- Autoimmune liver disease: encompasses autoimmune hepatitis, primary and autoimmune sclerosing cholangitis. Some links with coeliac disease for these conditions has been established (Davison 2002).

It is not known if the types of liver disease described above are separate entities or if they fall on a pathological spectrum.

COW'S MILK ALLERGY

Cow's milk allergy is primarily a disease of childhood and affects an inexactly determined number of the population, but it has been suggested that the figure can be estimated as 1–3% of the general population and 3–5% of bottle-fed infants. There is an increased prevalence in infants in whom there is history of prematurity, atopy or other gastrointestinal disorders (Bahna 2002). Cows milk protein comprises of two major fractions – casein and whey – in a proportion of approximately 80:20. Casein and the β-lactoglobulin component of whey are the most allergenic, with varying degrees of sensitivity shown in affected individuals. Sensitivities are manifest in specific gastrointestinal symptoms or severe systemic and life-threatening reactions. The most hypersensitive individuals can react not only to ingested proteins but also if there is skin contact.

Aetiology

Hypersensitivity to cows milk can be mediated by one of four immunlogic reactions (Bahna 2002):

- Type I (anaphylactic or intermediate): most common, mediated by IgF antibodies.
- Type II (cytotoxic): least common, IgM, IgG or IgA antibodies activate complexes.
- Type III (arthus type): second most common, formation of immune complexes that comprise antigen, involves IgA, IgG, IgM and occasionally IgE.
- Type IV (delayed): mediated by sensitised T lymphocytes.

Diagnosis

Whereas type 1 reactions are relatively easy to clinically evaluate, the other three types are more difficult. Assessment particularly addresses the relationship between the ingestion of cows milk protein and manifest symptoms. However, all possible symptoms are shared with other disorders. Specific diagnosis therefore rests most conclusively with measuring serum IgE antibodies for specific foods.

Management

Ideally, management should be considered from the proactive and preventive viewpoint. There is evidence that food allergies may be related to early exposure to food allergens. In some cases, exposure may be via maternal breast milk. In terms of general protection against a range of food allergies there is evidence that breast-feeding contributes to prevention, but this protection may be lessened where there is high maternal fat intake (Hanson et al 2003). There is also evidence that early gut colonisation with Gram-negative organisms lessens the incidence of food allergy developing. Current hygiene practices (enthusiastically rigorous) in early infant care detract from this early colonisation process. The practice of supporting early neonatal feeding with cows milk formula, before establishing breast-feeding, may contribute to cow's milk allergy developing in early childhood. Studies so far do not suggest that restricting maternal diet in pregnancy mediates against cow's milk allergy (Fiocchi et al 2003).

Once the problem exists effective management requires introduction of alternatives to cows milk protein. Soya food products and soy formulas are usually well tolerated, but other options are hydrolysed cow's milk protein formula, e.g. Pregestcmil.

LACTOSE INTOLERANCE

The terms 'cow's milk allergy' and 'cow's milk intolerance' are often used interchangeably and it is important to note that they are two distinct entities.

Whereas cows milk allergy is an immunologically mediated reaction to cow's milk proteins, characterised by local and systemic reactions that can be fatal, cow's milk intolerance refers to problems with the digestion, absorption or metabolism of components of cow's milk, which are non-immunological. Cow's milk allergy primarily affects infants and young children and the majority of those affected will experience spontaneous resolution, whereas cow's milk intolerance tends to have its onset in later childhood or young adulthood, and persists. The exception to this is when it develops secondary to acute gastroenteritis in infancy or early childhood, when it is usually a transient problem. Lactase (β-galactosidase) is required to hydrolyse lactose (carbohydrate component of mammalian milk) into the monosaccharides glucose and galactose. If insufficient lactase is produced to complete this process, lactose with water passes on to the colon where it undergoes a fermentation process, producing hydrogen, carbon dioxide and lactic acid. This causes the symptoms of bloating, flatulence, abdominal pain and watery diarrhoea. Severity of symptoms is variable dependent on individual degrees of insufficiency. The problem has racial prevalence, with the highest incidence in races with darker skins and the least affected being the very fair skinned. Primary lactose intolerance is rare in infants and may be an inherited autsosomal trait.

Diagnosis

Various tests support diagnosis, including blood glucose monitoring post-ingestion of a measured 'dose' of lactose. The simplest test is to measure hydrogen levels in exhaled breath, as the hydrogen produced in the colon is excreted via the lungs. Definitively, individuals whose symptoms resolve on introduction of a lactose-reduced diet can have diagnosis confirmed.

Management

Dietary exclusion of lactose, as the primary 'milk' source will be effective in controlling symptoms. Other than in infants with primary intolerance, most individuals can tolerate some lactose, particularly in live yoghurts and non-pasteurised cheeses where the lactose-digesting enzymes produced by the lactobacillus aid its digestion. Infants can be swapped to a soybean formula (Bahna 2002). Of interest is the finding of Fiocchi et al (2003), whose small study found that even children with hypersensitive reactions of cow's milk proteins were not intolerant of lactose.

INFLAMMATORY BOWEL DISEASE

Crohn's disease and ulcerative colitis are distinct forms of inflammatory bowel disease (IBD). Although their histology differs, they share many symptoms and have a similar impact on the child and family's life. Studies suggest that their incidence has increased since the 1980s, although it is not clear whether this is a true increase or due to better diagnosis (Jenkins 2001). The incidence of newly diagnosed cases seems now to have settled, which would lend support to the increase being due, at least in part, to increasing skills in diagnosis.

Currently, the British Paediatric Surveillance Unit (BPSU) identifies incidence as 5.3 cases per 100,000 children under the age of 16. This equated to 700 new cases per annum in the UK. Average age at diagnosis is 11–12, with 13% of cases occurring in children under 10. Crohn's disease is twice as common as ulcerative colitis and there appears to be a higher than average incidence in the Asian and Afro-Caribbean population

Aetiology

Research to date is unable to offer any definitive causes for IBD. There appears to be a genetic predisposition with 'susceptibility' genes being located. However, findings are not consistent across different groups, suggesting the need for further studies. Environmental factors, which are likely to include specific infectious pathogens, dietary elements and common childhood infections, are also thought to trigger

the disease. The suggestion that the measles vaccine or virus is a predisposing factor has yet to be supported, and several studies have concluded that the there is no statistical support to link measles vaccine with either IBD or autism (Black et al 2002, Davis et al 2001). In affected individuals, immunologically mediated inflammatory responses in the intestinal mucosa are exaggerated

Evidence-based Practice

In recent years we have seen much published on the safety or otherwise of the MMR vaccination and its links with both gut disorders and autism. At the time of writing, the initial research (Wakefield 1998), which suggested the association between MMR and autism, has been largely discredited. The popularising of Wakefield's initial theories was largely via the non-professional press. Consider how you can ensure that children and their families can be helped to make decisions about their care and treatment, based on accurate interpretation of the evidence available.

Diagnosis

Some symptoms are shared between Crohn's and ulcerative colitis but there are differences, which are summarised in Table 29.4. Whereas diagnosis of IBD may be suspected on symptom history and initial blood testing, visual examination of the gut using endoscopy, radiological tests and gut biopsy is needed to confirm and differentiate diagnosis. More recently, magnetic resonance imaging (MRI) has been found to be an accurate diagnostic procedure (Laghi et al 2003).

Management

Physiological management approaches differ between ulcerative colitis and Crohn's disease, although the aims are shared, including the need to induce and maintain remission, secure a reduction in symptoms and promote normal physical social and emotional growth and development.

Currently, the preferred initial treatment choice for Crohn's disease in the UK is the use of enteral feeding. It is proving most successful in children where the disease is focused in the small intestine, but has been shown to improve outcomes for those with colon involvement. Enteral diets can be:

- true elemental
- semi-elemental
- polymeric.

The last, being palatable, can be taken orally rather than via naso- or intragastric tube systems. Elemental diets comprise

Table 29.4 Differences between Crohn's Disease and Ulcerative Colitis (Jenkins 2001, Metcalf 2002, Walker-Smith 2000)

Feature	Crohn's disease	Ulcerative colitis
Location	Can affect whole of GI tract but mouth, stomach and oesophagus rare	Ulceration confined to the colon
Diarrhoea	Type varies dependent on area of gut involved	Loose stools, blood
Pain	Present	Usually dull ache
Bleeding	Present	Present
Linear growth delay	May be most obvious feature prior to diagnosis	Less common, however diagnosis made earlier due to acute onset of gastro symptoms
Gut mucosal inflammation and ulceration	Present – patchy, plus may develop strictures	Present, diffuse
Mucous	Present in stool in Crohn's colitis	Depletion
Extra intestinal signs		
Anaemia		
Raised ESR and platelets	Present	Present
Increase in inflammatory mediators (cytokines, leukotrienes, prostaglandins	Erythema nodosum	
Skin manifestations		

ESR, erythrocyte sedimentation rate; GI, gastrointestinal.

of protein sourced from amino acids or short-chain peptides, with short-chain carbohydrates and added fats, minerals and vitamins. Semi-elemental diets include protein hydrosylate; polymeric diets contain whole proteins and fats.

Treatment protocols recommend enteral feeding for a period of 8 weeks, with only additional water allowed. This is followed by food introduction, re-excluding foods that are associated with symptom return. Results are proving favourable, with the majority of children achieving remission and enjoying a normal diet within a 4-month period. Unfortunately 30–50% relapse within 1 year but respond well to a further programme. One of the most positive advantages of this approach is the lack of the side effects seen when steroid treatment is used. Also, there tends to be an associated growth increase, whereas steroids often limit linear growth.

Enteral feeding is not recommended for those with severe disease or for children with perianal involvement. For children for whom the enteral feeding programme is unsuitable or for whom remission is not achieved, drug therapy is the treatment option. This includes corticosteroids, 5-aminosalicylic acid (5-ASA) agents, immunomodulators and monoclonal antibodies.

Surgery is an option in children who have not achieved remission with other treatments. It is most effective when the disease is quite localised, although it does not guarantee reoccurrence.

Activity

Using either web-based resources or pharmacology texts:
- Identify the different actions of each of the groups of drugs listed in the above text.
- How would you explain their actions to an 11-year-old child?

www

Useful web address:
- http://www. crohnsresource.com/about/drug.jsp

ULCERATIVE COLITIS

Dietary regimes are not helpful for children with ulcerative colitis. As with the treatment approaches for Crohn's disease, there is a three-phased approach:

- Mild cases are treated initially with 5-ASA agents, namely mesalazine and sulfasalazine. Drugs are continued for 2 years after induction of remission.

- More severe cases have high-dose oral steroids added to the 5-ASA therapy. Steroids are given for 4–6 weeks and then the dose is weaned and withdrawn.

- Patients who become steroid resistant may respond to azathioprine. If unsuccessful, or the patient is steroid dependent, surgery is indicated. Surgery is curative for ulcerative colitis, although a stoma will often be required, as children have not proved good candidates for ileoanal anastomosis and pouch formation (Walker-Smith 2000).

Some children may develop perianal lesions or proctitis, both of which are difficult to treat. Rectal water-soluble steroids or 5-ASA drugs may be used successfully for management of proctitis.

Emergency care is required for the child who develops severe colitis, including administration of intravenous fluids, electrolytes, antibiotics and steroids. Perforation is a risk and surgery may be required.

Arguably, physical care and management is clearly described, with specific protocols to follow. However, the potential impact of inflammatory bowel disease on the child and family, both socially and mentally, is worthy of consideration within nursing strategies. Some studies suggest that young adults who developed IBD as children have problems with self-esteem. The average age at diagnosis coincides with onset of puberty and adolescence.

Reflect on your Practice

How might the adolescent child with inflammatory bowel disease be supported, using a multidisciplinary approach, to minimise the threat to self-esteem? You may find it useful to read: Vitulano-Lawrence (2003).

CONSTIPATION

Constipation, which can be defined as delay or difficulty in defecation, is a common paediatric problem. Normal frequency of bowel movements varies from child to child, ranging from more than once per day to none for several days, and infrequency alone is not necessarily a problem. Causes of constipation are broadly differentiated into organic and non-organic. Organic causes are shown in Table 29.5.

However, for the majority of children presenting with constipation problems, the cause is non-organic. Non-organic causes include poor dietary management, including insufficient fibre, and dehydration, developmental problems that complicate toilet training, emotional abuse,

Table 29.5 Organic Causes of Constipation (Baker et al 1999)

Cause	Examples
Anatomic malformations	Imperforate anus Anal stenosis Pelvic mass
Metabolic and gastrointestinal	Cystic fibrosis Diabetes mellitus Coeliac disease Hypothyroidism
Neuropathic	Spinal cord problem Neurofibromatosis
Intestinal nerve or muscle disorders	Hirschsprung's disease Visceral myopathies and neuropathies
Abnormalities of abdominal muscles	Prune belly syndrome Gastroschisis Down syndrome
Connective tissue disorders	Systemic lupus erythematosus Scleroderma
Drugs	Opiates Phenobarbitone Antihypertensives Antidepressants
Miscellaneous	Lead poisoning Vitamin D overdose

depression and also inappropriate/punitive toilet training practices in the younger child. There are also those who have a familial tendency and sedentary lifestyle. In early years the most common cause of constipation is functional – meaning it exists in the absence of obvious cause. It is thought to commonly develop in response to the child experiencing unpleasant emotional experiences or pain associated with defecation. This results in the child deliberately holding faeces and actively working against the impulse to defecate. Ignoring the urge to defecate results in retention of faeces in the colon, fluid is reabsorbed and the faecal mass becomes, large dry and hard, termed 'impacted'. As a consequence, liquid faeces leak around the impacted mass, causing involuntary soiling (encopresis). The problem is progressive as the child becomes frightened, anticipating that the experience of defecation will be painful and difficult, and resisting the urge to defecate. Soiling is unpleasant and may create tension in the home, nursery or school, which can lead to social isolation and feelings of poor self-worth.

Soiling is usually involuntary but it may be a behaviour learnt after toilet training has been achieved. This is often indicative of stress or emotional upset; 80–95% of encopresis is associated with functional constipation.

Diagnosis

Functional non-organic constipation is diagnosed on the basis of medical and psychosocial history taking and physical examination. Initially, organic causes need to be excluded. Indicators of organic causes would include general malaise or other systemic signs such as weight loss, nausea/vomiting, and blood in the stools or abdominal distension. Rectal examination allows size of the rectum to be assessed and also amount and type of stool. The perineum and perianal area can be examined at the same time to assess for signs of trauma. If there is nothing of note and there is a history of toileting difficulties and stool-withholding behaviour, it is likely that the cause is functional. If it is inappropriate to conduct a rectal examination, for example if the child refuses or abuse is suspected, abdominal X-ray can be used to determine whether impacted faeces are present.

Reflect on your Practice

Consider the kind of questions that might be asked to establish the state of a child's bowel function (colour, shape, frequency, size, associated with pain...):
- How might some children and families find this interview?
- How can it be facilitated to be more comfortable?

Management

Baker et al (1999), based on a review of evidence and practice, suggested a staged approach to management. This is described as follows:

1. determine if there are impacted faeces
2. remove/resolve impaction
3. maintenance: using education, support, diet and medications
4. follow up.

Successful and complete disimpaction is arguably a precursor to successful ongoing management. Removal of impacted faeces can be achieved using oral or rectal medication or a combination of the two. Choice should centre on child and family preference. Oral medication may be perceived as less invasive.

Oral medications include electrolyte solutions, either alone or in combination with high-dose laxatives, for example lactulose or senna. Ideally, stool softeners, such as lactulose, should be used before stimulants to minimise the pain of passing a large, hard stool. Rectal preparations can also be used, including saline and phosphate enemas, and some success has been achieved using glycerol suppositories. Mineral oils, which act as stool lubricants, are also favoured in the US and Australia, and feature in practice guidelines developed by the North American Society for Paediatric Gastroenterology and Nutrition (NASPGN). Their use in the UK is not widely accepted because of concerns about aspiration pneumonias, gut changes and altered vitamin absorption. However, the evidence to support these concerns is insubstantial (Sharif et al 2001).

Having removed the impacted faeces, management moves to maintenance using a 'whole child' approach. Therapy includes dietary management, maintaining laxative therapy and also behaviour modification, focusing on making toileting and bowel evacuation into a non-stressful experience.

Dietary changes aim to increase fluids and include fruit, fibre and non-absorbable carbohydrates. Laxatives can include osmotic laxative, such as lactulose, docusate sodium and polyethylene glycol (Movicol). The latter has a limited licence for use with children, with restrictions on period of use. Softeners are combined with bowel stimulants, which include senna and sodium picosulphate. Rectal medication may be used with caution, given the associated unpleasant experiences it may engender. Medication programmes require use of dosage adequate to establish bowel function, which is regular and characterised by absence of straining, soiling or discomfort. Careful weaning from medication can then begin. Behaviour modification makes use of diary keeping, unhurried regular toileting, ideally shortly after meals to capitalise on the effect of the gastrocolic reflex, and also reward systems for successful evacuations (ERIC 2001).

A recent Cochrane review found that combining behavioural and/or cognitive interventions with drug therapies resulted in better outcomes at 6- and 12-month follow-ups (Brazelli & Griffiths 2004). During the treatment and management phases, close family support and education is required. Families need to understand the origins of the problem and where additional problems such as soiling have developed, make clear that this is likely to be non-intentional. Families may need support to set realistic objectives, in terms of outcomes over time, and to develop the ability to manage behaviour reinforcement using positive learning approaches. Education and encouragement to change the family diet to one that is more balanced may also be required.

WWW

The following websites offer further reading and management guidelines. You could consider to what extent guidelines are consistent between organisations and care teams:

- http://www.eric.org.uk
- http://www-lmec.chester.ac.uk/guide/const.htm
- http://www.london. nhs.uk/lempig/constipation.htm
- http://www. naspghan.org/PDF/constipation.pdf

Summary

This chapter has offered an overview of some of the major gastrointestinal problems likely to be encountered by children's nurses. Additional information can also be found on the Evolve website. Generally, acute problems can be managed effectively, with positive outcomes expected in most cases. However, there is an increase in the incidence of chronic illnesses in child health, some of which have been explored in this chapter. This is creating a need to focus on long-term family-centred care and to continue to develop strong links between ambulatory and acute care settings. Continuing to strengthen multiprofessional cooperation in care commissioning and delivery remains a child health professional responsibility. It is envisaged that this will continue to be a key challenge in child health care for the foreseeable future.

References

Augood C, MacLennan S, Gilbert R, Logan S 2003 Cisapride treatment for gastro-oesophageal reflux in children (Cochrane Review). The Cochrane Library, issue 3. Update Software, Oxford

Baker S, Liptak G, Colletti R et al 1999 Constipation in infants and children: evaluation and treatment. Journal of Paediatric Gastroenterology and Nutrition 29:612–626

Bahna S 2002 Cow's milk allergy versus cow's milk intolerance. Annals of Allergy Asthma and Immunology 89(6):56–60

Black C, Kaye J, Jick H 2002 Relation of childhood gastrointestinal diseases to autism: nested case control study using data from UK General Practice Research Database. British Medical Journal 325(7361):419–421

Brazelli M, Griffiths P 2004 Behavioural and cognitive interventions with or without other treatments for defecation disorders in children (Cochrane Review). The Cochrane Library, issue 1. John Wiley, Chichester

Catassi C 2002 Coeliac disease, an emerging problem in developing countries. Celiachia News Inglese. Online. Available at: http://www.celiachia.it.news/page33.html [accessed 3 November 2003]

Cystic Fibrosis Trust 2001 National consensus standards for the nursing management of cystic fibrosis. Cystic Fibrosis Trust, Bromley, Kent

Davis R, Karmarz P, Bohlke K et al 2001 Measles-mumps-rubella and other measles-containing vaccines do not increase the risk for inflammatory bowel disease: a case-control study from the vaccine safety datalink project. Archives of Pediatrics and Adolescent Medicine 155(3):354–359

Davison S 2002 Coeliac disease and liver dysfunction. Archives of Disease in Childhood 87(4):293–296

De Vizia B, Raia V, Spana C, Pavlisis C 2003 Effect of an 8-month treatment with omega-3 fatty acids (eicosapentaenoic and docosahexaenoic) in patients with cystic fibrosis. Journal of Parenteral and Enteral Nutrition 27(1):52–57

Dodge J 2000 Fibrosing colonopathy. Gut 46(2):152–153

ERIC 2001 Childhood soiling, minimum standards of practice for treatment and service delivery: benchmarking guidelines. ERIC, Bristol

Fiocchi A, Martelli A, de Chiara A et al 2003 Primary dietary prevention of food allergy. Annals of Asthma, Allergy and Immunology 91(1):3–13

Gale L, Wimalaratna H, Brotodiharjo A, Duggan JM 1997 Down's syndrome is strongly associated with coeliac disease. Gut 40(4):492–496

Hanson L, Korotova M, Telemo E 2003 Breast feeding, infant formulas and the immune system. Annals of Allergy, Asthma and Immunology 90(6):59–63

Holmes G 2001 Coeliac disease and type 1 diabetes mellitus—the case for screening. Diabetic Medicine 18:169–177

Jenkins H 2001 Inflammatory bowel disease. Archives of Disease in Childhood 85(5):435–437

Laghi A, Borrelli O, Paoloantonio P, Dito L 2003 Contrast enhanced magnetic resonance imaging of the terminal ileum in children with Crohn's disease. Gut 52(3):393–397

Metcalf C 2002 Crohn's disease: an overview. Nursing Standard 16(31):45–52

Miall L, Rudolf M, Levene M 2003 Paediatrics at a glance. Blackwell Science, Oxford

McVerry M 1999 Managing the child with gastroenteritis. Nursing Standard 13(37):49–52

Powers S, Patton S, Byars K, Mitchell M 2002 Caloric intake and eating behavior in infants and toddlers with cystic fibrosis. Pediatrics 109(95):75–79

Puntis J 2001 Nutritional support at home or in the community. Archives of Disease in Childhood 84(4):295–301

Royal College of Nursing (RCN) 2004 Good practice in infection control – guidance for nursing staff. RCN, London. Online. Available to RCN members at: http://www.rcn.org.uk

Sharif F, Crushell E, O'Driscoll K, Bourke B 2001 Liquid paraffin: a reappraisal of its role in the treatment of constipation. Archives of Disease in Childhood 85(2):121–124

Sicherer S 2003 Clinical aspects of gastrointestinal food allergy in childhood. Pediatrics 111(6):1609–1619

Smart J, Nolan T 2000 Paediatric handbook, 6th edn. Blackwell Science, Australia

Stapleton D, Gurrin L, Zubrick S, Silburn R 2000 What do children with cystic fibrosis and their parents know about nutrition and pancreatic enzymes? Journal of the American Dietetic Association 1000(12):1494–1500

Stark L, Mulvihill M, Jelalian E, Bowen M 1997 Descriptive analysis of eating behavior in school age children with cystic fibrosis and healthy control children. Pediatrics 99(5):665–670

Sullivan A 1999 Coeliac disease. Nursing Standard 14(11):48–52

Truby H, Paxton A 2001 Body image and dieting behavior in cystic fibrosis. Pediatrics 107(6):E92

Vitulano-Lawrence A 2003 Psychosocial issues for children and adolescents with chronic illness: self-esteem, school functioning and sports participation. Child and Adolescent Psychiatric Clinics of North America 12(3):585–592

Wakefield A et al 1998 Ileal-lymphoid-nodular hyperplasia, non-specific colitis, and pervasive developmental disorder in children. Lancet 351:637–641

Walker-Smith J 2000 Chronic inflammatory bowel disease in children: a complex problem in management. Postgraduate Medical Journal 76(898):469–473

Wong D 1999 Whaley and Wong's nursing care of infants and children, 6th edn. Mosby, St Louis

Chapter Thirty

30

Caring for Children with Cardiovascular Problems

Barbara V Novak

ABSTRACT

The purpose of this chapter and its companion PowerPoint presentation is to explore the advances in the knowledge of cardiovascular problems in infants and children and their impact on the delivery of informed, competent care based on the best available empirical evidence. The ranges of cardiovascular problems, the expanse of knowledge and the individuality of the child do not permit a full and comprehensive exploration of all the factors that can arise in these circumstances. Nevertheless, the intention is to focus on common principles that form the basis of knowledgeable and competent practice in a context of children's nursing.

Learning Outcomes

- Critically review the embryonic and fetal development of the cardiovascular system.

- Demonstrate understanding of the specific anatomical and physiological features of the cardiovascular system.

- Detail the nomenclature of congenital cardiovascular disease in childhood.

- Outline the nature of acquired cardiovascular problems in childhood.

- Outline the assessment of a child with suspected cardiovascular problem.

- Detail the strategy for evidence-based nursing care of a child with cardiovascular problems.

Introduction

Some of the most complex childhood health problems are related to the cardiovascular system. Most of these problems arise as a direct consequence of congenital cardiovascular defects. The direct cause of these congenital anomalies is not always known, although a range of contributing factors may play decisive roles. Many of these defects can be diagnosed in utero before birth. Other problems may be detected at birth largely due to the child manifesting persistent central cyanosis. Yet other forms of defects may not be detected until later in childhood. In most instances the clinical management of such defects will require specialist medical, surgical and nursing interventions.

Improved health care and better infection control have, in many instances, reduced the incidence of acquired cardiovascular disease such as bacterial endocarditis in childhood. Nevertheless, viral myocarditis, cardiomyopathies and secondary cardiovascular disease caused by metabolic problems can arise. Each of these problems will require very specific therapeutic and nursing interventions. Emphasis on evidence-based practice, as a basis for holistic nursing care, is crucial if the overall management of the child and support for the family are to be proactive.

The Embryonic Development of the Cardiovascular System

The perfectly developed cardiovascular system is an efficient transport network supported by a rhythmically pulsatile four-chambered heart. Its role is to transport blood within the closed circuit of semi-compliant vessels, delivering nutrients and metabolic substrate to the tissue and removing metabolic waste products from the tissue. This functional potential of the cardiovascular system is, however, dependent on the presence of a vast range of factors including appropriate genetic expression, sequential embryonic and fetal development and functional adaptation after birth.

Scenario

Christopher, a third-year child branch student nurse, reported to his seminar colleagues that a number of children had been admitted to his ward with a history of respiratory difficulties and cyanosis. The evidence drawn from the physical assessments suggests that these children are suffering from congenital cyanotic cardiac anomalies. The severity of the respiratory difficulties and cyanosis means that these children require specialist hospitalised care. Christopher asked that the seminar should focus on the normal embryonic development of the heart and then critically examine the anatomy and physiology of the cardiovascular system in children.

The Normal Circulatory System

The normal circulatory system can be divided into two functional compartments: the systemic circulation, which is supported by the left ventricle; and the pulmonary circulation, which is supported by the right ventricle. Both, the right and the left ventricle work in relative harmony. This ensures that the systemic circulation transports oxygenated blood and nutrients from the left ventricle through the aorta to the systemic arteries and capillaries. By contrast, the pulmonary circulation receives its deoxygenated blood from the right ventricle. This blood is then pumped through the pulmonary artery to lungs. Here a complex capillary bed surrounds the alveoli and facilitates gaseous exchange across the capillary–alveolar membranes. As a consequence of this efficient gaseous exchange, oxygenated blood is transported to the left atrium by way of pulmonary venules, which fuse, eventually giving rise to four pulmonary veins that attach to the posterior wall of the left atrium. The fundamental difference between the pulmonary and systemic circulation is the purpose of the circulating blood. The systemic circulation supplies blood to all organs supporting the metabolic requirements of the tissue, whereas the pulmonary circulation serves as an important part of the body's gas exchange system that ensures the return of oxygenated blood to the left atrium.

The Development of the Embryonic and Fetal Heart

The heart and its corresponding blood vessels develop from the splanchnopleuric mesoderm (embryonic tissue adjacent to the endoderm) in the cardiogenic region. The underlying endoderm contributes to this development by signalling to the primitive angioblastic cords to converge and form a pair of lateral endocardial tubes, which are then gradually fused and reshaped as the embryo grows and folds. The gradual fusion of these tubes shapes the single primitive heart tube, which is then remodelled by a sequential process of septation and folding that transforms the single lumen into the four chambers of the definitive heart. The initial chambers are, however, primitive, and will require considerable development.

Activity

Read Chapter 7 (Development of the heart, pp 151–188) and Chapter 8 (Development of the vasculature, pp 189–223) in:
- Larsen W 2002 Human embryology. Churchill Livingstone, Edinburgh.

Activity

Critically reflect on the embryonic developments of the heart and the blood vessels and discuss how such developments contribute to the shaping of the fetal circulation.

The Shaping of the Embryonic Cardiovascular System

The primitive heart tube consists of endothelium shaped to form a series of definitive expansions, shallow ridges and crevices (sulci), which outline the early framework of the heart. By the 22nd day a thick mass of splanchnopleuric mesoderm surrounds this heart tube, differentiating into the loosely organised myocardium and cardiac jelly, a layer of thick acellular matrix synthesised by the developing myocardium (Larsen 2001). The visceral pericardium lies externally to the myocardium. It evolves from mesothelial cells, which are derived independently from the splanchnopleuric mesoderm. These cells are believed to migrate onto the surface of the developing heart from the regions of the septum transversum or the sinus venosus.

From the 23rd day, the single heart tube begins to elongate, simultaneously loop, and fold. This displaces the bulbus cordis to the right and adjusts the position of the primitive ventricle to the left, allowing the primitive atrium to move in an upward direction. The complex cardiac folding is believed to be completed by the 28th day of embryonic life. According to Larsen (2001), this highly organised looping of the primitive heart tube may be intrinsically motivated. The assumption being that the state of hydration of the cardiac jelly, active migration and development of the primitive myocytes (cardiac muscle cells), and local haemodynamic forces initiated by the embryo's circulating blood could play a decisive role. This early cardiac morphogenesis includes the formation of the coronary vascular plexus, which later forms the coronary vessels.

The mesoderm, and its ability to synthesise mesodermal growth factors, is essential for the progressive cardiovascular development. Other growth factors are also transiently expressed in the developing myocardium, and differentially regulated during the course of atrial and ventricular development. Ambalavanan et al (1998) attributes the early configuration of the heart to the cardiac neural crest, which contributes to the formation of the primitive ventricular outflow tracts. Subsequent internal septation of the heart, and formation of the heart valves, is attributed to the development of the mesenchymal tissue at the atrioventricular and proximal outflow regions of the heart. Structural developments in the heart and blood vessels may play a role in regulating the functions of the cardiovascular system. For instance, marginal increases in blood pressure may contribute to the development of the myocardium as well as the muscle of the blood vessels and these developments could influence cardiac remodeling, especially in circumstances where the embryo has a congenital cardiac anomaly.

The primitive heart begins to contract on approximately the 22nd day (Larsen 2001). Blood begins to circulate through the primitive vessels within the next two days. The first blood cells found in the embryo's circulation are formed in the yolk sac, although normal embryonic and later fetal haematopoiesis occurs in the liver, spleen, thymus and, of course, eventually the bone marrow. The sustained rhythmic myocardial contractility may, in part, be dependent on myocardial hypertrophy, which is a basic adaptive response of the cardiac myocytes to an increasing workload. Ambalavanan et al (1998) argue, however, that myotropin (which might also play an important part in the pathogenesis of myocardial hypertrophy) may be an important primary modulator responsible for enhancing myocyte protein synthesis, cells growth and differentiation, essential to this normal development of the myocardium.

THE DEVELOPING ATRIA

Remodelling of the right atrium occurs during the 4th and 5th weeks of gestation. This initiates the gradual incorporation of the enlarged right sinus horn and the development of the venae cavae. A single pulmonary vein sprouts from the posterior wall of the left atrium and then divides to form the right and left pulmonary veins, which grow in the direction of the lung tissue, joining the smaller pulmonary veins that develop around the primitive bronchial tissue. The right and left pulmonary veins are eventually reconstructed forming, in most instances, four pulmonary veins.

The anatomical divisions between the atria and the common atrioventricular canal separate the systemic from the pulmonary circulation. This separation, however, also depends on the gradual fusion of the septum primum and the septum secundum. The septum primum establishes a firm interatrial muscle and the septum secundum contributes to the development of the foramen ovale, or oval widow. Throughout the embryonic and early fetal life, all septal structures form large openings that allow blood to flow in a specific direction. The foramen ovale is one of the most important of these openings because it permits shunting of blood from the right atrium to the left atrium. This mechanism allows the blood to bypass the right ventricle, the pulmonary artery and its tributaries. The foramen ovale normally closes soon after birth, partly because of the abrupt cessation of fetal circulation at birth, with the first breath and the eventual dilatation of the pulmonary vessels. These mechanisms reverse the pressure difference between the atria and push the flexible membranous part of the septum against the less conforming muscular septum thus closing the foramen ovale and blocking any shunting of blood from the right to the left atrium.

Division and shaping of the common atrioventricular canal by the septum intermedium (the middle segment of the intraventricular septum) into the right and left atrioventricular canals ensures that the right atrioventricular canal aligns the right atrium with the right ventricle and the left atrioventricular canal aligns the left atrium with the left ventricle. The division and reshaping of the common atrioventricular canal initiates the development of the primitive left ventricle, which establishes a firm contact with the proximal portion of the truncus arteriosus, a major vessel, which ultimately divides to form the future aorta and the main pulmonary artery. The four main cardiac valves begin to form in the 5th week of gestation, almost immediately following the division of the atrioventricular canal, and the septation of the truncus arteriosus, and is initially supported by growth and shaping of ventricular muscle from below. However, proliferating cells, which surround these orifices eventually, form the complex mitral and tricuspid valves respectively.

THE DEVELOPING VENTRICLES

The right and the left ventricle are composite structures. According to Larsen (2001) the right ventricle is derived predominantly from the inferior aspects of the bulbus cordis and the right aspect of the conus cordis. The left ventricle develops mainly from the primitive ventricle and the left wall of the conus cordis. The division of the two ventricles and the establishment of their corresponding outflow tracts, namely, the main pulmonary artery and the aorta, complete the morphogenesis of the heart and its major vessels. The intraventricular septum is formed by the developing right and left ventricular walls opposing one another (Collins 1995, Larsen 2001). The growth of this muscular septum is halted just before the superior edge meets the inferior membranous surface of the septum intermedium, the middle segment of the intraventricular septum. This arrest in growth allows for blood flow between the ventricles and prevents the left ventricle being occluded by its outflow tract. The flow of blood between these two chambers appears to contribute to the development of the ventricles. As the ventricular septum develops, the myocardium itself begins to enlarge forming characteristic ventricular trabeculae (ridges in the myocardium), which shape the ventricular chambers and their respective outflow tracts so that the heart can function as a competent mechanical pump.

The main cardiac outflow pathway, the truncus arteriosus, is divided by a septum and this shapes the distal aspects of the right and left outflow tracts for the two ventricles. The separation of the aorta from the main pulmonary artery is followed by the appearance, at their base, of three distinctive swellings. These swellings (tubercules) are believed to evolve, during the 6th week of gestation, into the characteristic semilunar valves, also known as the aortic and the pulmonary artery valves. Development of these valves is not thought to be complete until the 9th week of gestation (Larsen 2001), although they appear to be directing the intracardiac blood flow at an earlier stage.

The final stage in the intracardiac development involves the growth of the membranous interventricular septum, which is originally derived from the inferior endocardial cushion. The membranous septum fuses with the muscular interventricular septum to prevent any blood flow between the right and the left ventricles at about 8 weeks of gestation. The earlier development of the aorta and the pulmonary artery ensures that both ventricles can now function autonomously with respect to their own outflow tracts. Where complete fusion of these two important structures fails a membranous ventricular septal defect (VSD) will persist. This is the most common type of congenital cardiac anomaly that occurs in children.

THE DEVELOPMENT OF THE VALVES

The atrioventricular valves begin their development in the 5th week of gestation with the formation of the cusps within the atrioventricular canals. The free edges of these cusps attach to the sinew-like chordae tendineae, which in turn insert into the papillary muscles. The design of these valves ensures that, on folding back during diastole, blood flows uninhibited from the atria to the ventricles, but that on closing tightly during systole a backflow of blood into the atria is prevented. Generally, the left atrioventricular valve has only two cusps, which form the bicuspid valve, also known as the mitral valve. The right atrioventricular valve usually, but not always, develops three cusps, which shape the tricuspid valve.

CHAMBER AND VESSEL CONCORDANCE

Primitive blood vessels begin to appear in the splanchnopleuric mesoderm of the yolk sac on the 17th day. A similar aggregation of cells, also known as blood islands, appears in the embryonic disc on the 18th day. These cells initiate the formation of the embryo's blood vessels. The early development and subsequent reshaping of the endocardial tubes allows a pair of dorsal aortas to attach to their cranial axis and then form the first pair of aortic arches. Four additional aortic arches develop during the 4th and 5th weeks, connecting the rudimentary aortic sac (also known as the truncus arteriosus) to the dorsal aortas, which fuse later to form the median dorsal aorta. This complex network of the aortic arches is eventually remodeled to establish arteries within the upper thorax, neck and head. The dorsal aorta gives rise to three distinctive sets of arterial vessels (Collins 1995, Larsen 2001):

- the ventral arteries, which supply the gut
- the lateral arteries, which supply the retroperitoneal organs such as the kidneys and the gonads
- the intersegmental arteries, which supply, in part, the head, the neck and body walls.

The arteries supplying the gastrointestinal tract are derived from remnants of vitelline arteries and the vitelline duct, which anastomose with the paired dorsal aortae. The dorsal aortae in turn connect to the umbilical arteries, which carry blood from the embryo and later the fetus to the placenta.

The primitive venous system consists of three major components:

- the cardinal veins, which drain the head, neck, body walls and limbs
- the vitelline veins, which initially drain the yolk sac
- the umbilical veins, which carry oxygenated blood from the placenta to the embryo/fetus.

All three sets of veins initially drain into the right and left sinus horns but their extensive modification gives shape to a more defined systemic venous connection with the right atrium. The left sinus horn is eventually transformed into the coronary sinus and the oblique vein of the left atrium. The coronary sinus receives most of the venous blood returning from the coronary vascular bed. The vitelline venous system gives rise to the liver sinusoids and the portal system that transports venous blood from the intestinal tract to the liver. The vitelline system further subdivides within the liver establishing the ductus venosus, a small vessel that directs the embryonic/fetal blood from the umbilical vein directly into the inferior vena cava.

The complex arrangement of the heart is attained by the 55th day of gestation (Larsen 2001). The remaining period of gestation facilitates growth and relative maturation of the cardiovascular structures and corresponding haemodynamic adaptation. Myocardial cells proliferate in conjunction with the rapid accumulation of contractile proteins and metabolic substrates.

Activity

Read
- Chapter 22 (The circulatory system) in Hoffman (2003 pp 1745–1904).
- Chapter 21 (Blood vessels and circulation) in Martini (2004 pp 721–777).
- Critically review the anatomical and physiological characteristics of the fetal circulation.
- Give a reasoned account of the adaptations, which need to occur in the fetal circulation shortly after the birth of a child.
- Give a rationale for the differences between the fetal circulation and the assumed normal circulation of a 7-year-old child.

Developmental Changes in the Cardiovascular System

THE NORMAL POSITION AND SHAPE OF THE HEART

In children, the heart is a small, rounded, three-dimensional pyramid that lies in the mediastinal cavity more horizontally than in the adult. The apex of the heart is normally higher, and located in the fourth left intercostal space, extending only to the fifth intercostal space by 7 or 8 years of age. The base of the heart lies in an oblique position behind the sternum. It consists of the atria and their respective auricles (small appendages of each atrium). The two ventricles form the inferior aspect of the cardiac silhouette coming together to form the apex.

A mature heart weighs between 230 and 340 g, and this reflects the person's body size. However, according to Gabella (1995), this weight is achieved only between 17 and 20 years of age. In children, the normal heart is relatively small, the size varying with age and body surface area.

The heart is suspended in a pericardial sac by its attachments to the aorta and the pulmonary artery. This leaves the apex relatively free and allows the ventricles to move the apex forward to strike against the left side of the chest wall during contraction (systole). This characteristic thrust is best heard as the apex beat on auscultation and is frequently referred to as the point of maximal intensity.

Activity
- Name the three anatomically distinctive layers of the heart.
- Give a reasoned account of the functions of these distinctive layers.

THE PERICARDIUM

The fibrous pericardium encloses, and to some extent protects, the heart. It forms a continuum with the adventitia of the major veins and arteries that communicate with the heart. The serous pericardium is a double-layered membrane that consists of flat secretory epithelium, connective tissue and some adipose tissue, which is present in insignificant quantities in children. The two layers of the serous pericardium form a pericardial cavity, which holds a very small volume of serous fluid that acts as a lubricant preventing the occurrence of friction as the two membranes glide over each other during systole.

THE MYOCARDIUM

The myocardium is the contractile muscle of the heart, which is composed of highly specialised myocytes that contain a rich bed of sarcoplasmic reticulum. The myocardial mass increases fairly rapidly during fetal life as a result of the gradual increase in cell number. The composition of the myofibrils within the myocytes increases rather more slowly throughout fetal life and early infancy, giving rise to what is known as myocyte hypertrophy (i.e. an increase in the size of the myocytes). After birth, in children of all ages, the capacity for myocyte hyperplasia may be limited, although myocyte hypertrophy continues up to 20 years of age, under normal physiological conditions.

Sources of Chemical Energy for the Myocardium

The chemical energy for the contraction of heart muscle is derived from the metabolism of carbohydrates and fatty acids. However, because the amount of oxygen required for fatty acid metabolism is 11% more than that required for carbohydrate metabolism, to produce an equivalent quantity of adenosine triphosphate, fatty acids are not as efficient as glucose in terms of providing metabolic fuel or energy. Nevertheless, the adult myocardium has a strong preference for fatty acids. This contrasts with the preferences of the fetal and neonatal myocardium, which appears to be an obligatory user of carbohydrates or glucose. This may be clinically significant in circumstances of severe hypoglycaemia, when myocardial contractility and cardiac function in neonates (and possibly young children) may be affected adversely (Gluckman & Heymann 1996). There is no evidence suggesting the timing of this transition from the use of glucose to fatty acids as the dominant metabolic fuel, but it is possible that this transition is a gradual process influenced by dietary factors.

THE ENDOCARDIUM

The endocardium is composed of a specialised endothelium and a layer of fibroelastic connective tissue that lines the inner surfaces of the heart including the four cardiac valves. Characteristically, the endocardium is thicker in the atria than the ventricles and this may have a functional significance yet to be determined.

Electrophysiology: Functional Features of the Heart

The coordinated contraction of heart muscle provides the mechanical energy for the transportation of blood throughout the entire vasculature. The electrodynamic controls of the heart and the force of myocardial contractility are the consequence of the sophisticated cellular mechanisms, which bring about the rhythmic excitation–contraction coupling phenomena. In the fetus, the right ventricle ejects approximately 60% of blood while the left ventricle ejects only 40% of the total cardiac output (Hoffman 2003). As both ventricles pump blood against a similar vascular resistance, there is little difference in the thickness of the myocardium as the two ventricles develop. However, in some instances the right ventricular wall is slightly thicker than the left ventricular wall, and this persists for a considerable time after birth. Electrocardiographic (ECG) recordings reflect this phenomenon as a relative right ventricular dominance (Hoffman 2003 pp 1757–1762). The origin of this ventricular hypertrophy is physiological and can be attributed to the workload of the right ventricle and associated physical development of the myocardium during fetal life. However, a clear distinction must be made between this physiological right ventricular hypertrophy and a hypertrophy initiated by some form of pathophysiological changes that may affect the hearts of the neonates and children.

Activity

- Give a reasoned explanation for the significant differences in the normal ranges in children's heart beats identified in Table 30.1.
- Define bradycardia in the context of each of the age groups in Table 30.1.
- Define tachycardia in the context of each of the different age groups.
- In your view, is bradycardia or tachycardia more clinically significant in children; and why is this the case?

The faster heart rate in infants is largely attributed to the smaller size of the ventricular chambers, which are capable of ejecting only a small amount of blood, commonly referred to as the stroke volume, on each ventricular contraction. However, as the child's metabolic demands are high, and these have to be met by an effective cardiac output (the quantity of blood pumped by the left ventricle per minute), the potential deficits created by the small stroke volume are corrected by the higher heart rate. As children grow older, their hearts, and especially the ventricular chambers, become larger and the stroke volume increases, which contributes to the significant reduction of the heart rate. It is important, however, to appreciate that the normal heart rate and stroke volume in all children fluctuate with activity and crying.

The Cardiac Cycle

The cardiac cycle is defined as the time from the beginning of one heart beat to the beginning of the next. Each cardiac cycle is initiated and governed by an action potential generated within the sinoatrial node and conveyed rapidly to both

Table 30.1 Normal Range of Heart Rates in Children at Rest

Age of the child	Normal range (beats per minute)	Average (beats per minute)
Newborn–6 months of age	90–160	120
6–12 months of age	80–140	110
1–3 years	80–120	100
3–6 years	75–115	90
6–9 years	70–110	90
9–11 years	70–105	85
11–14 years	65–100	80

atria. The fractional delay in the transfer of the impulse from the atria to the ventricles ensures that the atria contract before the ventricles, as a result of which the blood is pumped by the atria into the ventricles, increasing the ventricular volume, which in turn raises the stroke volume.

The four phases of the cardiac cycle are commonly known as:

- contraction (phase I)
- ejection or systole (phase II)
- relaxation (phase III)
- filling or diastole (phase IV).

Although the rhythmic contraction of the heart is intrinsic (a mechanism frequently referred to as myogenic), the harmonising of the cardiac cycle, in terms of rate, force of contractility and volume output, is accomplished by the autonomic nervous system (Priebe & Skarvan 2000). The autonomic nervous system has a direct effect on the nodal tissue, the coronary vessels, atrial and ventricular myocardium and so, to some extent, augments and supports the adapting cardiac function. Physical activities or crying will also increase the child's heart rates significantly by, among other factors, increasing oxygen demand.

At the onset of ventricular contraction, the atrial and ventricular pressure are fairly equal. However, as the ventricular blood volume increases and the ventricular pressure rises initiating the closure of the atrioventricular valves. This gives rise to the first heart sound (called 'lub'). Because the pulmonary artery and aortic valves remain closed, the ventricles are said to be in isovolumetric contraction. This raises the ventricular pressure further and causes a bulging of both the semilunar and the atrioventricular valves. The semilunar valves open when the left ventricular pressure exceeds the aortic pressure and the right ventricular pressure exceeds the pulmonary artery pressure. The rapid expulsion of blood during the early phase of systole raises the ventricular pressures further establishing a maximum ejection point. This is followed by the last systole phase, which influences the gradual decline in the ventricular and aortic pressures, and the onset of ventricular diastole or early isovolumetric relaxation which culminates in the closure of the semilunar valves and the initiation of second heart sound ('dub').

The volume of blood ejected on each ventricular contraction is defined as the stroke volume. The cardiac output is defined as the amount of blood ejected by the heart during each minute (cardiac output = stroke volume × heart rate/min). The cardiac index takes into consideration the child's body surface area and is therefore a measure of the cardiac output per square metre of body surface area. In children, cardiac index values continue to rise to above 4.0 L/min/m^2 up to 10 years of age, and then declines, falling to a new lower normal value of about 2.4 L/min/m^2 (Guyton & Hall 2002). This phenomenon may be attributed to the normally high metabolic rate in younger children. Exercise and crying will also influence the child's stroke volume, cardiac output and cardiac index but this is usually transitory in contrast to the factors that have a more definitive effect on cardiac output such as the child's age, size, metabolism and body surface area.

While the function of the heart shows some degree of adaptability, four factors are perceived as critical to the ultimate control of the cardiac output. These are the:

- heart rate
- myocardial contractility
- preload (the volume of blood that returns to and stretches the ventricles prior to contraction)
- afterload (the resistance to the ejection of blood from the ventricle into the great vessels), and total peripheral resistance.

Although the heart rate and myocardial contractility are of cardiac origin both can be augmented by neural and humoral mechanisms. By contrast, the preload and afterload are dependent on blood volume, the size of the heart and the dimension of the blood vessels. There is, however, a cyclical nature to this, in that both preload and afterload are important determinants of cardiac output, which is influenced by the heart rate and myocardial contractility.

Scenario

Christopher's knowledge of the developmental aspects of anatomy and physiology of the cardiovascular system now leads him to focus on the nature of cardiovascular problems that can occur in infancy and childhood.

Determining the Origins and Extent of Cardiovascular Problems in Childhood

Children of all ages can present with signs and symptoms that suggest underlying cardiovascular problems that invariably require therapeutic intervention. However, it must be recognised that effective therapeutic and nursing care for a child with a cardiovascular problem is dependent on the precise diagnosis of the problem and competent delivery of care that is evidence based and carefully planned to meet the individual child's health needs.

Evidence-based Practice

The professional context

Children's nurses need to be fit for practice. This includes being knowledgeable about the:
- normal anatomical features of the child's heart
- normal functional scope of the child's cardiovascular system
- possible deviations from such norms and how these might affect a child.

It requires the nurse to be competent in:
- assessing such children for evidence of a cardiovascular problem
- monitoring the physical, physiological and behavioural changes that may appear as a consequence of an underlying cardiovascular problem
- communicating the findings to other practitioners in a professional manner
- using the empirical evidence in the formulation of diagnosis, therapeutic interventions and appropriate care
- communicating with the child and the parents in an informed and professional manner.

Knowledge of possible structural anomalies and functional problems is clearly indispensable in the competent assessment of a child with suspected cardiovascular problem. Such prior knowledge acts as a basis for critical reflection on the evidence collected during various assessments, and more invasive investigation, which such children must have.

Cardiovascular problems, which present in childhood, are commonly classified according to their congenital or acquired origins. The purpose of the systematic observation, assessment and investigation is to establish the structure and functions of the cardiovascular system, identifying in the process the precise nature of the problem. In general, children with acquired heart disease, such as myocarditis, commonly present with symptoms that suggests generalised ill health. By contrast, some children with congenital heart disease can be asymptomatic whereas others present with signs and symptoms that are confined to the cardiovascular and sometimes the respiratory system, at a very early. The most common features are cyanosis, failure to grow, a cardiac murmur, dysrhythmia and symptoms of congestive cardiac failure.

Activity

- Read Chapter 34 (The child with cardiovascular dysfunction) in Wong et al (2003 pp 1464–1529).
- Access the companion PowerPoint presentation and define congenital cardiovascular disease that occurs in children.
- Distinguish between the common features of acyanotic and cyanotic congenital cardiovascular lesions that occur in children.

- Distinguish between congenital cardiovascular disease and acquired cardiovascular disease that may occur in children.

The congenital cardiovascular problems can be classified into two distinctive groups: the acyanotic cardiovascular lesions and the more profound cyanotic cardiovascular lesions. The acyanotic cardiovascular lesions generally include structural problems such as patent ductus arteriosus, atrial septal defects and some ventricular septal defects. In general, children with these defects are initially asymptomatic. The first indication of an underlying cardiovascular problem may be the child's history of recurrent respiratory infection, failure to grow or poor exercise tolerance.

Ventricular septal defects are the most common congenital cardiovascular defects occurring in isolation or in association with other more complex cardiovascular anomalies. These defects are commonly classified according to their size and position in the interventricular septum. Defects are most common in the membranous part of the septum, although they do extend into the muscular part of the septum. A wide range of defects can also occur in the muscular part of the septum. The position, size and complexity of the defect (Hoffman 2003) determine the signs and symptoms with which the child presents. For instance, the size of the defect determines the magnitude of the shunting of blood from the left ventricle to the right ventricle. Larger defects tend to have a more profound effect on the right ventricle as a consequence of which infants present early with respiratory difficulties and congestive cardiac failure. Both problems are caused by an increase in pulmonary blood flow caused by the amount of oxygenated blood being shunted from the left ventricle across the defect into the right ventricle. This additional volume of blood is then directed to the lungs. This leads to pulmonary plethora as a consequence of which normal pulmonary ventilation and gas exchange may be compromised. In time, the haemodynamic disturbances caused by the abnormal inter-ventricular shunting of blood causes right ventricular hypertrophy, left atrial and ventricular dilatation (Hoffman 2003). This augments the normal shape of the heart, a feature that is observed on the child's chest X-ray.

Congenital cardiovascular lesions that cause the baby to be cyanotic from birth account for less than 25% of all congenital cardiac defects. Many of these defects are life threatening, such as, for instance, tricuspid atresia, and early diagnosis and therapeutic intervention is essential. The severity of the cyanosis is invariably determined by the restrictions to pulmonary blood flow, which has a compromising effect on pulmonary gas exchange. Transposition of the great arteries is one of the most common forms of cyanotic congenital cardiac defects that presents in neonates. It occurs more commonly in males than females with a ratio of 3:1 (Hoffman 2003).

The abnormality is confined to the ventricular–arterial connections in which the aorta is attached to the right ventricle and the pulmonary artery is attached to the left ventricle. This means that the pulmonary and systemic circulation run in parallel to each other, a process that interferes with the normal oxygenation of blood in the lungs, as a consequence of which the blood in the systemic circulation is oxygen poor and the baby suffers from severe cyanosis. In this instance, the baby's survival depends on the presence of other defects, such as a patent ductus arteriosus or atrial or ventricular septal defects, which permit mixing of blood between the pulmonary and systemic circulation. The presence of these associated defects and the degree of mixing between the two bloodstreams also determine the haemodynamic findings.

Most commonly, babies present with only a small patent foramen ovale, which does not facilitate adequate mixing between the pulmonary and the systemic blood, and thus contributes to severe cyanosis shortly after birth. As a consequence, such babies experience low PaO_2, which leads to metabolic acidosis and depression of myocardial function. The normal fall in pulmonary vascular resistance and the corresponding increase in pulmonary blood flow that occurs soon after birth leads to left atrial and left ventricular volume overload. The combination of metabolic acidosis with depression of myocardial contractility and volume overload may be contributing to heart failure and rapid deterioration in the infant's haemodynamic status.

Acquired cardiovascular disease is relatively uncommon in children in the developed world. Nevertheless, awareness of the existence of such problems is important if children are to receive the most appropriate treatment that their condition warrants. The acquired cardiovascular diseases can be grouped into those that are caused by:

- infection, as in endocarditis, myocarditis and pericarditis

- systemic metabolic problems, as in myocardial disease

- unknown factors, as in cardiomyopathy and cardiac tumours.

Depending on the primary cause, each of these conditions may affect the child in a very different way, for instance, the nature and virulence of the pathogen, the magnitude of the metabolic problem or the severity of the abnormal morphological change to the heart. It is therefore important to recognise that children affected by any of these problems can present acutely ill with severe haemodynamic instability and signs of low cardiac output. Alternatively, some children may experience more subtle forms of ill health and present with failure to grow, reduced exercise tolerance and occasionally cardiac dysrhythmias (Bristow 2003 p 1860) that if untreated may result in sudden death.

The common denominator in the acute and the more long-standing acquired form of heart disease is congestive

cardiac failure, which must be treated in conjunction with any treatment for the underlying cause of the primary disease. However, supportive therapeutic interventions culminating in a successful eradication of the primary disease is not always possible. Surviving children with myocardial disease may, in some circumstances, require cardiac transplantation as a means to enhancing their quality of life.

Reflect on your Practice

A 6-week-old baby is admitted to the cardiac unit with a short history of breathlessness, difficulties with feeding and increasing cyanosis, especially during crying. Following a thorough physical assessment and ultrasonic scan of the baby's heart and greater blood vessels, a diagnosis of ventricular septal defect is made. On arrival to the cardiac unit the baby is found to be in congestive cardiac failure and, therefore, will require swift therapeutic intervention and competent nursing care:

- How should this baby's care be managed to maximise the best therapeutic outcome?
- Give a systematic account of the nursing care that this baby will require.
- Give a reasoned account of the medical treatment that this baby will require.

CONGESTIVE CARDIAC FAILURE

The difference between the various kinds of congenital and acquired heart disease in childhood are determined, to a large extent, by the impact of the primary problem on the function of the cardiovascular and respiratory systems. Respiratory difficulties and hypoxia are common clinical features in children with altered pulmonary blood flow. Furthermore, as the myocardium is more oxygen dependent (Hoffman 2003, Wong et al 2003) in childhood, the hypoxia is likely to have a compromising effect on cardiac function eventually contributing to the development of heart failure.

Congestive cardiac failure occurs when the heart is unable to pump sufficient amounts of blood to the systemic (and pulmonary) circulation required to meet the metabolic demands of the body. Congestive cardiac failure is invariably the result of some structural or morphological defects in the cardiovascular system, which in time, give rise to characteristic haemodynamic changes that lead to:

- **Volume overload**: commonly caused by left-to-right intracardiac shunts that give rise to right ventricular hypertrophy and increased pulmonary blood flow.

- **Pressure overload**: commonly caused by obstructive lesions such as coarctation of the aorta and valve stenosis.
- **Impaired contractility**: caused by factors that affect myocardial contractility, such as cardiomyopathy, myocarditis, hypoglycaemia and low serum potassium, calcium or magnesium.
- **High cardiac output demands**: caused by such problems as septicaemia, in which peripheral vasodilatation allows an abnormal redistribution of the child's circulating blood volume away from the vital organs.

The pathophysiology of congestive cardiac failure can be viewed in terms of right ventricular failure and left ventricular failure. Right ventricular failure is characterised by suboptimal ventricular function. This leads to an abnormal rise in end-diastolic pressure, which in turn raises the central venous pressure and causes systemic venous engorgement. The ensuing systemic venous hypertension causes hepatomegaly and, in some instances, dependent tissue oedema. By contrast, left ventricular failure is characterised by abnormal increases in the left ventricular end-diastolic pressure, resulting in haemodynamic changes in the left atrium and the pulmonary veins. As a consequence, the lungs become congested with blood that then raises the pulmonary pressures and contributes to pulmonary oedema. However, because both sides of the heart depend on an adequate function of the other side, failure of one ventricular chamber invariably also causes reciprocal changes in the opposite chamber. This is particularly so in children whose hearts are small and functionally immature. Nevertheless, the cardiovascular system is capable of initiating compensatory mechanisms that result in a sustainable increase in cardiac output in keeping with the metabolic needs of the body. These compensatory mechanisms include activation of the sympathetic nervous system, increased heart rate, ventricular hypertrophy and dilatation. The failing heart and the compensatory mechanisms are responsible for the clinical features with which the child presents. The four most distinctive features that must be recognised in children are:

- impaired myocardial contractility
- pulmonary congestion
- systemic venous congestion
- fluid retention.

Each of these features must be critically and methodically evaluated. The intention being to ensure that the:

- severity of congestive cardiac failure is recognised
- primary cause is identified
- best therapeutic and caring interventions are utilized.

Diagnostic Assessment and Evaluation of the Child

The child's health and appearance frequently reflects the competence of the cardiovascular system, although this cannot always be assumed without careful physical assessment and evaluation. Therefore, a typical physical assessment should consist of inspection, palpation and auscultation. These will be followed by a range of more invasive assessments, such as evaluation of blood gases, echocardiography and cardiac catheterisation, which will provide more definitive evidence regarding the specific nature of the cardiovascular problem. The collected evidence must be documented and critically evaluated as part of the process of establishing the diagnosis.

INSPECTION

Inspection of the child's general appearance must include the body size, proportions, skin colour, visible pulsations and exaggerated shapes to the thorax. Assessment of the respiratory rate and pattern will also contribute to a better evaluation of the cardiovascular function. The child's response to stimuli and the surrounding environment will give an indication of the developmental milestones that have been reached. In health, a child's core body temperature is relatively constant at 36.0 to 37.5°C and the peripheral temperature is no lower than 34 to 35°C. However, if the peripheral skin temperature is found to be consistently lower it is important to distinguish between the possible contributing factors, such as low environmental temperatures or the child's compromised peripheral perfusion.

PALPATION

This involves tactile skills that contribute to the evaluation of the child's haemodynamic status. The pulse can be palpated in superficial arteries such as the brachial, radial, femoral artery and dorsalis pedis. The qualities of the pulse can be describes in terms of:

- frequency
- rhythm
- amplitude.

However, it must be appreciated that pulses may be difficult to feel in neonates and infants because of the relatively low arterial resistance to blood flow generated by the comparative thinness of the tunica media within the walls of the arteries and arterioles. For this reason, in children under 1 year of age, the heart rate should be recorded over the apex of the heart, using a stethoscope rather than by means of palpation of the radial pulse as it may not be possible to reliably feel the radial pulse. However, as the child grows older, the muscle fibres of the tunica media enlarge, augmenting the internal diameter of the arteries and raising the resistance to arterial blood flow, which in turn influences the magnitude of the pulse wave.

The intensity of a pulse can be rated on a scale of 0 to 4 as follows:

- An absent pulse is graded as 0.
- A palpable but weak and easily obliterated pulse is graded 1.
- A normal easily palpable pulse is graded as 2.
- A full pulse is graded as 3.
- A bounding pulse that is easily visible is graded as 4.

BLOOD PRESSURE

This term generally applies to the arterial pressure in the systemic circulation. Blood pressure fluctuates with each heart beat, between a maximum value (systolic pressure) achieved during cardiac systole and a minimum value (diastolic pressure) that reflects the diastolic phase. The blood pressure can be measured by invasive methods, which involve inserting a needle, attached to a monitoring device, into a peripheral artery. More commonly, however, blood pressure is measured externally, or is estimated by using an inflatable cuff on the upper arm or sometimes on the leg (below the knee). The accuracy of the measurement is dependent on the size of the cuff and this must be proportional to the length and diameter of the limb (two-thirds of the limb must be covered, e.g. on the upper arm this is two-thirds of the distance between the shoulder and the elbow). Alternatively, a Doppler percutaneous flow probe can be used to measure the systolic and a diastolic pressure. This device detects cessation of blood flow very accurately. The difference between the systolic and the diastolic pressure values is known as the pulse pressure. The major physiological factors that affect the pulse pressure are the stroke volume, the force of ventricular ejection and the compliance of the arterial vascular network. The greater the stroke volume, the greater is the amount of blood that must be accommodated in the arterial network. This produces a rise in the systolic pressure and a fall in the diastolic pressure, which will culminate in a wider pulse pressure.

Wide ranges of factors influence the child's blood pressure such as maturation of the autonomic nervous system, developments and maturation in the cardiovascular system and corresponding reflex mechanisms. Furthermore, there is some evidence to suggest that the intrauterine environment which influences low birth weight may also contribute to the development of hypertension in adulthood

(Barker et al 1993). In health, children's blood pressure parameters vary with age and under normal physiological conditions there should be a gradual increase in the systolic and diastolic pressures according to age (Table 30.2).

The physiological adaptation and maintenance of normal blood pressure is attributed principally to baroreceptors, which are present in the carotid and aortic bodies. These receptors are thought to augment and sustain the normal systemic blood pressure by reflex. However, in children with hypoxia, fluid retention and congestive cardiac failure the function of these baroreceptors could be compromised and so contributing to the changes in blood pressure that is sometimes observed in these children.

AUSCULTATION

This involves listening to the specific sounds generated by the heart as a consequence of the:

- systematic opening and closing of atrioventricular valves
- systematic opening and closing of the semilunar pulmonary artery and aortic valves
- vibration of blood against the walls of the heart and major blood vessels.

It is not uncommon for neonates and young children to present with a range of heart sounds and murmurs that are not always indicative of an underlying cardiovascular problem. Nevertheless, the presence of cardiac murmurs must be taken into consideration in the overall assessment of the child's cardiovascular system. The two distinguished heart sounds that must be heard are known as S_I and S_{II}. Under

Table 30.2 Blood Pressure in Childhood. Readings are the 50th Centile for Boys (Taken from Second Task Force on Blood Pressure Control in Children 1987)

Age	Systolic blood pressure (mmHg)	Diastolic blood pressure (mmHg)
Newborn	73	55
6 months	90	53
1 years	90	56
3 years	92	55
6 years	96	57
9 years	100	61
12 years	107	64
15 years	114	65

normal circumstances, S_I is louder at the apex of the heart in the mitral and tricuspid valve area. Conversely, S_{II} is best heard near the base of the heart in the pulmonary artery and the aortic valve area. Two further heart sounds may be audible and these are known as S_{III} and S_{IV}. S_{III} is though to be produced by vibrations caused during ventricular filling and may be heard in some children and young adults. By contrast, S_{IV} is generally attributed to the reduction in vibration initially caused by atrial contraction at the end of diastole. This sound is seldom heard and, when audible, further cardiovascular assessments should be considered. Cardiac murmurs are important sounds in neonates and young children, and must not be ignored, as they can suggest underlying cardiac or major blood vessel anomalies that will require further systematic screening and critical evaluation.

CHEST RADIOGRAPHY

This can determine the position of the heart, its size, shape, chamber and major vessel enlargement or hypoplasia. It depicts the anatomical size and shape of the trachea, the bronchi, and the lungs in relation to the heart. It provides considerable evidence regarding air entry and pulmonary ventilation and demarcates the extent of the pulmonary blood flow and pulmonary venous return. In children with cardiac problems such as congestive cardiac failure, chest radiography will help to establish the extent of the primary anatomical anomalies as well as the severity of path physiological problems such as cardiomegaly, pulmonary plethora and pulmonary congestion. In isolation, such evidence may be inconclusive; however, when considered in conjunction with other factors it can contribute to a definitive diagnosis.

ELECTROCARDIOGRAPHY

This records the changes in the electrical potentials during cardiac activity (Table 30.3). Such data also provide information about the anatomical orientation of the heart; the relative size of the chambers of the heart; heart rate, rhythm and origin of excitation; and the spread of the impulse. Disturbances in the normal conduction process can be suggestive of a primary cardiovascular problem.

Electrocardiography in children will also reflect some age related changes, which must be taken into consideration in the overall evaluation of the child's cardiovascular system. A summary of the age-related significant points may be detailed as follows:

- At birth, the thickness in the right ventricular muscle exceeds the thickness of the left ventricular muscle. This is a physiological phenomenon reflecting the right

Table 30.3 Electrocardiograph Recording of the Function of the Heart as a Pump

Electrocardiographic event	Corresponding physiological event in the heart
P wave	Depolarisation (excitation) of the atria prior to their contraction. The action potential (impulse) is initiated in the sinoatrial node. It spreads through the atrial muscle reaching the atrioventricular node
P-R segment	Atrial depolarisation and conduction of impulses through the atrioventricular node
QRS complex	Depolarisation (excitation) of the ventricles, the repolarisation (relaxation) of the atria is masked by the ventricular depolarisation
S-T segment	End of ventricular depolarisation and the beginning of the ventricular repolarisatuion
T wave	Repolarisation (relaxation) of the ventricles

ventricular workload during fetal life. However, the significant increase in the left ventricular workload, after birth, gradually augments this. Thus, the right ventricular dominance normally seen in neonates and young infants is gradually replaced by left ventricular dominance in later childhood. The ratio of left to right ventricular muscle mass in young adults is believed to average at 2.5:1 (Houston 1998, Park & Guntheroth 1987) and the electrocardiography recording reflects this ratio.

- The gradual increase in the chambers of the heart, in conjunction with the ongoing maturation of the myocardium, allows the heart to handle greater quantities of blood volume. In the healthy child this results in increasing stroke volume and cardiac output as a consequence of which the heart rate decreases.

- In conjunction with the decreasing heart rate all lengths and intervals (PR interval, QRS duration, QT interval) of the cardiac cycle increase (Houston 1998).

Existing cardiovascular problems can, however, interfere with the electrophysiological conduction throughout the atrial and ventricular myocardium, and these are then reflected in the electrocardiographic recordings.

ECHOCARDIOGRAPHY

This technique uses high-frequency sound waves to document detailed images, from which the atria, ventricles, the septal tissue, the atrioventricular and semilunar valves, and the great vessels can be identified and their dimensions measured. Most congenital cardiovascular defects and major myocardial changes may be identified using this technique. However, the correct diagnosis and therapeutic intervention is dependent on the precise measurement and critical evaluation of the size and complexity of the cardiovascular problem.

CARDIAC CATHETERISATION

This is the most invasive procedure that a child with a suspected cardiovascular problem may have to undergo. It involves inserting a radio-opaque catheter through a peripheral blood vessel into the respective chambers of the heart. This procedure is usually combined with angiocardiography in which a radio-opaque die is injected through the catheter into the circulation. Combined these procedures facilitate the collection of evidence regarding:

- oxygen saturation of the blood within the four chambers of the heart and the greater blood vessels
- haemodynamic pressure values within the four chambers and the greater blood vessels
- stroke volume and cardiac output values
- the position, size and complexity of the cardiovascular defects and anomalies.

Nursing Care Considerations

Children born with cardiovascular anomalies, and those that acquire cardiovascular disease, will require extensive diagnostic, therapeutic and nursing interventions. The specific range and sequence of interventions will be dictated by the severity of the cardiovascular problems with which the child presents. For instance, cardiovascular anatomical problems are likely to require surgical and supporting pharmacological interventions. By contrast, functional problems within the cardiovascular system, such as congestive cardiac failure, may be resolved by appropriate pharmacological interventions. In both instances, however, these children will require nursing care and their families will require support and education.

Evidence-based Practice

The nursing care of a child with a suspected cardiovascular problem can be challenging because such children do not consistently display symptoms until the child's energy expenditure exceeds the ability of the heart to meet the metabolic needs of the body. With the exception of children born with cyanotic cardiovascular disease, the onset of signs and

symptoms, in many children, is gradual and at times inconsistent requiring the nursing and medical staff to be vigilant in obtaining the appropriate clinically and socially significant evidence.

Methodical assessments of the child will enable the nurse to identify several nursing diagnoses that will require attention. All assessments must take into consideration the history of the child's physical growth, intellectual and psychosocial development, nutritional preferences and exercise tolerance. This information forms a critical part of the evidence about the child's general state of health and gives an indication about the kind of supportive nursing care and therapeutic interventions that the child may require.

In all circumstances, nursing interventions must be driven by the evidence collected during methodical assessments, or derived by critical evaluation of the child's:
- general physical appearance
- responsiveness
- behaviour
- restfulness and sleep
- vital signs: body temperature, heart rate/rhythm, respiratory rate/effort, blood pressure
- presence of hypoxia
- state of hydration
- elimination: extent of perspiration, urine output, emesis, faeces.

Activity
- Give a reasoned account as to why the above assessments are required.
- Critically evaluate the available evidence and demonstrate how this evidence can be used in the overall management of this child.

Children with established cardiovascular disease, especially congestive cardiac failure, must be cared for in a manner that will ensure comfort, maximise rest and support cardiac, respiratory, digestive and renal function. Nursing and therapeutic interventions must be coordinated so as to ensure the child's energy expenditure is minimised. Positioning the child in a manner that promotes comfort, facilitates lung expansion and minimises cardiac workload is an important aspect of nursing. Allowing for frequent rest and sleeping periods will also reduce the workload of the heart and promote the child's healing and restoration of health where this is possible.

Invasive diagnostic procedures such as thoracic surgery are painful and frightening. These children will, therefore, require emotional and psychological support from their parents, siblings and the practitioners caring for them. It must also be recognised that the child's parents, siblings and significant others will find such situations justifiably stressful. Every effort must be made to support them by involving them in the decision-making process. They should be given explanations about the evolving symptoms and how these can impact on the child's well-being. Similarly, explanations must be offered about care and treatment options if the parents are to make informed decisions.

Children are not always able to communicate verbally their pain, discomfort or distress and every effort must be taken to monitor their emotional, physical and physiological state to ascertain that comforting interventions and appropriate analgesia are administered proactively. For instance, children who have undergone surgery may require continuous intravenous infusion of opioids such as morphine sulfate or fentanyl for a period of 24–48 hours. Providing the dosages are calculated carefully in relation to the child's body surface area, these drugs are considered as safe and effective in relieving severe forms of pain. However, milder forms of oral analgesia, such as paracetamol or ibuprofen, may be given at regular intervals or when required to control less severe forms of pain. Providing the child is haemodynamically stable, provision must be made to encourage active play and mobilisation. Children who are comfortable, pain free and happy are likely to make a quicker recovery in health.

Activity

Most infants with congenital or acquired cardiovascular problems develop, at some stage, congestive cardiac failure, which contributes to difficulties with feeding due to breathlessness caused by other factors such as ventilation-perfusion mismatch. Read:

- Chapter 34 (The child with cardiovascular dysfunction) in Wong D et al (2003 pp 1464–1526).

Give a reasoned account of the nutritional needs of such children and how these needs can be best met without causing due distress to the individual child.

Small, nutritious and appetising meals should be offered to these children. Infants should be offered small but frequent bottle feeds and, where this is not possible, nasogastric tube feeding may have to be considered, especially if the infant manifests respiratory distress or cyanosis. Managing the child's hydration is an important aspect of care and all fluid intake must therefore be monitored carefully to ensure that episodes of overhydration or dehydration are avoided.

Children with congestive cardiac failure frequently experience problems of systemic fluid retention and hepatomegaly, which may further aggravate the child's respiratory distress, cardiac workforce and ability to digest and absorb nutrients.

Activity

- Critically review the impact of systemic fluid retention and hepatomegaly on the child's ability to feed and absorb nutrients.
- Establish as to why hepatomegaly could have a compromising effect on the function of the diaphragm and the gastrointestinal tract.
- Explain why these children may be failing to grow.

The limited availability of nutrients combined with the child's greater respiratory effort can have a devastating effect on the child's metabolism and might ultimately lead to metabolic acidosis, hypoglycemia, electrolyte imbalance and inappropriate activation of the renin–angiotensin–aldosterone system.

Activity

- Give a reasoned account how each of these problems can be recognised.
- Explain why each of these problems could have a detrimental effect on the child.
- How can the above problems be avoided?

Congestive cardiac failure also augments cardiac output, which in turn reduces renal perfusion. This also activates the renin–angiotensin–aldosterone system, which leads to renal retention of sodium and water. The increasing retention of sodium and water may be contributing to pulmonary and systemic oedema and concomitant reduction in urinary output. The retention of fluid will in turn contribute to weight gain despite the child's reduced nutritional intake or vomiting. This phenomenon can mask the child's cachexic state.

Activity

- Outline the measures that can be taken to monitor the child's fluid intake and elimination.
- Give a reasoned account as to why the child's blood electrolyte values should be monitored.

Therapeutic Intervention

Even in the most difficult situation, the primary cause of congestive cardiac failure needs to be determined and if possible treated. Correctable problems must be resolved expediently. One of the most successful interventions of congestive cardiac failure is likely to consist of the use of medication such as furosemide (a loop diuretic), lanoxin (a cardiac glycoside) or spironolactone (a potassium-sparing diuretic). In some circumstances, such children may also be given potassium supplements to maintain physiologically desirable plasma potassium values.

Cardiac rhythm disturbances may occur in children. Some of these disturbances resolve spontaneously, although more persistent disturbances will require definitive therapeutic interventions. For instance, a child with persistent bradycardia caused by conduction problems will require a permanent pacemaker to sustain acceptable cardiac rhythm. By contrast, children with recurrent episodes of profound supraventricular tachycardia may require suitable antiarrhythmic drugs. The primary rationale for both therapeutic interventions is to normalise cardiac rhythm in order to sustain good cardiac output.

Activity

Read:
- Chapter 17 (The heart) and Chapter 18 (The vascular system) in Rang et al (2003 pp 264–284 and pp 285–305).

Reflect on your Practice

- How would this medication affect the child's congestive cardiac failure?
- Give a reasoned account of the improvements in the child's health as a consequence of the appropriate therapeutic intervention.
- Consider the kind of preparation the child and family will require in instances where surgical intervention is required in order to safeguard the child's quality of life and long-term survival.

KEY POINTS

Following a methodical assessment of the child and a critical review of the clinically significant evidence, every effort must be made to assist the child in a manner that will reduce the cardiac workload. Such therapeutic and nursing interventions must also make every effort to reduce the child's respiratory distress, improve cardiac output and assist in elimination of undesirable quantities of retained body fluids. Care must be taken to ensure that the child's hydration and nutritional intake meets the metabolic demands and that the child is showing signs of growth and development.

Major anatomical defects that present at time of birth in the form of cyanotic congenital heart defects will require palliative or corrective surgical intervention at the most clinically appropriate time. The central aim here is to reconstruct the heart and, where necessary, the blood vessels in a manner that will restore normal cardiovascular haemodynamics and avoid the long-term complications that are commonly associated with congenital heart disease. Functional problems, such as myocarditis, congestive cardiac failure and low cardiac output must also be dealt with as they arise. In these instances, swift diagnostic and therapeutic interventions consisting of inotropic agents and antifailure drugs, among others, are essential.

Activity

Critical reflection on theory and practice
- Review the therapeutic intervention that should be considered for a child with a known cyanotic congenital cardiovascular anomaly and evidence of congestive cardiac failure.
- Critically review the nursing diagnoses that will have to be considered in the planning of nursing care for a child with congestive cardiac failure.
- Critically examine the merits of evidence-based practice in your consideration of holistic nursing care for a child with congestive cardiac failure.

Evidence-based nursing interventions are fundamental in the overall management of the child and family. These interventions begin with a methodical assessment of the child, documenting the available evidence. A critical exploration of this evidence will inevitably lead to informed decisions regarding the specific care that a child with a cardiovascular problem may require. Proactive holistic care must take into consideration the child's need for comfort, rest, sleep and nutrition. The more technical aspects of care, such as monitoring the child's haemodynamic values and evaluating the child's response to planned therapeutic and nursing interventions, must also form an important part of competent nursing practice.

Summary

It is not possible to consider here the full extent of the complex nature of cardiovascular problems that are known to encroach on children's lives. Nevertheless, attempts have been made to draw attention to the embryonic and fetal developments of the cardiovascular system with a view to establishing a basis for understanding the normal cardiovascular function in children. This approach has in turn prepared the background for understanding some of the common congenital and acquired cardiovascular problems that some children present with. The therapeutic interventions must be decided according to the specific problems with which such children present. This suggests that the ethos of best practice requires children's nurses to collect and critically consider the evidence that will significantly influence the therapeutic and nursing management in a manner that will result in a more restful child with improved cardiac function.

References

Ambalavanan N, Mariani G, Philips J et al 1998 The role of peptide growth factors in cardiovascular development and remodelling. In: Polin R, Fox W (eds) Fetal and neonatal physiology. WB Saunders, Philadelphia, pp 814–826

Barker DJP, Osmond C, Golding J et al 1993 Growth in utero, blood pressure in childhood and adult life, and mortality from cardiovascular disease. In: Baker DJP (ed.) Fetal and infant origins of adult disease. British Medical Association Publishing, London

Bristow J 2003 Acquired cardiovascular disease. In: Rudolph C, Rudolph A, Hostetter M et al (eds) Rudolph's paediatrics, 21st edn. McGraw Hill, New York, pp 1860–1865

Collins P 1995 Neonatal anatomy and growth. In: Bannister L et al (eds) Gray's anatomy. Churchill Livingstone, New York, pp 343–375

Gabella G 1995 Cardiovascular system. In: Bannister L et al (eds) Gray's anatomy. Churchill Livingstone, New York, pp 1451–1605

Gluckman P, Heymann M 1996 Paediatrics and perinatology: the scientific basis. Edward Arnold, London

Guyton A, Hall J 2002 Textbook of medical physiology. WB Saunders, Philadelphia

Hoffman J 2003 The circulatory system. In: Rudolph C, Rudolph A, Hostetter M et al (eds) Rudolph's paediatrics, 21st edn. McGraw Hill, New York, pp 1745–1905

Larsen W 2001 Human embryology. Churchill Livingstone, London

Martini F 2001 Fundamentals of anatomy and physiology. Prentice Hall, New Jersey

Park M, Guntheroth W 1987 How to read paediatric ECGs. Mosby Year Book, Baltimore

Priebe HJ, Skarvan K 2000 Cardiovascular physiology. BMJ Books, London

Rang H, Dale M, Ritter J, Moore P 2003 Pharmacology. Churchill Livingstone, Edinburgh

Second Task Force on Blood Pressure Control in Children 1987 Normal blood pressure readings for boys. National Heart, Lung and Blood Institute, Bethesda, MD

Wong D, Hockenberry-Eaton M, Wilson D et al 2003 The child with cardiovascular dysfunction. In: Wong D et al (eds) Nursing care of infants and children, 6th edn. Mosby, St Louis, pp 1464–1529

Suggestions for Further Reading

Berne R, Levy M 2001 Cardiovascular physiology. Mosby, Baltimore
This text offers an invaluable account of cardiovascular physiology as seen in healthy adults.

Brawn W, Barron D 2004 Management and outcome in hypoplastic left heart syndrome. Current Paediatrics 14(1):26–32
This article provides an informative and well-illustrated account of problems associated with hypoplastic heart syndrome, including the options available as palliative therapeutic interventions.

Campbell A, McIntosh N 1998 Forfar and Arneil's textbook of paediatrics. Churchill Livingstone, New York
This textbook offers an invaluable account of knowledge and skills required in assessing newborn infants and children. It also provides a helpful account of common congenital cardiovascular pathophysiology.

Chien K 2000 Genomic circuits and the integrative biology of cardiac diseases. Nature 407:227–232
This article explores some of the complex interactions between possible genetic and environmental factors and how these could act as modifiers of human health, particularly cardiovascular disease. Considerable attention is given to the distinctions between the pathogenesis of congenital and acquired cardiovascular problem.

Kitchiner D 2004 Antenatal detection of congenital heart disease. Current Paediatrics 14(1):39–44
This article offers an informative account of the methods used to detect structural and functional cardiac anomalies that present in fetuses during the antenatal period.

Nolan G 1998 Transcription and the broken heart. Nature 392:129–130
This article offers an invaluable insight into some of the factors that may influence the development of the embryo's heart.

Seale A, Shinebourne E 2004 Cardiac problems in Down syndrome. Current Paediatrics 14(1):33–38
This article provides an excellent account of the spectrum of heart defects, therapeutic interventions and anticipated outcomes in children with Down syndrome.

Smith J, Ley S, Curley M et al 1996 Tissue perfusion. In: Curley M, Bloedel Smith J, Moloney-Harmon P (eds) Critical care nursing of infants and children. WB Saunders, Philadelphia, pp 155–245
This chapter provides an informative account of the many facts, which are known to influence tissue perfusion.

Srivastava D, Olson E 2000 A genetic blueprint for cardiac development. Nature 407:221–226
This article offers an invaluable insight into some of the genetic factors that may influence the development of the embryo's heart.

Walsh K 2004 Interventional cardiology. Current Paediatrics 14(1):45–50
This article gives an excellent account of the current ranges of therapeutic interventions, which should be considered when managing the care of a child with congenital cardiovascular problems.

Yaffe S, Avanda J 1992 Paediatric pharmacology: therapeutic principles in practice. WB Saunders, Philadelphia
This book provides an excellent account of a range of pharmacological principles that need to be taken into consideration when caring for a child with compromised cardiovascular function.

Caring for Children: The Role of the Immune System in Protecting against Disease

Maureen R. Harrison

ABSTRACT

The aim of this chapter is to provide an overview of immunology, in particular barrier defence, and therefore to increase the children's nurses' understanding of how this knowledge can relate to the prevention and process of infection in infants and children.

Learning Outcomes

- Be able to understand the different phases of the immune response.

- To identify how innate immunity provides the first line of defence in protecting against infections.

- Be aware of the physiological barriers that prevent infection occurring.

- To understand other factors of first-line defence, such as cell-mediated and humoral immunity, which enable most infants and children to respond to microbial attack.

- To apply knowledge of innate immunology to principles of nursing practice, in particular infection control.

- To outline the assessment of a child with acute infection.

Introduction

The efficiency of the immune system in protecting against infection is often taken for granted in countries such as the UK. Even the World Health Organization (WHO) has demonstrated that, in developed countries like the UK, death from infections is not as significant as other causes of death, being only fourth in ranking from the ten leading causes of death (Mathers et al 2002). However, in developing countries, six of the top ten causes of death have infectious and perinatal causes. Figure 31.1 demonstrates causes of death among children under the age of five worldwide. It is important to note that 54% of deaths are also associated with malnutrition.

As a significant number of children worldwide continue to die from diseases of an infectious nature, an understanding of the nature of the battle between humans and micro-organisms, and the role of the immune system in protecting children from infectious diseases, is important. This knowledge then needs to be linked to how the children's nurse can promote and optimise health.

Many infectious agents (bacteria, viruses, fungi and protozoa) would use any opportunity to utilise the human body as a means for growth and proliferation. However, the human body has developed a series of very effective defence mechanisms to establish immunity against infection (Roitt et al 2001). The word 'immunity' comes from the Latin word *immunitas*, meaning 'freedom from'. In most instances, the human body is very efficient at avoiding attack but at certain times the infectious agents win, the result being the development of an infection (Roitt et al 2001).

There are many interindividual variations in how the immune system functions such as genetics, age, gender, diet, history of infections and vaccination (Clader & Kew 2002), and Figure 31.1 demonstrates the importance of nutrition; however, this chapter is concerned predominantly with the main process of immunity. The immune system has three phases in the overall response to attack:

- phase 1: immediate response – innate immunity.

- phase 2: the inflammatory response.

- phase 3: the adaptive immune response.

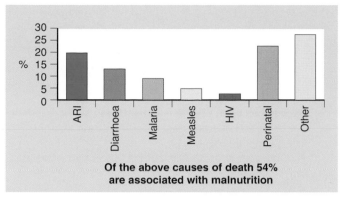

Fig. 31.1 • Proportional mortality among under fives worldwide, 2001. Of the causes of death shown, 54% of deaths are associated with malnutrition (from WHO 2003).

Each of these phases has its own unique strategies of warfare. However, only the first and second phases will be discussed with particular application to the developing immunity in a child. This will then be linked to the relevance of certain aspects of care for children.

Phase 1. The Immediate Response to Infection: Innate Immunity

At birth, most infants have the capacity to develop a very efficient immune system, as is demonstrated by the majority of infants who survive their first year of life without suffering from major life-threatening infections. Indeed, from as early as 20–26 gestational weeks, the fetus has been observed to be capable of mounting a sophisticated immune response, as evidenced by those fetuses who were infected with rubella during pregnancy (Warner 2004) and were shown to have antibodies against the rubella in their blood. However, the immune system is not fully developed at birth, and certain 'units' need to undergo learning programmes that will eventually enable them to recognise and destroy the huge dimension of immunogens (agents that are harmful to the human host) (Stiehm 1996). That part of the immune system involved in learning is referred to as the 'adaptive immune response' and includes the development of specific immune cells, lymphocytes, and the production of antibodies (immunoglobulins) against all harmful micro-organisms. This arm of the immune system will be not be discussed in any depth in this chapter, although aspects of it will be referred to.

The first means of defence against micro-organisms that would cause harm to the body is called 'innate immunity' or 'non-specific immunity' and previous exposure to these organisms is not needed to provide protection against infection. In other words, this part of the immune system does not need to learn how to destroy or render inactive these organisms because the ability to know how to fight against them is inherent, and from birth most babies have these fundamental immunological capabilities. The three main mechanisms of innate immunity are (Fig. 31.2):

- barrier mechanisms.
- cell-mediated mechanisms.
- humoral mechanisms.

These non-specific resistance mechanisms are responsible for the major part (> 95%) of host defence, the 'host' being the human body; they will therefore be studied in detail in this chapter (Zinkernagel 2003).

BARRIER MECHANISMS

Many of the essential components of the immune system develop very early in fetal life and most healthy newborn babies are prepared to deal with antigen challenges (Janeway et al 1999, Newell & McIntyre 2000). An antigen is any molecule that can stimulate an immune response, in particular a response that mobilises the adaptive immune system. The first lines of defence against infection are the external systems, which are commonly described as the barrier mechanisms. These are so called because they protect individuals by stopping harmful micro-organisms from entering the body, and inhibit colonisation of the same.

Skin

The skin is the largest organ in the young baby and it provides an intact, dry surface that is resistant to the penetration of micro-organisms. Not all micro-organisms are harmful

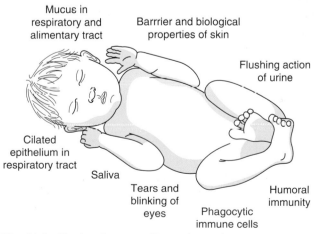

Fig. 31.2 • The key features of innate immunity.

and the skin of children and adults is normally host to a number of bacteria, such as harmless diphtheriods, Gram-positive cocci and yeasts, which are called commensal micro-organisms (Greenwood et al 2002). They are called 'commensal' because they have been 'permitted' to live on the skin and they provide some protection by taking up space and competing for nutrients that cannot then be used by more harmful disease-causing bacteria. They also produce by-products that inhibit the growth of other organisms (Greenwood et al 2002).

At birth, the skin is sterile because it has been contained within amniotic fluid. A biological advantage of an infant being nursed in close skin-to-skin contact with the mother immediately after birth is to encourage the rapid colonisation of the infants previously sterile skin, with the mothers harmless commensal bacteria and fungi (Coleman et al 1992, Inglis 2003).

Nurses must remember that they also carry commensal bacteria on their skin. In most instances the bacteria on their skin will remain harmless if transferred to children by contact. However, stringent infection control measures are paramount to reduce transfer of potentially harmful pathogens through skin contact.

Activity

Review the following online course on infection prevention, in particular with relation to hand washing:
* http://www.engenderhealth.org/ip/

Also go through the publication *The management and control of hospital acquired infections in acute NHS Trusts in England* (National Audit Office 2000):
* http://www.nao.org.uk/publications/nao_reports/9900230.pdf

Analyse the implications for your own practice.

An example of a commensal bacterium is *Staphylococcus aureus*, which is found in 20–30% of the noses and skin of normal healthy people and spread predominantly by contact. Most strains of this bacterium are sensitive to antibiotics, and infections such as dermatitis and pneumonia can be effectively treated, However, some strains of *S. aureus* are resistant to antibiotics containing methicillin, and are referred to as methicillin-resistant *Staphylococcus aureus* or MRSA (Gray 2004, van Belkum 2001). New strains of epidemic MRSA, EMRSA-15 and EMRSA-16, have emerged and spread to almost every hospital in the UK and there is growing concern over the increasing incidence of healthcare-associated infections with MRSA in children with underlying conditions predisposing to infection with *S. aureus*. Previously, MRSA outbreaks tended to be confined to adult and elderly areas but there have been reported outbreaks among children with cystic fibrosis and

in neonatal units (Isaacs et al 2004). The following case scenario presents the policies and treatment protocols for a child infected with MRSA (Gray 2004).

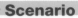

Scenario

Khaleda has been admitted with infected atopic dermatitis and microbiology reports indicate that her skin is infected with MRSA.
* From your understanding of the barrier properties of innate immunity, identify why she is more prone to developing an infection in her skin.
* Discuss how you will manage her care. To inform your discussion these are topics you must address:
  * infection control procedures
  * risk factors for developing MRSA
  * the rationale behind presenting symptoms
  * treatment strategies
  * the evidence base for treatment.

The National Audit Office (2000) has identified that the very young are particularly vulnerable to hospital acquired infections (HAI) but that adequate hand-washing has proven to be one of the most effective preventative measures against HAIs (Bissett 2003, Parker 1999, Ward 2000).

Non-compliance with hand-washing policies is a well-known problem and Ng et al (2004) found that a technique of hand rub with alcohol preparations and the wearing of non-sterile gloves led to a considerable reduction in infection episodes. Although this procedure can be monitored more overtly than straightforward hand-washing, it cannot fully replace the need to adequately wash the hands before any procedure involving an infant and child.

Serious bacterial infections in infants are not solely attributable to hand-washing and the mode for infection spread can also include nasopharyngeal colonisation and through penetration of micro-organisms into the blood (Brook 2003). These organisms can gain access to the blood through microscopic tears in the skin, such as those caused by intravenous access devices (Inglis 2003). Organisms cited as the most responsible for early onset neonatal sepsis are the group B streptococcus, *Escherichia coli* and *Staphylococcus epidermidis*, all of which are both commensal and nosocomial organisms, and most can be eliminated by meticulous hand-washing (Ballot 2000, Nenstiel et al 1997).

The skin controls the numbers of commensal bacteria through various secretions such as sweat and sebum. There are two types of sweat gland, one of which – the eccrine glands – are functional at birth. Apocrine sweat glands, which are found mainly in the axillae, groin, face and scalp are stimulated by the sex hormones and therefore do not become fully functional until puberty (McCance & Huether 2002). Sweat contains mostly water, salts, traces of metabolic wastes and some immunoglobulin A (IgA). Immunoglobulins are produced by B lymphocytes, very specialised immune cells and part of the adaptive immune system, which are produced from the lymphoid lineage in the bone marrow (Parham 2005). In the newborn infant, IgA antibodies in sweat are quite limited, but fortunately the concentration of salt and a fairly acidic pH 4–6 is inhibitory or lethal to the survival of many microorganisms (Rennie & Roberton 1999, Whaley & Wong 1995).

The sebaceous glands, which also produce sebum, are stimulated by maternal androgens and become very active in the last trimester and early infancy. In utero, these produce vernix caseosa, a white, waxy substance that gives an additional layer of protection in terms of its antimicrobial and mechanical properties (Clark 1991, Greenwood et al 2002, Marchini et al 2002). Following the birth of the baby, the mother is advised not to wipe away vernix caseosa because not only does it protect the skin against microorganism attack, it is one of nature's most efficient emollients. Many mothers worry about the white spots on their babies faces and they need to be assured that these are not acne but the final remnants of vernix in the skin pores.

The skin is also protected by mechanical means, which is the thickness of the skin and the hardness of keratinised cells, however the delicate neonate's skin lacks the hard extra layers of the skin of an older child. In the very low birthweight infant the stratum corneum is absent or deficient (Bautista et al 2000, Marchini et al 2002), therefore awareness of these infants' lack of the immunological barrier properties of the skin is crucial.

In fully developed skin, cells divide rapidly, the top layers constantly being renewed and dead cells sloughing away. An example of how proliferate the sloughing action is can be seen in the dust that relentlessly collects on furniture, most of which is dead skin cells. This sloughing action provides protection, because any harmful bacteria that are starting to colonise the skin will be sloughed away (Janeway et al 1999). Regular cleansing of an infant and child's skin not only facilitates the sloughing action but the massaging action stimulates the blood supply to the skin, which protects the skin immunologically and encourages growth of new cells.

Cleansing is of particular importance in the nappy area, because the combination of microorganisms and urine together in a damp environment will encourage the growth of certain organisms, and in turn, their by-products will contribute to skin breakdown.

The final means of the skin providing protection is through Langerhans cells (immature dendritic cells) and macrophages, which are found in the dermis. These cells arise from the myeloid lineage of cells produced in the bone marrow (Parham 2005), all of the cells from this line providing innate protection. The role of dendritic cells, Langerhans cells and macrophages is to recognise, ingest and destroy antigens, presenting them later to T and B lymphocytes, for future recognition. Most of the cells from the myeloid lineage release lysozymes and cytokines from granules within their cytoplasm. Lysozymes are enzymes that damage and cause the death of bacteria by splitting the sugars found in their cell walls, thus destroying the bacterial cell wall. Cytokines will be discussed later but they are protein messengers that affect the behaviour of other cells (Parham 2005).

Like all soldiers, Langerhans cells need to be fully equipped for killing and to have the ability to recognise the enemy before they can attack. Mature Langerhans cells, which are ready for attack, can be found from the 5th month of gestation, but some of their action is limited until well after birth, owing to their lack of opportunity to have previously met and therefore recognised antigens in utero (Ballot 2000, Rennie & Roberton 1999). This final means of control is vital, especially when the top epidermal layer of the skin is broken by small cuts or erosions, and it is another reason why nurses must be aware that skin damage in a very young baby, even through a tiny venepuncture site, will render the infant more prone to attack, invasion from microorganisms and the development of infection (Janeway et al 1999).

Activity

Basic hygiene care

Prepare written guidelines for new parents on the hygiene needs and principles of care for their baby. Identify actions required in a step-by-step approach and provide a simple rationale for each action taken.

Activity

Reflecting on practice

Review the guidelines in caring for the skin of premature and low birthweight infants in Storm & Lund Jensen (1999):

1. Due to the immaturity of the skin of the preterm infant, it is particularly susceptible to damage.
2. Adhesives for attaching probes, etc. should be used as little as possible and should be removed with great care.
3. Bathing is not recommended for very low birthweight babies for at least 7 days after birth.

Are there variations in the way these recommendations have been implemented in your experience of neonatal care?

A summary of the protective properties of skin is shown in Box 31.1.

Respiratory Tract

Mucous lines the surface of many areas in the body, such as the respiratory tract. To some extent, these areas are more prone to infection than skin, because their moist and sticky

Box 31.1

Summary of Protective Properties of Skin

Intact skin resistant to micro-organsms
Presence of commensal organisms
Skin secretions such as sweat and sebum
Thickness of skin
Sloughing off of old skincells and rapid replacement of new skin cells
Presence of immune cells within the dermis of skin
Presence of immune proteins such as antibodies and complement

surface provides a good breeding environment to bacteria (Janeway et al 1999). In the respiratory tract, micro-organisms and unwanted dust particles that have been inhaled are trapped in the mucus, which is constantly being driven upwards, by the action of cilia, towards the pharynx. The mucus, with all its debris, is then either coughed out or swallowed. Cough and swallow reflexes have been demonstrated as early as 12 weeks' gestation (McIntosh et al 2003), and are therefore well developed in a full-term healthy neonate. These reflexes are both efficient means of expelling unwanted invaders to the body.

However, the ability of the entire respiratory tract to produce mucus is reduced in infancy (McIntosh et al 2003) and breach of this fine layer of mucus through a number of factors (Rona 2000, Schwartz 2004, von Mutius 2000) will cause a breach in the protective properties and render the infant very prone to colonisation by airborne micro-organisms or antigens (Janeway et al 1999). Viruses in particular are very quick to take advantage of this reduced protection in the young baby, hence the relatively frequent occurrence of symptoms of 'snuffles', caused in response to viral attack.

The antibody, immunoglobulin A (IgA) is secreted into the mucous linings. Two of the roles of IgA are to inhibit the adherence and proliferation of any antigens, such as bacteria, on epithelial surfaces. In the infant, IgA is one of the last immunoglobins to reach competent levels, therefore the neonate has relatively less protection against infection from those parts of the body where micro-organisms can gain such easy entry, such as the respiratory tract (Newell & McIntyre 2000). However, IgA protection can be provided from the mother as discussed later.

It has been found that those children who have enhanced responsiveness to allergens (produce more immunoglobulins) in the neonatal period (Warner 2004) have been associated with a later risk of developing allergies such as asthma. These infants produce IgE instead of IgA. Subsequent exposure to the allergen that has resulted in the production of IgE, causes binding of the allergen to the IgE on the mast cell. This triggers the inflammatory response, which can vary in severity and, in some circumstances, produce life-threatening reac-

tions such as severe asthma or anaphylaxis. Unfortunately, the damage caused by the allergic reaction is out of proportion to the threat posed by the allergen.

Eyes

The eyes are potentially an area where micro-organisms can gain access into the body. Protection is provided by the conjunctiva, which is covered by a film of tears, and the constant blinking of the eyes flushes and cleanses the eye surface. Tears contain antibacterial products such as lysozyme but tear glands do not normally function until the child is 2–4 weeks old. Because of their narrow lumen, the tear glands are liable to blockage, which prevents the properties of tears from washing the eyes and renders the small baby prone to invasion by micro-organisms that can cause conjunctivitis (Clark 1991, Greenwood et al 2002, Kreir & Mortensen 1990). Parents should be shown how to clean their babies eyes by taking a damp piece of soft material from the area nearest the nose, the caruncle, and then across to the other side. This action helps to clear the tear ducts.

The Gastrointestinal Tract

The large surface area of the gastrointestinal tract is covered by a single layer of columnar epithelium and mucus, which allows for absorption of nutrients but also for entry of microbial pathogens (Garside & Mowat 1999). Within moments of birth, the gastrointestinal tract is challenged by myriads of bacterial and food antigens. There is evidence to suggest that even before birth the gastrointestinal tract is exposed to some antigen challenges as the fetus swallows amniotic fluid (Warner 2004). These swallowed antigens are met by antigen-presenting cells (APCs, e.g. macrophages and dendritic cells) in the fetus's gastrointestinal tract. For lymphocytes from the adaptive immune system to recognise antigens, they must first be presented by these antigen-presenting cells and the gastrointestinal tract is one of the only organs in the newborn infant with mature antigen-presenting cells.

The adaptive immune system, which allows for the formation of immune memory, is prominent at the mucosal site within the gastrointestinal tract. There are two subsets of memory T cells, natural and aquired. The natural memory T cells are self-specific, responding to self-antigens such as stressed and worn out epithelial cells. The acquired memory T cells gain their memory from antigens presented by antigen-presenting cells (Cheroutre & Madakamutil 2004). They then stimulate B cells to produce immunoglobulins specific to the antigens, such as IgA and IgG. In most cases, the presence of those immunoglobulins induces tolerance to those antigens within the gastrointestinal tract (Warner 2004) by neutralising the antigen and rendering it harmless. Unfortunately, there are instances when the antigen introduced to the gastrointestinal tract becomes immunogenic, meaning that it will cause a reaction including inflammation of the local tissues within the gastrointestinal tract. The result of this reaction is once again because of the production of IgE rather than IgA and IgG. Examples of this are those babies who develop intolerance to the proteins, carbohydrates or fats in manufactured baby milks, or the immune responses to gluten in patients with coeliac disease.

Seminar discussion topic

Read the article by Sicherer (2003). This article discusses a range of food allergies seen in infants and children:
- Discuss the common symptoms demonstrated by food allergies.
- Differentiate between what is an allergy and a hypersensitivity.

Many food intolerances do resolve in time but management of children's diets can be a problem for parents. Choose a couple of the more common disorders and identify what the problems might be and the advice you would give to parents regarding dietary management.

There is a huge network of immune tissue called gut-associated lymphoid tissue (GALT), which acts as a selective barrier to prevent the entry of these antigenic or infectious material into the body. The gastrointestinal tract is therefore considered the largest 'immune organ' in the body, with more than 70% of immune cells, both innate and adaptive, located there (Garside & Mowat 1999, Grönlund et al 2000).

Neonates have a limited amount of GALT but this develops rapidly over the first 2 years of life and certainly feeding is associated with the maturation of gut-associated lymphoid tissue (Flidel-Rimon et al 2004). Immunological protection is also provided by secretory IgA, which is quantitatively and functionally defective for a variable period after birth (Flidel-Rimon et al 2004). The number of IgA plasma cells (B lymphocytes) in the duodenal mucosa reaches that of adults by 2 years of age, whereas the level of mucosal secretory IgA antibodies reaches adult levels only at the age of 6–8 years (Grönlund et al 2000). Owing to the undeveloped mucosal immunological protection, there is higher vulnerability to infection and possibly more sensitisation to dietary antigens (MacDonald 1994, Warner 2004).

The saliva in the mouth has protective properties, which include IgA, lysozymes, mucopolysaccharides, which block some viruses, and glycolipids that compete with bacterial cell wall products for attachment to the mucus membranes (Coleman et al 1992, Greenwood et al 2002, Janeway et al 1999).

The newborn infant is unable to gain the full protective benefits of saliva because saliva production is limited in comparison to the amount produced later in life. However, this is compensated for as the different shape of the mouth and oral cavity facilitates efficient sucking and allows milk to be swallowed almost immediately. As milk does not stay in the mouth long, saliva is not needed for its protective action. Breastfeeding counteracts most of the immunological deficiencies because the IgA concentrations found in breast milk are very high in the first few months of feeding (Weaver et al 1998). Other protective properties of breast milk include lysozyme and lactoferrin, which is an iron-binding protein that has a bactericidal effect on E. coli. Breast milk also contains macrophages and lymphocytes, which play a vital role in the immune response (Cushing et al 1998, Howie et al 1990, Oddy et al 2003, Wilson et al 1998, WHO 2002).

Early introduction of enteral feeding in preterm infants is recommended (Flidel-Rimon et al 2004, Okada et al 1998) owing to the reduced risk of nosocomial infection, maintenance of the intestinal barrier and development of competent mucosal immunity.

The production of saliva is only noticeably increased around 4 months. Around about this time, as the child starts weaning, the shape of the mouth changes, food is kept in it for longer periods and production of saliva is noticeably increased through the baby drooling (Weaver et al 1998). The salivary glands continue to increase in size while the child is undergoing the oral phase of development. In their attempts to understand the world better, children will put almost anything into their mouth to be sucked or chewed and the protection the saliva affords is very advantageous (Greenwood et al 2002).

Saliva can protect the mouth from many micro-organisms but an organism that is particularly resistant to the effects of saliva is Streptococcus mutans, an organism that has been very closely linked to cause dental caries and has been found in the saliva of infants even as young as 1 year old (Radford et al 2000). Studies have suggested that mothers are the principal source of S. mutans to their infants (Li & Caufield 1995). Because of this, the practice of mothers sucking their infant's dummy (pacifier) to 'clean' it is not to be recommended! Saliva has the capabilities of protecting the infant from those organisms that would have attached to the dummy after rolling on the floor!

The pH of the stomach in older babies is between 1.5 and 3.5, which is not conducive to the survival of many micro-organisms (McCance & Huether 2002). However, in the first week of life it has been found that the gastric pH is often higher than pH 4, and the acidity is not increased until the establishment of feeds at 2 week (Sonheimer et al 1985). Again, this is not a problem for breast-fed infants, but is a factor to be considered for those who are bottle fed.

The large intestine contains a substantial and diverse population of commensal bacteria that are important for health (Fingold et al 1983). These bacteria have a protective function in that they secrete bacteriocins, which are substances that inhibit the growth of other pathogens that cause disease, and they stimulate the maturation of the adaptive immune system and IgA-secreting cells (Grönlund et al 2000). It is very important that, soon after birth, bacteria that are beneficial rather than harmful to health colonise the colon. Beneficial genera include *Bifidobacterium* spp, *Bacteroides fragilis* and *Lactobacillus* spp. Breast milk contains 'bifidus factor', which promotes the growth of *Bifidobacterium*, which is a significant contribution that breastfeeding provides against gut infections. Only one feed of commercial milk can upset the very delicate balance of beneficial versus harmful bacteria in the first week of life (McKay & Perdue 1993). There is a recommendation for premature infants to commence enteral feeds early because failure to use the gut has been shown to lead to an alteration in gut flora allowing the overgrowth of enteropathogenic species. These render the intestine prone to increased permeability and allow bacteria to be translocated in the bloodstream (Flidel-Rimon et al 2004), increasing the potential for neonatal sepsis and or necrotising enterocolitis.

The movement of faeces also helps to clear the intestinal tract and prevent adherence of harmful pathogens to the intestinal mucosa and the shorter colonic transit times in young children (Arhan et al 1981, Kreir & Mortensen 1990).

A summary of the protective properties of the gastrointestinal tract is shown in Box 31.2.

Box 31.2

Summary of Protective Properties of Gastrointestinal Tract

Presence of mucus
Huge numbers of innate immune cells such as macrophages and dendritic cells
Large quantities of IgA and IgG produced from B cells
Gut-associated-lymphoid tissue (GALT)
Saliva
Protection from breast feeding
Hydrochloric acid in stomach
Commensal bacteria
Movement of faeces

Evidence-based Practice

Evidence suggests that the most common enteric pathogens causing gastroenteritis are caused by self-limiting viral infections, notably rotavirus, adenovirus, adenovirus, astrovirus, Norwalk-like viruses and bacterial agents such as salmonella and campylobacter (McIver et al 2001).

Young children are vulnerable to dehydration owing to profuse diarrhoea and in most cases the treatment recommended is oral rehydration therapy to replace lost fluids, continuation of breastfeeding and early reintroduction of food when vomiting has stopped (Candy 1987).

Administration of the oral rehydration therapy via a nasogastric tube is a reliable and safe method of managing mild to moderate dehydration (Armon et al 2001, Callaghan et al 2003).

On recovery, recommended treatments include the introduction of live microbial food supplements (probiotics) such as foods containing bifidobacteria and lactobacteria to re-establish the intestine's natural defence barrier (Isolauri et al 2002).

Urogenital Tract

The urinary tract is protected primarily against microorganisms by being flushed by sterile urine, and babies and toddlers who wear nappies certainly void more frequently than older children. Urinary stasis and bacterial virulence are risk factors for bacterial invasion, resulting in urinary tract infections. This problem is demonstrated in children with congenital, structural abnormalities that prevent complete emptying of urine from the genitourinary tract (Jakobsson et al 1999, Smellie et al 1998).

CELL-MEDIATED MECHANISMS OF INNATE IMMUNITY

If microbes succeed in breaching the external barrier defences, protecting the blood are a group of immune cells called monocytes, which eventually enter the tissues and become macrophages. From the same myeloid lineage there are also polymorphonuclear leucocytes (PMNs); the most numerous polymorphonuclear leucocyte is the neutrophil. Neutrophils, and a variety of antimicrobial substances found in the blood and body fluids, can be rapidly mobilised to enter any site of infection (Parham 2005).

From the lymphoid lineage comes a group of highly specialised innate cells called the natural killer (NK) cells. NK cells are very important in the defence against viral infections (Roitt et al 2001, Ward 2000). They are almost absent during fetal life and their numbers are seen to rise considerably 3 weeks after birth, reaching peak activity by 8 weeks of age, after which their activity slows down (Stiehm 1996).

Polymorphonuclear leucocytes have a variety of functions, one of which is phagocytosis – a feeding process whereby the phagocytic polymorphonuclear leucocytes engulf and digest particles recognised by them as foreign to the body. Many of these particles are antigens, which stick to the surface of the phagocyte and are then engulfed within the cell by a process in which parts (pseudopods) of the polymorphonuclear leucocyte surround the antigen. Once inside the polymorphonuclear leucocyte, the antigen is enclosed in a vacuole so that it cannot harm the cell, lysozyme then fuses with the vacuole and destroys the antigen (Fig. 31.3) (Roitt et al 2001).

Some micro-organisms can be very 'slippery', making it difficult for phagocytic polymorphonuclear leucocytes to grab and keep hold of them. To overcome this problem, the polymorphonuclear leucocytes coat the micro-organisms with antibodies (immunoglobulins) and with a group of proteins called complement.

Phagocytosis in the neonate is often impaired because there is diminished attachment of the micro-organism to the polymorphonuclear leucocytes (McIntosh et al 2003). Also in the neonate, once inside the polymorphonuclear leucocyte, killing of micro-organisms can be depressed by the poor production of oxygen free radicals, which are essential in the destruction process. These functions are further depressed when the infant is stressed and otherwise compromised physiologically (McIntosh et al 2003).

INNATE HUMORAL DEFENCE MECHANISMS

A number of antimicrobial proteins are present in the tissue and body fluids. These are collectively known as humoral defence mechanisms, which are used predominantly to prevent attachment by microbes to cell and tissue surfaces (Clark 1991). 'Complement' is a generic term encompassing a very complex group of about 20 serum proteins that have the ability to lyse (break down) red blood cells, and destroy Gram-negative bacteria. Complement proteins interact with each other, and with antibodies, together greatly assisting in the war against harmful micro-organisms by inducing opsonisation (i.e. preparing the micro-organisms to be 'eaten') and therefore aiding phagocytosis (Janeway et al 1999, Kreir & Mortensen 1990, Roitt et al 2001) (Fig. 31.4).

There are decreased complement levels in the neonate, however, the complement system matures more rapidly than any other innate immune systems, and, within weeks of birth, complement levels in a baby are comparable to adult levels (McIntosh et al 2003).

Other humoral factors include antibodies (immunoglobulins) from B lymphocytes and plasma cells. Antibodies produce precipitation, agglutination and neutralisation of many antigens, including bacteria and viruses, and they also enhance phagocytosis considerably (Roitt et al 2001). Immunoglobulin M (IgM) and IgG protect against antigens in blood and the lymphatic system, and IgA protects mucosal membranes, as already discussed. During gestation and after birth, the developing fetus and infant are relatively immunoincompetent and very dependent on maternal antibodies transferred transplacentally (IgG) and through breast milk (IgG and IgA). These maternal antibodies attenuate systematic infections when the infant's own antibodies are slowly being produced and eventually providing effective protection on their own by 3–6 months of age (Zinkernagel 2003).

Many tissues synthesise proteins that can be referred to as basic polypeptides, which help to destroy micro-organisms by inhibiting cellular respiration, inhibiting the synthesis of DNA and RNA and increasing the permeability of bacterial cell membranes. The liver also produces a protein called C-reactive protein (CRP), which stimulates the complement cascade, enhances the release of cytokines, and activates phagocytic cells that bind to and disrupt the cell wall of certain micro-organisms (Cermak et al 1993). C-reactive protein is synthesised within 6–8 hours of exposure to a pathogen and it can increase a 1000-fold during the inflammatory response, hence it is a very useful diagnostic marker (from a blood sample) for the presence of infection. Unfortunately, the delay in the synthesis of CRP can mean the early detection of an infection using this CRP marker can be a problem (Da Silva et al 1995, Ng et al 1997).

Cytokines

Cytokines are glycoproteins that are rapidly synthesised by many immune cells, in response to any antigen. Cytokines are 'cellular messengers'. They have different names depending on where they originate. They not only have an effect on the cells of the immune system, they also gener-

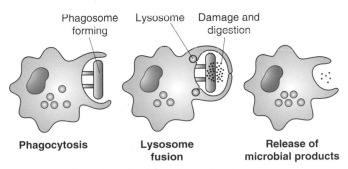

Phagosome forming   Lysosome   Damage and digestion

Phagocytosis   **Lysosome fusion**   **Release of microbial products**

Fig. 31.3 • The action of polymorphonuclear lymphocytes.

Complement is activated

Complement protein C3b binds to the surface of a pathogen, a disease causing microbe

PMNs are recruited   Pathogens are opsonised   Perforation of pathogen cell membrane

Death of cell membrane

Fig. 31.4 • The role of complement.

ate a response with many other physiological systems. Each cytokine that has been identified has its own function(s). Collectively, their functions include the stimulus and activation of cells of the immune system. An example is interleukin-1, a cytokine known for its fever-producing properties and also its ability to stimulate white cell production in the bone marrow (Ballot 2000).

Cytokines are partially responsible for many of the symptoms that are recognised as a deviation from health (National Audit Office 2000, Parker 1999, WHO 2003) and their role is very important in the next stage of immune protection, the inflammatory response (Fig. 31.5).

Having identified many of the factors in innate immunity, this section has shown the diverse ways that foreign substances are dealt with so efficiently. If bacteria or viruses manage to avoid all the barrier and innate mechanisms of protection, the body is still able and ready to fight against the invading organisms by bringing into play another very sophisticated means of protecting itself, ensuring that infants and children do not succumb to every infection.

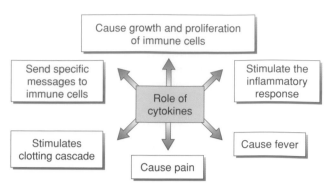

Fig 31.5 • The role of cytokines.

Activity

Neonatal sepsis

The main bacterial causes for infections in children under 1 month are group B streptococcus, *Escherichia coli*, *Listeria monocytogenes*, *Streptococcus pneumoniae*, *Haemophilus influenzae*, *Staphylococcus aureus*, *Staphylococcus epidermidis*, *Neisseria meningitidis* and *Salmonella* spp (Brook 2003). Signs and symptoms of infection in the very young infant include (McIntosh et al 2003):

- lethargy
- poor feeding, vomiting, abdominal distension
- apnoea and respiratory distress
- pallor
- temperature instability
- seizures
- prolonged capillary refill time
- mottling of skin.
1. What procedures would you undertake to detect the source of infection?
2. What other factors (other than barrier functions) would predispose a newborn to infection.

Phase Two. The Inflammatory Response: The Response after Microbial Attack

In the first part of the chapter, various strategies used by the body to prevent infection occurring were discussed.

In the above activity, you would have described symptoms that are caused by the inflammatory response.

Over the years, certain micro-organisms have evolved very clever strategies to avoid the body's attempts to prevent their entrance and, once they have gained entrance, they then resist the cells which can destroy them. Once micro-organisms have become established in the body, they will start multiplying. Fortunately, the body is ready for such subterfuge and within minutes of any invasion by micro-organisms through the body's defence barriers, a highly sophisticated series of events takes place. This protective, healing response involves inflammation, and it is put into motion by a number of immune cells such as dendritic cells, macrophages, neutrophils, T and B lymphocytes and mast cells, through the cytokines that they release.

The classical signs of this stage – the inflammatory response – are heat, swelling, redness, pain and loss of function (McCance & Huether 2002). To briefly summarise, this response is as follows. After micro-organisms have gained entrance into tissues, heat in the area is caused by localised vasodilatation, which is an opening up of arteries or capillaries that allows increased amounts of blood to flow into the area. In the innate response it was identified that blood contains many components that are vital to the war against micro-organisms. Heat is also caused by the increased amount of cellular and metabolic activity in the area. The local blood capillaries become permeable, which means leakier than normal, allowing plasma proteins, phagocytic cells and leucocytes to exude out from the blood into the extracellular spaces where the microbes have become established. The end result of the extra flow of blood and blood products to the area causes swelling and redness to tissues.

During the inflammatory response the pain is caused by pressure on the nerve endings in the swollen tissue and the effects of prostaglandins released from locally damaged cells.

The whole of the inflammatory response however is far more complex, and this detail will be discussed in the context of an infection, under the following headings (Kreir & Mortensen 1990):

- micro-organisms that are successful in breaking the defence barriers
- the changes in blood circulation in the inflamed area
- the effects of inflammatory mediators
- the effect of inflammation on the whole body: the febrile response.

MICRO-ORGANISMS THAT ARE SUCCESSFUL IN BREAKING THE DEFENCE BARRIERS

Many micro-organisms, such as bacteria, have evolved mechanisms aimed at avoiding some of the innate defences of the human body and some pathogens even have genes devoted to this purpose (Parham 2005). The whole immune response to any pathogen involves complex molecular and cellular reactions whereby immune cells recognise the bacteria through the proteins, some of which are antigens, on the bacterial cell wall. Many of these antigens are complex carbohydrate and protein structures. If the structure of these antigens becomes slightly changed through evolution, the body's immune system will not recognise the antigen as quickly as it previously did and action taken against the bacteria is delayed. Another common method of pathogenic bacteria avoiding is the synthesis of an outer capsule, which is very hard for phagocytic cells to attach to (Roitt et al 2001). An example of the effects of evolution on *Staphylococcus aureus* is the development of methicillin-resistant *Staphylococcus aureus* (MRSA) discussed earlier (Gray 2004, van Belkum 2001).

Viruses are good examples of the ability to genetically mutate. The common cold and influenza virus passed from person to person through coughs and sneezes is destroyed by antibodies that bind to its outer envelop. It takes 1–2 weeks for the immune system to produce these antibodies and, once produced, the virus is soon cleared and symptoms subside. However, in the meantime the virus might have spread to a large number of individuals, causing an epidemic. Over a period of time new viral strains are produced that have slightly different molecules on the viral envelope. These are therefore not immediately recognised by the immune system and there are not specific antibodies within the system against these new strains. Therefore, if these new strains manage to evade defence systems, once again an individual will have cold and influenza symptoms (Parham 2005).

Having avoided phagocytosis, once in the tissues, micro-organisms will rapidly reproduce and increase their num-

bers. Despite the genetic mutations to avoid detection, once in the tissues these agents will soon be met by dendritic cells and macrophages. Molecules on the outer surface of micro-organisms are characteristic of pathogens but absent from human cells. Examples of these are lipopolysaccharide (LPS), peptidoglycan, lipoteichoic acid and flagellin (Bochud & Calandra 2003). Complement binds with these molecules, allowing opsonisation and phagocytosis. Macrophages also have sensors (Toll-like receptors, TLR) on their surface for pathogenic components and, when macrophages come into contact with these components, they secrete cytokines (Bochud & Calandra 2003, Parham 2005). The cytokines then recruit other immune cells, in particular neutrophils into the infected area, initiating and continuing the inflammatory response until all the micro-organisms have been destroyed.

The degree of inflammation is usually associated with the success with which the organism has established itself; the greater the numbers of bacteria or virus, the greater the inflammation. Until the inflammatory response has been fully initiated, there will be very few symptoms to affect and warn the child of the presence of the bacteria.

CHANGES IN BLOOD CIRCULATION IN THE INFLAMED AREA CAUSED BY CYTOKINES

Cytokines produced by activated macrophages include interleukins (IL) such as IL-1, IL-6, IL-8 (also known as CXCL8), IL-12 and tumour necrosis factor alpha (TNF-α) (Fig. 31.6). Other molecules are released by macrophages and mast cells include histamine, bradykinin, prostaglandins, oxygen radicals, nitric oxide, leukotrines and platelet activating factor (PAF). Collectively, these substances are called

Fig. 31.6 • The role of cytokines released from macrophages.

inflammatory mediators because they all contribute to tissue damage and inflammation.

On their release, these substances cause the local blood capillaries to relax, dilate and become permeable 'leaky'. This increases the blood flow to the area, resulting in redness and plasma and immune proteins leaking from the vessels causes swelling of the tissues. The neutrophils can leave the circulation by adhering to blood vessel walls and then squeezing through the walls by a process called diapedesis. The process of attraction is called chemotaxis (Janeway et al 1999).

Once at the site of infection and inflammation, neutrophils and tissue macrophages work very quickly to fight against the microbes through phagocytosis. The site of inflammation becomes a real battleground, where cells from both sides of the conflict die. The accumulation of white blood cells, dead tissue cells, fluids leaked from the circulation and microbes, all contribute to 'pus'.

Typical examples of the inflammatory response can be seen in the inflamed skin in dermatitis and in tonsillitis. If the tonsils were examined they would look more red and swollen than normal with spots of pus. The child with tonsillitis may have a difficulty in swallowing owing to increased pain. Eventually the body will get rid of the pus via the lymphatic system or by using tissue macrophages to remove it.

Tonsillitis is an example of 'local' inflammatory responses and in most instances the effects of cytokines are contained within tissues. However, if the infection is more widespread in the body (systemic) and is bacterial, the effects of the inflammatory response are seen throughout the body. Inflammatory reactions vary slightly dependent on the type of bacteria, whether they are Gram positive or Gram negative, but it has been clearly demonstrated that if TNF-α is released into the circulation, the effect of vascular dilatation and permeability can lead to severe shock (Cohen & Abraham 1999).

As the cytokines are produced at the start of the inflammatory response, their presence in blood samples can be indicative of an infection. Even though preterm and term infants have immature inflammatory responses, it has been demonstrated that they display a higher percentage of IL-6 and IL-8 (Ng 2004) and high plasma levels of IL-6, Il-10 and TNF-α often signify severe infection. IL-6 is an important cytokine because it coordinates the body's response to infection. For example, with IL-1, IL-6 is responsible fir resetting the hypothalamic thermostat to raise body temperature. It also stimulates the liver to produce C-reactive protein and it mobilises neutrophils to enhance their phagocytic activity. Recently, IL-6 has been used as a marker with a sensitivity of up to 89% in detecting infection early in neonates (Ng 2004). Unfortunately, soon after the initial inflammatory response and if a child receives antibiotic therapy, IL-6 levels fall and become almost undetectable after 24 hours (Ng 2004).

A summary of the protective properties of inflammation is shown in Box 31.3.

Box 31.3

Summary of Protective Properties of Inflammation

Changes in blood circulation causing:
   Heat
   Swelling
   Redness
   Pain
Further moblisation of innate and adaptive defence mechanisms
Resetting of the thermoregulatory centre resulting in fever
Activation of the sympathetic nervous system to aid in the increase in temperature
Symptoms associated with sympathetic nervous system activation: nausea and vomiting
Lethargy and malaise to promote rest

THE EFFECTS OF OTHER INFLAMMATORY MEDIATORS

Histamine and serotonin are some of the cytokines released from granules within damaged mast cells. Other substances are manufactured from arachidonic acid, a molecule found within the cell walls of mast and local tissue cells. These substances are prostaglandins and leukotrienes. They are responsible for the pain that comes with inflammation. They cause pain by further increasing the vascular permeability, therefore increasing the swelling, which produces pressure on the nerve endings. Prostaglandins also intensify pain by sensitising nerve receptors.

Bacteria that enter into tissues will damage the lining of blood vessels exposing collagen. On contact with collagen, a plasma protein, factor XII (the Hageman factor), is activated and initiates the clotting cascade: platelets start adhering to each other, forming tiny clots within the local vessels and in the blood products at the site of inflammation. At the same time, the damaged endothelial cells release platelet-activating factor, a cytokine that encourages platelet aggregation. Clots help to immobolise microorganisms and prevent them entering the blood and lymph tissues, as well as preventing significant blood loss from the blood capillaries, which have been made permeable. During the clotting process, platelets release prostaglandins, which further promote inflammation and the start of tissue healing (Parham 2005).

THE EFFECT OF INFLAMMATION ON THE WHOLE BODY: THE FEBRILE RESPONSE

Inflammation in any localised tissue can, and often does, result in a response by the whole body, such as fever, tiredness and general malaise.

Fever, as mentioned, results following the release of IL-1, IL-6 and TNF-α, endogenous pyrogens (fever-producing substances) released by macrophages and, through the release of prostaglandins, produced by tissue cells and neutrophils. These fever-producing substances have a direct action on the hypothalamus, causing the hypothalamus to reset the thermoregulatory set point, so instead of the normal body temperature of between 36.0 and 37.2°C, the new set point will be at a higher rate. The new set point is determined by the number of endogenous pyrogens in the circulation, the more pyrogens, the higher the set point and the resulting body temperature (Klugger 1995).

To facilitate the rise in temperature, the hypothalamus stimulates the sympathetic nervous system, causing vasoconstriction, whereby the arteries in the body's peripheries become narrowed. This helps to conserve any body heat that might be lost through radiation from the skin surfaces. The sympathetic nervous system raises the metabolic rate and glycogen stores are mobilised to provide extra fuel for the energy and heat produced from increased metabolism. Oxygen demands are increased because it is also a fuel needed by cellular metabolism, therefore the child's respiratory rate will increase; the heart rate will also increase to deliver the oxygenated blood to the cells and remove the by-products of metabolism.

The additional heat created by the enhanced metabolic rate is retained by the body, causing an increase in body temperature.

While the body temperature is rising, the child will look pale and will often feel anorexic and tired, both effects of the sympathetic nervous system. The observant mother or a nurse would notice an increase in respiratory and pulse rate. The child's trunk might feel warmer than normal, but the peripheries will feel cool. The child might be shivering, an attempt of the body to create more heat through muscular activity. At this point the kindest treatment would be to tuck the child up in bed to let him or her sleep and allow the body to wage war against the bacteria. Once the raised hypothalmic temperature point has been reached, the body will commence its cooling-down process. Only in extremely rare conditions (associated with altered fluid and electrolyte balance) does the body temperature keep rising relentlessly. In most instances, once the raised hypothalamic set point has been reached the body will start cooling itself and the child will kick off the covers.

Fever is thought to have many beneficial effects for the host because it accelerates many of the innate and acquired or specific immune reactions. Fever causes a reduction of the iron and zinc levels in the blood, both of which are needed for bacterial growth. Fever increases the movement of neutrophils and lymphocytes into the war zone and, on its own, fever can kill or dramatically reduce the ability of bacteria to function and reproduce. Many bacteria cease to function at temperatures of 38°C and above. However, the negative aspects of fever are discomfort of the child and potential dehydration. Dehydration in the case of tonsillitis would result from the child not drinking, owing to the discomfort in the throat, and increased loss of insensible fluids as the temperature rises, and possibly vomiting.

When caring for a child all these factors must be considered, and it must be remembered that fever is a very important diagnostic sign and need therefore not be actively reduced. It is generally considered that the benefits of fever far outweigh the disadvantages. If the child is well hydrated, antipyretics need not be given, however, if the resulting inflammatory response has caused many symptoms of malaise and the child is in a lot of discomfort, it is better to consider the administration of these medications for their analgesic rather than their antipyretic properties.

Summary

Having identified the events of the inflammatory process, it is easy to liken it to the body being at war against an unwelcome and unwanted invasion of enemies. If the body fails to meet the challenge, bacterial invasion would soon overwhelm the body and the prognosis of recovery would be poor. The fact that so many children survive infections is credit to their very efficient immune systems. The reaction of the body to the enemy results in some unpleasant side effects, such as fever, but they usually serve the important purpose to cause the individual to rest to allow the immune army and other body systems, such as the sympathetic nervous system, to win the battle.

References

Arhan P, Devroede G, Jehannin B et al 1981 Segmental colonic transit time. Disease of the Colon and Rectum 24(8):625–629

Armon K, Stephenson T, MacFaul R et al 2001 An evidence and consensus based guideline for acute diarrhea management. Archives of Diseases in Childhood 85:132–145

Ballot DE, Neonatal Sepsis, Newell ML, McIntyre J 2000 Congenital and perinatal infections. Cambridge University Press, Cambridge, pp 321–336

Bautista MIB, Randall Wickett R, Visscher MO et al 2000 Characterisation of vernix caseosa as a natural biofilm: comparison to standard oil based treatments. Pediatric Dermatology 17(4): 253–260

Bissett L 2003 Interpretation of terms used to describe handwashing activities. British Journal of Nursing 12(9):536–542

Bochud P-Y, Calandra T 2003 Pathogenesis of sepsis: new concepts and implications for future treatment. British Medical Journal 326:262–266

Brook I 2003 Unexplained fever in young children: how to manage severe bacterial infection. British Medical Journal 327:1094–1097

Callaghan S, Hughan J, Johnson L 2003 The use of a nasogastric tube for rehydration therapy in the dehydrated paediatric patient with gastroenteritis: a clinical audit of adverse events associated with its use. Neonatal and Paediatric Child Health Nursing 6(1):13–17

Candy CE 1987 Recent advances in the care of children with acute diarrhea: giving responsibility to the nurse and parents. Journal of Advanced Nursing 12(1):95–99

Cermak J, Key NS, Bach RR et al 1993 C-reactive protein induces human peripheral blood monocytes to synthesis tissue factor. Blood 82:512–520

Cheroutre H, Madakamutil L 2004 Acquired and natural memory T cells join forces at the mucosal front line. Nature Reviews. Immunology 4(4):290–300

Clader PC, Kew S 2002 The immune system: a target for functional foods? British Journal of Nutrition 88 (Suppl 2):S165–S177

Clark W R 1991 The experimental foundations of modern immunology, 4th edn. John Wiley, Singapore

Cohen J, Abraham E 1999 Microbiologic findings and correlations with serum tumor necrosis factor alpha in patients with severe sepsis and septic shock. Journal of Infectious Diseases 180:116–121

Coleman RM, Lombard MF, Sicard RE 1992 Fundamental immunology. WC Brown, Dubuque

Cushing AH, Samet JM, Lambert WE et al 1998 Breastfeeding reduces risk of respiratory illness in infants. American Journal of Epidemiology 147:863–870

Da Silva O, Ohlsson A, Kenyan C 1995 Accuracy of leukocyte indices and C-reactive protein for diagnosis of neonatal sepsis: a critical review. Pediatric and Infectious Diseases 14:362–366

Fingold SM, Sutter VL, Mattisen GE 1983 Normal indigenous intestinal flora. In: Hentges DJ (ed.) Human intestinal microflora in health and disease. Academic Press, New York

Flidel-Rimon O, Friedman S, Lev E 2004 Early enteral feeding and nosocomial sepsis in very low birthweight infants. Archives of Diseases in Childhood. Fetal and Neonatal edition 89:F289

Garside P, Mowat AM 1999 Oral tolerance in disease. Gut 44: 137–142

Gray JW 2004 MRSA: the problem reaches paediatrics. Archives of Diseases in Childhood 89:297–298

Greenwood D, Slack RCB, Peutherer JF 2002 Medical microbiology: a guide to microbial infections, 16th edn. Churchill Livingstone, Edinburgh

Grönlund M-M, Arvilommi H, Kero P 2000 Importance of intestinal colonization in the maturation of humoral immunity in early infancy: a prospective follow up study of healthy infants aged 0–6 months. Archives of Diseases in Childhood. Fetal and Neonatal edition 83:F186–F192

Howie PW, Forsyth JS, Ogston SA et al 1990 Protective effect of breast feeding against infection. British Medical Journal 300:11–16

Inglis TJJ 2003 Congenital and neonatal infections. In: Inglis TJJ (ed.) Microbiology and infection: a clinical core text for integrated curricula with self assessment, 2nd edn. Churchill Livingstone, Edinburgh, pp 159–169

Isaacs D, Fraser S, Hogg G 2004 Staphylococcus aureus infections in Australasian neonatal nurseries. Archives of Diseases in Childhood. Fetal and Neonatal edition 89:F331

Isolauri E, Kirjavainen PV, Salminen S 2002 Probiotoics: a role in the treatment of intestinal infection and inflammation? Gut 50:iii54–iii59.

Jakobsson B, Jacobson SH, Hjalmas K 1999 Vesico-ureteric reflux and other risk factors for renal damage: identification of high and low-risk children. Acta Paediatrica 431 (Suppl):31–39

Janeway CA, Travers P, Walport M, Capra JD 1999 Immuno-biology: the immune system in health and disease, 4th edn. Churchill Livingstone, London

Klugger MJ 1995 The mechanism of fever. In: David TJ (ed.) Recent advances in paediatrics. Longman, Harlow, p 13

Kreir JP, Mortensen RF 1990 Infection, resistance and immunity. Harper and Row, New York

Li Y, Caufield PW 1995 The fidelity of initial acquisition of mutans streptococci by infants from their mothers. Journal of Dental Research 74(2):681–685

MacDonald TT 1994 Development of mucosal immune function in man: potential for GI disease states. Acta Paediatrica Japan 36:532–536

Marchini G, Lindow S, Brismar H et al 2002 The newborn infant is protected by an innate antimicrobial barrier: peptide antibiotics are contained in the skin and vernix caseosa. British Journal of Dermatology 147:1127–1134

Mathers CD, Stein C, Mafat D 2002 Global burden of disease; version 2. Methods and results. Global programme on evidence for health policy. Discussion paper no. 50. World Health Organization, Geneva

McCance KL, Huether SE (eds) Pathophysiology: the biological basis for disease in adults and children, 4th edn. Mosby St Louis

McIntosh N, Helms PJ, Smyth RL 2003 Forfar and Arneil's textbook of pediatrics, 6th edn. Churchill Livingstone, Edinburgh

McIver CJ, Hansman G, White P et al 2001 Diagnosis of enteric pathogens in children with gastroenteritis. Pathology 33:353–358

McKay DM, Perdue MH 1993 Intestinal epithelial function: the case for immunophysiological regulation. Digestive Diseases and Sciences 38(8):1377–1387

Mowat AM, Viney JL 1997 The anatomical basis of intestinal immunity. Immunology Reviews 156:145–166

National Audit Office 2000 The management and control of hospital acquired infection in acute NHS Trusts in England. HMSO, London

Nenstiel RO, White GL, Aikens T 1997 Handwashing a century of evidence ignored. Clinical Reviews 7:55–58, 61–62

Newell ML, McIntyre J 2000 Congenital and perinatal infections.Cambridge University Press, Cambridge

Ng PC 2004 Diagnostic markers of infection in neonates. Archives of Diseases in Childhood. Fetal and Neonatal edition 89:F229–F244

Ng PC, Cheng SH, Chui KM et al 1997 Diagnosis of late onset neonatal sepsis with cytokines, adhesion molecules, and C-reactive protein in preterm, very low birth weight infants. Archives of Diseases in Childhood. Fetal and Neonatal edition F221–F227

Ng PC, Li K, Wong RPO et al 2003 Proinflammatory and anti-inflammatory cytokine responses in preterm infants with systemic infections. Archives of Diseases in Childhood. Fetal and Neonatal edition 88:F209–F210

Ng PC, Wong HL, Lyon DJ et al 2004 Combined use of alcohol rub and gloves reduces the incidence of late onset infection in very low birthweight infants. Archives of Diseases in Childhood. Fetal and Neonatal edition 89:F336

Oddy WH, Sly PD, de Klerk NH et al 2003 Breast feeding and respiratory morbidity in infancy: a birth cohort study. Archives of Diseases in Childhood 88:224–228

Okada Y, Klein N, van Saene HK et al 1998 Small volumes of enteral feedings normalise immune function in infants receiving parenteral nutrition. Journal of Pediatric Surgery 33:16–19

Parham P 2005 The immune system, 2nd edn. Garland Science, Abingdon

Parker LJ 1999 Importance of hand washing in the prevention of infection. British Journal of Nursing 8(11):716–720

Radford JR, Ballantyne HM, Nugent Z et al 2000 Caries associated micro-organisms in infants from different socio-economic backgrounds in Scotland. Journal of Dentistry 28(5):307–312

Rennie JM, Roberton NRC (eds) Textbook of neonatology, 3rd edn. Churchill Livingstone, Edinburgh

Roitt I, Brostoff J, Male DK 2001 Immunology, 6th edn. Mosby Books, Edinburgh

Rona RJ 2000 Asthma and poverty. Thorax 55:239–244

Schwartz J 2004 Air pollution and children's health. Pediatrics 113(4):1037–1043

Sicherer SH 2003 Clinical aspects of gastrointestinal food allergy in childhood. Pediatrics 111(6):1609–1616

Smellie JM, Prescod NP, Shaw PJ et al 1998 Childhood reflux and urinary infection: a follow up of 10–41 years in 226 adults. Pediatric Nephrology 12:727–736

Sonheimer JM, Clark DA, Gervaise EP 1985 Continuous gastric pH measurement in young and older healthy preterm infants receiving formula and clear liquid feeds. Journal of Pediatric Gastroenterology and Nutrition 4(3):352–355

Stiehm RE 1996 Immunologic disorders in infants and children, 4th edn. Harcourt Brace, New York

Storm K, Lund Jensen T 1999 Skin care of preterm infants: strategies to minimise potential damage. Journal of Neonatal Nursing 5(2):13–15

van Belkum A 2001 40 years of methicillin-resistant Staphylococcus aureus. British Medical Journal 323:644–645

von Mutius E 2000 The burden of childhood asthma. Archives of Diseases in Childhood 82(Suppl II):ii2–ii5

Ward D 2000 Hand washing facilities in the clinical area: a literature review. British Journal of Nursing 9(2):82–86

Warner JO 2004 The early life origins of asthma and related allergic disorders. Archives of Diseases in Childhood 89:97–102

Weaver LT, Arthur HML, Bunn JEG et al 1998 Human milk IgA concentrations during first year of lactation. Archives of Diseases in Childhood 78:235–239

Whaley LF, Wong DL 1995 Whaley and Wong's nursing care of infants and children, 5th edn. Mosby, St Louis

Wilson AC, Stewart Forsyth J, Greene SA et al 1998 Relation of infant diet to childhood heath: seven year follow up of cohort of children in Dundee infant feeding study. British Medical Journal 316:21–25

World Health Organization (WHO) 2002 Infant and young child nutrition: global strategy on infant and young child feeding. 55th World Health Assembly, Geneva, April 2002, A55/15

World Health Organization (WHO) 2003 Child and adolescent health development: overview. Online. Available at: http://www.who.int/child-adolescent-health

Zinkernagel RM 2003 On natural and artificial vaccinations. Annual Review of Immunology 21(1):515–542

Chapter Thirty Two

32

Caring for Children and Adolescents with Malignant Disease

Beth Sepion

ABSTRACT

Cancer is a group of malignant diseases that are rare in childhood and adolescence. The aim of this chapter is to give an overview of the care of the children/adolescents with a malignant disease. It will begin with a brief explanation of what cancer is and an overview of shared care. The main focus will be on the challenges, physical and psychological, facing children's nurses when caring for a child/adolescent and his or her family as they undergo treatment. The majority of children/adolescents with cancer experience care over a period of months or years, in regional centres, district general hospitals and the community. Few nurses, therefore, will experience caring for a child and their family from the time of diagnosis to the completion of treatment. The concept of the illness trajectory, identified by Corbin & Strauss (1991), has been used to offer an insight into the journey, physical and emotional, that these families travel and the variety of healthcare professionals they will encounter during their individual journeys.

The companion PowerPoint presentation provides the background information about the common treatment modalities, side effects and management strategies.

Learning Outcomes

- Identify common childhood malignancies.

- Describe the different treatment modalities and common associated side effects.

- Discuss the impact of a cancer diagnosis on the patient and different members of the family.

- Discuss the role of the nurse caring for the child with a malignancy and his or her family throughout the illness trajectory.

- Identify the skills required to work with children/adolescents with cancer and their families.

- Discuss the strategies that different families develop to cope with cancer and its treatment throughout the illness trajectory.

- Discuss interdisciplinary and transdisciplinary care for the child with cancer and the family.

Introduction

Childhood malignancies are considered to be a chronic illness and, although rare, nurses may care for these children/adolescents in a variety of healthcare settings. It is important, therefore, to have an understanding of the disease, its treatment and the impact this can have for the children/adolescents and their family as they undergo intensive and complex treatment regimens.

Malignancy/Cancer/Tumour

The terms cancer, tumour and malignancy are often used synonymously. Cancer is a name given to a group of diseases that share common characteristics of uncontrolled cell growth following a genetic mutation. In childhood, in particular, there is invasion to local tissue with spread to distant sites via the lymphatic and blood system. The names of the specific cancers signify the tissue of origin, e.g. nephroblastoma, a malignant tumour of the kidney.

Activity

- What is the more common name for a tumour of the kidney?

A tumour is a swelling; it can be benign or malignant. Benign refers to a swelling that does not invade its surrounding tissue, it causes damage by local pressure and/or obstruction.

Malignant tumours are invasive, they cause damage by invading surrounding tissue and they have the ability to establish new tumours at distant sites (metastases). Cancer (from the Greek work *karkinos*, meaning crab) was described by Hippocrates as growths that invaded other tissues.

Malignancies in childhood are rare. There are approximately only 1470 new cases each year in the UK (2004 data available at: http://www.statistics.gov.uk). However, despite the dramatic improvement in the cure rate over the past 25 years (60–70%), cancer remains one of the most feared diagnoses (Parry 2003). The improvement in success rate is due to a greater understanding of the nature of childhood malignancies, including refined diagnostic and prognostic investigations, knowledge of treatment modalities, supportive care and the establishment of regional centres where participation in multicentre trials is acknowledged as being essential (United Kingdom Children's Cancer Study Group (UKCCSG) 1987).

PowerPoint

Access the companion PowerPoint presentation to learn more about the common childhood cancers:
- List the common presenting signs and symptoms for each of the diseases.

Shared Care

Many of the children/adolescents diagnosed with cancer will participate in a system of care known as 'shared care'. Within this approach, the individual may receive care at the regional oncology centre, the district general hospital and at home from the primary healthcare team and, in some areas, paediatric oncology outreach nurses.

The concept of shared care is not unique to cancer but its adaptation within childhood cancer services has had to embrace the challenges of developing a countrywide transdisciplinary service for patients with rare diseases. In the 1970s, the UKCCSG recognised the need to treat children/adolescents in regional oncology centres to develop specialist knowledge and a multidisciplinary team with specific skills to care for this group of patients (UKCCSG 1997). Twenty-two regional centres within the UK were created. This meant that many patients had to travel significant distances, which in turn meant disruption for other family members, potential lack of family support for the patient and family at the hospital, and financial implications.

It also resulted in the deskilling of staff at the district general hospitals in relation to care of the patient with cancer (Patel et al 1997). However, as mortality and morbidity rates improved, it was decided to assess the feasibility of children/adolescents with acute lymphoblastic leukaemia receiving part of their treatment at their local district hospital. Muir et al (1992) demonstrated that 'sharing care' was safe practice and the service, for children/adolescents with other malignancies as well as acute lymphoblastic leukaemia, has continued to develop. However, it is not without its problems, especially the need to educate staff in the shared care centres, community and regional centres, about caring for, and working with this group of patients (Patel et al 1997).

The Calman–Hine report (Department of Health (DoH) 1995) identified shared care as an important approach for the care of patients with cancer. Having been established within paediatric oncology since the early 1990s, the NHS Cancer Plan (DoH 2000) acknowledged the childhood cancer services success in developing such a service.

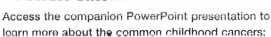

Activity

Read Sepion (2004) to discover how some parents felt about participating in shared care.

However, if families are to participate in shared care they require contact names, telephone numbers and information regarding the roles of the shared care centre, the regional centre and in some cases the paediatric oncology outreach nurses. Patient/parent held records have been developed to facilitate resolution of some of the problems associated with all the information that the parents require. They provide resources for the parents when they get home and help with the communication between regional centres, shared care and the community (Hooker & Williams 1996).

The Illness Trajectory

PRE-DIAGNOSIS

The illness history for a child with a malignancy may be relatively short; parents may take their child to the GP with a history of a persistent infection, as with Jonathan in the following case scenario. GPs are usually the first professional encountered by the family. A common investigation for children/adolescents with a history of recurrent infection, abnormal bruising or bleeding, lethargy or abnormal lumps is a blood count for the assessment of their haemoglobin, platelets and white cell count including a differential.

Scenario

Jonathan, aged 6 years, was taken to his GP with a chest infection; he was treated with antibiotics for a week. As his chest infection did not improve after the course of antibiotics his mother returned to the GP with Jonathan. The GP requested a chest X-ray and a full blood count. That evening, Jonathan's parents were telephoned by the GP, who explained to them that as Jonathan's blood count was abnormal, they needed to take him to their local hospital immediately. On arrival at the hospital, Jonathan's parents were advised that his blood results were indicative of leukaemia and the next morning, following a blood transfusion overnight, he would be transferred to a regional cancer unit where he would undergo investigations for leukaemia.

His blood results were haemoglobin 6.8 g/dL, platelets 48×10^9, and total white cell count 25.4×10^9. The differential showed 95% blast cells.

Activity

- What are the normal ranges for a full blood count and differential?
- What do the terms anaemia, neutropenia, thrombocytopenia and pancytopenia mean?

GPs are likely to see only one or two cases of childhood malignancy in a 20-year practice but education regarding the signs and symptoms of these conditions and the need for prompt intervention has seen a significant improvement in GPs' responses to such symptoms over the last 30 years (Pinkerton et al 1994).

It is likely that the admission to the district general hospital will be for a short period of time, in some cases just an overnight stay while arrangements are made for transfer to the regional paediatric oncology centre where the diagnosis and prognosis will be confirmed and treatment commenced. Transfer to another centre will raise the patient's and parents' anxiety levels. They require written details and an explanation of how to get there, the name of the ward and staff that are expecting them. It is also useful to be able to advise them what to expect when they arrive at the centre. This can help the parents prepare themselves and their child to face a children's ward where they will see children/adolescents who are undergoing treatment and who have altered body images such as alopecia.

Information booklets about the regional cancer unit are useful for the patient and family to enable them to prepare for the transfer.

Activity

Discover the number and location of regional centres in the UK at:

- http://www. ukccsg.org

Many families may well have to travel a significant distance away from home to their nearest centre. Make a list of the advantages and disadvantages for the patient and family members when being transferred to a regional oncology centre.

REACHING A DIAGNOSIS

Due to a greater knowledge about childhood malignancies, the confirmation of the diagnosis is rarely a medical emergency. However, for the child/adolescent and parents it will be a time of great emotional distress and uncertainty (Pinkerton et al 1994). It is vital, therefore, that the investigations are planned to cause the minimum amount of physical and psychological stress for the child and family. However, due to the neutropenia, children/adolescents can become acutely ill very quickly, therefore nurses need to be able to identify children/adolescents at risk of developing septic shock, recognising subtle changes in their condition, and be able to prioritise appropriate emergency care.

Activity

- What are the normal ranges of observations for Jonathan?
- List the signs and symptoms of septic shock?

Establishing venous access is often the first priority, both for assessment of blood values and to facilitate the administration of medications, hydration and the correction of haematological and electrolyte abnormalities prior to further investigations being carried out. The type and variety of investigations required will be decided upon depending on the suspected diagnosis. Bone marrow aspirates and trephines are carried out to confirm and determine the type of leukaemia (acute lymphoblastic leukaemia and acute myeloid leukaemia), lumbar punctures are required to identify the presence of leukaemia cells in the cerebral spinal fluid. Children/adolescents with solid tumours are likely to undergo a combination of:

- X-rays
- computerised tomography (CT) scans
- radioisotope scans, e.g. bone scans, renal function scans
- magnetic resonance imaging (MRI) scans.

Effective communication between the different departments involved in the investigative procedures is essential. It is also important to remember, however, that the patient may have to experience the investigations numerous times throughout treatment, the preparation for the procedures is, therefore, crucial.

Consideration for the use of pharmacological interventions, such as sedatives or anaesthesia and non-pharmacological methods such as distraction, play, hypnosis, for procedures that are invasive, painful or that require the patient to remain still should be given (Christensen & Fatchett 2002). Assessment and intervention by the play therapist is valuable as relationships are just beginning to be established. Carrying out as many procedures under one anaesthetic or sedative requires expert planning and negotiation skills. If the investigation is deemed not to be invasive or painful, or the patient is considered to be able to comply with instructions, it will still be necessary to assess that the patient is free from physical and/or emotional pain/discomfort and establish appropriate therapeutic interventions where required (Pinkerton et al 1994).

This is an extremely difficult time for the patient, parents, other family members and the members of the healthcare team. Effective communication is vital to minimise additional stress and to establish trusting relationships that are essential to assist the child and family as they start this journey.

Parents see themselves as advocates for their child (Holm et al 2003), making medical decisions, limiting the actions of healthcare professionals and learning about their child's condition. Their education in order to participate, therefore, is paramount.

Activity

- List the different healthcare professionals that the patient and parents are likely to come into contact with or require the services of during the diagnostic phase of their illness.
- What are the advantages and difficulties for the parents and child meeting all these people?
- Having done this, now think about the role of the nurse, what skills will the nurse require to minimise the additional stress for the child and family?

CONFIRMING THE DIAGNOSIS

The confirmation of the diagnosis will bring many mixed reactions and emotions. The family whose child has had a short history of a mild illness may find it difficult to accept that their child has a life-threatening illness, whereas for the family who have encountered a delay or complications in the confirmation of diagnosis and whose child's condition has continued to deteriorate, it may come as a relief in that

they can now begin treatment. Buckman (1992) advises that, although specific details of what was said will be forgotten, the way in which the news of the diagnosis is given to the family will be remembered. It is important, therefore, that the confirmation of the diagnosis is a planned event. Privacy, an appropriate environment, time and honesty are key issues. Parents will search for a cause for their child's illness and a meaning of the illness (Ruccione et al 1994). Parents feel responsible for their child, yet at this stage they lack knowledge, authority and power to participate in healthcare decisions. It is important that they receive the right amount of information and feel listened to (Clarke & Fletcher 2003). Interestingly, Clarke-Steffen (1993) identified that once parents felt they had been told the details of the worst things that could happen to their child, they felt more able to trust the professionals to be honest with them about subsequent information or news.

It is recommended that children/adolescents are informed of their diagnosis, treatment and prognosis (Eiser et al 1994). However, many factors need to be taken into consideration, such as the existing communication strategies within the family, cultural and religious beliefs, and the child's age and level of development.

Activity

Read *The private worlds of dying children* by Myra Bluebond-Langner (1978), who was one of the first people to research the informational needs of children with a life-limiting illness. How have attitudes changed over the past 25 years?

It must be remembered that parents will react in different ways depending on their coping strategies, previous experiences, relationships and culture. The grief that the families experience when they hear the diagnosis has been likened to Kubler Ross's (1969) model of grief.

Activity

Describe why theories of grief and loss are applicable to the parents of children/adolescents following a diagnosis of cancer.

Although it is recognised that children/adolescents have a right and a need to know their diagnosis (Eiser et al 1994), negotiation with the parents will help to decide the best way this is carried out for their child. Parents may need time to come to terms with the diagnosis first, but delay in confirming the diagnosis with the child/adolescent might result in finding out via an alternative source, which can subsequently lead to difficulties in establishing trusting relationships. Telling the patient and family together may be valuable for some families, for others the parents may prefer to break the news themselves. Price (2003 p 38) identifies the following strategy to assist information giving to children:

C = consider age and cognitive development stage carefully.

H = highlight and establish child's current level of understanding.

I = include other members of the multidisciplinary team (MDT) as appropriate, e.g. play specialist.

L = language that is simple and age appropriate should be used.

D = discuss with and involve parents.

R = restrict the time of the session: remember a child has limited attention.

E = employ a range of strategies, e.g. play, stories, etc.

N = necessary to elicit feedback and evaluate effectiveness.

It is recognised that the confirmation will come as a shock and the ability to remember information will be reduced, it is vital, therefore, that the patient and parents feel reassured that they can ask staff to go over information as often as is required for them (Pinkerton at el 1994).

Activity

Do an internet search and discover how many different sources of information regarding childhood tumours are available. Think about how you might guide parents to use this source and variety of information.

COMMENCEMENT OF TREATMENT

An outcome of the establishment of the UKCCSG in 1978 and the organisation of the 22 regional centres has been the increase in the number of children/adolescents that are entered into clinical trials, which evaluate current treatments, test new drugs or test existing drugs in different dosages, ways of administration or combinations.

PowerPoint

Access the companion PowerPoint presentation for the section on clinical trials.

www

Log onto the following website for information regarding current trials:

• http://www. ukccsg.org

Although recruitment of adults with cancer into trials is low (approximately 30%) the figures for children/adolescents is much higher; 90% of children/adolescents with a malignant disease are registered with the UKCCSG, 80% of these are eligible for entry onto trials and 70% actually participate in trials (more details are available at: http://www.cancerresearchuk.org). As previously mentioned, the rarity of childhood cancer makes this vital because the significance of findings would be difficult to evaluate if the numbers entered onto trials was low.

The aim of treatment is to remove or to kill the malignant cells and achieve a cure. The term 'cure' refers to the patient who can be expected to have the same life expectancy as any other child/adolescent who does not have a malignancy. Quality of life (QoL) for patients is an important consideration when deciding upon treatment approaches. QoL for cured patients is also very important and will be discussed in more depth in the cure/survivorship section. Cure usually refers to patients that have not been receiving treatment for 5 years and have no evidence of disease.

The main treatments for childhood malignancies are:

• chemotherapy

• radiotherapy

• surgery

• biotherapy/ immunotherapy.

Chemotherapy

Chemotherapy is a systemic treatment and is widely used in childhood malignancies as the tumours have a high rate of proliferation and dissemination (metastatic spread). A helpful analogy for children/adolescents is that chemotherapy is like a space ship that boldly goes where other treatments cannot go.

An interesting information guide for children/adolescents undergoing chemotherapy is an interactive cartoon character, called Captain Chemo, which was created by a patient.

www

Log onto the following website and follow the links to patient information and the adventures of Captain Chemo:

• http://www. royalmarsden.org.uk

Chemotherapy may be used in the following way:

• Definitive/primary: when it is used as the sole treatment.

• Adjuvant: when it is administered following the removal of a primary tumour to destroy any remaining micrometastases.

• Neoadjuvant: when it is used to shrink a tumour prior to surgery.

- Salvage: when it is administered to a patient who has relapsed following treatment using a different modality.
- Palliative: when it is administered to manage symptoms in patients with advanced/incurable disease.

Chemotherapy attacks rapidly reproducing/dividing cells. Three systems in particular are affected: the haemopoetic (bone marrow; BM), the gastrointestinal (GI) and the skin. These are often the most common and most well known associated side effects. Key issues of these more common side effects will be explored following the outlines of the different treatments.

Activity

Using the three headings above, make a list of the potential side effects and symptoms that may occur when cells are destroyed or damaged. You could have up to seven side effects for the GI tract, three for the BM and up to four for the skin.

As previously mentioned, children/adolescents will face repeated courses of chemotherapy and it is important, therefore, to aim for the first one to be a positive experience in order to prevent anticipatory problems with subsequent courses.

Radiotherapy

Radiotherapy is the use of ionising radiation. To begin to understand the principles of radiation, it is necessary to undertake some physics revision, in particular the atom, which can be found on the companion PowerPoint presentation. The different types of radiotherapy used in the treatment of childhood malignancies are also described.

Activity

Read Faithfull (2001), who describes what radiation is, how it occurs naturally or is made and how it is used in the treatment of malignancies. Carry out her analogy of the process of ionisation likened to the game of playing marbles.

Like chemotherapy, radiation has different uses, it may be used for:

- the eradication of the disease, e.g. cure
- the control of symptoms: this may be as a planned treatment or as an emergency, e.g. for children/adolescents with raised intracranial pressure

- imaging
- treatment.

Another useful resource for staff, patients and their families is a video *It's all in the zap* made by a group of teenagers who had received radiotherapy.

PowerPoint

View the extract from the video *It's all in the zap* on the companion PowerPoint presentation.

WWW

A web page has also been created for information and communication. Log on and read the information provided by the teenagers for other patients:
- http://www.allinthezap.com

Members of the public and healthcare professionals are frightened of radiation because it is invisible and is highly technical. Parents and patients require up-to-date information and supportive advice to help them through this treatment. The majority of children/adolescents will receive radiotherapy as an outpatient, the treatment is usually daily, Monday to Friday, and can last for a period of 2 to 6 weeks. Families often feel isolated during this time, as the radiotherapy department may not be in the hospital where they are receiving the other treatment. It is useful, therefore, to ensure that the families have contact names and telephone numbers of appropriate personnel to enable them to seek help, reassurance and advice. They may also require financial help or other social support to manage the impact of daily outpatient trips to the radiotherapy department.

Surgery

Surgery for childhood cancer was the only treatment until the 20th century, when radiotherapy and subsequently chemotherapy became available; cure rate at this time was

Activity

Explain why surgery in childhood/adolescent cancer is rarely used as a single treatment modality.

very low. These have risen considerably since multimodality treatment approaches have been developed.

Surgical services for childhood malignancies have developed over the past 25 years and now include important roles such as:

- aiding a diagnosis, e.g. biopsy
- aiding treatment, e.g. central venous line, gastrostomy tube
- a treatment, e.g. complete resection, partial resection
- assessing response to treatment, e.g. bone marrow aspirates and trephines
- limb conservation surgery, e.g. endoprosthesis
- the management of metastasis.

It is almost inevitable that children/adolescents with a malignancy will undergo a surgical procedure in some form and although it may appear to be the most straightforward of all the treatments it may, as Hollis (1997) identifies, result in loss of function, a cosmetic insult or both, for example a teenager with an osteosarcoma who undergoes limb amputation as part of a treatment protocol.

Activity

As children/adolescents with a malignancy undergoing surgical procedures may have received chemotherapy, what investigations would be undertaken to ensure that it is safe for the procedure to be carried out? You will have to revisit your notes on the side effects of chemotherapy.

Throughout their treatment, children/adolescents will encounter repeat investigations and procedures to assess the response of the treatment. For example, patients with leukaemia will undergo repeated bone marrow aspirates and trephines, and lumbar punctures. Assumptions may be made that because this is the 5th or 10th time, the patient will be used to it and the appropriate psychological care and support may not be offered. Models of nursing such as family-centred care, primary nursing or named nurse (Bishop 2000) offer the opportunity to establish therapeutic relationships that facilitate nurses' understanding of the coping strategies used by individual patients. This also applies to knowledge of how the parents cope as their child undergoes yet another general anaesthetic.

It is also worth remembering that major surgery, such as orthopaedic surgery, may be carried out in specialist units, possibly even in other centres. This again adds to the patient and families' need for appropriate advice and information. Once more, the patient and parents may be faced with meeting yet another group of healthcare professionals, establishing relationships and learning to trust them.

The nurse has a major role to play in ensuring that the patient is prepared, physically and emotionally for the procedure.

Another important consideration is the outcome of the surgical procedure. This may determine the long-term outcome for the patient, is he or she cured or is yet more treatment required? In addition to being worried about surviving the procedure, and perhaps the potential of altered body image, par-

ents and the patient will be anxious to know whether the tumour was completely removed, whether further treatment will be needed or if there is a viable next option.

Biotherapy

Biotherapy refers to the manipulation of the immune system to treat diseases. Other terms used to describe this approach are biologic response modifiers and immunotherapy. The common biotherapy used in childhood/adolescent malignancy treatment is granulocyte colony stimulating factor (GCSF), which is used to support patients going through intensive chemotherapy regimens and peripheral stem cell transplants.

COMMON SIDE EFFECTS OF TREATMENT

Children/adolescents undergoing treatment for a malignancy are likely, therefore, to receive a combination of therapies, which may last for months or, in the case of leukaemia, years. Some patients will undergo long periods of hospitalisation, others will receive much of their treatment as outpatients, attending both the regional centre and the shared care hospital. The effective management of side effects, therefore, is vital.

Effective management incorporates the physical and psychological care for the patient and the psychological care of family members. Symptom management for a patient undergoing treatment for a malignant disease requires nurses to have knowledge of the:

- disease and its symptoms
- treatments and their side effects
- management of both of the above.

Nurses must be able to prioritise their care and show flexibility in the way that the care is delivered (Pinkerton et al 1994). Many of the skills that nurses demonstrate will be carried out by the parents once the patient is discharged and, therefore, negotiation and education are key aspects of care.

Activity

- List the body's normal defence mechanisms.
- Why is the patient with a malignant disease, who is receiving treatment, at risk from infection?

Neutropenia

The treatment of a malignant disease attacks the body's normal defence mechanisms directly and indirectly. The direct effects are on the white cells and the immune system. The indirect effects are through the methods of administration, e.g. via long lines that puncture the skin, other procedures such as venepunctures, bone marrow aspirates and lumbar punctures, which increase the risk of infection. In addition, poor nutritional intake due to nausea and/or vomiting has an effect, as does the use of antibiotics, which damages normal flora. For the children/adolescents who have received chemotherapy, the greatest risk is of developing septicaemia. However, they are also susceptible to haemorrhage, anaemia and anorexia leading to cachexia.

The prevention and early detection of infection is, therefore, a priority. Regular observations of temperature, pulse, respirations and blood pressure and an accurate fluid balance are essential for the patient who is neutropenic. The nurse also needs to be able to recognise subtle changes such as skin colour, position, the patients' interest in ward activities, even personality traits which may indicate the need to initiate repeat observations or other investigations. Recognition of the early signs of septicaemia is essential to prevent septic shock. Oral hygiene, skin integrity and nutritional intake must also be regularly evaluated.

Reflect on your Practice

Nursing tip

The definition of neutropenia is the absence of neutrophils. Neutrophils are white cells and, therefore, when observing for the classic signs of infection, patients who are neutropenic will not produce pus!

Management of neutropenia regarding where the patient is nursed will vary depending upon local policy. In regional centres, neutropenic patients are unlikely to be isolated as there are insufficient facilities. However, in district general hospitals they may be routinely isolated because of other infections on the ward. The most important aspect for the prevention of infection is hand washing (Pinkerton et al 1994).

Nausea and Vomiting

Nausea and vomiting are immediate side effects of chemotherapy but they can persist for several days following administration of the drug, especially nausea. Children have identified nausea as being worse than vomiting, and assessment, which includes the patient and family, is therefore essential. Various rating scales have been developed (Le Baron et al 1988) but as yet they have not been seen universally in practice. There are debates about young children's ability to accurately report their feelings. Zelter et al (1988) recommend that children as young as 5 years are able to use a rating scale, whereas Abu-Saad (1993) does not fully agree.

Knowledge of the emetogenic potential of the chemotherapy drugs and combinations of antiemetic drugs can be found on the companion PowerPoint presentation.

Hawthorne (1995) suggested that the best approach is prevention rather than control once it has occurred. Some patients experience anticipatory nausea and vomiting, this is a complex reaction that triggers memories, thoughts, images from previous experiences. It could be a particular smell, such as disinfectant, food or a nurse's perfume, a particular room, generally something that the patient associates with nausea and/or vomiting.

Pharmacological, non-pharmacological and complementary methods all have a role to play in establishing individualised approaches.

Scenario

Pete, aged 16 years, felt nauseous as soon as the car turned into the drive of the hospital. He was treated with Nabilone (a cannabinoid) taken the evening prior to admission. This helped him sleep better on the night before admission and prevented the experience of nausea as he arrived at the hospital.

Activity

Read Pearman (2002), who explores the management of nausea and vomiting from a health promotion base

Stomatitis

There is conflicting evidence as to the number of children who experience oral complications – stomatitis – following chemotherapy (Aitkin 1992, Holmes 1991). However, as with nausea and vomiting, prevention is better than cure. The term 'stomatitis' refers to inflammation of the oral mucosa. It occurs as a direct effect of the chemotherapy and is indirectly complicated by the decreased myeloproliferation of the bone marrow. The clinical picture is one of ulceration, swelling, pain, dry, cracked bleeding lips, desquamation of the gums and palate (Hooker & Palmer 1999). This can have a direct effect on the patients' quality of life, affecting the ability to eat, drink, communicate and, in severe cases, even swallow saliva. Some patients require continuous morphine analgesia to control pain and facilitate oral care (Pinkerton et al 1994).

Although it is recognised that oral care is essential, there is again conflicting evidence as to oral care regimens. The principles are identified in Box 32.1.

How this is achieved is strongly debated. Although there is no disagreement regarding assessment being the first vital step in planning effective care (Campbell et al 1995), the type of oral assessment guide for children is an issue where there is conflicting evidence (Holmes & Mountain 1993).

Box 32.1

Aims of oral care

To maintain oral function and promote patient dignity, comfort and well-being by maintaining:
- a clean and healthy oral cavity
- moist mucosa
- mucosal integrity.

And preventing:
- plaque
- infection
- dry cracked lips.

Activity

Read Gibson & Hayden (2004) for a description of the development of an oral assessment tool by Great Ormond Street Hospital for Children. This tool is based on Eilers et al's (1988) tool and the discussion includes an analysis of the predominantly adult-based evidence with regard to the applicability of the equipment and solutions for use with children.

Constipation

As previously identified, many of the side effects that the patients experience are compounded by the combination of direct and indirect effects. Constipation is another example of this. Patients in hospital are often at an increased risk of developing constipation because of inactivity and a change in their diet and fluid intake, this may then be complicated by medications such as analgesics, especially opioids and some of the chemotherapy drugs. For example, vincristine, a drug commonly used in the treatment of leukaemia, causes autonomic neuropathy. Educating the patient and family about the importance of appropriate nutrition and hydration and the monitoring of bowel actions is essential. Initiating, maintaining and evaluating accurate fluid, diet and bowel records is a responsibility of the nurse, even if parents decide to participate by carrying out the documentation.

Activity

- With reference to the side effects of chemotherapy, what are the potential risks for a patient who develops constipation?

Nursing tip: patients who are prescribed opioids for pain relief should always receive laxatives to prevent constipation

Anorexia/Cachexia

The importance of adequate nutritional intake has been highlighted several times already but it is important to recognise the challenges for the patient and his or her family. Once again, there are compounding issues. The treatment is likely to result in the patients' nutritional intake being altered, through nausea (with or without vomiting), stomatitis, anorexia and taste alteration, or food restriction prior to procedures. Working with the dietitian, identifying at-risk patients, initiating flexible meal ordering, and facilities for parents to cook or to bring food in are ways of preventing or minimising severe problems (Pinkerton et al 1994).

Steroids, used as part of a treatment protocol or as an antiemetic, can also affect the appetite of patients. Patients with tumours of the central nervous system who may be receiving steroids to reduce raised intracranial pressure often experience problems associated with weight increase. Children/adolescents with leukaemia receive pulses of steroids, which can alter their eating habits. Parents require advice and support to enable them to cope with the impact of having a child whose interest in food varies from waking in the night because they are hungry to one who has no interest in food at all.

Pain

Patients may experience pain as a result of their disease, the investigative procedures, facilitation of treatment, treatment and side effects. Effective assessment and management is essential because, as previously mentioned, many of the patients will experience some or all of the above repeatedly throughout their illness trajectory.

Effective pain strategies have been discussed elsewhere in this book, as has the use of pharmacological, non-pharmacological and complementary approaches, but it is important to remember spiritual pain. These patients will be exposed to other children/adolescents with malignant disease, they will observe them at different stages of their illness trajectory and may well see those suffering painful experiences (Pinkerton et al 1994). They may be aware of, or even witness, death – possibly the death of a close friend, a friendship that has developed through the camaraderie of sharing the same illness and therefore, the same or similar experiences. It is vital, therefore, to acknowledge this and to work with the patient to develop coping strategies. Effective communication, which is an essential part of transdisciplinary working, becomes vital.

Fatigue

Cancer-related fatigue (CRF) has been recognised as a distressing and debilitating symptom in the adult cancer arena for over a decade but has only recently been explored in children/adolescents (Gibson et al 2004a). Fatigue has been identified in adolescents as being multidimensional and multifactorial (Edwards et al 2003, 2004). It can affect the patient's ability to cope with the disease and treatment, participate in normal activities of daily living and can have long-lasting impact. Coping strategies suggested by patients include medical interventions such as blood transfusions, nutrition, sleeps/naps and distraction.

Activity

Think about the ward environment and the activities that nurses carry out and identify factors that may contribute to the patients experiencing fatigue.

Altered Skin Integrity

This is particularly relevant to children/adolescents receiving external beam radiation. The reaction is likened to having sunburn. The first sign is redness, the skin then becomes dry and flaky (dry desquamation) and can proceed to being wet and flaky (moist desquamation). The key principles are to promote comfort, prevent infection and minimise trauma. Faithfull (2001) discusses current evidence on the prevention and management of skin side effects, whilst it is adult based it is applicable with adaptation for children and adolescents.

Altered Body Image

Children/adolescents are concerned about their appearance, and it is important to be able to look and dress like their peers. Treatment, as already identified, can result in undesirable physical changes that make them look and feel different (Thompson 2001). Although it is important to stress the temporary nature of side effects such as alopecia and weight gain/loss, patients and other family members will require help from the multidisciplinary team to develop coping strategies to deal with these, especially for permanent side effects such as amputation or surgical scars.

Other body changes may not be visible, such as infertility, but can have a major impact for males as well as females. Again, psychological support to develop coping strategies is essential. Two cancer charities, the Teenage Cancer Trust and Teencancer, have developed web pages that give adolescents the opportunity to share experiences of coping with these and other problems.

Activity

Log onto the following websites. List the facilities that are available for teenagers. Identify the common questions asked by this group of patients:
- http://www. teencancer.org
- http://www. teenagecancer.org

PSYCHOLOGICAL CARE

In the 1980s, when improvements in the remission and cure rates were becoming evident, new problems for the psychological care of the patient and family were being identified. Koocher & O'Malley (1985) interviewed survivors and their families who described the problems of living with cancer. One of the key factors identified was the need for the preparation to be able to live with cancer. For the parents, it included advice and support to let their child live as 'normal a life' as possible and to be able to facilitate all members of the family to live with the impact of the disease and treatment.

More recent research by Clarke-Steffen (1997) explored how current families managed 'living' with childhood cancer. She identified the concept of 'reconstructing reality', which consisted of the strategies in Box 32.2.

Box 32.2

Reconstructing reality (from Clarke-Steffen 1997 p 281)

- Managing the flow of information.
- Reorganising roles.
- Evaluating and shifting priorities.
- Changing future orientation.
- Assigning meaning to the illness.
- Managing the therapeutic regimen.

Clarke-Steffen (1997) explains the stages that the parents, patient and family members go through to develop the above strategies. She begins with the impact of the potential diagnosis and uses the analogy of being in 'limbo', when the patient, parents and family members are waiting to know the diagnosis, and are experiencing feelings of vulnerability and helplessness. When the diagnosis is confirmed, there is a new daily routine to adjust to and with this are feelings of uncertainty, and a change in the way that life is viewed. Reconstructing reality provides evidence of the challenges that the family faces and the importance of the role of the members of the professional healthcare team. An interesting finding from this qualitative study was that parents appreciated nurses 'being there'. Being there when families are in 'limbo' requires very special skills.

Activity

Imagine how it would feel to be with the parents of Jonathan as they waited for the confirmation of his diagnosis. How would you feel, what would you say, and what would you do?

Sadly, nothing we can say will make it better but, as mentioned earlier, the way that we say things and the courage to stay with the family – just 'being there' – can make a memorable difference.

Quality of Life

Quality of life (QoL) for children/adolescents with cancer is now being researched (Eiser & Morse 2001, Gibson et al 2004b, Hicks et al 2003) and the following issues are being explored:

- physical well-being and symptoms
- psychological well-being
- social well-being
- spiritual well-being.

Recently, Hicks et al (2003 p 192) identified the following five themes, which can have an effect on the psychosocial well-being of the patient and subsequently the ability to become well adjusted survivors:

- fatigue
- effect on activities
- medication and treatment effects
- relationship changes
- hair loss.

The philosophy for treatment in the 1960s and 1970s, when cure was rare, was cure at whatever cost. The philosophy is now cure with the least cost (Pinkerton et al 1994).

As previously mentioned, children/adolescents will receive multimodal therapy and, therefore, may experience some or all of the side effects identified. Healthcare professionals, therefore, require knowledge of the compounding factors associated with the treatments and the appropriate skills to identify at-risk patients, initiate appropriate assessment strategies, implement effective management plans and evaluate all aspects of the care. Some patients will receive treatments during which intensive or high doses of chemotherapy and/or radiotherapy are used. These treatments will result in an increase in the severity of the side effects, both from the symptoms themselves and also the length of time they persist. As the risk of complications increases with the intensity of the treatment, the skill and role of the health care professional must also be extended and developed.

GOING HOME

Scenario

Jonathan was in the regional centre for 10 days. On discharge his white cell count was 1.9×10^9 with 30% neutrophils, haemoglobin 10.9 and platelets 68×10^9. He had started his first course of chemotherapy, which was to be completed as an outpatient at his local hospital. He had a skin-tunnelled catheter in situ.

Activity

List the information that Jonathan and his family require to facilitate a smooth and safe transition to home?

It has already been identified that once the diagnosis of a malignancy has been confirmed, the ability to remember details about the disease and treatment is reduced. When planning the discharge, providing the information is only a small part of the process. Nurses caring for these families need to be able to negotiate with them to provide information at an appropriate and convenient time, in a format that is acceptable and as frequently as is required by individual families (Cox 2000). The families will require information and advice regarding:

- identification of infection (including temperature monitoring)
- medication administration
- care of the central venous device
- nutrition
- oral hygiene
- contact names and numbers/ who to call in an emergency
- how to recognise an emergency
- outpatient appointments
- details of shared care.

Several of these require the parents to be proficient in new skills, for example, caring for the central venous device and administering cytotoxic medication, as well as managing all the information and coping without having knowledgeable, supportive people, such as staff and other parents, around.

Although it is acknowledged that discharge planning begins on admission, the planning and timing of patient and parent education must be negotiated in a way that acknowledges and recognises the impact that the diagnosis may have had.

Activity

- Write a detailed plan of how you would structure the teaching for Jonathan and his parents.
- What factors will you take into consideration when planning the timing?
- What specific nursing skill is central to the success of your plan?

REMISSION

Remission is the term used to describe no evidence of disease. It is most commonly used in the leukaemias to describe the amount of blast cells in the bone marrow.

A remission marrow will have less than 5% blast cells (blast means immature), it is normal for bone marrow to have up to 5% blast cells present, therefore a remission marrow is one that has less than 5% blast cells.

Once in remission, patients with acute lymphoblastic leukaemia will commence the treatment phase known as maintenance therapy. This is to maintain the remission and minimise the chance of relapse, i.e. the disease returning. Boys will undergo a 3-year maintenance protocol, whereas girls have 2 years of maintenance therapy.

Protocols for acute myeloid leukaemia and the solid tumours last for months rather than years. The chemotherapy is more intensive, requiring frequent and/or extended hospitalisation and inpatient supportive care.

RELAPSE/RECURRENCE

Parents in Koocher & O'Malley's (1985) study likened the threat of relapse as the sword of Damocles. Even after being pronounced 'cured', the fear did not disappear. Relapse rates vary with individual diseases and depend on prognostic features and the stage of the disease at diagnosis.

Relapse brings with it the need for information regarding confirmation and extent of the spread of recurrent disease and the possibility of further treatment. This may include the opportunity to gain second opinions.

Having experienced them once, it is important that the patients' feelings regarding QoL issues are taken into consideration when treatment opportunities are being discussed. This poses the potential for ethical debates regarding the use of experimental treatments.

www

Read Dyer (1995) and Entwistle et al (1996) on the case of child B, and the surrounding media coverage, at:
- http://www.bmj.com

Previous knowledge of how the patient has coped with treatment will be useful but it is essential that a trusting and supportive relationship be established at the time of relapse. As a decision is reached, the family needs to feel supported by all members of the healthcare team.

If further treatment is not an option, discussion about the provision of appropriate palliative care will be required. Parents will need support and advice regarding communicating the results and their implications to the patient. Harris & Curnick (2000) recommend that parents are given time to assimilate the information before they can begin to discuss it with the patient. Bluebond-Langner (1992) suggests that openness within a family is more likely if the parents feel supported. The skills and approaches used at the time of diagnosis will be required again, incorporating the knowledge gained through the previous treatment experience. At this time, however, parents may feel the need to protect their child from the pain of facing death.

Activity

In *The private worlds of dying children*, Bluebond-Langner (1978) identified the concept of 'mutual pretence':
- In the current climate where 'openness' is recommended, list the difficulties for nurses working with a family where mutual pretence may be utilised as a coping strategy.

PowerPoint

Access the companion PowerPoint presentation for information relating to the incidence of patients developing a second malignancy

PALLIATIVE CARE AND DEATH

Although cure rates are improving, cancer is the highest cause of death due to illness in the UK (2004 data available at: http://www.statistics.gov.uk). The majority of children/adolescents dying from cancer are cared for at home with the support of appropriately experienced nurses (Hunt 1996). A small number, however, will die in hospital. Some of these will be anticipated deaths, when the parents and/or patient haven chosen to receive palliative care in hospital or when a decision is reached that further active treatment is no longer appropriate but the patient is too ill to be transferred home. Rarely, unexpected death due to oncological emergencies such as septic shock, an allergic reaction to medication, haemorrhage or tumour lysis syndrome, can occur.

PowerPoint

Access the companion PowerPoint presentation to learn more about oncological emergencies.

Sudden death prevents the establishment of effective palliative care, the opportunity to prepare for the death and the chance to say goodbye. Black (1991) advocates that managing and coping with sudden death requires specific skills, especially the ability to communicate effectively and offer appropriate support. Sudden death can impact on normal grieving and can exacerbate grief reactions.

Activity

Read Curnick & Harris (2000) for issues related to the child dying with cancer.

WWW

The following are the websites of charity organisations that develop advice and information for healthcare professionals, patients and families preparing for and coping with bereavement. Log on to both sites and view the facilities available:

- http://www.childbereavement.org.uk
- http://www. winstonswish.org.uk

Long-term Survivors

The introduction of multimodal treatment has seen an improvement in survival rates to almost 70% (2004 data available at: http://www.statistics.gov.uk). This has posed new challenges for the healthcare team in the prevention, recognition and management of long-term side effects. The UKCCSG has developed guidelines for long-term follow-up care (UKCCSG 1995). Specialists in paediatric respiratory, endocrinology, cardiology, neurology and psychology are part of the long-term follow-up team.

Long-term side effects are related to the combination and dosage of drugs used, multimodal therapies can exacerbate any toxicity. The body systems where toxicities are anticipated include the:

- lungs
- heart
- renal system
- liver
- gonads: fertility
- endocrine: growth and puberty
- hearing
- central nervous system
- skin
- skeletal
- eyes.

Chesterfield (1999) advocates the nurse's responsibility of facilitating survivors' adaptation to the physical and/or psychological disabilities they may have. However, for some patients this may be a life-long challenge. For children/adolescents who have missed a significant amount of schooling and have received treatment such as cranial irradiation, which has detrimental effects on some aspects of intellect (Anderson et al 1994), the choice of further education/employment may be restricted.

The decision-making skills of adolescents who had received treatment for cancer were explored by Hollen & Hobbie (1996). They concluded that, for some, the ability to make decisions was affected by the combination of treatment and the impact of hospitalization, which had resulted in them missing out on normal developmental interaction. This is particularly important when the role of the nurse as health promoter is considered. Giving advice about not smoking to a teenager who has received lung irradiation may not be enough for patients who have difficulty in making decisions. The context in which they may be tempted to smoke – being out with their peers when perhaps they are the only one not smoking – needs to be considered. Advice on strategies to prepare them to be able to say no are also required.

Health promotion regarding sexual health for adolescents may present challenges for some parents and healthcare professionals. Information regarding safe sex, for example the use of condoms, may prevent difficulties in families where the parents may be unaware that their son/daughter is sexually active. Adolescents who may have been told that their fertility has been impaired, may decide to experiment without the use of contraception and are therefore at risk of an unwanted pregnancy as well as of developing life-threatening infections. Support groups with other survivors and interactive internet networks, such as the http://www.allinthezap.com, http://www.teencancer.org and http://www.teenagecancer.org have been developed by young people to help each other.

ADOLESCENTS AND YOUNG ADULTS

Adolescents and young adults have very specific needs in relation to achieving their unique developmental tasks (Taylor & Muller 1995) and adapting to their disease, its treatment and the restrictions that may result as a direct consequence. Their ability to comprehend the illness and its implications, the restrictions made by the treatment and the physical changes, can lead to lowered self-esteem and depression (Ritchie 1992) and increase their sense of personal vulnerability (Eiser 1996). To help them cope and maintain hope, Hooker (2004) identified the need for accurate, truthful information that enables them to participate in decision-making, assess the threat of the illness and gain a sense of control. There is debate as to the most appropriate place for this group to receive treatment (Whelan 2003). They have been described as being at the edge of no-man's land by Hollis & Morgan (2001) and in need of dedicated services. Morgan & Hubber (2004) describe the challenges of establishing such a service, identifying the problems associated with acting as the mediator between the patients, their families and the adult and paediatric healthcare professionals.

Activity

Read Morgan & Hubber (2004). Identify the key issues for nurses caring for this age group when dedicated facilities are not available.

Surviving Cancer and Cure

The treatment of cancer is often depicted as a battle, with patients either winning the battle or losing the fight. Survival could, therefore, be associated with winning the battle. Lozowski (1993) proposes that survival begins at the time of diagnosis, with the patients surviving the many components of cancer and its treatment, living with their cancer through periods of remission and relapse. However, as the definition of cure is that there is no evidence of disease 5 years after completion of treatment, there are children/adolescents who are survivors but who are not cured, they have won the battle but not necessarily the war.

Significantly, Van Eys (1991) suggests that as well as biological cure, psychological and social cure is also required and, therefore, biological cure alone could be viewed as only part success if the patient is left with psychological and/or social needs.

Research by Eiser & Jenney (1996) has identified a correlation between duration and intensity of treatment and the prevalence of psychological late effects. Medical interventions such as venepuncture or side effects affecting body image, such as alopecia or altered weight, can affect the patient's psychological well-being, reiterating the importance of managing the procedure effectively.

Earlier in the chapter, Clarke-Steffan's (1997) model of family adjustment identified the important role that parents have in managing the flow of information regarding the treatment and the day-to-day care of the patient. Children/adolescents with cancer have to cope with being different, of living a different type of life to that of their healthy peers, and this can leave them with feelings of abandonment, loneliness and loss of control. Time away from school may leave them with different career choices, perhaps being dependent on their parents when their peers are experiencing and enjoying their growing independence.

Interestingly, a recent study of school-age children with acute lymphoblastic leukaemia by Dowling et al (2003) explored the relationship between childhood cancer stressors and the psychological adjustment to cancer and identified a direct correlation. Although the authors acknowledge limitations with the study and recommend further research, it does raise questions regarding personal factors that may help children/adolescents cope with the stressors of cancer and its treatment and hypothesises whether personal traits such as humour, resilience, hardiness and optimism can be learnt and developed.

The role of parents, peers and schools in providing psychosocial support has also been explored by Suzuki & Kato (2003). A review of the literature identified a variety of resources available to facilitate the education and skill development of the parents, peers and schools to help the patient adjust and cope. The internet and video games were particularly useful for education and provided an opportunity to practice or rehearse communications with the patient.

Hicks & Lavender (2001) promote the development of psychosocial support interventions to facilitate improvement of QoL regardless of the eventual outcome of the illness. Acceptable QoL is linked to rehabilitation by Bradwell & Hawkins (2000), who advocate that rehabilitation begins at diagnosis. Although this is important, Selekmans' (1991) suggestion of a revision of the concept of rehabilitation for children is compelling in that she advocates the philosophy of habilitation. This recognises the need to continue normal development to prevent developmental delay. She advocates supporting children to achieve levels of development as yet unknown to them. For patients facing months of hospitalisation, isolation from peers, school and social activities, this is an important aspect of care.

The child/adolescent with cancer, and the family, face many hurdles as they try to reconstruct reality (Clarke-Steffan 1997). The patient will miss school, peers and social activities, and might have to cope with altered body image and come to terms with uncertainty about the future, even as a survivor.

Siblings also have to adjust to the change in their life brought about by the reconstruction. The impact of this depends on their age and relationship with the ill sibling. Initially, it may be separation from the family (Foley et al 1993) followed by non-negotiated routine changes and altered family plans for holidays, etc. as a result of adaptation to the treatment and its restrictions. They experience the same fears and incomprehension as the parents but often they do not have someone to talk to or confide in (Faulkner et al 1995). Parents require guidance to meet the needs of all family members throughout the illness trajectory, but especially at times of crisis. They may feel that they are protecting their healthy children/adolescents but they may be adding to their burden by making them feel excluded, unable to participate in the care and decisions. Simms et al (2002) advocate involving them in the care of their sick sibling.

Summary

Childhood malignancy has been described as a chronic illness. It is essential, therefore, that children/adolescents receive comprehensive care that encompasses their physical, psychological and psychosocial well being within a philosophy of family-centred care, preparing and supporting them as they live with cancer, its treatment and the side effects (Langton 2000). Working with this group of patients, whether in a regional centre, shared care or primary health care environment can be very rewarding but is also stressful (Bulley 2000). Maintaining clear professional boundaries when working closely with families can be difficult, but it is essential because the patient and family need professional care and, to continue to provide this care, nurses are required to identify and develop their own coping strategies.

The concept of the illness trajectory (Fig. 32.1) (Corbin & Strauss 1991) has been used to identify the challenges that a child/adolescent with cancer, and his or her family, will face as treatment is undergone. The number of health-care professionals and care environments they may encounter on this journey has also been highlighted. Many nurses will see the patient and family in the context of only one healthcare setting and it is important, therefore, to have an understanding of the challenges facing these families as they receive transdisciplinary care. The Cancer Plan (DoH 2000) identified a seamless approach to care, which is difficult when care is shared between different healthcare professionals and environments.

However, the last three decades have seen remarkable improvements, both in the approach to the care of the child/adolescent with a malignant disease and in the success of treatments. The enthusiasm and determination to deliver improved evidence-based care for the child/adolescent and their family continues.

Activity

Read Thompson (2004).

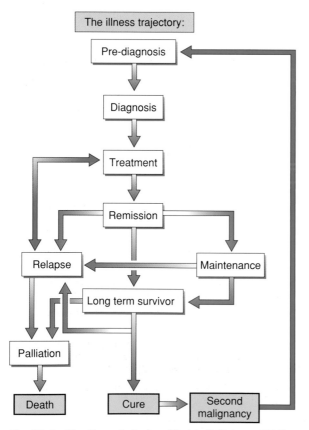

Fig. 32.1 • The illness trajectory (Corbin & Strauss 1991).

References

Abu-Saad H 1993 Paediatric pain management. An intervention study. Paper presented at Royal College of Nursing 1st International Conference in Paediatrics, Cambridge, UK

Aitkin TJ 1992 Gastrointestinal manifestations in the child with cancer. Journal of Pediatric Oncology Nursing 9(3):99–109

Anderson V, Smibert E, Ekert H, Godber T 1994 Intellectual, educational and behavioural sequelae after cranial irradiation and chemotherapy. Archives of Diseases in Childhood 70:476–483

Bishop J 2000 Partnership in care. In: Langton H (ed.) The child with cancer: family centred care. Baillière Tindall, London

Black K 1991 Sudden unexpected death: caring for the parents. Paediatric Nursing 17(6):571–574

Bluebond-Langner M 1978 The private worlds of dying children. Princeton University Press, Princeton, NJ

Bluebond-Langner M 1992 Children and death: directions for the 90s. Princeton University Press, Princeton, NJ

Bradwell M, Hawkins J 2000 Survivorship and rehabilitation. In: Langton H (ed.) The child with cancer; family centred care in practice. Baillière Tindall, London

Buckman R 1992 How to break bad news. A guide for health care professionals. Papermac, London

Bulley S 2000 Impact of treatment on the nursing team. In: Langton H (ed.) The child with cancer; family centred care in practice. Baillière Tindall, London

Campbell ST, Evans MA, MacTavish P 1995 Guidelines for mouth care. The Paediatric Oncology Nurses Forum, Royal College of Nursing, London

Chesterfield P 1999 Late effects of chemotherapy. In Gibson F, Evans M (eds) Paediatric oncology acute nursing care. Whurr, London

Christensen J, Fatchett D 2002 Promoting parental use of distraction and relaxation in pediatric oncology patients during invasive procedures. Journal of Pediatric Oncology Nursing 19(4):127–132

Clarke JN & Fletcher P 2003 Communication issues faced by parents who have a child diagnosed with cancer. Journal of Pediatric Oncology Nursing 20(4):175–191

Clarke-Steffen L 1993 Waiting and not knowing: the diagnosis of cancer in a child. Journal of Pediatric Oncology Nursing 10(4):146–153

Clarke-Steffen L 1997 Reconstructing reality: family strategies for managing childhood cancer. Journal of Pediatric Nursing 12:278–287

Corbin JM, Strauss A 1991 A nursing model for chronic illness management based upon the trajectory framework. Scholarly Inquiry for Nursing Practice: An International Journal 5:154–174

Cox A 2000 Discharge – a planned event. In: Langton H (ed.) The child with cancer; family centred care in practice. Baillière Tindall, London

Curnick S, Harris A 2000 The dying child. In: Langton H (ed.) The child with cancer: family centred care in practice. Baillière Tindall, London

Department of Health (DoH) 1995 A policy for commissioning cancer services. A report by the expert advisor on cancer of the Chief Medical Officers of England and Wales (the Calman–Hine report). HMSO, London

Department of Health (DoH) 2000 The cancer plan. DoH, London

Dowling JS, Hockenberry M, Gregory RL 2003 Sense of humor, childhood cancer stressors, and outcomes of psychosocial adjustment, immune function, and infection. Journal of Pediatric Oncology Nursing 20(6):271–292

Edwards J, Gibson F, Richardson A et al 2003 Fatigue in adolescents with and following a cancer diagnosis; developing an evidence base for practice. European Journal of Cancer 39(18):2671–2680

Edwards J, Gibson F, Sepion B 2004 Cancer-related fatigue in teenagers: a journey of discovery. In: Gibson F, Soanes L, Sepion B (eds) Perspectives in paediatric oncology nursing. Whurr, London

Eilers J, Berger AM, Petersen MC 1988 Development, testing and application of the oral assessment guide. Oncology Nursing Forum 15:325–330

Eiser C 1996 The impact of treatment: adolescents' views. In: Selby P, Bailey C (eds) Cancer and the adolescent. BMJ Publishing, London

Eiser C, Jenney MEM 1996 Measuring symptomatic benefit and quality of life in paediatric oncology. British Journal of Cancer 73:1313–1316

Eiser C, Morse R 2001 A review of measures of quality of life for children with chronic illness. Archives of Diseases in Childhood 84:205–211

Eiser C, Parkyn T, Havermans T, McNinch A 1994 Parents' recall of the diagnosis of cancer in their child. Psycho-oncology 3:197–203

Faithfull S 2001 Radiotherapy. In: Corner J, Bailey C (eds) Cancer nursing care in context. Blackwell Science, Oxford

Faulkner A, Peace G, O'Keefe C 1995 When a child has cancer. Chapman & Hall, London

Foley GV, Hochtrian D, Hardin Mooney K 1993 Nursing care of the child with cancer. WB Saunders, Philadelphia

Gibson F, Hayden S 2004 Development of an oral care protocol. In: Gibson F, Soanes L, Sepion B (eds) Perspectives in paediatric oncology nursing. Whurr, London

Gibson F, Edwards J, Sepion B 2004a Cancer related fatigue in teenagers: a journey of discovery. In: Gibson F, Soanes L, Sepion B (eds) Perspectives in paediatric oncology nursing. Whurr, London

Gibson F, Soanes L, Sepion B 2004b Perspectives in paediatric oncology nursing. Whurr, London

Harris A, Curnick S 2000 Care in the community. In: Langton H (ed.) The child with cancer: family centred care in practice. Baillière Tindall, London

Hawthorne J 1995 Understanding the management of nausea and vomiting. Blackwell Science, Oxford

Hicks MD, Lavender R 2001 Psychosocial practice trends in pediatric oncology. Journal of Pediatric Oncology Nursing 18(4):143–153

Hicks J, Bartholomew J, Ward-Smith P, Hutto CJ 2003 Quality of life among childhood leukaemia patients. Journal of Pediatric Oncology Nursing 20(4):192–200

Hockenberry-Eaton M, Hinds PS 2000 Fatigue in children and adolescents with cancer. Evolution of a programme of study. Seminars in Oncology Nursing 16:261–272

Hollen P, Hobbie W 1996 Decision and risk behaviours of cancer surviving adolescents and their peers. Journal of Pediatric Oncology Nursing 13(3):121–134

Hollis R 1997 Childhood cancer into the 21st century. Paediatric Nursing 9(3):12–15

Hollis R, Morgan S 2001 The adolescent with cancer – at the edge of no-man's land. Lancet Oncology 2(1):43–48

Holm KE, Patterson JM, Gurney JG 2003 Parental involvement and family centred care in the diagnostic and treatment phases of childhood cancer: results from a qualitative study. Journal of Pediatric Oncology Nursing 20(6):301–313

Holmes S 1991 The oral complications of specific anticancer therapy. International Journal of Nursing Studies 28(4):343–360

Holmes S, Mountain E 1993 Assessment of oral status: evaluation of three oral assessment guides. Journal of Clinical Nursing 2(1):35–40

Hooker L 2004 Teenagers' information needs. In: Gibson F, Soanes L, Sepion B (eds) Perspectives in paediatric oncology nursing. Whurr, London

Hooker L, Palmer S 1999 Administration of chemotherapy. In Gibson F, Evans M (eds) Paediatric oncology acute nursing care. Whurr, London

Hooker L, Williams J 1996 Parent-held shared care records: bridging the communication gaps. British Journal of Nursing 5(12):738–741

Hunt J 1996 Paediatric oncology outreach nurse specialist: the impact of funding arrangements on their professional role. Paediatric Oncology Nurses Forum, Royal College of Nursing, London

Koocher GP, O'Malley JE 1985 The Damocles syndrome. McGraw Hill, London

Kubler Ross E 1969 On death and dying. MacMillan, New York

Langton H 2000 The child with cancer-family centred care in practice. Ballière Tindall, London

Le Baron S, Zeltzer LK, LeBaron C et al 1988 Chemotherapy side effects in pediatric oncology patients; drugs, age, sex as risk factors. Medical and Pediatric Oncology 16(4):262–268

Lozowski S 1993 Views of childhood cancer survivors. Selected perspectives. Cancer 71 (Suppl):3354–3357

Morgan S, Hubber D 2004 Setting up an adolescent service. In: Gibson F, Soanes L, Sepion B (eds) Perspectives in paediatric oncology nursing. Whurr, London

Muir KR, Parkes SE, Boon R et al 1992 Shared care in paediatric oncology. Journal of Cancer Care 1:15–17

Parry C 2003 Embracing uncertainty: an exploration of the experiences of childhood cancer survivors. Qualitative Health Research 13(1):227–246

Patel N, Sepion B, Edwards J 1997 Development of a shared care programme for children with cancer. Journal of Cancer Nursing 1:1–4

Pearman K 2002 Chemotherapy-induced nausea and vomiting: a health promotion resource. Paediatric Nursing 14(6):30–32

Pinkerton CR, Cushing P, Sepion B 1994 Childhood cancer management: a practical handbook. Chapman & Hall, London

Price J 2003 Information needs of the child with cancer and their family. Cancer Nursing Practice 2(7):35–38

Ritchie MA 1992 Psychosocial functioning of adolescents with cancer. Oncology Nursing Forum 19:1947–1501

Ruccione K, Waskerwitz M, Buckley J et al 1994 What caused my child's cancer? Parents' responses to an epidemiology study of childhood cancer. Journal of Pediatric Oncology Nursing 11(2):71–84

Selekman J 1991 Pediatric rehabilitation from concepts to practice. Pediatric Nursing 17(1):26–27

Sepion B 2004 Shared care. In: Gibson F, Soanes L, Sepion B (eds) Perspectives in paediatric oncology nursing. Whurr, London

Simms S, Hewitt N, Vevers J 2002 Sibling support in childhood cancer. Paediatric Nursing 14(7):20–22

Suzuki LK, Kato PM 2003 Psychosocial support for patients in pediatric oncology: the influences of parents, schools, peers and technology. Journal of Pediatric Oncology Nursing 20(4):159–174

Taylor J, Muller D 1995 Nursing adolescents: research and psychological perspectives. Blackwell Science, London

Thompson J 2001 The needs of children and adolescents. In: Corner J, Bailey C (eds) Cancer nursing in context. Blackwell Science, London

Thompson J 2004 Preface. Personal reflections on the development of paediatric oncology nursing as a speciality. In: Gibson F, Soanes L, Sepion B (eds) Perspectives in paediatric oncology nursing. Whurr, London

United Kingdom Children Cancer Study Group (UKCCSG) 1987 Report on cancer services for children. UKCCSG, London

United Kingdom Children's Cancer Study Group (UKCCSG) Late Effects Group 1995 Long term follow up therapy-based guidelines. UKCCSG, Leicester

United Kingdom Children Cancer Study Group (UKCCSG) 1997 The resources and requirements of a UKCCSG treatment centre. UKCCSG, London

Van Eys J 1991 The truly cured child. Pediatrician 18:90–95

Whelan J 2003 Where should teenagers with cancer be treated? European Journal of Cancer 39(18):2573–2578

Zelter LK, LeBaron S, Richie M et al 1988 Can children understand and use a rating scale to quantify somatic symptoms? Journal of Consulting and Clinical Psychology 56(4):567–572

Useful Websites

http://www.allinthezap.com

http://www.bmj.com

http://www.cancerresearchuk.org

http://www.childbereavement.org.uk

http://www.royalmarsden.org

http://www.statistics.gov.uk

http://www.teenagecancer.org

http://www.teencancer.org

http://www.ukccsg.org

http://www.winstonswish.org.uk

Chapter Thirty Three

33

Caring for a Child with Neurological dysfunction

Joanna Smith

ABSTRACT

The aim of this chapter and companion PowerPoint presentation is to provide an overview of neurological problems in childhood. This will be achieved by introducing the nervous system and the principles of caring for a child with a neurological dysfunction, and outlining common childhood neurological disorders.

Learning Outcomes

- Understand the basic functions of the nervous system

- Understand the general principles of caring for a child and family, where the child has a neurological disorder.

- Appreciate the range of neurological disorders in childhood and the potential impact on the child and family.

- Describe the common neurological disorders of childhood.

Introduction

Nervous system malformations account for approximately 75% of fetal and 40% of infant deaths (Padgett 2002). Approximately 15–20% of hospitalised children have a neurological problem either as the sole or associated complaint. Diseases of the neurological system have a profound affect on the lives of the child and family and are probably the most disruptive of all ailments. Caring for these children and their families is challenging because the outcome is often uncertain, many disorders are rare and the family will have expert knowledge of the child's needs, which can lead to frustration for parents and feelings of inadequacy for healthcare professionals. Traditional models of care focusing on the disease process (illness, dependence and treatment) are inappropriate. Although key principles can be applied, care must be individually designed, have a developmental focus and influenced by encouraging the child to reach their full potential.

The Role, Structure and Function of the Nervous System

The nervous and endocrine systems are the main regulatory systems of the body. The nervous system is the most rapid means of maintaining homeostasis, which is achieved by reacting and responding to internal and external stimuli. The nervous system is descriptively divided into the central nervous system (CNS) and the peripheral nervous system (PNS) (Sugerman 2002). The CNS consists of the brain, the control centre for the entire nervous system, and the spinal cord. The PNS consists of the nerve networks, which link the CNS with the periphery.

The PNS has two main subdivisions, the somatic nervous system (SNS) and the autonomic nervous system (ANS). Actions carried out by the SNS are voluntary and sensations are perceived consciously, whereas actions carried out by the ANS are involuntary and generally not perceived consciously. The ANS has sympathetic and parasympathetic divisions and is primarily concerned with the innervation and control of visceral organs, smooth muscles and secretory glands. Where there is both sympathetic and parasympathetic nerve innovation their actions have an antagonistic effect, for example sympathetic activity increases the force of contraction of cardiac muscle and the heart rate, whereas parasympathetic activity reduces the force of contraction and decreases the heart rate.

EMBRYOLOGY

Many neurological problems result from malformations occurring during embryological development (Padgett 2002). One of the three primary germ layers, the ectoderm, forms nervous tissue, ear, eye and epidermis. Between 3 and 4 weeks after fertilisation, the dorsal midline of the ectoderm thickens forming the neural plate, which folds and fuses creating the neural tube. By the 5th week of gestation the rostral portion of the neural tube enlarges and differentiates into the forebrain (cerebrum), midbrain and hindbrain (pons, cerebellum and medulla oblongata) (Fig. 33.1).

In addition to structural developments, cells organise themselves into zones, which allows for specialization and results in the typical appearance of the brain: an outer layer of grey mater (cell bodies) and an inner layer of white matter (nerve tracts). Epidermal cells, precursors of both supporting (glial) cells and specialist (nerve) cells, increase in number and migrate through the layers of previously formed cells, adding to the expanding cerebral cortex. During the final stages of specialisation, nerve cells lose the ability to divide, and therefore do not increase in number after birth. Glial cell proliferation and nerve myelination increase the weight and size of the brain, particularly during the first year of life. Nerve myelination occurs from 22 weeks of gestation and is probably not complete until adult life (Padgett 2002).

CELLS OF THE NERVOUS SYSTEM AND THEIR FUNCTION

Glial cells form the connective tissue of the nervous system; astrocytes provide mechanical support and help maintain the blood brain barrier, microglia correspond to brain phagocytes, oligodendroglia and Schwann cells form myelin in the CNS and PNS respectively, and ependymal cells form the epithelial linings.

The neuron has a specialised structure that facilitates the transmission of electrical impulses (Fig. 33.2). A stimulus of sufficient strength applied to a dendrite receptor site generates a nerve impulse, which is transmitted along the dendrite to the cell body. The impulse exits via the main axonal process (nerve fibre) ending at the terminal boutons. These contain chemical transmitters capable of stimulating adjacent neurons or affector organs. Generating and conducting a nerve impulse is based on the neuron's ability to maintain a difference in the ion concentration outside and inside the cell membrane. Disruption of the ion concentration causes an ionic current flow, which is conducted along the entire neuron, is independent of any further stimulus and is unidirectional. The speed of the nerve impulse increases (Longstaff 2000):

- if temperature increases
- the diameter of the fibre increases
- myelin is present.

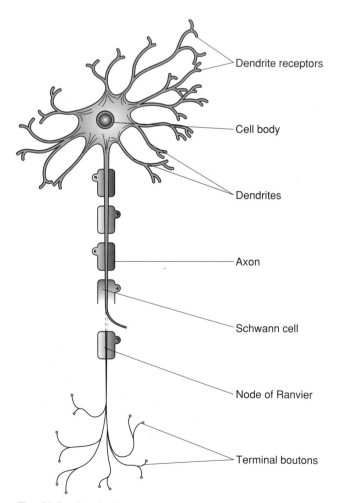

Fig. 33.2 • A typical motor neuron.

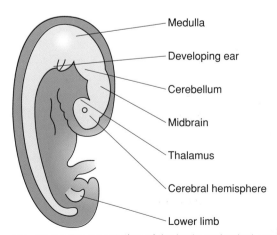

Fig. 33.1 • Representation of the brain and spinal cord at 5 weeks' gestation.

Information passes between neurons at junctions (synapses). When a nerve impulse arrives at the terminal bouton, neurotransmitters such as noradrenaline or acetylcholine are released. These cross the synapse and bind with the receptor site on the adjacent dendrite. Calcium ions are necessary to facilitate this process. Neurotransmitters stimulate or inhibit postsynaptic dendrites, allowing impulses either to proceed or be inhibited. Once the neurotransmitter binds with the receptor site it is rapidly deactivated by enzymes in the postsynaptic junction.

ANATOMY OF THE BRAIN

The brain consists of the cerebrum (two cerebral hemispheres), diencephalon, brainstem and cerebellum (Fig. 33.3).

The cerebral hemispheres are divided into important functional areas (Fig. 33.4) joined at the base by the corpus callosum (a sheet of nerve fibres allowing communication between the hemispheres). The topographical representation of the cerebral cortex relates different functions to specific areas (Fitzgerald & Folan-Curran 2002):

- The frontal lobe contains the primary motor cortex responsible for controlling movement, the speech area and higher functions including personality and behaviour.
- The parietal lobe contains the primary somatosensory cortex where sensations such as touch, pressure, pain and temperature are consciously perceived.
- The occipital lobe contains the visual cortex.
- The temporal lobes contain the auditory cortex, and areas involved in memory and emotions.

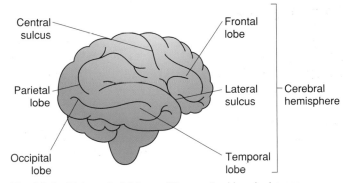

Fig. 33.4 • Major subdivisions of the cerebral hemispheres.

Decussation of fibres at the medulla oblongata results in each hemisphere communicating with the opposite side of the body.

The diencephalon consists of specialist structures such as the thalamus and hypothalamus. The thalamus is a relay and integration centre. The hypothalamus coordinates homeostatic mechanisms and has autonomic, neuroendocrine and limbic functions.

The brainstem collectively describes the midbrain, medulla oblongata and the pons. The midbrain contains part of the auditory system. Most nerve fibres transcend the medulla and midbrain, which function as important relay and integration centres. The medulla contains nuclei that are important for the regulation of blood pressure, respiration, maintenance of arousal and initiation of sleep. Like the medulla, the pons contains many functional structures but also acts as a relay centre between the cerebrum and cerebellum.

The cerebellum sits in the base of the cranial cavity in an area known as the posterior fossa. It is important in the

Fig. 33.3 • Cross-sectional view of the brain.

coordination of muscular functions such as tone and posture, and operates at an unconscious level.

THE VENTRICULAR SYSTEM

The ventricular system contains cerebrospinal fluid (CSF) and consists of four chambers: two C-shaped lateral ventricles situated within the cerebral hemispheres; the third ventricle situated in the diencephalon; and the fourth ventricle situated between the brainstem and the cerebellum. CSF circulation begins in the lateral ventricles flowing through the foramina of Monro to the third ventricle, continuing via the aqueduct of Sylvius to the fourth ventricle. CSF leaves the fourth to circulate around the brain and spinal cord via the subarachnoid space (Fig. 33.5). CSF is reabsorbed into the bloodstream via capillaries on the surface of the cerebral hemispheres.

CSF helps maintain the cerebral chemical environment by supplying nutrients and removing toxic substances, is a shock absorber, contributes to maintaining the blood–brain barrier, and gives the brain buoyancy. CSF has high sodium, chlorine and bicarbonate levels and low potassium, urea, glucose and amino acid levels, and a negligible protein content (Sugerman 2002).

BLOOD SUPPLY

The brain requires a continual input of glucose and oxygen, with 20% of the cardiac blood flow reaching the brain each minute (Sugerman 2000). The internal vertebral and carotid arteries, and their subsidiaries ensure the brain has a rich blood supply. These vessels form a system of interconnecting arteries in the base of the brain, known as the circle of Willis. The principle being that in the event of damage to one of the arteries supplying the brain there is the potential for compensation from the other arteries, offering some protection from ischaemic damage.

Venous blood primarily returns to the circulation via the superficial veins draining into the venous sagittal sinus that eventually flows into the internal jugular vein. The deep veins of the cerebral hemispheres drain into the vein of Galen and then into the sagittal sinus.

The composition of the brain's extracellular fluid needs to be regulated because circulatory chemicals are toxic to neurons. This is achieved by the blood–brain barrier, a complex process that is the consequence of specific characteristics of the cerebral capillaries resulting in a highly selective exchange of substances across their endothelial end plates.

PROTECTION AND COVERINGS

The brain is supported and protected by the skull and the membranous coverings collectively known as the meninges. The bones of the skull are separated at birth, allowing for brain moulding during delivery and rapid growth within the first year of life. Complete ossification occurs at about 8 years of age, and the sutures (Fig. 33.6) cannot be separated even in the presence of raised intracranial pressure after 12 years of age (Padgett 2002).

NEURON REGENERATION

The brain's limited capacity to regain function following damage is a result of the association of discrete body functions with specific structures and the inability of neurons to divide (Stephenson 1996). However, neurons can survive damage, regenerate new axons and form new synaptic connections (Stephenson 1996). This process of reactive synaptogenesis may result in the recovery of function, but can form aberrant connections resulting in abnormal recovery. Recent studies suggest latent areas within the brain may be able to assume the functions of damaged areas (Rose et al 1997).

Fig. 33.5 • Cerebrospinal fluid flow through the ventricular system.

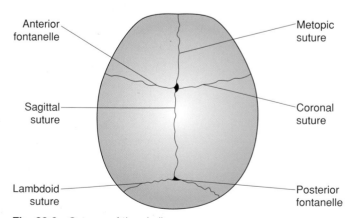

Fig. 33.6 • Sutures of the skull.

Activity

Revisit your knowledge and add more depth by accessing the Evolve website:
- File chapter 9 test your knowledge (brain teasers).
- File chapter 9 PowerPoint teachings (overview of anatomy and physiology of the brain, embryology and cells of the nervous system).

The textbooks by Crossman & Neary (2000) and Fitzgerald & Folan-Curran (2002) might also be useful.

The Range of Neurological Disorders in Childhood

The range of neurological disorders in childhood is vast, terminology is complex and many children who present with a neurological dysfunction may never have a definitive diagnosis (Table 33.1). This can be confusing for the child and family, who often find a lack of diagnosis in particular difficult. The outcome of neurological disorders is extremely variable. It is essential the child and family are viewed as

Table 33.1 Range of Childhood Neurological Diseases

	Features	Example
Congenital malformations	Disruption to normal CNS development, usually occurs early in gestational period Often multifactorial genetic transmission	Hydrocephalus Agenesis of the corpus callosum Microcephaly
Neurocutaneous disorders	Errors occurring in early ectodermal cell proliferation results in a group of disorders, which present with combined CNS, ophthalmic and skin abnormalities	Tuberous sclerosis Sturge–Weber syndrome
Vascular disorders	A diverse group of disorders with various aetiologies from structural anomalies to spontaneous intracranial bleeds	Arteriovenous malformations Intracranial arterial aneurysms Moyamoya disease
CNS infections	Common cause of acute neurological disorders Despite improved preventative programmes through vaccination and improved antimicrobial agents remain a challenge with significant morbidity	Meningitis Intracranial abscesses Encephalitis (measles, herpes simplex, mumps)
Neoplastic disorders	Most common solid tumours in children Often difficult to treat	Medulloblastoma Astrocytoma Brainstem glioma Craniopharyngioma
Progressive degenerative disorders	Includes the many neurometabolic disorders, which although individually rare, collectively are an important group of disorders Most follow a autosomal recessive Inheritance pattern Two major groups are the neuronal storage diseases and the leucodystrophies	Tay-Sachs disease Battens disease Niemann–Pick disease Krabbe's disease
Non-progressive brain damage	Persistent disorder as a result of brain insult during early development The underlying problem is static but subsequent development is affected	Cerebral palsy
Neuromuscular disorders	Normal muscle functioning is dependent upon effective muscle and nerve functioning. Children with this group of disorders present with hypotonia and increasing muscle weakness	Duchenne muscular dystrophy Myasthenia gravis Guillain–Barré
Learning disabilities	A wide range of learning disabilities exist from very specific skill deficiencies to complex disorders affecting the ability to carry out activities of living and achieve independent living Aetiology is often due to hereditary and environmental factors	Fragile-X syndrome Down syndrome Autism Asperger's syndrome

unique with individual needs. Genetic counselling is vital in assisting the parents in decisions relating to planning future children.

WWW

Develop your knowledge of these conditions by accessing the following websites:

- Association for Spina Bifida and Hydrocephalus: http://www.asbah.org.uk
- Association for Tuberous Sclerosis: http://www.tuberous-sclerosis.org.uk
- Children's Hemiplegia and Stroke Association: http://www.hemikids.org
- Meningitis Trust UK: http://www.meningitis-trust.org.uk
- Scope (focuses on providing supporting for people with disabilities, primarily with cerebral palsy): http://www.scope.org.uk
- Muscular Dystrophy Campaign: http://www.muscular-dystrophy.org/

Principles of Caring for a Child with a Cerebral Dysfunction

Understanding the principles underpinning the management of the child with both acute and long-term neurological dysfunction is essential to ensure safe and appropriate care. However, neurological disorders have a unique effect and care must be based on assessment and meeting individual needs. General principles need to be adapted to each situation, and the child and family's needs. Seizure management is covered in Chapter 24.

DIAGNOSTIC PROCEDURES

The child and family require detailed explanation and effective preparation prior to investigative procedures. Consent must be obtained. The type of diagnostic investigations will vary depending on the child's presentation but may include:

- Blood profiling, including urea and electrolytes, metabolic and immunological assays, and genetic screening.
- Lumbar puncture performed to collect CSF samples in order to detect the presence of bacteria or tumour deposits, and the measurement of CSF pressure. Performing a lumber puncture in a child with a high intracranial pressure may cause brainstem compression with fatal consequences.
- Neuroimaging; X-rays, computerised axial tomography (CT), magnetic resonance imaging (MRI).

- Specialised physiological imaging techniques such as positron emission tomography (PET) and single-photon computed emission tomography (SPECT), assist with evaluating cerebral metabolic functioning and cerebral blood flow.
- Cerebrovascular studies such as angiography, used to identify cerebrovascular abnormalities such as aneurysms and arteriovenous malformations.
- Electroencephalogram (EEG) records the electrical activity of the brain primarily used to detect changes in brain activity during seizures. Often used as a continuous monitoring procedure with video recording to correlate a child's presentation with EEG changes (video telemetry).
- Electromyography (EMG) conduction studies are used to measure electrical activity and velocity times in muscle fibres. Particularly useful in assisting in the diagnosis of neuromuscular and peripheral nerve disorders.
- Muscle biopsies measure a range of muscle enzymes. Useful in identifying whether a problem is neurogenic or myogenic in origin, assisting in the diagnosis of neuromuscular conditions.

Many of these procedures are available only in specialised centres.

Activity

Common imaging techniques are widely available; therefore all nurses must have appropriate knowledge of associated care related to these procedures:
- Think about the advantages, disadvantages and care needs of the child who requires an X-ray, CT scan or MRI scan.

You might want to add more depth to your knowledge by accessing the Evolve website:
- File chapter 9 imaging techniques.

RAISED INTRACRANIAL PRESSURE

Intracranial pressure (ICP) is the pressure exerted by the cranial contents on the skull. Typical values are 5–15 mmHg in older children and 3–7 mmHg in infants and young children (Chitnavis & Polkey 1998). The rigidity of the skull results in the intracranial volume being fixed:

$$\text{Intracranial volume} = \text{Vol}_{brain} + \text{Vol}_{CSF} + \text{Vol}_{blood}$$

Maintaining a state of equilibrium requires any change in one component to be reciprocated in another, known as the Monro–Kellie doctrine (Chitnavis & Polkey 1998). However, there is little ability to significantly reduce any of these components and an increase in intracranial volume results in a rise in ICP (Fig. 33.7).

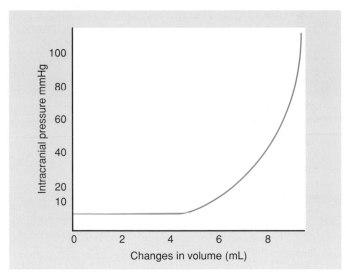

Fig. 33.7 • Volume/pressure curve.

Raised intracranial pressure (RICP) is usually described as an ICP above 20 mmHg sustained for 5 minutes or more (Miller & Dearden 1992), causes include:

- increased volume (tumour, abscess, haematoma, cerebral oedema)
- Increased blood volume or obstruction to venous outflow
- increased CSF (hydrocephalus).

The signs and symptoms of RICP include (Hazinski et al 1999):

- alteration in conscious levels; irritability, lethargy, confusion, decreased responsiveness
- dilated pupils, decreased response to light
- abnormal motor activity or reflexes
- headaches, nausea and vomiting
- Cushing's response (increased blood pressure with a compensatory bradycardia) and apnoea are late and ominous signs.

The signs and symptoms of RICP in an infant, prior to fusion of the skull sutures, usually occur late because increased volume forces the membranes between the skull bones to splay, accommodating pressure changes. There will be more insidious signs such as irritability, poor feeding, general developmental delay, large and tense anterior fontanelle even when the infant is in the sitting position, and increased head circumference (Brett & Harding 1997a).

Once the intracranial pressure starts to rise a cycle of events occurs: ICP increases, cerebral blood flow (CBF) decreases, leading to tissue hypoxia resulting in cerebral

vasodilation and oedema, causing further increases in ICP. The brain will shift from the area under pressure to an area of less pressure, resulting in compressed, traction and shearing of brain structures. Eventually, downward shifts occur, resulting in brainstem herniation with vital centres becoming compressed. Management of RICP is based on the need to prevent cerebral ischaemia by maintaining cerebral perfusion pressure (CPP) between 70 and 80 mmHg (Rosner & Daughton 1990), with care best provided in paediatric intensive care unit.

Evidence-based Practice

Evidence-based guidelines relating to the management of RICP (Bullock et al 2000) recommend:
- Maintaining oxygenation (ventilatory support).
- Minimising the brain's metabolic needs, sedation and analgesic infusions and paralysis may be required.
- Monitoring ICP levels and wave patterns.
- Maintaining an adequate systemic mean arterial pressure, necessary to maintain an adequate cerebral perfusion pressure (inotropic support).
- Avoiding extreme flexion, which will impair venous drainage, and optimising cerebral venous return by nursing with the head 30° above the body and in a midline position.
- Maintaining normal fluid and electrolyte balance with precise fluid management, preventing over or under hydration, and considering diuretic therapy (mannitol is the usual drug choice).
- Maintain normothermia.
- Managing seizures (monitor EEG).
- Preventing abnormal tone and posture by avoiding supine lying and promoting the use of side lying, if the supine position cannot be avoided support knee and elbow joints to minimise extensor tone.
- Considering the frequency of endotracheal suctioning which can dramatically cause an increase in ICP. However, maintaining a patent airway and reducing respiratory complications are essential in preventing atelectasis, which may result in hypoxia and consequently compromise cerebral perfusion.
- Avoiding noxious stimuli for example painful procedures, loud noises and sudden movements, which increase ICP. Plan care appropriately, consider minimising the duration of care and allowing sufficient rest periods.
- Include family members, their presence and the effect of gentle touch may be beneficial and it is vitally important that the family become involved in the care of their child at an early stage.

NEUROLOGICAL ASSESSMENT

Accurate neurological assessment and skilled observations are essential if changes in neurological function are to be detected.

Reflect on your Practice

Think about the last time you performed neurological observations on a child. What was their purpose? How did you use the information gained in subsequent care delivery?

The purpose of a neurological assessment includes (Hickey 2003a):

- providing a baseline and identifying the child's normal parameters
- identifying the presence and effects of neurological dysfunction
- detecting life-threatening situations
- identifying changes promptly through serial observations
- influencing management decisions by monitoring overall improvement or deterioration
- assisting predicting eventual outcomes.

Neurological observations include; assessment of conscious levels, pupillary reactions, motor functioning and other parameters including the presence of seizures and changes to vital signs. The frequency of undertaking observations will depend on the initial assessment, the stability of the child and the underlying problem. In the acute situation ½–1-hourly observations seem to be the norm (Ferguson-Clark &

Williams 1998). Unless a full assessment is carried out, unconsciousness cannot be distinguished from normal sleep.

Activity

Write down the meanings of the following words:
- consciousness
- coma
- stupor
- disorientated
- confused.

Assessment of Consciousness

Consciousness, a cerebral cortical function, is a sensitive indicator of neurological functioning (Hickey 2003a). The terminology used to grade levels of consciousness is unsatisfactory because of differing interpretations of the meaning of words such as confusion, lethargy and stupor. Teasdale & Jennett (1974) developed the first, and most frequently used numerical scale for assessing consciousness levels. The Glasgow Coma Scale (GCS) assesses three parameters – eye opening, verbal response and motor response – with a numerical score given for the best response within each parameter (Table 33.2).

No response to an auditory stimulus or light tactile pressure requires application of a painful stimulus. To test for localisation of pain, central pressure, for example over the supraorbital area, should be applied (Teasdale & Jennett 1974). Sternal rub, although a central stimulus, can poten-

Table 33.2 The Glasgow Coma Scale (Teasdale & Jennett 1974)

Parameter	Score	Components
Eye opening	4	Eyes open spontaneously in response to normal environmental activities
	3	Eyes open in response to direct commands
	2	Eyes open in response to a painful stimulus
	1	Absence of eye opening despite application of a painful stimulus
Verbal response	5	Answers appropriately to questions
	4	Converses but confused
	3	Makes little sense
	2	Incompressible sounds
	1	No verbal response to deep pain
Motor response	6	Obeys commands
	5	Localisation of a painful stimulus is a purposeful movement in an attempt to locate the stimulus and remove it
	4	Withdrawal from painful stimuli is an attempt to move away from the stimulus but it is not a purposeful movement and implies further depression of neurological function
	3	Flexion response
	2	Extension to painful stimuli implies an even further impairment of neurological function
	1	Flaccidity, there is no detectable movement or change in tone of the limbs despite repeated and varied stimulation

tially damage soft tissues (Hickey 2003a). Nail bed pressure may elicit a flexion reflex response. Supraorbital pressure is not appropriate to elicit eye opening because it causes grimacing, and simultaneous eye closing. Under 6 months the normal motor response to stimulation is flexion (Brett & Kaiser 1997).

It is usual practice to summate the scores of the three parameters, giving a numerical value to the whole assessment. This provides an overall reference guide when reviewing the child's condition but can conceal the whole picture, where a number of combinations will result in the same score (Watson et al 1992). Coma is often defined as a score of 8 or less (Kraus et al 1987), unless a modified paediatric scale – which may be inappropriate in children – is used, when the best score for their stage of development may be 9.

The GCS has undergone several adaptations for use in children, including the James' adaptation (James & Trauner 1985) and the Adelaide Scale (Reilly et al 1988). The National Paediatric Neuroscience Benchmarking group (Tatman et al 1997, Warren 2000) and the National Institute for Clinical Excellence (NICE 2003) advocate using the James' adaptation because it is easy to use, the scoring system (a maximum of 15 and minimum of 3) is internationally recognised and it takes into account the developmental level of the child. The addition of the grimace score makes it suitable for use in intensive care settings (Warren 2000) (Table 33.3). The normal verbal response will depend on the linguistic and cognitive developmental stage of the child and, where possible, should be ascertained from the child or carer prior to undertaking the first assessment. This will enable the child's optimal score to be documented; deviation from the child's normal will assist in determining the child's conscious level.

Motor Strength

This is not the same as assessing the motor response in the GCS. The aim is to obtain a general overview of limb functioning in terms of: muscle strength (normal, mild weakness, severe weakness); and whether movements are spontaneous or in response to painful stimuli or flaccid, in each of the four limbs independently. Abnormal posture and movements should be documented. The neonate's normal response to stimulation is flexion (Brett & Kaiser 1997).

Pupil Reactions

The response of the pupils to light is dependent on intact cranial nerves II and III, which transmit nerve impulses from the retina to the midbrain and from the midbrain to the pupillary muscles, respectively. Assessment of their function provides valuable insights into the physiology of the brainstem. Assessment of pupils should include size, equality and reactivity to light (Hickey 2003a). Pupils are usually between 2 and 6 mm in size, but there may be slight discrepancies between the two pupils. Extremely small pupils can indicate narcotic overdose or direct lower brainstem compression. The size of the pupil is either recorded as pinpoint, small, moderate or dilated, or on a scale ratio of 1:8. Drugs that either constrict or dilate the pupils should be accurately recorded.

The normal response to a direct light stimulus is an immediate brisk constriction of the pupil, and a brisk dilation of the pupil once the light source is removed (Hickey 2003a). Although each eye is examined independently, the response should be observed in both eyes. Light directed into one eye will constrict the pupil in the opposite eye due to the consensual light reflex. The pupillary response is graded and recorded descriptively in terms of brisk, sluggish or non reactive (fixed). A dilated fixed pupil is an ominous finding and suggestive of a terminal state (Hickey 2003a).

Vital Signs

Changes in vital signs can indicate pathophysiological changes within the brain, particularly the brainstem. Cardiovascular observations are particularly important

Table 33.3 Verbal Component of the Neurological Assessment Adapted for Use in Children (Warren 2000)

Score	Infant/young child	Verbal response Older child/adult	Grimace–all ages
5	Alert, babbles, coos, words or sentences, usual ability	Orientated	Spontaneous normal facial/ oro-motor activity
4	Less than usual ability or spontaneous irritable cry	Confused	Less than usual spontaneous or only response to touch stimuli
3	Cries inappropriately	Inappropriate words	Vigorous grimace to pain
2	Occasional whimpers/moans	Inappropriate sounds	Mild grimace to pain
1	No response	No response	No response

because of the relationship between cerebral haemodynamics and cerebral functioning (Hickey 2003a). Compromise to cerebral blood flow (CBF) will result in a vasomotor response, with blood being diverted from other body systems in order to maintain adequate cerebral perfusion. The resultant rise in arterial blood pressure is known as Cushing's reflex or response (Hickey 2003a). Tachycardia will initially occur as a result of mild hypoxia. Significant compromises to cerebral blood flow cause further increases in blood pressure resulting in a compensatory bradycardia, suggestive of a dangerously high intracranial pressure and potential catastrophe.

Changes in respiratory rate and rhythm can occur with neurological dysfunction. Alterations to normal respirations such as hyperventilation, shallow breathing or irregular breathing should raise concerns. Rapidly expanding lesions such as intracranial haemorrhage, direct medulla damage or brainstem herniation are likely to cause respiratory arrest (Hickey 2003a).

Alterations in body temperature; both hypo- and hyperthermia can be manifestations of neurological impairments. Hyperthermia is probably more common (Hickey 2003a) and can be due to infective and non-infective conditions. Central fever due to neurogenic aetiologies are typically associated with brain tumours, trauma and following neurosurgery.

Neurological assessment should include observation of the adequacy of the cough and gag reflex, which can become depressed following widespread brain damage. Brain insults have the potential to cause seizures requiring appropriate monitoring and management because of the resultant hypoxia, which will compound existing problems.

Reflect on your Practice

Think back to neurological observations that you have performed.
- Was the chart sufficiently flexible to accommodate all age ranges of children?
- How easy did you find the process?
- How did you apply painful stimuli?
- How and why did you act on any changes in the child's condition?

CARE OF THE UNCONSCIOUS CHILD

Unconsciousness is a lack of awareness of self and the environment and an inability to respond to sensory stimuli (Hickey 2003b). There is a myriad of neurological conditions that result in unconsciousness, with the depth and duration lasting for seconds for example during a seizure to months for example following major head trauma.

Activity

Sally is 14 years old and has suffered a cerebrovascular accident necessitating emergency craniotomy and resulting in a prolonged period in paediatric intensive care. She is now stable and able to maintain her own airway. Her nutrition is primarily maintained via gastrostomy feeding. She remains unresponsive and dependent on carers for all her needs. Her family, primarily her mother, although not resident, is actively involved in Sally's care.
- Identify Sally's actual and potential problems.
- Write a detailed nursing care plan outlining how Sally's needs will be met.

Children with impaired levels of consciousness due to acute cerebral dysfunction, who are unable to maintain their own airway, at risk of hypoxia or hypercarbia, associated shock or respiratory failure will require intensive care facilities, intubation and management of RICP (Hazinski et al 1999).

Many children who are unconscious do not require intensive care facilities, but are dependent on having their needs met by the healthcare team. The major goals in caring for these children are; to ensure activities necessary to sustain life are maintained, prevent complications relating to immobility, maximise the restoration of functions and offer support to the family. Table 33.4 outlines the child's needs in relation to maintaining essential activities of daily living and preventing complications.

NURSING CARE OF THE CHILD UNDERGOING NEUROSURGERY

Activity

Jamie is 6 months old and has been admitted for insertion of a ventricular shunt.
- Write a care plan outlining the principles of the pre- and postoperative care Jamie and his family will require.

The principles that apply to every child requiring surgery are also important for the child undergoing cranial surgery. In general there are few specific preoperative requirements. The child will require preoperative blood sampling, including cross-match, because of the potential for blood loss during surgery. The child and family must be prepared for the immediate postoperative period, including the possibility of being nursed in intensive care, the child's appearance including descriptions of the wound/bandages, drains, facial swelling, and the range and function of monitoring equipment. It is usual practice to undertake skin preparation and hair removal after induction of the anaesthetic. However, it is essential the child and family are prepared for hair removal.

Table 33.4 Caring for the Unconscious Child

Actual/potential problems	Nursing interventions
Altered neurological functioning due to cerebral dysfunction	Monitor neurological functioning through regular assessment Manage alterations in sleep patterns and periods of irritability through structuring activities appropriately, having planned rest periods, using relaxation techniques such as aromatherapy and massage Ensure stimulation activities are planned and appropriate for the child's age and condition Drugs such as melantonin may be prescribed for sleep disturbances – review their use regularly Assess and manage pain appropriately
Risk of altered respiratory function due to underlying cerebral dysfunction, inability to maintain airway and immobility	Assess respiratory function and identify risk of airway obstruction, ensure position does not compromise the airway, use airway aids and suctioning as appropriate Appropriate monitoring such as respiratory rate and effort, colour, peripheral perfusion and pulse oximetry
Potential problem of atelectasis and chest infection	Assess gag and swallow reflexes (often undertaken by speech and language therapist). Nil by mouth until these reflexes have returned Regular chest physiotherapy, position changes and passive movements Monitoring temperature, change in secretions (amount and colour)
Unable to maintain nutritional intake and hydration Potential problems of malnutrition, anaemia and electrolyte disturbances, gastric ulcers	Assess nutritional status, including monitoring weight Provide good nutritional intake by appropriate methods that meet the needs of the child, enteral feeding via a nasogastric or gastrostomy tube is the norm Ensure nutritional intake reflects increased calorific intake, liaison with a dietitian to ensure the correct composition and volume of feed Monitoring intake and output, observing for signs of undernourishment and dehydration Where possible encourage oral food and fluids. The reintroduction of oral feeding may need to be supplemented by enteral feeding because neurological problems may result in oral-motor difficulties, reduced alertness and increased fatiguability contributing to inadequate nutritional intake Consider the child's needs in relation to positioning and supportive seating, taste and textures, likes and dislikes, choice of utensils, and effective age-appropriate communication
Unable to maintain self-care needs	Ensure care is appropriate in meeting individual needs and considers usual family practices Assess mucous membranes, particularly eyes and oral cavity for dryness, take appropriate action to keep clean and moist Corneal dryness will require instillation of appropriate eye drops Provide protective eye patching if the child is unable to completely close the eyes Ensure frequent teeth brushing, consider the need to use suction techniques to prevent aspiration
Potential complications of immobility include: • skin breakdown • muscular skeletal deformities, muscle wasting, contractures peripheral nerve impairment, poor muscle tone • poor circulation, inadequate lung functioning • infections particularly chest and urine infections • constipation	Assess risk of skin breakdown by undertaking an assessment using a recognised tool Ensure correct positioning is used at all times for children with immobility problems Liaise with the physiotherapist to establish individual positioning regimes. Principles include maintaining head in neutral position, with the spine and hips positioning in alignment with the head, maintaining flexion of the limbs and preventing extension of the ankles Undertake passive exercises and regular position changes in order to improve circulation, relieve pressure, facilitate lung expansion, prevent urinary stasis, improve gut mobility and minimise muscle atrophy Minimise the risk of infection, by nursing child in nappies or incontinence pads and ensuring meticulous skin care Assess for risk of infection by observing colour, smell and concentration of urine and measurement of body temperature. Monitor bowel motions and manage constipation appropriately including high fibre diet or supplements, adequate hydration and use of suppositories For older children consider anti-coagulant therapy and using anti-embolic stockings.

The child's postoperative care must consider the potential complications of all surgical procedures, and those specific to neurosurgery, including cerebral haemorrhage (subdural, epidural, intracerebral and intraventricular), RICP, seizures, cerebrospinal fluid leakage, pneumocephalus, hydrocephalus, meningitis, metabolic imbalances and a range of neurosurgical deficits (diminished levels of consciousness, communication difficulties, motor and sensory deficits, diminished swallow and gag reflexes and visual disturbances) (Hickey 2003c). The immediate postoperative needs of the child following cranial surgery are outlined in Table 33.5.

Any neurological deficits that occur as a result of surgery may require the child to have a programme of care that shifts from managing acute surgical needs to one of rehabilitation.

Preparation for discharge must consider the advice the child and parent will require; specific advice to the neuro-

Table 33.5 Immediate Postoperative Care Following Cranial Surgery

Actual/potential problems	Nursing interventions
Potential airway obstruction/inadequate oxygenation due to depressed consciousnesss levels and the effects of prolonged anaesthesia	Maintain airway Assess and monitor respiratory effort and oxygen saturation levels Maintain adequate oxygen, consider ventilatory support
Potential cardiac and respiratory instability due to neurological depression and effect of prolonged anaesthesia	Assess and monitor respiratory effort, oxygen saturation levels and vital signs Consider ventilatory support and invasive blood pressure monitoring
Altered neurological functioning due to potential risk of RICP as a result of oedema and heamorrhage	Neurological assessment Follow RICP management guidelines Monitor for signs of excessive blood loss including observing wound bandages/wound drains if present, changes in consciousness levels, raised pulse, falling blood pressure, changes in peripheral perfusion Administer blood transfusion therapy as required Consider surgical control of bleeding
Potential fluid and electrolyte disturbances due to inability to take oral fluids Maintaining fluid and electrolytes is a balance between ensuring adequate circulatory blood volume to maintain good cerebral perfusion and preventing over-hydration, which will add to cerebral oedema	Fluid intake and output must be monitored Management of fluids in terms of the type and amount of fluid will be specific to each child's needs and urea and electrolyte profile Monitor blood profile (including serum osmolality). Perform circulatory assessment (pulse, blood pressure, capillary refill, temperature gradient difference between core and periphery) Unless there is potential damage to the 9th and 10th cranial nerves, which may affect swallowing, the child may begin oral fluids as soon as consciousness is regained
Potential problem of inappropriate antidiuretic secretion or diabetes insipidus following surgery to the posterior fossa area	Measure and monitor urine output, test and record specific gravity
Potential inability to maintain normal thermoregulation Hyperpyrexia can be a result of hypothalamus dysfunction and/or irritation of cerebral tissues such as the presence of blood	Regular temperature recording Manage pyrexia appropriately because any increase in core temperature increases cerebral metabolic rate, increasing cerebral perfusion and potentially adds to any rises in intracranial pressure
Vomiting, as a direct result of pressure from RICP and the effects of anaesthetic agents	Administer antiemetics Continue intravenous fluids If prolonged undertake a nutritional assessment Ranitidine may be prescribed to prevent gastric irritation
Pain from wound incision, positioning in theatre, stretching of the meninges and RICP	Assess pain Administer regular analgesia Intravenous narcotic may further compromise respiratory effort, oral or rectal codeine may be a suitable alternative

Table 33.5 Immediate Postoperative Care Following Cranial Surgery—cont'd

Actual/potential problems	Nursing interventions
Potential for the development of seizures due to cerebral inflammation/irritation	Observe for signs of seizure activity In the unconscious child this may require continuous EEG monitoring Follow seizure management guidelines
Promote wound healing following surgical incision Potential wound infection	Maintain universal infection control measures Wound bandages are usually present for the first 48–24 hours and assist in reducing swelling at the wound site and help secure drains that may be present Consider prophylactic antibiotics Observe wound for redness, hardness and presence of exudates, which may indicate presence of infection Monitor temperature Clips are often used to secure the wound and usually removed 7 days postoperatively

RICP, raised intracranial pressure.

surgical procedure and, where appropriate, a clear indication of subsequent healthcare interventions.

EMOTIONAL AND PSYCHOLOGICAL NEEDS OF THE CHILD AND FAMILY

Seminar discussion topic

Donna is a third-year nursing student undertaking a specialist placement on a neurosciences ward. She is enjoying her placement and has been learning to care for children with complex needs, particularly enhancing her practical skills in areas such as tracheostomy and gastrostomy care.

Donna has been caring for Amy, 14 months old, who has a progressive degenerative disease. Amy's development has always been slow and she did not achieve independent sitting. Recently, her condition has deteriorated, with a loss of abilities, recurrent seizures and increased spasticity.

Donna feels able to care for Amy in relation to ensuring all physical needs are met. However, she is finding it difficult to accept that Amy has an undiagnosed condition, with a short life expectancy. She finds it hard to communicate with Amy's parents.

- What issues do you think are important to discuss in relation to this scenario within Donna's learning set?

The diagnosis of a neurological disorder is devastating for the child and family, having far-reaching effects that can potentially affect physical, cognitive and affective (behaviour, personality) functions (Hickey 2003d). Changes in cognitive and affective functions can be particularly difficult for the family to accept, having the potentially to alter all dimensions of family life and changing the anticipated expectations parents may have for their child. It is vital that the emotional and psychological needs of the child and family are considered and incorporated into care because normal coping abilities may become ineffective. The presence of nurses over the 24-hour care period often results in emotional and psychological care becoming a nursing responsibility. The range of situations that the child and family may have to come to terms with include (Hickey 2003d):

- Threat to the survival of the child.
- Threat to quality of life of the child:
  - motor paralysis
  - bowel and bladder dysfunction
  - communication difficulties
  - sensory deficits
- Behavioural problems.
- Future ability of the child to live independently.
- Future ability of the child to form relationships.
- Future education and career prospects.
- A dependent child may require the parents to review current care arrangements, which may result in a reduction of income and alteration in lifestyles.
- Reaction and needs of siblings.

The family will have many questions in relation to the child's condition, why and how it has happened, and they may be experiencing feelings of guilt. These feelings may be compounded in situations when there is no definitive diagnosis or the child's condition is life threatening; parents my feel frustrated and isolated. Extensive investigations and unpleasant treatments will add to the general despair. The family may be angry that vague signs and symptoms have gone unnoticed. There will be fears in relation to the prognosis and long-term outcomes. The family may be experiencing difficulty in accepting the changes in their child and grieving for the child they know, love and who has been an integral part of their lives. These emotions will affect the family's ability to comprehend information given to them.

It is essential to establish the usual coping strategies and support systems used by the child and family. Long-term support should be aimed at supporting and developing existing mechanisms. Nursing interventions, which form an integral part of everyday practice, in supporting the emotional and psychological needs of the child and family include:

- Ensuring the family is given enough opportunity to ask questions and that responses are clear, accurate and honest.
- Providing and reinforcing information regularly, keeping the family updated. Essential information should be communicated effectively between the whole multidisciplinary team, to ensure a consistent approach to care.
- Including the child in discussions at a level appropriate to their age and stage of development.
- Providing support by listening to the family's anxieties and concerns.
- Ensuring a non-judgemental approach to care respecting the cultural, religious and spiritual beliefs of the family.
- Assisting the family to make realistic goals in relation to their child's care.
- Ensuring care is family centred, all aspects of care are discussed and care planning is negotiated with family, and child where appropriate.
- Recognising that there will be extreme anxiety if a child requires care in different settings, ensure systems allow for smooth transfers.
- Recognising when there is a need to refer to other members of the multidisciplinary team.

REHABILITATION

Traditional models of care focusing on the disease and its treatment are not always appropriate for a child with a neurological problem. The philosophy of rehabilitation focuses on enabling an individual to circumvent impairments in order to minimise disability (Neumann 1995). Programmes of care must be individually designed and strongly influenced at encouraging the child to reach his or her full potential, working within a developmental context to integrate the children back into the family, school and community (Roffe 1989). This can only be achieved through a structured, caring and safe environment with all members of the multidisciplinary team adopting a child- and family-

orientated approach to care. The care given will be provided for by a variety of disciplines, the team must have common goals with care integrated into the child's daily routines.

Nurses are a vital component of the multidisciplinary team and their roles include: assessment of the child particularly in relation to actual or potential problems relating to activities of living, coordination of care and maintaining effective links with all team members, providing technical and physical care, integrating therapies initiated by other professionals into every day care, providing emotional support, and involving the family in care (Long et al 2002). If the child is to be successfully integrated back into the family, the family must be involved and understand the process of rehabilitation, be involved in goal setting and monitoring of their child's progress.

Overview and Principles of Managing Selected Neurological Conditions in Childhood

This section will provide an overview of selected neurological conditions. Meningitis is covered in Chapter 40, abnormalities in physical development including cerebral palsy in Chapter 25 and learning disabilities, including Down syndrome, in Chapter 47.

BRAIN TUMOURS

Brain tumours are the most common solid tumour and the second most common malignancy in children (leukaemia being more prevalent). Approximately 300 children are diagnosed with a brain tumour every year within the UK (Cancer Bacup 1999). Progress in the management of these children has reduced the overall mortality (Stewart & Cohen 1998) but morbidity, in terms of physical and intellectual sequelae, remains significant (Duffner et al 1993). Tumours in general are divided into malignant or benign, referring to the ability of the tumour to spread and the sensitivity to treatment. With brain tumours, factors that determine outcome are less clear and influenced by the anatomical position of the tumour and age of presentation. The accessibility of the tumour for surgical treatment influences management options, therefore potential outcomes.

Aetiology

The causes of brain tumours are unclear; contributing factors include (Strother et al 2002):

- exposure to ionising radiation
- association with other cancers, or their treatments

- underlying immunosuppression syndromes
- a family history of brain tumours, bone cancer, leukaemia and lymphoma
- familial clustering of embryonal tumours
- potential link to environmental carcinogens.

Classification of Brain Tumours

Figure 33.8 shows the anatomical position of the common brain tumours in children:

- Medulloblastomas: part of a group of embryonic tumours collectively known as primitive neuroectodermal tumours (PNETs), which arise from neuroepithelial cells and usually occur within the posterior fossa. The tumour cells have no clear line of demarcation from normal tissue (Brett & Harding 1997b) and often permeate along the CSF pathways resulting in spinal cord deposits (Halperin et al 1994).
- Astrocytomas: found throughout the brain, arising from astrocyte cells (Ryan-Murray & McElwain Peticcione 2002) and have a tendency to form large cysts. Astrocytomas are graded from I to IV, grade I indicates a benign slow growing lesion and grade IV a highly malignant tumour. The majority in children are graded I or II.
- Ependymomas: originate from the ependymal tissue within the ventricular system (Shiminski-Maher & Shields 1996). The histology varies from benign through to highly malignant. There are many similarities with medulloblastomas, including a tendency to metastasise along the CSF pathways (Brett & Harding 1997b).
- Brainstem gliomas: have varied histology. A definitive diagnosis is not always possible because the position of the tumour within the brainstem may not be conducive

to obtaining a biopsy (Brett & Harding 1997b). Most are high-grade astrocytomas, fast growing, diffuse and highly malignant, with extensive branching and a poor response to treatment (Ryan-Murray & McElwain Petriccione 2002).
- Craniopharyngiomas: benign, slow-growing tumours arising from epithelial cells within the pituitary gland. Diagnosis can be time consuming and often delayed because signs and symptoms are vague and insidious (Greenwood 1992). The effects are significant because the tumour is difficult to treat due to the anatomical location and the abnormal tissue adhering to surrounding tissues, preventing normal function and associated endocrine dysfunctions (Strother et al 2002).

Presentation

Symptoms occurring within a short time span suggest a rapidly growing or aggressive tumour, with gradual symptoms more likely to be caused by a low grade or benign tumour (Stewart & Cohen 1998). Most childhood brain tumours are associated with signs of RICP. In addition there will be specific signs and symptoms related to the altered function/compression of structures within the direct vicinity of the tumour. Children with a medulloblastoma, cerebellar astrocytoma or brainstem ependymoma typically present cerebellar signs such as ataxia, coordination and gait disturbance (Fenichel 1997a, Worrall 1999). Any spinal cord involvement may result in neck stiffness. Compression of the optic nerves resulting in visual field defects, a low basal metabolic rate resulting in fatigability, a low blood pressure, disruption to pituitary functioning causing delayed skeletal growth and sexual maturation, and hypothalamic disturbances causing obesity and diabetes insipidus suggests a

Fig. 33.8 • Common brain tumours: position and frequency (adapted from Vernon-Levett & Geller 1997).

craniopharyngioma (Brett & Harding 1997b). Tumours within the posterior fossa can obstruct CSF flow resulting in hydrocephalus. The specific presentation of supratentorial tumours is directly related to function of the cerebral cortex where the tumour is located (Strother et al 2002) (see Fig. 33.4).

Diagnosis

Diagnosis is often difficult because the presenting symptoms can be vague and non-specific or similar to those of more common childhood illnesses (Stewart & Cohen 1998). Diagnosis will be made following a detailed neurological examination and confirmed by a MRI or CT scan. Children with medulloblastoma will require imaging to determine spinal metastasis.

Treatment and Management of Children with Brain Tumours

Many children will require multimodal therapy: surgery, radiotherapy, chemotherapy and symptom management (Walker at al 1999). Surgery aims to remove or reduce the size of the tumour, control ICP, obtain a biopsy to establish a definitive diagnosis and re-establish patent CSF pathways (Walker at al 1999). Total surgical removal improves survival (Shiminski-Maher & Shields 1995) but may be contraindicated with deep-seated tumours or where there is attachment to vital structures.

The general care of the child requiring neurosurgery has been outlined. Posterior fossa syndrome is a potential complication following posterior fossa tumour resection, with the symptoms causing additional anxieties for the child and family (Kirk et al 1995). Symptoms usually present 72 hours postoperatively and include cranial nerve palsies, dysphagia, motor weakness, mutism or speech disturbances and emotional liability (Dailey 1995, Kirk et al 1995).

Radiotherapy is used (Turini & Redaelli 2001):

- for inoperable tumours
- to treat tumours only partially removed at surgery
- to destroy any remaining tumour seeds post surgery
- to reduce the tumour size in order to relieve acute symptoms prior to surgery
- to treat secondary brain metastasis.

Radiotherapy targets and disrupts the action of deoxyribonucleic acid, which is essential for cell division (Shiminski-Maher & Shields 1995). Radiation primarily affects cells during division; therefore rapidly growing tumour cells are especially sensitive to radiation exposure. The aim is to deliver therapeutic doses of radiation that causes tumour cell destruction and inhibits cell division

but minimises toxic effects to surrounding healthy tissue. Linear accelerators and computer-assisted equipment have made radiotherapy more precise by ensuring accurate delivery to the tumour site (Lew & LaVally 1995, Moore 1995). Radiotherapy is inappropriate for children less than 3 years of age because of the high susceptibility of the immature developing brain to radiation damage resulting in growth failure and cognitive dysfunction (Lew & LaVally 1995).

Ideally radiotherapy is administered five times a week for approximately 6 weeks, 2–3 weeks following surgery or diagnosis (Walker et al 1999).

Treatment planning is vital because the child requires immobilising within an individually constructed mould, essential for ensuring precise and consistent positioning of the treatment area during every radiotherapy session (Lew & LaVally 1995). Children with posterior fossa tumours may be required to lie face down to allow the radiation to be directed to the posterior base of the skull, which can be distressing for the child. It may be necessary to consider either sedation or general anaesthesia if the procedure is extremely distressing, to reduce psychological stress. The decision should not be taken lightly as both procedures have potential risks. Play therapists are invaluable in preparing and supporting the child during radiotherapy.

Acute toxicity may occur during or immediately following radiotherapy as a result of acute inflammation at the tumour site, which can cause a significant rise in ICP, requiring monitoring of the child's neurological status (Moore 1995). Other immediate side effects include nausea, vomiting, headaches, loss of appetite, fluid and electrolyte disturbances and localised skin irritation (Moore 1995). Children receiving radiotherapy are at risk of developing radiotherapy somnolence weeks to months after the completion of treatment, characterised by excessive lethargy, up to 20 hours a day and general malaise (Moore 1995) but is usually self-limiting.

Chemotherapy rarely provides a cure but offers an opportunity to limit tumour expansion in the young child until radiotherapy can be delivered (Duffner et al 1993), and has increased the long-term survival rates of children with brain tumours (Shiminski-Maher & Shields 1995). The difficulties in using chemotherapy for the treatment of brain tumours is poor drug penetration across the blood–brain barrier, due to the tight junction between endothelial cells in the brain capillaries. This impermeability can be overcome by multidrug combinations, adjuvant therapies such as the administration of mannitol, which disrupts capillaries/endothelial junctions, administrating high doses of chemotherapeutic agents such as methotrexate in combination with a rescue therapy such as folic acid (Turini & Redaelli 2001). There are no standard or proven chemotherapy regimes for the treatment of childhood brain tumours (Walker et al 1999). Therefore, all children should be cared for in a UK Children Cancer Study Group accredited centre, where treatment protocols are adapted to incorporate the current evidence, and outcomes can be monitored (Lashford & Walker 1997).

In addition to the knowledge and skills required to ensure both the physiological and psychological needs of the child with a brain tumour are being met, the principles of caring for a child having chemotherapy must be applied (see Chapter 32). The nurse will need to be proactive in minimising the risk of and treating the side effects of chemotherapy including vomiting, sore mouth, pain, bone marrow suppression and increased risk of infection (Vernon-Levett & Geller 1997). Good communication between differing specialities and understanding an overview of all the treatment modalities are essential in order to meet the needs of the child and family.

Symptom management will be necessary to reduce the side effects of treatments and where palliation is the main aim of care (Walker at al 1999). Corticosteriods, primarily dexamethasone, usually prescribed as a short course of treatment, may reduce cerebral swelling and provide temporary relief from symptoms at diagnosis and where there is acute radiotherapy-induced inflammatory response (Walker et al 1999). Low-dose steroids may help to reduce the symptoms of delayed radiation induced toxicity (Walker et al 1999). Persistent symptomatic hydrocephalus may require the insertion of a ventricular shunt.

Long-term Outcomes

Long-term survival is often accompanied by deficits including motor and sensory dysfunction, delays in neurobehavioural function, cognitive and learning disabilities, visual and hearing deficits and chronic endocrine deficiencies (Lew & LaVally 1995). Many children will require special educational assistance (Mulhern et al 1998). Radiotherapy in particular has been linked to long term developmental deficits (Stewart & Cohen 1998) and can cause subcortical white matter degeneration, diffuse slowing of electroencephalogram, ophthalmic and auditory damage, and is linked to alterations in intellectual functioning (Moore 1995). Endocrine dysfunction, particularly growth hormone deficiency and hypothyroidism necessitating hormone replacement therapy, may occur as a result of pituitary and hypothalamic damage following irradiation to the posterior fossa area (Cullen et al 2002). Radiotherapy can cause premature closure of growth plates resulting in precocious puberty (Stewart & Cohen 1998). Neurological disabilities as a result of the effects of the tumour and/or treatments will require the child to have a thorough assessment involving all members of the multidisciplinary team and early initiation of a rehabilitative programme. It is vital that the emotional and psychological needs of the child and family are met as previously discussed.

WWW

Develop your knowledge in relation to children with cancer including brain tumours by visiting the following websites:
- United Kingdom Children's Cancer Study Group: http://www.ukccsg.org.uk
- Cancer Bacup: http://www.cancerbacup.org.uk

Evidence-based Practice

You may wish to review evidence-based guidelines relating to improving the outcomes of patients with tumours of the central nervous system by accessing the NICE website:
- http://www.nice.org.uk

CRANIOSYNOSTOSIS

Craniosynostosis describes children who presented with premature fusion of one or more of the skull sutures, affecting approximately 1 in 2000 children (Sarnat & Menkes 2000, Warren et al 2001). Simple craniosynostosis is a primary synostosis of a single suture with no involvement of the facial skeleton. Complex craniosynostosis is a primary synostosis of one or more sutures with involvement of the facial skeleton, and includes a plethora of craniosynostotic syndromes, where craniosynostosis is a predominant feature (Cohen & Maclean 2000), Apert's and Crouzon's being the most well known.

Actiology

Most cases are sporadic, with the cause unknown. However, craniosynostosis syndromes probably have a genetic mode of inheritance:

- Primary craniosynostosis may be due to a single gene defect.
- If a parent and child have craniosynostosis, or two siblings have craniosynostosis with normal parents, the risk of another child developing the disorder increases.
- There may be an X-linked mode of inheritance, particularly with sagittal synostosis which is much more common in males.

Predisposing factors include:

- male predominance
- plural birth
- older maternal and/or paternal age
- low birthweight infants
- white Caucasians
- drug teratogenicity
- maternal excesses of vitamin A and D and ethanol
- intrauterine compression.

Presentation

In the newborn the cranial sutures are separated by membranous spaces several millimetres wide (see Fig. 33.6). Early closure of a suture inhibits normal perpendicular brain expansion and the skull is forced to grow in a direction parallel to the fused suture (Sarnat & Menkes 2000). The fused bones remain small and underdeveloped, the non-affected bones enlarge to compensate, thus allowing brain growth. The characteristic head shape that results depends on which suture or sutures fuse (Fig. 33.9). Craniosynostosis may be apparent at birth but the deformity is usually diagnosed in early infancy when the abnormally shaped head becomes more pronounced (Panchal & Uttchin 2003). Diagnosis is usually made by visual inspection of the skull and palpitation of the sutures (Fenichel 1997b). Skull X-rays will show a band of increased bone density at the site of the prematurely closed suture (Fenichel 1997b) and a CT scan will reveal the extent of the premature fusion.

Fig. 33.9 • Types of craniosynostosis and characteristic features (Adapted from May 2001, Johnston 2001, Panchal & Uttchin 2003).

Type of Synostosis	Characteristic Skull Shape
Sagittal synostosis: - fusion of the sagittal suture - most common form of craniosynostosis - accounts for 50–55% of cases	Scaphocephaly 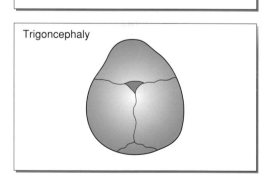
Coronal synostosis: - fusion of one or both of the coronal sutures - accounts for 20–25% of cases	Brachycephaly
Metopic synostosis: - fusion of the metopic suture - accounts for approximately 10% of cases	Trigoncephaly
Lambdoid synostosis: - fusion of one or both of the lambdoid suture - rare, accounting for 3–5% of cases	Plagiocephaly 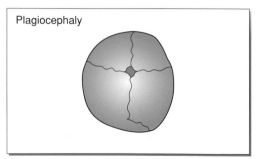

Premature closure of all the cranial sutures can occur. This is sometimes referred to as crainiostenosis or oxycephaly, with the child in danger of having extremely high RICP, which may lead to impaired mental and motor functions, optic nerve atrophy and death and is associated with cerebral malformations and hydrocephalus (Sarnat & Menkes 2000).

Treatment and Management Options

Operative correction of the deformity is the treatment of choice and the general consensus of opinion is that it should be undertaken early, preferably within the first year of life (Johnston 2001, MacKenzie 1990). Within this timeframe the deformity has not progressed, the bones are more malleable and correction will allow subsequent brain growth to promote a normal shape resulting in greater cosmetic improvements. Early treatment potentially minimises later complications such as visual, nasal, phonetic and dental problems (Panchal & Uttchin 2003). If left untreated, skull deformities become permanent and there is increased risk of raised intracranial pressure (Moos & Hide 1993). Prior to surgery, psychometric assessment is necessary to establish developmental delay, which will aid in predicting the outcome of surgery (Panchal & Uttchin 2003).

Surgery can range from excision of the fused suture, for example in sagittal synostosis, to complex craniofacial surgery involving the repositioning and reshaping of the skull and facial bones (Kershner & Claussen 1986). Correction of craniofacial syndromes requires surgery throughout childhood, with future procedures determined by alterations to cranial–facial structures as the child grows (Panchal & Uttchin 2003). Although, paediatric neuroscience is regarded as a specialist field of practice (Department of Health (DoH) 2002), complex craniofacial surgery is further identified as a subspeciality (Society of British Neurological Surgeons 2001). The management of these children must occur within designated centres, with care delivered by an experienced team of healthcare professionals.

The general care of the child requiring neurosurgery has been outlined. It is particularly important to prepare parents for the significant postoperative swelling that will occur and that the child will not be able to open his or her eyes. Blood loss may be significant and the child must be monitored for cardiac instability. Blood loss must be assessed through monitoring of drains, clinical condition of the child and haematological blood profiling and may require the administration of whole blood. Hyperpyrexia, which is common during the first 3–4 days postoperatively, must be controlled, continued pyrexia may indicate wound infection (Panchal & Uttchin 2003). Parents will require support and advice in positioning and handling their child

postsurgery and should be advised not to lay the child prone for 1 week.

Long-term Outcomes

The child's long-term care needs depend on the severity of the condition, severity of raised intracranial pressure and the prognosis of any associated syndrome. The child may have physical impairments ranging from problems with vision and hearing, facial dysostosis and prognathism and there may be associated psychosocial and psychomotor development delay, with many children having learning difficulties (Sarnat & Menkes 2000). The child and family will require psychological support to assist and support them in dealing with their emotional stresses, especially alterations to body image.

EPILEPSY

Epilepsy is an umbrella term used to describe a range of conditions characterised by recurrent, unprovoked seizures. A seizure is a symptom of a disease rather than a disease itself. It has been estimated 1 person in 2000 is diagnosed with epilepsy each year, but the risk increases to 1 in 500 in children less than 1 year of age (Heaney et al 2002), with an estimated prevalence of 1 in 200 (Royal College of Paediatrics and Child Health 2000) (Fig. 33.10). Epilepsy is more prevalent in families who are socio-economically disadvantaged (Heaney et al 2002).

Aetiology

The two main causes of epilepsy are irreversible brain damage, which provides a focus for seizure activity (trauma brain injury, CNS infections, perinatal hypoxia, perinatal intraventricular haemorrhage, tumours) and malformations during cerebral development (Appleton & Gibbs 1995).

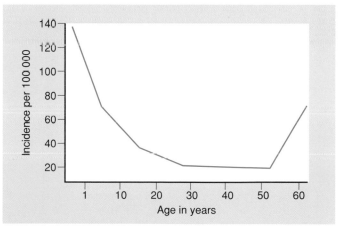

Fig. 33.10 • Incidence per 100,000 people related to age (Appleton 1995).

Epilepsy is also associated with neurodegenerative disorders. However, in the majority of cases no known cause will be identified (but are probably genetic in origin) and are best termed cryptogenic.

Classification

There are two main classification systems:

1. International League Against Epilepsy (ILAE) Seizure Classification (Commission on Classification and Terminology of the International League Against Epilepsy 1981): based on whether the seizure onset is focal (partial) or generalised. Partial seizures are subdivided into whether consciousness is retained (simple partial) or lost (complex partial) (Fig. 33.11) and can progress to a generalised seizure. In generalised seizures there is widespread nervous disruption across both hemispheres that can result in a range of seizure manifestations:
   - absences: staring and blinking
   - myoclonic: repeated jerking movements
   - tonic-clonic: typical image of a seizure (increased muscle tone results in rigidity followed by rhythmical movements)
   - atonic: loss of tone results in typical falling to the ground (drop attacks).

The classification system has been criticised for overreliance on EEG findings, not considering pathophysiological changes and ictal symptoms, and confusing terminology, which can result in misdiagnosis of the type of epilepsy (Engel 1998).

2. Semiological Seizure Classification (Lüders et al 1998) is based on presenting signs and symptoms, which are divided into six categories:
   - auras: including abnormal sensations, visual hallucinations or illusions, auditory, taste or smell hallucinations
   - autonomic seizure: palpitations, hot flushes
   - dialeptic seizure: alterations of consciousness
   - motor seizures: including myoclonic (muscle contractions—jerks), tonic, spasms, clonic, tonic-clonic, versive (eye or head movement to one side)
   - special seizures: atonic drop attacks, astaic seizures, hypomotor seizures, aphasic seizures
   - paroxysmal events: non-epileptic seizures.

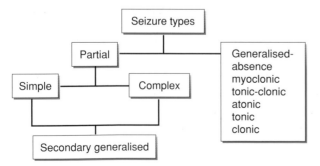

Fig. 33.11 • ILEA seizure classification.

More than one of these categories can be used to describe the seizure. The classification is helpful when nurses are describing a seizure for example a visual aura followed clonic movements of the left hand, which last briefly before a tonic-clonic seizure occurs.

In addition to the outlined classification systems for epilepsy, many epileptic syndromes exist. These syndromes have characteristic seizure patterns, signs and symptoms, which are suggestive of a particular condition, examples include infantile spasms (West syndrome), Lennox–Gaustaut syndrome and juvenile myoclonic epilepsy.

Rare types of epilepsy include sleep seizures and photosensitive epilepsies.

Presentation

A diagnosis of epilepsy is usually only made if two or more seizures have occurred. Accurate diagnosis is dependent on a good history, and detailed description of the seizure activity (Appleton & Gibbs 1995). Classifying the type of epilepsy needs to consider, the age of onset of the first seizure, the types of seizure activity, presence of underlying neurological problems, family history and EEG findings.

Treatment and Management Options

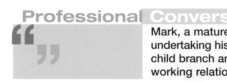

Professional Conversation

Mark, a mature student, is undertaking his first placement within child branch and has built up a good working relationship with Jane.

Jane has had epilepsy for many years, which has been well controlled with medication. However, she has had several acute admissions following seizures when at school. Jane has confided to Mark that she hates taking her medication at school and in front of her mum's new boyfriend. She resents having to care for her younger brother after school but accepts her mum has to work. Jane's mum had indicated to the nursing staff that she is concerned about Jane's failure to comply with medication, which has always been successful, and that her behaviour has changed with Jane becoming sullen and withdrawn.

Issues affecting the relationship between Jane, her mother and the staff

What issues do you think are important for Mark to discuss with his mentor in relation to Jane and her family?

The first-line treatment for epilepsy is antiepileptic drugs, with the aim being to use a single drug in the lowest possible dose to control seizures while minimising side effects. A wide range of antiepileptic drugs are now available and choice will depend on the type of seizures and underlying diagnosis, with monotherapy being successful in the majority of children (Camfield et al 1997). Despite limited evidence to guide the decisions on which drug to prescribe, sodium valproate appears to be the first choice for generalised seizures and carbamazepine for partial seizures (Marson et al 2003). However, newer antiepileptic drugs such as vigabatrin and lamotrigine are becoming well established. Parents need to understand the action of the drugs, side effects, drug toxicity monitoring and possible drug interactions (including over the counter drugs).

Intractable epilepsy occurs in 4% of children with epilepsy (Camfield et al 1997). It is difficult to manage often not responding to multiple drug therapy and occurs primarily in children with complex neurological problems (Camfield et al 1997). Treatment options, which may offer opportunity to reduce seizure activities in these children, include:

- Ketogenic diet: thought to have a therapeutic effect by producing ketones that may have anitepileptic properties. To maintain a sufficient level of ketones the body must utilise fat as the main energy source. The diet consists of high fat with restricted carbohydrates.

- Surgery: requires accurate diagnosis and a focal site for seizure activity. Surgical procedures include corpus callosotomy, which aims to prevent seizure activity affecting both hemispheres, cerebral resections (focal or unilateral hemispherectomy), which aims to remove focus of the seizure activity in uncontrolled localised epilepsy.

- Vagal nerve stimulation: a stimulator is surgically placed under the skin in the left upper chest, with electrodes attached to the vagal nerve used to stimulate the nerve. The exact reasons for a reduction in seizure activity remain unclear.

There is no reliable evidence to support these treatments but they appear successful for some children.

Evidence-based Practice

The Cochrane Library has a range of systematic reviews relating to treatment options for epilepsy. The Cochrane Library can be accessed at the following:
- http://www.cochrane.co.uk

or via the National Electronic Library for Health:
- http://www.nelh.nhs.uk

Evidence-based guidelines relating to the diagnosis and management of epilepsy in children and adults were published in 2004 by NICE:
- http://www.nice.org.uk

Nursing care of the child with epilepsy involves supporting the child and family during diagnosis and in the management and understanding of treatment modalities. For children with severe epilepsy the family will require additional support in relation to activities of daily living and promoting social, motor and cognitive functioning. Increased metabolism during frequent seizures and disruption to normal eating patterns may put the child at risk of undernourishment. Parents, other carers and schoolteachers need to be taught the skills required to maintain the child's safety during a seizure and ensuring a safe environment without putting undue restrictions on the child. Children with epilepsy may have altered cognitive functioning that may affect the perception of dangers. Healthcare professionals will need to access appropriate government guidelines in relation to immunisation schedules.

Adolescence is a time of turbulence and peer pressure, and personal challenges will be increased for the adolescent with epilepsy. The adolescent will need support and advice in relation to lifestyle choices such as career opportunities, learning to driving, socialising and maintaining a healthy lifestyle, the need to continue medication and advice in relation to treatment options, contraception and planning a family.

WWW

A wealth of lifestyle and practical advice relating to epilepsy is readily available on the following web sites:
- Epilepsy Action (British Epilepsy Association): http://www.epilepsy.org.uk [search for seizure-first aid]
- National Society for Epilepsy: http://www.epilepsynse.org.uk [search for first aid for epilepsy]

Evidence-based Practice

Current immunisation information is available at the following websites:
- http://www.immunisation.nhs.uk
- http://www.doh.gov.uk/greenbook/index.htm

Long-term Outcomes

The mortality rate for people with epilepsy is 2–3 times greater than the general population, with the most common reason being sudden unexpected death associated with seizures (Hanna et al 2002). The effectiveness of antiepileptic drugs achieves protracted remission in 70% of people with epilepsy (Hanna et al 2002). The remaining 30% have a chronic disabling condition with the overall prognosis dependent on the type and severity of the epilepsy and coexisting neurological disorders. Many of these children will have complex care needs and will require physical, emotional and social support in order to maximise their potential.

HYDROCEPHALUS

Hydrocephalus comprises a highly diverse group of disorders that have little in common except the increased volume of CSF within the intracranial fluid spaces. It is generally accepted that the overall incidence of hydrocephalus is approximately 3–4 per 1000 live births (Carey et al 1994).

Aetiology

The majority of cases have an identifiable cause, predictably a result of congenital malformations for example aqueduct stenosis, Arnold–Chiari malformations and Dandy–Walker syndrome, with aqueduct stenosis, accounting for about 15% of all cases of hydrocephalus (Brett & Harding 1997a).

Other causes of include:

- Tumours that obstruct the flow of CSF.
- Infections such as meningitis can cause adhesion between the epithelial linings of the CSF spaces, obstructing CSF flow.
- Intraventricular heamorrhage in premature infants can cause an initial blockage within the ventricles and secondary obstruction due to scarring.
- Associated with spinal bifida.
- Rare causes of hydrocephalus include arteriovenous malformations, obstruction of venous sinuses (intracranial hypertension), craniosynostosis or hypersecretion of CSF.

Classification

There are several systems of classifying hydrocephalus:

- 'Communicating hydrocephalus'/'non-communicating hydrocepalus' where the blockage of CSF flow either occurs outside the ventricular or within the ventricular system respectively.
- Congenital/acquired hydrocephalus.
- Age of occurrence.

Presentation

The effects of an increased CSF volume will depend on the compliance of the skull. In newborn babies and infants the skull is expandable because the skull sutures have not yet fused, and a rise in CSF levels will not cause a rapid rise in ICP like it does in older children and adolescents (Brett & Harding 1997a). Hydrocephalus in an infant will result in a rapidly increasing head circumference, tense anterior fontanelle, splayed skull sutures, scalp vein distension, loss of upward gaze and neck rigidity (Kirkpatrick et al 1989). The infant often has a characteristic appearance with a small face in comparison to head size and the eyes have a typical sun-setting appearance (the sclera is not visible below the iris) and nystigmus, with vomiting and irritability important additional symptoms (Kirkpatrick et al 1989). Older children may display the more classic signs of RICP.

Diagnosis

Prenatal diagnosis can be made as early as the 13th week of gestation, when ultrasound scanning can detect ventricular enlargement. However, accurate diagnosis will require amniocentesis in order to obtain samples for alpha-feta protein levels and to identify chromosomal abnormalities. If severe brain dysfunction is suspected termination may be offered. Postnatal diagnosis is usually made following an increase in head circumference (in infants) and neurological examination, with CT scanning confirming the diagnosis.

Treatment and Management

The management of hydrocephalus will depend on the cause and severity of the CSF obstruction. Very rarely hydrocephalus can arrest of its own accord. However, the risk of delaying treatment must be balanced with the potential of compromising normal development. Conservative management is generally not effective and rarely an option with perhaps the exception of premature infants post intraventricular haemorrhage (Chumas et al 2001). Ventricular shunts in these acutely sick infants are difficult to place and often become dysfunctional (possibly due to high CSF protein levels) and infections are common. Drug therapy has traditionally included the use of diuretics (furosemide and acetazolomide), which are known to decrease CFS production. However, the International PHVD Drug Trial Group (1998) does not advocate the use of diuretics, which are associated with increased neurological morbidity.

Making an opening through the third ventricle and chiasmatic cistern, which facilitates CSF flow, can treat hydrocephalus due to aqueduct stenosis. This obviates the need for a shunt. Success rates following third ventriculostomy are variable because there may be associated problems contributing to the hydrocephalus such as poor CSF absorption (Chumas et al 2001).

The vast majority of children are managed by the surgical insertion of a shunt that diverts excess CSF from the ventricles into another body cavity. A catheter is inserted into the ventricles (the proximal catheter) through a burr hole made in the temporal bone of the skull, just behind the ear. This catheter is attached to a unidirectional valve system situated over the skull. The valve is attached to a second catheter (the distal catheter), which is placed into a body cavity such as the peritoneum (ventriculoperitoneal shunts) or the left atrium (ventriculoatrial shunts). Ventriculoperitoneal shunts (Fig. 33.12) are usually the first

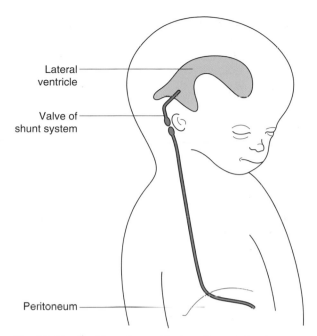

Lateral ventricle

Valve of shunt system

Peritoneum

Fig. 33.12 • Position of a ventriculoperitoneal shunt.

choice because they are easier to insert, catheters can be of sufficient length to allow for growth, good absorption of CSF occurs across the peritoneum and there is not the added potential of septicaemia, bacterial endocarditis and shunt nephritis, associated with ventriculoatrial shunts.

Shunts systems operate on the same principle; the valve offers resistance to the flow of CSF with a threshold pressure difference, below which the valve remains closed and above which the valve opens allowing CSF to flow through the shunt system. Different valve systems have different resistant pressures: low pressure (5 cmH$_2$O), medium pressure (10 cmH$_2$O) and high pressure (15 mmH$_2$O) (Drake & Kestle 1996). One of the major functional problems with shunt valves is overdrainage of the ventricles due to gravitational effects with upright posture (Pudenz & Foltz 1991), which creates a larger pressure differential between the head and abdomen due to the effects of gravity, resulting in CSF flowing at a higher rate than when a child is lying flat.

A trouble-free shunt is a desirable but elusive goal and unfortunately there are numerous potential complications with intraventricular shunts. Shunt failure is a major issue with reported failure rates of 39% during the first year following insertion and a further 14% during the second year following insertion (Drake et al 1998). Complications can be broadly divided into three groups: infection, mechanical failure and functional problems (Table 33.6).

The care of the child and family must be specific to current health needs. Initially, the emphasis of care will be directed towards assisting the parents (and older child) to understand and come to terms with the condition and supporting them to care for their child while waiting for surgery. For an infant this may include supporting parents to

Table 33.6 Main Complications of Ventricular Shunts

Complication	Examples
Infection (colonisation of shunt system by bacteria causing blockage)	Meningitis Wound infection Peritonitis (VP shunts) Septicaemia (VA shunts)
Mechanical failure (can result in malfunction or blockage of system)	Proximal obstruction due to catheter becoming lodged in tissue such as choroid plexus, brain tissue Distal obstruction due to catheter becoming lodged in tissues, kinking Catheter misplacement intracranial, intra-abdominal, intravascular Fractures of catheters and disconnections Migration of catheters into hollow viscera such as bladder or inguinal canal
Functional failure	Overdrainage Underdrainage

Miscellaneous problems affecting shunt functioning

Intracranial hypotension
Post-shunt pericerebral collections
Slit ventricle syndrome

VA, ventriculoatrial; VP, ventriculoperitoneal.

comfort an irritable child, assisting with feeding and positioning techniques.

The principles of care for the child requiring insertion or revision of a ventricular shunt revolve around an acutely ill child with RICP, due to a rapidly developing hydrocephalus or blocked existing ventricular shunt and the immediate dangers of cerebral herniation with its potential life-threatening consequences. Neurological changes must be detected promptly, through systematic neurological assessment and observations. In addition care will be primarily aimed at preparing the child for investigations (CT scan) and theatre in an organised and structured manner, while offering support to the child and family. The child who has been vomiting as a result of RICP will require intravenous fluids to correct dehydration.

The immediate potential postoperative complications following insertion of a ventricular peritoneal shunt are primarily intraventricular haemorrhage, blockage of the shunt and subdural haemorrhage (due to rapid overdrainage of the ventricles). Positioning of the child is an important consideration and will be influenced by the type of shunt; nursing staff must ensure they have clear postoperative instructions.

There is no specific care relating to the shunt once inserted, avoiding lying on the shunt site may prevent skin breakdown, particularly in the immediate postoperative period. The child and family will require detailed advice and support in relation to detected signs and symptoms of shunt failure. The Association of Spina Bifida and Hydrocephalus (ASBAH) offers an effective support network and a range of information for children and their families.

 WWW

A wealth of lifestyle and practical advice relating to hydrocephalus is readily available on the following website:
- Association of Spina Bifida and Hydrocephalus (ASBAH): http://www.asbah.org.uk

Long-term Outcomes

The child's long-term care needs depend on the reasons for hydrocephalus and the presence of addition association conditions. The majority of children with hydrocephalus will attend mainstream school. However, 40% of children will have associated physical, cognitive and behavioural difficulties (Casey et al 1997). These children will require appropriate multidisciplinary team input to ensure they reach their full potential.

TRAUMATIC BRAIN INJURY

Acquired brain injury can result from both traumatic and non-traumatic insults to the brain. Trauma is the main cause of acquired brain injury, due to an external force, which may produce a diminished or altered state of consciousness. The survival rate following traumatic brain injury has increased due to medical and technological advances.

Aetiology

Traumatic brain injury is the leading cause of mortality and morbidity in children and accounts for one-third of accidental deaths in children (Kraus et al 1987, Mahoney et al 1993). The dramatic increase in the number of children sustaining a head injury over the last 30 years is primarily due to increased motorisation. Causes of traumatic brain injury in children include (Henry et al 1992)

- Road traffic accidents: account for approximately 57% of traumatic brain injury, with the majority resulting from a child pedestrian hit by a moving car.
- Falls: account for approximately 22% of traumatic brain injury; severe head trauma is rare in home accidents.
- Non-accidental injury is the most common cause of severe head injury in children under 1 year.

Associated factors include (Henry et al 1992, Kraus et al 1987):

- Higher incidence in boys because they develop distance and spatial interpretation later than girls and are more likely to participate in risk-taking behaviours.
- Seasonal, with the peak incidence occurring during spring/summer and between 2 p.m. and 10 p.m.
- Increased risk in poor socio-economic areas and urban residences.
- Increased risk with previous head injury.
- Other variables may influence a child's vulnerability to traumatic brain injury, such as the presence of visual or hearing deficits, learning deficits.

Classification

1. Primary injury: occurs at the time of injury. The range of injuries include:
   - Closed head injury due to rapid acceleration or deceleration forces. Diffuse axonal brain injury as a result of stretching, twisting and tearing of nerve fibres. Shearing and compression of tissues on the bony ridges inside the skull can result in damage to arteries and veins causing haemorrhage.
   - Rotational forces add to the shearing effect particularly where structures are mobile such the brainstem and corpus callosum, common in shaken babies.
   - Open or penetrating injuries involve the brain becoming exposed and damaged.

- Skull fractures can be linear, comminuted and depressed. Basal skull fractures are particularly important due to the danger of secondary CSF infection.
  - Localised contusions often occur on the crest of the gyri of the cerebral cortex, and although they may produce dramatic focal neurological signs, tend to have a good overall progress, scarring may result in post traumatic seizures.

2. Secondary injury: occurs after the initial impact as a result of cerebral hypoxia, ischaemic damage, continued haemorrhage or oedema. Oedema peaks 24–48 hours after the injury. Seizures and the development of CNS infection further may compound secondary injury.

Presentation

Minor head injuries are defined as injuries where there has been only brief loss of consciousness, no abnormal neurological signs, GCS above 13, and transient symptoms such as dizziness, confusion, headaches and vomiting (Satz et al 2001). Major injuries result in unconsciousness, potentially compromising vital functions and an inability to maintain the airway, which threatens life.

Treatment and Management

Minor head injury is common in children (Satz et al 2001). Admission to hospital is not always necessary but is often a precaution if there has been a seizure, a skull facture, a labile GCS or the cause is suggestive of serious injuries, and to manage persistent symptoms such as vomiting. The focus of care must be the detection of neurological changes by undertaking a through assessment and ongoing observations. The child and family will require appropriate support and detailed discharge advice.

The NICE (2003) guidelines relating to the triage, assessment and management of head injuries in infants, children and adults identify the initial priorities of care as: assessment and stabilisation of the airway, breathing and circulation, and assessment of neurological status. All children with a GCS less than 8 will require, after stabilisation, transfer to a tertiary paediatric intensive care facility.

The child and family progresses through four distinct phases following major traumatic brain injury (Singer 1996).

Phase 1

A head injury is a sudden unwanted event, with an unpredictable outcome and immediate disruption to family life, the initial impact of the injury is life threatening. Following initial stabilization, the aim of care is to prevent secondary ischaemic damage. Interventions include preventing hypoxia and hypotension, monitoring ICP/EEG and early surgical intervention where indicated (refer to the management of RICP). The principles of rehabilita-

tion (previously outlined) must be a feature of care from the outset.

Phase 2

Recovery is a gradual and variable process with fluctuating responses and ongoing uncertainty. Often parents feel hopeless during this phase. The agitated child is often difficult to manage and may be distressing for parents.

Phase 3

The child's level of awareness returns and there may be early motor and cognitive recovery. The full extent of injuries becomes apparent.

Phase 4

There is continued cognitive recovery but social–emotional recovery with changes in personality and behaviour may be difficult to cope with. Discharge from hospital is a difficult time for the family, transition to community care needs to be well planned if the child and family are to adjust to the injury's effects. Schooling issues and consideration of future needs become important. After major traumatic brain injury, children require detailed continual assessment to monitor development because later milestones may not be achieved or the child may grow into deficits.

WWW

Practical advice relating to head injury is available on the Headway National Head Injuries Association website:
- http://www.headway.org.uk

Evidence-based Practice

The NICE (2003) guidelines relating to triage, assessment and management of head injuries in infants, children and adults are available on the NICE website:
- http://www.nice.org.uk

Long-term Outcomes

Deficits associated with mild to moderate head injury include social disinhibition, intellectual impairment, psychiatric disorders, perceptual distortion, learning problems, sensory impairment, neuromotor deficits and severe economic implications.

Factors affecting the outcome of major traumatic brain injury include: age (with poorest outcome is in infancy, possibly due to age-specific response to trauma), severity and type of injury, extent of secondary damage, disruption of normal development and pre-existing conditions (Crouchman 1998). Long-term sequelae include impairments in attention, memory and motivation, which can result in significantly reduced levels of interaction with the child and the environment (Rose et al 1997). Cognitive, behavioural and psychological recovery (and future development) may not necessarily correlate with physical improvements.

Summary

Caring for the child and family where the child has a neurological problem can be particularly challenging but highly rewarding. The challenges relate to a lack of exposure to caring for children with rare disorders, the uncertain outcome of many conditions, and the potential of many conditions to cause dramatic changes in function, both cognitively and physically. This chapter has outlined the nervous system and general principles of care required for a child with a neurological problem. It is not a comprehensive guide to the management of the wide range of neurological conditions of childhood but does provide insight into the common conditions. There has been an emphasis on an interdisciplinary approach to care delivery, and the need to ensure care delivery is individually designed and strongly influenced by encouraging the child to reach their full potential. Links have been made with other chapters where appropriate.

References

Appleton R 1995 Epilepsy in childhood. Aspects of Epilepsy Issue 1.

Appleton R, Gibbs J 1995 Epilepsy in childhood and adolescence. Taylor and Francis, London

Brett EM, Harding BN 1997a Hydrocepahalus and congenital anomalies of the nervous system. In: Brett EM (ed.) Paediatric neurology, 3rd edn. Churchill Livingstone, London

Brett EM, Harding BN 1997b Intracranial and spinal cord tumours. In: Brett EM (ed.) Paediatric neurology, 3rd edn. Churchill Livingstone, London

Brett EM, Kaiser AM 1997 Neurology of the newborn. In: Brett EM (ed.) Paediatric neurology, 3rd edn. Churchill Livingstone, London

Bullock R, Chestnut RM, Clifton G et al 2000 Guidelines for the management of severe traumatic brain injury. Journal of Neurotrauma 17(6/7):451–553

Camfield PR, Camfield C, Gordon K et al 1997 If a first antiepileptic drug fails to control a child's epilepsy, what are the chances of success in a second? The Journal of Pediatrics 131(6):821–824

Cancer Bacup 1999 Children's cancers – brain tumours in children. Factsheet. Cancer Bacup, London

Carey CM, Tullous MW, Walker ML 1994 Hydrocephalus, eitiology, pathological effects, diagnosis and natural history. In: Check WR (ed.) Pediatric neurosurgery: surgery of the developing nervous system, 3rd edn. WB Saunders, Philadelphia

Casey AT, Kimmings EJ, Kleinlugtebeld AD et al 1997 The long-term outlook for hydrocephalus in childhood. Pediatric Neurosurgery 27:63–70

Chitnavis BC, Polkey CE 1998 Intracranial pressure monitoring. Care of the Critically Ill Child 14(3):80–84

Chumas P, Tyagi A, Livingston J 2001 Hydrocephalus – what's new? Archives of Diseases in Childhood, Fetal Neonatal edition 85(3):149–154

Cohen MM, Maclean RE 2000 Craniosynostosis: diagnosis, evaluation and management, 2nd edn. Raven, New York

Commission on Classification and Terminology of the International League Against Epilepsy 1981 Proposal for revised clinical and electroencephalographic classification of epileptic seizures. Epilepsia 22:489–501

Crossman AR, Neary D 2000 Neuroanatomy – an illustrated colour text, 2nd edn. Churchill Livingstone, Edinburgh

Crouchman M 1998 Traumatic brain injury. In: Ward Platt MP, Little RA (eds) Injury in the young child. Cambridge University Press, Cambridge

Cullen PM, Derrickson JD, Potter JA 2002 Radiation therapy. In: Baggott CR, Kelly KP, Fochtman et al (eds) Nursing care of children and adolescents with cancer, 3rd edn. WB Saunders, Philadelphia

Dailey AT 1995 The pathophysiology of oral pharyngeal apraxia and mutism following posterior fossa tumor resection in children. Journal of Neurosurgery 83(3):467–475

Department of Health (DoH) 2002 Specialist services for children – definitions. No.23. Online. Available at: http://www.doh.gov.uk

Drake JM, Kestle JRW 1996 Determining the best cerebrospinal fluid shunt valve design: the pediatric valve design trial. Neurosurgery 38(3):604–607

Drake JM, Kestle JRW, Milner R et al 1998 Randomized trial of cerebrospinal fluid shunt valve design in pediatric hydrocephalus. Neurosurgery 43(2):294–305

Duffner PK, Horowitz ME, Krischer JP et al 1993 Postoperative chemotherapy and delayed radiation in children less than three years of age with malignant brain tumors. New England Journal of Medicine 328(24):1725–1731

Engel J 1998 Classification of the international league against epilepsy: time for reappraisal. Epilepsia 39(9):1014–1017

Fenichel GM 1997a Ataxia. In: Fenichel GM (ed.) Clinical pediatric neurology. A signs and symptoms approach, 3rd edn. WB Saunders, Philadelphia

Fenichel GM 1997b Disorders of cranial volume and shape. In: Fenichel GM (ed.) Clinical pediatric neurology. A signs and symptoms approach, 3rd edn. WB Saunders, Philadelphia

Ferguson Clark L, Williams C 1998 Neurological assessment in children. Paediatric Nursing 10(4):29–35

Fitzgerald MJT, Folan-Curran J 2002 Clinical neuroanatomy and related neuroscience, 4th edn. WB Saunders, Edinburgh

Greenwood I 1992 A benign tumour with lifelong effects. Treatment and management of craniopharyngioma. Professional Nurse 7(6):358, 360–361

Halperin EC, Constine lS, Tarbell NJ et al 1994 Tumors of the posterior fossa of the brain and the spinal canal. In: Halperin EC, Constine lS, Tarbell NJ et al (eds) Pediatric radiation oncology, 2nd edn. Raven Press, New York

Hanna NJ, Black M, Sander JWS et al 2002 The national sentinel clinical audit of epilepsy-related deaths. Epilepsy – death in the shadows. The Stationery Office, London

Hazinski MF, Headrick C, Bruce D 1999 Neurological disorders. In: Hazinski MF (ed.) Manual of pediatric critical care. Mosby, St Louis

Heaney DC, MacDonald BK, Everitt A et al 2002 Socioeconomic variation in incidence of epilepsy: prospective community based study in southeast England. British Medical Journal 325:1013–1016

Henry PC, Hauber RP, Price M 1992 Factors associated with closed head injury in a pediatric population. Journal of Neuroscience Nursing 24(6):311–316

Hickey JV 2003a Neurological assessment. In: Hickey JV (ed.) The clinical practice of neurological and neurosurgical nursing, 5th edn. Lippincott, Philadelphia

Hickey JV 2003b Management of the unconscious neurological patient. In: Hickey JV (ed.) The clinical practice of neurological and neurosurgical nursing, 5th edn. Lippincott, Philadelphia

Hickey JV 2003c Management of patients undergoing neurosurgical procedures. In: Hickey JV (ed.) The clinical practice of neurological and neurosurgical nursing, 5th edn. Lippincott, Philadelphia

Hickey JV 2003d Behavioural and psychological responses in neurological illness. In: Hickey JV (ed.) The clinical practice of neurological and neurosurgical nursing, 5th edn. Lippincott, Philadelphia

International PHVD Drug Trial Group 1998 International randomised controlled trial of acetazolamide and furosemide in post-haemorrhagic ventricular dilation in infancy. Lancet 352:433–440

James HE, Trauner DA 1985 The Glasgow Coma Scale. In: James HE, Anas NG, Perkin RM (eds) Brain insults in infants and children. Grune and Stratton, Orlando, FL

Johnston S 2001 Calvarial vault remodeling for sagittal synostosis. AORN Journal (Official Journal of the Association of Operating Room Nurses) 74(4):632, 634–647

Kershner DD, Claussen JA 1986 Craniofacial reconstruction — perioperative care of the craniosynostosis patient. AORN Journal (Official Journal of the Association of Operating Room Nurses) 44(4):554–562

Kirk EA, Howard VC, Scott CA 1995 Description of posterior fossa syndrome in children after posterior fossa tumor surgery. Journal of Pediatric Oncology Nursing 12(4):181–187

Kirkpatrick M, Engleman H, Minns RA 1989 Symptoms and signs of progressive hydrocephalus. Archives of Diseases in Childhood 64:124–128

Kraus JF, Fife D, Conroy C 1987 Pediatric brain injuries: the nature, clinical course and early outcomes in a defined United States population. Pediatrics 79(4):501–507

Lashford LS, Walker DA 1997 Improved care for central nervous system tumours: a mood for change. Archives of Diseases in Childhood 76(2):88–90

Lew CM, LaVally B 1995 The role of stereotactic radiation therapy in management of children with brain tumors. Journal of Pediatric Oncology Nursing 12(4):212–222

Long AF, Kneafsey R, Ryan J et al 2002 The role of the nurse within the multi-professional rehabilitation team. Journal of Advanced Nursing 37(1):70–78

Longstaff A 2000 Instant notes – neuroscience. BIOS Scientific Publications, Oxford

Lüders H, Baumgarter C, Benbadis S et al 1998 Semiological seizure classification. Epilepsia 39(9):1006–1013

MacKenzie N 1990 Craniofacial surgery. Paediatric Nursing 2(6):24–25

Mahoney WJ, D'Souza BJ, Haller JA et al 1993 Long-term outcome of children with severe head trauma and prolonged coma. Pediatrics 71(5):756–762

Marson AG, Williamson PR, Hutton JL et al on behalf of the Epilepsy Monotherapy Trialists 2000 Carbamazepine versus valproate monotherapy for epilepsy (Cochrane Review). In: The Cochrane Library, issue 4. Update Software, Oxford

May L 2001 Craniosynostosis. In: May L (ed.) Paediatric Neurosurgery: a handbook for the multidisciplinary team. Whurr Publishers, London

Miller JD, Dearden NM 1992 Measurement, analysis and the management of raised intracranial pressure. In: Teasdale GM, Miller JD (eds) Current neurosurgery. Churchill Livingstone, Edinburgh

Moore IM 1995 Central nervous system toxicity of cancer therapy in children. Journal of Pediatric Oncology Nursing 12(4):203–211

Moos KF, Hide R 1993 Craniofacial surgery—surgical correction of congenital deformities. Surgery 11(8):457–465

Mulhern RK, Kepner JL, Thomas PR et al 1998 Neuropsychologic functioning of survivors of childhood medulloblastoma randomized to receive conventional or reduced-dose craniospinal irradiation: a pediatric oncology group study. Journal of Clinical Oncology 16(5):1723–1728

Neumann VC 1995 Principles and practices of treatment. In: Chamberlain MA, Neumann VC, Tennant A (eds) Traumatic brain injury rehabilitation services, treatment and outcomes. Chapman and Hall, London

NICE 2003 Head injury. Triage, assessment, investigation and early management of head injury in infants, children and adults. NICE, London

Padgett K 2002 Alterations of neurological function in children. In: McCance KL, Huether SE (eds) Pathophysiology: the biological basis for disease in adults and children, 4th edn. Mosby, St Louis

Panchal J, Utchin V 2003 Management of craniosynostois. Plastic and Reconstructive Surgery 111(6):2032–2048

Pudenz RH, Foltz EH 1991 Hydrocephalus: overdrainage by ventricular shunts – a review and recommendations. Surgical Neurology 35:200–202

Reilly P, Simpson DA, Sprod R et al 1988 Assessing the conscious levels of infants and young children: a paediatric version of the Glasgow Coma Scale. Children's Nervous System 4:30–33

Roffe J 1989 The role of the nurse in paediatric rehabilitation. Paediatric Nursing 1:11–13

Rose FD, Johnson DA, Attree EA 1997 Rehabilitation of the head injured child: basic research and new technology. Pediatric Rehabilitation 1(1):3–7

Rosner MJ, Daughton S 1990 Cerebral perfusion pressures, management in head injury. Journal of Trauma 30:933–940

Royal College of Paediatrics and Child Health (RCPCH) 2000 A national approach to epilepsy management in children and adults. RCPCH, London

Ryan-Murray J, McElwain Petriccione M 2002 Central nervous system tumors. In: Baggott CR, Kelly KP, Fochtman D et al (eds) Care of children and adolescents with cancer, 3rd edn. WB Saunders, Philadelphia

Sarnat HB, Menkes JH 2000 Neuroembryology, genetic programming and malformations of the nervous system. In: Menkes JH, Sarnat HB (eds) Child neurology. Lippincott, Williams and Wilkins, Philadelphia

Satz P, Zaucher K, McCleary et al 2001 Mild head injury in children and adolescents: a review of studies 1970–1995. Psychological Bulletin 122(2):107–131

Shiminski-Maher T, Shields M 1995 Pediatric brain tumors: diagnosis and management. Journal of Pediatric Oncology Nursing 12(4):188–198

Singer GHS 1996 Constructing supports. In: Singer GHS, Glang A, Williams JM (eds) Children with acquired brain injury. Paul H Brooks, Baltimore

Society of British Neurological Surgeons 2001 Safe paediatric neurosurgery 2001. Society of British Neurological Surgeons, London

Stephenson RC 1996 Therapeutic consistency following brain lesions. Professional Nurse 11(11):738–740

Stewart ES, Cohen DG 1998 Central nervous system tumors in children. Seminars in Oncology Nursing 14(1):34–42

Strother DR, Pollack IF, Fisher PG et al 2002 Tumors of the central nervous system. In: Pizzo PA, Poplack DG (eds) Principles and practices of pediatric oncology, 4th edn. Lippincott Williams and Wilkins, Philadelphia

Sugerman RA 2002 Structure and function of the neurological system. In: McCance KL, Huether SE (eds) Pathophysiology: the biological basis for disease in adults and children, 4th edn. Mosby, St Louis

Tatman A, Warren A, Williams A et al 1997 Development of a modified paediatric coma scale in intensive care clinical practice. Archives of Diseases in Childhood 77(6):519–521

Teasdale G, Jennett B 1974 Assessment of coma and impaired consciousness – a practical scale. Lancet 2:81–83

Turini M, Redaelli A 2001 Primary brain tumours: a review of research and management. International Journal of Clinical Practice 55(7):471–475

Vernon-Levett P, Geller M 1997 Posterior fossa tumors in children: a case study. American Association of Critical Care Nurses (AACN) Clinical Issues 8(2):214–226, 285–286

Walker DA, Punt JAG, Sokal M 1999 Clinical management of brain stem glioma. Archives of Diseases in Childhood 80(6):558–564

Warren A 2000 Paediatric coma scoring researched and benchmarked. Paediatric Nursing 12(3):14–18

Warren SM, Greenwald J A, Spector JA et al 2001 New developments in cranial suture research. Cranial Suture Research 107(2):523–540

Watson M, Horn S, Curl J 1992 Searching for signs of revival: uses and abuses of the Glasgow Coma Scale. Professional Nurse 7(10):670–673

Worrall L 1999 Medulloblastoma. In: Miaskowski C, Buchel P (eds) Oncology nursing – assessment and clinical care. Mosby, St Louis

Chapter Thirty Four

34

Caring for Children with Diabetes and other Endocrine Disorders

Philomena Morrow

ABSTRACT

This chapter aims to review the range of problems that may present for the child and family as a result of hormone dysfunction. Care of the child and family with reference to health promotion/education will be significantly addressed in relation to the endocrine disorders presented. Active participation is encouraged throughout to increase and further develop knowledge and understanding. The Evolve website will provide an opportunity for revision of the production and function of hormones in the body and their effect on the growth and development of the child.

Learning Outcomes

- Understand the role and function of the endocrine system.

- Appreciate how disordered function affects the child.

- Understand the care requirements of the child and family in relation to specific endocrine disorders.

- Understand the specialist nature of caring for a child with diabetes.

- Recognise the importance of health promotion/education in the care of the child and family with an endocrine disorder.

- Appreciate the need for continuing care and support required by the child and family with an endocrine disorder.

Endocrine System

The endocrine system is a chemical communication system that provides the means to control a number of physiologi-cal processes within the body. As it is a communication network, the endocrine system contains transmitters, signals and receivers that are called hormone-producing cells, hormones and receptors.

The endocrine system consists of a number of distinct glands and some tissues in other organs. The endocrine glands (Fig. 34.1) are:

- pituitary gland
- thyroid gland
- four parathyroid glands
- two adrenal glands
- pancreatic islets (also known as the islets of Langerhans)
- pineal gland
- thymus gland
- two ovaries in the female
- two testes in the male.

Endocrine glands secrete hormones directly into the bloodstream, whereas exocrine glands pass their secretions directly into body cavities. The hormones released by endocrine glands are carried in the bloodstream to their target organ, where they are active. The activity of a number of endocrine glands is regulated through the activity of the hypothalamus.

THE HYPOTHALAMUS

Nine different substances have been identified as hypothalamic hormones that either stimulate or inhibit the release of anterior and posterior hormones (Table 34.1). These hormones are formed in the median eminence of the

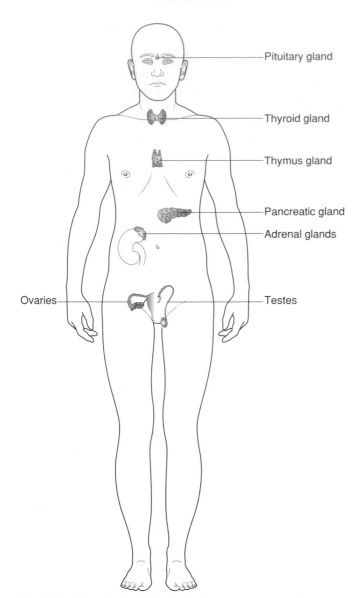

Fig. 34.1 • The glands within the body.

Labels: Pituitary gland, Thyroid gland, Thymus gland, Pancreatic gland, Adrenal glands, Ovaries, Testes

Table 34.1 The Hypothalamic Hormones

Hypothalamus

Synthesis of posterior pituitary hormones and transport via nerve axons	Hypothalamic hormones carried in hypothalamohypophyseal portal system

Pituitary gland

Posterior pituitary (neurohypophysis)	*Middle lobe*	*Anterior lobe (adenohypophysis)*
Oxytocin	Melanocyte-stimulating hormones	Trophic hormones: ACTH, adrenal cortex hormone
Vasopressin (antidiuretic hormone)		
Thyroid stimulating hormone (TSH)		
Growth hormone (GH)		
Follicle stimulating hormone (FSH)		
Luteinising hormone (LH)		
Prolactin (PRL)		

hypothalamus (the area that is connected to the pituitary gland by the pituitary stalk).

PITUITARY GLAND

The gland develops from the merging of different tissues (Fig. 34.2).

Anterior Pituitary Gland

Originates from an upgrowth of glandular epithelium from the pharynx and is known as the adenohypophysis. This is only linked to the brain via the venous hypothalamohypophyseal portal system. This network transports blood from the hypothalamus to the anterior pituitary, thereby transporting releasing and inhibiting hormones secreted by the hypothalamus. These hormones influence secretion and release of other hormones formed in the anterior pituitary (Fig. 34.3):

- corticotropin-releasing hormone: controls release of tropic hormones, such as adrenocorticotropic hormone (ACTH)
- thyrotropin-releasing hormone (also known as thyroid-stimulating hormone)
- growth-hormone-releasing factor
- gonadotropin-releasing hormone
- somatostatin-releasing hormone (also known as growth-hormone-release inhibiting factor)
- prolactin-inhibiting factor
- melanocyte-stimulating hormone (MSH).

Posterior Pituitary Gland

This is derived from a downgrowth of nervous tissue from the base of the brain and is known as the neurohypophysis. It has nervous connections with the hypothalamus, down which the antidiuretic hormone (ADH) and oxytocin pass. ADH and oxytocin are synthesised in the nerve cell bodies of the hypothalamus, transported along the axons, and then stored and secreted by vesicles within the axon terminals.

Fig. 34.2 • The pituitary gland.

Their release is triggered by nerve impulses from the hypothalamus.

Disorders Affecting the Pituitary Gland

Disorders affecting the pituitary gland result in disruption in regulation of hormone secretion. Symptoms vary depending on the location of the disorder, and are related to a disturbance in production of a specific hormone or group of hormones and relate to the role they play in maintaining health and development.

Hypopituitarism

This term denotes subnormal pituitary hormone production (Parks 2002). It is generally a result of disorders of the anterior pituitary and may involve one or more of the hormones produced (Table 34.2). Deficiencies of anterior hormone production are due to primary disease or disorder of the anterior pituitary. Secondary hypopituitarism, which is attributed to dysfunction of the hypothalamus, affects the synthesis and release of releasing hormones and release inhibiting hormones.

Factors contributing to pituitary hyposecretion include congenital hypopituitarism due to genetic abnormalities or other developmental defects. Congenital hypopituitarism is mainly related to growth hormone deficiency.

Disordered pituitary hormone secretion that develops after birth is referred to as acquired hypopituitarism (Parks 2002). This may have resulted from central nervous system trauma, meningitis or encephalitis, vascular abnormalities or haemorrhage, brain tumours, pituitary tumours and/or radiation therapy.

Hyperpituitarism

Pituitary tumours that secrete hormones produce characteristic symptoms of excessive hormone levels. Symptoms may range from complaints such as listlessness or restlessness to more severe symptoms such as headaches, vomiting or dizziness. In addition, problems due to an increase in any of the hormones produced may give rise to growth, adrenal or sexual dysfunction. (see Table 34.2).

Hormonal abnormalities occurring as a result of pituitary tumours or defects will be discussed under specific headings.

Growth Hormone Deficiencies

Growth hormone deficiency exists when growth hormone is absent or is produced in inadequate amounts to support normal growth. If growth hormone deficiency occurs in combination with one or more other pituitary hormone deficiencies the condition is related to hypopituitarism, as described earlier.

Growth hormone deficiency can be congenital, resulting from deficiency of hypothalamic growth hormone releasing hormone that may be associated with defects such as septo-optic dysplasia or primary pituitary disorders such as defects in the growth hormone gene. Most congenital cases of growth hormone deficiency are currently considered idiopathic (Cuttler 2002), which is the most common form, accounting for approximately 50–70% of cases (NICE 2002). Fetal growth is growth hormone independent and therefore infants with congenital growth hormone deficiency are born normal size and weight. However, growth hormone deficiency may present in the newborn

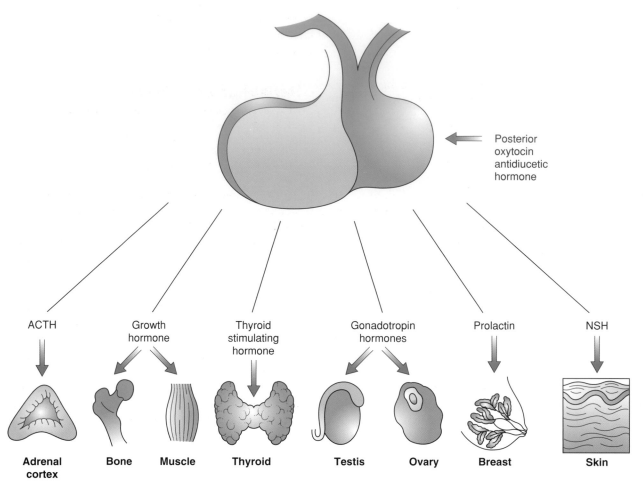

Fig. 34.3 • Anterior pituitary hormones.

Table 34.2 Disorders of Pituitary Hormones

Hypopituitarism	Hyperpituitarism
Anterior pituitary gland	
Growth hormone: somatic growth retardation	Somatic growth acceleration Adrenal hyperfunction
Adrenocorticotropic hormone (ACTH): adrenal hypofunction	Hyperthyroidism Precocious puberty/retarded sexual development
Thyroid hormone: hypothyroidism	
Follicle stimulating and luteinising hormone: absence/regression of secondary sex characteristics	Prolactin: stops menstruation
Prolactin	
Posterior pituitary gland	
Antidiuretic hormone: diabetes insipidus	

period with hypoglycaemia, and prolonged jaundice. These symptoms are often significant early diagnostic features. Growth hormone deficiency becomes evident only during the first years of life, when linear growth begins to slow.

Acquired growth hormone deficiency may be the result of injury, infection, radiation or tumours of the pituitary gland and/or the hypothalamus; it may become evident during infancy or childhood. Failure to grow normally may also be a key feature of other underlying medical conditions, e.g. chronic renal insufficiency, Turner syndrome, Prader–Willi syndrome. Among children who are of very short stature (i.e. at least 3 standard deviations below the population mean), 25% have growth hormone deficiency (NICE 2002).

PowerPoint

Access the companion PowerPoint presentation and refer to the discussion on growth hormone for detailed information on assessment and diagnosis in relation to family history, child's history, radiographic and imaging findings, and laboratory findings.

Principles of Nursing Care and Management

Care and management will be based on the assessment of individual needs of the child and in collaboration with the child and family (Table 34.3).

In children with growth hormone insufficiency, exogenous (biosynthetic) growth hormone (somatropin) is administered by subcutaneous injection; the dose is increased during the period of adolescence. The recommended dose varies according to the child's condition and is self-administered at home 6–7 times a week. Biosynthetic human growth hormone has been licensed for use in the UK for long-term treatment of children who have growth failure due to inadequate secretion of normal endogenous growth hormone (NICE 2002). A variety of growth hormone preparations and devices are available, knowledge of which is important if the nurse is to help the child and family choose the most suitable product and device. Although treatment enables many children to reach their adult height potential, this may mean many years of treatment for the child. Establishing and maintaining optimum therapy both at the outset and over what may be a long period of time may be extremely challenging for many families (Nairn & Moore 2002). Treatment is generally continued until attainment of final height. The initial and ongoing education of the child and family and the monitoring and maintenance of long-term compliance to achieve the best possible outcomes are important aspects within the role of the children's nurse.

Evidence-based Practice

Growth hormone therapy can increase short-term growth and improve (near) final height (Bryant et al 2004).

Activity

Children and parents need to understand the importance of complying with treatment regimes and to

be competent in administration. This requires that the child and family are educated regarding the rationale for treatment and adverse effects.

Reflect on your Practice

- Explain to a parent the technique required to administer a subcutaneous injection.
- Review the advice regarding proper injecting technique for growth hormone at: http://www.heightmatters.org.uk

Side effects of growth hormone therapy are rare but can include headache, visual problems, nausea and vomiting, fluid retention (peripheral oedema), arthralgia, myalgia, paraesthesia, antibody formation, hypothyroidism and reactions at injection site. Particular attention should be paid to treating children with risk factors associated with diabetes mellitus and slipped capital epiphyses.

Storage and preparation of medication, as well as choosing and alternating the injection site are important aspects of the education process. Timing of administration of growth hormone may be dependent on family routines. The evening is usually the recommended time as this mimics the pattern of normal production of growth hormone. (Hockenberry et al 2003). Compliance to treatment may be enhanced by enabling the child take control over administration of growth hormone, which may be achieved by the use of the pen injector.

Activity

Review the section on needle phobia on p 547.

Child and Family Resources

Raising awareness of the guidance on the use of human growth hormone in children with growth failure (NICE 2002; website: http://www.nhsdirect.nhs.uk) and encouraging parents to discuss this guidance with their doctor will provide further encouragement to comply with treatment.

Table 34.3 Nursing Care and Management of Growth Hormone Deficiencies

Characteristics of child with growth hormone deficiency	Nursing considerations
Short stature	Accurate assessment and monitoring of height and weight
Delayed growth of all body parts	Accurate recording/plotting height and weight on appropriate
Delayed skeletal maturation	growth chart
Immature facial appearance	Early recognition of deviation in height and weight pattern
Increased subcutaneous fat	Accurate detailed assessment of child's health and health problems
In prolonged growth failure the child	Assessment of family history
will be shorter than children of the same age	Referral for medical consultation and assisting and supporting the
Hypoglycaemia may be present particularly in young children	child/family during medical examination, radiological surveys and endocrine studies

The Human Growth Foundation is a national organisation of parents who provide education and guidance on the physical, psychological and social development of children with growth problems. This resource may be beneficial in providing parents and children with additional support and advice. Good nutrition and adequate rest is vital when promoting growth. A well-balanced diet with appropriate calorie and protein intake needs to be encouraged.

Children's nurses have a significant role in the routine monitoring of growth and the assessment of growth disorders. The development of good history-taking skills and an accurate, repeatable measurement are central to the success of growth assessment and evaluation. Measuring height is subject to error as a result of poor technique, variations between instruments and observers and diurnal variation (Hall 2000).

Evidence-based Practice

Height is greatest on getting up in the morning – up to 2.0 cm can be lost over the whole day. Measurements made at different times of the day can significantly affect the measured height and, thus, the estimated rate of growth (Hall 2000).

Activity

Review a growth chart for a boy and a girl from birth to 18 years. Identify the nurse's responsibilities in relation to the assessment of the following:
- weight
- standing height
- supine length
- head circumference.

Review the PowerPoint presentation for measurement technique for standing height (Hall 2000).

During therapy, the child's growth needs to be monitored against expected growth on standard growth charts to assess ongoing response to treatment (Table 34.4). Expected growth may be based on parental height. It is rec-

Table 34.4 Normal Growth Rates for Height in Children (Desrosiers 2002)

Age	Growth in height
0–6 months	18–26 cm/year
6–12 months	15–18 cm/year
1–2 years	10–13 cm/year
2–3 years	7–10 cm/year
3–4 years	5–8 cm/year
4–10 years	5 cm/year

ommended that treatment should be discontinued if the child's growth velocity is less than 50% from baseline in the first year of therapy, i.e. if extra height gain is not at least half the height gain in the year before treatment began. Persistent and uncorrectable problems with adherence to treatment should also be taken into account as part of the re-evaluation process (NICE 2002).

Recognition of the complexity of problems experienced by the child and family in relation to growth deficiency and/or short stature is necessary if physical and psychosocial dilemmas are to be overcome. Children who are small for their age may have problems with friends, teachers and parents, who tend to treat them as though they were younger and have reduced expectations of them. In turn, children may not act their age because it is not expected from them and thus experience problems with self-esteem and ability to interact appropriately with others. Those involved in the care of these children should be aware of the importance of emphasising abilities and strengths rather than physical size.

PowerPoint

Access the companion PowerPoint presentation and revise your knowledge on the production and regulation of secretion of the thyroid hormones before proceeding to the next section of this chapter on disorders of thyroid function.

DISORDERS OF THYROID FUNCTION

Disturbance in the secretory pathway of the thyroid hormones may result in an increase or decrease in production. Hypothyroidism is a result of a deficiency in secretion of thyroid hormones and may be congenital or acquired (juvenile hypothyroidism). Congenital hypothyroidism may be due to aplasia or hypoplasia of the thyroid gland (Fig 34.4), or hereditary defects in thyroid hormone synthesis that may be associated with maternal administration of antithyroid drugs during pregnancy (McCance & Huether 1998).

Juvenile hypothyroidism may be primary or secondary. Primary causes include:

- defective hormone synthesis resulting from acute thyroiditis caused by bacterial infection
- subacute non-bacterial inflammation associated with viral infections
- autoimmune (circulating antithyroid antibodies) thyroiditis occurring as a result of Hashimoto disease is the most common cause of juvenile hypothyroidism in children (Roth et al 1997)
- an endemic of iodine deficiency or antithyroid drugs, or loss of thyroid tissue can be contributory factors in hypothyroidism.

Thyroid gland

Fig. 34.4 • The thyroid gland.

Secondary hypothyroidism is due to insufficient stimulation of the thyroid gland by thyroid stimulating hormone as a result of hypothalamic or pituitary disorders.

Nursing Assessment and Diagnosis

In children under the age of two, the symptoms may not be as clear as those associated with hypothyroidism therefore nursing assessment and ongoing monitoring of the neonate with presenting problems is vital to ensure early diagnosis of the condition. Presenting symptoms depend on extent of dysfunction and age at onset. However, if undetected and left untreated in early childhood, permanent defects can arise, for example, mental retardation, deafness, deceleration in growth and other nervous system disorders. At birth there may be difficulty in identifying hypothyroidism. Hypothermia, delay in passing meconium and neonatal jaundice may be significant signs and require to be investigated immediately. Newborn screening programmes within 10 days of birth have helped aid early diagnosis and treatment, which have resulted in a reduced number of children affected by the condition.

 WWW

Review the UK process measures, standards and supporting implementation guidelines for newborn blood spot screening. These are available on the website of the UK Newborn Screening Programme Centre at:

• http://www.ich.uc/.ac.uk

Clinical manifestations of hypothyroidism may not be evident until after 4 months of age. Signs and symptoms may include difficulty eating, hoarse cry, protruding tongue caused by myxodema of oral tissue and vocal cords. The child may present with constipation and abdominal distension due to hypotonia of abdominal muscles. A subnormal temperature, excessive sleeping, slow pulse and a cold, mottled skin may be present. Often the baby is seen as being a 'good' baby. Skeletal growth may be decelerated due to impaired synthesis of protein, poor absorption of nutrients and lack of bone mineralisation. Enlargement of the thyroid gland, known as goitre, may be evident, particularly in older children. If the condition remains undiagnosed and untreated, the child will be dwarfed with short limbs (cretinism) as well as presenting with mental retardation.

Care and Management

Once diagnosis is confirmed, treatment is replacement therapy, which is prescribed according to the child's hormonal levels. Treatment is required on a life-long basis. Regular estimates of hormone levels are essential to prevent development of hyperthyroidism. In addition, regular monitoring of growth and development is necessary.

 WWW

Obtain further information on thyroxine and recommended dosages at:

• http://emc.medicines.org.uk

Parent information is available at:

• http://www.ivillage.co.uk

Information for children is available at:

• http://www.childrenfirst. nhs.uk/kids/health/illness/thyroid problemss.html

Hyperthyroidism

Hyperthyroidism is a condition in which the thyroid hormones exert greater than normal responses. Generally there is excess secretion of thyroid hormones, which might be associated with acute, subacute, or chronic thyroiditis, tumours of the thyroid, or other tumours of the pituitary (which secretes thyroid-stimulating hormone). Specific diseases that cause hyperthyroidism include Graves' disease and toxic multinodular goitre.

Graves' disease is the most common cause of hyperthyroidism in children. Although the exact cause is unknown, it is thought to be associated with autoimmune abnormalities that cause enlargement and thus hyperfunction of the thyroid gland.

Assessment and Diagnosis

Hyperthyroidism is four times more common in girls than boys and most frequently presents in childhood between ages of 12–14 years. The condition usually presents with a history in deterioration in school performance. Other symptoms mimic the opposite effects of hypothyroidism.

Scenario

June, a 12-year-old who presented with a history of weight loss, anxiety, disturbance in sleep and mood changes, was diagnosed as having Graves' disease.
- When undertaking June's nursing assessment, what specific information would you be required to obtain?
- What specific requirements would need to be considered when planning June's care?

A discussion of this scenario appears at the end of the chapter.

PowerPoint

Access the companion PowerPoint presentation and review regulation of adrenal and renal function before proceeding with the next section of this chapter on disorders of adrenal function.

DISORDERS OF ADRENAL FUNCTION

Disorders of the adrenal cortex (Fig. 34.5) are related to either hyperfunction or hypofunction (Table 34.5).

Activity

With reference to the care of a child receiving steroid therapy, explain the likely symptoms that may present in a child with Cushing's syndrome.

A discussion of this activity is presented at the end of the chapter.

Congenital Adrenal Hyperplasia

Congenital adrenal hyperplasia is a group of disorders of adrenal steroid synthesis. Excessive secretion of androgens by the adrenal cortex may occur as a result of a number of conditions of the adrenal gland. However, the most common disorder affecting children is congenital adrenogenital hyperplasia, an inborn deficiency of various enzymes necessary for the biosynthesis of adrenal steroidogenesis (Hockenberry et al 2003). Interference with the biosynthesis of glucocorticoids in fetal life results in cortisol secretion been diminished and an increased production of adrenocorticotropic hormone, which stimulates hyperplasia of the adrenal gland. There is an increased production of various adrenal hormone precursors, including androgens. Deficiency of enzymes necessary for biosynthesis of mineralocorticoids may result in diminished secretion of aldosterone.

Fig. 34.5 • The adrenal gland.

In its severe form, excess adrenal androgen production beginning in the first trimester of fetal development results in virilisation of the female infant and life threatening hypovolaemic, and hyponatraemic shock (adrenal crisis) in the newborn.

Assessment and Diagnosis

In the female with potentially normal ovaries and uterus, virilisation occurs and sexual development is therefore along

Table 34.5 Disorders of Adrenal Function	
Hyperfunction of adrenal cortex	**Hypofunction**
Cushing's syndrome: increased levels of circulating cortisol	Acute adrenocortical insufficiency
	Chronic adrenocortical insufficiency (Addison's disease)
Congenital adrenal hyperplasia: increased secretion of adrenal androgens and oestrogens leading to virilisation or feminisation Primary hyperaldosteronism Hyperfunction of adrenal medulla Phaeochromosytoma: increased secretion of catecholamines	

heterosexual lines. The abnormality of the external genitalia may vary from mild enlargement of the clitoris to complete fusion of the labioscrotal folds, forming a scrotum, a penile urethra, a penile shaft, and enlargement of the clitoris to form a normal-sized gland. Signs of adrenal insufficiency (salt loss) may be present during the first days of life. When the enzyme defect is milder, salt loss may not occur. If untreated, growth rate and skeletal maturation are accelerated. Pubic hair appears early, acne may be excessive and voice may deepen. Excessive pigmentation may develop as a result of melanocyte stimulation by excessive production of adrenocortotropic hormone (Kappy et al 2003).

In males, sexual development proceeds normally. Male infants may appear normal at birth but present with salt-losing crisis in the first 2–4 weeks. The infant may present with vomiting, poor weight gain, poor feeding and electrolyte imbalance. The older male child who was not losing sodium may present with rapid growth and precocious sexual development.

Hormonal studies are essential for accurate diagnosis. Adrenal ultrasonography, CT scanning, and MRI may define pelvic anatomy or enlarged adrenals or indicate the presence of an adrenal tumour. Pelvic ultrasonography may help in delineating the internal anatomy of a newborn with ambiguous genitalia.

Nursing Care and Treatment

Initially, the recognition of ambiguous genitalia in the newborn requires to be attended to immediately in relation to informing the parents and commencing investigations to confirm sexual identity.

Early diagnosis and treatment is crucial. Aims of treatment consist of normalising growth velocity and skeletal maturation using the smallest dose of glucocorticoids that will suppress adrenal function. Mineralocorticoid replacement helps to sustain normal electrolyte homeostasis, although excessive use may result in hypertension.

Evidence-based Practice

Puberty imposes greater difficulty in achieving and maintaining adrenal suppression despite optimal doses of substitution therapy (Charmandari et al 2002):
- Discuss.

Patient education is necessary as has been described for other endocrine disorders. Parents should understand the child's need for life-long therapy and the side effects, as well as signs of underdosage and requirements during illness. The need for compliance requires to be stressed and the importance of the child carrying appropriate identification. Surgical intervention may be necessary for reconstruction of the female genitalia as soon as possible during infancy in an effort to support ongoing

physical and psychological development. Multiple surgical procedures may be necessary, which will require ongoing psychological support for the child and parents. They require ongoing support as they come to terms with the sex of the baby and decisions that they may have to make regarding the need for surgical interventions. Reassurance regarding surgical interventions and the future care and treatment, which will be a lifelong commitment, need to be discussed.

Ambiguity in relation to the sex of the newborn can have a devastating effect on parents and other siblings. At this time, anticipation of parental reaction, which may be likened to the process of bereavement and loss, may enhance the nurse's ability to engage in a more therapeutic way at this time. Parents need to have information in relation to the infant's condition reinforced while at the same time been provided with the opportunity to express their own sorrow, loss and disappointment.

As the hereditary form of adrenogenital hyperplasia is an autosomal-recessive disorder, parents should be referred for genetic counselling.

Activity

Review Chapter 46 on caring for a child requiring palliative care:
- Discuss how this information may be relevant to the care of the child and family in the above situation in relation to bereavement and loss.

Chronic Adrenocortical Insufficiency (Addison's Disease)

Adrenal insufficiency (Table 34.6) may be the result of:

- hereditary enzymatic defects (congenital adrenal hyperplasia)
- loss of adrenal function due to autoimmune destruction of the gland (Addison's disease)
- pituitary hypothalamic tumours
- irradiation of the hypothalamus.

Chronic adrenal insufficiency typically occurs when 90% of adrenal function is lost (Miller 2002).

Acute Adrenocortical Insufficiency (Adrenal Crisis)

Acute adrenal insufficiency (adrenal crisis) is most common in the child with undiagnosed chronic adrenal insufficiency who is exposed to additional severe stress, such as major illness, trauma or surgery. Some of the aetiological factors include haemorrhage into the gland from trauma, which may be caused by a prolonged, difficult labour; fulminating infections, such as meningococcaemia, which results in haemorrhage; and necrosis (Waterhouse–Friderichsen

Table 34.6 Causes of Adrenal Insufficiency

Characteristics of glucocorticoid deficiency	Characteristics of mineralocorticoid deficiency	Nursing considerations
Poor weight gain, weight loss, anorexia	Hyponatremia Hyperkalemia	Assessment of dietary intake to avoid obesity
Hypoglycaemia Weakness/fatigue	Nausea Gastrointestinal complaints	Prevent episodes of hypoglycaemia
Increased levels of adrenocorticotropic hormone and melanocyte stimulating hormone give rise to hyperpigmentation of skin and mucous membrane	Hypotension Tachycardia	Ensure additional sodium intake (as in table salt) – increase intake in event of sweating, vomiting, diarrhoea Assessment and ongoing monitoring of cardiovascular status Frequent monitoring of vital signs, blood pressure Monitor compliance to treatment of replacement therapy of glucocorticoid and mineralocorticoids on long-term basis Assessment and monitoring for signs of overtreatment: • monitor growth and development and observe for signs of cushingoid features • regular follow-up and provision of ongoing support and education • encourage child to wear medic alert bracelet

syndrome). Other factors include abrupt withdrawal of exogenous sources of cortisone or failure to increase dosage during stress (Campbell & Glasper 1995).

This condition is rapid in onset. All symptoms as identified in chronic adrenocortical insufficiency are exaggerated. The child may present with circulation collapse, confusion or coma and therefore requires emergency interventions. Nursing care is focused on:

- fluid and electrolyte resuscitation
- intravenous administration of glucocorticoids until oral therapy becomes possible
- administration of mineralocorticoids when oral intake is tolerated
- treatment of the underlying illness.

Prolonged care and treatment, as for the child with chronic adrenocortical insufficiency, will be required.

Activity

Review Chapter 45 on caring for a critically ill child:
- Discuss how this information is relevant to the care of the child with acute adrenal insufficiency.

Primary Hyperaldosteronism

Primary hyperaldosteronism may be caused by a benign adrenal tumour or by adrenal hyperplasia. This condition results in increased sodium levels with water retention, and potassium depletion. Thus the condition is characterised by paraesthesia, tetany, weakness, polyuria, nocturnal enuresis, periodic paralysis, low serum potassium, elevated sodium levels, hypertension, metabolic acidosis, and production of a large volume of urine with a low specific gravity. Plasma and aldosterone levels are elevated, but other steroid levels are variable.

Treatment is with glucocorticoids or spironolactone, which blocks the effects of aldosterone, thereby promoting the excretion of sodium and water and preserving potassium (Hockenberry et al 2003). Subtotal or total adrenalectomy for hyperplasia may be necessary, and surgical removal of a tumour, if present.

The role of the nurse in relation to providing holistic care and treatment from the stage of diagnosis to long-term management of primary hyperaldosteronism is similar to that for other endocrine disorders. When surgery is indicated then involvement in pre- and postoperative care becomes the priority.

Phaeochromocytoma

Phaeochromocytoma is a tumour of the adrenal medulla but may be located wherever chromaffin tissue is present, e.g. sympathetic ganglia and carotid body. Physical manifestations are generally caused by excess secretion of catecholamines. Symptoms may include:

- increased anxiety, such as perspiration and headaches, palpitations tachycardia, hypertension and hyperglycaemia
- dizziness, weakness, nausea and vomiting with diarrhoea
- weight loss and anorexia
- blurring of vision and dilated pupils
- papilloedema, retinopathy and enlargement of the heart
- in severe cases, signs of congestive heart failure may be evident
- nervousness, excitability and overactivity.

Nursing Assessment and Diagnosis

A careful history of the onset of symptoms and association with stressful events is helpful in distinguishing between an organic and a psychological cause for the problem (Wong 1995).

Serum catecholamines are elevated, particularly when the child is symptomatic. Urinary excretion of catecholamines parallels serum levels. The tumour may be identified on CT scan or MRI.

Nursing Care and Management

Surgical removal of the tumour is the treatment of choice. Prior to surgery, the child's physical condition must be adequately stabilised. Manipulation of the tumour may cause sudden and profound, potentially fatal changes in blood pressure. Hypertension with associated tachycardia may be the result of excessive release of catecholamines during removal of the tumour. Hypotension may occur as a result of catecholamine withdrawal. A preoperative preparation requirement involves the administration of medication, aimed at inhibiting the effects of catecholamines. The major group of drugs used is the α-adrenergic blocking agents. β-adrenergic blocking agents may be required when α-adrenergic blocking agents are ineffective in controlling release of catecholamines alone. The wanted effect of preoperative drug administration is to lower the blood pressure and minimise the symptoms the child has previously presented with.

During the preoperative period, frequent recordings of clinical observations are required to monitor blood pressure and heart and respiratory rate in an effort to detect hypertensive episodes and observe for signs of congestive heart failure. Daily blood glucose monitoring is required to observe for signs of hyperglycaemia.

The child is likely to remain in hospital in the weeks prior to surgery because of the necessary preoperative preparation and monitoring. The effects of prolonged hospitalisation may increase emotional distress for the child and thus aggravate symptoms. Parental presence and involvement in the child's care must be encouraged. Parents must be fully informed about the child's condition so that they can promote an environment for the child that is as restful and as stress free as possible. They require detailed information regarding the child's surgery and complications that may arise as a result.

The child may require admission to the intensive care unit following surgery until the condition is stable postoperatively.

WWW

Review the Department of Health's *Guidelines in good practice in consent* at:
- http://www.doh.gov.uk/publications

THE GONADS: OVARIES AND TESTES

A variety of abnormalities in chromosomal distribution, gonadal differentiation, gonadal function, testerone synthesis and action, or adrenal function can lead to aberrant development of internal or external genital structures as described under the section congenital adrenal hyperplasia.

PowerPoint

Access the companion PowerPoint presentation and review:
- abnormalities in female pubertal development and ovarian function.

Before proceeding with the next section of this chapter, on diabetes mellitus, review:
- endocrine regulation of blood glucose.

Diabetes Mellitus

Diabetes comprises a group of disorders with many different causes, all of which are characterised by a raised blood glucose level. This is the result of a lack of the hormone insulin and/or an inability to respond to insulin. There are two main types of diabetes, type 1 and type 2:

- Type 1: characterised by a cessation of insulin production in the pancreas.
- Type 2: caused by an inadequate production of insulin necessary for the body's needs. The cells in the body not being able to respond to the insulin that is produced often accompanies type 2 diabetes.

In childhood, the incidence of type 1 is greater than type 2 and is therefore more likely to be encountered in practice.

However, the incidence of type 2 is increasing at all ages and across races, and may now account for between one-fifth and one-third of all new cases of diabetes. Peak ages of presentation are 12–14 years (DoH 2001).

Type 1 Diabetes

The aetiology of type 1 diabetes is not completely understood. It is thought to be the result from a cellular-mediated autoimmune response of the insulin-producing cells of the pancreatic islets (Fig. 34.6). This response results in recruitment of cytoxic lymphocytes and production of anti-insulin and anti-islet cell antibodies, which progressively destroy the beta cells of the islets of Langerhans in the pancreas. Susceptibility to immunological damage has been associated with strong genetic determinants in combination with environmental factors. Environmental triggers of this immune process that have been proposed include viruses, cows milk protein and chemical toxins.

ASSESSMENT AND DIAGNOSIS

The classic presenting symptoms of diabetes are polyuria, polyphagia, polydipsia, weight loss and lethargy. Onset may be acute, precipitated by the stress of an acute illness, or chronic and insidious over weeks or months. The diagnosis is made by finding glucosuria on routine urinalysis. Diabetes is increasingly diagnosed at an earlier stage of illness and, as a result, the symptoms of ketonuria, ketonaemia and secondary acidosis have become less common. However, severe vomiting, dehydration, abdominal pain, hypovolaemic shock, hyperventilation due to acidosis, drowsiness and coma are signs and symptoms of later stages of the illness.

Diagnosis is usually confirmed in a symptomatic child by finding a markedly raised random plasma glucose (> 11.1 mmol/L), glycosuria and ketonuria (Lissauer & Clayden 1998). A fasting blood glucose level over 7 mmol/L and/or a raised glycosylated haemoglobin (HbA1c) will help clarify the diagnosis. Glycohaemoglobin is formed when glucose is bound non-enzymatically to free amino groups of the haemoglobin molecule. The percentage of glycohaemoglobin correlates with the mean blood glucose over the life span of the red blood cell thus glycaemic control over the proceeding 8–16 weeks can be determined.

NURSING CARE AND MANAGEMENT

The goals of treatment and nursing care aim to avoid episodes of severe hypoglycaemia and to prevent chronic complications associated with type 1 diabetes. The five fundamental aspects of treatment necessary to obtain safe and effective metabolic control are:

1. establishing the appropriate insulin dosages and regimes
2. establishing appropriate diet
3. exercise
4. stress/illness management
5. blood glucose and urine ketone monitoring.

Establishing Appropriate Insulin Dosages and Regimes

Initial Care and Management
The initial management will depend on the child's clinical condition. Those in advanced diabetic ketoacidosis require urgent hospitalisation for treatment. Most newly presenting children can be managed on subcutaneous insulin, but intravenous fluids and an insulin infusion is required if the child is vomiting or is dehydrated. Newly presenting children not requiring intravenous therapy may not require admission to hospital. A child presenting with moderate hyperglycaemia without acidaemia, who is clinically stable and can take fluids orally, may be managed at home with the support of medical and nursing diabetic specialists.

PowerPoint

Access the companion PowerPoint presentation and review the section on insulin therapy: Requirements of new-onset diabetes for more detailed information.

Establishing the correct dosage of daily insulin requires adjustments to be made based on food recently eaten or to be eaten and forthcoming exercise in addition to blood

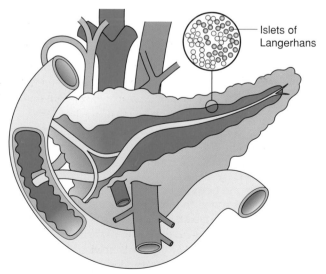

Islets of Langerhans

Fig. 34.6 • The pancreas.

glucose levels. In adolescence, due to insulin resistance, insulin requirements increase. These higher doses are reduced at the end of growth and puberty.

After the initial correct dosage of insulin is achieved, daily adjustments are usually not needed. However, small decreases may be made for heavy activity. Most children receive at least two injections of insulin daily. However, some children and families are willing to undertake multiple injections per day. In this case, the evening dose of insulin is often split, with the fast-acting insulin being administered before dinner and the longer-acting insulin administered at bedtime. The most common combinations are mixtures of a short and intermediate or longer-acting insulin. Insulin via subcutaneous injection can be administered by pen injector or by needle and syringe, if preferred by the child.

Needle Phobia

Some children and young people with diabetes present with needle phobia. This can pose a real difficulty in that it may affect treatment and thus diabetic control as the child or young person may forget or omit injections and blood testing or refuse to go on to a multidosing regime because it means more injections. Needle phobia is a defined medical condition, the cause of which is not entirely known (Hamilton 1995). It may be the result of previous unpleasant experiences relating to injections or venepuncture. Children and young people with needle phobia may be more sensitive to pain during these procedures. However, many may be needle phobic as a combination of fear, strange environment and the pain of injection.

Nursing Assessment of Needle Phobia

It is important that needle phobia is recognised as a very real problem and that assumptions are not made that the child or adolescent is simply being non-compliant. The children's nurse needs to recognise the significance of the symptoms that present and are associated with anxiety:

- dry mouth
- palpitations
- sweating
- trembling
- overbreathing
- dizziness
- feeling sick
- fainting.

Developments in injection technology have produced shorter, finer needles, which has resulted in less discomfort associated with frequent subcutaneous injections (Birkebaek et al 1998). To help with needle phobia a simple device such as Penmate hides the needle from view (Fig. 34.7).

Fig. 34.7 • The Penmate (top) with needle hidden; the Novo Pen (bottom) has a 6-mm needle.

The systems of insulin delivery must be discussed, demonstrated and practiced, and the chosen method must be acceptable to the child and adolescent. Alternative methods of insulin delivery are currently being explored, for example, use of needle-free injection methods that deliver insulin and other medication (growth hormone) under pressure from a gas cartridge. Other approaches include the use of insulin inhalers (Wallis 2003).

Children and young people who present with psychological problems associated with needle phobia may benefit from the support of a clinical psychologist because they need to be encouraged to communicate their fears. Play interventions should be undertaken by a play specialist or a children's nurse who has attended a needle phobia workshop and has demonstrated competency in practical assessment.

Activity

Review stages of needle play at:
- http://www.nahps.org.uk/needle.htm

Evidence-based Practice

To ensure the most reliable and consistent absorption of insulin, injections should be made into subcutaneous adipose tissue. There is a difference in absorption rate and duration of different insulins when injected into subcutaneous fat and muscle. Intramuscular injection speeds up absorption and can lead to unexpected hypoglycaemia (King 2003, Polak et al 1996, Strauss et al 2002, Thow et al 1990).

Before mixing insulin in the same syringe, there is a need to establish that this procedure does not change the pharmacokinetics of both types of insulin, otherwise the practice should obviously be avoided. Cartridges (Fig. 34.8) and vials containing predetermined mixtures of insulin need to

Fig. 34.8 • An insulin cartridge.

be adequately mixed prior to administration. Insulin is absorbed at different rates from different sites, so routine is required for consistent absorption. Injections into the arms or stomach is recommended in the morning, and into the legs and buttocks in the evening (Hayes 2003). In addition, sites used need to be rotated, otherwise fat atrophy will develop, making insulin absorption erratic.

Continuous subcutaneous infusion is an alternative method for insulin administration using a small, battery-powered pump.

Blood Glucose Monitoring

Frequent blood glucose determinations allow:

- more accurate adjustment of insulin dose
- enhanced patient education
- identification of emergency situations.

Realistic goals for blood glucose monitoring need to be agreed with the child, with compromises reached about the frequency of monitoring (Fig. 34.9).

PowerPoint

Access the companion PowerPoint presentation and review the section on blood glucose monitoring for more detailed information.

Fig. 34.9 • Blood glucose monitoring equipment.

Urine testing is always recommended when a high blood glucose level is suspected or when there is difficulty with blood glucose monitoring. Urinary ketones should be checked during intercurrent infection or when control is poor.

The measurement of glycosylated haemoglobin (HbA1c) is particularly helpful as a guide to overall control over the previous 6 weeks and should be checked every 2–3 months.

Diet

Nutritional requirements for the diabetic child should be individualised, with consideration given to cultural eating habits and other lifestyle matters. Children need sufficient calories to satisfy the requirements for growth and development, as well as achieving the best possible blood glucose control.

Meal times need to correspond with the timing and action of insulin administered. Meals and snacks must therefore be consumed according to the peak action of insulin, and the total number of calories and nutrients must be consistent from day to day. Approximately 55–60% of calories should be derived from unrefined carbohydrates, less than 30% should be derived from fats, and 15–20% should be derived from proteins. A meal plan based on the individual child's usual food intake should be determined and used as a basis for integrating insulin therapy into the usual eating and exercise pattern (McCance & Huether 1998). The constant release of insulin into the circulation makes the child prone to hypoglycaemia between the three main meals unless a snack is taken between meals and at bedtime. The distribution of calories should be calculated to suit the activity pattern of the child. A larger snack is required when the child is expected to engage in additional physical activity. More flexible meal planning is an option for those receiving multiple injections or insulin via continuous infusion.

WWW

Visit Diabetes UK website for nutritional guidelines for diabetes healthcare professionals at:

- http://www.diabetes.org.uk

Exercise

Regular daily exercise is important for children with diabetes because it:

- fosters a sense of well being
- helps insulin sensitivity
- helps maintain proper weight, blood pressure, and blood fat levels
- helps promote optimal physical and psychosocial growth and development.

Hypoglycaemia during exercise, or in the 2–8 hours after exercise, should be prevented by careful monitoring of blood sugar before, during and after exercise. This may be achieved by reducing the dosage of insulin that is expected to peak at the time of exercise and by taking extra snacks. The longer and more vigorous the activity, the more food should be eaten before exercising (Chase & Eisenbarth 2003) and the use of drinks containing dextrose should be available during the period of exercise.

COMPLICATIONS OF TYPE I DIABETES

Hypoglycaemia

See Table 34.7.

Diabetic Ketoacidosis

Diabetic ketoacidosis is a condition requiring emergency medical treatment and nursing care. The condition occurs most often in children with type 1 diabetes, however the increasing incidence of childhood obesity in the UK and the inevitable rise in type 2 diabetes from an early age may present with the associated risk of ketoacidosis and ketonuria (Drake et al 2002). Episodes of ketoacidodis usually result from:

- missed insulin injections, therefore giving rise to an increased blood glucose level
- excessive glucagon
- excessive glucocorticoids
- infection or other illness
- vomiting trauma, burns, surgery
- stress.

All of these conditions result:

- In a lack of insulin, which means that glucose in the blood cannot be taken up into the cells, fat is broken down to provide energy.
- Fat is broken down rapidly and incompletely, producing ketone bodies in excess of the tissue cells' ability to metabolise them.
- Alterations in liver metabolism leads to further ketone production, which is accelerated when glucagon levels–rise.
- Muscle tissue is unable to utilise these organic acids, which further contributes to an accumulation of these acids and acetone in the blood that will eventually result in acidosis with low bicarbonate levels—ketoacidosis.
- Ketones have two other effects in addition to acidosis: they have a central action giving rise to nausea and vomiting.
- Ketone excretion in the urine gives rise to osmotic diuresis resulting in loss of Na^+, K^+ and Cl^-.
- High blood glucose gives rise to glycosuria and osmotic diuresis increasing cellular dehydration and renal hypofusion.
- In addition, moderate or large amounts of ketones may be detected in the child's urine. Ketonuria, if untreated, may progress to ketoacidosis, which may be accompanied by deep breathing (Kussmaul respirations) and excessive weakness.

Characteristics of Diabetic Ketoacidosis

There is insidious onset over several days. Presenting symptoms include:

Table 34.7 Characteristics of Hypoglycaemia

Characteristics	Nursing considerations
Blood glucose < 3.3 mmol/L	Requires immediate administration of fast-acting sugar to raise blood glucose
Hunger, weakness, shaking, sweating	If a meal is not anticipated within the next hour a snack—carbohydrate, fat and protein is
Drowsiness at unusual times	recommended (Finberg & Kleinman 2002)
Headache, behavioural changes	Check blood glucose level after 30 minutes
Loss of consciousness	Assess the need for additional carbohydrate or possibility of hyperglycaemia
Convulsions	If child presents with seizure or in a coma administer subcutaneous glucagon as directed –
	may cause nausea and vomiting so need to administer oral carbohydrate when child is awake
	Check consistency in routine
	Check that correct insulin dosage is being administered
	Encourage regular blood glucose monitoring
	Encourage controlled snacking
	Encourage child/family compliance
	Ensure all involved with the child on a daily basis is educated and trained in recognition and
	treatment of hypoglycaemia

- polyuria, thirst, glycosuria and general weakness
- anorexia, nausea, vomiting
- deep/rapid respirations (Kussmaul)
- abdominal pain and muscle cramps
- dry skin and mucous membrane
- dark and sunken eyes due to dehydration
- hypotension, weak pulse
- hypothermia due to peripheral vasodilation
- drowsiness and coma are late signs.

Management and Nursing

Management and nursing care of diabetic ketoacidosis consists of rapid assessment and treatment which is based on four physiological principles:

1. restoration of fluid volume
2. inhibition of lipolysis and return to glucose utilisation
3. replacement of body salts
4. correction of acidosis.

WWW

Review calculations for fluid and insulin requirements in the guidelines produced by Diabetes UK (*Guidelines for the management of diabetic ketoacidosis*) and the British Society of Paediatric Endocrinology and Diabetes at:
- http://www.diabetes.org.uk
- http://www.bsped.org.uk/dka.htm

Nursing care requires ongoing assessment and monitoring of:

- neurological status: to observe for early signs of cerebral oedema
- respiratory function: record respiratory rate and depth and SaO_2 to identify need for O_2 administration
- blood for blood gas analysis, blood sugar, urea and electrolyte estimation
- cardiovascular functioning: ECG monitoring observe for flat T wave, which may indicate hypokalaemia
- regular blood pressure and pulse monitoring
- gastrointestinal problems: if child is vomiting there may be a need to pass a nasogastric tube to ensure safety and comfort as well as enabling a more accurate record of total fluid output
- monitoring the administration of insulin, and administration of intravenous fluids and electrolyte supplements as prescribed (Fig. 34.10)
- accurate intake and output, observe for levels of glycosuria and ketones

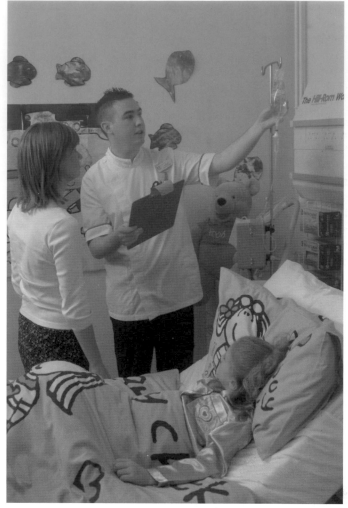

Fig. 34.10 • 8-year-old girl requiring intravenous therapy.

- regular monitoring of blood glucose to ensure that insulin requirements are adjusted accordingly.

The child's condition should continue to be monitored until blood glucose returns to normal and the urine is free from ketones and oral feeding is established. Any concerns regarding the child's condition must be reported immediately to a senior doctor. The evaluation of all nursing interventions must be accurately reported on and recorded. Throughout this period attention is required to hygiene and comfort needs of the child. Child and parents require to be supported and reassured and explanations for all interventions need to be provided.

Chronic Complications

Chronic complications are associated with chronic hyperglycaemia and include retinopathy, nephropathy, neuropathy, hyperlipidaemia and hypertension. Improvement in glycaemic control will help reduce these risks. All young people with diabetes will receive regular surveillance for long-term complications (DoH 2001).

ADOLESCENCE AND TYPE I DIABETES

Normal adolescent physical, psychosexual and developmental maturation is affected by diabetes (Lissauer & Clayden 1998). In addition, diabetes is often more difficult to control due to hormonal changes of puberty as well as the emotional difficulties associated with adolescence. For some, this stage of development will present with behavioural changes such as denial, indifference or depression about their illness. In addition, there may be an unwillingness to conform to treatment regimes, which may give rise to conflict with family and health professionals. There may be a tendency to avoid aspects of their diabetic management, e.g. omit insulin injections or manipulate the regime, and ignore dietary needs. Blood glucose monitoring may not be carried out or results may be falsified. Many teenage girls experiment with crash diets at some time, which is likely to cause major problems in diabetic control.

This is a time when the young person should be encouraged to take increasing control for their diabetes. It may be helpful to identify short-term goals for them and ensure that effort to improve their control is communicated promptly and enthusiastically. A united team approach, with agreement of the essentials they wish to promote and clear, unambiguous guidelines for health and diabetic management is necessary. Peer group pressure may be utilised to promote health, especially in relation to smoking and alcohol consumption. Holiday camps provide opportunities for young diabetics to meet and learn about their diabetic management.

CHILD AND FAMILY EDUCATION

The primary goal in caring for children and young people with diabetes is to enable them and their families to manage their own lifestyle and condition, by providing support and structured education as well as drugs and treatment (DoH 2001). Therefore, a coordinated, multidisciplinary team approach to care and management in partnership with the child and family is essential if the following long-term outcomes are to be achieved:

- normal growth and development
- maintaining as normal a home and school life as possible
- good diabetic control, appropriate knowledge, good technique and self-reliance
- avoidance of hypoglycaemia
- prevention of long-term complications.

This will be reflected in the child's personal record that contains the clinical record of care, treatment and management. A personal diabetes record should include the following:

- An agreed care plan, including education and the personal goals of the child and family in relation to care and treatment.
- Information as to how the child's diabetes is to be managed until the next review to foster greater understanding and ownership of the goals of diabetes care.
- Identification of social and educational needs, how they will be met and who will be responsible.
- Identification of the named contact (DoH 2003).

Central Role of the Nurse

The children's nurse has a central role in the assessment and planning of care aimed at meeting the holistic needs of the child and family during the initial stages following diagnosis through to long-term care and management. As such, the nurse will be able to determine the process by which education about diabetes for all family members might be best achieved. The care plan should consider the need for involving siblings in the care and thus reflect a family centred approach whereby collaboration and facilitation and thus partnership is evident. The children's nurse may be the person who acts as the named contact person for the child and family, helping them to access the services available to help and support them and enabling them to see other members of the multidisciplinary team as appropriate. This team should include a paediatrician with training in diabetes, paediatric dietitian with an interest in diabetes, and specialised support obtained from adolescent psychology and psychiatry services. Effective management of diabetes and increases life expectancy and reduces the risk of complications developing (Diabetes UK 2003a).

Activity

Review Chapters 44 and 45:
- How does the knowledge of both chapters relate to the care of the child with diabetes?

The child and all caregivers need to learn about diabetes and how to give insulin injections and perform home glucose monitoring, as well as monitor dietary requirements and recognise signs of hypoglycaemia or hyperglycaemia. This requires commitment and active involvement and support from the children's nurse and other members of the multidisciplinary team.

WWW

Topics to be covered in an educational programme have been included in the National Service Framework for Diabetes: Delivery Strategy (DoH 2003):
- http://www.goh.gov/planning2003-2006/index.htm
Familiarise yourself with the four main areas of this programme: nature of diabetes, day-to-day management of diabetes, specific issues in relation to diabetes, living with diabetes.

Home management at the time of diagnosis provides immediate opportunities for the children's nurse to educate the child, parents and others in relation to diabetes. Education requirements should be adopted to suit the needs of the child and family and provided at a rate that is in keeping with what suits them (McEvilly 2003). The stress imposed on the family around this time may lead to feelings of shock, denial, sadness, anger, fear and guilt. These feeling may be greatly intensified when the reality that diabetes is a life-long chronic condition that impacts almost every aspect of life is recognised. At this stage, the child and family may require only the essential information and skills to be learned with more intense information been provided later. Books, teaching aids and website addresses might enhance the learning process and provide guidance for child and parent in the absence of the nurse (Fig. 34.11). Opportunities should be made for child and family to explore their perceptions of the impact of diabetes on their lives and the implications of care required by the child, and the immediate problems they envisage. Meeting with other parents and children with diabetes may provide additional support.

Parents need to understand the positive support their child will need throughout childhood and into adolescence to optimise physical, psychological, intellectual, educational and social development. This must include a period of independence that the young person may be enabled to take on the responsibility and develop the confidence to be self-caring (McEvilly 2003).

The provision of education for school staff and others involved in the school day has been identified as one of the key interventions in the National Service Framework for Standards in Diabetes (DoH 2001). It is essential that they receive information and support to enable them to understand the importance of regular mealtimes, requirements to undertake physical activity and to recognise the signs of hypoglycaemia and to know what action is required.

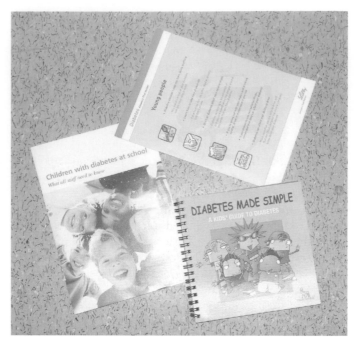

Fig. 34.11 • Examples of information available for child, family and others.

Type 2 Diabetes

This form of diabetes is generally associated with obesity and usually presents at the time of puberty. Failure of adequate insulin secretion over time implies either pancreatic exhaustion or a genetic defect in insulin secretion unmasked by the increasing insulin resistance of progressive obesity. Visceral fat produces a cytokine hormone called tissue necrosis factor (TNF), which desensitises the insulin receptor to insulin (Qi & Pekala 2000). The increase in type 2 diabetes in adolescents mirrors the epidemic of obesity at all ages in developed countries and in nations with emerging economies. The incidence of type 2 diabetes is increasing in children as the prevalence of childhood obesity continues to increase. Lack of exercise (a sedentary lifestyle) is recognised as a risk factor for obesity and diabetes mellitus. Ahn et al (2003) have suggested that diabetes is significantly less common in the physically fit population. Excessive nutrition combined with decreased activity contributes to obesity. Studies associating behaviour, especially eating and drinking, with health outcomes suggest an association with cardiovascular disease, cancer and diabetes (Parlimentary Office of Science and Technology 2003, Williams et al 1999). However, there appears to be a high prevalence of type 2 diabetes in African, Hispanic and Asian populations.

Type 2 diabetes thus presents with a major public health issue with profound implications for health because of the unfavourable activity of high blood insulin levels, which cause major problems for the person with insulin resistance (Howdle & Wilkin 2001). These problems include a varying degree of hyperglycaemia, hypertension, coronary heart disease and other vascular complications.

ASSESSMENT AND DIAGNOSIS

Clinical findings may be similar to type 1 diabetes mellitus in childhood, or they may be milder and develop more slowly and thus be unrecognised as type 2 diabetes. Whereas type 2 diabetes can mimic type 1 with ketones at presentation, it is distinguished by the presence of insulin resistance. Hyperglycaemia leads to glysuria with osmotic diuresis and symptoms of polyuria and polydipsia. Increased appetite and weight loss occur. If early symptoms are not recognised, diabetic ketoacidosis can occur, with symptoms of nausea, vomiting, abdominal pain, tachypnoea and lethargy (Finberg & Kleinman 2002). The clinical presentation between type 1 and type 2 diabetes mellitus may be indistinguishable. However, as the number of children with type 2 diabetes increases, it becomes increasingly important to classify their diabetes correctly so that appropriate therapy may be instituted (American Diabetic Association 2000).

Diagnosis is confirmed if fasting blood glucose concentrations are greater than 7 mmol/L on two separate days, or if random glucose concentrations are 11 mmol/L on two separate occasions. Urinalysis may reveal ketonuria and glycosuria.

NURSING CARE AND MANAGEMENT

There is a limited amount of evidence on which to base treatment strategies due to type 2 diabetes being a relatively new phenomenon in children's nursing (Howdle & Wilkin 2001).

Some children with type 2 diabetes can be managed effectively with a diet that is sufficiently balanced to meet the needs for normal growth but moderately restricted in calories and low in fat with increased physical activity. The benefits of exercise have been highlighted under care and management of type 1 diabetes.

Evidence-based Practice

Structured programmes of lifestyle change which emphasise weight loss (5–7% of body weight) by reduced energy and fat intake and increased physical activity can reduce the risk of overweight people with impaired glucose intolerance developing type 2 diabetes (Diabetes UK 2003b).

If this regime is not sufficient to achieve adequate glycaemic control then oral hypoglycaemic drugs will be required. These drugs appear to not have been tested for safety and efficacy in children. If glycaemic control is still not achieved then the child will be commenced on insulin. Care and management is similar to that for type 1 diabetes.

Due to the nature and presentation of type 2 diabetes, which contribute to long-term complications, preventative measures need to be developed whereby children in at-risk families, a positive family history of type 2 diabetes, obese children, children of certain race or ethnic group or those who present with signs of insulin resistance need to be screened. The American Diabetic Association (2000) recommends that a fasting blood glucose is carried out every 2 years, starting at age of 10 years or at the onset of puberty if it occurs at a younger age.

Those involved in care of children have an obligation to encourage lifestyle modification that might delay or prevent the onset of type 2 diabetes. Prevention and management of obesity requires a range of coordinated policies to improve diet and physical activity level in early years, at schools, and in families and communities.

As type 2 diabetes is likely to become increasingly common, it is essential that nurses appreciate the risk of unrecognised type 2 diabetes associated with obesity because early investigation and appropriate treatment may delay the onset of complications (Drake et al 2002).

Maturity Onset Diabetes of the Young (Mody)

MODY is a rare form of diabetes in the children occurring as a result of gene abnormalities and has four main characteristics:

- Diabetes presents at a young age.
- Runs in families through several generations: a parent with MODY has a 50% chance of passing it on to their child. This is called autosomal dominant inheritance.
- Children with MODY do not always need insulin treatment and can often be treated with oral glycaemic therapy or meal planning alone.
- Children with MODY do not produce enough insulin. This is different to type 2 diabetes, where the individual produces sufficient insulin but does not respond to it.

The clinical spectrum is broad, ranging from asymptomatic hyperglycaemia to a severe acute presentation. MODY has been reported in all races and ethnicities.

Diagnosis is based on molecular testing, currently not available to all. Until such testing becomes commonplace, children with MODY should be classified as having the type of diabetes that best fits their clinical picture and which requires appropriate care, management, education and ongoing support and follow up.

Discussion of the Scenarios

JUNE: GRAVE'S DISEASE

Observations necessary to assess June's need to plan her nursing interventions include:

- Vital signs of temperature, pulse and blood pressure may be elevated and June may complain of palpitations due to hyperthyroid state.
- Observation of skin for warmth, moistness and flushed appearance.
- Respiratory difficulties may present as a result of hypervascularity and enlargement of the thyroid gland.
- Enlargement of the thyroid gland may be evident.
- Enlargement and protrusion of the eye balls leading to irritation, pain, lacrimation, photophobia and blurred vision.
- Monitoring of height may indicate a degree of accelerated growth and development.
- Monitoring weight may indicate a loss despite having an increased appetite.
- June may complain of excessive weakness and lack of ability to engage in usual activities.
- Observation of her emotional state, nervous excitability and mood stability is necessary as there may be associated hyperactivity of the sympathatic division of the autonomic nervous system.

June's Specific Care Requirements

The symptoms of hyperthyroidism may fluctuate with spontaneous remissions and exacerbations. Mild cases may require no treatment. The condition is generally treated with medical interventions and/or radiation therapy.

Bed rest is advisable at the beginning of medical treatment. This treatment is aimed at controlling symptoms of nervous instability, tachycardia, and hypertension that may require the administration of β-adrenergic blocking agents (propranolol, atenolol). Continual monitoring of vital signs is necessary to evaluate effectiveness of interventions and monitor for early signs of complications.

Drugs that interfere with thyroid hormone synthesis, namely carbimazole or propylthiouracil may be prescribed according to the individual needs of the child. Treatment with antithyroid drugs must be continued for at least 2–3 years, with the smallest drug dosage that will produce a symptom-free state in the child.

When response to medical treatment is not achieved then radiation therapy with radioactive iodine may be considered. In some cases, radioiodine is the initial treatment of choice considered (Kappy et al 2003).

In hypothyroidism and hyperthyroidism, the aim of care is to achieve an optimal level of thyroxine that will enable growth and development, including enhancement of intellectual ability. June and her parents need to understand the nature of the condition, the aims and different types of treatment, including dosages of prescribed medication and repeat prescriptions, as well as the signs of under and over treatment The consequences of non-compliance needs to be discussed. As with all other conditions the provision of literature and appropriate website addresses as identified may enhance understanding.

Attendance at clinics is essential to:

- monitor June's response to medication
- assess growth and development
- provide the opportunity for June and her family to discuss their fears or problems associated with the care and management of the condition
- enable them to meet other families who have been caring for their children with similar problems which for some may prove beneficial.

The children's nurse can remain as the named contact person and through assessment in collaboration and negotiation with the child and family can plan the education and ongoing support required.

Activity

Review Chapter 46:
- Discuss how this information may relate to the care of the child with hyperthyroidism or hyperthyroidism.

CUSHING SYNDROME

Cushing syndrome results from prolonged exposure of the tissues to glucocorticoids. It may be caused by primary dysfunction as a result of neoplasm or adenoma of the adrenal cortex, or by hypersecretion of adrenocorticotropic hormone as a result of a pituitary tumour. In addition, Cushing-like syndrome may be an adverse effect from long-term exogenous administration of cortisone used in the treatment of allergic, autoimmune, neoplastic, haematologic, skin and other diseases.

Clinical Manifestations

Cushing syndrome is an uncommon syndrome in children and young people (Boscaro et al 2002). However, the resulting hypercortisol causes considerable morbidity in childhood and adolescence (Storr et al 2003). The earliest and most common signs in almost all presenting with the condition are:

- Generalised obesity, which is characterised by facial rounding (moon face) and 'buffalo hump' (Fig. 34.12). These results from accumulation of adipose tissue in the trunk, facial and cervical areas.

- Transient weight gain from sodium and water retention may occur due to the mineralocorticoid effects of cortisol.

- Growth retardation or complete arrest of growth is present in all but 10% of affected children (Chrousos 2002).

- Other clinical manifestations include sleep disturbance, irritability and depression.

- Muscle weakness and fatigue, due to protein wasting is caused by the catabolic effects of cortisol.

- Loss of protein matrix leads to osteoporosis, with pathological fractures.

- Loss of collagen also causes weakening and thinning of the skin through which capillaries become visible. These

changes, together with fluid retention, account for the characteristic purple striae.

- Loss of collagenous support makes blood vessels more susceptible to rupture, leading to bruising. Thin atrophied skin is easily damaged and leads to skin breaks and ulceration (McCance & Huether 1998).

- Hyperpigmentation is associated with high serum levels of adrenocorticotropic hormone, which is thought to increase melanotropic activity. Thus skin, mucous membrane and hair acquire a characteristic bronze colour.

- Hypertension due to increased vascular sensitivity to catecholamines, which are increased as a result of increased levels of cortisol.

- Elevated levels of cortisol also cause suppression of the immune system, which increases the child's susceptibility to infection and poor wound healing.

- Amenorrhoea, advancement or arrest of pubertal development may be encountered.

- Glucose intolerance occurs because of cortisol-induced insulin resistance and increased gluconeogenesis and glycogen in the liver.

Assessment and Diagnosis

Confirmation of excess cortisol levels may be obtained indirectly by ascertaining fasting blood glucose levels for hyperglycaemia, and serum electrolyte levels for hypokalaemia and alkalosis (Campbell & Glasper 1995).

Elevated levels of urinary free cortisol and plasma cortisol obtained in the evening will further aid confirmation of diagnosis.

A dexamethasone (cortisone) test may be used to confirm the diagnosis and confirm the cause. Administration of exogenous cortisone normally suppresses production of adrenocorticotropic hormone. Cortisol levels remain elevated in children with Cushing syndrome. This helps differentiate between children who are obese and those who appear to have Cushingoid features (Campbell & Glasper 1995).

Computed tomography (CT) or magnetic resonance imaging (MRI) may be carried out when an adrenocorticotropic-hormone-secreting adenoma of the pituitary is suspected.

Care and Management

Treatment is specific according to the cause for hyperadrenocorticosteroid levels. Therefore differentiation among pituitary, adrenal and other causes is essential for effective treatment. For adrenal and pituitary causes, treatment generally involves surgical, irridiation and postoperative replacement of cortical hormones.

When Cushingoid features are a result of steroid therapy, the effects may be lessened by administration of the drug in

Fig. 34.12 • Cushing syndrome.

the morning, as this maintains the normal diurnal pattern of cortisol secretion. In addition, an alternate day schedule allows the anterior pituitary an opportunity to maintain more normal hypothalamic–pituitary–adrenal control mechanisms (Campbell & Glasper 1995).

Activity

Review Chapters 18, 45 and 46:
- Discuss how this information is relevant to the care of the child with Cushing syndrome.

Summary

This chapter has presented an overview of the endocrine system and associated problems that may present for the child and family. Care of the child and family with reference to health promotion and education has been significantly addressed. Development of knowledge and understanding has been enhanced through active participation and the companion PowerPoint presentation.

Acknowledgements

Thanks to James Davis, Graphic Designer, Media Services, Queen's University Belfast for his work in producing diagrams of the endocrine system and outline of a child with Cushing Syndrome. Thanks to Paul Morris, Clinical Skills Technician, School of Nursing, Queen's University Belfast for photographic support and also for allowing his daughter to be involved.

Thanks also to my colleague Patricia McNeilly, Teaching Fellow, and Michael Ward, student nurse, for involvement in photographic evidence. Finally, thanks to Kevin Campbell, Clinical Skills Technician, School of Nursing, Queen's University Belfast for allowing his daughter to participate.

References

Ahn NC et al 2003 Insulin densitivity in physically fit and unfit children of parents with type 2 diabetes. Diabetic Medicine 21:59–63

American Diabetic Association 2000 Type 2 diabetes in children and adolescents. Diabetic Care 23(3):381–389

Birkebaek N et al 1998 Cutis/subcutis thickness at insulin injection sites and localization of simulated insulin boluses in children with type 1 diabetes mellitus: need for individualization of injection technique. Diabetic Medicine 15(11):965–971

Boscaro M, Nicoletta S, Scarda A et al 2002 Anticoagulant prophylaxis markedly reduces thromboembolic complications in Cushing's syndrome. Journal of Clinical Endocrinology and Metabolism 87(8):3662–3666

Bryant J, Care C, Milne R 2004 Recombinant growth hormone for idiopathic short stature in children and adolescence (Cochrane Review). Cochrane Library, issue 1. Wiley, Chichester. Online. Available at: http://www.update-software-com/abstracts

Campbell S, Glasper EA 1995 Whaley and Wong's children's nursing. Mosby, London

Charmandari E, Brook CGD, Hindmarsh PC 2002 Why is management of patients with classical congenital adrenal hyperplasia more difficult at puberty? Archives of Diseases in Childhood 86(4):266–269

Chase HP, Eisenbarth GS 2003 In: Hay WW, Hayward AR, Levin MJ, Sondheimer JM (eds) Current pediatric diagnosis and treatment, 16th edn. McGraw-Hill, London

Chrousos GP 2002 In: Finberg L, Kleinman RE (eds) Saunders manual of pediatric practice, 2nd edn. WB Saunders, London

Cuttler L 2002 In: Finberg L, Kleinman RE (eds) Saunders manual of pediatric practice, 2nd edn. WB Saunders, London

Department of Health (DoH) 2001 National Service Framework for Diabetes: Standards. Department of Health, London

Department of Health (DoH) 2003 National Service Framework for Diabetes: delivery strategy. Department of Health, London

Desrosiers P 2002 Online. Available at: http://www.magicfoundation.org/divisions/ftt.htm

Diabetes UK 2003a CREST: report of the Northern Ireland Task Force on Diabetes. Diabetes UK, London

Diabetes UK 2003b Guidelines for the management of diabetic ketoacidosis in children and adolescents. Diabetic medicine. 20:786–807. Online. Available at: http://www.diabetes.org.uk

Drake AJ, Smith A, Betts PR et al 2002 Type 2 diabetes in obese white children. Archives of Disease in Childhood 86:207–208

Finberg L, Kleinman RE (eds) 2002 Saunders manual of pediatric practice, 2nd edn. Elsevier Science, London

Frid A, Linde B 1993 Clinically important differences in insulin absorption from the abdomen in IDDM. Diabetes Research in Clinical Practice 21:2–3, 137–141

Hall DMB 2000 Growth monitoring. Archives of Diseases in Children 82:10–15

Hamilton JG 1995 Needle phobia: a neglected diagnosis. Journal of Family Practice 41(2):169–175

Hayes P 2003 In: Barnes K (ed) Paediatrics. A clinical guide for nurse practitioners. Butterworth Heinemann, London

Hockenberry MJ, Wilson D, Winkelstein ML, Kline NE 2003 Wong's nursing care of infants and children, 7th edn. Mosby, London

Howdle S, Wilkin T 2001 Type 2 diabetes in children. Nursing Standard 15(18):38–42

Kappy MS, Steelman JW, Travers SH, Zeitler PS 2003 In: Hay WW, Hayward AR, Levin MJ, Sondheimer JM (eds) Current pediatric diagnosis and treatment, 16th edn. McGraw-Hill, London

King L 2003 Subcutaneous insulin injection technique. Nursing Standard 17(34):45–51

Lissauer T, Clayden G 1998 Illustrated textbook of paediatrics. Mosby, London

McCance KL, Huether SE 1998 Pathophysiology. The biologic basis for disease in adults and children, 3rd edn. Mosby, London

McEvilly A 2003 In: Barnes K (ed) Paediatrics: a clinical guide for nurse practitioners. Butterworth Heineman, London

Miller WL 2002 In: Finberg L, Kleinman RE (eds) Saunders manual of pediatric practice, 2nd edn. WB Saunders, London

Nairn J, Moore BJ 2002 The role of nurses in providing educational support to growth hormone deficient children, adolescents and their families. Neonatal, Paediatric and Child Health Nursing 5(1):10–13

National Institute for Clinical Excellence (NICE) 2002 Guidance on the use of human growth hormone (somatropin) in children with growth failure. NICE, London

Parks JS 2002 In: Finberg L, Kleinman RE (eds) Saunders manual of pediatric practice. WB Saunders, London

Parlimentary Office of Science and Technology 2003 Childhood obesity. Postnote, September, Report 205

Polak S et al 1996 Subcutaneous or intramuscular injections of insulin in children. Are we injecting where we think we are? Diabetes Care 19(12):1434–1436

Qi C, Pekala PH 2000 Tumor necrosis factor-alpha-induced insulin resistance in adipocytes. Proceedings of the Society for Experimental Biology and Medicine 223(2):128–135

Roth C, Scortea M, Stubbe P et al 1997 Autoimmune thyreoiditis in childhood. Experimental and Clinical Endocrinology and Diabetes 105(4):66–69

Storr HL, Plowman PN, Caroll PV et al 2003 Clinical and endocrine responses to pituitary radiotherapy in paediatric Cushing's disease. An effective second line treatment. Journal of Clinical Endocrinology and Metabolism 88(1):34–37

Strauss K et al 2002 A pan-European epidemiologic study of insulin technique in patients with diabetes. Practical Diabetes International 19(3):71–76

Thow J, Home P 1990 Insulin injection technique: depth of injection is important. British Medical Journal 301(22):3–4

Wallis S 2003 http://www.diabetesuffolk.com

Waugh A, Grant A 2001 Ross and Wilson: anatomy and physiology in health and illness. Churchill Livingstone, London

Williams J et al 1999 Studies associating behaviour, especially eating and drinking with healthy outcomes suggest an association with cardiovascular disease, cancer and diabetes. Journal of Clinical Epidemiology 52:329–335

Wong DL 1995 Whaley and Wong. Nursing care of infants and children, 5th edn. Mosby, London

Useful Websites

ACTH Association: http://www.cushingsacth.co.uk

British Thyroid Foundation: http://www.btf-thyroid.org

British Society of Paediatric Endocrinology and Diabetes: http://www.bsped.org.uk

CREST website: http://www.crestni.org.uk

Diabetes Nursing: http://www.diabetesnursing.com

Diabetes UK: http://www.diabetes.org.uk

Diabetes National Service Framework: http://www.doh.gov./nsf/diabetes

National Institute of Child Health and Human Development: http://www.nichd.nih.gov/publications/pubs/pit.htm

The Endocrine Society: http://www.endo-society.org

The Hormone Foundation: http:// www.hormone.org

Child Growth Foundation: http://www.heightmatters.org.uk

Chapter Thirty Five

35

Caring for Children with Orthopaedic Disorders

Brian Silverwood

ABSTRACT

The aim of this chapter is to give the reader a basic introduction to the speciality of orthopaedics in relation to the child with common bony injuries/disorders and the medical and nursing care they may receive. The word 'orthopaedic' is derived from the Greek *orthos pais* and means 'straight child'. The specialty has expanded from correcting disorders in children to include all areas of musculoskeletal surgery and conservative management (Danby & Edwards 1999).

Caring for children with an orthopaedic injury provides the nurse with a challenging and rewarding experience. Unlike most other paediatric specialties, the child admitted to the orthopaedic ward is usually well and active and requires, apart from attention to the bony injury/surgery, planning and interaction to provide him or her with play and distraction to prevent boredom. Many children's and emergency nurses care daily for children with bony injury and therefore require a sound knowledge base to deal both with the injury and reassure the anxious child and parent.

Learning Outcomes

- Describe bone structure, formation and resorption and the core functions of the skeleton, joints and muscles.

- Outline common childhood fractures and methods of management.

- Understand the pathophysiology of common childhood conditions and the medical/surgical treatments available.

- Devise an individualised plan of nursing care for a child who faces a period of immobility.

- Discuss the importance of discharge planning.

Glossary

Abduction:
  Moving a body part away from the body.
Adduction:
  Moving a body part towards the body.
Artho:
  Prefix meaning relating to a joint.
Congenital:
  Present at birth.
Distal:
  Situated further away from the area of consideration.
Dorsiflexion:
  Movement of hand or foot towards the dorsal surface.
Dysplasia:
  Abnormal development of skin, bone or other tissues.
Entonox:
  A self-administered inhaled pain relieving agent consisting of 50% nitrous oxide and 50% oxygen.
Equinovarus:
  The foot points downwards and inwards.
Equinus:
  The foot points downwards.
Extension:
  Straightening a joint.
Flexion:
  Bending a joint.
Hyperextension:
  Excessive extension.
Intramedullary:
  Within the medullary (inner) cavity of a long bone.
Inversion:
  Downwards and inwards movement of the foot.
Lateral:
  Situated away from the midline of the body.

Macrophage:
A large scavenger cell that wanders between cells and removes bacteria and other foreign bodies from blood and tissues.

Medial:
Near to the midline of the body.

Proximal:
Situated close to the point of origin or attachment.

Osteoblast:
A bone-forming cell.

Osteoclast:
A large cell that resorbs bone.

Osteocyte:
A basic bone cell.

Osteomyelitis:
Inflammation of the bone due to infection.

Osteotomy:
A surgical cut across the bone.

Rotation:
Turning about an axis.

Sclera:
Whites of the eyes.

Subluxation:
Partial dislocation.

Valgus:
A limb deformity in which the extremity is more away from the body's midline.

Varus:
Opposite of valgus.

Bone Biology

THE FUNCTION OF THE SKELETAL SYSTEM

The musculoskeletal system consists of 206 bones with their surrounding muscles. The main functions of the bones of the skeleton are to support and give shape to the body, to protect vital organs and to provide a system of levers that enables the body to make movements. In addition, bone serves as storage sites for certain minerals such as calcium and is also responsible for the production of red and white blood cells, a function performed by the red bone marrow. Yellow bone marrow acts as a storage site for lipids.

Activity

Using a suitable anatomy and physiology textbook, or suitable online source, identify and name the different bones of the body. Examine the relative significance of each bone in relation to its main function and location within the human skeleton.

BONE STRUCTURE

Bones are extremely strong and can withstand considerable forces. Bone is very resilient and can return to its normal shape after the removal of the force that caused the misshape. This tensile strength and resilience is due to the framework of interwoven fibres within bone called collagen, which is a tough, white, slightly flexible material. Bones are made up of two types of tissue (Fig. 35.1):

- Compact or cortical bone: is the dense and hard part of the bone that gives the bone its shape and strength. It is made up of many rods, known as the Haversian system. These have a central canal, which contains blood vessels and nerve fibres, and is surrounded by several sheets of bone tissue called lamellae. The Haversian canals branch and interweave, giving bone great strength along lines of stress.

- Cancellous or spongy bone: is composed of fine bars of bony tissue that interlace with one another to give a honey-comb appearance. These bars of tissue are known as the trabecular bone and are strong, light and provide an excellent structure to absorb stress. The space within the trabeculae is filled by the red blood marrow.

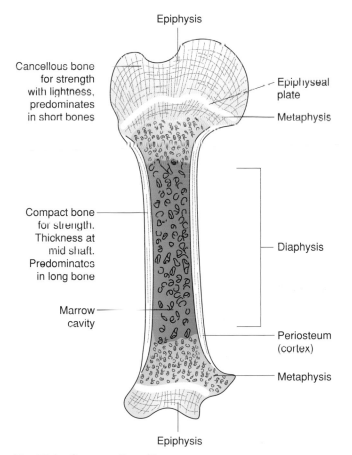

Fig. 35.1 • Cross-section of bone.

All bones are covered by a layer of fibrous tissue called periosteum, which protects the bone and allows the circumference of the bone to grow.

BONE GROWTH, FORMATION AND RESORPTION

Bone is constantly remodelling and adapting to the daily stresses placed on our skeleton (Silverwood 2003) (Fig. 35.2). From infancy through to adolescence, bones are actively growing in length, width and density (Table 35.1).

Bone remodelling is regulated by several factors including:

- Mechanical loads arising from muscle forces regulate the process of bone formation and resorption. For example, a tennis player's racket arm is typically stronger and wider than a non-player's arm because the remodelling bone has adapted to the increased daily strain and loading experienced when serving the ball.

- Calcium: this is the most abundant mineral found within the body. It is arranged around the matrix of collagen, which gives bone its strength and rigidity. Calcium is stored in the bone and released when serum calcium levels are low. A normal serum calcium level is required to allow adequate muscle contraction, transmission of impulses across nerve cells, activities of some enzymes and the building of strong bones.

- Parathyroid hormone (PTH): controls distribution of calcium. When serum calcium concentrations are low the hormone causes increased calcium absorption from the intestines, calcium reabsorption by the kidneys and increased bone resorption. Parathyroid hormone also regulates the synthesis of the active metabolites of vitamin D, which also enhance absorption of calcium from the intestine.

- Sex hormones: oestrogen and testosterone provide a 'control' over bone resorption and keeps bone remodelling in homeostasis.

FRACTURE REPAIR AND BONE HEALING

The fractured ends of the bone bleed and form a clot. The inflammatory healing process commences and the dead tissue and clot is removed by macrophages. The initial strands from the blood clot begin to change into osteoid tissue, which develops and forms callus around the fracture site; osteoclasts remove necrotic bone and osteoblasts develop new bone (Apley & Solomon 2001). Between 6 and 12 weeks, as the callus hardens, the bone regains some mechanical strength. Further callus maturity occurs between 12 and 26 weeks. By 1–2 years bone remodelling has occurred (see Fig. 35.2) and normal bone shape has been restored. Unlike adults, children can restore bony deformity resulting from a significant (up to 30°) malalignment through bone remodelling (Danby & Edwards 2001).

JOINTS

A joint or articulation is where two or more bones are in close contact with each other. Joints are classified according to their mobility and structure into fibrous, cartilaginous or synovial. Fibrous joints exist between bone and cartilage. The surfaces are simply joined by fibrous tissue and there is little or no movement. Cartilaginous joints allow a small degree of movement and are covered by layers of cartilage linked by a thick pad of tissue, for example, between vertebral bones. Synovial joints, which include all limb joints, permit a great deal of movement and are the most common type of joint. Hyaline cartilage covers the articulating surfaces to prevent friction and a fibrous capsule encloses the joint and helps hold the bones in place. A synovial membrane lines the capsule, which secretes synovial fluid to lubricate the structure.

Table 35.1 Skeletal Development (Gallo 1996)	
Infancy	Rapid growth in proportion and size as calcium is added to cartilage-like bones Calcium content in relation to body size increases faster than any other stage of life
Childhood	Growth continues Bone density and thickness increase Bone formation outpaces resorption
Adolescence	Growth accelerates Bone growth peaks around ages 12–17 in boys and ages 11–15 in girls Bone density and thickness increase Bone formation outpaces resorption
Age 20	90% of peak bone mass achieved
Age 35	Peak bone mass achieved *Note:* Peak bone mass is about 30% higher in men than women
Age 40+	Bone resorption begins to outpace formation Adult bone loss occurs at a rate of 6–8% per decade

Activity

Identify the differing types of joint within the human skeleton and justify the joint type in relation to its function and location.

Bone Resorption
At random the lining cells of bone become activated by substances including PTH & calcitriol, change from a pancake shape to a cubiod shape. The cells then secrete ODF (osteoclast differentiating factor) which allows the cells to fuse and differentiate into mature multinucleated osteoclasts (bone eating cells).

The osteoclast resorb (munch) away at the bone. New osteoclasts are activated and start resorption as the remodelling moves across the area of bone requiring repair. This resorption lasts around 2 weeks then the osteoclasts undergo apoptosis (programmed cell death).

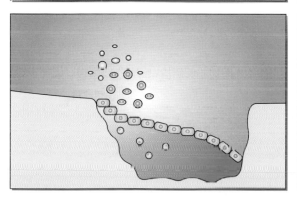

Bone Formation
Osteoblasts (bone forming cells) are derived from marrow stromal cells. They are attracted by bone derived growth factors and the remains of the self destructed osteoclasts.

The secreting osteoblasts then make layers of osteoid and slowly refill the cavity. The osteoblasts secrete a range of growth factors including osteocalcin and other proteins. The osteiod mineralises as the cavity fills.

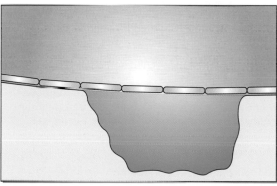

Over a period of around 3–4 months the crystals of mineral become closely packed together and the density of the new bone increases. The final osteoblasts turn into lining cells which participate in the release of calcium from the bone. Some osteoblasts turns into osteocytes (bone cell) which remain in the new bone and are connected by long cell processes which can sense mechanical stresses to the bones

Fig. 35.2 • Bone remodelling (Silverwood 2003.)

SKELETAL MUSCLE

The skeletal muscles are known as voluntary muscles because they produce movement under voluntary control.

These muscles are composed of large elongated cells known as muscle fibres, which are bound together by connective tissue into small bundles and are further bound into larger bundles forming the muscle. Each muscle is enveloped in a sheet of fibrous tissue known as the fascia, which is continuous with the tendon. Tendons are composed of bands of fibrous tissue, which attach muscles to bones.

Muscle activity is coordinated and most muscles work in pairs or groups; muscle tissue is capable of contraction and relaxation and may be stimulated by nervous, chemical, electrical or thermal stimulation.

Fractures

A fracture is quite simply a break in the continuity of bone. Most fractures are diagnosed from the description of the injury and the physical appearance of the limb, confirmed by plain X-ray. Physical signs and symptoms of a fracture may include (Danby & Edwards 2001, Pagdin 1996):

- Pain, which may be throbbing or localized: the pain is often aggravated by active or passive movement.
- Impaired or loss of function due to pain and the nature of the fracture.
- Swelling at the fracture site caused by oedema/haematoma formation. Usually increases in the first 12–24 hours following injury.
- A deformity may be seen or felt.
- Abnormal movement in a particular limb due to movement at the fracture site.
- Tenderness and/or bruising at the fracture site.
- Crepitus (grating) heard or felt when the ends of the broken bone are un-deliberately rubbed together.

TYPES OF FRACTURE

There are many descriptions of fractures, depending on the nature of the injury and the force that causes the fracture (Fig. 35.3).

In children, a fracture through the epiphyseal (growth) plate may result in interference or complete cessation of bone growth of that long bone, which will produce a limb length discrepancy. These fractures are known as epiphyseal fractures. Salter and Harris classified these fractures into five types (Fig. 35.4).

Other Descriptions of Fractures

A fracture may be displaced or undisplaced. An undisplaced fracture is one in which the bone ends are lined up, whereas in a displaced fracture the bone ends or fracture fragments are out of alignment and will require correction.

Open (compound) fractures are fractures in which the soft tissue and skin envelope have been disrupted by, for example, the acute angulation of the fracture which breaks through the skin. Such fractures are in immediate danger of infection and risk development of osteomyelitis. Most fractures do not break through the skin and are called closed fractures.

Intra-articular fractures may present where the fracture involves the joint surface. If there is a step or gap in the joint surface this may need surgery to correct it.

FRACTURE COMPLICATIONS

There are many potential associated complications with fractures including:

- Infection: in open fractures, a wound infection may spread from the skin and soft tissues and infect the underlaying bone. Often, children are at increased risk due to the activity at the time of fracture, which may involve dirt, grit or grass. The child with an open wound should have the wound cleaned and be commenced on systemic antibiotic therapy. If the wound is very dirty it will be left open, dressed appropriately and then closed later on.
- Malunion: this is when the fracture heals in the wrong position/alignment. This may be due to poor reduction or the result of an unstable fracture that slips following reduction. It is important that all children with fractures are seen afterwards as frequently as needed to ensure the bone heals in the right position.
- Delayed union: this complication occurs for a variety of reasons. It may be because the blood supply to the fracture is poor or the fracture is inadequately immobilised. The fracture heals but takes longer than expected.
- Non-union: the fracture fails to heal. This may be due to infection, trapped soft tissues or local bone necrosis.
- Avascular necrosis: the blood supply becomes disturbed to the bone fragments causing failure to heal. It may not present until some time following the injury.
- Fat embolism: a fat deposit originating from the bone marrow at the fracture site may enter the blood stream and block a blood vessel. This may have potential fatal consequences if the blockage is caused in a major organ, for example, the lungs.
- Damage to structures: in severe fractures other structures may be affected, for example, ischaemia to blood vessels, nerves, organs.
- Compartment syndrome: the fascial compartments within the upper and lower limbs are at risk when bleeding occurs into them from the fracture. The closed non-elastic space fills with blood and increases the pressure on the venous drainage thereby raising the pressure in the compartment. This starves the muscle

Transverse

Usually the result of a bending injury caused by direct impact and the fracture lies across the shaft of the long bone.

Oblique

Usually the result of a combination of a bending and twisting injury and lies across the shaft of the bone.

Spiral

Usually the result of a pure twisting injury. The fracture line spirals around the shaft of the bone.

Comminuted

Occurs when the bone is broken into more than two fragments. Usually the result of severe force.

Greenstick Fractures

Greenstick fractures are only found in children where the bone has not completely calcified and is more elastic. Therefore, a direct blow to the bone will cause it to bend but not completely break. The bone is said to resemble a green twig which never breaks cleanly.

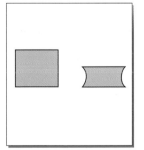

Crush fractures

Examples of crush fractures may be seen when the bone is pathologically weak due to disease. For example, children with moderate/severe osteogenesis imperfecta will have several crush fractured vertebrae.

Fig. 35.3 • Types of fracture.

Type I

Injuries occur when the fracture line is along the plane of the growth plate. If the fracture is undisplaced it may be missed due to the absence of a fracture line on x-ray. Pain on weight bearing will be the main symptom.

Type II

Injuries occur when the fracture is along the plane of the growth plate but extends into the metaphysis (the growing portion of a long bone) on one side. This gives the appearance of the "triangle sign" on x-rays.

Fig. 35.4 • Epiphyseal fractures.

Type III
Injuries occur when the fracture line is along the plane of the growth plate, but extends into the epiphysis (bone end) on one side.
Type IV
Injuries occur where the fracture extends from the epiphysis through the growth plate into the metaphysis.
Type V Injuries involve a crush injury to the growth plate. This may not be obvious on X-ray but the clinical signs will suggest a serious injury.

cells of oxygen and they die. The circulation can also be disturbed by a bone fragment or very tight plaster cast. The signs and symptoms of compartment syndrome in an upper limb may include:

- painful clawing of the fingers with increasing pain on passive extension of the fingers
- altered sensation, including a burning sensation or patchy loss of sensation
- the pulse is weak, intermittent or absent
- the fingers are cold and bluish
- weak ability to flex the fingers.

Many texts describe these signs of compartment syndrome as the five P's:

- pallor
- paraesthesia
- paralysis
- pain
- pulselessness.

The main symptom to note is pain, which is out of proportion to the injury and which is intractable. This condition needs to be recognised early because it is limb-threatening and prompt surgical attention can save the limb.

NEUROVASCULAR OBSERVATIONS

When a child enters the hospital with a fracture, the neurovascular status should be assessed initially, then half hourly for 4 hours, then hourly for 12–24 hours prior to and following repair of the fracture. This involves assessing colour, sensation, temperature, pulse and movement of the limb. Any alteration of these observations should be reported immediately to the orthopaedic team.

Professional Conversation

Yesterday we had a young boy who had a supracondylar fracture to his left elbow. I observed when checking neurovascular observations that his fingers were very dusky and when I tried to extend his fingers he was screaming out in pain. I was very concerned but didn't really feel very confident so I went to ask the ward manager but she was busy with a parent. I remembered what my preceptor had told me so I contacted the orthopaedic registrar. He came to the ward immediately and within 20 minutes the child was being escorted to theatre for a fasciotomy to release the pressure on his brachial artery. Later the registrar came and thanked me. He said I had probably saved the boy from developing Volkmann's ischaemia or losing his arm. I am really glad I listened to my preceptor and now really do realise the importance of neurovascular observations.

Failure to recognise a compartment syndrome of the forearm may result in the child developing Volkmann's ischaemic contracture caused by progressive muscle necrosis. The muscle is replaced by scar tissue leading to flexion contractures and clawing of the fingers. The result of this condition involves operations to release forearm flexors, muscle slide and tendon lengthening. Prevention through diagnosis would be attained by restoration of blood flow through reduction of compartmental pressure.

TREATMENT OF FRACTURES

The five R's summarise the five main aims of fracture treatment:

1. Resuscitation: the child with a fracture should rarely require fluid resuscitation, but the nurse should be aware of the signs and treatment necessary for shock. In fractures, shock may be related to pain and blood loss.

2. Reduction: describes the realignment of the fractured bone ends. The best reduction will take place under general anaesthesia where the surgeon can manipulate the bone and observe the correction using an image intensifier. This is especially relevant to children in whom it would not be acceptable to attempt reduction using sedation in the casualty department. Alignment may be acceptable in children with greenstick fractures.

3. Restriction: after the fracture has been manipulated into a good position it needs to be held until bony union occurs (usually 6 weeks in children). The methods used to hold the fracture will depend on the bone affected and the nature of the injury and will include one of:

- plaster cast
- traction
- internal or external fixation.

The aim of restriction is to prevent any deformity and allow bone growth to proceed normally.

4. Restoration: when a limb is immobilised there is a risk that the muscles and joints will stiffen and lose some function. Therefore it is important that the child is encouraged to exercise all joints and muscles except that affected by the injury. For example, a child with a fractured distal radius who has an above elbow cast can be encouraged to exercise all digits, which keeps the fingers nimble, encourages the muscle to move within the cast and promotes venous return.

5. Rehabilitation: when the method of restriction has been removed the limb must be exercised to restore normal ranges of movement. Children are quick to return to normal activity but may require the help of a physiotherapist.

Activity

A child presents with head injury and an open fractured femur following a road traffic accident.
- What immediate nursing and medical approach should be taken to resuscitate this 7-year-old child who has deteriorating consciousness and in hypovolaemic shock?
- Prioritise and analyse each intervention in relation to how it will stabilise the child's condition.

METHODS OF HOLDING FRACTURES

Plaster Casts

Plaster casts hold a number of advantages for the child with a fracture, including:

- allowing the child to mobilise and perform most activities of daily living
- low cost and readily available
- light and porous, which allows the skin to breathe
- relatively easy to use and apply
- strong, providing protection
- permeable to X-rays.

Disadvantages may include:

- It may cause discomfort including itching and feel heavy and warm and a child will be tempted to push toys and small objects down the cast leading to pressure sores.
- It may hide developing problems:
  - a poorly applied cast may cause pressure on the skin and encourage the development of a pressure ulcer
  - a surgical wound following an open reduction may develop sepsis.
- It is not waterproof.

Reflect on your Practice

Consider what education and skills you need to be competent in the application of a plaster cast.

In what way does this relate to your professional accountability and the recommendations of the British Orthopaedic Association (BOA)?

Plaster Casts – Nursing Care

Prior & Miles (1999) considered the following when caring for an inpatient with a plaster cast:

- Care should be taken not to apply pressure to the cast during the drying period to avoid causing dents in the cast (plaster of Paris takes 24–48 hours to dry; synthetic, fibreglass casts take around 30–60 minutes). The limb should be supported on a pillow to provide even pressure along the cast which prevents undue pressure on bony prominences.

- Elevation of the limb may be necessary to help reduce the amount of swelling which, within a cast may cause constriction and neurovascular impairment.

Plaster Casts – Observations

- The cast should be observed regularly for cracking, softening or breakdown.

- If a child has had an open reduction, the cast should be observed for blood loss, which will stain the cast. A line drawn around the cast illustrates any further blood loss.

- Neurovascular observations should be performed, see p 568.

- When the child has recovered and appears stable the cast may need trimming to improve comfort. Hip spica casts will need protection around the edges to prevent contamination by urine and faeces.

Before a child is discharged home, the parent and child should receive advice regarding care of the plaster (sample discharge advice in companion PowerPoint presentation). See p 578 for nursing and discharge care for a hip spica cast.

Activity

Examine your hospital's plaster care advice sheet given to the patient on discharge:
- Can you think of ways of improving the information provided and could it be made more child friendly?

Plaster Casts – Cast Bracing

Cast bracing is commonly used following internal fixation of a femoral or tibial fracture. The cast brace comprises plaster casts on the upper and lower limb, which are connected by hinges. These allow a greater degree of mobility to help prevent joint stiffness and allow the child to mobilise with partial weight-bearing, which encourages bone healing.

Traction

Traction is a pulling force. It is used to reduce and maintain alignment of fractures, to immobilise inflamed or injured joints, relieve pain, correct mild deformities and reduce muscle spasm. Traction is either fixed or balanced:

- Fixed traction is achieved by exerting a pulling force on the point splinted between two fixed points.

- Balanced traction exerts a pulling force on the part held between two mobile points, and works by using the patient's weight against the applied load.

Common forms of balanced and skin traction used with children include:

- Thomas splint traction: fixed traction that works against the force of the body (Fig. 35.5). It is used in the treatment of femoral fractures usually as a means to hold and pull the fracture until the swelling subsides before internal or external fixation.

- Gallows traction: works by the body's weight being balanced by an applied load. Is frequently used in babies and infants with femoral fractures to allow the swelling to subside prior to the application of a hip spica (Fig. 35.6).

- Simple skin traction (Fig. 35.7): commonly used to rest the affected limb or joint prior to surgery and to reduce pain/muscle spasm. It involves applying adhesive strips of material to either side of the affected limb. The limb is then bandaged, taking care to leave the knee free. The cord allows a pull to be exerted on the strips, which is transmitted from the material and skin to the underlying tissues and bone. Only a moderate amount of pull can be exerted using weights and the bed end is then elevated to provide counter traction.

- Skeletal traction: now rarely used in paediatrics because of the advances in surgical techniques. It may be used if the alignment of the fracture is difficult to achieve and maintain and internal fixation not possible. It involves the insertion of a sterile pin through an area of strong bone, such as the femoral condyles, tibial tuberosity or calcaneum. A metal stirrup is then attached to the pin ends and cord fastened to it. Weights are attached to the stirrup and hang over a pulley; they are then left free hanging over the elevated bed end. Skeletal traction is

Fig. 35.5 • Thomas splint traction.

Fig. 35.6 • Gallows traction.

also used following trauma, such as when the integrity of the skin is damaged and the application of skin traction would be difficult.

- Slings traction: used for children with hip conditions who require a combination of bed rest and allows the physiotherapist to teach the child a range of exercises performed on the hip and lower limbs.

NURSING CARE OF THE CHILD ON TRACTION

Once traction has been applied, the child's pain and discomfort is usually relieved but analgesia may still be required. The nurse should be aware of the following observations and care when nursing children on traction.

The Position of the Patient

Often, the position required for successful traction will cause difficulty with the activities of daily living including eating, drinking, washing, elimination and learning.

Assistance with these activities are essential, as well as maintaining the privacy and independence of the patient.

Once over the initial discomfort of an injury, the child will become frustrated and bored due to loss of mobility. The school-age child may display poor behaviour. This should be dealt with sensitively but firmly to prevent general disruption to the ward. The nurse should employ the full skills of the play specialist and ward teacher, and encourage full parental participation in their child's care. Once adjustment, has been made the child will quickly establish a rapport with the ward team.

Fig. 35.7 • Simple skin traction.

The child is at risk from the usual complications of bed rest including:

- Pressure ulcers: bony prominences, including the buttocks and heels, are at risk of pressure ulcers as the result of the constant pressure between the skin surface and the hard mattress. Frequent cleansing, minor alterations in position and the use of pressure-reducing mattresses or polymer gel pads (Fig. 35.8) will lessen the risk of pressure sore development.

- Kidneys: urinary stasis may result in kidney stones or a urinary tract infection leading to difficulty passing urine therefore the child should be encouraged to drink plenty of fluids.

- Bowel: significantly reduced exercise and the decrease of roughage can lead to constipation, therefore the child's diet should include increased fibre and fluid. Laxatives may be prescribed.

Reflect on your Practice

Look at the National Institute for Clinical Excellence (NICE) guidelines on the use of pressure-relieving devices at:

- http://www.nice.org.uk

What sort of pressure-relieving devices do you have in your area and do they meet the needs of your patients?

Bandages

Constriction of the limb by bandages used with traction may cause disturbance to the circulatory system, muscles, joints and nerve supply. Bandages should be applied firmly, but not tightly, and removed each span of duty to check skin integrity/sensitivity due to adhesive skin traction (Box 35.1).

Fig. 35.8 • Polymer gel pad.

Box 35.1

Application of skin traction (Huband & Twigg 2000 p 298)

- Skin traction can be a painful procedure for a child and careful preparation must therefore be given, including a detailed explanation and appropriate analgesia, before the procedure is commenced, to gain the child's cooperation and trust.
- Privacy should be maintained throughout the procedure.
- The limb should be cleaned prior to applying the adhesive skin traction, to prevent the risk of infection.
- The ankle joint is kept free allowing normal movement of that joint.
- The patella is left free and the leg placed in slight flexion, thus preventing deformity and stiffness.
- Pressure on bony prominence should be avoided or pressure sores may occur.
- Folds and creases in the strapping should be avoided to prevent discomfort or sores.
- The temperature and colour of the limb is checked to ensure the tension of strapping is correct.

Powerpoint

Access the PowerPoint presentation for a detailed description of the mechanics of traction and a step-by-step guide on applying skin traction.

INTERNAL FIXATION (FIG. 35.9)

The many types of internal fixation devices include plates, screws and intramedullary nails/rods. Internal fixation allows accurate reduction of the fracture and stabilisation of the reduced position. It allows the child to mobilise and avoids joint stiffness by encouraging prompt rehabilitation. It encourages good bone union and reduces the time spent in hospital. Complications include the risks associated with a general anaesthetic, the potential of infection and other postoperative complications. Further surgery is required to remove the

Fig. 35.9 • Internal fixation.

device. When possible, the surgeon will remove the fixation device at 6–12 months, although removal may not always be possible and the device may be safely left in situ.

EXTERNAL FIXATION

A fracture may be held by transfixing screws, which pass through the bone above and below the fracture. The screws are held together with a rigid frame or lockable sliding bar. External fixation is particularly useful for fractures with severe soft tissue damage, fractures with nerve or blood vessel damage, unstable comminuted fractures that can be held to length until bone healing occurs and infected fractures where internal fixation may be unwise (Apley & Solomon 2001). The fixation device is left in place until bone healing occurs. Older children may remove the screws themselves by using Entonox in outpatients (Pickup & Pagdin 2000), avoiding further general anaesthesia. Complications occurring from external fixation are pin site infections and occasionally delayed union. Occasionally a stress fracture may occur at the site of one of the screws following removal. External devices (Fig. 35.10) are used in limb reconstruction and leg lengthening treatments throughout the UK.

✚ Evidence-based Practice

Skeletal pin site care

There remains little consensus regarding the correct management of skeletal pin sites (Bernardo 2001, Rowe 1997, Sims & Whiting 2000). The surgical literature often describes the prevalence of pin site infections and nursing literature describes pin care techniques. The Royal College of Nursing's Focus for Research in Orthopaedics Group (RCN 2003) has a pin site project team whose aim is to achieve consensus toward evidence-based pin site care. Lee-Smith et al (2001) have published summary guidelines and a Cochrane Review is in progress (RCN 2003). Until evidence-based practice based on a significant multicentre trial is published, individual centres should review the literature themselves to reach local multidisciplinary consensus.

◆ Scenario

Charlotte is a second-year adult branch student nurse who is on allocation within the local general hospital A & E department.

A 4-year-old boy is brought to the A&E department by emergency ambulance and is taken immediately to the resuscitation room. The child appeared pale, was immobilised with a hard collar around the neck and had a splint around his leg with a large blood-stained dressing.

Later, after the child is transferred to the nearest children's hospital, Charlotte asks her mentor why aspects of the child's assessment and stabilisation were different and why the child was rushed to another hospital when all the 'hard work' had been done. The mentor responded by explaining how the management of polytrauma (multiple injuries) is different between children and adults.

Fig. 35.10 • External fixation (Ilizarov frame).

Polytrauma

Trauma is the most common cause of death in childhood. The most common causes of multiple trauma in children include road traffic accidents, falls from height and physical child abuse. Initial assessment and management of children with multiple injuries should be carried out within a dedicated resuscitation room according to the guidelines of advanced paediatric life support (APLS) and advanced trauma life support (ATLS) as recommended by the Royal College of Surgeons (Bell 2002, Glasgow & Kerr Graham 1997). Initial stabilisation should be followed by transfer to a specialist paediatric centre with the necessary paediatric intensive care unit, specialist neurological, anaesthetic, orthopaedic, radiological and medical teams.

Within an adult orientated centre it is important to remember that during initial assessment children present specific anatomical differences from the adult:

- The head and tongue are large whereas the face and oral cavity are small. This may present difficulties with endotracheal intubation and the large head increases the risk of cervical spine injuries during the time of the accident.

- Regarding the airway, infants are obligate nose breathers, nasal passages are narrow and therefore easily obstructed and children between the ages of 3 and 8 years commonly present with adenotonsillar hypertrophy. The differences in the anatomy of the epiglottis and larynx require a different intubation technique. Ribs are more horizontal in appearance, elastic in structure and breathing diaphragmatic, leading to considerable lung injury without fracture.

- Blood volume varies according to age. Bearing in mind the smaller circulating blood volume in relation to age and size a femoral fracture may produce enough blood loss leading to haemorrhagic shock/cardiac decompensation. The pulse rate of children is higher and blood pressure lower and is more prone to the effects of anxiety. Cardiac output is largely dependent on the heart rate as the stroke volume is small and fixed meaning bradycardia is poorly tolerated.

- Abdominal organs are more vulnerable as the abdominal wall is thin and the diaphragm more horizontal.

- Children's bones have growth plates, injury to which may cause permanent growth arrest of that bone leading to short limbs.

STRUCTURED APLS AND ATLS APPROACH

On arrival in the casualty department, ATLS advises four steps in the management of the child presenting with polytrauma:

1. initial assessment
2. resusitation
3. secondary survey
4. definitive care.

Steps 1 and 2 are performed simultaneously.

Initial Assessment (Primary Survey) and Resuscitation

Assesses vital functions and consists of five steps:

A = Airway patency and cervical spine control: if the gag reflex is absent or of doubt the child's airway will be maintained by utilising a oropharyngeal (Guedel) airway or endotracheal intubation. The trauma team will assume that cervical spine injury will have occurred so a rigid collar will be applied.

B = Breathing adequately to maintain oxygenation: assessment will be made of reduced respiratory effort and for potential life threatening emergencies such as tension pneumothorax, haemopneumothorax and pericardial tamponade.

C = Circulation and control of bleeding: the aim here is to detect the presence of circulatory shock (Table 35.2) and sites of blood loss which, where possible, should be controlled. Intravenous access is paramount; however, access is often difficult in children due to peripheral shutdown. Intraosseous needles (special needles designed to be screwed into the lumen of the bone) may used until a central line is accessed later. Shock is managed by rapid fluid bolus/replacement and administration of high concentration oxygen through bag and mask or reservoir mask.

D = Disability (neurological assessment): the central nervous system is examined only after completion of ABC and resuscitation. Initial assessment will determine if the child is:
- **A** = **a**lert
- **V** = responds to **v**oice
- **P** = responds to **p**ain
- **U** = **u**nresponsive.

  During the secondary survey the child will be scored using the Glasgow coma score.

E = Exposure: to fully examine front and back; secondary survey.

Secondary Survey

Following the initial assessment and resuscitation, strong analgesia such as morphine will be considered to lessen pain. The child will undergo radiological examination of the cervical spine, pelvis and chest (other X-rays may depend on the history and initial assessment) and a thorough head to toe, front and back examination. Vital signs of ABCD will be continually checked and interventions to deal with other, less life-threatening, injuries. For example, a nasogastric tube may be passed to relieve gastric dilatation and a urinary catheter passed to prevent urinary retention and allowing accurate recording of fluid balance. The secondary survey may take place within the secure environment of a paediatric intensive care unit where definitive care will commence.

Orthopaedic Definitive Care in Polytrauma

- As bone is more elastic in children than in adults, pelvic fractures require increased high-energy trauma to occur. Most pelvic fractures rarely cause difficulties and unite well with minimal intervention.

- Children are at increased risk of spinal cord injury. The cervical spine area must be protected with a hard collar and the child log-rolled until detailed examination and investigation has ruled out spinal cord injury.

- Fractures of the long bones should be stabilised as soon as possible. In the short term, a femoral fracture will be stabilised using splintage; however, it is preferable to stabilise all long bone fractures through internal or external fixation (Fig. 35.10) because it aids nursing care and provides secure stabilisation. Neurovascular assessment should take place as soon as the child's initial resuscitation as the risks of compartment syndrome is increased in children with multiple injuries.

- Most compound or open fractures are caused by high-energy road traffic accidents. The presence of an open fracture often suggests other injuries. Open fractures are classified as shown in Table 35.3.

Open fractures may require immediate intervention through an operative procedure to stabilise, clean and close the wound to prevent the development of sepsis. The injury will require copious irrigation to clean the wound. Vascular repair may be performed immediately following stabilisation of the fracture. A plastic surgeon may be required to perform complex free flap skin grafts in the most serious cases. The child will be commenced on broad-spectrum intravenous antibiotics.

Advances in paediatric medical and surgical management ensure the child with multiple injuries often makes a full recovery. However, every attempt should be made to reduce the risk of potential fatal injury through education, car safety, traffic calming and suitable children's play areas.

www

Visit the resuscitation council UK for the latest advanced paediatric resuscitation guidelines at:
- http://www.resus.org.uk/pages/pals.htm

Osteogenesis Imperfecta

DESCRIPTION

Osteogenesis imperfecta (OI), commonly known as 'brittle bone disease', is a hereditary disorder characterised by bones that break easily (Silverwood 2001). The defective gene affects the body's collagen in one of two ways, underproduction of otherwise normal collagen fibres (mild OI; type I) or abnormal or 'bent' collagen fibres, giving more severe forms. The defect interferes with bone turnover, leading to an inability to accumulate bone as healthy children would (Hill et al 2003). The characteristic features of osteogenesis imperfecta vary immensely between each child. The classification now in general use was proposed by Sillence et al in 1979 and is based on genetic, clinical and radiological features (Table 35.4).

The incidence of osteogenesis imperfecta in the UK population is estimated to be around 6000, based on a prevalence of 1:10,000. Around 1200 of these are children, with around 200 children severely affected (Bishop 1999a). Children with severe osteogenesis imperfecta may be diagnosed in

Table 35.2 Recognition of Stages of Shock			
		Assessment of % blood loss	
Sign	**<25**	**25–40**	**>40**
Heart rate	Tachycardia +	Tachycardia ++	Tachycardia ++ or bradycardia
Systolic blood pressure	Normal	Normal or decreasing	Decreasing
Pulse volume	Normal/reduced	Reduced +	Reduced ++
Capillary refill time (normal < 2 s)	Normal/Increased	Increased +	Increased ++
Skin	Cool, pale	Cold, mottled	Cold, pale
Respiratory rate	Tachypnoea +	Tachypnoea ++	Sighing
Mental state	Mild agitation	Lethargic, Uncooperative	Reacts only to pain

Table 35.3 Classification of Open Fractures (Bell 2002)

Type I	An open fracture with a wound <1 cm long and clean
Type II	An open fracture with a laceration >1 cm long without excessive soft tissue damage, flaps or avulsions
Type III	Massive soft tissue damage, compromised vascularity, severe wound contamination, marked fracture instability
Type IIIA	Adequate soft tissue coverage of a fractured bone despite extensive soft tissue laceration or flaps or high-energy trauma irrespective of the size of the wound
Type IIIB	Extensive soft tissue injury loss with periosteal stripping and bone exposure; usually associated with massive contamination
Type IIIC	Open fracture associated with arterial injury requiring repair

Table 35.4 Classification of Osteogenesis Imperfecta (OI)

Type	Description
I	Most common and mildest form of OI Fractures occur occasionally, especially before puberty Normal or near normal stature Sclera often blue Bone deformity is minimal or absent Brittle teeth (dentinogenesis imperfecta); hearing loss Collagen structure is normal but the amount is less than normal
II	Most severe form Lethal at birth, or shortly following birth, due to complex respiratory problems Growth retardation in utero Numerous fractures, long bones crumpled and bowed, ribs appear beaded Collagen abnormal
III	Bones fracture easily. Fractures often present at birth, plain X-rays may show partially healed fractures. Several crush fractured vertebrae Short stature Sclera may be blue, but may lighten with age Brittle teeth and hearing loss common Barrel shaped rib cage. Respiratory problems possible Triangular face Bone deformity severe. Spinal curvature present Collagen abnormal
IV	Bones fracture easily, especially in infants and children Shorter than average stature. Crush fractured vertebrae May have bowing of long bones and develop spinal curvature White sclera. Brittle teeth and hearing loss possible Collagen abnormal

utero using ultrasound, or at birth when the baby presents with 'classic' features including a triangular face and several new and healing fractures of long bones. However, children with milder forms may face a long road towards diagnosis. Many parents have to endure investigation by the authorities of suspected child abuse (Mahoney 2000).

TREATMENT

The management of osteogenesis imperfecta focuses on minimising fractures and maximising function and independence. This is achieved through a combination of coordinated surgical and medical management with physiotherapy and occupational therapy (Silverwood 2001).

Medical Management

This includes the administration of a bisphosphonate (intravenous pamidronate or oral risedronate). They are based on the chemical structure of a naturally occurring substance within the body called pyrophosphate (Bishop 1999b) and bind very strongly to bone reducing the actions of osteoclasts.

The beneficial effects of pamidronate include:

- a substantial increase in bone mass
- a reduction in fracture frequency
- increase in height of previous crush-fractured vertebrae
- a reduction of chronic bone pain and fatigue
- improved mobility and reduced dependence on mobility aids
- increase in thickness in the tube walls of long bones.

The treatment is given in combination with multidisciplinary care. The physiotherapist deals with improving mobility and physical function and the occupational therapist maximises the child's independence of performing the activities of daily living.

Surgical Management

The mainstay of surgical management is intramedullary rod fixation. The aim of rodding long bones is to correct and prevent bony disorders. Rods are either fixed length or expanding. Expanding rods are telescopic and expand as the bone grows in length. These hold a number of advantages over fixed rods, not least because the child requires less frequent change of the rod and when the rod requires revision; only the expanding part of the rod is changed (Stockley et al 1989). Complications may include infection, migration or separation of the rod and a bent rod following fracture (Wilkinson et al 1998). Although the operation may appear complicated, the average length of the admission lasts only 3–4 days. The perioperative period lasts around 1–2 hours, the child returns to the ward with an intravenous infusion (until diet and fluids are re-established) and a patient-controlled analgesia (PCA) to ensure adequate pain control. A lightweight cast or a cotton/crepe bandage will protect the limb for 4–6 weeks.

NURSING CARE

The nursing care of osteogenesis imperfecta is outlined in Table 35.5.

 WWW

For further information regarding osteogenesis imperfecta visit:
- http://www.oif.org
- http://www.brittlebone.org

Developmental Dysplasia of the Hip

DESCRIPTION

Developmental dysplasia of the hip (DDH) is a recent term used to describe a dislocation of the hip joint occurring at birth (congenital) or during the first year of life (Benson & Macnicol 2002). The head (ball) of the femur does not sit true in the acetabulum (socket). There are varying degrees of dislocation including:

- Unstable: the shape of the head of the femur and acetabulum are normal or near normal. Using manipulation the head of the femur may be moved in and out of the acetabulum.

- Subluxed: the head of the femur is only in partial contact with the acetabulum. The acetabulum is not of a normal shape.

- Dislocated: the head of the femur lies completely out of the joint. Usually the shape and size of the joint is abnormal and will deteriorate further if left out of the joint.

Incidence varies between different countries but is estimated to be 1.5 per 1000 in European countries (Danby & Edwards 2001). Incidence is higher in girls than boys, and in first-born babies. The cause of DDH is unclear but it is believed that there may be a genetic factor because it tends to run in families. Other examples of contributory

Table 35.5 Nursing Care of Osteogenesis Imperfecta (OI)

Parents	Listen to what the parents have to say about the handling of their child. Regard them as colleagues because they are experts in their child's routine care
Babies and infants	Toys should be soft and easy to handle
Lifting	Head, trunks and buttocks should be evenly supported when the baby is lifted Make your movements slow, methodical and gentle
Changing nappies	Avoid lifting by the ankles Change the nappy by lifting under the buttocks and place the nappy with the other hand
Dressing	May suffer excessive sweating. Use cotton clothing Position/set out clothes next to the baby Openings should be generous. Slip your hand up the sleeve and pull the baby's arm through
Positioning	Babies with OI can develop flattening of the head Reposition frequently on alternate sides and supine Support the position with soft rolled sheets
Feeding	Often a poor feeder Small, frequent feeds Hold the child to give comfort, utilising a soft pillow
Constipation	Ensure adequate hydration Advice on diet, including fibre and fruit
Transporting around hospital	Traditional methods, i.e. in the cot, are satisfactory. Consider using a car seat, which provides a comfortable protective environment
Older children	Very independent Regarded as above normal intelligence (Wacaster 1996) and appreciate normal adult conversation

factors include lax ligaments, which is caused by increased levels of oestrogen during pregnancy, overdue pregnancies and breech deliveries. Environmental causative factors have been shown in the North American Indian and Eskimo population where babies are carried with their legs straight.

The classic signs of DDH may include the paediatrician observing a 'hip click' during routine postnatal checks.

Other signs may include: the thigh showing a partial lateral rotation, flexion and abduction, asymmetry of the hips and a flattening of the buttock. The baby will be referred to a paediatric orthopaedic surgeon who will perform ultrasound scanning to establish the severity of the condition.

TREATMENT

Treatment will depend on the time of diagnosis, but may be divided into conservative and surgical treatments.

Conservative

The aim is to hold the legs abducted and flexed so that the head of the femur falls naturally into the acetabulum. The constant pressure of the ball of the femur helps to mould the acetabulum and therefore stabilise the hip. This may be achieved in a young baby by the wearing of double nappies or the wearing of a special splint shaped in the form of an 'X' or 'H'. This fits around the thighs of the legs and wraps over the shoulders to maintain position. Examples include the Cambridge splint, Pavlik harness and von Rosen splint. The splint will be worn constantly for a minimum of 12 weeks and is removed only for examination.

Traction was, until a few years ago, the treatment of choice for babies whose treatment had failed with splints or for a baby diagnosed later. The hip is reduced by gradually abducting the hips over a 4–6-week period before being held in plaster. A popular example was the Japanese frame. Plaster fixation is commonly used following manipulation of the hips under anaesthesia. The types of plaster casts used include a double hip spica or a frog plaster. The baby is reviewed in clinic at 6 weeks where the hips are reassessed for hip stability. Plaster treatment may last for 6–9 months and the family requires support and advice during this period.

Surgical

Surgical treatments are used when either conservative method has failed or the diagnosis is made late. Common procedures include:

- Tenotomy: the groin tendon is lengthened. This releases a tight tendon that had prevented satisfactory reduction of the hip.
- Open reduction: allows the femoral head to be surgically placed in the acetabulum. The position is maintained by plaster cast.
- Femoral derotation osteotomy: a surgical break of the bone used to return the femur to a normal anatomical position following open reduction of the hip. The break is held in place by a blade plate until bone healing has occurred and the plate is removed between 6 and 12 months. A hip spica cast is used to maintain position during the first 6–8 weeks.
- Salter's osteotomy: may be performed in a late diagnosis where poor development of the acetabulum has occurred. This involves surgical reconstruction of the acetabulum to prevent further dislocation.

Nursing Care of a Child with a Hip Spica Cast

Hip spicas are cumbersome and uncomfortable for the child and parents, who have to carry a largely immobile child in a heavy cast, although young children soon learn to drag themselves around the floor despite the hip spica. Parents must be taught how to lift and carry the child before discharge. Parents should be made aware of the signs of wound infection under the plaster – usually identified by an unpleasant smell from the plaster combined with a pyrexia. If this occurs, or if the cast cracks or softens, the parent should contact the hospital promptly.

HYGIENE

The plaster edges must be examined for rough edges, which can cause skin breakdown. A daily sponge-down replaces bathing. Talcum powder should be used sparingly around the plaster because it can cause excessive irritation to the skin under the cast. Hair washing can be a problem and usually requires two people, one to hold the child over the bath, the other to wash. Nappy cares require some thought. A larger disposable nappy is usually required, nappies should not be tucked under the cast, which could result in the risk of pressure ulcers and excessive dampening.

SLEEPING

Younger children are less likely to be affected by the plaster, although wind can be troublesome, therefore winding after feeding is important. Children in casts may sleep for only short periods and often become restless. Disturbed nights can result from itching and an inability to turn over. A child in a spica takes up much more room than one without therefore the width of the bed may require thought; placing the mattress on the floor can be useful and also removes the fear of the child falling out of bed. Supporting the child in a comfortable position can be done with foam or pillows but care must be taken to prevent pressure points or strain on the cast. The child may require fewer bed clothes – the plaster acts as insulation.

TRANSPORT

This is often a major problem for the family with a child in a hip spica cast but the ability to get out of the home is important for the parent and child. Smaller babies will often fit into a push chair with some extra support from pillows. Transporting a child in a cast by car is difficult, as children cannot be safely strapped into car seats; special harnesses are sometimes available. An occupational therapist will advise the parent regarding safe transport.

EATING AND DRINKING

Some children are able to eat and drink lying on their tummies, others require support in an upright position either strapped in a normal high chair or using a bean bag. There are also designs available of specific 'hip spica' chairs. A closed cup or straw is the best method of drinking and preventing too many accidents.

CLOTHING

Usually larger sizes are required, these can be split and then applied using tapes, poppers, velcro or zips.

PLAY

Play and activity should be encouraged as much possible to allow the child to develop as normal and to provide him or her with a means of releasing the tension experienced while in plaster. Physical and very active play will be almost impossible. The child will have to rely on imaginative or 'craft' types of play. A child in a plaster can become isolated from friends and peers. Contact should therefore be encouraged, although games should not be allowed to become too boisterous.

Activity

Devise some play activities for the following children on the ward:
- A 10-month-old on gallows traction.
- Two 8-year-old boys with Thomas splint traction.
- A 14-year-old girl on bilateral skin traction.

Talipes (Clubfoot)

DESCRIPTION

Congenital (present at birth) talipes (ankle and foot) equinovarus (pointing downwards and inwards) is the most common congenital abnormality of the feet, which are malformed and irregularly positioned. It varies in type and severity. The cause is unknown, although there may be a hereditary or genetic component. It has been associated with other congenital conditions and it may be caused by the position of the foot in utero. Incidence is 1 per 1000 births (Catteral 2002). Diagnosis is usually made at birth but increasingly through prenatal ultrasound scanning. The aims of treatment are to have a functional, pain-free, plantigrade foot and able to get into normal footwear.

TREATMENT

Conservative Treatment

This includes physiotherapy on newborn babies: the parent is taught to stretch the ligaments and tendons. Adhesive strapping is applied around the foot, up the sides of the legs and anchored around the knee in an overcorrected position. Plaster cast fixation involves the foot being manipulated by the surgeon into an overcorrected position, with the knee flexed to prevent the cast slipping off. The cast is changed regularly due to rapid growth of baby and the foot is re-manipulated. This acts by stretching the soft tissues. A more recent treatment known as the Ponseti technique involves serial progressive casting with tendo-achilles tenotomy.

Surgical Treatments

These vary widely in type and will depend on the severity of the talipes and the child's age. Surgical intervention is usually started at 9 months, with the aim of achieving correction in time for walking. Examples include soft tissue releases followed by a period in plaster through to bony procedures of the foot. An increasingly popular treatment is to correct the abnormality by using an external circular frame (Ilizarov frame), which allows the position of the foot to be altered slowly by both stretching the soft tissues and distracting osteotomies in the bones of the foot. When a normal position is achieved the frame is 'locked' until bone healing has occurred. The whole period of treatment may take around 6 months followed by a period in plaster.

Perthes' Disease

Perthes disease, also known as Legg–Calve–Perthes' disease, after Legg (an American), Calve (a Frenchman) and Perthes (a German), was first described around 1910. It is characterised by a loss of circulation to the head of the femur leading to avascular necrosis. This is followed by a period of revascularisation lasting 18 months to 2 years. During this period the bone is soft and revascularisation often results in fracture and or collapse of the femoral head. The resulting non-spherical shape causes the child to have stiffness and pain. The cause of Perthes' disease is unknown; statistics show that it is more common in boys than girls around ages 3 to 8.

The child often presents with an acutely painful hip due to inflammation of the hip joint. There is often a painful obvious limp that has appeared merely over a few hours. The condition is usually diagnosed through X-ray following other investigations to rule out conditions that cause similar symptoms, for example, epiphyseal dysplasia.

TREATMENT

Conservative/Surgical Treatment

Traditionally, these children were placed on periods of prolonged bed rest and non-weight-bearing on the affected hip because it was thought weight bearing caused the head to collapse. Treatment approaches now suggest maintaining the head within the acetabulum. These is achieved conservatively through casting and bracing or surgically by a femoral rotational osteotomy or pelvic osteotomy. If the hip shows tightness on examination the child may already have flattening of the femoral head and the outcome will be less favourable. In such cases a period of traction and physiotherapy is given to release tightness usually followed by surgical hip adductor releases.

It is known that diagnosis before the age of 4 years leads to a good outcome irrespective of treatment, and in all ages at least 70% of affected children do well with no long-term disability.

Discharge Planning

Effective discharge planning for the child who undergoes orthopaedic surgery should begin at preadmission clinic or on admission to the ward. The family should receive information about care of a plaster cast and or the importance of cleansing pin sites daily for external fixators. They need to be able to recognise potential complications of surgery, including the signs of infection and the difference between 'routine' discomfort and severe pain. Parents should be encouraged to follow the exercises given by the physiotherapist to maintain joint mobility. The nurse must act as the coordinator to ensure the family receives multidisciplinary ongoing care in the community, including the community nursing team, social services, occupational therapy and physiotherapy. For example, an older child going home with

a broomstick or spica cast may require home assessment by the occupational therapist, who will need to arrange for the child to have a urinal, bed pan or even a hoist to enable transfer from the bed to a wheelchair. A number of support groups supply advice, support and information for families of children with specific conditions.

It is outside the scope of this chapter to provide a detailed review of the many childhood orthopaedic conditions. Review the references and further reading sections of this chapter or use the many online sources.

WWW

For further information about support groups, visit:
- http://www.steps-charity.org.uk/home.html

WWW

Read about common childhood orthopaedic conditions online at:
- http://www.orthoseek.com

or:
- http://www.orthoteers.co.uk

References

Apley AG, Solomon L 2001 Concise system of orthopaedics and fractures, 2nd edn. Edward Arnold, London

Bell MJ 2002 Polytrauma in children. In: Benson MKD et al (eds) Children's orthopaedics and fractures, 2nd edn. Churchill Livingstone, London, pp 579–586

Benson MKD, MacNicol MF 2002 Developmental dysplasia of the hip. In: Benson MKD et al (eds) Children's orthopaedics and fractures, 2nd edn. Churchill Livingstone, London, pp 359–383

Bernardo LM 2001 Evidence based practice for pin site care in injured children. Orthopaedic Nursing 20(5):29–34

Bishop NJ 1999a Osteogenesis imperfecta – current perspectives and treatment. The European Calcified Tissue Society. Online. Available at: http://www.etcsoc.org/reviews/002_bish.htm

Bishop NJ 1999b Drug treatment of children with OI. Brittle Bone Society Newsletter, issue 70, November

Catteral A 2002 Early assessment and management of the club foot. In: Benson MKD et al (eds) Children's orthopaedics and fractures, 2nd edn. Churchill Livingstone, London, pp 464–477

Danby DJ, Edwards DJ 2001 Essential orthopaedics and trauma, 3rd edn. Churchill Livingstone, London

Gallo AM 1996 Building strong bones in childhood and adolescence: reducing the risk of fractures in later life. Pediatric Nursing 22(5):369–374

Glasgow JFT, Kerr Graham H 1997 Management of injuries in children. BMJ Publishing, London

Hill C, Hampshire D, Silverwood B, Bishop NJ 2003 Recent advances in the management of osteogenesis imperfecta. Current Paediatrics 13:151–157

Huband S, Twigg E 2000 Practices in children's nursing: guidelines for hospital and community. Churchill Livingstone, London

Lee-Smith et al 2001 Pinsite management. toward a consensus: part 1. Journal of Orthopaedic Nursing 5:37–42

Mahoney C 2000 Handle with care. Nursing Times 96(1):24–26

Pagdin J 1996 The musculoskeletal system. In: McQuaid L et al (eds) Children's nursing. Churchill Livingstone, London, pp 239–262

Pickup S, Pagdin J 2000 Procedural pain: Entonox can help. Paediatric Nursing 12(10):33–36

Prior MA, Miles S 1999 Casting: part one. Nursing Standard 13(28):49–53

Rowe S 1997 A review of the literature on the nursing care of skeletal pins in the paediatric and adolescent setting. Journal of Orthopaedic Nursing 1:26–29

Royal College of Nursing (RCN) 2003 Pinsite care project. Focus for research in orthopaedics group. Online. Available at: http://www.man.ac.uk/rcn/ukwide/frogpinsite.htm

Sillence DO et al 1979 Genetic heterogeneity in osteogenesis imperfecta. Journal of Medical Genetics 16:101–116

Silverwood B 2001 Osteogenesis imperfecta – care and management. Paediatric Nursing 13(3):38–42

Silverwood B 2003 Building healthy bones in children. Paediatric Nursing 15(5):27–29

Sims M, Whiting J 2000 Pin-site care. Current evidence for best practice in preventing infection when using external fixators to stabilise bones. Nursing Times 96(48):46

Stockley I et al 1989 The role of expanding intermedullary rods in osteogenesis imperfecta. Journal of Bone and Joint Surgery 71-B:3

Wacaster P 1996 Managing osteogenesis imperfecta: a medical manual. Osteogenesis Imperfecta Foundation. Gaithersburg, MD

Wilkinson JM et al 1998 Surgical stabilisation of the lower limb in osteogenesis imperfecta using the Sheffield telescopic intramedullary rod system. Journal of Bone and Joint Surgery 80-B:6

Further Reading

Benson MKD et al 2002 Children's orthopaedics and fractures, 2nd edn. Churchill Livingstone, London, pp 464–477

Glorieux FH, Bishop NJ et al 1998 Cyclic administration of pamidronate in children with severe osteogenesis imperfecta. New England Journal of Medicine 339(14):947–952

Kanis KA 1996 Textbook of osteoporosis. Blackwell Science, London, pp 74–78

McCarthy GT 1992 Physical disability in childhood. An interdisciplinary approach to management. Churchill Livingstone, London

McRae R, Esser M 2002 Practical fracture treatment, 4th edn. Churchill Livingstone, London

Miller M, Glover C 1999 Wound management: theory and practice. NTBooks, London

Miller M, Miller JH 1985 Orthopaedics and accidents illustrated. Hodder & Stoughton, London

Royal College of Nursing (RCN) 1992 A practical guide to casting. Royal College of Nursing Society of Orthopaedic Nursing and Smith & Nephew, London

Saleh M, Scott BW 1992 Pitfalls and complications in leg lengthening: the Sheffield experience. Seminars in Orthopaedics 7(3):207–222

Staheli LL 2003 Fundamentals of pediatric orthopedics, 3rd edn. Lippincott Williams Wilkins, Philadelphia

Young ID 2002 Genetics for orthopaedic surgeons. Remedica Publishing, London

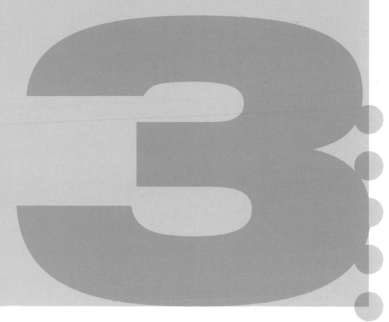

36 Prevention of childhood injuries 581
37 Information is the key to empowerment 591
38 Inherited conditions and the family 607
39 Health problems of the neonate 623
40 Health problems during infancy 637
41 Health problems in early childhood 665
42 Health needs of middle childhood 686
43 Child and adolescent mental health: the nursing response 700

Chapter Thirty Six

36

Prevention of Childhood Injuries

Jo Sibert, Donna Mead, Jim Richardson

ABSTRACT

The primary aim of this chapter and its companion PowerPoint presentation is to explore accidents in childhood. This will include consideration of mechanisms of injury and risk factors. The specific risks for children and causes of their vulnerability in this respect will be examined. Finally, a full analysis of measures that children's nurses can take to reduce morbidity and mortality will be made. The significance of this can be seen in the fact that accidents remain the single most frequent cause of death in children over the age of one.

Learning Outcomes

- Explore strategies for reducing the incidence and severity of childhood accidents.

- Describe and evaluate effective health education and promotion measures in relation to accident prevention.

- Examine specific accidents, their associated aetiology and their incidence.

Introduction

The prevention of injuries is an important issue for all those working with children because of the scale of the morbidity and mortality they cause.

Injuries are unlikely to be prevented by campaigns covering all types of injury: the aetiology and preventative solu-

www

You can find information and tables about the scale of the problem of accidents in childhood at:

- http://www.dti.gov.uk/ccp/topics1/pdf1/hass032002 data.pdf

tions are far too complex for that. However, a well-researched multidisciplinary action on individual types of accidents can be successful.

In preventing a particular injury, a methodological approach is needed: looking first at the size and nature of the problem, then deciding what preventive solutions are possible, implementing them on a small scale and then introducing them more widely when they have proved to be effective. There are three main strategies for injury control:

- education of children and parents
- changing the environment
- enforcing changes in the environment by law.

This approach of education, environment, and enforcement has become known as the 3 E's strategy. The introduction of child-resistant containers for medicines and household products is an example of a change in the environment that has reduced the incidence of accidental poisoning. Likewise, the reduction of the speed limit through enforcing local speed management strategies (particularly around schools, town centres and residential areas) has reduced both the incidence and severity of road traffic accidents. Teaching children to swim is an example of an education intervention that can reduce death from drowning. However, whereas all three strategies have had some success in reducing the incidence of childhood accidents, most successes have followed environmental changes. Educational campaigns by themselves are of only limited value. However, they do have a role and this is explored in detail further in the chapter.

What Can a Practitioner Do?

Possible roles of the practitioner in injury prevention are:

- as an advocate for children
- working with local authorities and non-governmental organisations on safe community activities
- working with families to ensure that the safety focus is firmly on the individual child
- encouraging a safe environment for children during the child surveillance programme
- opportunistic education
- responding to local issues.

Activity

Children's nurses working in the trauma area of an inner city hospital have noted that, in the summer months, many more children are admitted with serious trauma following road traffic accidents with the child as pedestrian:
- Using the 3 E's approach outlined above, make a list of proposals for action that might reduce the number and seriousness of the accidents.

AS AN ADVOCATE FOR CHILDREN

Before environmental measures are introduced by legislation, campaigns are needed to encourage the voluntary uptake so that ergonomic and effectiveness evaluation can be undertaken. Education can result in a change in public opinion, and the nurse can act as advocate and empower parents to lobby for environmental change. For instance, parents can be educated that safe playground equipment is needed for their children. They can then pressure the local authority to act.

In 1977, the Child Accident Prevention Trust (CAPT) was formed in England. The Trust brings many disciplines together to foster research and action on accidents to children. There are similar, but less well funded, groups in Wales (Child Safe Wales; Diogelu Plant Cymru), Scotland (Child Safe Scotland) and in other parts of the world. Similar groups exist throughout the word, e.g. Kidsafe in Australia, which claims to have halved childhood accidents since its inception in 1979.

WWW

For details on Kidsafe, go to:
- http://www.greenweb.com.au/kidsafe/

For details on CAPT, which includes Child Safe Wales:
- http://www.capt.org.uk/Publications/default.htm

ENCOURAGING A SAFE ENVIRONMENT FOR CHILDREN DURING THE CHILD SURVEILLANCE PROGRAMME

A number of studies (Schlesinger et al 1966, Sibert & Williams 1983) have shown that, by themselves, mass education campaigns to prevent accidents to children are ineffective. However, there is evidence to suggest that health visitors visiting the home and giving specific one-to-one attention to accident prevention can make a difference in the way that families behave, in particular with regard to the installation of safety equipment (Roberts et al 1996).

One of the problems is that it is extremely difficulty to establish firm cause and effect between safety interventions and reduction in incidence of severity of accidents. For example, a paper by Kendrick and colleagues (1997) reports on a randomized controlled trial of an intervention package of safety education in primary care assessed by the frequency of minor injuries. The intervention package was not effective in reducing the frequency of minor unintentional injuries in children at home. This is perhaps not surprising with such a difficult outcome measure where attendance in Accident Department is dependent on so many factors apart from the severity of the injury and when severe injuries (the ones we want to prevent) are not common enough to assess in this way.

Activity

A health visitor is undertaking a safety review for a family comprising a single, unsupported mother with three children aged 6 months, 18 months and 2.5 years:
- Consider each child's characteristics and stage of development together with the physical layout of the home and social determinants.
- Make notes on the areas that the health visitor and mother will look into and proposals for improving safety in each of those areas.

The Child Surveillance Programme is an excellent example of an initiative that stresses injury prevention through the various editions of *Health for all children*. This has become the basis for work with children in primary care. It stresses injury prevention.

WWW

More information on the Child Surveillance Programme can be found at:
- http://www.healthforallchildren.co.uk

WORKING WITH LOCAL AUTHORITIES AND NON-GOVERNMENTAL ORGANISATIONS ON SAFE COMMUNITY ACTIVITIES

The least effective way, in the long-term, of tackling the problem of childhood accidents is for locally derived actions to develop haphazardly. Strategies need to be within a national strategy, which encompasses epidemiology, legislation and evaluation, and with appropriate resource allocation. Once the overall strategy is in place, coordinated local activities can set the direction. In 1996, a public health team from the Karolinska Institute in Stockholm developed the concept of local action through safe communities. The first World Injury Control Conference (1989) approved a manifesto for safe communities: *Safety – a universal concern for all*. The second World Conference in Atlanta, Georgia, confirmed this.

WWW

For details of road safety strategies in Wales and Scotland, visit:
- http://www.wales.gov.uk/subitransport/content/consultation/saferoads/index.htm#top
- http://www.scotland.gov.uk/cru/kd01/blue/r-acc00.htm

Experience with Safe Child Penarth (Sibert & Stone 1998) showed that safe community projects on an individual child basis are possible but difficult to assess. Problems in demonstrating causal relationships between preventative intervention and outcomes such as reduction in overall injury presentation are problematic. It is very difficult to establish with any certainty whether the change that is observed was brought about by an intervention or by some other factor in the child's life and experience. Similarly, an increase in presentation at accident and emergency departments does not necessarily mean a failed intervention. However, a paper by Sibert et al (1999) looking at preventing injuries in public playgrounds showed that there has been some success with limited projects involving one type of injury such as playground injury. Throughout the UK there are small groups undertaking community projects.

Much is done on a low budget or voluntary level. One should not expect too much from community projects and it not reasonable to expect them not only to show that an injury prevention method works but also that the method of applying the method works. One of the problems of small-scale community projects is sustainability, in that interest often lapses over time. It is essential that sustainability is incorporated into the design of initiatives.

Overall, practitioners should take the opportunity for opportunistic safety education. A randomised trial by Clamp & Kendrick in 1998 showed that GP advice coupled with access to low-cost equipment for low-income families resulted in increased use of safety equipment and other safe practices. These findings are encouraging for provision of injury prevention in primary care.

Scenario

Children and families in some communities have a tradition of cooking with an open fire. The following factors are important:
- flammable clothing
- young women and female children undertaking cooking wearing loose clothing
- the high incidence of accidents resulting in burn injuries.

Activity

Propose a set of information which could be used to give to these families that would help them to reduce the risk of burn injuries in this situation.

Risk Factors for Injury

SOCIAL GRADIENTS

Among children aged 0–14 in England and Wales, fires are the second leading cause of accidental death. There is a steep social class gradient in the risk of fire-related death, due in part to social class differences in the prevalence of risk factors for residential fires, such as lone parenthood, financial difficulties and living in rental accommodation or poor quality housing.

Difference in smoke alarm ownership might also help to explain this social class gradient. Households least likely to have alarms include lone parent and low-income households and rental accommodation.

Activity

Consider the advantages and disadvantages of fire alarm giveaway schemes, targeted at high-risk households in a densely populated, multicultural, materially deprived community.

Social factors are important in childhood injuries. Road traffic injuries to children are five times more common and deaths in house fires 16 times more common in materially disadvantaged families. Similar social class gradients are seen in other injuries to children with the disadvantaged children having more injuries. The reasons are complex. Poorer families usually live in more dangerous environments, for example, it is much easier for a child to have a road accident if the house opens straight onto a main road in the inner city than if it is a detached house with a garden. Psychosocial stress factors are also involved in the aetiology of many childhood injuries, particularly road traffic injuries and accidental childhood poisoning.

PERSONALITY

The question of personality in childhood accidents and whether children can be injury prone is difficult. It is much more likely that injury proneness is related to the environment, both physical and social, rather than to personality factors. It is probably more correct to speak of an injury-prone community than an injury-prone child. Nevertheless, the characteristics of the child as a person will have a role to play. For example, adolescence is a particularly vulnerable time because children of this age are striving to become independent, are inclined to ignore rules and are prone to thrill-seeking and risk-taking behaviour.

 WWW

For details of the European Parliament's Injury Prevention Programme, go to:
- http://europa.eu.int/comm/health/ph_determinants/ environment/IPP/ipp_en.htm

Details of British activity in this field can be found at:
- http://www.rospa.com/CMS/index.asp

Specific Accident Types

ROAD TRAFFIC ACCIDENTS

Pedestrian Road Traffic Injuries

Pedestrian road traffic injuries are particularly common in the inner city and in children from socially deprived families. Fatality rates are correlated with the prosperity of the area. Psychosocial stress is an important factor in road traffic injuries and the interaction of a poor environment with stress is probably involved in many injuries.

Children, particularly boys under 10 years, are particularly at risk from pedestrian road traffic injuries. Parents may overestimate the ability of their children to handle traffic and let them go out on the road unsupervised. Sharples et al (1990), looking at deaths from head injuries in the northern region, found that 72% of these deaths occurred between 3 p.m. and 9 p.m. and mostly to boys playing after school.

Environmental Change and Child Pedestrian Road Traffic Injuries

The most effective means of preventing pedestrian road traffic accidents is by modifying the environment. Residential areas can be redesigned to give priority to pedestrians and to separate them from traffic. The speed of traffic can be reduced by speed humps and safe crossings can be provided. There is now good evidence that area-wide engineering schemes and traffic-calming schemes reduce injuries (Towner et al 2001). The provision of play areas will reduce the number of children on dangerous streets. The Safe Community approach is a way of introducing traffic calming.

Education and Child Pedestrian Road Traffic Injuries

It is possible to teach some children pedestrian skills. One approach is designating safer routes to school. Two randomized trials (Thomson et al 1992, Thomson & Whelan 1997) have showed improvements in children's finding safe places to cross the road. However, there is little evidence that these programmes have actually gone on to prevent injuries. Roberts (1994) concluded that safety and traffic education are unlikely by themselves to prevent road traffic injuries. School-based traffic clubs have not been shown to be effective.

Passenger Accidents

The protection of children in cars from serious injury and death must be an important part of any child safety programme. A major part of such protection is the development of child-restraint systems and seat belts.

The campaign group Belt Up School Kids (BUSK) has been campaigning since 1993 for the introduction of seat-belts on minibuses and other vehicles used by school children.

 WWW

For details on BUSK go to:
- http://www.ldv.co.uk/main_site/busk_about.htm

Much of the research on seat belts has been on adult passengers. There is good evidence that seat belts are effective in preventing death and serious injury. The Transport and Road Research Laboratory found that no child died in a 2-year period when in a restraint whereas 264 non-restrained children were killed in that period. Child-restraint systems have the unexpected bonus of improving children's behaviour and this probably improves driving standards. The problem is getting children to use them.

In young children and babies the barrier to the use of child restraints has in many cases been cost, and child-restraint loan schemes have been developed to help poorer families. They appear to be an effective strategy to increase the number of children safely transported in cars (Towner et al 2001). However, a randomized controlled trial demonstrating restraint use did not appear to increase correct use (Christopherson et al 1985).

Educational campaigns used to persuade children to wear seat belts have had mixed results. Miller & Pless (1977) found no significant differences in seat belt use, although Macknin et al (1987) found a campaign effective in the short term. Most countries have believed that legislation is needed to ensure seat belt usage. Serious injuries fell by 20% following the 1983 legislation in the UK compelling the wearing of seat belts in front seats. A systematic review (Towner et al 2001) of nine studies in the US evaluating seat belt legislation concluded that it was associated with reductions of injuries and death and increases the numbers of children using restraints. Many children remain unrestrained, however.

Cycle Helmets

The story of cycle helmets illustrates the international evolution of an environmental solution to a problem. Analysis by Clarke & Sibert (1986) of accident and emergency admissions shows that a significant number of children sustained severe head injuries after a cycle accident. Research-based evidence includes at least five case control studies (Thompson et al 1989, Spaite et al 1991, McDermott et al 1993, Thomas et al 1994, Malmaris et al 1994) that show the effectiveness of cycle helmets in preventing head injury. Work from Seattle (Rivara et al 1994) found that cyclists had an 85% reduction in their risk of head injury by wearing helmets. In addition to this compelling evidence there is also evidence in papers from 1994, by Cameron et al and Pitt et al, of a reduction in injuries following increases in cycle helmet use. These studies followed the introduction of safety legislation. State legislation regarding cycle helmets has been introduced sporadically in Australia and USA. Its effect continues to be monitored. No such action has been taken in the UK and, despite the research evidence, arguments continue as to whether cycle helmets are the solution to the problem. One centre, in Reading (cited in Lee et al 2000), has had some success in getting older children to use helmets but elsewhere experience is much less encouraging.

It is likely that the optimum way to reduce cycle injuries to children consists of a combination of designated cycle tracks, cycle proficiency education and cycle helmet legislation. The government's THINK website offers further advice.

WWW

For details on THINK go to:
- http://www.thinkroadsafety.gov.uk/

SMOKE DETECTORS AND HOUSE FIRES

Fires and flames are a significant cause of accidental death in childhood second only to road traffic accidents in many countries in Europe. The majority of children die in conflagrations in private dwellings, often in conditions of poverty. Many children die from gas and smoke inhalation rather than from direct heat. There have been striking changes in the number of children who have died from fire in recent years. Despite this, the death rate from fires is unacceptably high. A major component of the reduction has been the fall in the number of deaths from the ignition of clothing following flame proofing regulations and the reduction of open fires. House fires are a particular problem in poor families and are 16 times more common in social class V than social class I.

Smoke detectors are widely used in several countries. Reports by the US Fire administration (1980) and the Council for Scientific Affairs (1987) found them to be effective, particularly for children, as shown in DiGuiseppi et al (1998). Roberts (1994) indicates that they are becoming more established in the UK. They have an important role in the prevention of conflagrations and their use should be enforced both in public and private housing.

The effectiveness of education programmes to use smoke alarms has been less clearly established. In a recent systematic review of controlled trial interventions to promote smoke alarms, DiGuiseppi & Higgins (2000) suggest only modest potential benefits from education to promote smoke alarms. Smoke alarm promotion through the child surveillance programme may be more effective. Most effective of all would be regulations to have wired alarms in all housing, particularly in housing for the poor. This is because a major problem is that neither giving away smoke alarms nor enacting legislation will necessarily increase the prevalence of functioning alarms (Roberts & DiGuiseppi 1999)

● Seminar discussion topic

'Every family receiving state benefits should receive free smoke alarms, assistance to fit them and 6-monthly checks to ensure that they are working satisfactorily.'

SCALDS

Scalds are among the most distressing injuries a child can receive. They do not often cause the death but they do cause considerable pain, they often need prolonged treatment and they often result in life-long scarring. This scarring and deformity may result in considerable emotional difficulties that can affect the child's whole life. Clearly it would be much better if we could prevent these concerning injuries rather than have to treat them. Sadly, evidence from Wales (Green et al 1984, Eadie et al 1995) suggests that there had been no reduction in the numbers of scalds to children since 1956. There has been a change in the pattern of these injuries. Hot water from teapots caused a fifth of the injuries in 1956. This has declined to very few cases in 1991. However, hot liquids from cups now cause almost half the scald injuries compared with less than one case in ten 35 years ago. People are now making hot drinks with instant coffee and tea bags in the cup rather than in the pot.

The most common cause of scalds – those from the cup – presents particular difficulties for prevention. It is difficult to see how an environmental solution such as an especially designed cup would be practicable or acceptable. More encouragingly, there may be preventive solutions to these injuries that involve environmental modification that may be successful with kettle and bath scalds. The usual mechanism of a scald from a kettle is the child pulling the flex that overhangs the work surface. A preventive answer to this has been the use of coiled or short flexes. Recently there has been a change in European Consumer Standards. Flexes (coiled or otherwise) should now be no longer than 80 mm. This hopefully will result in a reduction in scalds.

The majority of bath scalds are caused when the child falls in the water (Yeoh et al 1994). A reduction in the temperature of tap water entering the bath should prevent these scalds. Although standards for gas and electricity recommend 60°C maximum for thermostats, many households have water temperatures above 60°C (Murray 1988). Even at this temperature, a partial thickness burn to a child will result in 10 seconds (Lawrence & Bull 1976). There may be considerable consumer resistance to the altering of thermostats. A study in New Zealand (Waller et al 1993) evaluated an educational programme to reduce the temperature of hot tap water in homes. They found that there were significant decreases in tap water temperature in their study population but that the majority of households still had a temperature above 55°C. A more easily acceptable solution should be the use of thermostatic mixer taps for the bath set at 43°C. This is the answer that is now accepted practice in the NHS Estates (Health Guidance Note 1982). High cost is at present a key factor in their more widespread introduction.

WWW

Further details on scalding can be found at the Department for Trade and Industry's website:
- http://www.cst.gov.uk/homesafetynetwork/bs_intro.htm

DROWNING

Drowning is the third most common cause of accidental death in children in the UK and in Europe. When the problem was reviewed in 1992 (Kemp & Sibert 1992), each site of drowning incident has a definite age range and corresponds to a stage in child development:

- babies who cannot protect themselves when they fall in bath water
- toddlers who wander off and drown in accessible water (garden ponds in the UK, drainage ditches in the Netherlands and domestic swimming pools in southern Europe).
- older children who die when swimming unsupervised.

Drowning deaths in the UK were again reviewed for 1998–9 (Sibert et al 2002). There was a reduction by a third in deaths over the 10 years (however, garden ponds were a particular problem).

Prevention of Drowning

- **Supervision**: there is evidence that supervision of swimming and water activity should prevent drowning. In the UK only one child dies a year in municipal pools where there is clear observation of swimming enforced by the Health and Safety Executive, whereas many die in rivers, lakes and canals where there is no supervision. Certainly, there has been an overall fall in the number of deaths of children from drowning, which has coincided with better supervision. Some European countries have a clear emphasis on the supervision of swimming.

- **Drowning in hotel pools**: there is clear evidence from work by consumer organisations and from press reports that children drown in hotel pools while on holiday. These deaths are likely to be preventable if these pools could be supervised. Progress could be achieved by action by tour operators.

- **Provision of safety fences in domestic pools**: in affluent, warm countries, drowning in swimming pools is a common cause of death in toddlers. There is evidence from Australia that fencing domestic pools can prevent drowning. Pearn & Nixon (1977) compared drownings in private swimming pools in Brisbane and in Canberra. Fencing has been introduced by regulation in parts of Australia, South Africa, New Zealand and parts of the United States (Pearn & Nixon 1977, Langley 1983, Orlowski 1989).

- **Garden ponds**: just as Australian toddlers drown in swimming pools, British children drown in garden ponds. The numbers are small but they are preventable deaths. No home with children under five should have an open garden pond. This should be clearly stated in the Child Surveillance Programme.

WWW

Advice on water safety can be found at:
- http://www.lifesavers.org.uk/

Activity

Devise a leaflet to give new parents information aimed towards preventing babies drowning in baths.

FALLS

Falls cause some deaths in childhood but are also the most common cause of presentation to the accident and emergency department. They have a varied aetiology. They may be on one level, such as falling on the pavement, at home or in the school playground. Younger children may be dropped, fall from furniture or fall down the stairs. Older children fall from trees, cliffs and mountains, play equipment and buildings. Poor window catches and design allow a number of accidents, particularly in high-rise flats. The introduction of safety catches or window guards will reduce these. In New York City a programme providing free window guards (The Children Can't Fly Program) has been successful in preventing window falls in a poor area of New York (Spiegal & Lindaman 1977).

Falls downstairs are a particular problem for toddlers. Much can be done to prevent them, by better stair design and stair gates. The use of stair gates can be encouraged by the health visitor, and a Safe Community programme. Open stairs with wide gaps between balustrades may be aesthetically beautiful but are dangerous for young children. In 1985, UK building regulations were changed to make certain that a 100 mm sphere could not be passed through any opening or guard to a flight of stairs.

Baby Walkers

The danger of falls from baby walkers has been highlighted by a number of studies throughout the European Union:

- In Greece, Petridou et al (1996) identified the incidence of baby walkers injuries as 3.5/1000 per year. They also identified that these do not have any benefit for child development.

- In the UK, Glendill et al (1987) identified baby walkers as a major hazard without benefit. Kendrick & Marsh (1998) identified baby walker use as common across all social groups and as being associated with other unsafe practices such as not using stair gates or fireguards. They believed that health professionals should support campaigns to limit the sale of baby walkers but, in addition, they should ascertain each family's reasons for walker use and try to find acceptable alternatives. They should also make the family aware of the importance of properly fitted stair gates and fireguards and help the family to obtain and use such items of safety equipment.

Baby walkers offer risks of injury but no benefit to children. There are EU regulations on baby walkers but many do not comply with them. There is a clear argument that they should be banned. They should be discouraged in any health promotion programme with families with young people.

Activity

Using the 3 E's approach, introduced earlier, plan health education strategies to discourage the use of baby walkers.

FARM INJURIES

Agriculture is an essential part of the work of the UK within the European Union. Recently, much attention has been paid to bovine spongioform encephalitis, however many more people have died from agricultural injuries than from new variant CJD.

Agriculture is unique in that a significant component of the work force is made up from children under the age of 16, especially at times of peak activity in the farming year. For children, the most significant feature in considering farm-related accidents is that the farm is perceived as a place of excitement and adventure. For many, the farm is often also the home, or the place where holidays are taken. There have been a number of studies:

- In 1989, Doyle and colleagues in Ireland reviewed farm injuries. They also found significant unrecognised problems.

- Schelp (1992) in Sweden found that the dominant types of injuries were falls, crushes and eye injuries.

- In the UK, Cameron et al (1992) reviewed the problem of farm accidents among children by a 12-month prospective study of farm accidents involving children in the county of Dyfed and found that one child in 50 living on a farm presents with a farm-related accident in a year. None of these non-fatal cases had been reported to Health and Safety Executive, although they should have been by law. There is also legislation to prohibit the driving of tractors by children under the age of 13 and to prohibit the riding of any persons as passengers on tractors, trailers, or other field implements. This has been in place for many years but is often ignored. A safe community approach is being tried in some places, for example Ceredigion, Wales.

- In the USA, a study from 1990 to 2003 into fatal and non-fatal injuries, found 8 deaths per 100,000 child farm residents per year.

Farm safety should be an integral part of the Child Surveillance Programme in rural areas.

PLAYGROUND INJURIES

Play is vital for children in their physical development and their ability to make social relationships. Although children play at home and in organized groups, many play in playgrounds provided by local authorities and private organisations. Playgrounds provide an alternative to playing in dangerous places such as the road and need to be as safe as possible. Professionals will wish to influence playground safety in their districts by lobbying the local authority. There has been much work developing safer equipment and surfaces and producing acceptable safety standards. This has been done in Europe, America and Australia. These standards and safety features in modern playgrounds have been developed in the laboratory using road crash adult cadaver data on head injury. They include safety surfaces, modifying equipment and maintenance.

Injuries to children in playgrounds are a complex subject. They are influenced by many factors, including the environment of the playground, the behaviour of the child and the frequency of use. There is a potential conflict between safety and play value. The quality of the literature is not high and there are few intervention studies. Many of the studies that have investigated playground injuries have described overall injuries. This may have resulted in insufficient focus on the injuries that really matter: those to the head and fractures. A historical review implies that there were serious head injuries before the introduction of modernisation and safety surfacing. Indeed, the prevention of head injuries was the reason why safety surfacing was introduced. There are very few serious head injuries now in modern playgrounds. We believe that safety surfacing is important to prevent head injuries and should be continued. These and other safety measures such as swing design should not prevent children getting play value out of equipment in modern playgrounds. Play can be exciting but not unnecessarily dangerous.

 WWW

The Royal Society for Prevention of Accidents has factsheets on playgrounds at:
- http://www.rospa.co.uk/cms/

There is also evidence that safety surfacing has prevented overall injuries, although there is no evidence that fractures of the arm have been prevented by safety surfacing; indeed, the rate of fractures is remarkably constant of all presentations throughout the literature. There are biomechanical reasons for this. We need now to be developing surfaces that are protective against fractures while not compromising safety against head injury. There are difficulties in implementing intervention studies to prevent playground injuries. Despite these difficulties we really must be looking to perform more of these studies if safety is going to progress. The key to this is ongoing surveillance in partnership between health professionals and the local authority.

POISONING

Accidental poisoning is predominantly seen in children under the age of 5 years but older children may be involved if they are developmentally delayed. The peak age is between 1 and 4 years. This is a key area because of the preventive value of child resistant containers and packaging.

Children may take a variety of substances accidentally. These are conveniently divided into medicines (prescribed and non-prescribed), household products and plants. The majority of children who take poisons do not have serious symptoms. Medicines may be of low toxicity, e.g. the oral contraceptive pill or antibiotics; intermediate toxicity, which may cause symptoms in young children, or of potential high toxicity (Sibert & Routledge 1991). Many of the household products children take may be relatively non-toxic, however a few such as caustic soda, soldering flux and paint stripper may cause serious harm.

Child-resistant Containers and Packaging

Dr Jay Arena in Durham, North Carolina, first suggested child-resistant containers (CRCs) in 1959. These containers were evaluated in a community in the US by Scherz (1970) and found to be successful. They were then introduced with successful results into the US for aspirin preparations (Walton 1982). Following this work in the US, child-resistant closures were progressively introduced in some countries in Europe. There have been few studies evaluating these changes.

In the UK, CRCs were introduced by regulation in 1976 for junior aspirin and paracetamol preparations. This resulted in a fall in admissions of children younger than 5 years after salicylate poisoning (Sibert et al 1977, Jackson et al 1985). In 1982, a voluntary agreement between the British government and the Royal Pharmaceutical Society ensured that all prescribable solid dose medication would be placed in CRCs or safety packaging with exceptions only for the elderly and infirm. In 1985 Department of Trade and Industry regulated for a number of household products to be sold in CRCs. Now many medicines are dispensed in opaque unit packaging.

Information on child-resistant container and packaging regulations from the 15 countries in the European Union has been collected. Some countries appear to have no regulations at all, some have regulations for some household products and some have regulations for some medicines and some household products. There is good evidence that child-resistant containers and packaging prevent childhood poisoning. There is also evidence that their use is very variable across the European Union. Regulations that involve consumer products should be harmonised throughout the European Union.

Summary

The range and mechanisms of the most common accidents to children as well as the changes in incidence of different forms of accident over time offers a good range of insights. Strategies for keeping children safe can be discerned and action planned following a framework such as:

- education
- environment
- enforcement.

The field of child safety and accident prevention provides examples of how health education can be delivered opportunistically. This is an area where children's nurses can help families to improve the safety and well-being of children. Every encounter between nurse and family is an opportunity to give useful information.

References

Arena JM 1959 Safety closure caps. Journal of the American Medical Association 169:1187–1188

Ball D 2002 Playgrounds: risks, benefits and choices. Contact research report 426/2002. Health and Safety Executive, London

Cameron D, Bishop C, Sibert JR 1992 Farm accidents in children. British Medical Journal 305:23–25

Cameron MH, Vulcan AP, Finch CF 1994 Mandatory bicycle helmet use: an evaluation. Accident Analysis and Prevention 26:325–327

Christopherson E, Sosland-Edelman D, LeClaire S 1985 Evaluation of two comprehensive infant car seat loaner programs with one-year follow-up. Pediatrics 76:36–42

Clamp M, Kendrick D 1998 A randomised controlled trial of general practitioner safety advice for families with children under 5 years. British Medical Journal 316:1576–1579

Clarke AJ, Sibert JR 1986 Why child cyclists should wear helmets. Practitioner 230:513–514

Council for Scientific Affairs 1987 Preventing death and injury from fires with automatic sprinklers and smoke detectors. Journal of the American Medical Association 257:1618–1620

DiGuiseppi C, Higgins JP 2000 Systematic review of controlled trials of interventions to promote smoke alarms. Archives of Diseases of Childhood 82:341–348

DiGuiseppi C, Roberts I 1998 Smoke alarm ownership and house fire death rates in children. Journal of Epidemiology and Community Health 52:760–761

Doyle Y, Conroy R 1989 Childhood farm accidents; a continuing cause for concern. Journal of the Society of Occupational Medicine 39:35–37

Eadie PA, Williams R, Dickson WA 1995 Thirty-five years of paediatric scalds: are lessons being learned? British Journal of Plastic Surgery 48:103–105

First World Conference on Accident and Injury Prevention (Stockholm) 1989 Manifesto for safe communities. World Health Organization, Geneva

Glendill DNS, Robson WV, Cudmore RE, Tavistock RR 1987 Baby walkers – time to take a stand. Archives of Diseases of Childhood 62:491–494

Green AR, Fairclough J, Sykes PJ 1984 Epidemiology of burns in childhood. Burns 10:368–371

Health Guidance Note 1982 Safe hot water and surface temperatures. NHS Estates, HMSO, London

Illingworth C, Brennan P, Jay A et al 1975 200 injuries caused by playground equipment. British Medical Journal 4:332–334

Jackson RH, Craft AW, Lawson GR, Sibert JR 1985 Changing pattern of poisoning in children. British Medical Journal 287:1468

Kemp A, Sibert JR 1992 Drowning and near drowning in children in the United Kingdom. Lessons for prevention. British Medical Journal 304:1143–1146

Kemp A, Sibert JR 1996 Preventing scalds to children. British Medical Journal 311:643–644

Kemp A, Gibbs N, Vafidis G, Sibert JR 1998 Safe Child Penarth: experience with a Safe Community strategy for preventing injuries to children. Injury Prevention 4:63–68

Kendrick D, Marsh P 1997 Injury prevention programmes in primary care: a high risk group or a whole population approach. Injury Prevention 3:170–175

Kendrick D, Marsh P 1998 Baby walkers: prevalence of use and relationship with other safety practices. Injury Prevention 4:295–298

Kendrick D, Marsh P, Fielding K, Miller P 1999 Preventing injuries in children: cluster randomised controlled trial in primary care. British Medical Journal 318:980–983

Langley J 1983 Fencing of private swimming pools in New Zealand. Community Health Studies 7:285–289

Lawrence JC, Bull JP 1976 Thermal conditions which cause skin burns. Engineering in Medicine 5:61–63

Lee A, Mann NP, Takriti R 2000 A hospital-based promotion campaign aimed to increase bicycle helmet wearing among children aged 11–15 living in West Berkshire 1992–98. Injury Prevention 6:151–153

Macknin M, Gustafson C, Gassman J, Barich D 1987 Office education by pediatricians to increase seat belt use. American Journal of Diseases in Children 141:1305–1307

Malmaris C, Summers CL, Browning C, Palmer CR 1994 Injury patterns in cyclists attending an accident and emergency department: a comparison of helmet wearers and non-wearers. British Medical Journal 308:1537–1540

McDermott FT, Lane JC, Brazenor GA, Debney EA 1993 The effectiveness of bicycle helmets: a study of 1710 casualties. Journal of Trauma 34:834–844

Miller J, Pless I 1977 Child automobile restraints: evaluation of health education. Pediatrics 59:907–911

Milliner N, Pearn J, Guard R 1980 Will fenced pools save lives? Medical Journal of Australia 2:510–511

Mott A, Rolfe K, James R et al 1997 Safety of surfaces and equipment for children in playgrounds. Lancet 348:1874–1876

Murray JP 1988 A study of the prevention of hot tap water burns. Burns 14:185–193

Norton C, Rolfe K, Morris S et al 2004 Head injury and limb fracture in modern playgrounds. Archives of Diseases in Childhood 89(2):152–153

Oliver TI, MacFarlane JP, Haigh JC et al 1981 Playground equipment and accidents. Australian Paediatric Journal 17(2):100–103

Orlowski JP, 1989 It's time for pediatricians to 'rally round the pool fence'. Pediatrics 83:1065–1066

Pearn JH, Nixon J 1977 Are swimming pools becoming more dangerous? Medical Journal of Australia 2(21):702–704

Petridou E, Simou E, Skondras C et al 1996 Hazards of baby walkers in a European context. Injury Prevention 2:118–120

Pitt RW, Thomas S, Nixon J et al 1994 Trends in head injuries amongst cyclists. British Medical Journal 308:177

Rfidah EI, Casey PB, Tracey JA, Gill D 1991 Childhood poisoning in Dublin. Irish Medical Journal 84:87–89

Rivara F 1997 Fatal and non-fatal farm injuries to children and adolescents in the US 1990–3. Injury Prevention 3:190–194

Rivara FP, Thompson DC, Thompson RS 1994 The Seattle children's bicycle helmet campaign: changes in helmet use and head injury admissions. Pediatrics 93:567–569

Rivers RP, Boyd RD, Baderman H 1978 Falls from equipment as a cause of playground injury. Community Health 9:178–179

Roberts I 1994 Smoke alarm use: prevalence and household predictors. Injury Prevention 2:263–265

Roberts I, DiGuiseppi C 1999 Smoke alarms, fire deaths and randomised controlled trials. Injury Prevention 5:244–246

Roberts I, Kramer M, Suisa S 1996 Does home visiting prevent childhood injury? A systematic review of randomised control trials. British Medical Journal 312:29–34

Schelp L 1992 The occurrence of farm–environmental injuries in a Swedish municipality. Accident Analysis and Prevention 24:161–166

Scherz RG 1970 Prevention of childhood poisoning. Pediatric Clinics of North America 17:713

Schlesinger ER, Dickson DG, Westaby J et al 1966 A controlled study of health education in accident prevention: the Rockland County child injury project. American Journal of Diseases in Children 111:490-4-96

Sharples PM, Storey A, Aynsley-Green A, Eyre JA 1990 Causes of fatal childhood accidents involving head injury in northern region, 1979–86. British Medical Journal 301:1193–1197

Sibert JR, Kemp AM 2003 Safe communities for children: only models of good practice or ways through practical difficulties in injury prevention? Child: Care, Health and Development 28:439–442

Sibert JR, Routledge P 1991 Accidental child poisoning – can we admit fewer children with safety? Archives of Diseases in Childhood 66:263–266

Sibert JR, Stone D 1998 Injury prevention in the UK – the European dimension. Injury Prevention 4(Suppl):S34–S41

Sibert JR, Williams H 1983 Medicine and the media. British Medical Journal 286:1893

Sibert JR, Craft AW, Jackson RH 1977 Child resistant packaging and accidental child poisoning. Lancet ii:289–290

Sibert JR, Lyons RA, Smith BA, et al 2002 Safe water information monitor collaboration. Preventing deaths by drowning in children in the United Kingdom: have we made progress in 10 years? Population-based incidence study. British Medical Journal 324(7345):1070–1071.

Sibert JR, Mott A, Rolfe K et al 1999 Preventing injuries in public playgrounds through partnership between health services and local authority: community intervention study. British Medical Journal 318:1595.

Sibert JR, Norton C, Nixon J 2004 Playground injuries to children: play value or safety or both? Archives of Diseases in Childhood 89(2):103–108

Spaite DW, Murphy M, Criss EA et al 1991 A prospective analysis of injury severity among helmeted and non helmeted bicyclists involved in collisions with motor vehicles. Journal of Trauma 31:1510–1516

Spiegal CN, Lindaman FC 1977 Children can't fly: a program to prevent childhood morbidity and mortality from window falls. American Journal of Public Health 67:1143–1147

Sundstrom M, Svanstrom L 1996 Criteria for the Safe Community Network. WHO Collaborating Centre, Karolinska Institute, Stockholm

Thomas S, Acton C, Nixon J et al 1994 Effectiveness of bicycle helmets in preventing injury in children: a case control study. British Medical Journal 308:173–176

Thompson R, Rivara FP, Thompson DCA 1989 case control study on the effectiveness of bicycle safety helmets. New England Journal of Medicine 320:1361–1367

Thomson J, Ampofo-Boeteng K, Pitcairn T, Grieve R 1992 Behavioural group training of children to find safe routes to school. British Journal of Educational Psychology 62:173–183

Thomson J, Whelan K 1997 A community approach to road safety education using practical training methods. The Drumchapel Project. Road Safety Report No. 3, Department of Transport, London

Towner E, Dowswell T, Mackereth C, Jarvis S 2001 What works in preventing unintentional injuries in children and young adolescents? An updated systematic review. NHS Health Development Agency, London

US Fire Administration 1980 An evaluation of residential smoke detectors under actual field conditions. Final report, EMW-C-002. US Fire Administration, Washington DC

Waller AE, Clarke JA, Langley JD 1993 An evaluation of a program to reduce home hot tap water temperatures. Australian Journal of Public Health 17:116–123

Walton WW 1982 An evaluation of the poison prevention act. Pediatrics 69:363–370

Yeoh C, Nixon J, Dickson W et al 1994 Patterns of scald injuries to children in the bath. Archives of Diseases in Childhood 71:156–158

Chapter Thirty Seven

37

Information is the Key to Empowerment

Tom C A Hain, E Alan Glasper

ABSTRACT

The primary aim of this chapter and its companion PowerPoint presentation is to consider the role of information in empowering children and their families in health care. Key background documents are discussed, the role of the children's nurse in providing information is considered, and issues explored around ensuring such information is accurate, relevant and communicated clearly for the child and his family.

Learning Outcomes

- Define empowerment in the context of health promotion.
- Consider the importance of providing information to support family-centred and self-care.
- Understand key issues raised in the Bristol Inquiry related to information giving.
- Review current initiatives in the field of consumer health information.
- Identify quality criteria for health information.
- Appreciate the role of NHS Direct Online.

Introduction

There is growing recognition in the UK of the need for healthcare professionals to improve the way they communicate with patients and the public. There is also acknowledgement that written and other information resources play an increasingly important role in modern health care, with a focus on empowering service users. Such information needs to be developed with users of services, and to the highest standards. The report of the Bristol Inquiry (Department of Health (DoH) 2001), which is perhaps the most in-depth analysis of a modern health service and its systems, made a number of key recommendations for improving communication. As a consequence, many national initiatives have emerged.

Empowerment

The term 'empowerment' has become somewhat of a buzz word, yet it is often misunderstood or used as a euphemism for any strategy that saves nursing time. The term stems from the Latin word *potere*, meaning 'to be able' and is also linked to the word *potent*, meaning 'powerful, cogent, persuasive and having or exercising a great influence'.

However, the rhetoric of empowerment is somewhat different from the concreteness of strategies of empowerment that purport to enable people to make health-related decisions. Although the pursuit of empowerment strategies by nurses is a relatively recent phenomenon, it has become an integral component of advocacy. The term 'empowerment' is appealing perhaps because it conjures up images of power and independence. The nursing profession has embraced advocacy as a method of promoting family-centred care but the methods of achieving its implementation have changed considerably over the years. From a position of interceding or pleading a case for families, children's nurses now act as guardians, for their rights to autonomy and free choice. Indeed, current health promotion ideology accepts empowerment as enabling and supporting people to set their own health agendas and to take control of their health status through skills development and critical consciousness-raising (Glasper & McWilams 1998).

Although there have been many innovations in patient advocacy, and empowerment is a real force within the field of child care, it has to be stressed that patients and families are sometimes passive bystanders in the process and this results in inequalities in the healthcare professional–family relationship.

Gann (1991) has stated that information giving is the key to empowerment and if this is true, the provision of information will enhance the relationship between the professional and the family.

Patient-centred Care

When considering the role of health information, it is important to place this in context within a framework for patient-centred care. In the late 1970s, the Planetree organisation, based in Connecticut, USA, pioneered a model for patient-centred care that is widely used today (Planetree 2003). Planetree states that its model is holistic and considers healing in all dimensions – mental, emotional, spiritual and social, as well as physical. It aims to maximise healthcare outcomes by integrating complementary medical therapies such as mind/body medicine and therapeutic massage with conventional medical therapies. Within the Planetree model a strand has developed that focuses on empowering patients through information and education. This is achieved through a variety of initiatives, including production of information tailored for the individual, collaborative conferences for patients and experts and the development of patient care pathways. Many similar initiatives based on Planetree have since emerged in the UK.

THE BRISTOL ROYAL INFIRMARY INQUIRY (2000)

Close to 200 recommendations were made following the national, public 'Bristol Inquiry' (DoH 2000a). Many of the key recommendations relate to the means through which information is obtained and communicated to children and their families (Box 37.1). It is important to consider these in context. The main issues leading to the national public inquiry are clarified in the summary document itself.

 WWW

Read the summary of the Bristol Inquiry report online at:
• http://www.bristol-inquiry.org.uk/final_report/Summary.pdf

In the summary report, specific references are made to characteristics of the information made available to the families represented in the inquiry.

 Box 37.1

Key messages from the Bristol Inquiry

• Patients must be involved in decisions about their treatment and care, wherever possible (recommendation 1)
• Health professionals must adopt the notion of partnership, where the patient and professional meet as equals with different expertise (recommendation 3)
• Information about treatment and care should be given in a variety of forms, be given in stages and be reinforced over time (recommendation 4)
• Information should be tailored to the needs, circumstances and wishes of the individual (recommendation 5)
• Information should be based on the current available evidence and include a summary of the evidence and data, in a form which is comprehensible to patients (recommendation 6)
• Various modes of conveying information, whether leaflets, tapes, videos or CDs, should be regularly updated, and developed and piloted with the help of patients (recommendation 7)
• The public should receive guidance on those sources of information about health and health care on the internet which are reliable and of good quality: a kitemarking system should be developed (recommendation 9)
• Patients must be given such information as enables them to participate in their care (recommendation 12)
• Before embarking on any procedure, patients should be given an explanation of what is going to happen and, after the procedure, should have the opportunity to review what has happened (recommendations 13, 16)

Such information as was given to parents was often partial, confusing and unclear . . . Patients should be able to gain access to information about relative performance of a hospital, or a particular service or consultant.

This illustrates the need for healthcare professionals to ensure all information is complete and clearly communicated. Nurses should be in a position to respond appropriately when asked by families for details of a hospital's performance (such information may be provided within a Commission for Health Improvement report) as well as details related to clinicians' performance.

Another key issue raised in the Bristol report is whether staff have the skills to communicate effectively:

All healthcare staff who treat children should be trained in communicating with young people and parents.

This statement implies that the content of basic and postgraduate training courses for many healthcare staff should be reviewed in light of the findings from the Bristol Inquiry. A number of communication-related training initiatives have since emerged. For example, the new NHS University is developing a communication skills module within its induction programme for all new NHS staff (NHSU 2004).

The Bristol Inquiry recommendations suggest that a range of information is usually required by the child and family, not only information about treatment and care, but also information that supports the child and family to deliver care for themselves. All information should be discussed face-to-face and information supporting such discussion should be made available, at least in written format. Where multimedia resources exist, these may add considerably to the usefulness of the resource (for example, a video/DVD demonstrating the use of a piece of equipment such as an inhaler can be a very useful aid).

Following the Bristol Inquiry report, other key initiatives illustrate the stronger focus for information provision in the context of empowerment and advocacy. Included are the Children's National Service framework (DoH 2003) and the Welsh Children's Commissioner's report *Telling concerns* (Children's Commissioner for Wales 2003).

CHILDREN'S NATIONAL SERVICE FRAMEWORK (2003)

In April 2003, the DoH published the Children's National Service Framework for hospital standards (DoH 2003). It is recognised within this document that children and their parents should be given support and information to enable them to understand and cope with the illness or injury, and the treatment needed. The document indicates that there will be a greater focus on delivering better information: for children, young people and their parents on health and health services, and how to access them; about children receiving care, through support of an integrated care pathway; to support clinical practice; and for monitoring and continual improvement of services.

CHILDREN'S COMMISSIONER FOR WALES REPORT (2003)

The *Telling concerns* report (Children's Commissioner for Wales 2003) considers how far systems for complaints, whistle blowing and advocacy are effective in safeguarding and promoting the rights and welfare of children in Wales. Relating to complaints and representation of children, the report recommends that local authority social services should continue to involve children and young people in the review and future design of information material (recommendation 3.7). In relation to advocacy, the report states that local authority social services, in partnership with the advocacy provider, should continue to involve children and young people in the production of any publicity materials (recommendation 5.17).

The Growth of Consumer Health Information as a Specialism

Patient organisations have in many ways been leading the development of health information services for a number of years, responding particularly to information needs unmet by the NHS. Sophisticated information services will provide a range of information in a variety of formats and often in different languages. A number of national information services have developed rapidly over the last decade. When supporting the child and family in obtaining current information to support health needs, the nurse is now able to draw upon a number of services available nationally. Examples of these services are summarised in this chapter, starting with a synopsis of the work of the Help for Health Trust, birthplace of both The Centre for Health Information Quality (http://www.chiq.org/chiq) and NHS Direct Online (http://www.nhsdirect.nhs.uk), and considered by many to be the lead organisation in the field of consumer health information.

THE HELP FOR HEALTH TRUST

To help people become active partners in their own health care by improving the provision of quality information (mission statement of the Help for Health Trust)

The Help for Health Trust (website: http://www.hfht.org) began as a British-Library-funded research project into information about self-help groups. During the 1980s, with funding initially from Hampshire Area Health Authority, and then from Wessex Regional Health Authority, the Trust established itself as one of the first consumer health information services, based at Southampton General Hospital. Later in the 1980s, the Trust was active in early consumer health information work on HIV/AIDS and waiting times for treatment. The Trust's database of self-help groups and publications, Helpbox (http://www.hfht.org/Helpbox%20 Ad.htm), was also launched at this time. In 1991, the implementation of the Patient's Charter saw the requirement on all Regional Health Authorities to set up a helpline based on the Help for Health Trust's model. The Trust worked closely with the NHS Executive to develop the national freephone Health Information Service (Help for Health Trust 1997) and provided central support to all health information service providers with funding from the DoH. Additionally, as part of the Patient's Charter (DoH 1991), the Trust was commissioned to produce a user guide to the health service, the *NHS A–Z* (http://www.hfht. org/nhs%20atoz.htm), which is still supplied as an online database.

During the 1990s the Trust continued to develop its services, with the establishment of a research unit with a specialism in research into dissemination of treatment information to consumers. The Trust also provided information to public health professionals through a contract with the Wessex Institute for Health Research and Development. In 1996, the Trust was awarded the contract to set up The Centre for Health Information Quality, funded by the DoH to promote the production of high-quality, evidence-based information for patients. Between 1998 and 2001, the Trust managed the Support Unit to the Standing Group on Consumers in NHS Research (now known as Involve; website: http://www.invo.org.uk). The Trust was a lead partner in NHS Direct Hampshire and was responsible for setting up, running and developing NHS Direct Online, which was launched by the Prime Minister in December 1999. Both *NHS A–Z* and Helpbox have been supplied to NHS Direct Online and to a number of other key providers, including Primary Care Trusts.

As well as supporting its database services and The Centre for Health Information Quality, the Help for Health Trust is also a Forum Support Organisation for the Commission for Patient and Public Involvement in Health (http://www.cppih.org), providing support for local Patient and Public Involvement Forums. The Trust also promotes community engagement through the development of online communities such as 'Engage', which is designed for Primary Care Trusts (see: http://www.kingstonpct.nhs.uk).

PATIENT ORGANISATIONS AND SELF-HELP GROUPS

Patient organisations and self-help groups have a rich history of providing combined information services for specific target audiences. For example, people with cancer can use specialist telephone advice services provided by CancerBacup (http://www.cancerbacup.org.uk) or Macmillan Cancer Relief (http://www.macmillan.org.uk). Through such services, users can access further information in leaflet format or via the internet. However, although the aforementioned services are recognised as leaders in their field, the quality of similar services can be variable and the nurse should take time to review exactly what is being provided before recommending such services to families.

TELEPHONE SERVICES

The telephone, mainly through NHS Direct, now plays a very significant role in healthcare provision throughout the UK. Nurses can develop telephone skills that will allow them to give information, communicated clearly to a client at the other end. There are currently 22 NHS Direct call centres across the UK, providing a round-the-clock national telephone advice service. Some 6 million calls are taken

through this service each year, a figure that is expected to rise to around 15 million.

INTERNET SERVICES

NHS Direct Online was launched by the Prime Minister in December 1999. A range of databases covering health topics is available 24 hours a day, and receives more than 450,000 visitors each month. Users of NHS Direct Online are able to access a number of databases to obtain information about health and health services and current health news items. In the future, users will also be able to develop personal space for information.

 WWW

Visit the NHS Direct Online website and consider how the information available may be of use to a child (and his or her family) that you are currently looking after:

- **http://www.nhsdirect.nhs.uk**

NHS DIRECT ONLINE
(http://www.nhsdirect.nhs.uk)

NHS Direct Online is a website providing high-quality health information and advice for the people of England. It is unique in being supported by a 24-hour nurse advice and information helpline. NHS Direct Online is viewed as the public interface with the NHS, providing health information, advice and appropriate use of NHS resources (Jenkins & Gann 2001).

NHS Direct Online has become one of the most popular websites in the UK, with around half a million people now visiting the website each month. It has established itself as Europe's leading health website (Jenkins & Gann 2003). This was recognised in May 2003 when it won the eHealth Europe award for empowering citizens in management of health and well-being at the European Commission in Brussels.

History

The government introduced *The NHS Plan* as a plan for investment with sustained increase in funding to reform the NHS. The vision was to give the people of Britain a health service fit for the 21st century: a health service built around the needs of the patient (DoH 2000b). The need for a knowledge (information)-based NHS is a political imperative. The national strategic programme (DoH 2000c) is concerned with major developments in the use of information technology within the NHS, including development of services using electronic communications. The government's vision is for information and IT to connect delivery of *The NHS Plan* with the capabilities of modern information technologies. As a result, December 1999 saw further diversification of the services provided by NHS Direct with the launch of NHS Direct Online (http://www.nhsdirect.nhs.uk). The aim of this site is to provide a gateway to high-quality and reliable health information and advice (for clients and public in England) on the internet (Nicholas et al 2002). NHS Direct Online provides multichannel access and is made up of several components, which aim to deliver information with a high level of user involvement.

NHS Direct Online provides public access to a variety of topics and users can benefit from information services including:

- Online encyclopaedia: this is a comprehensive guide to over 600 common medical conditions. The encyclopaedia contains sections on diagnosis and treatments along with explanatory diagrams and images.

- Self-help guide: an interactive, easy-to-use guide to treating common health problems at home. A 'body key' helps you identify your symptoms, then by answering simple step questions, you will be advised what to do next. The guide is also available in book form and is distributed through a variety of routes including pharmacies, doctors' surgeries, supermarkets, and 'new mother' packs.

- Local NHS services: a searchable database of hospitals and community health services, GPs, dentists, opticians and pharmacies in England. Addresses, telephone numbers, opening times and location maps are just some of the details provided. There are also contact details for all Health Authorities and NHS Trusts in England.

- Other links: this section hosts a directory of links to selected websites and other resources for a range of medical conditions where the user can seek further advice and information.

- Audio clips: for users who would like to listen to information, there is a selection of the College of Health's audio files in RealAudio format. To access this type audio clip into the search box.

- Hot topics: this section offers up-to-date information on the latest health issues. NHS Direct Online provides an important role in disseminating information to the public in the event of a health scare.

- Health information enquiry service: this is a very practical and popular health information enquiry service. The user completes a simple form, which is then researched by a health information professional. To maintain confidentiality, the user is allocated a password and, within 5 working days, is notified by e-mail that the information is ready. The user can access the information they requested by entering their previously allocated password.

- FAQs: this section contains the site's most frequently asked questions about health and health care. The most frequently asked questions and answers on child health include:
  - feeding/weaning
  - childhood vaccinations
  - how to reduce the risk of cot death.

- HealthSpace: this is a personal 'health organiser' created in a secure environment on the internet, in which users can record key personal health information (e.g. blood group, medication, allergies, appointments) and care wishes (e.g. organ donation, birth plans). HealthSpace can act as a 'postbox' for health news of interest to the user and for responses to health information requests submitted to the website's online enquiry service. Password permission to a user's HealthSpace could be shared with a partner, carer or doctor if they wished. NHS Direct Online is now working with the national programme for IT to develop HealthSpace as a web portal through which patients can access their electronic NHS records (Gann 2003).

- NHS Direct digital TV: this health information service in the interactive area on digital TV became available at the end of 2004. It offers information about:
  - the NHS Direct services, details of local NHS services, national bodies, voluntary organisations and patient groups
  - health information on illnesses and conditions, tests, treatments and operations, self-care advice and medicines
  - healthy living
  - hot topics on current health issues.

The NHS Direct digital TV service will continue to develop and expand over time, and subject to successful piloting, may offer transactional services such as ordering repeat prescriptions.

The DoH has appointed the new media agency, MMTV Ltd, to develop and run the NHS Direct digital TV service. The NHS Direct board will be responsible for the overall strategic direction. This service is being developed to expand the choice of ways in which people can access health information.

Activity

Explore the NHS Direct Online 'body key'. Do you find it easy to use?

Clinical Governance

To maintain the information on the site, topics are regularly reviewed and updated. The NHS Direct Online Editorial Board acts as a single editorial board for NHS Direct Online content whether in a web, information point, digital TV or print format. The editorial board is responsible for:

- a consistent editorial policy across NHS Direct Online
- prioritising content development
- commissioning content from third parties
- quality assurance of content
- reviewing users' suggestions for new content
- ensuring consistency with other NHS websites
- ensuring synergy with the NHS Direct telephone service.

The 21st-Century Patient

Nurses have a long history of 'being there' for people who are in need of health care (Cudney & Weinert 2000) and there is an opportunity for nurses to reach those people who may be isolated. Although the internet is not a new medium, it can be considered contemporary for the delivery of nursing/health care and is an innovative way of providing support, education and reassurance. There are many websites and chat environments where people exchange ideas and opinions on health related issues, however, their validity and reliability could be open to question and depends on the 'ownership' of the chat platform. As NHS Direct and NHS Direct Online are extensions of the NHS, they can instil confidence and trust.

Activity

Access the NHS Direct Online site and challenge it with a number of child-health-related questions. Discuss how efficient you thought the system was in your learning group:

- http://www.nhsdirect.nhs.uk

TELEVISION SERVICES

In 2001, the DoH piloted information services, delivered by television, to explore the use of new interactive technologies (Dick 2001, Hain 2001). The pilot services included:

- Appointment booking: where viewers can book appointments with their GP via the TV.
- Text service: where thousands of pages of health information can be accessed, working in a similar way to a conventional teletext service.
- Health videos: seven half-hour programmes for pregnant women and new mothers are all screened daily. Each programme deals with a different stage of pregnancy. The viewer is able to see the video relevant to her specific period of pregnancy.
- Online consultation: where a viewer can see and talk with a NHS Direct nurse. The nurse can then

display multimedia information to support the consultation.

All of the pilot TV services underwent extensive evaluation and the DoH began rolling-out a national service in 2004 (NHS Plan 2000).

INFORMATION KIOSKS

An increasing number of information kiosks are available to the public. These are located in public areas, often libraries or hospital waiting areas. Kiosks allow the user access to health information databases through a user-friendly interface.

COMMERCIALLY PRODUCED INFORMATION

Some excellent health information resources are produced commercially, in print and electronic format. However, there is also much that is of dubious quality and the nurse should review each on an individual basis. Information to look out for is that which carries the Centre for Health Information's Quality TriangleMark or NHS logo, but even these can be subject to abuse and no information should be taken at face value.

Professional Conversation

John, a registered children's nurse on Part 15 of the professional Nursing and Midwifery Council register, is discussing information giving with a recently qualified colleague.

Getting better information to parents

Until recently, I had been uncertain how to go about guiding parents to good information. I had heard a great deal about information on the internet not being trustworthy. I got some good advice from one of the staff in my PALS service, which is rather like a Citizen's Advice Bureau specifically for health issues. I also discovered that there is an organisation called CHIQ (apparently this stands for The Centre for Health Information Quality). This organisation tests health information to help ensure it is accurate, clear and relevant for patients and the public. I know there are a number of producers of health information who work with CHIQ and carry their mark of quality – the TriangleMark. Now when parents and children need health information, I suggest they look out for the TriangleMark on information. The CHIQ website is http://www.chiq.org/chiq. The NHS Direct Online website also has some good information: http://www.nhsdirect.nhs.uk.

Face-to-Face with Families

PATIENT AND PUBLIC INVOLVEMENT FORUMS

There should be a Patient and Public Involvement Forum (PPIF) in every Primary Care Trust and NHS Hospital Trust in England. Members of these forums play an active role in decisions relating to health (more details are available at: http://www.cppih.org). The forums are part of a national network to promote patient and public involvement in health and health services. More details of these services will be available from your local Patient Advice and Liaison Service (PALS).

The Commission for Patient and Public Involvement in Health (http://www.cppih.org) was established on 1 January 2003. Its primary mission is to advocate for the involvement of the public in all aspects of their local NHS. The establishment of this commission is mandated under section 11 of The Health and Social Care Act 2001, which places a duty on NHS Trusts, Primary Care Trusts and Strategic Health Authorities to develop and put in place structures for involving patients and the wider public in service planning, operation, and the development of proposals for changes to health provision. It is important to note that such structures will be audited to ensure compliance. It is not yet clear how children will be involved. However, there is no doubt that involving certain patient groups, such as children and young people, will be challenging. Although the Bristol Inquiry catalogued a whole series of misdemeanours that resulted in a climate of poor practice, there has been a paucity of advice on how to capture the views of children and young people. Children's nurses will have to explore every opportunity to give children and young people a strong voice in determining the future of their health service.

The future symbiotic relationship between the Commission for Health Audit and Inspection (CHAI) and the Commission for Patient and Public Involvement in Health is exemplified in the review of Birmingham Children's Hospital in 2002, in which one of the key areas highlighted was the need to consult adequately on the patient and public involvement strategy and to engage staff and stakeholders in the development of the long-term strategic vision for its services. This is a powerful message of what is to come, and individual Trusts will ignore children and young people at their peril.

Although there is intense pressure on healthcare professionals to include the voice of the child in all aspects of care, it should be remembered that the views of parents need to be sought in their own right. However, parental views are but one facet of family satisfaction with health care and reliable and valid instruments need to be developed to optimise the voice of the child and young person.

Children's nurses are in a unique position with their over-arching philosophy of family-centred care to help in eliciting the voice of all families in the health service. The Association of Chief Children's Nurses is working with the commission to ensure that the voice of the child patient is represented on the patient forums.

PATIENT ADVICE AND LIAISON SERVICES (PALS) (http:www.doh.gov.uk/patientadviceandliaisonservices)

In responding to increasing demand for information, the development of new information services should be seen as significant. One major and rapidly emerging service is that provided by the Patient Advice and Liaison Services (PALS), which provides service users with access to skilled information-giving staff.

The NHS Plan announced the commitment to establish Patient Advice and Liaison services in every trust by 2002. PALS are central to the new system of patient and public involvement. They are complementary to existing services, such as mental health and learning disability advocacy. In providing information and on the spot help for patients, their families and carers, they will be a powerful lever for change and improvement. PALS aim to:

- advise and support patients, their families and carers
- provide information on NHS services
- listen to concerns, suggestions or queries
- help sort problems quickly on behalf of patients and the public.

PALS act independently when handling patient and family concerns, liaising with staff, managers and, where appropriate, relevant organisations, to negotiate immediate solutions and to bring about changes to the way that services are delivered. If necessary, they can also refer patients and families to specific local or national support agencies.

PROVIDING INFORMATION TO FAMILIES

The exchange of information takes place during any and almost every interaction between a health professional, the child and a member of the child's family. The children's nurse has a critical role in ensuring the child and his family has access to adequate, high quality information. Children's nurses are among the best communicators in healthcare, ideally experienced to inform, educate and advise.

There are information points at each stage of the child's journey through the healthcare system. The nurse should be aware of these, and be in a position to provide additional information as required. Whereas some parents prefer not to have any information, the majority expect to have as much as can be made available. The four main information points in the journey for the family with a hospitalised child are: preadmission, on admission, during the hospital stay and after discharge.

Preadmission

Information provided before the child arrives in hospital should cover details about how to get to the hospital; travel issues, such as parking and cost of parking (often a significant concern to parents); how to get to the relevant department once inside the hospital; and details of key members of hospital staff. There should be a standard introductory leaflet to cover these issues, to accompany personalised information. The hospital's web address should be included.

On Admission

The nurse admitting the child is likely to be using a standardised admission sheet, which, if set out well, will provide an ideal framework for exploring the immediate information needs of the family. It is particularly important here to explain the hospital's own signage system. For example, colour-coded directional signs and long place names such as 'paediatric rheumatology clinic', can be confusing.

During the Hospital Stay

Leaflets giving details of any investigations should be read through with the child and family. The nurse should explain any unfamiliar terms. The family should be given the opportunity to think about and write down any questions they may need answering. In addition to discussing these issues with appropriate staff, the family may require back-up with leaflets, or printed information from the hospital's own information systems or the internet (local hospital policy on internet usage should be checked; some hospitals do not allow staff access to the internet). When internet usage is permitted, the nurse will ideally have an opportunity to take the family through some of the most common NHS-approved websites for health information. The nurse should be appropriately trained in knowing where to get hold of useful information, and how to be critical of its quality. Also, the nurse should be aware of others inside and outside the clinical team who can help. In other words, if the nurse doesn't know, he or she will know how to get hold of someone who does. There are key informants within the hospital team with whom the nurse may need to liaise to ensure that the most useful and appropriate information is obtained: the PALS lead and/or the local healthcare librarian. The clinical governance lead and the clinical effective-

ness lead will also be responsible for ensuring that a range of reliable information is readily available. These and other key information leads are identified in Box 37.2.

Box 37.2

Key information leads

- Patient Advice and Liaison Service (PALS) manager
- communications director
- clinical directors
- clinical governance/effectiveness leads
- healthcare librarian
- information management and technology team
- family information nurse

Activity

Identify your hospital's policy dealing with internet usage:
- Are there any issues to be resolved if you want to be able to use the internet to get information for your families?

After Discharge

When a child is discharged from hospital, the nurse could provide business cards that give the telephone number on which the nurse can be reached. When 24-hour nursing advice service is not available, a telephone linked to voice-mail is now standard practice to ensure calls can be followed up. In addition, written information should be provided and the family should be aware of who to contact once the child is back at home. This is likely to include the relevant member of the multidisciplinary team but additional details of patient support groups and organisations should also be given. An increasing number of excellent support services are available to families, although families should be encouraged to scrutinise these carefully before giving any personal details. In addition, the family will have a variety of services that they can access through the telephone, internet, information kiosks and TV, etc. However, it is possible for families to drown in a sea of information and not actually access the key facts they need to continue to care for their sick children.

The children's nurse is in an ideal situation to ensure information is provided at a rate and volume appropriate to the needs of the family. Often, family members will ask when they need to know something but the nurse should get into the habit of checking that information needs are being met. It is also important to check that the family understands the information that is given; levels of illiteracy and low adult reading ages should not be underestimated. The child will not always ask for information and neither will the child's parents/carers. A key service where face-to-face consultation and the provision of written and other resources are combined are Centres for Health Information and Promotion (CHIP), such as the Southampton Family Information Service, the Family Information Centre at The Hospital For Sick Children, Great Ormond Street and the service provided at 'Sick Kids' in Toronto, Canada.

www

Go to the Sick Kids website and visit health information for parents. Select an information leaflet and discuss its features in your learning group:
- http://www.sickkids.on.ca/chip/

THE FAMILY INFORMATION SERVICE

Hospitals such as the University Hospital of Southampton provide information to many families attending with sick children. This ranges from preadmission information to specific information related to illness (Glasper et al 1995).

The wide variety of clinics offered within the outpatient department at Southampton, coupled with a busy Accident and Emergency department, catering for large numbers of children, generates an increased need for family-centred information. In addition, the hospital provides a range of inpatient services for children. The paediatric population is, therefore, diverse by nature.

The introduction of the Patient's Charter, and subsequently the findings of the Bristol Inquiry, have highlighted the responsibility of hospitals to provide health information to families, not only to meet their needs but also to promote family involvement in care. In addition, the shift of resources from tertiary to primary health care increasingly encourages hospitals to focus more broadly on health promotion. In Southampton, for example, there has been a proliferation of materials provided to families attending the hospital, and all members of the multidisciplinary team have been involved. As part of a move towards a coordinated strategy, a specialised information service was developed. In 1995, an experienced paediatric nurse was appointed at 'F' Grade level to develop the concept under the facilitation of the clinical leader, to act as a Family Information Nurse (FIN). The role of the FIN is to coordinate information for families for sick children throughout all areas where children are cared for. Funding was made available to build a purpose-designed Centre for Health Information and Promotion (CHIP) within the outpatient department.

The aim of a CHIP is to provide specialist materials for carers and children to help them understand and cope with health and health- and illness-related family concerns. They are located in large tertiary hospitals and concentrate on families with sick children, although they also promote healthy lifestyles for all. The role of a CHIP is to augment and support information provided by healthcare staff to families. In many ways a CHIP is similar to a PAL service and, in some hospitals (such as the Hospital for Sick Children, Great Ormond Street), they are combined within one structure.

The fundamental component of a CHIP philosophy is the sharing of complete and unbiased information to families in an appropriate and supportive manner. This is a response to the increasing reality that parents seek-out health information as a way of coping positively with new or difficult child health situations.

The provision of a CHIP within a busy area of the hospital allows nurses to be much more assertive in the promotion of health information and opportunistically involve even those families who, under normal circumstances would prove passive in the pursuit of health information. Most parents want to understand their children's medical condition and give appropriate explanations to their children.

CHIPs employ a number of strategies to achieve their aims. These are:

- The organisation of materials designed to provide families with information appropriate to the care of children.
- The promotion of partnership in care.
- The creation of an infrastructure that allows members of the multidisciplinary team to communicate with one another and individual families through the utilisation of appropriate technologies

Producing Local Information

Prewritten leaflets are unlikely to satisfy all potential clients and staff may wish to develop their own. Writing a family information leaflet may, on the surface, appear easy but the reality is that they cannot be generated one evening at home. Although they can be designed and produced using easily available desktop publishing software, the actual contents require rather more skill.

The Centre for Health Information Quality (CHIQ) recommends that, for effective consumer health information, members of the target audience, experts in the subject area and professional communicators should all be involved in the production process.

Activity

Access the companion PowerPoint presentation to see photographs of family information centres.

Reflect on your Practice

You are keen to develop a leaflet for a child you are looking after:
- How can you find out if such a leaflet already exists?

- Who should be involved with the development of the leaflet?
- Where and how could they meet together?
- What issues should they be made aware of in relation to national/local information policy?

Improving the Quality of Health Information

READABILITY FORMULAE

Readability formulae can help the writers of patient information leaflets to assess how well their writing can be understood by the reader. However, such formulae are not a panacea to correct the inadequacies of badly written information (Glasper & Burge 1992).

Many tools have emerged over the last half a decade to help writers and editors improve the way their messages are presented. The Flesch index (Flesch 1948) and Fog index (Gunning 1952, 1968) use mathematical formulae to test how easy writing is to understand. Similarly, the SMOG (Standard Measure of Gobbledegook; McGlaughlin 1969) can be used to measure the readability of information leaflets, for example for patients with asthma (Smith et al 1998).

Activity

Access the companion PowerPoint presentation to learn more about SMOG.

Read Smith et al (1998) online at:

- http://www.pubmedcentral.nih.gov/articlerender. fcgi?articl=28620

Services such as the Write Stuff (http://www.writestuff. com) and CHIQ (http://www.chiq.org/chiq) provide a range of tools, guides and tips. One of earliest and most celebrated tools is the Ten Principles of Clear Statement, which was developed in America (Gunning 1952). This has been adapted by The Centre for Health Information Quality, and is presented in Box 37.3.

Box 37.3

Ten principles of clear writing (CHIQ 2003, after Gunning's Ten Principles of Clear Statement)

1. Keep sentences short
2. Use simple, rather than complex explanations
3. Use familiar words where possible
4. Avoid unnecessary words
5. Put action into verbs used
6. Write like you talk
7. Use terms your reader can picture
8. Link in with your readers' experience
9. Use a wide variety of writing techniques
10. Write to express, not impress

Writing Patient Information Leaflets

Family information leaflets should be:

- Comprehensible: does the reader understand the text?
- Usable/readable: can the reader apply the information?
- Accessible: can the reader find the information easily (or is it lost in a sea of ambiguous text)?

Before rushing to your computer to produce your patient information leaflet:

- Know your purpose: what is it you want to achieve?
- Know your target audience: who are you writing for? (The child or carer or both?)
- Know your subject: do you have the knowledge to write the material?
- Know the setting under which the target audience will read the leaflet.

When writing information leaflets, make sure that they contain:

- Awareness information: which allows the reader to relate to the contents of the information leaflet.
- How to information: which allows the reader to optimise the purpose of the leaflet.
- Principles information: which gives real concrete information on why for example certain drugs actually work.

Healthcare professionals are not always the best people to write the information leaflets, and skilled as they are, may not have the particular skills to write for different patient groups. Seeking advice from organisations such as the Help for Health Trust and librarians will help to ensure that the final product is useful.

WHAT STYLE TO USE FOR PATIENT INFORMATION LEAFLETS

- Use informative not descriptive headings: for example, 'Commuter disease' (not very inspiring), 'What is commuter disease?' (better), 'Living with commuter disease' (best of all).
- Try to personalise the leaflet by using personal pronouns such as 'I', 'we', 'us' or 'you'.
- Use decisive language, which is clear and unambiguous.
- Describe actions positively. For example, 'Do not administer unless the patient is developing a temperature' (bad), 'Give only when the patient has a

temperature above 38 degrees centigrade' (much clearer).

- Use familiar words: 'Your child has fractured his or her leg' (not good), 'Your child has broken his or her leg' (better). Do not assume that the general public understands medical jargon.
- Use short paragraphs with strong topic sentences.
- Use simple visual images.
- Use at least 12-point type (larger if possible) for younger readers.

 Activity

Access the companion PowerPoint presentation to see examples of patient information leaflets.

THE CENTRE FOR HEALTH INFORMATION QUALITY

In the UK, it was recognised that there needed to be a national resource to facilitate the production of patient information (DoH 1996). In response to this, the Centre for Health Information Quality (CHIQ) was established. The Centre was opened in 1997 as an expert resource for NHS staff and patient representative groups seeking to produce or procure high-quality patient information resources (DoH 1998, Gann 1998, Hain 2002). Since then, key national documents such as *The NHS Plan* (DoH 2000b) have continued to stress the importance of communicating well with patients and their families. Recommendation 8 of the Bristol Inquiry called for the development of a system for accrediting patient information materials. CHIQ works to meet these national objectives. It is hosted by the Help for Health Trust, an independent charity that is recognised internationally as a lead organisation supporting the field of consumer health information.

Principles of Quality

Based on the findings of extensive consultation and research through key partner organisations, CHIQ identified three overarching themes and defined good-quality consumer health information as that which is: evidence-based, clearly communicated and involves the consumer in its production.

NHS and other patient organisations engage and work with CHIQ to ensure these issues are fully addressed within the production and dissemination of health information for the public. Producers and providers of health information contact CHIQ, using either telephone or e-mail enquiries, or by visiting CHIQ in Winchester. Databases support these services, referring enquirers to key research articles and projects. The internet has rapidly become the primary source for enquiries and, as a result, online resources have been developed, including the Hi-Quality

website, to provide a comprehensive guide to the quality issues for consumer health information. CHIQ news items and other articles are available from CHIQ's main website (http://www.hfht.org/chiq). The topic bulletins consider the principles of quality assurance in detail.

Quality Tools and Appraisal Processes

Key quality assessment tools were developed with input from CHIQ, including the DISCERN tool (Charnock & Shepherd 1998), led by the Oxford Health Services Research Unit, and the King's Fund's POPPI Guide (Duman & Farrell 2000). Subsequently, CHIQ produced guidelines for assessing and producing information (CHIQ 2003). Other resources include Quick for children (which was developed with the then Health Education Authority) and HiQuality, both of which are online educational tools.

 www

Visit the Quick website at:
- http://www.chiq.org/chiq/Quick%20website/docs/index.html

There are two types of appraisal of health information. In the archaeological approach, information is tested against quality criteria once it has been published. Using the architectural approach, assessment is based on research and editorial processes adopted from the outset of production of the information. In both approaches, appraisal is carried out by an appropriately trained and experienced assessor.

Training

A short course – entitled 'An introduction to producing health information' – was developed and piloted by CHIQ. This course is available for anyone new to health information and/or the NHS. The workshop has a considerable focus on the practical application of CHIQ guidelines.

Patient Advice and Liaison Services (PALS) are rapidly emerging within the NHS, as front-of-house information services. CHIQ workshops have been developed and piloted with PALS staff to facilitate the link between policy and good practice, with a key focus on issues around information quality.

 Reflect on your Practice

'All healthcare staff who treat children should be trained in communicating with young people and parents.'
Consider what training you have had in:
- face-to-face communication with children and their families
- developing written information.

Are there areas that you feel you would like further training?

Accreditation in Practice

Health Information on the Internet

The national database linking users to tested patient information became available, and was immediately the most popular resource on NHS Direct Online, when this service was launched by the Prime Minister in December 1999. Hundreds of patient information leaflets were tested retrospectively by CHIQ expert appraisers, using the DISCERN tool. Trained appraisers gave the leaflets a star rating and these formed the majority of content for NHS Direct Online's database 'conditions and treatments'.

Public Versions of Clinical Guidelines

In 2000, public versions of national clinical guidelines were developed by CHIQ as part of a key programme for the National Institute for Clinical Excellence (NICE). This ensured that patients had access to accredited information, developed in parallel with the version for health professionals.

Health Information through Digital TV

Based on the architectural approach, CHIQ developed and implemented a quality assurance programme across all public-facing NHS digital TV pilot services (Dick 2001, Hain 2001), for a project led by the DoH. This ensured all the pilot services were adopting the same dedicated and agreed standards from the outset. As a result, users of the interactive services would know that mechanisms were in place to ensure:

- sources of information were clear to the viewer
- accuracy of information was regularly reviewed, and
- consumers were involved in the development of the service.

A simple framework for quality assurance emerged from this, easily transferable into any information services environment, and comprising three phases:

1. Developing standards: developed and agreed by a group of stakeholders, including appropriate consumer representation.
2. Training and support for staff: ensuring health information appraisal skills were available within production teams.
3. Monitoring progress towards the standards: to ensure standards were being adopted and developed, taking into account, for example, feedback from trainees.

Recently, CHIQ has taken forward key work programmes for the DoH , identifying key resources for cancer information, information for children and their families, and providing administrative support to PALS services across England.

CHIQ recommends that members of the target audience, experts and communicators should always be involved in the production of health information. In other words:

- When members of the target audience have been involved, the information is more likely to demonstrate **relevance**.
- When experts in the topic area have been involved, the information is more likely to demonstrate **accuracy**.
- When a skilled health communicator has been involved, the information is more likely to demonstrate **clarity**.

The following sections are taken from the CHIQs guidelines for producers (CHIQ 2003). They explore some of the additional key issues that need to be considered in order to ensure that health information provided to children and their families is relevant, accurate and clearly communicated.

MAKING SURE INFORMATION IS RELEVANT

Involving Consumers

Consumers should be involved at some stage during the production of good-quality health information to ensure information is relevant and accessible. Health information consumers may be patients, families, carers, service users or any member of the general public. Consumers should be involved to identify relevant issues, provide balance against professional opinion and encourage consumer ownership. The involvement of consumers in producing health information may also avoid wasting resources. Consumers might choose to become involved for a variety of reasons, for example, to improve information, to be able to influence services and to identify areas of need. Three key ways in which consumers can be involved in the production of health information are: consultation, collaboration and user control.

Consultation

Consumers are asked for their views, which may or may not be adopted in full. It is important that all contributions are acknowledged so consumers do not feel their time has been wasted.

Collaboration

Collaboration involves a more active, ongoing partnership between consumers and producers. This can increase the likelihood that outcome measurements, assessment criteria and evaluation have greater relevance.

User Control

Here, consumers design and undertake the project. This results in increased consumer involvement throughout the project and is likely to address questions that may not have been considered important by the producers. Consumers should be involved before, during and after the information has been produced. It is important to build feedback mechanisms into resources so that consumers can continue to feed in their comments and suggestions. It is also important to ask consumers to evaluate information, in order to measure how effective it is.

Some useful websites for more information on consumer involvement are:

- Involve (formerly Consumers in NHS Research): http://www.invo.org.uk/
- The Patients Forum: http://www.thepatientsforum.org.uk/default.asp

MAKING SURE INFORMATION IS CLEAR

Communicating Clearly

Communicating health messages clearly is an essential principle for producing consumer health information. Well-presented and easy-to-read information is vital for everyone. Three key areas of communication can be identified: format, content and language:

- Format: is the information communicated via an appropriate and accessible medium?
- Content: is the message clearly communicated?
- Language: is the choice and style of language appropriate?

Format

Information should be made available in the most appropriate format to meet the user's needs. You can use multiple formats, for example a leaflet supported by online resources. If you use a variety of formats, make sure they complement each other, for example an online resource can offer direct links to other sources of information.

Think about translating information into different languages so that ethnic minorities can access it. Consider any cultural implications this may have.

It is also important to consider how easy it is for the users to find their way around the information, i.e. is the navigation method clear? For example, does it have a glossary and clearly defined headings, is there a contents list, etc.?

For improved legibility of printed materials, use at least 12-point type. Dark type on a pale background is recommended, as is a basic font such as Arial. For further advice on legibility see:

- Plain English Campaign: http://www.plainenglish.co.uk
- RNIB clear print guidelines: http://www.rnib.org.uk
- Basic Skills Agency website: http://www.basic-skills.co.uk

Content

The content should be relevant to the target audience. The material should state who it is aimed at and the source of the information should be made clear to the consumer, as should the name of the author, the date and the copyright owner. It should also be clear if the publication has been sponsored by a commercial company. The information should be balanced and up-to-date, giving clear signposting to other references and links.

Repetition should be used to good effect, to reinforce the most important parts of the information.

Language

The pitch, tone and choice of language should be considered. Language should be pitched at a level that will be familiar to your target audience. Give advice rather than orders. Use 'we' and 'our' and address the reader as 'you'. Absolute statements should also be avoided. So, for example, instead of saying 'You will experience particular symptoms', say 'You may experience . . . '. Avoid using jargon or abbreviations that people may not recognise, or make sure that they are clearly explained. Language should be non-discriminatory (for gender and race).

It is recommended that any organisation producing consumer health information develops a house style (grammar, abbreviations, font, titles, colours, etc.) to ensure consistency across all publications, and also a list of preferred terms, again to ensure consistency and to avoid causing offence.

It is important to note that many of the clearest and easy-to-use information resources emerge from the field of child health.

Activity

Pick up a patient information leaflet and test it against the CHIQ checklist for quality. Can you identify good and bad examples of practice?

- What issues around *accuracy* have and have not been addressed?
- What issues around *clarity* have and have not been addressed?
- What issues around *relevance* have and have not been addressed?

MAKING NATIONAL INFORMATION AVAILABLE

A number of key national resources should be made available to families (see above). In addition, a number of producers and providers have their information regularly assessed for quality by expert appraisers at the Centre for Health Information Quality. These include:

- Macmillan Cancer Relief: together with CHIQ, Macmillan Cancer Relief has produced the 4th edition of a *Directory of information materials for people with cancer*. All entries to the directory have been tested using an assortment of appraisal tools (see: http://www.chiq.org/macmillan).

- Discovery Health: provides a range of services, including games and features, news headlines, and a TV guide that complements an interactive TV service. There are different sections, including those for men's health, and women's health (see: http://www.discoveryhealth.co.uk).

- StartHere: this system provides a range of health and social care information. Of particular note is a user-friendly interface, where text on the screen is kept to a minimum and navigation is assisted with large icons representing buttons (see: http://www.starthere.co.uk).

- Patient.co.uk: this website has more than 500 leaflets available online, covering a range of health and disease topic areas. Most general practitioners in the UK have access to these same leaflets to print out for patients and carers (see: http://www.patient.co.uk).

- The Brain and Spine Foundation: has published 27 booklets on a variety of neurological conditions and procedures. A related helpline service was launched in 1998 and has since responded to more than 18,000 calls; a website receives more than 3000 users a month (see: http://www.brainandspine.org.uk).

- Midirs (Midwives Information and Resource Service): produces a series of leaflets called 'Informed Choice', which provides fully referenced content for consumers and health professionals on a range of health issues around pregnancy and birth (see: http://www.midirs.org).

- EIDO Healthcare: produces procedure-specific, medicolegal documents to support the consent process. Recent research indicates that patients find these very easy to understand (see: http://www.eidohealthcare.com).

- BUPA (British United Provident Association): produces a range of health information resources, including factsheets, healthy living articles and news items (see: http://www.bupa.co.uk).

- National Knowledge Service (NKS): with many databases supporting health care in the UK produced nationally, the DoH is developing the NKS to coordinate development and provide access to these through one website. The NKS is piloting quality assurance techniques broadly similar to the CHIQ Partners concept (see below).

Probably the best-known component of NKS is NHS Direct Online, which provides a range of online health services, including a health encyclopaedia. CHIQ has recently undertaken projects on behalf of NHS Direct Online, identifying those consumer health materials which are most widely used in the fields of cancer, and presently, children's and maternity health care (see: http://www.nks.nhs.uk and http://www.nhsdirect.nhs.uk).

- The Child Health Specialist Library: an indispensable resource that is now available from the National Electronic Library for Health (see: http://www.nelh.nhs.uk/childhealth).

Activity

Take a virtual tour of the Child Health Specialist Library:
- http://www.nelh.nhs.uk/childhealth

LINKING LOCAL INFORMATION STRATEGY TO NATIONAL STRATEGY

A key responsibility on the part of whoever leads on patient information is to ensure that local strategy fits with national strategy. Much of this may be achieved by working closely with those staff identified in Box 37.2. Patient information leads within an organisation should identify a lead and meet regularly, taking forward and developing local strategy with the support from the highest level. A nurse with a patient information role must have an appreciation of the current national strategy documents including National Service Frameworks, the Clinical Negligence Scheme for Trusts and review instruments from the Commission for Health Audit and Inspection

National Service Frameworks (NSFs)

- NSFs set national standards and identify key interventions for a defined service or care group.
- NSFs put in place strategies to support implementation.
- NSFs establish ways to ensure progress within an agreed timescale.
- NSFs form one of a range of measures to raise quality and decrease variations in service.

The Commission for Health Audit and Inspection

The Commission for Health Audit and Inspection (CHAI) is the independent inspection body for the NHS. CHAI publishes reports on NHS organisations in England and Wales. It highlights where the NHS is working well and the areas that need improvement. CHAI reviewers inspect healthcare services against national standards; this includes assessment of information services (Sweeting & Hain 2002).

Clinical Negligence Scheme for Trusts

You can find out about the information requirements under the Clinical Negligence Scheme for Trusts (CNST) from the NHS Litigation Authority's website (http://www.nhsla.com).

MAKING SURE INFORMATION IS ACCURATE

Working with Evidence

Evidence-based health care is a particular focus for the UK government: 'The government is determined that the services and treatment that patients receive across the NHS should be based upon the best evidence of what does and does not work' (DoH 1998). This same principle applies to health information in that all health information should be based upon the best, reliable evidence. It is essential to appraise critically the evidence on which health information is based.

There are three broad bands of originators of evidence: the State, the commercial sector and non-State or voluntary organisations. These different originators are motivated by different factors to produce the evidence that informs patient information. The State is motivated by political demands, a public-service ethos, professional interest and cost efficiency. The commercial sector is motivated by competition, the direct influence on consumers and sales/profit. The non-State and voluntary sectors are motivated by the service to their members, competition for funding, profile and income. It is therefore very important to recognise the motivation behind the evidence.

All evidence is of value, whether it comes from systematic research or individual opinion. Therefore the most important issue of including the evidence base in patient information is always to state where the information comes from so that consumers can make their own objective decisions.

CHIQ recommends a five-point checklist for objectivity when researching the evidence base:

1. Where does the evidence come from?
2. Is it up-to-date?
3. Is it relevant to your target audience?
4. Does it detail other options?
5. Does it detail the risks and benefits?

In addition, there are three basic principles for producing evidence-based patient information:

1. Always specify the evidence source.
2. Always balance the evidence: use a combination of patient opinion and expert research/opinion.
3. Always ensure evidence is up-to-date and current.

Summary

There is a growing recognition of the importance of providing information to the child and his or her family throughout all phases of the child's healthcare journey. A number of key national initiatives directly support children and their families with their information needs. A number of different services are available to support healthcare professionals to meet these information needs. The information needs to be accurate, relevant and communicated well, and reinforced over time. The children's nurse plays a crucial role in ensuring family understanding of key health messages, both through face-to-face communication and by providing appropriate guidance on where to access high-quality health information resources when face-to-face consultation is not practical.

ACKNOWLEDGEMENTS

The section of NHS Direct Online was contributed by Aideen M Tarpey, Clinical Adviser (Nursing), NHS Direct Online.

References

Centre for Health Information Quality (CHIQ) 2003 Guidelines for producers and reviewers of health information. Online. Available at: http://www.hfht.org/chiq/guidelines.htm [accessed 31 December 2003]

Charnock D 1998 The Discern handbook: quality criteria for consumer health information. Radcliffe Press, Oxford

Children's Commissioner for Wales 2003 Telling concerns: report of the Children's Commissioner for Wales' review of the operation of complaints and representations and whistleblowing procedures and arrangements for the provision of children's advocacy services. Online. Available at: http://www.childpolicy.org.uk/Document/ DocumentDownload.cfm/Telling%20Concerns.pdf?DType= DocumentItem&Document=Telling%20Concerns%2Epdf [accessed 31 December 2003]

Commission for Patient and Public Involvement in Health 2003 Online. Available at: http://www.cppih.org [accessed 31 December 2003]

Cudney S, Weinert C 2000 Computer-based support groups, nursing in cyberspace. Computers in nursing 18(1):35–43

Department of Health (DoH) 1996 Patient partnership: building a collaborative strategy. DoH, London

Department of Health (DoH) 1998 The new NHS: modern and dependable. DoH, London

Department of Health (DoH) 1999 Patient and public involvement in the new NHS. DoH, London

Department of Health (DoH) 2000a Final report of the Bristol Royal Infirmary inquiry. Online. Available at: http://www.bristol-inquiry.org.uk/final_report/index.htm [accessed 31 December 2003]

Department of Health (DoH) 2000b NHS Plan: a plan for investment, a plan for reform. DoH, London

Department of Health (DoH) 2000c Delivering 21st century IT support for the NHS. National strategic programme. The Stationery Office, London

Department of Health (DoH) 2001 The patient's charter. DoH, London

Department of Health (DoH) 2003 Getting the right start: National Service Framework for Children. Online. Available at: http://www.doh.gov.uk/nsf/children/index.htm [accessed 31 December 2003]

Dick P 2001 Towards NHS Direct TV. The British Journal of Healthcare Computing & Information Management 18(9):22–24

Duman M, Farrell C 2000 The practicalities of producing patient information. King's Fund, London

Flesch P 1948 A new readability yardstick. Journal of Applied Psychology 32:221–233

Gann B 2003 Enabling patient access and expertise. In: Dean K (ed.) Connected health thought leaders: essays from health innovators. Premium Publishing, London pp 8–15

Gann R 1991 Consumer health information: the growth of an information specialism. Journal of Documentation 47(3):284–308

Gann R 1998 Centre for Health Information Quality. Health Libraries Review 15:295–299

Glasper A, Burge D 1992 Developing family information leaflets. Nursing Standard 6(25):24–27

Glasper EA, Lowson S, Manger R, Phillips L 1995 Developing a centre for health information and promotion. British Journal of Nursing 4(12):693–697

Glasper EA, McWilliams R 1998 Developing a Centre for Health Information and Promotion. In: Glasper EA, Lowson S (eds) Innovations in paediatric ambulatory care. Macmillan, Basingstoke

Gunning R 1952 The technique of clear writing. McGraw-Hill, New York

Gunning R 1968 The Fog Index after twenty years. The Journal of Business Communications 6:3–13

Hain T 2001 A quality assurance programme for NHS Digital TV services. Health Expectations 4(4):260–262

Hain T 2002 Improving the quality of health information: the contribution of CHIQ. Health Expectations 5:270–273

Help for Health Trust 1997 Health information service, central support 1997–1998. Summary of contract with NHS Executive. Online. Available at: http://www.hfht.org [accessed 31 December 2003]

Help for Health Trust 2003 Online. Available at: http://www.hfht.org [accessed 31 December 2003]

Jenkins P, Gann B 2002 Developing NHS Direct as a multichannel service. British Journal of Healthcare Computing and Information Management 19(4):20–21

Jenkins P, Gann B 2003 NHS Direct Online in 2003. British Journal of Healthcare Computing and Information Management 20(6):25–27

McLaughlin GH 1969 SMOG grading: a new readability formula. Journal of Reading 12:639–646

NHS Executive (NHSE) 1996 Patient partnership: building a collaborative strategy. NHSE, Leeds

NHS Executive (NHSE) 1998 Information for health: an information strategy for the modern NHS. NHSE, Leeds

NHS University (NHSU) 2004 Online. Available at: http://www.nhsu.nhs.uk/learning/progcat.html [accessed 17 February 2004]

Nicholas D, Huntington P, Williams P et al 2002 NHS Direct Online: its users and their concerns. Journal of Information Science 28(4):305–319

Planetree 2003 Creating patient-centered care in healing environments. Online. Available at: http://www.planetree.org/PDF/brochure.pdf [accessed 31 December 2003]

Smith H, Gooding S, Brown R, Frew A 1998 Evaluation of readability and accuracy of information leaflets in general practice for patients with asthma. Online. Available at: http://bmj.bmjjournals.com/cgi/content/full/317/7153/264 [accessed 31 December 2003]

Sweeting A, Hain T 2003 Monitoring health information services: a new tool for information quality review. Health Expectations 6:182–186

Chapter Thirty Eight

38

Inherited Conditions and the Family

Maggie Kirk, Emer Parker

ABSTRACT

This chapter and its companion PowerPoint presentation aims to help you in your understanding of the impact of genetic conditions on family life and to gain an awareness of the implications of advances in genetics for children and their families.

Learning Outcomes

- Appreciate the impact that a genetic illness may have on family life.

- Apply basic genetic principles to understand how genetic conditions can be passed on in families.

- Evaluate the role of the children's nurse in helping families to access genetic information and supporting the decision making based on this.

- Appreciate some of the ethical issues surrounding the application of genetic technologies of relevance to children and their families.

Glossary

Alleles:
The different forms that a gene may have at one particular position (or locus) on a chromosome.

Autosome:
An 'ordinary' or non-sex chromosome.

Carrier:
An individual who has a copy of a disease-causing gene, but does not have the disease. Such individuals are usually heterozygous for a recessive condition.

Dominant:
A characteristic that is evident in an individual even when there is only one altered copy of a particular gene present.

Expressivity:
The severity or extent to which a disease or condition is expressed.

Gene:
The unit of inheritance, composed of a sequence of DNA that codes for one or more proteins. It is estimated that we have about 26,000 genes, which direct the development, growth and function of every cell in the body, its tissues and organ systems.

Genetic testing:
The analysis of a specific gene, its product or function, or other DNA and chromosome analysis to detect or exclude an alteration likely to be associated with a genetic disorder (Harper & Clarke 1997).
Different types of genetic tests include:
(a) Diagnostic: carried out on individuals who either have, or are suspected of having, a particular condition because of clinical signs or symptoms.
(b) Presymptomatic: carried out on individuals at high risk of an adult-onset condition, where an abnormal test result indicates that development of the condition is almost inevitable.
(c) Predictive or susceptibility: aims to identify individuals at increased risk of developing a condition, where the increased risk of the condition developing may be substantial but is not necessarily certain.
(d) Carrier: identifies healthy individuals at risk of having a child affected by a genetic condition.

Genome:

All of the genetic information contained in the 26,000 or so genes carried on an individual's chromosomes. The normal human genome comprises 23 pairs of chromosomes, 22 pairs of autosomes, and one pair of sex chromosomes.

Genotype:

The genetic make-up of a person.

Heterozygote:

An individual who has two different forms of a particular gene.

Homozygote:

An individual who has the same form of an allele on both chromosomes.

Karyotype:

The chromosome makeup of an individual.

Multifactorial:

Traits or conditions that are the result of interactions between different genes, and between genes and the environment.

Penetrance:

The proportion of a population with a particular genotype that actually express that genotype. A condition that is not always expressed, even though the individual has the associated genotype, is said to have reduced penetrance.

Pharmacogenetics:

The study of how different people respond to drugs due to their genetic makeup, in order to identify new, more specific and more effective drug targets with fewer side effects.

Phenotype:

The observed characteristics of an individual.

Recessive:

A characteristic that is expressed in an individual only when it is not masked by a dominant allele. Thus it is seen in the homozygous state (i.e. when both copies of the particular allele have been inherited), or in the hemizygous state (such as the genes on the X chromosome in the male).

Sex chromosomes:

The X and Y chromosomes in humans.

Introduction: The Genetics Revolution

The interest that we have in how characteristics are passed down through the generations is demonstrated at a typical family gathering following the birth of a new baby. We like to identify who the baby most resembles, what features he or she may have inherited from a particular 'side' of the family. As the child grows and develops, the attribution of characteristics may be broadened from the mainly physical (he has his mother's eyes) to include aspects of tempera-

ment (she has her father's quick temper). With the advances in knowledge and understanding of the role that inheritance plays in our health and development, we have the potential to become more specific about the contribution of each parent to the features observed in their children. The range of features for which we can identify a genetic component will also increase, such as musicality, reading ability, or sports performance. Of course parents (and grandparents) take pride in the positive attributes but how do they feel when a child has inherited a less desirable characteristic, such as an illness?

With the 'genetics revolution' we are beginning to appreciate far more the extent of the role that genes play in health and illness – and it is far more extensive than most people imagined, and more complex. Genes and environment interact along a continuum, with relatively rare disorders at the one end where genes alone will dictate the existence of disease, and at the other end, a few diseases in which environmental factors only play a part. Most diseases, though, represent the outcome of the interactions between different genes, and between genes and the environment. Alongside our growing understanding of the nature and function of these genes and their interactions, we are also gaining knowledge of the role of some genes in protecting against disease, and of others in influencing our responses to medicines.

What is behind the genetics revolution is the Human Genome Project, the first phase of which was completed in 2003, two years ahead of schedule. This ambitious international project has deciphered the sequence of the chemicals that make up the DNA within the human blueprint (genome), paving the way for the next phase as our 26,000 or so genes are identified. Such advances in knowledge will have a profound impact on health care, with an increasing focus on individualised preventive medicine based on genetic risk, informed by environmental risk assessment. Bell (1998) outlined how genetics research would lead to:

- **A new disease classification:** based on the molecular mechanisms that cause disease rather than the clinical manifestation, e.g. in type 2 diabetes with the identification in particular of the maturity onset diabetes of the young (MODY) subtypes, based on the particular gene involved. There is also now a range of subsets of childhood leukaemia based on gene expression, chromosomal and molecular abnormalities. This will go alongside a better understanding of the pathological mechanisms of disease, and of the influence of environmental factors.

- **The possibility of earlier detection of disease, with an increasing range of genetic tests:** currently there are tests for around 200 of the 10,000 or so single gene disorders, and this number will grow as more and more genes are identified that account for these conditions. Genetic tests are also being developed to identify the genetic component of common diseases, and these will help identify people who may be at greater risk. Some genetic tests may become available commercially, as is already seen for example, for cystic fibrosis (CF).

- **Greater opportunities for prevention:** by identifying individuals and sub-populations who might be more at risk, and identifying ways of modifying or preventing this risk.

- **Better targeted and more effective treatments:** using genotype to identify subtypes of populations who are more likely to display an enhanced response or increased toxicity. Those with the MODY subset HNF1α mutation are very sensitive to sulfonylureas for example.

- **New types of treatment:** with rational drug development based on an understanding of the pathogenesis, with a longer-term focus on gene therapy. Gene therapy trials are already being conducted worldwide for a range of conditions, including cystic fibrosis and cancers.

 WWW

Read more about the Human Genome Project and related topics at:

- http://www.yourgenome.org
  This site is produced by the Wellcome Trust Sanger Institute and offers information tailored for basic, intermediate and advanced levels of knowledge.

The implications of all these for individuals, families and professionals are far-reaching. Iredale (2000) reminds us that with earlier genetic testing and more prompt, targeted and improved treatments, including the potential for gene therapy, some diseases that were once fatal are being considered more as chronic. Thus children with such conditions are being seen not only by nurses in paediatric intensive care but in ambulatory paediatric and adolescent care settings.

The potential for misuse of new knowledge and technologies has also to be considered. We are in a unique position of knowing ahead of time the potential impact and in the UK new initiatives are already underway to help the health professional workforce to prepare for these advances.

The Genetics White Paper

The publication of the UK government's White Paper *Our inheritance, our future* signalled very clearly how it intends to maximise the opportunities presented by genetics and meet the challenges it poses (Department of Health (DoH) 2003). It makes a powerful statement on the anticipated advantages:

The new genetics knowledge and technology has the potential to bring enormous benefits for patients: more personalised prediction of risk, more accurate diagnosis, safer use of medicines and new treatment options (DoH 2003 p 22)

 WWW

Read the genetics White Paper on line:

- http://www.doh.gov.uk/genetics/whitepaper.htm
  What are the four key action strands? Which do you think has the potential to impact most on your professional practice?

The existing specialist genetics centres will continue to play a leading role in maximising the benefits of this new knowledge, and these services are being strengthened accordingly to cope with the increasing demand. Other healthcare workers will have to become involved as genetics moves increasingly into mainstream services, and education in genetics of the professional workforce has become an important issue.

The White Paper acknowledges that the exact timing of the different advances is uncertain – this is not an overnight revolution, but it is already underway. One of the first major developments will be the increasing range of genetic tests, facilitating a more accurate diagnosis. This will affect not only children and families with new conditions, but also those with pre-existing conditions where previously no diagnosis was available. What will this mean for families and what do we know already about how genetic diseases can affect family life?

The Impact of Genetic Disease on the Family Life

Family functioning is affected when a child becomes ill because of the usual stresses and practical problems associated with this. If the illness becomes prolonged, or if the child has a chronic condition, in particular one that is degenerative, these stresses are exacerbated. What part might the fact that a disease is 'genetic' play in this? Does it make any difference to the family?

The question of whether genetic conditions bring added stresses is an important one. Over the next decade there will be an increase in the number of children for whom a genetic diagnosis becomes possible, not only for children newly affected by a condition but also for those with existing, previously undiagnosed conditions, as genetic discoveries are made. Depending on the current policies surrounding the testing of children, there could also be an increase in the number of children for whom presymptomatic and predictive testing would reveal a high risk of developing a condition.

A mother's account of her experiences following the diagnosis of two of her sons with adrenoleucodystrophy offers a powerful insight into how genetic diseases can impact on family life (McGowan 1999). Adrenoleucodystrophy is a degenerative metabolic disorder inherited as an X-linked condition; the variable range of symptoms is associated with a build up of fatty acids. McGowan says: 'The diagnosis of an inherited condition can drop a bombshell into family relationships' (p 197). She states earlier that: 'We now take nothing for granted, such as the simple hopes that our sons will become teenagers or adult men' (p 195).

Whyte (1992) studied four families caring for children with cystic fibrosis. As well as describing the stresses associated with the 'chronic burden of care', she analyses the part that the genetic nature of the illness plays and concluded that it has a profound effect. The assault on self-image and self-esteem of parents who feel they are unable to produce healthy children can be devastating, and the implications of this for future childbearing are keenly felt. Related to this are the tough decisions that parents may have to face about their reproductive options. This is especially challenging when parents may be considering an option to terminate a pregnancy following prenatal diagnosis. If they have an existing child with the condition, there may be worries that this could devalue that child, and explanations to the child could be difficult.

Activity

What circumstances can you think of where genetics will have an impact on family life? Make a list of the instances and compare these with those shown in the companion PowerPoint presentation.

So how do families with children affected by, or at risk of, genetic conditions adapt to the situation? Canam (1993) describes the tasks that parents have to face in adapting to chronic childhood illness:

- accept the child's condition
- manage the condition on a day-to-day basis
- meet the normal developmental needs of the child
- meet the developmental needs of other family members
- cope with continuous stress and periodic crises
- assist family members to manage their feelings
- educate others about the child's condition
- establish a support system.

We will consider each of the stages in relation to genetic diseases.

ACCEPTING THE CONDITION

Canam (1993) identifies acceptance as the first phase in the process. Seeking answers and a reduction of uncertainty are integral to this but a definitive diagnosis is not always available, particularly if the condition is rare. If the condition is one that is already 'in the family' the difficulties can vary. Many families may be accepting, with an established support system, but other parents have to cope with accusations of 'irresponsibility'.

One factor that can have an impact on accepting a condition is its visibility. The shock of a major physical abnormality can be profound and the reactions of others on first meeting the child serve as a reminder of this. Lack of visibility can also make it more difficult for the family and others to accept. When the condition is associated with behavioural problems (such as autism or Tourette syndrome) its physical invisibility frequently presents problems with acceptance and understanding from others, both within and outside the family.

Fanos (1999) reported how acceptance by siblings may be influenced by the visibility of a condition in an affected brother or sister. She noted that the visibility of ataxia telangiectasia (a recessive condition characterised by unsteady gait and involuntary movements) caused less resentment of the time given to the child, less guilt, and less tendency to idealize the affected sib, than children with cystic fibrosis. However, it was associated with more embarrassment and shame.

MANAGE THE CONDITION ON A DAY-TO-DAY BASIS

The problems of coping with the practical matters of everyday living when a child (or any family member) has a chronic illness have been widely reviewed (see Chapter 44). A crucial factor in dealing with the problems are resources, including time, energy, money and social support systems, and the availability of all of these over an extended time. The extent of the resources needed will vary according to the specific condition. With a condition such as cystic fibrosis, for example, the child will need daily physiotherapy, regular visits to clinics, careful supervision of diet and may require frequent periods of hospitalisation. Medication will need to be given and regular supplies maintained. The extra workload may make full- or even part-time employment impractical for one parent. In managing the condition on a day-to-day basis, then, the parent may have to adjust to reduced career prospects, loss of role, and problems with self-esteem. The latter may be a factor of the feelings of guilt at having passed on a condition to the child.

MEET THE NORMAL DEVELOPMENTAL NEEDS OF THE CHILD

The nature of the condition and how debilitating it is will clearly be a significant factor in how well the developmental needs of the child can be met. The instinctive desire to protect the child can be further fuelled by feelings of guilt, predisposing to 'spoiling' and children may take advantage of this. Labelling of the child by the family or by others can further compromise the situation.

Professional Conversation

This was Ella's second baby, a little boy. I'd been to see her on the 3rd day and mum and baby were doing well. On the 5th day I popped in again, and was pleased to see that her breastfeeding was settling down nicely. I told her that I'd be back the day after next to do the heel prick test (Guthrie) and asked if she'd read the little leaflet about the test that we give out at antenatal clinics. Ella hadn't, and looked a bit embarrassed when she said she'd lost it. We had a laugh as I said she probably had enough to do with the baby and a toddler without searching for it, and I gave her another one.

When I went back on the 7th day, I asked Ella if she'd read the leaflet and she said yes, so I asked her to sign the consent form. I told her the tests were routine, and that the diseases were all very rare, but it helps if we pick them up early enough. I said that it took about 3 weeks for the labs to do the tests, and they only contact us if there's a problem, so not to worry if she didn't hear any more. The baby screamed of course when I did the heel prick – that always upsets the mums! Ella's husband Rob came home just as I was leaving, so I told him what a gorgeous son he had. I remember how proud he looked.

When the results came back to us a few weeks later, I was really shocked to hear that the baby had tested positive for Duchenne's. Something like this had never happened to me before. I went back with the health visitor to give Ella the results. I felt awful. Ella and Rob looked grey as they listened. The health visitor explained how it only affects little boys from about the age of two, and that his muscles would get gradually weaker. Ella got up and went over to the baby's carry cot and looked down at him and said 'You know, I thought he wasn't kicking his legs as

strongly as Sophie did when she was a baby. Do you think he's showing signs of it now?'

It really hit me then that this test really means something. I mean, something that changes people's lives. I just felt like, well, we'd taken away the babyhood of this little boy for his family.

When we got back to the car, I just sat there and cried.

MEET THE DEVELOPMENTAL NEEDS OF OTHER FAMILY MEMBERS

Fanos (1997) reminds us that the accessibility of a parent for the psychosocial support of a child is a crucial factor in its well-being. If the condition is an autosomal dominant one, a parent may already be trying to cope with his or her own illness, or that of the partner. With one (or more) children affected by a condition, the accessibility of the parents will be compromised – more so when they are grieving the death of an affected child. With frequent hospital stays, the availability of a parent on a day-to-day basis will also be severely limited. In a later study of the impact on siblings of boys with severe combined immunodeficiency disorder, most expressed distress over the prolonged absence of the mother during hospitalisation of the ill brother (Fanos & Puck 2001). They concluded that parents need help in balancing the needs of well sibs with those of an affected one.

Professional Conversation

The Bradley family was well known to me – various members had been back and fore to the cystic fibrosis clinic over the years. Teresa was just 15 when she came and asked me about carrier testing for cystic fibrosis. Her cousin has the condition and her mum, older sister and another cousin are carriers, as well as her aunt and uncle of course. The family has always talked openly about cystic fibrosis and Teresa said she felt it was now her turn to be tested. I was a bit concerned because of her age, although she is quite mature and sensible, but also because I wondered how she might feel if she turned out not to have the gene. With so many of her family being carriers (in fact, all of the older females and the uncle) a negative result might exclude her from 'the gang'. I don't think the family had registered this and I know they would not knowingly exclude her but the potential for her to feel left out needed to be raised.

COPE WITH CONTINUOUS STRESS AND PERIODIC CRISES

Sickle-cell disease and cystic fibrosis (both of which are recessive conditions) are typical examples of how the pattern of the illness is one of continuous stress, managing the condition on a daily basis with a regime of medication and other therapy, interspersed with crises, usually triggered by infection. Chest infection in children with cystic fibrosis, and sickle-cell crisis (where the abnormally shaped red blood cells can cause infarction and necrosis) require prompt hospitalisation and aggressive clinical intervention.

The day-to-day fluctuations in condition and the uncertainty this brings make a major contribution to stress (Locker 1991). To this symptomatic uncertainty is added the trajectory uncertainty of being able to predict the course and outcome of the disease. This is not only because of individual variation in gene expression, but also because of advances in management in a fast-moving research field, underpinning hopes for more effective treatments or even cure (through gene therapy) in the future.

Activity

Read Merry France-Dawson's story about her experiences of living with sickle-cell disease in *The troubled helix* (Marteau & Richards 1996). She recalls overhearing her father being told she would not survive the night as a young girl in ITU over 30 years ago, and describes how she then 'lived by instalments'.

MANAGING THE FAMILY'S FEELINGS

It is important to acknowledge the positive contribution that the child makes to the family, irrespective of the nature of the condition. Kearney & Griffin (2001) conceptualise the experiences of parents of children with developmental disability as being a dynamic between joy and sorrow. Although there are undoubtedly negative experiences, these can be balanced by positive feelings such as hope and humour. As McGowan expresses it: 'My sons are special people, beyond their genetic flaw . . .' (McGowan 1999 p 199).

Nonetheless, the sorrows can be profound and long-lasting, and other feelings such as guilt, blame, anger, fear, anxiety and depression can also be difficult to cope with. One factor that may be more apparent in families with a child affected by a genetic condition is the feeling of guilt. This can take the form of 'survivor guilt' in unaffected family members, including children. In one study examining the long-term psychological effects of genetic testing for a hereditary colorectal cancer, some children with a negative result and a positive-testing sibling demonstrated an increase in symptoms of anxiety at follow-up (Codori et al 2003).

The guilt that parents can feel can be overwhelming. In his book about his daughter Alex, Frank Deford recounts eloquently the impact of genetic disease on family life (Deford 1983). Alex had cystic fibrosis, and she lived until she was 8 years old. The story of Alex's life, of the family's struggle with her disease, and of her death is indescribably moving and essential reading for any children's nurse. Deford captures some of the feelings that many parents may experience in this situation:

Ultimately, whether in my dealings with Carol [his wife], with Alex herself, with anyone involved with the disease – or with myself, for that matter – the major emotion pressing upon me was the feeling of inadequacy . . . And I could not explain how I felt, because of the shame, nor could I ever escape, because of the guilt (Deford 1983 p 96)

He goes on to say:

When our child was dying – when she was dying because of the genes we passed on to her – no matter how irrational it may have been to flagellate ourselves, there were times, in the mustiest corners of self-awareness, when we had to. Had to. I could not forgive Carol any more than I could forgive myself. After all, we quickly enough assume credit for the genes that make our children attractive and bright – she takes after me. It's only human nature, then, that we also accept the responsibility when we pass on genes of destruction (Deford 1983 p 94)

Of course, such feelings are not the prerogative of parents in this situation. Many parents will blame themselves for contributing in some way to their child's condition. However, with genetic disease, particularly the single gene disorders and chromosomal conditions, the cause may be clearly attributable to one or both parents. Furthermore, as the condition may be passed on to future generations, this may be accompanied by ongoing guilt and fear that subsequent children will also inherit it.

EDUCATE OTHERS

There are thousands of single gene disorders and most are rare. However, even the more common ones are unfamiliar to most health professionals outside the specialist genetics service. The families tend to become the experts, demonstrating knowledge and understanding of the condition and using this to educate others involved in the care of the child.

ESTABLISH A SUPPORT SYSTEM

With any chronic illness, the healthcare system becomes a major part of the family's environment and they need to become socialised into it. The success of this depends in part on the quality of information available and on accessible and effective multiagency communication. Support groups can thus be life savers.

● Seminar discussion topic

The NHS encourages involvement of user groups in the education of health professionals and there is a call for easier access to information about particular conditions. Many support groups now host websites and produce their own literature. What are the benefits of this and what might be the drawbacks if the information has not been assessed beforehand?

Problems can arise if a professional provides contact details and has not evaluated the information available. Those in support groups may be related to a child more severely affected by a condition – the parents of a child who is mildly affected by the same condition may not feel the need for membership of such a group. The information available may not then reflect the experiences of all families across the spectrum.

How can children's nurses make best use of user groups as a source of information?

The phases of adaptation we have described can be 'worked through' by families, with time and support. However, it is important to note that individuals within a family will progress at different rates, and the progress itself may not be linear as individuals move back and forth between the stages. Whyte (1992) identifies that a crucial aspect of the process is the synchrony with which partners move through these phases.

Many of the challenges facing families that we have outlined so far apply to other diseases, and not just genetic disease, but the distinction between these is becoming blurred as advances in genetics research increasingly are revealing the genetic component of common diseases. The next section explains how genes can be passed on through the generations and how 'faulty' genes may lead to disease and ill health.

It Runs in the Family: The Role of Genetic Factors in Disease

There are over 4000 simply inherited serious genetic disorders, such as cystic fibrosis, sickle-cell disease and Duchenne muscular dystrophy. Together with the chromosomal abnormalities such as Down syndrome, they account for about 10 to 20 cases of genetic disease per 1000 population. However, by the age of 60, about 60% of the population is likely to have been affected by a disease that is partially genetically determined. Our genes, at least in part, determine nearly all of our characteristics, including how we respond to infection, and so they play a fundamental role in our health. But what are genes and how can they lead to ill health that can be passed on through the generations?

GENES

Almost every cell of the body contains a complete set of genes, each one representing a chemical instruction to make proteins for different cell functions, guiding development from embryo to adult. There are genes that control other genes, switching them on or off according to the cell type and the functions it performs. For example, in the pancreas, the gene providing the instructions for the manufacture of insulin might be turned on, whereas genes for making keratin, a structural protein, would be switched off. There are also genes that control cell growth; faults in these genes can lead to different types of cancers.

Genes are Made up of DNA

The genes themselves are carried on the chromosomes, each chromosome being made up of two enormously long strands of DNA, tightly coiled into a double helix. The genes are spaced along the DNA molecule, and are an integral part of it.

If we use the analogy of imagining that a chromosome is a C90 cassette, then the DNA is the tape inside, tightly coiled and packaged in an organised way. The genes would represent the songs recorded onto the tape, an average gene taking up about 3 cm of the 135-m tape.

The DNA consists of building blocks of chemical bases (nucleotides), of which there are only four different types, A, C, G and T. A single gene has thousands of these bases, some, like the dystrophin gene (associated with Duchenne muscular dystrophy), have millions. If the DNA molecule that comprises one chromosome was likened to a tower of Lego®, then the tower could be built using only four colours of Lego® blocks but the tower could be about 100 million blocks high!

It is the order or sequence of the four nucleotides within a gene along the length of a DNA molecule that contains the instructions to make specific proteins, in the form of a chemical code. A block of three nucleotides (a triplet) represents the code for one amino acid, the building blocks of proteins. Essentially, each gene is made up of a series of three-letter words (using a four-letter alphabet), which, when deciphered, gives us a sequence of amino acids.

ALTERATIONS TO THE GENETIC MAKE-UP

The sequence of the chemical bases that make up the DNA in each of the 23 pairs of chromosomes is the same in every person, for about 99% of the human genome. However, there are variations in the remaining genetic material and it is these variations that make us unique.

Some of the variations occur by chance, and although many such mutations are repaired, some are not. Of these, some may confer an advantage to the genome but others may be harmful, particularly if the number of mutations increases with increasing age and exposure to environmental hazards. These mutations are effectively gene errors. Mutations that occur in the sex cells can be passed on to future generations.

The nature of the gene error can also vary. Some arise when a single nucleotide from an entire gene sequence is accidentally replaced by a different nucleotide. The mutation associated with sickle-cell disease is a classic example of this type of 'point' mutation. Sickle-cell disease is the most common of the haemoglobinopathies, affecting about 1 in 300 people of Afro-Caribbean origin, with about 1 in 10 being carriers of the disease. Carriers are more resistant to malaria for a short time.

Haemoglobin is formed from four chains of amino acids, two α chains, and two β chains, each of which is associated with a haem group that binds with oxygen. In sickle-cell disease there is a mutation in the gene on chromosome 11 that provides the code for the β chains. A single base (A) within the gene is replaced by a different base (T). This alters the code so that the amino acid valine is manufactured instead of glutamine, and this single alteration is sufficient to change the normal β-globin structure of haemoglobin (Fig. 38.1). The result is that the red blood cells become abnormally shaped in conditions of reduced oxygen levels, such as during an infectious illness. The sickle-shaped cells can block capillaries, causing painful infarctions at times of such crises, and the disturbances to blood flow can also cause leg ulcers. Internal organs are compromised, and splenomegaly may be apparent. Premature destruction of the abnormally shaped cells also leads to anaemia, and a loss of immune function predisposes the child to infection.

Fig. 38.1 • The sickle-cell mutation.

If the mutation has an effect that is so marked that it is always seen, the alteration is said to be dominant, and it will mask the effect of the allele on the other chromosome. On the other hand, it could have an effect that is apparent only when both alleles of a chromosome pair are the altered version, in which case the mutation is said to be recessive. Sickle-cell disease is caused by a recessive mutation, although people with one altered gene ('carriers') may show some signs of the disease under extreme conditions of low oxygen.

An analogy can be drawn with a fluorescent light containing two tubes. When functioning normally, the tubes together provide a steady illumination. If one tube is faulty, so that it flickers constantly, the effect can be so irritating as to mask the effect of the other tube. On the other hand, if the fault resulted in the tube being unable to function, so long as the other tube worked effectively, the light itself would still be functional, albeit with a reduced intensity; this is analogous to a recessive mutation. If both tubes have the same fault, the light will not work.

HOW GENES ARE PASSED ON THROUGH FAMILIES

Mutations that occur within a gene (known as the single gene disorders) show characteristic patterns of inheritance as they are passed on through generations, depending on whether they are dominant or recessive, and located on an autosome or the sex chromosomes (Table 38.1).

Because an autosomal dominant trait is invariably expressed in the affected person, the family tree shows someone affected with the condition in each generation, and with both sexes affected (Fig. 38.2). Each child of an affected parent has a 1 in 2 or 50% chance of inheriting the faulty gene but unaffected parents do not transmit it.

Table 38.1 Examples of Single Gene Conditions Seen in Childhood

Autosomal dominant	Autosomal recessive	X-linked recessive
Achondroplasia	Cystic fibrosis	Haemophilia A and B
Marfan syndrome	Sickle-cell disease	Alport syndrome
Osteogenesis imperfecta	Thalassaemia	Fragile X
Tuberous sclerosis	Phenylketonuria	Red–green colour blindness
Neurofibromatosis type 1	Spinal muscular atrophy (Werdnig-Hoffman disease)	Duchenne muscular dystrophy
Gilles de la Tourette syndrome (Tourette's)	Congenital deafness	Glucose 6-phosphate dehydrogenase deficiency

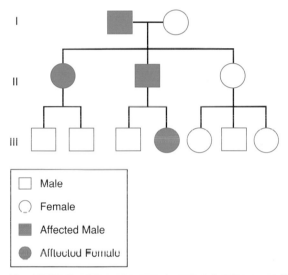

Legend:
- □ Male
- ○ Female
- ■ Affected Male
- ● Affected Female

Fig. 38.2 • Family tree for an autosomal dominant condition.

In contrast, an autosomal recessive trait can be carried through generations 'hidden' from view, because carriers show no symptoms. Often, the first indication of the condition being 'in the family' is when an affected baby is born of parents who are both carriers. The chances of this happening are usually quite rare, but higher when parents are related — such as first cousins. Some conditions are associated with a higher carrier frequency in particular populations, such as cystic fibrosis in white northern Europeans (in the UK, this frequency is approximately 1 in 25). When parents are both carriers, with each conception there is a 1 in 4 or 25% chance that the baby will be affected by the condition, and a 1 in 2 or 50% chance that the baby will be a carrier.

When the gene under question is located on the X chromosome, the pattern (known as X-linked inheritance) is somewhat different. As males have only one X chromo-some, genes located on that chromosome will always be expressed even if recessive, as they do not have the partner chromosome to compensate. Males are thus said to be hemizygous for X-linked genes. X-linked inheritance can be either recessive or dominant, although the latter is much rarer. Male-to-male transmission is not seen but all daughters of affected males will inherit the faulty gene (Fig. 38.3). Women who are carriers have a 50% chance of passing on the faulty gene to their sons (who will then be affected) and their daughters will have a 50% chance of being carriers themselves.

The characteristic features of the three types of inheritance can be summarised as shown in Table 38.2.

There are occasions when a family history does not seem to follow the typical pattern. Alterations to mitochondrial DNA show a mother-to-child inheritance. New mutations in the sex cells of a parent can account for the appearance of a dominant trait in a family. Some dominant traits can also be affected by penetrance and expressivity. Traits associated with a reduced penetrance may not be expressed in

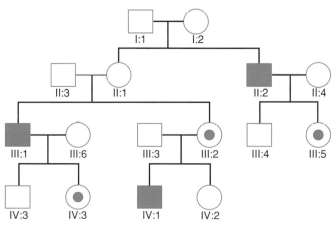

Fig. 38.3 • X-linked inheritance.

Table 38.2 The Family Tree: Characteristic Features of Classically Inherited Diseases

Dominant inheritance	Recessive	X-linked
Usually more than one successive generation affected	Usually only one generation affected	More than one generation affected
People of both sexes affected	People of both sexes affected	Males affected more severely than females
Male to male transmission evident	Offspring of two healthy parents affected	No male to male transmission

an individual, and when they are expressed, the severity of expression may also vary. Neurofibromatosis is a dominant condition with variable expression such that it may have gone undetected in an individual at first and thus appear to 'skip' a generation in affected families. However, closer examination would reveal, for example, some of the characteristic pigmented patches (café au lait spots) on the skin. Finally, non-paternity can also account for an otherwise puzzling family tree, and this situation has to be dealt with sensitively.

DNA IS PACKAGED INTO CHROMOSOMES

Chromosomes are the more visible elements of inheritance, tightly packed coils of DNA. Cells have 23 pairs of chromosomes, one member of each pair being inherited from the mother and one from the father. We inherit one set of 23 chromosomes, and thus one set of genes, from each parent, passed on through the egg and sperm cells. The total chromosome number of 46 is restored with the fusion of the egg and sperm to form the embryo.

When the chromosomes are examined in the laboratory, they are set out in a systematic way, according to their matched pairs, arranged in order of size, and aligned with the shorter arm of the chromosome (designated p) above the longer one (q). This arrangement is the karyotype (Fig. 38.4).

Members of a pair of chromosomes are referred to as being homologous, and each member of the pair will have the same genes in the same order. However, the form of a particular gene may be a little different on each chromosome – these different forms are known as alleles. For example, a gene that provides instructions for making eye pigments occurs at the same position (locus) on each chromosome of the pair. If both chromosomes have the same allele (e.g. brown eye pigment) the person is homozygous for (brown) eye colour. If the alleles are different (e.g. one brown and the other blue) the person is heterozygous for eye colour.

As well as errors that occur in the DNA sequence, at 'gene level', we can also have errors at the level of the chromosome, involving part or whole chromosomes. Such errors account for more than 50% of all spontaneous first trimester losses, 20% of second trimester losses, and occur

Fig. 38.4 • A normal male karyotype.

in about 1 in 160 live births. The errors involve alterations either to the number or structure of chromosomes.

Alterations to chromosome number are the most common. Polyploidy is the term given to cells that contain a multiple of 23 chromosomes. In humans, triploid (69 chromosomes) and tetraploid (92 chromosomes) conceptions can occur, but are incompatible with survival. An embryo that is aneuploid has missing or additional chromosomes, most commonly one additional chromosome (trisomy). The general rule is that we can tolerate additional genetic material more readily than a loss, so monosomy (loss of one chromosome) is not compatible with life. The exception to this is Turner syndrome, a condition seen only in girls where there is a loss of one X chromosome.

The most common form of aneuploidy is trisomy and whilst most trisomic fetuses are spontaneously aborted, some survive to term and beyond. Down syndrome, and its association with increased maternal age, is the most well known (Fig. 38.5). Trisomies of the sex chromosomes (XXX female, XYY male, or XXY Klinefelter male) have much less severe consequences, and many people with this condition may be undiagnosed until after puberty, or at fertility clinics.

Structural alterations occur when chromosome material becomes rearranged following breakage and abnormal reconstitution. Parts of a chromosome may become detached and lost, duplicated, or rearranged (Table 38.3).

Fig. 38.5 • Trisomy 21 karyotype (Down syndrome).

47,XY, +21

46,XX,t,(6;7)(q16.2;q34)pat

Fig. 38.6 • Karyotype of a reciprocal translocation. Genetic material has been exchanged between one of each pair of chromosomes 6 and 7 (arrowed).

Table 38.3 Some Examples of Chromosome Rearrangements

Numerical	Example	Karyotype
Gain of a whole chromosome	Down syndrome (Trisomy 21)	47,XX (or XY) +21 Gain of an autosome (Chr 21)
	Klinefelter syndrome	47,XXY Gain of a sex chromosome
Loss of a whole chromosome	Turner syndrome	45, X Loss of a sex chromosome
Structural		
Translocation	Balanced Robertsonian translocation	45,XY t(14;21) Chr 14 and 21 have fused to form one chromosome
Deletion	Cri du chat	46,XX (or XY)5p- Partial deletion on short arm of Chr 5
Microdeletion	22q	46,XX (or XY)22q- Microdeletion on long arm of Chr 22

Breaks can be caused spontaneously, or by certain viruses, drugs or radiation. The effects of these depend on the nature of the rearrangement and whether there is an overall loss or gain of genetic material.

A translocation occurs when there is an exchange of material between two different (non-homologous) chromosomes (Fig. 38.6). These are the most clinically significant of the structural chromosome rearrangements. In most cases, there is no net loss or gain of chromosomal material during the exchange process, and the translocation is thus said to be 'balanced'. It is estimated that 1 in 500 individuals have a balanced translocation, usually with no health consequences for the individual. However, problems arise during the formation of the egg or sperm cells, and some may carry unbalanced chromosomes, often causing early pregnancy loss or multiple abnormalities in the infant.

GENE TESTING

Cystic fibrosis provides a useful example to illustrate how 'finding' the gene can help in understanding the underlying disease mechanism and in providing a direct genetic test (Box 38.1).

Understanding how genes that contribute to ill health can be inherited, how they can then be detected to inform a diagnosis and then communicating this and other information to parents and children is part of the role of professionals within the genetics service. However, with the integration of genetics into mainstream services and increasing demand for genetic information, there is a growing need for all health professionals to develop competence in this area. The next section looks at the role of the children's nurse in relation to this.

Genetic Counselling and the Family Journey: The Role of the Children's Nurse

Genetic counselling is 'a communication process between the counsellor and the individual or family which deals with

Box 38.1

Gene testing

The gene for the cystic fibrosis transmembrane regulator protein (CFTR) was identified in 1989. The normal protein helps to control the flow of chloride ions across cell membranes and so produces good quality mucus secretions. If this flow is compromised, sodium and water balance will also be affected leading to abnormal secretions and a build up of thick mucus. Most mutations in Europe (70%) show a deletion of 3 bases at position Δ508 of the CFTR gene: This results in the loss of the amino acid phenylalanine from the protein product

Segment of normal DNA coding for CFTR gene:

... AAT ATC AT**C** **TT**T GGT GTT ...

Segment of mutated DNA with deletion of three base pairs at position Δ508:

... AAT ATC AT T GGT GTT ...

This deletion may be detected using direct analysis of DNA obtained from mouthwash samples. The fragments of DNA of interest may be isolated and then identified in the laboratory using specially 'marked' DNA fragments. The fragments separate according to size when subjected to an electric current, and these can then be compared with control fragments of known size and DNA sequence.

Mutated (508) fragment

Normal gene fragment

A   B   C   D

In the diagram above, individuals A and B have two normal gene fragments and so are normal homozygotes for the CFTR gene. Individual C has one normal fragment and one Δ508 fragment, and so is a heterozygous carrier for cystic fibrosis. Individual D has two Δ508 fragments and is thus homozygous for cystic fibrosis.

the medical and other implications associated with the occurrence, or the risk of occurrence, of a genetic disorder in a family' (DoH 2003 p 91). In the UK, families are referred to the specialist genetics service most commonly by their GP or paediatrician. They are seen by a consultant clinical geneticist and/or a genetic counsellor at outpatient clinics, although home visits are often also made.

Barr & Millar (2003) argue that genetic counselling should be seen as an integral part of the adaptation process that parents and other family members journey through. The role of the children's nurse is then to journey with the family, helping family members 'prepare for, engage in and move on' irrespective of the information provided at the genetic clinic. To do so effectively, the nurse has to be equipped with sufficient knowledge and understanding of genetics to be able to support the family, placing genetics information into context as a part of that journey.

The extent of the knowledge and skills required in genetics by all nurses in the UK has been set into a competency framework and described in a report (Kirk et al 2003b). The authors worked with stakeholders (including professional and client groups) to identify the knowledge, skills and attitudes in genetics that nurses should demonstrate.

www

Read the report online:
- http://www.glam.ac.uk/socs/research/gpu/FinalReport.pdf
  Discuss in your learning group if you think the competencies are relevant for children's nurses.

Seven competence standard statements have been constructed, representing the minimum standard that should be achieved by nurses at the point of registration (Box 38.2).

Box 38.2

The seven core competence standard statements

All nurses, midwives and health visitors, at the point of registration, should be able to:
1. Identify clients who might benefit from genetic services and information:
   - through an understanding of the importance of family history in assessing predisposition to disease
   - seeking assistance from and referring to appropriate genetics experts and peer support resources
   - based on an understanding of the components of the current genetic counselling process.
2. Appreciate the importance of sensitivity in tailoring genetic information and services to clients' culture, knowledge and language level:
   - recognising that ethnicity, culture, religion and ethical perspectives may influence the clients' ability to utilise these.
3. Uphold the rights of all clients to informed decision making and voluntary action:
   - based on an awareness of the history of misuse of human genetic information
   - understanding of the importance of delivering genetic education and counselling fairly, accurately and without coercion or personal bias
   - recognising that personal values and beliefs may influence the care and support provided to clients during decision-making.
4. Demonstrate a knowledge and understanding of the role of genetic and other factors in maintaining health and in the manifestation, modification and prevention of disease expression, to underpin effective practice.
5. Demonstrate a knowledge and understanding of the utility and limitations of genetic testing and information:
   - including the ethical, legal and social issues related to testing and recording of genetic information

- the potential physical and/or psychosocial consequences of genetic information for individuals, family members, and communities.
6. Recognise the limitations of one's own genetics expertise:
   - based on an understanding of one's professional role in the referral, provision or follow-up to genetics services.
7. Obtain and communicate credible, current information about genetics, for self, clients and colleagues:
   - using information technologies effectively to do so.

The report also suggests learning outcomes and practice indicators for each competence statement, and indicates how the competency framework may be adapted for more experienced practitioners.

Reflect on your Practice

- Do you think you could demonstrate these competencies in your practice?
- How can you address any deficit you identify in your skills?

Although the competencies apply to all nursing professionals, the situations in which children's nurses in particular need to use genetic knowledge and skills have been outlined by the Association of Genetic Nurses and Counsellors (2002). These include where the children's nurse would need to:

- provide supportive, informed communication at the time of diagnosis or receipt of definitive results

- act as a trusted and informed carer for children growing up with genetic conditions (such as muscular dystrophy or cystic fibrosis), as they may be probing increasingly for information about the condition, its prognosis and effect on life plans

- help parents deal with feelings of anger, guilt or blame as they acknowledge their own genetic contribution to the child's illness or consider prenatal diagnosis in a future pregnancy

- enhance awareness of conditions which may mimic non-accidental injury or abuse, such as osteogenesis imperfecta or conditions that result in failure to thrive

- facilitate referral to local genetic services when appropriate.

Evidence-based Practice

Barr & Millar (2003) describe the expectations and experiences of parents of children with learning disabilities in relation to genetic counselling. They found that parents largely felt unprepared for their appointment with the genetic consultant and that this could mean that parents hold unrealistic expectations about the appointment. The authors recommend that priority should be given to gaining an understanding of the expectations of clients prior to the first appointment.

The need for clear and accurate information, delivered sensitively and at a pace and level appropriate to the understanding and needs of family members is fundamental, but this is not always achieved (Chapple et al 1997, Fallowfield & Jenkins 2004, McGowan 1999). The family nurse can help in 'going over' information with the family, working with them at their own pace – and is in the ideal position to recognise that individuals within the family may be at different stages of adaptation. Preparing families for genetic counselling, helping them to have realistic expectations, is an important aspect of placing genetic information into context.

Skirton (2001) stresses the importance of certainty in the family's quest for a diagnosis, but there will be many times when a diagnosis is not available. It is worth noting here that as more genetic tests become available, there will also be circumstances where families who had not previously been given a diagnosis will be recalled, and a definitive diagnosis may become possible. These families may well experience a readaptation, particularly where a genetic cause can now be attributed to one or both parents.

Part of giving reliable information includes the need to avoid false reassurance, but at the same time provide a balanced perspective, helping the family to maintain hope. Support groups can be particularly helpful, but information about these needs to be delivered at an appropriate time, and the nurse needs to be aware of the type and quality of information available.

Evidence-based Practice

The importance of providing good quality information for parents and families is widely acknowledged, but how is this defined? Mitchell & Sloper (2002) used four focus groups of parents and one of professionals to explore how parents preferred to receive information, and their views on best practice. They propose a model that takes a three-dimensional approach, combining good-quality information that offers a review of local resources and more in-depth material, with personal guidance from a 'key worker' such as a community-based professional.

Reflect on your Practice

- Do you think you provide 'three-dimensional information' for your families? Are you confident that you do not over-rely on one source, such as leaflets?
- How do you check that your families have understood the information you have provided?

At the heart of effective communication is the relationship that the nurse has with the family. Trust is central to this, developed through open, honest communication and practice within an ethical framework as indicated by the competence standard statements. Some of the ethical issues surrounding the application of genetic technologies are of particular relevance to children's nurses.

Professional Conversation

" Geraldine is a registered children's nurse.

Recognise the limitations of one's own genetics expertise
For me, the most important competency is knowing when to say I don't know and then getting help from someone who does! I think this was brought home to me last year. I'd been talking to a mum who had brought her daughter to clinic for an unrelated problem. She was obviously a bit down and told me that she'd had a termination of pregnancy a few weeks earlier after an abnormality (a neural tube defect) was picked up on scan – she'd had an amniocentesis but that had been OK. She and her husband wanted to try for another baby, but were scared of the same thing happening again. I told her the chances of it recurring were a million to one. And then without really thinking it through, I reassured her that as well, she could have an earlier genetic test by chorionic villus sampling. She asked how that would show up anything if the amnio didn't. Of course at that point I realised I was out of my depth and said I'd check it out and get back to her. When I contacted our local genetics nurse, she was very helpful but I was embarrassed when I learnt that in fact the mum's chance of a recurrence was actually 1 in 20 (5%). Maybe I shouldn't have said anything, but it's natural to want to reassure families. I was able to liaise with the genetics nurse though about getting back to the mum, and I am more careful now about what I say.

- Whose role was it to provide information for this mother? Should it be the role of any one professional group?

Ethical Issues for Children's Nurses

Although the benefits that new genetic technologies may bring to help people with or at risk of a genetic disease are to be welcomed, there are also concerns about potential harms. An increase in genetic testing may challenge personal privacy, undermining the 'right not to know'. Some authors voice concern that it has the potential to promote discrimination, and devalues the existence of people with a disability (see, for example, Ward 2002). Newell (2000) claims that the prediction that an embryo is at risk of an increasing number of 'defects' is regarded as a standard basis for a decision to terminate the pregnancy on 'therapeutic' grounds.

The application of new genetic technology in reproductive decision-making provokes fierce debate on occasion. One aspect of this is the selection of embryos during in vitro fertilisation, on the basis of its genotype, for the purposes of helping an existing child. This could potentially help families such as McGowan's, where a bone-marrow transplant from a sibling with appropriate genotype could help her sons. She states that 'At this stage, my husband and I have rejected such options as we feel it is not right for us to have a child for such reasons . . . I really believe that people should be valued for more than just their genes' (McGowan 1999 p 197).

Activity

Yasmin and Michael have a happy, stable relationship. They are about to decide whether to start a family. Draw a decision tree (like a flow diagram) for the couple, starting with the question 'shall we have children?' and assuming that their initial decision is that they will. Work through all the subsequent decisions they have to make, up until the final decision of 'shall we have another child?'

Try and include all possible options, incorporating your knowledge of current reproductive technologies. What decisions might they have to make in the pre-conceptual and antenatal periods? What decisions might they face in the immediate postnatal period? Which do you think might be the most difficult? Once you have done this, you might like to draw another decision tree, but this time think of a couple facing this decision back in the 1950s. How has the nature of reproductive decision-making changed? Does increased choice bring greater freedom?

Certainly, a common concern is about whether and where a line should be drawn between using genetic information to prevent harm (negative eugenics) and to promote desirable characteristics (positive eugenics). Iredale (2000) reviews these issues and concludes that nurses need to play an active role in promoting good genetic health, underpinned by an appreciation of the history of genetics and the eugenics movement. Professional practice also has to incorporate the ethical principles of privacy, confidentiality, informed consent and non-discrimination

● Seminar discussion topic

Read *Stamping out short people* by Gregory Stock, accessed online at:

- http://www.com/wired/archive/11.11/view_pr.html

Describing the 'official recognition' by the Food and Drug Administration (FDA) agency in the US of the use of growth hormone for healthy but short children, the author supports the use of enhancement technology to make us 'stronger, smarter and faster'. He argues that 'The biggest risk isn't that we'll make mistakes or create a race of superhumans. It's that we'll proceed too cautiously with health enhancements that would benefit us all.'

- Is it a fundamental human right to be able to access new technologies to improve our inherited characteristics?
- Do parents have the right to enhance the characteristics of their children?
- What about unborn children? Do they have a right to inherit an 'un-enhanced' genome?

One of the key ethical issues for children's nurses is the genetic testing of children, in particular predictive testing for conditions of early and later adult onset, and carrier testing. Early identification of at-risk children might facilitate earlier surveillance and treatment, and would remove uncertainty (Carmichael et al 1999) but there are potential disadvantages. This issue is reviewed by Clarke (1997), who notes that many professional groups recommend caution. He outlines grounds for caution in carrying out predictive testing of healthy children for late-onset disorders on four counts:

- The child loses its autonomy as an adult to make its own decisions.

- Loss of confidentiality because the child's genetic status is known to its parents.

- The psychosocial consequences for the child, which might include labelling, fatalism, damage to self-esteem, and alteration to family dynamics

- Although the parents may make the decision they feel will be best for the child, they will do so from a hypothetical perspective. The child, faced with the reality, may see things differently. Clarke uses Huntington's disease as an example to illustrate this. Ahead of the gene being identified, the majority of at-risk families stated that they would seek testing once this became possible. In reality, when the gene was found,

the majority of at-risk adults chose not to be tested, preferring to retain uncertainty.

Fanos (1997) makes a further point when she states that:

The very children and adolescents most at risk for being tested for genetic disorders are those who have grown up in a world where the illness has already made a very real appearance. Parents may not be emotionally available to help their children with the impact of testing procedures or results because of their own illness or guilt over issues of inheritance (p 27)

Professional Conversation

I was asked to go and see Rebecca at home because the neonatal screening test on her baby Amy had revealed her daughter to be a carrier for cystic fibrosis. Of course, this meant there were quite a few implications for the family. Either Rebecca or her partner (or both) could be a carrier of the condition, and their siblings could also, so it would be important to make sure that Rebecca understood this, and understood how she might want to take this into account for further reproductive decisions. I would also need to make sure that Rebecca understood what being a carrier would mean for Amy in terms of her health, and the implications for Amy when she was old enough to have children. Lots to tell her – lots to ensure she understands. The headache for me is that Rebecca is only 13 years old herself.

This issue is likely to come to the forefront once again as the UK government examines the potential of genetic profiling at birth (DoH 2003). It proposes that participation would be voluntary and that individuals would retain the right to withdraw their information at any time. The role of the children's nurse, acting as advocate, will be central to upholding these rights.

Summary

The advance in genetics knowledge and related technology is transforming health care, moving a hitherto specialist subject, with its focus on rare conditions, into mainstream services. Understanding how genetics can affect families is increasingly important for children's nurses as they support families in their care. Being able to interpret and communicate information about genetics accurately, honestly and sensitively is a central feature of the role. A wider appreciation of the ethical issues that may arise, not only for children and their families, but also for wider society, is also important.

References

Association of Genetic Nurses and Counsellors (AGNC) Education Working Group 2002 Education in genetics for health professionals not working in specialist genetic units. Report E, Reports for the Genetics Policy Unit Department of Health. AGNC, Birmingham

Barr O, Millar R 2003 Parents of children with intellectual disabilities: their expectations and experience of genetic counselling. Journal of Applied Research in Intellectual Disabilities 16:189–204

Bell J 1998 The new genetics in clinical practice. British Medical Journal 316:618–620

Canam C 1993 Common adaptive tasks facing parents of children with chronic conditions. Journal of Advanced Nursing 18:46–53

Carmichael B, Pembrey M, Turner G, Barnicoat A 1999 Diagnosis of fragile-X syndrome: the experience of parents. Journal of Intellectual Disability Research 43(1):47–53

Chapple A, Campion P, May C 1997 Clinical terminology: anxiety and confusion amongst families undergoing genetic counselling. Patient Education and Counseling 32:81–91

Clarke AJ 1997 The genetic testing of children. In: Harper PS, Clarke AJ (eds) Genetics, society and clinical practice. BIOS, Oxford, pp 15–29

Codori AM, Zawacki KL, Petersen G et al 2003 Genetic testing for hereditary colorectal cancer in children: Long-term psychological effects. American Journal of Medical Genetics 116A:117–128

Deford F 1983 Alex. The life of a child. Viking Press, New York

Department of Health (DoH) 2003 Our inheritance, our future. Realising the potential of genetics in the NHS. The Stationery Office, London

Fallowfield L, Jenkins V 2004 Communicating sad, bad and difficult news in medicine. Lancet 363:312–319

Fanos J 1997 Developmental tasks of childhood and adolescence: implications for genetic testing. American Journal of Medical Genetics 71:22–28

Fanos J 1999 'My crooked vision': the well sib views ataxia telangiectasia. American Journal of Medical Genetics 87(5):420–425

Fanos J, Puck J 2001 Family pictures: growing up with a brother with X-linked severe combined immunodeficiency. American Journal of Medical Genetics 98(1):57–63

France-Dawson M 1996 Some observations about my life with a sickle cell condition. In: Marteau T, Richards M (eds) The troubled helix. Cambridge University Press, Cambridge, pp 47–50

Harper PS, Clarke AJ 1997 Genetics, society and clinical practice. BIOS, Oxford

Iredale R 2000 Eugenics and its relevance to contemporary health care. Nursing Ethics 7(3):205–214

Kearney PM, Griffin T 2001 Between joy and sorrow: being a parent of a child with developmental disability. Journal of Advanced Nursing 34(5):582–592

Kirk M, McDonald K, Longley M et al 2003a Fit for practice in the genetics era: defining what nurses, midwives and health visitors should know and be able to do in relation to genetics. University of Glamorgan, Pontypridd

Kirk M, McDonald K, Anstey S et al 2003b Fit for practice in the genetics era: a competence-based education framework for nurses, midwives and health visitors. University of Glamorgan, Pontypridd

Locker D 1991 Living with chronic illness. In: Scambler G (ed.) Sociology as applied to medicine. Ballière-Tindall, London, pp 81–92

McGowan R 1999 beyond the disorder: one parent's reflection on genetic counselling. Journal of Medical Ethics 25:195–199

Mitchell W, Sloper P 2002 Information that informs rather than alienates families with disabled children: developing a model of good practice. Health and Social Care in the Community 10(2):74–81

Newell C 2000 Biomedicine, genetics and disability: reflections on nursing and a philosophy of holism. Nursing Ethics 7(3):227–236

Skirton H 2001 The client's perspective of genetic counselling – a grounded theory study. Journal of Genetic Counselling 10(4):311–329

Ward L 2002 Whose right to choose? The new genetics, prenatal testing and people with learning difficulties. Critical Public Health 12(2):187–200

Whyte D 1992 A family nursing approach to the care of a child with a chronic illness. Journal of Advanced Nursing 17:317–327

Further Reading

Marteau T, Richards M (eds) 1996 The troubled helix: social and psychological implications of the new human genetics. Cambridge University Press, Cambridge

Skirton H, Patch C 2002 Genetics for healthcare professionals. A lifestage approach. BIOS, Oxford

Useful Websites

Essentially an online textbook on genetics: http://www.usd.edu/med/som/genetics/curriculum/TableofContents.htm

Public Health Genetics Unit, Cambridge: a good all-round resource with a regular 'round up' of current papers and events: http://www.medinfo.cam.ac.uk/phgu

An interactive website with some useful teaching and learning resources: http://gslc.genetics.utah.edu/

The Genetics Observatory website has short articles exploring genetics and ethics: http://www.ircm.qc.ca/bioethique/obsgenetique/

The GeneTests website offers detailed information about particular conditions and tests with an illustrated glossary: http://www.geneclinics.org

This Genetics Home Reference site provides clear information and a good glossary: http://ghr.nlm.nih.gov/

Health Problems
of the Neonate

Mary Brophy, Clare Barrow

ABSTRACT

The primary aim of this chapter and its companion PowerPoint presentation is to provide insight into the health problems of the neonate. Although it is not possible to cover every problem or potential problem the most pertinent problems to nursing management are addressed. Main areas to be covered are hypothermia, hypoglycaemia, neonatal nutrition, neonatal infection, pain, jaundice, respiratory illness and attachment.

Learning Outcomes

- Recognise a potentially ill neonate.

- Understand the rationale for interventions.

- Apply knowledge of potential problems to minimise distress of neonate and their parents.

- Evaluate and assess the care provided for an ill neonate.

Glossary

Extremely low birth weight (ELBW):
  An infant with a birth weight below 1 kg.
Intrauterine growth retarded (IUGR):
  An infant with a symmetrical low birth weight below the 10th percentile.
Low birth weight (LBW):
  An infant with a birth weight below 2.5 kg.
Nasogastric feeding:
  The practice of feeding an infant via a tube which is inserted through the nose and advanced to the stomach and normally left indwelling for up to a week.

Neonate:
  Describes an infant from birth to 28 days.
Orogastric:
  As with nasogastric but sited via the mouth.
Post-term:
  An infant born after 42 weeks.
Preterm:
  An infant born before 37 weeks gestation.
Small for gestational age (SGA):
  An infant with an assymetrical birth weight below the 10th percentile.
Very low birth weight (VLBW):
  An infant with a birth weight below 1.5 kg.

Introduction

The history of neonatology began with French midwives and obstetricians. Even after specialised neonatal care began to develop in the USA in the 1950s and 1960s, the approach to care was primarily from an obstetric and anaesthetic viewpoint. Specialist neonatologists and neonatal nurses have evolved to care for the most vulnerable of the paediatric population.

WWW

For more on the history of neonatology look up:
- http://www.neonatology.org/tour/history.html

Specialised neonatal units often in large university hospitals have evolved over the last 40 years to offer highly technological support to care for ill neonates. Preterm infants as young as 23 weeks gestation, and weighing <500 g, to term neonates with respiratory, surgical or cardiac problems are cared for on these neonatal units. Environmental adaptation is necessary for survival (Warren 2002). Recently, the focus of care has been the relationship between neonatal nursing practice and long-term developmental outcomes (Turrill, 2003). Studies have shown that developmental outcomes are influenced by both the infant's physiological stability and by the neonatal environment. This has implications for nursing practice.

WWW

Read National Service Framework documents at:
• http://www.doh.gov.uk/nsf/neonatal.htm

Neonatal Hypothermia

Hypothermia is a significant cause of morbidity and mortality in the neonate (Roberton & Rennie 2001). Humans attempt to maintain their body temperature within a certain range to maintain metabolic functions. The normal temperature range for term neonates is 36.5–37.5°C per auxilla and in preterm neonates 36.4–37.1°C (Mertenstein 2002).

DEFINITION OF HYPOTHERMIA

Hypothermia is the cooling of the body's core temperature to below 35°C (Campbell & Glasper 1999). Neonates are at risk of hypothermia primarily because of their size because, although small, they have a large surface area in proportion to body weight, a large head size (through which heat is lost) in relation to the rest of the body and an immature hypothalamus resulting in poor vasomotor control.

Those neonates primarily at risk of cold stress are (Crawford & Morris 1994):

• preterm infants (born less than 36 weeks)
• infants who are small for gestational age or with intrauterine growth restriction
• infants with respiratory distress
• infants in shock
• infants with congenital anomalies
• infants with convulsions
• infants with bleeding problems.

TEMPERATURE REGULATION

Temperature regulation is a complex process. The hypothalamus, which is located at the base of the brain, is responsible for temperature regulation. Receptors in the skin, abdomen, spinal cord and internal organs provide the hypothalamus with information to maintain temperature balance. The hypothalamus produces hormones in response to temperature imbalance and, together with the autonomic and sympathetic nervous systems, regulates temperature (Hackman 2001). For example, if the neonate is subject to reduction in body temperature, cold stress stimulates thermoreceptors to send impulses to the heat-promoting control centre in the hypothalamus, which in turn triggers responses to retain body heat. Vasoconstriction reduces heat loss through the skin. The adrenal medulla releases hormones that increase cellular metabolism and the thyroid gland releases thyroid hormone, which increases metabolic rate. Significantly, this requires an intact central nervous system. Furthermore, temperature regulation requires oxygen because it is an aerobic process. Glucose is also needed to carry out this aerobic process for heat production.

Non-shivering thermogenesis is a significant and unique form of heat production in the neonate (Klaus & Faranoff 1993). Neonates generate most of their heat from the breakdown of brown fat. 'Brown fat' refers to the deeply red, highly vascularised areas surrounding an infant's scapular, clavicular and sternal areas. It is rich in fats and glycogen. The full-term infant has sufficient storage of brown fat to maintain temperature for up to 4 days. Heat is generated by hydrolysis of triglycerides in brown fat utilising oxygen in the process. The responses to cold of neonates in a hypoxic state will be jeopardised. Non-shivering thermogenesis is inhibited by drugs, intracranial haemorrhage and hypoglycaemic states.

HEAT LOSS

There are four main routes of heat loss: evaporation, convection, conduction and radiation (Avery 1987). Evaporative heat loss occurs when water is converted to water vapour during perspiration or respiration. Neonates, wet from amniotic fluid and delivered into a cool labour ward can loose heat at a rate 0.25°C/minute (Roberton 1992). It is therefore important to dry the neonate thoroughly with warmed towels and dress him or her promptly. Convective heat loss occurs when the infant's heat is lost to surrounding cooler air, which is why it is important to dress infants and to keep them out of draughts.

Conductive heat loss occurs when the infant comes into direct contact with a cool surface. One way to prevent this would be to prewarm anything in contact with the neonates skin. Finally, radiative heat losses occur when the infant radiates heat to a cold exposed surface such as a window. In this case the neonate should be nursed away from windows and a constant environmental temperature maintained (Sheeran 1996).

EFFECTS OF COLD STRESS

The effect of cold stress is well documented. Constriction of skin blood vessels occurs in response to cold in neonates. The effect of peripheral vasoconstriction is to increase the core skin temperature gradient. Increased metabolic rate leads to increased oxygen consumption, lactic acid production, hypoglycaemia, and in very low birthweight infants decreased surfactant synthesis and secretion. Blood coagulopathies also occur leading to increased capillary permeability, and haemorrhage.

NEUTRAL THERMAL ENVIRONMENT

The neutral thermal environment (NTE) is the provision of an environmental temperature that minimises oxygenation consumption. The neutral thermal environment varies according to the maturity of the neonate and whether the infant is nursed in an incubator or a radiant heater and is dressed or not. Optimal weight gain and normal physical development occur when a neonate is cared for in a neutral thermal environment appropriate to his or her age and weight. Neonates should be nursed in a neutral thermal environment that maintains the neonate's peripheral temperature at 36.5° C.

WWW

Up-to-date reviews of comparative thermal care are available at:
- http://www.nichd.hih.gov/cochrane/cochrane.htm

NURSING MANAGEMENT

Initially, a thorough assessment of the neonate and history are required. Does the neonate look pale? How does the infant feel? Is the infant cool to touch? Is there a difference between central and peripheral temperatures? A hypothermic infant may appear pale and is cool to touch. This is primarily due to vasoconstriction. Is there associated acrocynosis, a bluish discolouration around the mouth? Is the infant tachypneoic or in respiratory distress? A hypothermic infant may develop respiratory distress secondary to the bodies attempt to maintain a normal temperature consuming oxygen in the process. How does the infant handle? Is the infant irritable or lethargic? Behavioural changes may occur as cold stress continues.

A history should be taken to assist with assessment. Maternal history is important because infants of diabetic mothers are at higher risk of hypothermia due to rapid depletion of glycogen stores. Drugs that mother have received during labour may affect the infant after birth. Side effects of sedatives include hypothermia, hypoglycaemia, lethargy and respiratory depression.

An unstable temperature may indicate infection. If infection is suspected a full blood count with differential will reveal elevated white cells and a positive result on blood culture analysis. Neurological sequelae, such as absent or poor temperature control and fitting may be significant and a head scan may reveal an intraventricular haemorrhage.

Neonates requiring specialist care should be initially nursed in a prewarmed incubator (38° C). Incubators prevent heat loss through radiation and convection. Radiant warmers similarly prevent heat loss and allow easier access. Care to prevent overheating is vital as hyperthermia can lead to dehydration, hypernatraemia, hyperbilirubinaemia, and increased metabolic demands.

Preventive measures are initiated to maintain a normothermic state from delivery onwards. Neonates are initially dried with a warm towel and placed on the mother's abdomen, or dried and dressed. However, ill neonates less than 32 weeks gestation are placed immediately in a plastic bag to reduce heat loss. A hat is applied prior to transferral to a neonatal unit in an incubator. Minimal handling of an ill hypothermic neonate is important to minimise cold stress.

REWARMING

Slow rewarming of a mildly hypothermic neonate is advocated about 1° C/hour. However, in neonates with extreme hypothermia, defined as a core temperature less than 35°C, rapid warming is advised to avoid the deleterious effects of metabolic acidosis and prolonged asymptomatic hypoglycaemia.

TEMPERATURE MEASUREMENT

Although rectal temperature recording has been described as the gold standard for core temperature assessment, there are potential problems with this method for example, bowel perforation and cross-infection (Roberton 1992). Intermittent axilliary measurement is the most commonly and frequently used method in neonatal care. Accuracy depends on consistent and universal measurement for a duration of 3 minutes at the same site (Sheeran 1996). Continuous skin and core temperature measurements are recorded in critically ill neonates. A temperature gradient is significant determining tissue perfusion.

Activity

On your ward placement at the neonatal unit describe measures taken to:
- Prevent cold stress.
- Warm up a cold infant.

WWW

Read the following report:

* http://www.neonatology.org.classics/mj1980/ch03.html

Neonatal Hypoglycaemia

Hypoglycaemia in the neonate is one of the most common clinical care issues facing the paediatric nurse. Increasing evidence suggests that neonatal hypoglycaemia may have long-term neurological effects (Cowett & Loughead 2002). Care is complicated by inconsistent definitive laboratory values of hypoglycaemia and by variable clinical signs and symptoms in term and preterm neonates.

DEFINITION OF HYPOGLYCAEMIA

Hypoglycaemia is described as a low blood sugar. Neonatal values for low plasma blood sugars vary from below 1.7 mmol/L to below 2.6 mmol/L (Fleming et al 1991). Significant hypoglycaemia depends on the infant's age, weight and clinical status. Neonates are at risk of hypoglycaemia because of a lack of glycogen and fat stores.

GLUCONEOGENESIS

In response to adaptation to extrauterine life, the healthy neonate creates fuel from glycogen and fat. While postnatal hormones mediate this response certain conditions predispose the neonate to hypoglycaemia. There are two main reasons for hypoglycaemia in neonates, the increased utilisation of glucose and the decreased production of glucose stores.

Glucose is obtained from two sources: glycogenolysis and gluconeogenesis. Initially, hepatic and muscle glycogen stores are broken down to form glucose and are rapidly utilised in the first 24 hours. The process of converting glycogen back into glucose is known as glycogenolysis (Tortora & Gabrowski 1993).

In gluconeogenesis, glucose is formed from the breakdown of fats ands proteins. Glucocorticoid hormones of the adrenal cortex mobilise proteins and thyroid hormones mobilise proteins and fats thus making glycerol available (Tortora & Gabrowski 1993). Gluconeogensis is regulated by changes in insulin and glucose ratios, catecholamine release, fatty acid oxidation and activation of liver enzyme production (Stables 1999). Prior to stabilisation of at an average blood glucose level of 3.6 mmol/L, neonatal blood glucose levels fall to their lowest level between 2 and 6 hours of age (Stables 1999).

NEONATES AT RISK OF HYPOGLYCAEMIA

* Small for gestational age (intrauterine growth retarded).
* Preterm infants.
* Hypoxic infants.
* Infected infants.
* Infants of diabetic mothers.
* Hypothermic infants.
* Infants with congenital heart disease.

Infants primarily at risk of hypoglycaemia are small for gestational age (SGA) neonates. Reduced glycogen stores combined with increased glucose utilisation account for hypoglycaemic states. Preterm infants are also at risk of hypoglycaemia. In the low birthweight infant, reduced enteral or parenteral intake may explain low plasma glucose levels. Immature hepatocytes, impaired gluconeogensis and glucogenolytic enzyme activity suggest that preterm neonates are dependent on continuous exogenous nutrition. Hypoxic neonates utilize glucose at an increased rate and are therefore at risk of hypoglycaemia. The main problem is the reduced rate at which glucose is formed during anaerobic glycolysis. The problem is compounded by the fact that the neonate is unable to feed in the regular way due to hypoxic state (Brooks 1997).

Hypothermic infants are also at risk of hypoglycaemia. In an attempt to maintain temperature with normal levels the neonate utilises glycogen and plasma glucose levels fall. Therefore early recognition of the effects of cold stress should involve consideration for administration of glucose intravenous infusion. Infants of diabetic mothers are one of the most common groups of neonates to experience hypoglycaemia. This is due to impaired glucose production and excessive insulin levels from prolonged intrauterine exposure to elevated blood sugar levels.

Infected infants frequently present with hypoglycaemia. Although this could be associated with inadequate calorie intake it is mainly as a result of sepsis-induced increased metabolic rate. Inborn errors of metabolism may give rise to a defective gluconeogenesis.

CLINICAL SIGNS AND SYMPTOMS OF HYPOGLYCAEMIA

* Abnormal cry.
* Apnoea.
* Cardiac arrest.
* Coma.
* Convulsions.
* Cyanosis.

- Hypothermia.
- Hypotonia.
- Jitteriness.
- Lethargy.
- Tachypnoea.
- Tremors.

SEQUELAE OF HYPOGLYCAEMIA

A significant feature of neonatal hypoglycaemia is that an infant can have extremely low blood sugars without any signs or symptom. Although short-term neonatal hypoglycaemia will not cause CNS damage, prolonged neonatal hypoglycaemia has serious consequences. Neuroglycopenia, the CNS depletion of glucose, can develop with apnoea leading to depression of consciousness and/or convulsions. In the long term, severe hypoglycaemia can lead to severe developmental abnormalities (Roberton & Rennie 2001).

NURSING MANAGEMENT OF THE HYPOGLYCAEMIC INFANT

Nursing management is dependent on a thorough assessment of the potentially hypoglycaemic neonate. Knowledge of the causes of hypoglycaemia (hypothermia, poor feeding history), a thorough history to include maternal risk factors (infant of a diabetic) and difficulties during or after delivery (prolonged labour, birth asphyxia), signs (intrauterine growth retarded infant) and symptoms and a plasma glucose level are important. Care centres on prevention of hypoglycaemia. Avoidance of risk factors is essential. The greatest risk factors are cold stress and poor feeding. Therefore it is important to nurse an infant in a neutral thermal environment. Unless contraindicated due to respiratory illness or birth asphyxia, early feeding is advocated.

Infants at risk of hypoglycaemia should have blood glucose levels monitored 4–6-hourly. If a Haemacue reading is less than 3.0 mmol/L, or YSI of below 2.6, a plasma glucose sample is obtained for analysis. If this result is lower than 2.6 mmol/L, the neonate is fed smaller amounts of milk more frequently by bolus intermittently or continuously via a nasogastric or orogastric tube. Fluid volumes are increased accordingly, usually calculated a day ahead of requirements. A hypoglycaemic neonate should be nursed in a warmed incubator or on a radiant warmer. Hypoglycaemic neonates with an apparently normal temperature may be working excessively to maintain their temperature within normal limits, thereby utilising glucose stores. Therefore it is important to monitor the infant's temperature closely. The neonate is monitored for symptomatic hypoglycaemia and for signs of respiratory distress. A repeat blood sugar level within an hour will indicate the need for further treatment. If the readings are consistently low, intravenous therapy is commenced.

Activity

Amy is an intrauterine growth retarded infant with a plasma glucose of 2.2 mmol/L. Her mother is an insulin-dependent diabetic:
- Describe how you would explain to Amy's breastfeeding mum the importance of feeding Amy via nasogastric tube and nursing her in an incubator.

Neonatal Nutrition

Meeting the nutritional needs of a sick and/or premature neonate is vital to his or her recovery and growth. Oral feeding is the desired outcome, however, depending on the age and severity of illness of the neonate, parenteral and enteral routes may have to be considered. An essential component of nursing management is to individualise nutritional requirements.

GROWTH AND DEVELOPMENT

Physically growth of the intestine and maturation of intestinal absorption continue to develop. At birth, the intestine is approximately 250 cm long and the stomach has a capacity of 90 mL (Kanneh & Davies 2000). Neonates tolerate small amounts of milk and feed frequently. There is a well coordinated suck and swallow reflex. This suck and swallow reflex develops from 34 weeks gestation onwards. This has implications for feeding preterm infants, although some preterm infants can develop this reflex earlier. In terms of intestinal absorption, pancreatic function is immature hence there are limited enzymes for fat and carbohydrate breakdown. Therefore neonates are at risk of malabsorption characterised by intolerance to feeds. Inadequate liver enzymes can lead to physiological jaundice a common treatable illness of infanthood. Intestinal mucosal immunoglobulin levels are low and neonates are at increased risk of infection, therefore care of feeding equipment is essential. Glycogen stores are depleted in periods of extreme stress of hypoglycaemia and hypothermia. In neonates gluconeogenesis is impaired thereby limiting compensatory responses to adverse conditions of illness. This highlights the importance of adequate nutritional support. In addition to intestinal growth and maturation, the motility function of the gut continues to develop. A measure of gastrointestinal motility is the passage of stools in the first

24 hours of life, however, the more premature the infant the greater the delay in defaecation. Enteral feeding promotes gastric emptying and the release of hormones that can stimulate peristalsis in term and preterm infants (Mertenstein 2002). In neonates, however, the rate of gastric emptying is prolonged.

NUTRITIONAL REQUIREMENTS

Ideally, the healthy preterm neonate should gain 15 g /kg/day in weight, 1 cm in length per week and 1 cm in head circumference per week, whereas the term neonate is expected to gain 20–30 g/day (Berseth 2002). Accurate calculation of feeds is essential to ensure the correct volume fluid, on average 150 mL/kg/day and calorific intake, on average 115 mL/kg/day (Kanneh & Davies 2000). Insensible losses are taken into account. Neonates are weighed on admission and twice weekly thereafter, depending on clinical stability and diagnosis. Weights and head circumferences are plotted on graphs called percentile charts. For example, infants on the 10th percentile or graph line means that 10% of the population of infants are smaller and 90% are bigger. Typically, neonates lose 5–10% of their bodyweight in the first week of life. Preterm infants have a higher body water content so may appear to lose more. Infants should have regained their birth weight by 2 weeks of age.

FEEDING

The way in which adequate nutritional intake is achieved depends primarily on neonatal well-being and level of maturity. In a well neonate, oral feeding – by breast or bottle – is initiated as soon as possible after delivery and infants are fed on demand. Healthy, low birthweight infants should have a nasogastric tube passed and feeding commenced. Breastfeeding is recommended nutritionally because human milk provides easily digestible protein, fat, carbohydrate and water for normal growth in the term infant (Mertenstein 2002). In terms of anti-infection, breast milk provides immunoglobulins (IgA), leucocytes, complement, lactoferrin and lysozome, which protect the infant from neonatal infections and reduces the incidence of necrotising entercolitus (Yeo 1998). Breast milk also contains growth hormones and minerals and trace elements necessary for organ maturation and growth. Apart from the nutritional benefits of breast-feeding, the physical and emotional benefits have been well documented, especially for ill or preterm infants. Mothers are encouraged to express breast milk for ill neonates. Expression of breast milk will initiate and maintain lactation. Successful breast expression depends on thoughtful patience and guidance. Breast

pumps (electrical or hand) and a breastfeeding room are widely available on neonatal units. Initially, mothers are encouraged to express every 3 hours to stimulate milk production. Breast milk can be frozen for up to 3 months. Once defrosted, it should be used within 4 hours.

Although breast milk is the preferred source of neonatal nutrition, it should be noted that infections such as cytomegalovirus , herpes, hepatitis B and HIV can be transmitted through breast milk. Expressed breast milk samples are routinely sent for culture and sensitivity to detect contamination. Furthermore, certain drugs are excreted in breast milk and women taking these drugs should therefore not express milk. Breast milk given to very low birthweight infants will need to be supplemented because infants weighing less than 1.5 kg require a higher protein and calorific intake. These infants are also at risk of hyponatraemia and therefore need sodium supplements. Calcium and phosphorous supplements reduce the risk of bone growth disorders of prematurity such as ricketts. Iron stores of infants born at 32–34 weeks or less are deficient and therefore supplemental iron is given with feeds. Folic acid and vitamins are given also (Roberton & Rennie 2001).

Standard infant formulae have been modified to imitate breast milk. Special preterm formulae have been developed to meet high protein and mineral requirements of low birthweight infants. Accurate calculation of fluid requirements is essential to promote infant well-being.

 WWW

Read about the Department of Health (DoH) infant feeding report at:
- http://www.doh.gov.uk/pdfs/infantfeedingreport.htm

PROBLEMS WITH ORAL FEEDING

Prolonged oral ventilation can interfere with the normal function of the mouth and swallowing. Speech therapists play an important role in assisting infants to develop a suck and swallow technique.

Oral disorders can interfere with feeding. The normal negative pressure of feeding is impaired in infants with unilateral and bilateral cleft lip and palate; a prosthetic palate will alleviate feeding difficulties. Pierre–Robin syndrome is characterised by poor muscular development and retromicronathia. Feeding is problematic but this can be overcome with the use of soft, elongated teats. Tongue-tie can prevent breastfeeding and will require surgical intervention.

ENTERAL NUTRITION

Infants who have difficulties with sucking or who are unable to suck can be fed into the stomach orogastrically, nasogastrically or transpylorically into the small intestine. Gastric feeding may be continuous via syringe pump or intermittently by hourly to 4-hourly bolus feeds. Assessment for complications is essential. Feeds should be discontinued:

- if gastric aspirate every 3–4 hours is greater than the volume of feed
- if there are signs of intestinal obstruction for example, abdominal distension, the presence of bile-stained aspirates or vomitus and failure to pass faeces or passage of blood-stained stools
- if feeding triggers apnoeic attacks
- if the infant has necrotising enterocolitis
- postoperatively.

Non-nutritive sucking is the practice of giving the neonate a dummy during feeding to help the infant associate sucking with the feeling of having a full stomach and improves the sucking reflex.

PARENTERAL NUTRITION

Total parenteral nutrition is the administration of total nutritional requirements intravenously to the infant unable to feed for more than 3 days. It is characterised by the gradual increase in fluid, proteins, fats and glucose concentrations to promote normal growth (Table 39.1). Electrolytes

Table 39.1 Intravenous Feeding Guidelines for the Neonatal Unit (University Hospital of Wales)

| | Total daily fluid intake (mL/kg per 24 h) | | | |
Day	Weight <1.5 kg	Weight >1.5 kg	Nitrogen	Intralipid 20% (mL)
1	90	60	–	–
2	110	90	–	–
3	130	110	0.06	–
4	150	140	0.12	2.5
5	170	150	0.18	5.0
6	180	160	0.24	7.5
7	190	170	0.30	10.0
8	200	180	0.30	12.5
9	200	180	0.30	15.0

Reproduced from Yeo (1998).

are monitored on a daily basis and adjusted accordingly. Light-sensitive vitamins and trace elements are also added to the intravenous solution. During administration, the solution is contained in a light impermeable covering. Total parenteral nutrition can be given via a peripheral venous line, however, due to the vein sclerosing nature of highly concentrated solutions central venous lines are the preferred method of administration.

Reflect on your Practice

What feeding related advice would you give to a first-time mother of a severely ill neonate?

Infection in the Neonate

Neonates are susceptible to infection due to an immature immune system. Infection of the neonate can be contracted prenatally such as seen in congenital infections, during delivery due to prolonged rupture of membranes (> 24 hours) or maternal infection for example and in the neonatal period either as superficial (umbilical) or systemic infections.

IMMUNITY

There are two types of lymphocyte-mediated immunity in the neonate:

- Cellular immunity, produced by B cell and T cell lymphocytes, enables the infant to produce some antigens in response to infections.
- Humoral immunity, produced by Immunoglobulins, offers protection from viruses and bacteria.

Initially, the neonate is protected by maternal immunoglobulins that cross the placenta in utero. Immunoglobulin G (IgG), which is present at birth, carries specific antigens to diseases that the mother has encountered and therefore the infant can produce antibodies in response. IgG potentially offers protection against tetanus, diphtheria, measles, rubella, mumps, as well as common strains of streptococci (Yeo 1998). IgM produced by the fetus offers protection from Gram-negative bacteria such as *Escherichia coli*. IgA is present in breast milk and protects the infant from gut infection.

NURSING CARE

Nursing care centres on prevention of infection and assessment and early diagnosis of sepsis. Ways to prevent infection are adherence to strict hand washing techniques and wearing gloves (Ramsey & Moules 1998). Infected infants should be nursed in isolation. Equipment should be cleaned regularly. Mothers should be encouraged to provide breast milk for their infant and parental education on the importance of prevention of infection is advocated.

Frequent assessment of neonate is vital to identify early signs of infection. Signs of infection in the neonate are often subtle. Is the infant quiet? How does the infant look: pale, mottled, jaundiced, presence of a rash? How does the infant handle: irritable, lethargic? How does the infant feel: hot, cool? How is the infant's breathing: fast, slow, using accessory muscles of respiration, nasal flaring? How does the infant feed: slowly, disinterested, vomiting, large aspirates? A septic infant's condition can deteriorate rapidly due to limited compensatory mechanisms.

Pain in the Neonate

For paediatric nurses, one of the most challenging situations is managing pain in the patient who cannot speak. It is well established that the neonate can feel pain (Franck 2002). Compared with older children neonates are more sensitive to pain and vulnerable to its long-term effects (Anand 2001).

PHYSIOLOGY OF PAIN

Nociception, i.e. pain perception, is transmitted via pathways in the peripheral and central nervous systems and is fully established by 37 weeks. Research has shown that pain inhibitory pathways are immature at birth, suggesting a developmental hypersensitivity to pain (Franck et al 2000). This means that preterm infants may be at greater risk of pain than the term infant. Behavioural and physiological responses to pain are observed to determine levels of pain in the neonate.

Facially, an infant in pain has a furrowed brow, eyes are closed tightly, nostrils flare, a mouth is unnaturally opened and a grey pallor to face. In terms of movement, an infant in pain will initially display sharp, tense movements and will withdraw the affected limb. As pain intensifies or is prolonged, the infant will lie still with clenched fists, altered breathing and little eye movement. Fingers and toes will be held tightly curled and the infant will cry almost all of the time. The nature of the cry is important. A prolonged, intense, high-pitched cry indicates severe pain. The severity of pain may compromise the infant's respiratory status. A mewing pitiful cry together with apnoea indicates a pre-respiratory failure state. Physiologically, there is increased heart rate, blood pressure is also raised, oxygen saturations fall and there is evidence of palmar sweating (Kanneh & Davies 2000).

Activity

During your placement on the neonatal unit, make a list of the painful procedures that you have observed. Note the infant's response and how the pain was controlled.

NURSING CARE

The aim of nursing care is to prevent pain and to minimise discomfort in neonates. Therefore infants should be assessed using an appropriate neonatal pain scale, for example the Liverpool Infant Distress Scale (Horgan & Choonara 1998). Currently, audit of pain tools are advocated (Royal College of Nursing (RCN) 2002). Non-pharmaceutical methods are incorporated into the nursing care plan to minimise environment-induced distress. For example, the care of neonates should be consolidated to avoid continuous disturbance. Infants should be handled gently with prewarmed hands and equipment, and offered gentle reassurance. Minimal handling of ill infants is advocated. Quiet periods during the day should be observed to promote rest. A daytime/night-time pattern should be established. Infants should be shielded from bright lights. Noise levels should be kept to a minimum and alarms attended to promptly. Infants should be contained within soft boundaries to promote a sense of security. Thoughtful use of electrodes and tape is important. Physical pain during blood sampling or intravenous cannulation can be minimised with the administration of oral sucrose via pacifier (Boyd 2002). Also, breastfeeding effectively reduces pain in term neonates undergoing minor invasive procedures (Carbajal 2003). In terms of pharmaceutical management of pain, effective pain relief is essential if indicated. Fentanyl or morphine is administered frequently; paracetamol is also administered. Regular administration of analgesia is important in pain management.

WWW

For further definitive reading, see:
- http://www.cirp.org/library/pain/anand

For guidelines for recognition and assessment of pain in neonates, see:
- http://www.rcn.org.uk

For prevention and management of pain stress in the neonate, see:
- http://www.guideline.gov/summary/summary.aspx?doc_id=2597&nbr=1823

Neonatal Respiratory Problems

The most common reason for admission to a neonatal unit is for respiratory difficulties. Respiratory difficulties can be present at delivery, requiring prompt resuscitation and admission to the neonatal unit for further treatment, but they can also occur during the postnatal period.

CLINICAL SIGNS OF RESPIRATORY DYSFUNCTION

- Cyanosis: the infant becomes 'blue' due to lack of circulating oxygen.
- Tachypnoea: the breathing rate is in excess of 60 breaths per minute.
- Sternal and intercostal recession: this becomes evident as the work of breathing becomes harder. It is more pronounced in preterm infants who have a more pliable rib cage.
- Grunting: infants expel air explosively over a partially closed glottis to attempt to retain some function residual volume so as to maintain alveolar distension.

Activity

Discover how neonatal staff monitor infants for these signs of respiratory difficulties.

RESPIRATORY DISTRESS SYNDROME

The most common respiratory difficulty in preterm infants is respiratory distress syndrome. The more preterm an infant is, the worse the condition is likely to be. In the very preterm infant, the disease is usually present at delivery and needs immediate treatment. In infants of greater gestational age, the disease can be seen to worsen gradually over a period of several hours. All of the clinical signs of respiratory distress are seen.

Respiratory distress syndrome is a disease directly resulting from the fact that the lungs are underdeveloped and the normal system of gaseous exchange is disturbed. One of the main problems is that the squamous epithelial type 2 cells producing surfactant are too immature and so insufficient amounts of surfactant are produced. Surfactant is necessary to reduce the surface tension of the alveoli, allowing continuous partial distension, and thus maintenance of functional residual capacity.

Diagnosis is usually assumed when an X-ray, performed when the infant is at least 4 hours of age, shows a typical 'ground glass' appearance. Duration of this disease is usually 5–7 days.

 www

For guidelines of respiratory disease management in newborns, see:
- http://www.rcpch.ac.uk/publications/neonatal-dataset.pdf

TREATMENT

- The severity of the disease can be reduced significantly by the use of antenatal steroids.
- Artificial surfactant is given to any infant with respiratory distress syndrome who is intubated.
- Inspired oxygen is given to maintain oxygen saturations between 90 and 93%.
- Continuous positive airways pressure (CPAP) or intermittent positive pressure ventilation (IPPV) can be used to maintain functional residual volume and to ensure that adequate gaseous exchange is maintained.

Activity

Discover how continuous positive airways pressure works and how it is administered.

TRANSIENT TACHYPNOEA OF THE NEWBORN

The most common condition causing respiratory difficulties in the term infant is transient tachypnoea of the newborn (TTN). This condition is most often seen in infants who are delivered by Caesarean section. The infant absorbs pulmonary alveolar fluid during labour and delivery. This loss of physiological function with Caesarean section is thought to be very significant because the presumed aetiology of tachypnoea of the newborn is transient pulmonary oedema (Kenner et al 1993). All five clinical signs of respiratory distress may be seen, depending on the severity of the condition.

The chest radiograph may show increased perihilar interstitial markings and increased plural fluid, especially in the minor fissure. The duration of the condition is usually 1–3 days.

TREATMENT

- Inspired oxygen to maintain oxygen saturations above 95%.
- Continuous positive airways pressure or intermittent positive pressure ventilation if maximal inspired oxygen fails to maintain adequate gaseous exchange.

NEONATAL PNEUMONIA

Pneumonias may occur at any gestational age. They may be congenital, i.e. onset from birth to 48 hours or age, or nosocomial, i.e. onset after 48 hours of age. They are usually caused by bacteria or a virus. The poorly developed immune system of the neonate makes them more prone first to contracting pneumonia and second to a rapid acceleration of the condition. Pneumonias are even more likely to occur in ventilated neonates (Roberton 1992).

The chest radiograph may show consolidation, interstitial infiltration or, particularly in group B streptococcus pneumonia, a 'ground glass' appearance. The diagnosis of pneumonia is also made by blood cultures, white blood cell count and C-reactive protein count. The duration of the disease is likely to be 5–7 days but may occasionally be prolonged – up to 3 weeks.

Treatment

- Broad-spectrum antibiotics for all infants with any clinical signs of respiratory difficulties: usually benzylpeniccillin, gentamicin and/or cefotaxime.
- Specific antibiotic treatment once the organism/sensitivity is known.
- Inspired oxygen to maintain oxygen saturations appropriately.
- Continuous positive airways pressure or intermittent positive pressure ventilation may be used if maximal oxygen fails to maintain adequate gaseous exchange.

Activity

- Name two bacteria and two viruses that cause neonatal pneumonia.
- What is a normal white cell count from birth to 1 week of age?

Principles of Nursing Management for Infant with Respiratory Distress

- Ensure continuous positive airways pressure or ventilation endotracheal tubes are in the correct position to promote effective ventilation. Secure tubes to minimise trauma to the infant's face.
- Observe for signs of deterioration in condition and report to medical team promptly.
- Maintain oxygen saturations between 90 and 93% in preterm infants and greater than 95% in term neonates.
- Administer analgesia as prescribed; observe for signs of pain.
- Reposition the infant 6-hourly.
- Ensure minimal handling of infants.
- Educate parents to care for their infant.

PERSISTENT PULMONARY HYPERTENSION OF THE NEWBORN (PPHN)

- Prolonged constriction of pulmonary blood vessels causes pulmonary hypertension.
- Idiopathic or secondary to:
  - meconium aspiration
  - congenital diaphragmatic hernia
  - sepsis
  - acidosis.
- Treatment:
  - ventilation and oxygen
  - inotropes
  - nitric oxide
  - ECMO.

MECONIUM ASPIRATION SYNDROME

- Meconium passed at or before delivery and inhaled in the presence of hypoxia.
- Chemical pnuemonitis:
  - interstitial oedema
  - small airway obstruction
  - concomitant persistent pulmonary hypertension of the newborn.
- Treatment:
  - ventilation and oxygen
  - antibiotics
  - surfactant
  - treatment for persistent pulmonary hypertension of the newborn.

JAUNDICE

Physiological Jaundice

Red blood cells have a life span of approximately 120 days. As the life of these red blood cells ends, they need to be destroyed. When red blood cells are destroyed in the liver and the spleen via the reticuloendothelial system, the globin is preserved for reuse and the haem is further broken down. This process produces bilirubin in a fat-soluble, water-insoluble form called unconjugated bilirubin. It cannot be excreted in bile or urine and must be further converted in the liver so that a conjugated, water-soluble bilirubin is produced that can be excreted by the body (Kelner & Harvey 1987).

The bilirubin is carried to the liver for conjugation in the circulating blood. Binding sites on the albumin carried in the plasma and the bilirubin binds to these sites until it is passed into the liver cells (the hepatocytes). Once in the hepatocyte, uridine diphosphate-glucoronal transferase joins the bilirubin with a water-soluble glucuronide to create bilirubin monoglucuronide. This is called conjugated bilirubin; this structure is water soluble. It is transferred into the bile for excretion in the stool.

In the neonate, several factors combine to overload this normal function:

In utero the fetus has a high haemoglobin level of 18–22 mg/dL as a result of the high number of circulating red blood cells. This allows sufficient transport of oxygen from maternal to fetal cells. At birth these cells are no longer required and must be destroyed. This is helped by fetal red blood cells having a life span of 80–100 days. The increased number of red blood cells being broken down means that there are increased amounts of unconjugated bilirubin.

The mechanisms for the transfer and breakdown of bilirubin, ex utero, can take several days to become fully activated. The more preterm the infant, the longer this process can be delayed. This adds to the amount of unconjugated bilirubin.

Once bilirubin has been conjugated and transferred to the intestine, it can be broken down by bilirubin gluconidase, an enzyme found in the small intestine. In the neonate, the passage of stool is slow for the first few days of life and this allows more breakdown by the enzyme. Normal gut flora inhibits this process but it is several days before normal gut flora is present. Also, in breastfed infants there is a continued lack of normal gut flora, which also allows more breakdown. This often causes what is known as 'breast milk jaundice'.

These combined factors result in more unconjugated bilirubin than there are binding sites. Some of this bilirubin can be stored in the skin, which is what gives the infant their yellow colour. There is a limit to how much can be stored in the skin and the excess is carried in the circulating blood with nothing to bind to. This is called 'free' bilirubin. Free bilirubin passes easily through the blood–brain barrier, where it is transferred into the brain cells. This can result in 'kernicterus', which causes brain damage. It is for this reason that it is necessary to provide treatment to restrict the amount of free bilirubin in the circulating blood.

Any infant who appears jaundiced will have a blood test taken to measure the serum bilirubin level. If the level is high, treatment will be given. The serum bilirubin level will be tested regularly. Once it falls to low levels, treatment will be discontinued. Assessing whether the levels are high enough for treatment can be done by plotting the level against a universal chart or by multiplying the infant's gestational age by 10 and treating for as long as the serum bilirubin level remains above this number.

Treatment with phototherapy is invariably successful. This is the use of a specific wavelength of light onto the skin. This light wavelength causes a chemical reaction in the bilirubin stored in the skin. This reaction changes the stored unconjugated bilirubin into conjugated bilirubin, which can be excreted.

One of the side effects of phototherapy treatment is that it accelerates the digestive process, resulting in diarrhoea. This actually enhances the reduction of bilirubin because it allows less time for bilirubin gluconidase to breakdown the conjugated bilirubin. The light can be delivered by a lightbox placed over the cot or incubator. This means that the infant must be naked for the light to fall on the skin. Infants may need to be transferred to an incubator if they are unable to maintain their core temperature when naked. Phototherapy can also be given via a 'biliblanket': a fibreoptic light source is used to provide the appropriate wavelength of light into a specially developed small rectangular 'blanket', which can be wrapped around the infant's torso and used underneath the clothes. This causes less disruption to the infant and is more acceptable to parents. Treatment usually lasts for 3–7 days.

Non-physiological Jaundice

The most common cause of non-physiological jaundice is incompatibility of blood groups. This problem used to be more common than it is now because the Rhesus blood proteins are highly antigenic, causing severe jaundice. The introduction of anti-D for any antenatal event and post-delivery for women whose partner has a different blood group has reduced the incidence of this condition significantly.

ABO incompatibility is probably more common than Rhesus incompatibility but is usually mild and does not require treatment other than phototherapy. However, in some instances the condition is very severe and requires prompt and efficacious management.

The best treatment commences antenatally with all pregnant women being screened for blood group and for antibodies. Sometimes there is no indication of problems until hydrops is seen on scan. It is possible for some fetuses to have in utero transfusions to maintain the pregnancy until viability. Fetuses are affected to varying degrees. In the most severe cases, there is fetal anaemia, cardiac failure, oedema and hydrops. The prognosis is poor and only immediate exchange transfusions provide any hope of survival.

In less severe cases, the infant may appear normal at birth but signs of clinical jaundice become apparent within hours of delivery. Jaundice is never a normal finding before 24 hours of age and if there is any doubt a serum bilirubin level must be measured. If there is any indication of problems blood for a Coombs test should be taken at delivery.

Activity

- Find out which method of assessing for treatment is used in your local neonatal unit.
- What kinds of problem are associated with kernicterus?

Phototherapy will be given in the first instance. There is no evidence to support the theory that double phototherapy is more effective as this process is rate-limited. If the level rises too high then an exchange transfusion will be given. This procedure aims to remove the affected blood and replace it with blood that has normal erythrocytes and a normal bilirubin level. Thus it will relieve anaemia and help to prevent kernicterus. Assessing whether an exchange transfusion is required can be done by plotting the serum bilirubin level against a universal chart, or by multiplying the gestational age of the infant by 10. If the serum bilirubin level is above this number then an exchange transfusion should be given.

In severe cases, several exchange transfusion may be required before the infant's condition becomes stabilised.

WWW

For current British Neonatal Practice, see:
- http://www.neonatal-nursing.co.uk

Activity

- Describe what a Coombs test is and why it is helpful?
- What other tests can be used?
- What are the principles of undertaking an exchange transfusion?

NURSING CARE ISSUES

- Undressing infants can lead to hypothermia, requiring incubator care.

- The use of the phototherapy lamp can increase the ambient temperature surrounding the infant. The set incubator temp should be reduced by 1° for all infants already being nursed in an incubator.

- Care should be taken that infants are changed regularly to avoid skin problems.

- Nappies should be used to ensure gonads are protected at all times.

- Eye shields must be used at all times to prevent the slight risk of retinal damage.

- Feeding and interaction with parents should be actively encouraged. Up to 4 hours in 24 hours out from under the phototherapy lamp does not affect treatment levels as treatment is rate-limited.

- Attention to good nutrition and adequate fluids are essential to avoid dehydration and/or weight loss.

- Constant reassurance of family members is usually required.

PARENTS

Parents feel a sense of loss for the interrupted pregnancy or an unexpected outcome. They may feel a sense of isolation from others and each other. The inability to produce a healthy infant, coupled with the inability to protect an ill neonate from invasive and sometimes painful procedures, leaves the parents feeling inadequate. In essence, parents are not only the mourning the loss of their perfect infant but anticipate the grief for the potential loss of their newborn. The birth of an ill or premature neonate has an overwhelming destabilising effect on parents. Many parents of newborns go through identifiable behaviours similar to a grief response. Parents' initial reaction to the birth of an ill infant is one of acute shock, characterised by irrational behaviour, feelings of despair and crying. Parents may feel guilty and blame themselves or each other for the unexpected outcome. Feelings of guilt are followed by feelings of anger and resentment, which can be internalised or directed towards healthcare professionals. With empathetic care parents can learn to cope and adapt as they are taught how to care and become increasingly involved in their infant's life. Psychosocial meetings provide a forum to discuss current and anticipated problems that may arise during provision of neonatal care. Healthcare professionals endeavour to promote attachment between the infant and family in a supportive and nurturing environment.

ATTACHMENT

Since the 1970s it has been acknowledged that the interaction between newborn infants and their families is essential in establishing good family dynamics. However, it has taken a long time to break down the barriers to interaction and integration, and the art of promoting family interaction is still one of the most challenging areas of neonatal nursing today. Often, the neonatal nurses can be the greatest barrier to parenting in the neonatal intensive care unit because they are seen as the gatekeepers to the infants (Griffin 1990).

Currently, most neonatal units encourage parents to visit their infant/infants whenever they choose. However, any indication by the staff that parents are interfering with the routine of the unit or that the nurses are too busy to speak to them will result in parents staying for a minimum of time and they will be reluctant to return. When families are given restricted visiting times or have restrictions on who may visit without good explanations, this can make the whole family, including the parents, feel unwanted and unwelcome in the unit.

Neonatal units are busy, noisy, bustling places, caring for a range of infants, some of whom are very ill and require constant, highly technical care. This environment is very frightening for parents and can make them reluctant to visit their infant at all and reluctant to touch or cuddle their infant, because they are frightened that this may make their condition worsen. In fact, research has shown that affectionate touch is essential to good developmental outcomes.

It is therefore imperative that neonatal nurses are proactive in ensuring that contact and interaction are initiated as soon as possible after admission and are sustained until discharge (Harrison et al 1996).

Being welcoming and making as much time for parents as they want or need seems very simple but it is important because it allows parents to relax and spend time getting to know their new infant. One of the most important aspects of this care is to include parents in plans and decisions about the care of their infant, by ensuring that they are fully informed and that their views are sought. As much written information as possible should also be given as verbal information is soon forgotten in stressful situations. Recognition of the mother by the infant is said to occur after eye contact over a 72-hour period. In infants without health problems, mothers spend many hours cuddling and gazing at their infant. This recognition is established within a few days but is delayed when an infant is ill. Therefore the neonatal nurse should encourage cuddling and gazing whenever possible to establish early recognition.

Kangaroo care, where parents spend extended time cuddling their infant with skin-to-skin contact has been proven to improve the condition of the infant in the short term and to improve developmental outcomes in the long term and should be encouraged.

WWW

For information on neonatal death see:
- http://www.uk-sands.org

Summary

Neonatal nursing is as challenging as it is rewarding. As neonatal care continues to evolve it is important for paediatric nurses to develop evidence-based practice and to keep abreast with changes. A neonate's outcome rests in nurses' hands.

References

Anand JKS 2001 Consensus statement for the prevention and management of pain in the newborn. Archives of Pediatrics and Adolescent Medicine 155:297–303

Avery GB 1987 Neonatology. Pathophysiology and management of the newborn, 3rd edn. Lippincott, Philadelphia

Berseth CL 2001 Feeding methods for the preterm infant. Seminars in Neonatology 6:417–424

Boyd S 2002 Sucrose analgesia: a realistic alternative to conventional pharmacology for pain relief in neonates. Journal of Neonatal Nursing 8(6):184–190

Brooks C 1997 Neonatal hypoglycaemia. Neonatal Network 16(2):15–21

Campbell S, Glasper EA (eds) 1999 Whaley and Wong's nursing care of infants and children, 6th edn. Mosby, St Louis

Carbajal R 2003 Analgesic effect of breastfeeding in term neonates: randomised controlled trial. British Medical Journal 326:13–15

Cowett RM, Loughead JL 2002 Neonatal glucose metabolism: differential diagnosis, evaluation and treatment. Neonatal Network 21(4):9–18

Crawford D, Morris M 1994 Neonatal nursing. Chapman and Hall, Bury St Edmunds

Fleming PJ, Speidel BD, Marlow N 1991 A neonatal vade mecum, 2nd edn. Edward Arnold, London

Franck LS 2002 Some pain, some gain: reflections on the past two decades of neonatal pain research and treatment. Neonatal Network 21(5):37–41

Franck LS, Greenberg CS, Stevens B 2000 Pain assessment in infants and children. Pediatric Clinics of North America 47(3):487–512

Griffin T 1990 Nurse barriers to parenting the special care nursery. Journal of Perinatal Neonatal Nursing 4(2):56–57

Hackman PS 2001 Recognising and understanding the cold-stressed term infant. Neonatal Network 20(8):35–41

Harrison L, Olivet L, Cunningham K et al 1996 Effects of gentle human touch on preterm infants: pilot study results. Neonatal Network 15(26):35–42

Horgan MF, Choonara S 1998 The Liverpool infant distress scale. Paediatric and Perinatal Drug Therapy 2:14–16

Kanneh A, Davies F 2000 Physical characteristics and physiological features of the full term neonate: theory, practice integration. Part 1. Journal of Neonatal Nursing 6(1):4–8

Kelner JH, Harvey D 1987 The sick newborn baby, 2nd edn. Baillière Tindall, London

Kenner C, Brueggemeyer A, Gunderson LP (eds) 1993. Comprehensive neonatal nursing: a physiologic perspective. WB Saunders, Philadelphia, p 304

Kenner C, Wright Lott J (eds) 1998 Comprehensive neonatal nursing, 2nd edn. WB Saunders, Philadelphia

Klaus MH, Fanaroff AA 1993 Care of the high-risk neonate, 4th edn. WB Saunders, Philadelphia

Merienstein GBM 2002 Handbook of neonatal intensive care, 5th edn. Mosby Year Book, St Louis

Ramsey T, Moules J 1998 The textbook of children's nursing. Stanley Thornes, Cheltenham

Roberton NRC 1992 (ed.) Textbook of neonatology, 2nd edn. Edward Arnold, London

Roberton NRC, Rennie J 2001 Neonatal intensive care, 4th edn. Edward Arnold, London

Royal College of Nursing (RCN) 2002 Clinical practice guidelines. The recognition and assessment of acute pain in children. Audit protocol. Royal College of Nursing, London

Sheeran MS 1996 Thermoregulation in neonates. Journal of Neonatal Nursing 2(4):6–9

Stables D 1999 Physiology in childbearing with anatomy and related biosciences. Baillière Tindall, Edinburgh

Tortora GJ, Grabowski SR 1993 Principles of anatomy and physiology, 7th edn. Harper Collins, New York

Turrill S 2003 A focus of care for neonatal nursing: the relationship between neonatal nursing. Practice and outcomes. Paediatric Nursing 15(5):30–34

Warren I 2002 Facilitating infant adaptation: the nursery environment. Seminars in Neonatology 7:459–467

Yeo H 1998 Nursing the neonate, 1st edn. Blackwell Science, Oxford

Further Reading

BAPM 1996 Standards for hospitals providing neonatal intensive care. BAPM, London

Chapter Forty

40

Health Problems During Infancy

Kathy Scanlon, Anna-Lisa Sorrentino

ABSTRACT

Infancy is a period of remarkable growth and development. Between 1 month and 12 months of age the infant will undergo major changes in physical development. Motor skills, cognition and social skills develop at a rapid pace during this period. The roles of nature and nurture contribute to the growth and development of the infant in both positive and negative ways. Nature, or heredity, has significant influence on general growth and development correlating around related family size and patterns of maturation. Nurture, or the environment, including diet, again plays a significant role for the developing infant. The infant remains dependent on adults to identify health needs and detect health problems.

This chapter will focus on the following four significant areas that influence the growth and development of the infant: nutrition, skin (and specifically atopic eczema), sleep and immunisation. These topics have been identified as significant because problems in these areas can impair the growth and development of the infant both in the short term and long term into later life.

Learning Outcomes

- Discuss the effects of nutrition on growth and development.
- Explain how skin conditions (e.g. atopic eczema) can affect the developing infant.
- Outline the role of sleep in an infant's development.
- Discuss the role of immunization for infant health.

Nutrition

Nutrition in the first year of life plays an important role in a child's development. An infant grows more in the first 6 months of life than at any other time. The early period of infancy is where important changes in diet and nutritional needs occur, e.g. weaning onto solid food. The importance of nutrition and how good nutrition can determine the growth and development of the child is clearly recognised. Research by Barker (1990), Barker et al (2002) and Eriksson et al (2001) suggests that nutritional status in infancy can be linked to ill health in adult life. Periods of nutritional deficiency during infancy have been linked with ischaemic heart disease, stroke, hypertension, and non-insulin diabetes mellitus in middle age. Adequate nutrition is also essential for intellectual development according to the Department of Health (DoH 1994), Mathieson (1995) and Singhal et al (2001).

MILK FEEDS

The DoH (2003) states that:

> *Breastfeeding is the best form of nutrition for infants. Exclusive breastfeeding is recommended for the first 6 months (26 weeks) of life as it provides all the nutrients a baby needs.*

When breast-feeding is discontinued, a commercial iron-fortified formula should be substituted. Not all mothers want to breastfeed and some find that they are unable to do it, therefore the use of formula milks is essential. Breast or formula milk will continue to be the primary source of nutrition during early infancy.

Unmodified cows milk should not be given as a main drink before 1 year of age, (DoH 1994) because it is low in iron and vitamin C. Also, the proteins in cows milk (predominantly casein) are more allergenic to some infants.

WWW

Read the DoH guidelines on breastfeeding at:
- http://www.doh.gov.uk

Milk Calculations

To calculate the correct quantity of milk feed for an infant who is full-term, and developing within normal parameters, it is important to consider expected weight gains and losses. Weight gain is expected to be in the region of 200 g per week during the first 3 months of life, although, as the infant first adapts to the environment, there is an expected weight loss within the first 2 weeks of life. This usually constitutes a loss of approximately 10% of body weight, i.e. if an infant weighs 3.5 kg at birth, there will be an estimated loss of 350 g.

Achieving Weight Gain

To achieve weight gain, the infant is offered 150 mL/kg of body weight every 24 hours, i.e. if the infant weighs 3.5 kg:

$$150 \text{ mL} \times 3.5 = 525 \text{ mL}/24 \text{ hours}$$

It is then necessary to divide this overall quantity into a set number of feeds. Under normal circumstances, an infant in the first month of life will be offered feeds approximately every 4 hours, which equates to six feeds in 24 hours:

$$525 \text{ mL}/6 = 87.5 \text{ mL}$$

Therefore one needs to prepare 90 mL of feed in each bottle (Hubbard & Trigg 2000).

Activity

- Use the above formula to calculate the quantity of feed an infant weighing 4 kg needs in 24 hours.
- Then calculate the amount required for each feed if six feeds are required per day.

Follow-on Milks

Follow-on milks are specially formulated to meet requirements not found in standard formula or breast milk. 'Follow-on' milks have higher protein and mineral content than standard infant formula. They are suitable for infants over 6 months old and are advertised as being more nutritious milk than cows milk. However, infants nutritional needs can also be met satisfactorily by increasing the introduction of a wide variety of foods, i.e. calcium and iron-rich foods when weaning plus use of standard formula milks.

Activity

- Identify the constituents of commercial iron fortified formula milk.
- Compare and contrast those constituents with breast milk.

WEANING

Weaning is the process of gradually changing an infant's diet from milk alone to a combination of milk and solids (DoH 1994). This also involves the process of giving up one method of feeding for another, which for infants usually refers to relinquishing the breast or bottle for a cup and spoon. It is a psychologically significant period because the infant is required to give up a major source of oral pleasure and gratification. Weaning is generally regarded as a major task for infants with the development of independence involving participation in the social activity of meal times. The major change in feeding is the addition of solid foods to the infant's diet.

When to Start Weaning

Weaning should start when the infant reaches 6 months of age (DoH 2003). Many parents according to Foote et al (2003), Hamlyn et al (2000) and Fewtrell (2003) choose to give solid foods before 6 months. However, parents should be encouraged to continue milk feeds until at least 4 months (17 weeks). Weaning should not commence before 4 months because the immature digestive and renal systems cannot cope with solid foods (DoH 1994, Scientific Advisory Committee on Nutrition 2003). Parents should be encouraged to view 4 months (17 weeks) as the earliest time to commence weaning.

It is imperative that individual circumstances are considered when health professionals are giving advice on the age for the introduction of solid foods. At 6 months of age infants reach a transition period. By this time the gastrointestinal tract has matured sufficiently to handle more complex nutrients and is less sensitive to potentially allergenic foods. Tooth eruption is beginning, which facilitates biting and chewing (DoH 1994, Hockenberry 2003).

Activity

- With the advent of the primary dentition, which teeth appear first?
- Which other aspect of infant development does the development of chewing aid?

Eating a weaning diet requires the infant to have a level of neuromuscular coordination that may not be achieved prior to 6 months, e.g. holding the head in an upright position, sitting up. Around 6 months of age, the tongue-thrust reflex, which causes food to be pushed out of the mouth, is reducing. Chewing motions and the ability to move food to the back of the mouth and swallow are developing (DoH 1994, Hockenberry 2003). Therefore, developmentally, the infant becomes ready to move into the weaning stage.

The weaning diet should consist of foods from all main food groups: carbohydrates, proteins, fats and oils, and sugars as well as fruit and vegetables (Table 40.1). However, when preparing foods for the infant, additional salt and sugar should be avoided due to the immaturity of kidneys and liver (DoH 1994).

New foods should be added to the infant diet one at a time. Infant cereal may be given mixed with modified formula milk in a bowl. If the infant is breast fed the cereal can be mixed with expressed breast milk or water.

Fruit juices can be mixed with the dry cereal – the vitamin C content of the juice enhances the absorption of iron. Vitamin C is destroyed by heat and juice should therefore not be warmed. Offer fruit juice from a cup rather than a bottle to prevent the development of dental caries.

WWW

Visit the DoH website and read the report on infant feeding:

- http://www.doh.gov.uk/public/infantfeedingreport.htm

Table 40.1 The Weaning Period		
Age	**Suggested diet**	**Developmental tasks**
6 months	Start weaning with bland foods The DoH (2003) recommends iron-enriched infant rice cereal as a starter food, e.g. baby rice. Smooth purées of vegetables, e.g. potato, swede, parsnip and fruit purées, e.g. pear, banana	Accustom infant to taking food from a spoon
From 7 months to 8–9 months	Introducing a variety of textures Purées of increasing variety of vegetables, meats, fruits Thicker purees gradually progressing to a lumpy texture, e.g. mashed vegetables As the infant progresses then move on to minced chicken, meat, fish or lentils and pulses like kidney beans Lumpier finger foods including chopped hard-boiled eggs, cubed or grated hard cheese, raw soft fruit and vegetables, e.g. tomato, banana Some wheat-based breakfast cereals and bread	Expose to different textures and different tastes Develop ability to chew and swallow Start 'finger' feeding Introduce cup
Around 9–12 months	Continue progression with textures Wholemeal breads, cereals and pasta Chopped meats, chicken, fish and liver Lightly cooked or raw vegetables and fruits A variety of textures for potatoes, noodles, and puddings, e.g. rice pudding Unsweetened orange juice as a drink with meals	Progress to a mature diet of 3 main meals with 2 or 3 snacks during the day
1 year	Adult texture Family meals: take the infant's portion out before adding salt and leave as adult texture, chop to bite size if needed Whole milk as a drink	Progress to self-feeding by continuing with finger foods Developing social skills by participating in family meals

FOOD INTOLERANCE

The terms 'food intolerance' and 'food allergy' are often used interchangeably. However, the conditions are very different.

Foods to Avoid

Common foods such as milk, eggs, soya, wheat, peanuts, tree nuts (e.g. hazelnuts), sesame seeds and, in older children, fish and shellfish, which form about 90% of cases of food allergy.

Cows Milk Intolerance

According to Fiocchi et al (2003), cows milk intolerance is a multifaceted disorder representing adverse systemic and local gastrointestinal reactions to cows milk protein. The hypersensitivity may be manifest through a variety of signs and symptoms. These may appear within 45 minutes of milk ingestion or after a period of several days, e.g. cows milk intolerance may be manifest as colic or sleeplessness in an otherwise healthy infant. The diagnosis is made after careful history taking.

Cows Milk Allergy

Allergy to cows milk affects 2–7% of infants under 1 year old. It is the most common food allergy in childhood (David 1993, Williams 1999). Children usually grow out of milk allergy by the age of three, but about 20% of these children will still be allergic to milk as adults.

Cows milk allergy is caused by a reaction to a number of allergens in cows milk. The protein in milk can be broken down into curds (casein), which form when milk sours. Whey is the watery part that is left when the curd is removed. A reaction can also be triggered by small amounts of milk received through the mother's breast milk from dairy products she has eaten, or, from feeding cows milk to the infant.

The symptoms of milk allergy are often mild and can affect any part of the body. In more severe episodes symptoms can include rashes, diarrhoea, vomiting, stomach cramps and difficulty in breathing. In a very few cases, milk allergy can cause anaphylaxis.

Process of Diagnosis

- A good history: including family allergic predisposition.
- Diagnostic tests: stool analysis for blood (frank and occult bleeding can occur from colitis), serum levels of immunoglobulin E (IgE) and skin-prick testing.
- Milk elimination: the most definitive diagnostic strategy is elimination of milk, followed by challenge testing after improvement of symptoms.

Therapeutic Management

- Simple exclusion diet: eliminate a single food or food constituent.
- Multiple food exclusion diet: elimination of all dairy products.

Infants fed cows milk formula are managed primarily by changing the formula to a casein or whey hydrolysate milk formula in which the protein has been broken down (or predigested) into its amino acids through enzymatic hydrolysis.

Soya-based formula is not recommended because as many as 20% of these infants are also allergic to soya (Fiocchi et al 2003). Goats milk and sheep milk are not appropriate substitutes either plus they are deficient in folic acid.

Infants who are breastfed but have symptoms of cows milk hypersensitivity (Table 40.2) are treated by eliminating all dairy products from the lactating mother's diet. These mothers need vitamin D and calcium supplementation. Infants are

Table 40.2 Cows Milk Intolerance: Generalised Signs and Symptoms

Digestive	Respiratory	Dermatological	Behaviour	Generalised
Diarrhoea	Sneezing	Eczema	Excessive crying	Failure to thrive
Vomiting	Coughing	Urticaria	Sleeplessness	Retarded growth
Colic	Chronic nasal discharge	Vascular	Hyperactivity	Malnutrition
Abdominal pain	Asthma	Facial pallor	Lethargy	
Haematochezia (bloody stools)	Bronchitis	Infraorbital oedema (swelling under the eyes)		
Malabsorption	Recurrent croup			
Enteropathy	Otitis media			
Constipation				
Anorexia				

maintained on the dairy-free diet for 1–2 years, after which time very small quantities of milk are reintroduced.

Differences Between Food Allergy and Food Intolerance

The differences between food allergy and food intolerance are shown in Table 40.3.

Activity

- How would you explain cows milk allergy to a parent/caregiver?

Implications for Nursing

The principle nursing objectives are assessment and identification of potential milk allergy and appropriate health education advice and counselling of parents regarding substitute milk feeds.

The protein-hydrolysed formulae are less palatable than milk-based formulae. Consequently, reluctance to accept the new formula by the infant may be a problem. This can be overcome by introducing the formula gradually over a period of days. Parents also need to be reassured that the infant will receive complete nutrition from the new formula and will suffer no ill effects from the absence of cows milk.

Once solid foods are started, parents require guidance in avoiding all associated milk products during weaning. This requires carefully reading all food labels to avoid potential addition of milk products to the prepared food.

Activity

When you next go shopping examine food labels for inclusion of milk products:
- Discuss your findings with your mentor.
- What information can you now give to parents following this activity?

Table 40.3 Food Allergy and Food Intolerance

Food allergy	Food intolerance
An immediate reaction	Often delayed reaction – from hours to days
Reaction is local	May affect remote organs
Usually IgE-mediated	Rarely IgE-mediated
Cause is normally easily detected	Often has multiple food causes Cause may be evident only after a period of avoidance

LACTOSE INTOLERANCE

Lactose intolerance is the reduced ability to digest milk sugars due to insufficient production of the enzyme lactase, which breaks down the sugar lactose for digestion. The resulting intolerance causes symptoms such as bloating, abdominal pain and diarrhoea shortly after ingesting milk products:

- Congenital lactose intolerance: appears soon after birth when the diet contains lactose from milk.
- Late-onset lactose intolerance: is similar to the congenital type but manifests later in life.

Milk from mammals including cows, goats, sheep and humans, contains lactose. This means that goats and sheep milk are not suitable alternatives to cows milk for infants and children with this condition.

Management

There is no medical treatment (Food Standards Agency (FSA) 2003) for lactose intolerance but the symptoms can be avoided by controlling the amount of lactose in the diet. This requires elimination of dairy products in the diet. In infants, a soya-based formula can be substituted for cows milk formula or human milk. As dairy products are a major source of calcium and vitamin D, supplementation of these nutrients is needed to prevent any deficiency.

Identification of sources of lactose is required, e.g. especially hidden sources such as bulk agents in certain medications. Check with the pharmacist regarding this possibility when ordering medications of any sort.

VEGETARIAN DIETS

The potential for nutritional deficiencies in vegetarian diets for infants cannot be overemphasised. Achieving a nutritionally adequate vegetarian diet is not difficult but requires careful planning and knowledge of nutrient sources.

The major nutrient deficiencies (Table 40.4) that may occur in the stricter vegetarian diets are inadequate protein required for growth, inadequate calories for energy and growth, poor digestibility of many of the natural, unprocessed foods, especially for infants. Deficiencies of vitamin B12, niacin, thiamine, riboflavin, vitamin D, iron, calcium and zinc (Hamlyn et al 2000, Savoi & Rioux 2002, Shaw & Pal 2002).

When solid foods are introduced, the safety and digestibility of the foods should be reviewed. Raw fruits with seeds and nuts are dangerous for infants because of the risk of aspiration. Beans, grain cereals and vegetables should be served well cooked and pureed or mashed to aid digestibility during infancy.

Table 40.4 Vegetarian Diets

Types of vegetarian diet	Foods included/excluded	Potential nutrient deficiencies
Lacto-ovovegetarian	Exclude meat from their diet but include milk, eggs, and sometimes fish	Protein intake needs monitoring
Lactovegetarian	Exclude meat and eggs but include and drink milk	Low in protein as well as iron
Vegan	Eliminate any food of animal origin, including milk and eggs	Low in protein, minerals, calcium
Macrobiotic	More restrictive than pure vegetarian diet. Cereals, especially brown or polished rice, are the mainstay of the diet	Low in protein, minerals, calcium

Activity

- Plan a healthy, nutritious diet for a lactovegetarian infant who has started weaning. Provide a rationale for your choices.

Ensuring the Right Foods

To ensure sufficient protein in the vegetarian diet, foods with incomplete proteins (those that do not have all of the essential amino acids) must be eaten at the same meal with other foods that supply the missing amino acids. The three basic combinations of foods consumed by vegetarians that generally provide the appropriate amounts of essential amino acids are:

- grains (cereal, rice, pasta) and legumes (beans, peas, lentils, peanuts)
- grains and dairy products (milk, cheese, yoghurt)
- seeds (sesame, sunflower) and legumes.

The best assurance of nutritional adequacy is to eat a variety of foods. Families need guidelines for selecting foods that provide essential nutrients without exceeding energy requirements. Nurses and health visitors involved in the care of infants play an important part in the health education process. By understanding the factors such as cultural and religious dietary needs that may influence the decisions parents make concerning weaning, health professionals can adapt recommended weaning guidelines appropriately for individual families (Shaw & Pal 2002).

Activity

Plan an appropriate weaning diet for an infant of the Islamic faith. Include halal meat in the diet.

GROWTH AND FAILURE TO THRIVE

Altered growth, or failure to thrive (FTT), refers to a state of inadequate growth from inability to obtain and or use calories required for growth. It is a symptom not a disease. Thorough assessment of nutritional intake, physiological growth parameters and family needs are necessary to develop plans of care to promote nutritional intake for growth and development (Wells 2002). There are two general categories of failure to thrive:

- Organic failure to thrive: can occur as a result of a physical cause. Examples of physical causes include congenital heart defects, neurological conditions, chronic renal failure, malabsorption syndrome, endocrine dysfunction, disease processes (as in cystic fibrosis and AIDS).

- Non-organic failure to thrive: most often the result of psychosocial factors unrelated to physical disease. Factors may include inadequate knowledge of nutritional needs of infants, stressors affecting the family, social problems (Krugman & Dubowitz 2003).

Assesssment

Growth measurements alone are not used to diagnose children with failure to thrive. The finding of persistent deviation from an established growth curve is cause for concern. Percentile charts should be used for all infants. If weight and height measurements fall off the percentile indicated by birth weight for that percentile then failure to thrive should be considered.

Activity

Examine a variety of assessment tools used to assess growth and development of infants.

Reflect on your Practice

- How were the growth and development charts used for the assessment of an infant with poor growth that you have nursed?
- Did the assessment tools provide all the necessary information needed to develop an appropriate plan of care?
- What other information was required?

Factors Leading to Inadequate Feeding

- Health education: i.e. inadequate nutritional health education for parents.
- Attachment disturbance: with maternal–child attachment relationships.
- Health beliefs: concerning the constituents of a healthy diet.
- Family stress: which may include financial worries, substance misuse, marital problems, mental health problems, e.g. depression.

The above factors require assessment and the infant may require hospitalisation for an assessment of physiological status. The needs of the family will also need to be assessed. The multidisciplinary team, including social workers, health visitors, dietitians, will play an important role in the assessment and planning of appropriate interventions to support the family in providing for the nutritional needs of the infant.

Eczema

ATOPIC ECZEMA

Infantile eczema is also known as atopic dermatitis or atopic eczema; the terms are often used synonymously. The term atopic eczema will used here.

Atopic eczema is an inflammation of a genetically sensitive skin (Cork 1999). Eczema is a symptom rather than a disorder. The condition is multifactoral and indicates that the infant is oversensitive to certain substances, called allergens, which can gain entry to the body via four methods:

- digestive tract: in foods
- inhalation: dust, pollen
- direct contact: wool, soap, strong sunlight
- injections: insect bites, vaccines.

Atopic eczema is rarely seen in breastfed babies until they begin to get additional food. The condition appears to have a definite familial tendency and emotional factors are often involved. Atopic eczema usually begins around 2–6 months of age and generally undergoes spontaneous remission by 3 years of age. The infant has a greater than normal risk of developing dry skin and eczema later in life.

Eczema may occur later in childhood at 2–3 years and in most cases the skin heals by age 5 years (Cork 1997). Preadolescent and adolescent eczema begins at about 12 years of age and may continue into adulthood. Some children develop the triad of atopic eczema, asthma, and hay fever.

Location and Development of Atopic Eczema

When atopic eczema occurs during infancy it affects each infant differently in terms of both onset and severity of signs and symptoms. A rash may first appear in patches around the cheeks and chin, combined with local vasodilation, which gives the rash a red appearance. This can progress to spongiosis (the breakdown of the dermal skin cells and the development of intradermal vesicles) (Spagnola & Korb 2002). This can be seen as red, scaling, oozing skin. Scratching can eventually produce a weeping skin. The skin may then become infected. Chronic scratching produces lichenification or coarsening of the skin folds.

Once the infant becomes more mobile and begins crawling, exposed areas, such as the inner and outer parts of the arms and legs, may also be affected. Atopic eczema may also affect the skin around the eyes, the eyelids, and the eyebrows and lashes. Scratching and rubbing the eye area can cause the skin to redden and swell. Rubbing also causes patchy loss of eyebrows and eyelashes. Over time, atopic eczema may lead to development of an extra fold of skin under the eyes.

An infant with atopic eczema may be restless and irritable because of the itching and discomfort of the disease (Table 40.5). Difficulty in sleeping can occur due to the nature of pruritus.

 Activity

Access the companion PowerPoint presentation. You will find a diagram of the skin: identify the areas of altered physiology as described below.

Altered Physiology

Researchers including Cork (1997) have observed differences in the skin of those with atopic eczema that may contribute to the symptoms of the disease.

The outer layer of skin, the epidermal layer, is divided into two parts: an inner part containing moist, living cells, and an outer part, known as the horny layer or stratum corneum, containing dry, flattened, dead cells. Under normal conditions, the stratum corneum acts as a barrier, keeping the rest of the skin from drying out and protecting other layers of skin from damage caused by irritants and infections. When this barrier is damaged, irritants act more intensely on the skin.

The skin of an infant with atopic eczema loses moisture from the epidermal layer, allowing the skin to become very dry and reducing its protective abilities. Thus, when

Table 40.5 Atopic Eczema

Feature	Dermatological description
Red and inflamed area	Erythema
Intense itching sensation	Pruritus
Hives (red, raised bumps) that may occur after exposure to an allergen, at the beginning of flares, or after exercise or a hot bath	Urticaria
Breakdown of dermal cells and the formation of intradermal vesicles	Spongiosis
Small raised bumps that may open when scratched and become crusty and infected	Papules
Small, rough bumps, generally on the face, upper arms, and thighs	Keratosis pilaris
Thick, leathery skin resulting from constant scratching and rubbing	Lichenification
An extra fold of skin that develops under the eye	Atopic pleat (Dennie–Morgan fold)
Eyelids that have become darker in colour from inflammation or hay fever	Hyperpigmented eyelids
Inflammation of the skin on and around the lips	Cheilitis
Dry, rectangular scales on the skin	Ichthyosis
Increased number of skin creases on the palms	Hyperlinear palms

Assessment of general health, past medical history, familial history plus specific assessment of skin should be carried out. In infancy, lesions are located on the:

- cheeks
- scalp
- trunk
- outer aspects of hands and feet
- skin folds.

Lesions can also be generalised, i.e. they can cover the entire body. The signs and symptoms of atopic eczema are shown in Box 40.1.

Box 40.1

Signs and symptoms of atopic eczema

Signs of atopic eczema
- Erythema
- Vesicles that weep
- Develop a dry crust
- Scaling
- Worse in winter
- Lesions easily infected by bacterial or viral agents
- Periods of temporary remission
- Laboratory studies may show an increase in IgE and eosinophil levels
- Extremes of temperature, humidity and sunlight can aggravate

Symptoms of atopic eczema
- Intense itching (pruritus)
- Scratching
- Irritable
- Unable to sleep
- May flare up following immunisations

combined with the abnormal skin immune system, the infant's skin is more likely to become infected by viruses (e.g. herpes simplex) or bacteria (e.g. *Staphylococcus* and *Streptococcus* spp.).

Immunoglobulin E (IgE) is a type of antibody that controls the immune system's allergic response. An antibody is a protein produced by the immune system that recognizes and helps fight and destroy viruses, bacteria, and other foreign substances that invade the body. Normally, IgE is present in very small amounts but levels are high in 80–90% of people with atopic eczema (Hanifin & Rajka 1980, Hoare et al 2000).

Assessment

Atopic eczema can present with a variety of symptoms. The symptoms can vary in intensity and also over time.

Exploration of any family history of allergies is necessary. Although atopic eczema runs in families, the role of genetics or inheritance is still not clear. It does appear that more than one gene is involved in the disease. Studies suggest that genetics play an important part in the inheritance of the disease (Spagnola & Korb 2002). Infants and children are at increased risk for developing the eczema if there is a family history of other atopic disease, such as hay fever or asthma. The risk is significantly higher if both parents have an atopic disease. In addition, studies of identical twins, who have the same genes, show that in an estimated 80–90% of cases, atopic disease appears in both twins. Fraternal (non-identical) twins are no more likely than two non-related people in a general population to both have an atopic eczema.

Major and Minor Features of Atopic Eczema

A preliminary diagnosis of atopic eczema can be made if the patient has three or more features from each of two categories: major features and minor features (Hanifin & Rajka 1980, National Eczema Society 2003).

Major Features

- Intense itching.
- Characteristic rash in locations typical of the disease.
- Chronic or repeatedly occurring symptoms.
- Personal or family history of atopic disorders (eczema, hay fever, asthma).

Minor Features

- Early age of onset.
- Dry skin that may also have patchy scales or rough bumps.
- High levels of immunoglobulin E (IgE).
- Numerous skin creases on the palms.
- Hand or foot involvement.

ALLERGIC SENSITIVITY

Allergens are substances from foods, plants, animals or the air (e.g. dust mites, pollens, moulds). They inflame the skin by causing the immune system to overreact. Inflammation occurs even when the infant is exposed to small amounts of the substance for a limited time. It is not yet certain whether inhaling these allergens or their actual penetration of the skin causes the problem. When infants with atopic eczema come into contact with an irritant or allergen they are sensitive to, inflammation-producing cells become active. These cells release chemicals – histamines – that cause itching and redness. As the infant responds by scratching and rubbing the skin, further skin damage occurs (Spagnola & Korb 2002).

Food Allergy

The most common allergenic (allergy-causing) foods are eggs, milk, peanuts, wheat, soy and fish. A recent analysis (Spagnola & Korb 2002) of a large number of studies on allergies and breastfeeding indicated that breastfeeding an infant for at least 4 months may protect the infant from developing allergies. Mothers with a family history of atopic conditions should be advised to avoid eating common allergenic foods during late pregnancy and breastfeeding.

Elimination Diets

A basic diet of hypoallergenic food is given to the infant initially. One new food at a time is added to determine the infant's reaction to it:

- If the infant is allergic to cows milk, a substitute such as soya bean milk can be used.

- Vitamin supplements may be needed, particularly if the infant is not taking fruit and vegetables.

IRRITANTS

Irritants are substances that affect the skin directly, causing it to become red and itchy or to burn. The substances that irritate and the effects of these irritants vary from one person to another. Over time, family members learn to identify the irritants causing infants the most trouble. Wool or synthetic fibres and rough or poorly fitting clothing can rub the skin, trigger inflammation, and cause the itch–scratch cycle to begin. Soaps and detergents may have a drying effect and worsen itching, and some perfumes and cosmetics may irritate the skin. Exposure to certain substances, such as solvents, dust, or sand, may also make the condition worse. Cigarette smoke can irritate the eyelids (Hockenberry 2003).

MANAGING THE INFANT WITH ATOPIC ECZEMA

The management of black skin is generally the same as white skin (National Eczema Society 2003). However, some differences in skin structure can lead to some specific problems. Changes in skin colour can occur when the pigment layer of the skin is disturbed by the disease process. Thickening of the skin (lichenification) is more likely in black skin. Once inflammation processes reduce, the skin will return to a normal colour, although this can take several months. Often, no explanation can be found for a particular flare-up of the condition, and many factors are probably working in combination at all times.

Family Needs

When an infant has atopic eczema, the family may have to cope with the stress and frustration associated with the disease (Campbell & Glasper 1995). The infant may be fussy and irritable and unable to keep from scratching and rubbing the skin. Sleepless nights also cause irritation to both infant and family. Distracting the child and providing activities that keep the hands busy are helpful but require much effort on the part of the parents or caregivers. Another issue family's face is the social and emotional stress associated with changes in appearance caused by atopic eczema

Activity

Reflect on your experiences caring for an infant who has atopic eczema:

- What were the contributory factors causing an exacerbation of the condition for that particular infant?

WWW

A wide variety of information for both adults and children/ young people is available on the National Eczema Society website:

• http://www.eczema.org

Principles of Care: Controlling Atopic Eczema

● Hydrate the skin.

● Relieve pruritus.

● Reduce inflammation and flare-ups.

● Prevent secondary infection.

Hydrate the Skin

● Give lukewarm, not hot, baths.

● Use emollient bath treatments.

● Apply emollient immediately after the bath to assist in trapping moisture and preventing moisture loss. If an emollient is not applied within 3 minutes of leaving the bath, evaporation causes excess drying of the skin (Spagnola & Korb 2002).

● *Safety point:* emollients can make surfaces slippery. Remain with the infant all times while in bath to prevent accidents, e.g. drowning.

● Avoid bubble baths and harsh soaps, which can cause irritation.

● Pat, do not rub the skin, dry.

Relieve Pruritus

● Prevent scratching or rubbing whenever possible.

● Attempt to distract the infant with activities to keep him or her from scratching.

● Keep fingernails cut short.

● Gloves and/or cotton socks may need to be placed over hands.

● Avoid fibres such as wool.

● Consider the use of prescribed sedating antihistamines to promote sleep and reduce scratching at night.

Reduce Inflammation and Flare-ups

● Protect skin from excessive moisture, irritants, and rough clothing.

● Avoid situations where overheating occurs.

● Consider potential irritants with toys.

● Select soft cotton fabrics when choosing clothing.

● Limit exposure to dust, cigarette smoke, pollens and animal dander.

● Recognize and limit emotional stress.

● Occasional flare-ups: may require the use of prescribed topical steroids to diminish inflammation.

● Acute flare-ups: may require the use of wet wraps.

Prevent Secondary Infection

● Learn to recognize skin infections and seek treatment promptly.

● Secondary skin infections can be managed with prescribed systemic antibiotics.

Emollients

Soaps and detergents are drying because they remove natural lipids from the skin surface. Emollients provide a barrier to prevent water evaporating from the skin and also foreign irritants from entering. Emollients can be applied in liberal amounts twice a day and whenever the skin feels dry and itchy.

Emollients are available in various forms, including creams, ointments, lotions, soap substitutes and bath additives. Twitchen & Lowe (1998) describe the action of emollients as hydrating, soothing and smoothing of the scales on the skin.

Medical Treatments

Corticosteroids

These can be administered locally or systemically. Topical corticosteroid creams and ointments are effective in suppressing inflammation and providing symptomatic relief (Cork 1999). Topical steroids should be applied sparingly and only to affected skin. Side effects of repeated or long-term use of topical corticosteroids can include thinning of the skin, infections, growth suppression in children, and stretch marks on the skin.

When topical corticosteroids are not effective, a systemic corticosteroid may be prescribed. This is taken orally instead of being applied directly to the skin. An example of a commonly prescribed corticosteroid is prednisone. This medication is only prescribed for short periods of time. The side effects of systemic corticosteroids can include skin damage, thinned or weakened bones, high blood pressure, high blood sugar, and infections (Devilliers et al 2002). Corticosteroids should not be suddenly stopped. It is very important that the doctor and family work together when reducing and completing the corticosteroid treatment.

Antibiotics

Antibiotics to treat skin infections may be applied directly to the skin in an ointment, as well as taken orally. If viral or fungal infections are present, the doctor may also prescribe specific medications to treat those infections.

Antihistamines

Antihistamines can reduce night-time scratching and allow more restful sleep when taken at bedtime. This effect can be particularly helpful for infants whose night-time scratching makes the skin lesions worse.

Wet-wrap Dressings

Wet-wrap dressings (Box 40.2) can be used when the atopic eczema does not respond to the first-line treatments of emollients and topical steroids. Wet-wrap dressings are an effective means of rehydrating and cooling the skin and reducing inflammation. The wet-wrap can also involve use of topical steroids for increased absorption, which in turn reduces the itch–scratch cycle (Hanifin et al 2003).

This treatment is usually commenced in the hospital setting. The technique can easily be taught for use at home (Twitchen & Lowe 1998).

Box 40.2

Wet-wrap dressings

A water-based emollient is applied all over the body. The emollients are covered with a double layer of wrapping of tubular bandages. The innermost wrapping is moistened with warm water. The outer layer is a dry layer of tubular bandage.

The benefits include the evaporation of water gradually from the wet layer causing a slight cooling of the skin, which partly relieves the itching. The moisture in the dressing helps to soften the skin, allowing better penetration of the topical corticosteroid, while the two layers of dressing can act as a mechanical barrier to scratching (Pei et al 2001).

By participating in making the decision to use wet-wraps, families with an infant with atopic eczema may feel they have gained some control over this condition. There are benefits to children of rehydrating the skin in this way, such as improvements seen in reduction of pruritus and improvements in sleeping patterns following the use of wet wrap dressings.

Frequency of Use

The bandages are usually left in place for up to 24 hours and the process is repeated daily until the skin is clear. However, as Donald (1997) found, wet-wraps are most effective during the first 8 hours of application and so are best used at night. This may prove a more acceptable way of incorporating the treatment into daily activities.

Once the skin state has responded to treatment, a maintenance regimen of bandaging may be required. Prolonged positive effects on the skin are achieved when occlusion is continued for a further 2 weeks to prevent skin dryness. Application of the wet-wraps may then be reduced to alternate nights, and further reduced until the skin state is maintained without occlusion. Twitchen & Lowe (1998) found the itch–scratch cycle seems to be broken more effectively this way.

Allergy

Some patients have allergic reactions to either the emollients, the topical steroids or the tubular bandaging used. Allergy may present as increased pruritus and exacerbation of the eczema. Treatment should be discontinued and reviewed for alternative management methods.

Temperature

Wet-wraps may cause the infant to feel very cold, resulting in shivering. Reducing the time wet-wraps are in situ, ensuring the home or hospital environment is warm, applying the treatment to localised areas only may surmount this difficulty. Alternatively, the bandaging may cause overheating, which can exacerbate pruritus. In such cases, it may have to be accepted that wet-wrap bandaging is simply not appropriate.

Other Methods of Treatment

Hoare et al (2000), in a systematic review of research into atopic eczema treatments, found there was insufficient evidence to make recommendations on treatments such as Chinese herbs, homeopathy, massage therapy, hypnotherapy and evening primrose oil.

WWW

Access the systematic review into atopic eczema treatments. The report is available on the DoH health technology assessment website:
- http://www.ncchta.org

Sleep and Rest

Infants and children have different needs for sleep and rest; the amount depends on their age and development. Bangura (1998) acknowledged that throughout the process of sleep maturation occurs, the pattern of sleep changes from frequent brief periods of sleep to a single prolonged uninterrupted sleep. An infant may expect to sleep for a period of 16 hours a day, compared with an older child who requires between 9 to 12 hours sleep per 24 hours.

Bennett (2003) described sleep as a complex natural phenomenon, common to all human beings. As sleep has a significant role in maintaining health, too little/too much sleep affects each individual's quality of life and well-being. Duxbury (1994) described sleep as the discrete state of reduced responsiveness to external stimuli whereby a person could be aroused if the stimulus is of significant magnitude.

PHYSIOLOGY OF SLEEP

Hogg (1998) proposed that sleep was a group of complex actions within the body sustained by the central nervous system. Other systems that influence sleep are the cardiovascular, respiratory, muscular and peripheral nervous systems. Bennett (2003) identified that studies using electroencephalography (EEG) discovered that there are distinct sleep patterns and levels. These are described as rapid eye movement (REM) sleep and non-rapid eye movement (NREM) sleep. Sleep commences with NREM, followed by REM, and this cycle continues throughout, alternating from one to the other. According to Finlay (1991) each cycle may eventually last up to 90 minutes.

Sleep is controlled by both internal and external factors, which are influenced by circadian rhythms. Hogg (1998) described these cyclic rhythms as being regulated by physiological and behavioural responses, each of the circadian rhythms ensues a 24-hour cycle.

Studies suggest that sleep is influenced by complex neurochemical reactions within the brain stem. These reactions are affected by the body's neurotransmitters such as noradrenaline and serotonin. The release of noradrenaline and other catecholamines causes wakefulness, whereas the release of seratonin causes sleep.

In infancy, REM tends to control a baby's sleep pattern; this is due to the rapid growth and development of the brain. Bangura (1998) recognised that sleep has an important effect on the body's immune system. Therefore, sleep proves to be of benefit to this system.

Bennett (2003) acknowledged that sleep provides the body with the ideal circumstances for biological growth and healing comprising protein synthesis, cell division increase enabling the recovery of tissues. Therefore, sleep has restorative properties.

ROUTINES AND BARRIERS TO SLEEP

By 3 weeks of age, most infants have established a pattern of sleep and have apportioned the times of sleep equally between day and night. At 3 months of age, most infants tend to sleep for 12 hours at night, i.e. 19:00 hours to 07:00 hours. Colic, crying and sleep disturbance have been suggested to be associated with the melatonin production, which codes the day length. Regular sleep patterns need to be promoted otherwise the infant maybe at a disadvantage and fail to distinguish appropriate signals for sleep.

THE BENEFICIAL EFFECTS OF THE SLEEP PATTERN

A bedtime routine is effective in promoting sleep patterns. A separate area for sleeping and allowing children to fall asleep by themselves should be encouraged. Established

positive sleep behaviour may prevent the development of irregular sleep in later life, and it will almost certainly reduce the possible effects of a tired and irritable child. In addition, a parent who has had little sleep may feel vulnerable and overreact in stressful situations. Hence, the quality of family life may be reduced.

Establishing Routines

As soon as it is possible, it is beneficial to establish a routine with a set bedtime, to enable the infant to differentiate between day and night. For example, a bath, bedtime story and darkening the room may induce sleep.

Reorganising areas for day activities and another to promote rest may be advantageous. If space is restricted, part of the room may be partitioned, enabling the cot to be visually separated from the rest of the living quarters. Parents need to establish whether the infant is too warm or too cold; if uncomfortable the baby is unlikely to sleep.

Behaviour Modification

- Minimal check: a system used to modify sleep patterns in infancy has been referred to as the 'minimal check programme'. This permits the parents to observe the infant briefly at regular intervals during the period if an infant is crying. The period of time between checking has ranged from 5 to 20 minutes; infant sleep patterns have been found to improve with this system.

- Parental presence programme: this is based on the concept that sleep disturbance in young children is due to the child's separation anxiety. Parents remain with the child during the first week of the programme, sleeping in the same room but in a separate bed, so that if the child wakes during the night interaction and involvement is withheld. After the allocated period the parent returns to a different room. The efficiency of this approach is minimal; sleep disturbance has continued to be portrayed.

- Graduated extinction and fading: this approach involves reducing the intensity of the parental response that is sustaining the undesirable behaviour. Graduated extinction involves in increasing the time before responding to bedtime crying (incremental graduated extinction) or decreasing the time spent with the infant on settling or on night awakening (decremental graduated extinction). Studies that have incorporated this method have resulted in marked improvements within the infant's sleep pattern.

The success of any modification programme depends on parental agreement and, where applicable, both parents need to have discussed the subject and are both prepared to undertake the chosen method.

Activity

- Reflect on your practice when nursing infants and preparation for sleep.
- Explore the rituals attached to preparation for sleep and consider the positive and negative aspects of the rituals you have observed.

SUDDEN INFANT DEATH SYNDROME

The *Medical nursing and allied health dictionary* (published by Mosby) defines sudden infant death syndrome (SIDS) as the unexpected and sudden death of an apparently normal and healthy infant that occurs during sleep and without evidence to suggest a disease. It is currently one cause of death in children between 2 weeks and 1 year of age. At present, statistical evidence suggests that the incidences are 1:300–350 live births. The origin is unknown but causative factors have been proposed, including inadequate biotin in the diet, mechanical suffocation, a defect in the respiratory mucosa, extensive apnoeas, a virus and immunoglobulin abnormalities. Sudden infant death syndrome occurs more often in infants aged between 10 and 14 weeks, especially those born prematurely, in boys more than girls and more often during the winter months. Evidence suggests that those infants who have experienced an upper respiratory tract infection may be predisposed to sudden infant death syndrome. The syndrome is neither infectious nor hereditary, although there may be a higher possibility of it occurring within the same family, which may imply genetic factors are involved.

Epidemiology of Sudden Infant Death Syndrome

Table 40.6 looks at the determinants of sudden infant death syndrome.

Activity

Examine Table 40.6. Discuss how and why the identified factors may cause a higher prevalence of sudden infant death syndrome.

Children at Greater Risk

In view of the research findings, some children are more at risk than others are. These include:

- Infants with a life-threatening condition needing cardiopulmonary resuscitation (CPR).
- Preterm infants who continue to experience apnoeic episodes at the time of hospital discharge.

Table 40.6 Sudden Infant Death Syndrome (Adapted from Wong 2001)

Determinant	Incidence
Frequency	0.6 per 1000 live births (1998)
Sleep patterns	Prone, soft bedding, overheating, co-sleeping with adults
Peak periods	2–4 months, 95% occur by 6 months
Feeding habits	Lower incidence in breast-fed infants
Males to females	Higher percentage of males affected
Siblings	Possibly greater
Maternal	Young age, cigarette smoker, poor prenatal care, alcohol and drug dependency
Time of death	During sleep
Socio-economic factors	Increased occurrence in lower socio-economic classes
Birth	Higher incidence in preterm infants, low birthweight infants Multiple births Neonates with low Apgar scores Infants with respiratory disorders

- Siblings of two or more sudden infant death syndrome victims.
- Infants with complex disorders or conditions, e.g. hypoventilation.

Equipment for monitoring within the home environment is recommended for these children, providing parents are aware of cardiopulmonary resuscitation techniques. At present there are no diagnostic tools to indicate which infants will live or die, but monitoring infants may alleviate parental anxiety.

Preventive strategies are directed at decreasing known risk factors, such as mothers requiring prenatal care, avoiding cigarette smoking and drug abuse both before and after the child's birth. The bedroom being at a suitable temperature (18°C) and the infant wearing suitable clothing helps to prevent sudden infant death syndrome.

The recommended health education messages to reduce the risk of cot death (these are available online at: http://www.sids.org.uk/fsid):

- Place your baby on his or her back to sleep.
- Place your baby with his or her feet to the foot of the cot, to prevent wriggling down under the covers.
- Do not let anyone smoke in the same room as your baby.
- Do not let your baby get too hot.

- Keep your baby's head uncovered.
- If your baby is unwell, seek medical advice promptly.

Whether subsequent siblings are at risk of sudden infant death syndrome remains unclear, but if home monitoring is an option this needs to be discussed with paediatricians, health visitors and nurses.

Ramifications for Nursing

Campbell & Glasper (2001) acknowledge that the loss of a child from sudden infant death syndrome presents the parents with a serious emotional matter, with which they must cope. In addition to grieving, the parents must face a catastrophic situation that was sudden, incomprehensible and unexpected.

Entering the Room and Finding the Child

It is usually one of the parents who discovers the child dead in the cot, with bedclothes disarranged and the blankets over the child's head. Often the parent can be alone in the house and must deal with the situation while coping with the emotional turmoil of shock, panic and grief.

The first of the personnel to arrive on the scene may be either the police or the paramedics. It is important to ask only essential questions in a non-judgemental manner when providing support and comfort for members of the family. Ambulance attendants should be educated to recognise the characteristic signs of sudden infant death syndrome and be able to inform the parents that the possible cause was sudden infant death syndrome, but that this cannot be predetermined. The compassion demonstrated by the ambulance attendants/police/health professionals in the first few minutes may help the parents to cope with the guilt and despair that accompany these types of situations.

Arriving at the Hospital

On arrival to the Accident and Emergency department, the nursing staff usually has first contact with the family and the infant is attended to by the doctor to certify death. As this period is emotionally charged, it is important to extract factual information from parents. This may include:

- What time was the infant found?
- How did the infant look?
- What position was the infant in?
- What assistance was provided?

Any questions that suggest responsibility should be avoided, such as was there any jealousy from other siblings?

It is necessary to determine the actual events: what happened when the parent/carer entered the infant's room, what resuscitation was attempted (this might have given rise to fractured ribs, internal bleeding and bruising, which

will need clarification). During this discussion, the doctor or nurse needs to approach the subject of a post-mortem, as the actual diagnosis of sudden infant death syndrome cannot be determined until this has been completed. Verbal and written information needs to be given regarding the post-mortem and funeral arrangements. Lawrence (1989) advised that mothers who were breastfeeding required accurate information regarding cessation of lactation.

Compassion towards the parents may consist of enabling them to say good-bye to their child, in privacy. Before this happens, the nurse needs to ensure that the infant appears tidy and the room is in order. As this maybe the last time the parents wish to see their child, they should be given as much time as needed, in peace and quiet.

The child's belongings needed to be returned to the parents. Contacting relatives or friends to take the parents home or a nurse escorting them to their car may be advisable.

At Home

Parents may receive a visit from their GP and health visitor, whereby issues of coming to terms with the infant's death may be explored. This may take more than one visit and consideration may need to address siblings and their grieving. A referral (and contact) details maybe given to the Foundation for Sudden Infant Death (FSID)

Dedicated charities, support groups and associations, can provide advice and help to families affected by sudden infant death syndrome. FSID provides information and a 24-hour helpline.

www

Access more information on the Foundation for the Study of Infant Deaths (FSID) website at:
- http://www.sids.org.uk

Activity

- Describe the grieving process.
- How can the primary healthcare team help the bereaved parents after the loss of an infant?

An important issue for many parents is later pregnancies, and concerns related to recurrent sudden infant death syndrome. Some parents may wish to re-establish their family within 12 months or so. One possibility of a subsequent child is that the infant may be a replacement for the previous one. If the pregnancy is a success, further anxiety may arise, especially near the time of the other infant's death, which maybe characterised by the parents being overprotective.

The health visitor can support the family in their decision for another child. The Care of the Next Infant (CONI) scheme allows the health visitor to provide effective support to prepare families for the birth of the next child.

APNOEA OF INFANCY

Apnoeic episodes can be defined as one of the following:

- central: absence of airflow and respiratory effort

- obstructive: absence of airflow but respiratory effort

- mixed: absence of airflow and respiratory effort followed
  by resumption of respiratory effort.

Short periods of central apnoea (15 seconds) are normal at
any age. Pathological apnoea refers to a respiratory pause
that is prolonged and may be accompanied with cyanosis,
pallor, hypotonia, and bradycardia. Apnoea of infancy (AOI)
occurs in infants greater than 37 weeks gestation. The clinical appearance of this disorder maybe classified as life
threatening. Apnoea of infancy may be associated with
many other disorders sepsis, convulsions, upper airway
abnormalities metabolic disorders and impaired regulation
of breathing during sleep or feeding.

Diagnosis

- Electroencephalogram (EEG).

- Electrocardiogram (ECG).

- Blood chemistry.

- Chest radiograph.

- pH study: to determine gastro-oesophageal reflux.

Ramifications for Nursing Practice

Confirmation of diagnosis needs to be discussed with parents before the provision of home monitoring. If monitoring is decided on, this may cause additional stress and
members of the nursing team are an ideal source of support
for the family. Parents need to be educated on the equipment, observation of the infant and immediate care in relation to cardiopulmonary resuscitation (CPR).

There are several types of home monitoring which are
available and most hospitals will choose a variety, which will
be used within the home environment. Guidelines for the
use of the apnoea monitors (adapted from Campbell &
Glasper 2001) are:

- Apnoea monitors have limitations, i.e. false alarms,
  however should be utilized.

- Do not adjust any settings to eliminate false alarms, this
  may reduce effectiveness.

- Place the monitors on an appropriate surface and not
  covered by sheets and blankets.

- Do not sleep in the same bed as a monitored infant,
  movement may reduce effectiveness.

- Pets and other children should be kept away from the
  monitor.

- Check the monitor several times a day to ensure that it is
  working, i.e. batteries and cord.

- Ensure that the caregiver can reach the infant in less
  than 10 seconds.

- Read the monitor's manual for usage carefully and report
  problems promptly.

- Prepare in advance for the event of an emergency by
  having telephone numbers next to the telephone.

- Health education is required in relation to recognising
  signs and symptoms of health problems and the need to
  communicate with health professionals.

- Education on when to initiate cardiopulmonary
  resuscitation.

 Activity

Design and develop written guidelines as supporting
material for parents using an apnoeic monitor for home
monitoring.

Immunisation

McCarthy (2001) suggested that immunisation programmes
within both the underdeveloped and developed world have
a significant and beneficial effect on children's health.
Vaccines are the products of the advancement with biotech-
nological techniques and ongoing research. Immunisations
need to be administered safely by professionals who are
competent and knowledgeable.

THE IMPORTANCE OF IMMUNISATION

In 1998, the Health Education Authority (now the Health
Protection Agency) defined immunisation as the process by
which immunity is produced against a variety of bacterial
and viral infections, which in effect cause immunity.

In England, epidemiological studies demonstrated that
outbreaks of measles, mumps, and rubella would occur if
education was not effective and not targeted at the most
vulnerable groups in society.

The World Health Organization (WHO 1984) adopted
the goal of eliminating measles, poliomyelitis, neonatal
tetanus, diphtheria and rubella by the year 2000. For this
to be achieved in England, a primary objective of a 90%

primary immunisation rate for all children under the age of 2 years had to be attained by 1995. This was met and, in 1992, a new target of 95% was introduced. Bedford (2003) supported these findings by acknowledging that for the vaccination programme to be effective, high levels of immunity are needed, to reduce and prevent the circulation of these illnesses.

The DoH (2003) released the statistics shown in Table 40.7 pertaining to measles. The figures suggest that there are still not enough children being vaccinated in the age group 1–4 years. This should be of concern to parents, the National Health Service and other allied organisations. Bedford (2003) acknowledged that to be given the equivalent of two injections of measles, mumps and rubella in the form of two separate injections takes at least 5 years, which leaves the child unprotected for an unnecessarily long period and might pose a risk to other individuals because herd immunity will fall, posing a risk to the community at large. Those who cannot be immunized, such as the immunosuppressed, neonates and pregnant women, will be at an increased risk of the disease.

Further reasons that contribute towards the high rate of notifications between 1 and 4 years may reflect the transient population, as well as mothers returning to work before the completion of the immunisation programme. Tudor-Hart (1971) suggested the inverse care law: that those who needed health care the most received the least and that those who would most benefit from the service are often less likely to use it, although children from the higher socio-economic classes were readily accepting the need for immunisation.

During the 1990s, concerns developed as to the efficacy and safety of the measles, mumps and rubella (MMR) vaccine. The government stated that this would be investigated, by reliable sources – predominantly the Health Protection Agency. If the threats to health were considered of significance action would be taken. In 2002, Uhlmann et al highlighted concerns about the combined vaccine resulting in autism and inflammatory bowel problems; by contrast, Dales et al (2001) demonstrated that the MMR vaccine continues to be used extensively in the US, and had been in use since 1972 without a correlation between use and the recently observed increase in autism. Bedford (2003) indicated that after a single-antigen vaccine had been advocated and used for a sustainable period of time,

many countries changed their strategy for controlling measles and began using the combined MMR vaccine so that children were protected from three of the most harmful infections. The aim was to eradicate measles, mumps and rubella; this was the first time that children had been offered protection from mumps. Bedford (2003) suggested that no vaccine was 100% effective. Ramsay et al (1994) indicated that following the initial injection of the combined MMR vaccine, approximately 10% of children within the population are not protected, suggesting that measles will occur amongst children who have been immunised. Following an outbreak of measles that occurred in Quebec in 1989, De Serres et al (1995) considered 62 siblings who developed measles: 41 had been vaccinated. This indicated that the vaccine had not been effective. However, further analysis demonstrated different findings: all 17 unvaccinated siblings acquired measles, whereas only 41 of 441 vaccinated siblings developed the disease. The results indicate that the vaccine has an efficacy of 91%; if the children had not been immunised, there would have been a further 400 cases.

Healthcare professionals whose speciality involves the administration of immunisations need to pursue non-attendees and actively involve parents in their decision to immunise. Nevertheless, parents in all socio-economic classes have their own justifications for not having their children immunized. Aston (1998) suggested that the reasons may be because of practical problems, or indifference. Crawford (1995) found the single most important factor that influenced most parents in favour of immunization were the knowledge, enthusiasm and confidence of the healthcare professional.

The presenting of information to parents by healthcare professionals needs to be undertaken impartially and the parents need to understand the importance of making the appropriate decision in the best interest of the child.

Activity

You are a student nurse. A parent tells you: 'I have read in the national press that there are risks associated with immunisations. My friend has refused the MMR vaccination for her child and I'm worried about what to do for my child.'
- What would you advise?

Table 40.7 Notification of Measles by Age Group (2001–03)							
Year	<12 months	1–4 years	5–9 years	10–14 years	15 years	Unknown	Total
2001	575	1127	298	86	140	24	2378
2002	751	1631	435	106	210	54	3187
2003	528	1275	429	111	164	22	2529

Activity

A parent asks: 'Should my children be vaccinated. My daughter is 2 months old and my son is 5 years old and has just started school?'
- Explain the advantages and disadvantages of vaccinations to this mother.
- Identify the evidence to support your answer. Refer to:
  - http://www.doh.gov.uk/policyandguidance
  - http://www.hpa.org.uk/infections/topics

Health Promotion

Health promotion and education contribute to providing parents and members of the public with information relating to immunisations for children. The importance of health promotion and education has been greatly emphasised over the past decade. *The health of the nation* (DoH 1992) and *Our healthier nation* (DoH 1998) emphasise the importance of good health for everyone from the young to the old. These documents recognise that individuals need to promote activities that have a beneficial consequence, and lessen those that cause significant harm and induce ill health.

The contribution of the nurse, the midwife and the health visitor has been extensive (DoH 2002, Hall 1996, Lindsey & Hartrick 1996). However, for health promotion programmes to be successful, it is important to consider the choice of target population so that the best possible results can be achieved. To improve health, communities need to gain more control over these systems through their full involvement in decision making, in order for this to be achieved health professionals need to empower, collaborate and provide resources to promote health. The ages at which the different immunisations should be given are shown in Table 40.8.

THE IMMUNE RESPONSE

Immunity may be either active or passive and involves the stimulation of antibodies. Active immunisation is provided by the stimulation of the host's antibodies, whereas passive immunisation involves the administration of antibodies. Passive immunity may be short term, whereas active immunity may be life long.

Passive Immunity

Passive Naturally Acquired Immunity
This method of immunity is acquired prior to birth, by the transfer of antibodies across the placenta to the fetus, and eventually to the baby in the form of breast milk. The variety of antibodies depends upon the mother's active

Table 40.8 Childhood Immunisations

Age	Immunisation	Notes
2 months: 1st dose	Diphtheria, pertussis, tetanus and polio	Three doses needed – primary course
3 months: 2nd dose	Hib	
4 months: 3rd dose	Measles, mumps and rubella	
12–15 months and 3–5 years	Booster: diphtheria, tetanus and polio Second dose: measles, mumps and rubella	Administered over the age of 12 months Three years after completion of primary course

Adapted from: http://www.doh.gov.uk/Policy/AndGuidance

immunity. The baby's lymphocytes are not effectual and the effects of the immunity are transitory.

Passive Artificially Acquired Immunity
In this form of immunity, the antibodies have been prepared, either by animal or human serum and are injected into the recipient. The source of the antibodies may be derived from an individual who is recovering from the infection or from animals – usually horses – that have been artificially actively immunised.

The immunoglobulins that have been obtained may be given prophylactically, to prevent the infection, or therapeutically after the infection has started. The proteins within the serum may cause the lymphocytes to be damaged most notably on subsequent occasions, which, according to Waugh and Grant (2003), may cause a severe reaction.

Active Immunity

Active immunity is created when an adjusted form of the infecting agent is administered, stimulating the production of antibodies. Active immunity is preferable to passive immunisation because of its duration. The manufacturing of vaccines is complex and requires a great degree of skill and knowledge. There is a fine line between ensuring that the antibody is effective and deactivating the antigen.

Active Naturally Acquired Immunity
Individuals can produce their own antibodies by the following:

- Having acquired the infection: Waugh & Grant (2003) suggested that during the illness B lymphocytes in the plasma cells produce antibodies in adequate quantities to engulf the infection. After recovery, the memory B cells maintain a specific ability to produce the specific antibodies to respond to a future infection by the same organism therefore immunity is bestowed.

- Having a subclinical infection for example a microbial infection, insufficient to cause a clinical disease but the memory B cells may be produced to create immunity.

Active Artificially Acquired Immunity

This form of immunity develops as a result of a response to the administration of dead or live artificially weakened microbes (Waugh & Grant 2003). These are referred to as vaccines or toxoids, they retain antigenic properties that stimulate immunity, but cannot cause the disease. These vaccines can prevent microbial diseases.

Activity

An infant has been admitted onto your ward for investigations. The mother informs you that she is pregnant, and one of her friends has told her that children do not require immunisations. To rectify misconceptions:

- What advice would you offer?
- Identify the literature that would provide the evidence base for the advice given to the parent.

Immunisation against certain diseases produces lifelong immunity. In other contractable diseases the immunity may last either years or weeks before a further vaccination is necessary. The loss of immunity may be as a result of a different strain of the same microbe, which causes the same clinical illness, e.g. the virus that causes the common cold.

DIPHTHERIA

Pathology

The *Medical nursing and allied health dictionary* (published by Mosby) characterises this condition as an acute contagious disease caused by the bacterium *Corynebacterium diphtheriae*. It causes the production of a systemic toxin and an adherent false membrane to the lining of the throat. The toxin that is produced is harmful to the tissues of the heart and central nervous system. The false lining to the throat can interfere with eating, breathing and verbal communications. The lymph glands within the neck swell and the neck becomes oedematous. If it remains untreated, the condition is fatal due to respiratory obstruction, heart or renal failure.

Children who are hospitalised are nursed in isolation, and given the diphtheria antitoxin (Box 40.3), antibiotics, bed rest and fluids. On occasions it may be necessary to perform a tracheotomy.

Box 40.3

Signs and symptoms of atopic eczema

Baker & Katz (2004) suggested that during the 1870s and 1880s diphtheria was one of the major diseases of childhood. The mortality rate was high, especially within cities. Baker & Katz (2004) identified that in New York fatalities ranged from 42 to 49%. Medical practitioners usually encountered a child experiencing difficulty breathing and who was asphyxiating, apart from surgical intervention and intubation by the 1880s there was little in the way of resources.

Emil von Behring was one of the first scientists to explore a vaccine to combat diphtheria; he combined an extract of the deadly disease toxins with antitoxins taken from healthy animals. In 1913, clinical trials established that children had conferred immunity without harmful side effects. Parish (1965) indicated that Bela Shick of the University of Vienna, in the same year had also identified a simple skin test that could determine whether an individual was immune to diphtheria.

These achievements were suddenly curtailed due to the First World War and proving the efficacy of the toxin–antitoxin became the responsibility of the Director of Hygiene Services – WH Park – who recruited more than 100,000 children within the American public school system for research, which eventually gave him acclaim as one of the leading advocates of this vaccine.

However, some countries did not advocate the use of toxin–antitoxin. In France, an effective vaccine was developed at the Pasteur Institute in the 1920s. The French Academy of Medicine approved this for children in 1927 and it begin to be used in France during the 1930s. This has become the preferred method of vaccination of children in developed countries.

PERTUSSIS (WHOOPING COUGH)

The American Centers of Disease Control and the UK Health Protection Agency (2003) have characterised pertussis as an acute infectious disease caused by *Bordetella pertussis*. The condition was first described in the 16th century and the organism was first isolated in 1906.

Before the start of immunisation in the 1950s, the average number of notifications in England and Wales was in excess of 100,000 (Health Protection Agency 2003). In 1972, immunisation approval was over 80% and, during that year, there were only 2069 notifications of whooping cough. Public anxiety increased regarding the safety of the vaccine after a report was published connecting a group of children who had been vaccinated with brain damage. By 1975, immunisation had fallen to 30%, which subsequently lead to epidemics in 1977 and 1981–83. This caused an extra 200,000 cases to be reported and 100 deaths. In the 1990s, public confidence in the pertussis vaccine steadily rose, due to professionals advocating the advantages, reaching 93% in 2002–03.

Despite the levels of vaccination being high, international reports suggest that there is reappearance of whooping cough. The Public Health Laboratory Service (PHLS) has been monitoring the condition and analysis of the information for

1995–97 indicates that the proportion of whooping cough in younger unvaccinated people is growing. The PHLS suggest that to cause a reduction within the condition in older age groups and reduce the spread of the communicable disease to infants too young to be fully protected may be achieved by introducing a booster before starting school; this was commenced in 2001.

Pertussis is commonly spread by droplet infection and the incubation period is usually 7–10 days (but see http://www.immunisation.org.uk, where it is suggested that the period of infection could be from 7–21 days after the initial onset of the paroxysms).

Signs and Symptoms

- Paroxysms of coughing.
- Loud whoop on inspiration.
- Viscid mucus maybe produced following the cough.
- Fever.
- Sneezing.
- Watery eyes.
- Vomiting.

Nursing Care

- Assess vital signs, temperature, respiratory rate, heart rate, blood pressure, oxygen saturation levels and record.
- Observe for any signs of cyanosis: administer prescribed oxygen as condition dictates.
- Promote rest—provide suitable toys and games.
- Encourage family-centred care/partnership in care.
- Provide oral fluids and diet as tolerated.
- Provide vomit bowls, tissues and encourage oral hygiene.
- Administer antibiotics as prescribed—although does not reduce the duration of the illness, stops the spread of the illness.

Potential Complications (as Determined by http://www.immunisation.org.uk)

- Bronchopneumonia.
- Weight loss: possibly related to nutritional intake.
- Brain damage: related to poor cerebral perfusion.
- Death.

TETANUS

Steimle et al (2002) defined tetanus as being caused by the bacterium *Clostridium tetani*. Although tetanus is prevent-able by the administration of a vaccine, tetanus is unique for it is not spread from person to person but entering the body through a wound. The bacterium associated with tetanus is found in environmental sources, which include soil, dust or faecal matter from animals with spores in their intestine.

A wound caused by a scratch or bite from an animal may lead to tetanus in individuals who have not been immunised. Steimle et al (2002) suggested that minor wounds have led to higher rate of tetanus cases, primarily due to the fact that a severe wound is usually treated within a healthcare setting, as opposed to a smaller wound being viewed as less harmful and consequently not requiring treatment. Tetanus may also occur following surgery, dental infection and termination of pregnancies in an unhygienic setting.

Clinical Signs and Symptoms

There are several forms of the infection localised, generalised, cephalic and tetanus neonatorum. However, Behrman & Kliegman (2002) indicated that the clinical examination of the wounds do not appear any different to an uninfected wound:

- Localised tetanus: uncommon in children, but causes pain, rigidity and spasms close to the wound site. The symptoms may last for weeks but resolve without complications.
- Generalised tetanus: this particular one causes gradual muscle rigidity, especially within the jaw, which may result in difficulty in swallowing. Convulsions may also be seen and contractions of various muscles. The airway may suddenly be compromised and as a result lead to respiratory insufficiency. The individual may be conscious but experience a great deal of pain. The duration of the illness may be from 2 to 6 weeks.
- Cephalic tetanus: this form may precede the former or be 1–2 days after otitis media, trauma to the face and head or due to the presence of a nasal foreign body according to Behrman & Kliegman (2002).
- Neonatorum tetanus: this usually starts 3–10 days after birth. Signs and symptoms include difficulty in sucking, swallowing, stiffness, excessive crying and contractions.

Pathology

The disease is as a result of exotoxins, tetanus toxin, or tetanospasmin and tetatanolysin, which may cause the tetanus toxin and result in muscle contraction, spasm and rigidity (Behrman & Kliegman 2002). The disease may also affect the neuromuscular junctions and cause paralysis. The toxins may proliferate, which may be characterised by tissues being inadequately oxygenated.

Signs and Symptoms

- Headache.
- Muscular stiffness in the jaw.
- Dysphagia.
- Stiffness in the neck.
- Rigidity in the chest, back and abdominal muscles.
- Sweating and fever.

Symptoms may start between 5 and 10 days after infection, but can range from 2 to 50 days (Steimle et al 2002).

Management of Care (Steimle et al 2002)

- It may involve an admission to intensive care unit (for respiratory management).
- Treatment of sepsis.
- Neutralising toxin before reaching the central nervous system.
- Cardiac instability may need to be treated.
- Determining urea and electrolyte and administering appropriate intravenous hydration.
- Treatment to entry or wound site – by debriding and irrigation.
- Monitoring pressure areas.
- Analgesia.

Complications

- Rigidity of the muscles of the face, neck and jaw.
- Muscle tears.
- Vertebral fractures.
- Respiratory problems: airway obstruction.
- Pneumonia.
- Septicaemia.
- Cardiovascular instability.

PowerPoint

Access the companion PowerPoint presentation.

Eradicating Tetanus

In industrialised countries, as the result of childhood immunisation programmes, the advancement of wound care, and improved farming practices, incidences of tetanus are infrequent. The PHLS (2000) suggests that the incidence is low in the UK; on average 6 cases were notified each year between 1990 and 1999.

The WHO (2001) identified that neonatal tetanus is a significant health issue in developing countries; in 1989 the World Health Assembly set an objective to eradicate the disease by 1995. However, most countries within the African region missed the goal. In 2001, WHO estimated that 124,000 cases and 93,000 deaths per year are principally due to tetanus in the African regions. A revised goal to eradicate neonatal and maternal tetanus globally has been set for 2005. To achieve this aim, support has to be given to the member states in the region to:

- achieve elimination of maternal and neonatal tetanus
- validate the achieved status of elimination
- implement strategies for maintaining the situation.

The planned implementation of national immunisation programme resulted in the Aftican region being divided into two categories:

- Category 1: countries that had eliminated or were close to eliminating neonatal tetanus and needed ongoing programmes.
- Category 2: countries with a high disease burden.

Steimle et al (2002) suggested that herd immunity is not a significant factor in the prevention of tetanus because it is an organism within the environment, which cannot be transferred from individual to individual. Therefore persons exposed to the bacteria need to have the antibodies in their blood at the time. Unless immunised they remain at risk of infection, contracting the infection does not provide immunity.

POLIOMYELITIS (POLIO)

This name comes from the Greek words *polio* (meaning grey) and *myelon* (meaning narrow – suggesting the spinal column). Polio has been described as an infectious disease, caused by a virus. Although the virus can cause an effect at any age, it predominantly affects children under 3 years of age (over 50 per cent of cases) (see http://www.polioeradication.org). One of the most significant effects of the disease is paralysis, which is almost always permanent. In severe cases the disease may lead to death by asphyxiation.

PowerPoint

Access the companion PowerPoint presentation for some historical information about polio.

The WHO (2002b) declared that 51 countries within the European region had been free of polio for over 3 years. There is a global initiative to eradicate polio by 2005. A coalition of four agencies includes:

- WHO
- Rotary International
- Centers for Disease Control and Prevention (CDC)
- The United Nations Children's Fund (UNICEF).

The objectives are:

- To stop the spread of the wild poliovirus as soon as possible and declare all WHO areas free by the end of 2005.
- To implement policies, include containment of the wild poliovirus and the development of post immunization policies.
- To organise systems, including strengthening routine immunisations and surveillance for communicable diseases.

The countries mainly affected by the poliovirus are in the developing world: Africa, south Asia, and areas which are affected by conflict with reduced healthcare systems and poor sanitation. To stop the transmission of the poliovirus will involve:

- Providing immunisation coverage to infants in the first year of life with four doses of the oral vaccine.
- Providing additional doses of the oral polio vaccine to children under the age of 5 years during national immunisation days.
- Surveillance for wild poliovirus through reporting mechanisms and laboratory testing, for children under the age of 15 years.
- Targeting a specific area when the wild poliovirus is within that area.

Pathology

The Centers for Disease Control and Prevention (2002) described the poliovirus as a member of the enterovirus subgroup. This particular type of virus is found within the digestive system and is stable at an acid pH. There are three serotypes – P1, P2 and P3 – within the poliovirus group. Immunity to one serotype may not produce considerable immunity to the others. The poliovirus is inactivated by heat, chlorine and ultraviolet light.

The virus enters the gastrointestinal system via the oral cavity and establishes itself within the pharynx and gastrointestinal tract. The virus may spread from the throat to be excreted via faeces; this may occur for several weeks after the onset of the illness. The poliovirus attacks the local lymphoid tissue, penetrates the bloodstream and then affects the central nervous system, where it infiltrates the nerve fibres and causes widespread destruction of the motor neurons.

Signs and Symptoms

- The intubation period is usually 6–20 days but may range from 3 to 35 days.
- May be asymptomatic but there is still a risk of emitting the virus to others.
- Non-specific illness: characterised by sore throat and fever nausea, vomiting and abdominal pain, influenza.

- Non-paralytic aseptic meningitis: rigidity within the neck, back and/or legs, abnormal sensation. Symptoms may last up to 10 days and there is a full recovery.
- Flaccid paralysis: paralysis generally begins 1–10 days after initial symptoms and continues for 2–3 days, although there is usually no further paralysis. When the temperature is within an acceptable range, sufferers may also experience loss of superficial reflexes, severe muscle pain and spasms. Strength returns and patients do not experience permanent loss of sensation or changes within levels of understanding.
- Paralytic polio: three classifications:
  - spinal polio: asymmetric paralysis often the legs are affected
  - bulbar polio: weakness of muscles supplying the cranial nerves
  - bulbospinal polio: combination of both of bulbar and spinal paralysis.

WWW

Find out more about the signs and symptoms of polio from the following websites:
- http://www.polioeradication.org/vaccines
- http://www.immunisation.org.uk

Epidemiology

The following may transmit the poliovirus infection according to the polio eradication programme:

- human: person to person
- faecal to oral.

In children who have not yet established urinary and bowel control, food or drink contaminated by faeces are ready sources of transmission. At first the disease circulates quietly, because of the way it affects the central nervous system, and the onset is insidious.

The Vaccine

The polio vaccine was developed during the 1950s and 1960s; the inactivated version was licensed in 1955 and was used until the 1960s. In 1963 the trivalent oral vaccine was permitted and licensed. The oral polio vaccine contains antibiotics and following administration the virus may be passed in faeces for up to 6 weeks. To acquire immunity against polio the schedule needs to be undertaken.

Until the introduction of the first vaccine in the 1950s, the poliovirus affected many young children. To ensure that countries remain clear of polio and its effects, healthcare professionals need to educate parents of the benefits of the vaccination and public health measures need to be monitored to maintain effective methods of cleanliness.

HAEMOPHILUS INFLUENZA

During the 1930s a prominent scientist – Margaret Pittman – demonstrated that haemophilus influenza could be isolated, and identified six forms or capsular types: a, b, c, d, e and f. Within the blood and cerebrospinal fluid, it was also found that in almost all the cases examined revealed capsular type b.

Before the advent of effective vaccines, the WHO (2003) suggested that haemophilus influenza type b (Hib) predominantly causes meningitis and pneumonia in children under 5 years of age and was a cause of concern both in developed and developing countries. In developing countries, Hib would mainly cause pneumonia, whereas in developed countries the primary cause would be bacterial meningitis. To reduce the incidence of these infections, a vaccination programme was required because antibiotics are essential for the treatment but resistance to antibiotics may result, therefore prevention was required and vaccination is the most effective public health strategy in reducing the spread of Hib.

Pathology

The WHO (2003) defined haemophilus influenza as a Gram-negative bacterium. The infection is attributed to strains carrying a polysaccharide capsule. Type b causes nearly all-systemic infections, 15% of children in non-vaccinated populations carry Hib in their nasopharynx. However, from this perspective a small percentage will develop the disease. The transmission of the infection is by droplet and, as a result, those individuals who are symptomatic are important in the distribution of the organism. In the USA, the Centers for Disease Control and Prevention (see http://www.cdc.gov) stated that the exact mode of causing a systemic infection is unknown but that a previous infection such as a viral or an upper respiratory tract may be a contributory factor.

Epidemiology

The prime periods for infections before the establishment of a vaccine were between September and December, and between March and May. Factors that may predispose the individual to exposure of the infection are overcrowding within the household, the size of dwellings, schools, children's nurseries, older siblings attending school and socio-economic influence. Other factors may include whether or the not the individual has a chronic disease, may cause susceptibility to other infections.

Diagnosis

This is usually confirmed by laboratory testing and infected bodily fluid may show Gram-negative coccobacilli suggestive of haemophilus influenza.

Signs and Symptoms

- Meningitis: an infection that affects the meninges within the brain. Meningitis caused up to 65% of cases before the pre-vaccine era. An elevated temperature, altered conscious level and neck rigidity, are common clinical signs.

- Epiglottitis: this is as a result of an infection that causes swelling of the epiglottis, the tissue that prevents food entering the lungs. Epiglottitis affects the throat and causes airway obstruction, leading to a high risk of mortality if untreated.

- Septic arthritis (joint infections), cellulitus (an infection that may affect the skin) and pneumonia are clinical signs of a severe infection.

- Osteomyelitis: an infection that affects the skeletal system.

Medical Management

Haemophilus influenza type (b) requires the individual to be hospitalised and treated with intravenous antibiotics from the cephalosporin group (see http://www.cdc.gov). A 10-day course is usually required.

The Vaccine

The vaccine was developed and licensed in the USA in 1985. Initially it was not effective in children younger than 18 months. According to the WHO (see http://www.who.int), the vaccine in current usage is based on Hib polysaccharide conjugated to a protein carrier, such as the diphtheria toxoid-like protein (PRP-HbOC) tetanus toxoid (PRP-T) or meningococcal outer membrane (PRP-OMP). The conjugation of the PRP to the relevant protein causes a T cell response to the Hib polysaccharide.

The immunisation is usually given in infancy (minimum age 6 weeks) at intervals of 1 month. A booster dose is usually given at 12–18 months of age but in developing countries the disease usually occurs before this age.

In adults and children over 18 months a single dose encourages immunity.

Activity

A staff nurse tells you that he has been approached by a parent whose infant is to be discharged from the children's medical ward today. However, the mother has disclosed that her son has not received his primary course of immunisations because she was unsure of how to proceed with the amount of literature pertaining to the subject, of the advantages and disadvantages. The staff nurse poses the following questions to you:

- What information would you offer?
- Which resources would you provide to support your verbal information?
- How would you explain the method of administration of the Hib vaccine?
- Finally, where should vaccines be stored on the ward and at what temperature?

What do you reply?

MEASLES

Measles is a viral illness that can be spread by droplet infection; the virus is referred to as the paramyxovirus. Richardson (2001) suggested the initial symptoms appear after an incubation period of 6–19 days. The first signs before a rash include irritability, elevated temperature, cough, feeling generally unwell and conjunctivitis. Over the next few days, Koplik's spots develop (small red spots within the oral cavity) approximately 1–2 days before the rash. Bedford (2003) described the rash as being maculopapular (red and blotchy). It usually starts at the hairline and spreads to other areas of the body over a period of 3 days. After 3 or 4 days, the rash may become brownish in appearance and then become less evident. The fever that accompanies the illness usually subsides before the rash diminishes.

Affected infants experience a fever and tend to feel uncomfortable and irritable. Davies et al (2001) identified that infants may have loss of appetite, cough, cold and conjunctivitis. The period for which an individual remains infectious is unknown, although it is acknowledged that the 1–2 days before the rash develops the patient is infectious.

Within the general population, where immunisation has not been undertaken there is a higher threat of transmission. Measles is a notifiable disease once diagnosed.

Epidemiology

According to the WHO (2002a), in 2001 there were 745,000 deaths from measles, and 30–40 million cases. The WHO suggested that many of the deaths could have been prevented by the use of a vaccine. The infection is more prevalent in areas where the population are disadvantaged, this usually applies to the developing countries.

Bedford (2003) suggests that in the UK before the routine administration of the vaccine in 1968, 90–95% of children under the age of 10 years had been infected. Miller (1964) suggested that a greater proportion infected were aged 3–5 years. After 1968, the incidence of measles fell by 98%.

Diagnosis

The illness is usually construed by clinical examination. Bedford (2003) implied that the PHLS has increased monitoring and provided the NHS with equipment to test saliva for measles-specific IgM from cases notified to the Office for National Statistics, thus providing actual confirmation.

Treatment

Children who do not experience complications can be managed within the home environment. The treatment of measles is symptomatic, which includes providing medication to alleviate an elevated temperature, which may be in the form of paracetamol or brufen elixir, and the encouragement of oral fluids to prevent dehydration. Some children may develop photophobia and need to be nursed in a darkened room with minimal light.

Complications

The complications that may result tend to be seen in individuals who are malnourished or immunosuppressed. Bedford (2003) indicated that concerns are as a result of ear infections (otitis media), pneumonia, croup, seizures and encephalitis. Atypical complications include idiopathic thrombocytopenia. During pregnancy, measles may result in premature labour.

The American Academy of Pediatrics (1993) illustrated a connection between low levels of vitamin A and the rise in morbidity and mortality. The administration of supplements of vitamin A has shown to improve the outcome, although clarification is needed to determine whether supplements can prevent measles in developed countries.

Prevention

The first vaccine to be successful against the virus that caused measles was made available in the USA in 1963, and in the UK in 1968. It stimulated the production of antibodies.

In 1988, the British government had a change of policy in relation to single-antigen vaccines, and began to use the combined measles, mumps and rubella (MMR) vaccine a single injection, which provides greater protection against the three diseases. For the first time there was a vaccine for mumps and a single immunisation for rubella, which enabled prepubescent girls to be vaccinated, thus reducing the transmission of the virus during pregnancy to the unborn fetus. Since the advent of this strategy the number of cases of rubella has fallen.

The aim of this programme is to eliminate the diseases and 95% of the public need to be vaccinated to stop the spread of the measles (Bedford 2003). The initial dose of the vaccine is given at the age of 12–15 months, and this is followed by a second dose before starting school. The latter dose is essential to safeguard children who did not have the first dose, creating an opportunity to implement the programme of achieving a high rate of protection and 99% are seen with a primary and secondary vaccination schedule as suggested by Hennessey et al (1999).

Side Effects

The MMR is a live vaccine, which means that side effects are possible. These include fever, irritability, cough or cold, and drowsiness. Side effects are less common with the second dose.

The MMR vaccine contains a small quantity of egg; as a result there has been concern whether or not children who have an allergy to egg should be given the vaccine because of the risk of an acute reaction. Although there is evidence to suggest it is safe, the DoH (1996) issued guidelines for safe practice, suggesting that it may be advisable to undertake the procedure in a hospital setting. Bedford (2003) indicated that most professionals would advise this course of action providing that the child had experienced an anaphylactic reaction, but those who had not experienced this type of reaction could be immunised without any specific precautions.

Activity

Access the companion PowerPoint presentation for information on the debate concerning MMR vaccine:
- Explore the controversial issues surrounding the MMR vaccine and make notes.
- Examine and discuss the concerns surrounding single vaccines.

www

Refer to the WHO (2002b) initiative for vaccine research:
- http://www.who.int/vaccine research/diseases/measles/en

MUMPS

Moses (2004a) defined mumps as being caused by a paramyovirus, which affects the parotid glands. In 2003, the Health Protection Agency stated that '. . . humans are the only known host of the mumps virus, and that it is a notifiable disease', suggesting that when it is suspected by law, it has to be reported (see the HPA website at: http://www.hpa.org.uk).

Mumps is a common childhood infection and may occur at any age. The disease is transmitted either by direct patient-to-patient contact or is airborne, by infected droplets of saliva. The highest rate of occurrence is late winter and early spring. The virus is prevalent where there are a large number of children, for example, preschools and schools. According to the Health Protection Agency (2003), mumps was the cause of 1200 hospital admissions each year in England and Wales before the development of the MMR vaccine. Mumps was made a notifiable disease in 1988. In the year 2000 there were 2162 cases of mumps, with one of the last outbreaks being in the North of England mainly affecting secondary school children, who had either not received the MMR vaccine or had not completed the course and had received only one dose.

Signs and Symptoms

- Usually starts with a headache and an elevated temperature.
- Characterised by a swelling of the parotid glands, which may either be uni- or bilateral. However, the Health Protection Agency (2003) suggested that 30% of cases in children did not show any of the symptoms.
- The intubation period varies from 14 to 21 days.
- Can be transmitted several days before and after the swelling of the parotid glands.
- Individuals who have been exposed to the virus should consider themselves infectious from 12 to 25 days after contact.

Moses (2004a) suggested that patients also experience general malaise and anorexia. This is thought to be as a result of the pain and discomfort experienced when eating and drinking due to tenderness at the mandibular angle, and redness within the oral cavity at the opening of the parotid duct.

Treatment

The treatment of mumps is symptomatic and consists of bed rest, copious amounts of fluid and paracetamol for the discomfort and pain. Most people feel better after approximately 10 days (see http://www.surgerydoor.co.uk for details).

Complications

Complications comprise (Health Protection Agency 2003):

- aseptic meningitis: 15%
- orchitis usually unilateral: in up to 20% of postpubertal males; infertility rarely occurs
- oophritis in 5% of postpubertal females; rarely infertility
- deafness: 1:15000 cases, usually affects one ear
- encephalitis
- pancreatitis
- arthritis
- nephritis
- pericarditis.

Although there is no evidence to suggest that mumps may cause any fetal abnormalities, if infected during the first 3 months of pregnancy there is an increased possibility of a spontaneous abortion.

Prevention

Since the development of the MMR vaccine in 1988, the 3-yearly sequences associated with mumps have ended. No single vaccine that is effective against mumps is licensed in the UK.

The immunisation schedule involves administering a vaccine at 12–15 months of age and a further one at 4–5 years. However, the Health Protection Agency (2003) states that

Activity

With the aid of a diagram of the human body, illustrate the possible complications that may result from mumps. The following might help:
- http://www.hpa.org.uk/infections/topics_az/mumps/gen_info.htm

'. . . there is not an age limit' and, when necessary, the two doses can be given 3 months apart. Following the initial dose, 90–95% will become immune to mumps.

RUBELLA

The Centers for Disease Control and Prevention (2003) ascertained that rubella was originally derived from the Latin 'little red'. Rubella was initially thought to be a variant of measles and scarlet fever, and was referred to as the third disease. It was first described as a separate disease in Germany, in 1814, and consequently became known as 'German measles'. In 1938 the viral aetiology was confirmed, by the passing of the disease to children using nasal secretions from confirmed cases.

An epidemic occurred in 1940, the following year an Australian ophthalmologist – Norman Gregg – described 78 cases of infants acquiring congenital cataracts, following maternal exposure to the virus in early pregnancy. The virus was first isolated in 1962, and classifies as a rubivrus.

Pathology of the Illness

The Centers for Disease Control and Prevention (2003) suggested that the virus may replicate within the nasopharynx and regional lymph nodes. After 5–7 days, it proliferates to the tissues; it is at this stage that the fetus may become infected.

Epidemiology

The disease occurs throughout the world and is an infection that affects only humans. As it is not transferred by an animal source, infants who have contracted congenital rubella may continue to shed the virus for a considerable length of time; a true carrier state has not yet been confirmed.

The infection is transmitted via human contact, either by airborne transmission or secretions from the respiratory system of an infected individual. The Centers for Disease Control and Prevention (2003) state that it is not communicated to humans by insects. The infection is more prevalent during the late winter and early spring.

Since 1997, the Centers for Disease Control and Prevention (2003) has reported that the greatest number of infants born with congenital rubella syndrome in America were to women of Hispanic origins, mostly in Latin America or the Caribbean countries where the vaccine was not routinely used or the immunisation programme has only just been fully implemented.

Clinical Manifestations

Acquired Rubella

The period of incubation for rubella varies from 12 to 23 days. The symptoms are frequently mild and, according to the Centers for Disease Control and Prevention (2003), the infection may be non-apparent. Moses (2004b) suggested that in children, a rash may cover the soft palate and face. Older children may experience a mild fever, general feeling of being unwell, lymphadenopathy and an upper respiratory tract infection, prior to the rash. Both the Centers for Disease Control and Prevention (2003) and Moses (2004b) indicate that the rash starts on the face and generally spreads to all parts of the body. It usually lasts for 3 days and may be pruritic. A maculopapular rash may be evident for 2 weeks.

Complications arising from the infection are rare in children but comprise:

- Arthritis: which may affect up to 70% of adult women who contract rubella.

- Encephalitis: may affect more adults. Mortality statistic varies from 0 to 50%.

- Disorders affecting the blood: e.g. thrombocytopenia, which is characterised by a low platelet count, causing gastrointestinal or cerebral haemorrhaging.

The duration of these complications varies from days to months, but most individuals recover.

Congenital Rubella

Due to vaccine development, initially as a single vaccine and then incorporated as part of the triple vaccine MMR (Box 40.5), the objective is to prevent congenital rubella.

Box 40.5

The rubella vaccine

The rubella vaccine is a live attenuated virus. The vaccine was first developed in 1965 at the Wistar Institute. It is available in three sources: the single antigen, combined with the mumps vaccine or with the measles and mumps vaccine (MMR). In clinical investigations, the vaccine has proved to be 95% effective in persons aged 12 months or over after a single dose. The Centers for Disease Control and Prevention (2003) established that the vaccine is effective for at least 15 years against both to rubella and viraemia. Further studies have provided evidence suggest that one dose of the immunisation, provides long-term immunity, which is probably life long.

Vertical transmission, i.e. from the maternal blood to the fetus, may cause catastrophic effects, especially during the first trimester. The infection may affect all the organs and cause a variety of congenital defects. During this period the virus may cause spontaneous abortion (miscarriage) or premature labour.

Activity

Explore the effects that congenital rubella syndrome has on:
- the infant
- the family
- the National Health Service
- the Social Services department
- the education system.

Initially, the following websites may help your search:
- http://www.cdc. gov/nip/publications/pink/rubella.pdf
- http://www.who. int/vaccines/en/rubella.shtml

When you have found the necessary information pertaining to this subject, share the information with your colleagues and identify services in your area for an infant who has complex developmental needs.

The risk of congenital problems decreases as the pregnancy progresses beyond the 16th week and, if exposure during the last trimester occurs, the possibility of abnormalities is no higher than with uncomplicated pregnancies (Centers for Disease Control and Prevention 2003).

Diagnosis

The virus may be determined from nasal secretions, blood, urine and cerebrospinal fluid. However, serology is the usual method used to confirm diagnosis. Acute rubella virus may be confirmed by a significant elevation in rubella antibody titre in acute and recovery stages, by the serum specimens or by the level of serum rubella IgM (Centers for Disease Control and Prevention 2003). The sera needs to be obtained as soon as possible, which may be defined as 7–10 days, following the onset of the infection and 2–3 weeks later.

Other tests that might assist in confirmation of the diagnosis include:

- enzyme-linked immunosorbent assays
- haemagglutination inhibition test
- immunofluorescent antibody.

Treatment

The treatment of rubella depends upon a number of factors, including the severity and whether the woman is pregnant.

The mild cases may just need to be advised upon encouraging oral fluids, rest and analgesia with antipyretic properties to alleviate discomfort and fever. More severe cases may acquire hospitalisation and treated accordingly if complications arise, for example encephalitis may require treatment within an intensive care unit, for monitoring vital signs to initiating ventilatory support, in addition to intravenous medication.

If the woman is pregnant this will require, sensitive management and referral to other services for counselling, other members of the multidisciplinary team, and the administration of a rubella immunoglobulin, depending on the stage of pregnancy.

References

American Academy of Pediatrics (AAP) 1993 Vitamin A treatment of measles. Pediatrics 91(5):1014–1015

Anderson KN (ed) 2002 Medical Nursing and Allied Health Dictionary. Mosby, St Louis

Aston R 1998 Who wouldn't protect children? The Practitioner 242:503

Baer MT 1997 Pediatric nutrition assessment: identifying children at risk. Journal of the American Dietetic Association 97(10):S107

Baker JP, Katz SL 2004 Childhood vaccine development: an overview. Paediatric Research 55(2):347–356

Bangura K 1998 Dying for a snooze. Nursing Times 94(21):29–30

Barker DJ 1990 The foetal and infant origins of adult disease. British Medical Journal 301:1111

Barker DJP, Eriksson JG, Forsen T, Osmond C 2002 Fetal origins of adult disease, strength of effects and biological basis. International Journal of Epidemiology 31:1235–1239

Bedford H 2003 Measles: the disease and its prevention. Nursing Standard 17(24):46–55

Behrman RE, Kliegman RM 2002 Nelson's essentials of pediatrics, 4th edn. WB Saunders, Philadelphia

Bennett M 2003 Sleep and rest in PICU. Paediatric Nursing: Critical Care 15(1):3–6

Bentele K, Albani M 1988 Are these tests predictive of prolonged apnoea and SIDS? A review of epidemiological and functional studies. Acta Paediatrica Scandinavica 342 (Suppl):1

Black P 1993 Setting a regular pattern: encouraging socially acceptable habits in the young child. Child Health 1(4):154–157

Campbell S, Glasper EA (eds) 1995 Whaley and Wong's children's nursing, 5th edn. Mosby, St Louis

Campbell S, Glasper EA (eds) 2001 Whaley and Wong's children's nursing, 6th edn. Mosby, St Louis

Centers for Disease Control and Prevention (CDC) 2002 Epidemiology and prevention of vaccine preventable diseases, 7th edn. CDC, Atlanta, GA

Centers for Disease Control and Prevention (CDC) 2003 Rubella and rubella vaccine. Online. Available at: http://www.cdc.gov/nip/publications/pink/rubella.pdf

Connellan T et al 1993 COVER (Cover Of Vaccination Evaluated Rapidly). Cited in: Bedford H 2003 Measles: the disease and its prevention. Nursing Standard 17(24):46–55

Cork MJ 1997 The importance of skin barrier function. Journal of Dermatological Treatment 8.S7–S13

Cork MJ 1999 Taking the itch out of eczema: how the careful use of emollients can break the itch–scratch cycle. Asthma Journal 4:116–120

Crawford J 1995 Winning the fight against disease: a review of childhood immunisation. Child Health 2(5):187–191

Dales L, Hammer SJ, Smith NJ 2001 Time trends in autism and in MMR immunization, coverage in California. Journal of the American Medical Association 285: 1183–1185

David TJ 1993 Food and food additive intolerance in childhood. Blackwell Scientific, Oxford

Davies E et al 2001 Manual of childhood infections. Cited in: Bedford H 2003 Measles: the disease and its prevention. Nursing Standard 17(24):46–55

Department of Health (DoH) 1992 Health of the nation: a strategy for health in England. HMSO, London

Department of Health (DoH) 1994 COMA report on weaning and the weaning diet. HMSO, London

Department of Health (DoH) 1996 Immunisation against infectious diseases. Online. Available at: http://www.greenbook/index.htm

Department of Health (DoH) 1998 Our healthier nation. HMSO, London

Department of Health (DoH) 2002 About pertussis (whooping cough). Online. Available at: http://www.immunisation.org.uk

Department of Health. (DoH) 2003 NHS immunisation statistics. Online. Available at: http://www.dh.gov.uk/Policy/ions/topics

De Serres G et al 1995 Measles vaccine efficacy during an outbreak in a highly vaccinated population: incremental increase in protection with age at vaccination up to 18 months. Cited in: Bedford H 2003 Measles: the disease and its prevention. Nursing Standard 17(24):46–55

Devilliers AC, de Waard-van der Spek FB, Mulder PG, Oranje AP 2002 Treatment of refractory atopic dermatitis using 'wet wrap' dressings and diluted corticosteroids: results of standardised treatment in both children and adults. Dermatology 204(1):50–55

Donald S 1997 Know how: wet wraps in atopic eczema. Nursing Times 93(44):67–68

Duxbury J 1994 Understanding the nature of sleep. Nursing Standard 9(9):25–28

Edmond AM et al 1999 Haemoglobin and ferritin concentrations in infants at 8 months. Archives of Disease in Childhood 74:36–39

Eriksson JG, Forsen T, Osmond C, Barker DJP 2001 Early growth and coronary heart disease in later life: longitudinal study. British Medical Journal 322:949–953

Fewtrell M, Lucas A, Morgan JB 2003 Factors associated with weaning in full term and preterm infants. Archives of Disease in Childhood. Neonatal edition F296, F301, Ed 88

Finlay G 1991 Sleep and intensive care. Intensive Care Nursing 7:61–68

Fiocchi A, Restani P, Gualtiero L, Martelli A 2003 Clinical tolerance to lactose in children with cows milk allergy. Pediatrics 112(2):359

Fischer G 1996 Compliance problems in paediatric atopic eczema. Australia Journal of Dermatology 37(Suppl)1:S10–S13

Food Standards Agency (FSA) 2003 Food intolerance. Online. Available at: http://www.foodstandards.gov.uk

Foote KD, Marriott LD 2003 Weaning of infants. Archives of Diseases in Childhood 88:488–492

Hall M 1996 Health for all children. Oxford University Press, Oxford

Hamlyn B, Brooker S, Oleinikova K, Wands S 2000 Infant feeding survey 2000. BMRB International, London. Online. Available at: http://www.doh.gov.uk/public/infantfeedingreport.htm

Hanifin JM, Cooper KD, Ho VC et al 2004 Guidelines of care for atopic dermatitis. Developed in accordance with the American Academy of Dermatology (AAD)/American Academy of Dermatology Association 'Administrative Regulations for Evidence-Based Clinical Practice Guidelines'. Journal of the American Academy of Dermatology 50(3):391–404

Hanifin JM, Rajka G 1980 Diagnostic features of atopic dermatitis. Acta Dermatologica Venreologica 92:44–47

Health Development Agency (HAD) 1998 Effectiveness of interventions to promote healthy feeding of infants under one year of age. Health promotion effectiveness reviews. Summary bulletin 9. HMSO, London

Health Education Agency (HEA) 1998 A strategic programme. HEA, London

Health Protection Agency (HPA) 2003 Infections. Fact sheet for schools: wired for health. Online. Available at: http://www.hpa.org.uk/infections/topics

Hennessey K et al 1999 Measles epidemic in Romania 1996–1998: assessment of vaccine effectiveness by case control and cohort studies. Cited in: Bedford H 2003 Measles: the disease and its prevention. Nursing Standard 17(24):46–55

Hoare C, Li Wan Po A, Williams H 2000 Systematic review of treatments of atopic eczema. Health Technology and Assessment 4(37):1–191

Hockenberry MJ 2003 Wong's Nursing care of infants and children, 7th edn. Mosby, St Louis

Hogg G 1998 Sleep deprivation in a high dependency unit. Professional Nurse 13(10):693–696

Hubbard S, Trigg E 2000 Practices in children's nursing. Guidelines for hospital and community. Churchill Livingstone, London

Krugman S, Dubowitz H 2003 Failure to thrive. American Family Physician 68(5):879–884

Lanigan JA, Bishop JA, Kimber AC, Morgan J 2001 Systematic review concerning the age of introduction of complementary foods to the healthy full-term infant. European Journal of Clinical Nutrition 55:309–320

Lawrence RA 1989 Breastfeeding: a guide for the medical professional, 3rd edn. Mosby Yearbook, St Louis

Lindsey E, Hartrick G 1996 health promoting nursing practice: the demise of the nursing process? Journal of Advanced Nursing 23(1):106–112

Long A, Hartwell P 1947 Tetanus in the US army in World War II. Cited in: Steimle D, Aston R, Van Damme P (eds) 2002 Tetanus and diphtheria. Nursing Standard 16(22):33–35

Mathieson A 1995 Infant weaning: the COMA report. Nursing Standard 9(16):25–30

McCarthy H 2001 Childhood immunisation. Nursing Standard 15(44):39–44

Miller D 1964 Frequency of complications of measles 1963. Report on a national inquiry by the Public Health Laboratory Service in collaboration with the Society of Medical Officers of Health. Cited in: Bedford H 2003 Measles: the disease and its prevention. Nursing Standard 17(24):46–55

Moses S 2004a Mumps. Practice notebook.com, a family medicine resource. Online. Available at: http://www.fpnotebook.com/ID233.htm

Moses S 2004b Rubella. Practice notebook.com, a family medicine resource. Online. Available at: http:www.fpnotebook.com/ID233.htm

National Eczema Society (2003) Online. Available at: http://www.eczema.org

Parish HJ 1965 A history of immunisation. E and S Livingstone, Edinburgh

Pei AYS, Chan HHL, Ho KM 2001 The effectiveness of wet wrap dressings using 0.1% mometasone furoate and 0.005% fluticasone proprionate ointments in the treatment of moderate to severe atopic dermatitis in children. Pediatric Dermatology 18(4):343–348

Public Health Laboratory Service (PHLS) 2000 Cited in: Steimle D, Aston R, Van Damme P (eds) 2002 Tetanus and diphtheria. Nursing Standard 16(22):33–35

Ramsay M et al 1994 Measles vaccine: a 27-year follow up. Cited in: Bedford H 2003 Measles: the disease and its prevention. Nursing Standard 17(24):46–55

Richardson M et al 2001 Evidence base of incubation periods, periods of infectiousness and exclusion policies for the control of communicable diseases in schools and preschools. Pediatric Infectious Diseases Journal 20(4):380–391

Sachs A 1952 Modern views on the prevention of tetanus in the wounded. Journal of the Royal Society of Medicine 45:641–650

Savoie N, Rioux FM 2002 Impact of maternal anaemia on the infant's iron status at 9 months of age. Canadian Journal of Public Health 93:203–207

Scientific Advisory Committee on Nutrition 2003 Introduction of solid foods. DoH, London

Shaw NJ, Pal BR 2002 Vitamin D deficiency in UK Asian families: activating a new concern. Archives of Diseases in Childhood 86:147–149

Singhal A, Cole TJ, Lucas A 2001 Early nutrition in preterm infants and later blood pressure. The Lancet 357:413–419

Spagnola C, Korb JD 2002 Atopic dermatitis. eMedicine Journal 3(10)

Spencer NJ Coe C 2000 Parent reported infant health and illness in a whole year birth cohort. Child: Care, Health and Development. 26(6):489

Steimle D, Aston R, Van Damme P 2002 Tetanus and diphtheria. Nursing Standard 16(22):33–35

Tudor-Hart J 1971 The inverse care law. Lancet i:405–412

Twitchen LJ, Lowe JA 1998 Atopic eczema and wet-wrap dressings. Professional Nurse 14(2):113–116

Uhlmann V, Martin CM, Sheils O et al 2002 Potential viral pathogenic mechanism for new variant inflammatory bowel disease. Molecular Pathology 55:1–6

Wakefield A et al 1998 Ileal-lymphoid nodular hyperplasia, non-specific colitis and pervasive development disorder in children. Lancet 351(9103):637–641

Waugh A, Grant A 2003 Ross and Wilson anatomy and physiology in health and illness, 9th edn. Churchill Livingstone, London

Wells J 2002 Growth and failure to thrive. Paediatric Nursing 14(3):37–42

Williams M 1999 Food intolerance. Nursing Times 95(21):68–69

Wilson AC, Forsyth JS, Greene SA 1998 Relation of infant diet to childhood health; seven year follow up of cohort of children in Dundee infant feeding study. British Medical Journal 316:21–25

World Health Organization (WHO) 1984 Report of the working group on concepts and principles of health promotion. WHO, Copenhagen

World Health Organization (WHO) 2001 Vaccines, immunisation and biologicals: neonatal and maternal tetanus. Online. Available at: http://www.who.int/vaccines /en tetanus shtml

World Health Organization (WHO) 2002a Child and adolescent health and development. Cited in: Bedford H 2003 Measles: the disease and its prevention. Nursing Standard 17(24):46–55

World Health Organization (WHO) 2002b Initiative for vaccine research. Online. Available at: http://www-who.int/vaccine_research/diseases/measles/en

World Health Organization (WHO) 2003 Immunization, vaccines, biologicals. Online. Available at: http://www.who.int/vaccines/en/haeflub.shtml

Useful Websites

Polio eradication initative: http://www.polioeradication.org/vaccines/polioeradication/all/background/disease/asp

Information in relation to child health issues: http://www.cyh.com/cyh/parentopics/usr-srch 2.stm

Advice for parents regarding childhood illness: http://www.surgerydoor.co.uk

Chapter Forty One

41

Health Problems in Early Childhood

Arija Nikola Parker

ABSTRACT

Early childhood, as a period of growth and development, is a wonderful time in a child's life, characterised by the opportunity to explore a world that has a lot to offer in terms of exploration and discovery from a preschooler's perspective. Parents will have a similarly rewarding experience, observing through their own eyes the experiences of their offspring. However, the magic and wonder of this period can, in reality, be very different, depending on social, economic and political factors, and the lifestyles we have to pursue living in the 21st century. This might mean that this is a very stressful time for parents and children alike. In addition to the broader societal influences, health problems may occur by the very nature of the developmental stage the child is progressing through. Preschool children are constantly on the move, questioning and reacting to everything around them in the absence of the sophisticated cognitive ability to deal with the potential dangers that seem to be around every corner, even within the child's home itself. It is a period of life when a large percentage of this age group are socialised into nursery schools and see a wider world than that of home and family. As a result, they are influenced by their peer group and other significant adults such as nursery nurses and teachers.

Learning Outcomes

- Identify the health problems that may specifically affect the early childhood period.
- Link the problems to the preschool developmental stage of childhood.
- Utilise the brief discussions to expand and develop knowledge and understanding in relation to children's nursing practice.
- Acquire a basic understanding of how the Activities of Living (Roper et al 1996) apply to children's nursing practice.

Introduction

This chapter will address the health problems specifically related to preschool children, with the obvious exclusion of issues covered directly in other chapters. Each section, structured by a heading relating to Activities of Living [see Box 41.1 (Roper et al 1996)], will detail the developmental and physiological aspects that relate specifically to the preschool child. This is followed by a brief description of the health-related problem, its management and the implications for the healthcare professional, most usually a practice nurse, children's nurse, health visitor or community children's nurse. These implications relate particularly to the nurse's role in offering parental advice and education, ensuring that this chapter has a health promotion/education focus. The broad range of topics covered means that detailed information will have to be gained by reading the more specifically focused related chapters, utilising the companion PowerPoint presentation, consulting the related websites and further reading references evident at the end of the chapter.

PowerPoint

The companion PowerPoint presentation contains supplementary information and answers to questions posed within this chapter.

The overall aim is to take a tour around the child and family's daily life, identifying where health problems may occur that will bring them into contact with healthcare professionals and, more particularly, children's nurses and/or health visitors. In light of the need for a holistic approach to subject coverage and a felt requirement for this chapter to have a structure, the Roper–Logan–Tierney model of Activities of Daily Living (1996) will be used as subheadings to ensure subject coverage. Although this model is not utilised exclusively in the children's nursing world, its influence is evident in any piece of nursing documentation used in paediatric clinical areas. It is generally integrated into a framework to support the philosophy of family-centred care widely cited and utilised in the practice of children's nursing.

The model uses a framework of twelve activities (Box 41.1) of living used within the context of biological, psychological, sociocultural, environmental and politico-economic factors that will impinge and affect an individual's life in society today. The model of living incorporates the idea of lifespan from birth to death, however short or long an individual's life may be. The children's nurse is thus usually involved in her client's care for only one stage of a person's lifespan and has a significant role in assisting child and family to reach adulthood by optimising health potential. The idea of a dependence/independence continuum, which is another element of the model, transfers readily to a children's health and social care setting, although the process of gaining independence is not motivated by the notion of being healthy or being ill but via the process of a developing child making the first steps to doing things on his or her own and gaining independence in activities of living. In the same way as with an adult patient, illness will scupper the drive for independence temporarily, where in a child's case re-learning skills barely learned should be achieved with relative ease. Thus the preschooler's dependence on parents/carers fluctuates as he or she starts learning to perform the activity of living tasks alone, although dependence on parents is high because of the need for constant supervision.

From the perspective of the children's nurse caring for a sick child during a period of illness, regression in skill acquisition may occur, which will cause great frustration to a child who is gaining independence, and confusion may arise in relation to a child's developing independence if, for example, a nurse may take on the caring role without understanding the roles the child is developing, i.e. dressing a child who usually, with minimal assistance, would work through getting dressed in the morning. Insight into the child's developmental stage and an appreciation of the family dynamics gained via questions triggered by such a model give the nurse valuable information regarding her client to then individualise care via the use of the nursing process (Roper et al 1996).

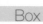

Box 41.1

Activities of living (from Roper et al 1996)

- Maintaining a safe environment
- Communicating
- Controlling body temperature
- Breathing
- Eating and drinking
- Eliminating
- Personal cleansing and dressing
- Mobilising
- Working and playing
- Expressing sexuality
- Sleeping
- Dying

Reflect on your Practice

- Are nursing models used in the clinical areas in which you have clinical experience?
- If so, which models are used?
- Do they improve the quality of care children and families receive?

Maintaining a Safe Environment

The preschool period of development is a time when a child has the opportunity to explore a world, which expands by the minute, hour and day as mobility increases and as, with growth in height and the ability to climb, different objects become more visible and new targets are more readily achievable. The need to climb higher, explore in greater detail and play more exciting games is a necessary stage in learning and developing limits and boundaries in relation to preventing harm and accidents during later years, although at this stage it means little to the person directly involved, namely the child him- or herself. It is the adult who has the responsibility of averting a potential accident seemingly at every minute of the day. This responsibility can be overwhelming and, even with the best intentions and correct interventions, accidents still happen.

The acceleration of gross motor skill acquisition means that a toddler at 20 months of age is throwing and kicking a ball quite effectively, although the direction and purpose of the act itself may be inconsistent. They climb with no fear of falling. At 2 to 3 years they are jumping, running and riding a tricycle with no problems and their abilities, from a fine motor and gross motor skills perspective, are developing at speed. At this time, cognitive abilities mean that, in Piagetian terms, the child is egocentric, i.e. unable to separate his or her own perspective from others: 'You see what I see, you think what I think', which will affect the child's perceptual and communication behaviour (Bukatko

& Daehlar 2004). Thus, the ability to predict what might happen as a result of his or her actions is limited. Using Piaget's theoretical terms, during the preoperational (or intuitive) period, language is developing, although intelligence is evident before starting to utilise words, as is evident by observing the way children act and behave in their environment. However, although children can link words together by the age of two it is clear that they cannot reason or make sense of the world in a logical way (Sylva & Lunt 1982).

When environmental factors, such as the houses we live in, the toys children play with and the areas children play in – all key components to modern living – are taken into account, it is not surprising that, even with the most safety-conscious and aware parents, accidents happen. In addition, inadequate adult supervision, the influence of stress and the size of the child are factors that contribute to an increased risk of accidents taking place.

These factors account for the fact that 500,000 children under the age of five attended A&E departments in 1999, and that in this year 90 children died as a result of accidents in the home in England and Wales. Although perceived as a place of safety, the home actually provides the necessary combination of obstacles and risks to ensure that the 0–4 age group is at a high risk of falls, strikings (i.e. bumping into static objects or being the victim of being hit by moving object), burns, foreign bodies in eye or other orifices, and so on. The vast majority of these will be dealt with in the Accident and Emergency department, as minor injuries, with no need for follow-up (Department of Trade and Industry (DTI) 2001). However, this is not to devalue the implications on child health and the important role of nurses in preventing such accidents. Thus the role of health visitors, children's nurses in health education and health promotion are key to preventing the health problems that may result due to accidents. According to information from the Royal Society for the Prevention of Accidents (ROSPA), in conjunction with the above statistics, falls account for the majority of non-fatal accidents and the highest numbers of deaths are due to fire. ROSPA argues that most accidents are preventable through increased awareness, improvements in the home environment and greater product safety.

www

The Royal Society for the Prevention of Accident's website contains fact sheets including one dealing with child safety in the home:

- http://www.rospa.com/CMS/index.asp

The nursing care of children who have sustained injuries as a result of accidents is discussed in the related chapters. What follows are additional statistics and recommendations

with regard to the nursing role as a health educator in some very specific areas related to the preschool child.

Accidental Poisoning

In 2000 the London National Poisons Information Service received around 200,000 calls from GPs and A&E departments. Cases involve intentional overdose in adults and adolescents, and accidental ingestion in children, which accounts for about 7% of all accidents (Pickford 2000). The most commonly implicated drugs are iron, methadone and tricyclic antidepressants, although, realistically, anything can be accidentally ingested by a child.

MANAGEMENT OF THE CHILD

The management will depend on the amount of drug ingested and how long it takes the child and parent to seek medical assistance. The care is based on advice offered by the Poisons Information Service. If attending A&E, the parents should take the container, packagig or part of plant/fungi with them and have an idea of time it was ingested. In the case of herbicidal poisoning it is important that the brand name as well as manufacturer's name is known so that the active ingredient and solvents can be identified by the poisons centre (Northall & Cullen 1999).

PowerPoint

Access the companion PowerPoint presentation and read the advice offered to parents with regard to preventing accidental ingestion.

IMPLICATIONS FOR THE HEALTHCARE PROFESSIONAL

Many strategies can be employed to prevent the accidental ingestion of many substances, which include controlling the child's access to poisons, making the environment safer and/or changing the child's behaviour (Pickford 2000). The main reasons for accidental ingestion are inappropriate storage of medicines, lack of safety awareness and insufficient supervision of children. Liquid preparations, purposely formulated to make them more palatable for children, add to the probability that, when children get access to these medicines, they are more likely to consume large amounts. For example, iron and vitamin preparations generally look attractive and taste good as well. Thus the health message involves ensuring safety of medicines within the home are out of reach and out of sight in child-resistant containers. Any chemicals, i.e. cleaning fluids like bleach, should be stored in their original containers and be out of reach and any unwanted medicines and chemicals should be disposed of accordingly.

Part of the developmental aspect of care involves educating the child with regards to encouraging them not to put things like berries in their mouths, in terms they will understand, as well as encouraging parents not to buy plants with poisonous leaves or berries or those that irritate skin. Toddlers put anything and everything in their mouths, so home safety is of prime importance.

In most localities in England, children presenting in A&E with accidental ingestion are followed up by their health visitor to prevent re-occurrence via a system of post-accident support visits (Cernik 1999a).

Reflect on your Practice

Jenny, aged 3, has been admitted to the ward having ingested an unknown quantity of her mum's iron tablets, which she takes because she has iron-deficiency anaemia due to pregnancy. Jenny's mum could not remember how many tablets were left in the bottle and Jenny, wanting to be like mummy, climbed onto a stool and helped herself to the container, which is kept in a kitchen cupboard.

- What are the risks of iron overdose to Jenny?
- What will be the nursing management of Jenny while admitted to the ward?
- What advice should be given to her mother on discharge?

The answers to these questions can be found in the PowerPoint presentation.

Choking

Anatomical aspects, including an obviously smaller airway, contribute to the problems children can experience when playing with certain toys. Children of this age persist in putting all sorts of things in their mouths. It is a problem that has the potential to lead to death, where almost anything can be inhaled including, obviously, food sources. Children aged 3 are more likely to have enlarged tonsils and adenoids, which also increases the risk of choking.

MANAGEMENT OF THE CHILD

The general advice regarding physical removal of the object from the mouth is to leave well alone unless it is clearly vis-

ible and easy to remove. The problem is likely to be exacerbated if the foreign body is pushed further down the airway. Diagnosis is not always very clear but the obvious signs of choking are respiratory compromise, which is accompanied by coughing, gagging and stridor. Evidence-based intervention should follow the Advanced Life Support Group guidance (2001) for managing a choking child, which utilises a basic life support approach, incorporating an algorithm that includes cycles of back blows and chest/abdominal thrusts to relieve the obstruction.

WWW

Look at this BBC interactive resource, which tests your first aid knowledge, as well as being of use for parents:
- http://www.bbc.co.uk/health/first_aid_action/hs_child/hs_choke.shtml

IMPLICATIONS FOR THE HEALTHCARE PROFESSIONAL

All children's nurses should be trained in basic and advanced life support and should be able to teach parents about basic life support and how to manage the choking child. Attendance on a first aid course should be encouraged for parents (and nurses) generally. For greater discussion and detail see the chapter on Respiratory illness in children.

Scenario

Peanuts are seen as the prime suspects in cases of preschool choking episodes. Why do they pose such a risk and what other food and objects could be a cause of concern, particularly for this age group?

WWW

The Ontario Sick Children's Hospital is an excellent resource for information giving for families. It includes a child physiology section, aimed at parents and caregivers, which will help you as a healthcare professional explain visually how and why choking is more likely to occur in this age group as well as discussing the mechanics of breathing more generally:
- http://www.sickkids.ca/default.asp

Burns and Scalds

In 1999, 47,000 children sustained a burn or scald. The most vulnerable group is the under 3s, in whom injury sustained is with hot fluids, steam, hot fat and boiling or hot water (DTI 2001). Other sources of burning are dry heat (contact with a hot surface such as an iron or directly from flames), chemicals, electrical appliances and radiation (i.e. overexposure to sunlight). Again, this age group has a particular vulnerability to physical damage due to physiological aspects, including the fact that they have proportionally more extracellular fluid than adults. As a result fluid loss is higher if burned or scalded. Children under 5 years of age account for nearly 45% of all severe burns and scalds and half of the accidents happen in the kitchen. The most likely suspects are cups of hot drinks, which are inadvertently placed where the child can reach up and pull them over themselves. Other causes include unsupervised children falling or climbing into a bath of hot water and accidents involving kettles, saucepans, fires and chip pans.

This subject area is a topic in its own right and thus is given the attention required in the related chapters. What will suffice here is the first aid advice that may be offered by health visitors, nurses and/or NHS Direct in the case of a child that has sustained a minor burn (i.e. sunburn) or scald in the home situation (Table 41.1).

 WWW

Look at the BBC interactive first aid website. Test your first aid knowledge in relation to burns and scalds:
- http://www.bbc.co.uk/health/first_aid_action/ es_scalds.shtml

 WWW

Look at PRODIGY guidance for the management of burns and scalds:
http://www.prodigy.nhs.uk

Table 41.1 The Immediate Management of the Scalded Child and the Role of the Healthcare Professional

Action	Rationale/evidence base	Additional information
Run the affected area under a cold water tap or in a bath for at least 10 minutes	Reduce the risk of further heat damage by cooling the affected area	Cold water should be applied even if a delay occurs
Remove bracelets, rings, watches and any other restrictive objects	Will cause constriction if swelling occurs	
After cooling remove clothing from affected area	To assess the extent of the damage and prevent further damage	Do not do immediately following injury – it may cause further damage and removal of skin
Apply cold compress if further relief needed and/or apply a dressing	To promote comfort and reduce distress to a child who might not want to see the burn/scald To protect the burn/scald from further damage Application of a dressing promotes moist healing	Do not advise application of adhesive, sticky or fluffy dressings The choice of dressing has to be guided by the fact that it should promote the maximum amount of movement of the affected area
Analgesia	To relieve pain In the home the analgesic of choice is paracetamol	
De-roof blisters or not?	The evidence base is unclear as demonstrated by the following comments for and against: The wound assessment process is clearer and joint movement is enhanced if you de-roof the blisters (Bosworth 1997) The blisters have a protective function and should be aspirated (as opposed to de-roofed) to reduce pressure only if necessary (Flanagan & Graham 2001, Gowar & Lawrence 1995)	

Sources: Taylor (2001), Prodigy (2001).

Non-accidental Injury

The issue of non-accidental injury within this age group is also relevant here. See Chapter 40 for a more in-depth discussion.

www

The NSPCC website offers information leaflets for parents, which are also relevant to healthcare professionals, identifying how to manage challenging toddler behaviour:

- http://www.nspcc.org.uk/html/home/informationresources/forparentscarers.htm

Mobilising

Again in this chapter we ignore the pre-existing health problems identified pre-, peri- or postnatally. The inquisitive nature of the child in relation to exploring his or her environment means that falls and many other accidents can occur, resulting in a range of injuries from simple bruising and sprains to complex fractures. Chapter 35, on orthopaedics, focuses on conditions that relate directly to this age group and gives detailed information of the nursing interventions and health promotion that should be offered to parents/carers and children.

Communicating

The acquisition of language and the whole process of a child's voyage from preverbal to verbal communication is complex and little understood. It is clear that a child's verbal communication increases with exposure to, and experience of, language. It is a healthy response to environmental stimulation, associated with normal development of hearing, neurological function and intellectual development (Woodfield 1999). The area of developing communication skills encompasses many factors, where the key to development is a healthy parent/child relationship. Again the use of developmental milestones, in the hands of community healthcare professionals working in partnership with parents and carers, will identify the very particular problems within the early childhood experience that can pose obstacles to development of effective communication skills.

During early childhood, the child will progress from speaking single words at 12 to 18 months to speaking in sentences, with a massive growth in vocabulary and the use of syntax – inflections, negatives, questions and passive voice – by the age of 5. The child also develops a sense of humour and starts to understand the pragmatics of a situation, i.e. the use of voice, form in sentence construction and choice of word in achieving a given end, for example, a

favourable response to question by the use of words like 'please' and 'thank you' (Bukatko & Daehlar 2004).

Again, community-nursing staff – especially health visitors – are at the forefront of identifying where potential problems are of issue. Any hearing problems will have been identified ideally within the first year of life via parental concerns and/or the distraction test which is performed by health visitors at 6–9 months via the usual child surveillance screening (Hall & Elliman 2003).

Developmental stages again define when children will display problems in hearing due to language development. The rate of speech and language acquisition varies from child to child and, if English is the child's second language, it can be difficult for an English-speaking healthcare professional to assess how language is developing (Cernik 1999b).

GLUE EAR

Glue ear (which can also be defined as chronic secretory otitis media or otitis media with effusion) is an inflammation of the mucous membranes that line the middle ear and is associated with malfunction in the drainage mechanism of the middle ear. The result is a build-up of fluid and increased pressure behind the tympanic membrane. The reason children are susceptible to this problem is the anatomically shorter, wider and more nearly horizontal Eustachian tubes and the frequent upper respiratory tract infections they seem to acquire. It is very much a preschool child problem, whereby one in four children under the age of ten will have an episode of acute otitis media, with a peak incidence of diagnosis between the ages of 3 and 6 (Scottish Intercollegiate Guidelines Network (SIGN) 2003).

Acute otitis media is caused by bacterial or viral infection, as opposed to glue ear, which usually has a non-infectious cause as described above. Glue ear is also associated with perennial and/or seasonal allergic rhinitis, enlarged adenoids, prolonged exposure to cigarette smoke, lack of breastfeeding in infancy and living in a household with many family members (Wong 1997).

PowerPoint

Access the companion PowerPoint presentation and find the diagram of the major parts of the ear. Test your knowledge by completing an unlabelled diagram.

The problem of otitis media is usually diagnosed by parents, perhaps in partnership with health visitors or the GP, because of problems with language development and speech. The child may present with other signs, including tugging at ear lobes due to pain and earache, discharging ears, and general tiredness and fatigue due to having to concentrate to hear, especially in social situations such as nursery. Other signs are deterioration in behaviour, obvious difficulty in hearing – the child asks for the television to be turned up – and speech difficulties generally, i.e. difficulties with pronunciations and shouting inappropriately (Wong 1997). The acute form of the disease will present with the characteristic signs of inflammation including earache, pyrexia and general irritability and may be preceded by a cough or other upper respiratory tract symptoms, whilst a child with glue ear may present only with the signs of hearing loss as discussed earlier (SIGN 2003).

Management of the Child

Pain and discomfort is treated with paracetomol and/or other analgesics and the infection, if present as an acute otitis media, is treated with antibiotics. With recurrent infections, i.e. more than four in 6 months, and in the case of a secretory otitis media, if the child is aged 3 and over and presents with speech and language problems, he or she will be referred to an otolaryngologist (SIGN 2003), which may result with an admission to a local hospital, on a day-case basis, for surgical intervention in the shape of myringotomy and grommet insertion. Surgical intervention remains controversial and the mainstay of glue ear management is the watch and wait approach (or 'watchful waiting'; SIGN 2003), and all forms of glue ear should improve spontaneously (Maw 2000). An alternative approach to managing glue ear is via autoinflation, which involves blowing a balloon with the nose, resulting in a raise in intranasal pressure, which opens up the Eustachian tubes. The evidence base is yet unclear and conflicting, but there may be some clinical benefit (Reidpath et al 1999).

 www

Useful website for users of healthcare services:
- http://www.patient.co.uk

More specifically, information about myringotomy and grommet insertion:
- http://www.patient.co.uk/ showdoc.asp?doc=23069159

Royal National Institute for the Deaf:
- http://www.rnid.org.uk

The RNID's leaflet relating to insertion of grommets:
- http://www.rnid.org.uk/ html/factsheets/med_glue_ear.htm

Implications for the Healthcare Professional

The role of the health visitor, midwife, practice nurse and community nurse in monitoring for problems in communication has already been mentioned. They perform a valuable function in health promotion and illness prevention, via advice to parents to stop smoking and promote breastfeeding.

 Activity

William, aged 2, has been admitted to a day-case ward for insertion of grommets:
- On recording his baseline observations what would you expect the normal ranges of observations be for a preschool age child?

See PowerPoint presentation for answers.

Breathing

This is the period of time, when starting nursery, attending playgroups or just socialising generally, when a runny nose seems to be a permanent feature of early childhood. It is not a very attractive or helpful addition to a child's development, but a requirement in developing immunity and resistance to infection. Life in the 21st century means that the need for childcare in this preschool age group is on the increase, especially where there is an economic need for the main carer to go out to work. Many studies have shown that care outside the home does contribute to acute respiratory illness in childhood and that these children experience these infections generally at an earlier age but fare better in the long term than children who are exposed to infection only when starting school. It has to be mentioned that there are no clear conclusions as to whether this is a risk or benefit overall (McCutcheon & Fitzgerald 2001). Physiologically, children aged 1–4 are more susceptible to respiratory illness due to immaturity of the respiratory system and, anatomically, they have narrower airways and as a result are more likely to have enlarged adenoids and tonsils.

UPPER RESPIRATORY TRACT INFECTIONS

Around 80% of respiratory infections involve only the nose, throat, ears and sinuses and cover a number of different conditions, such as common cold (coryza), sort throat, acute otitis media and sinusitis (Lissauer & Clayden, 2001). Thus a child will typically present with sore throat, fever, nasal blockage and discharge and earache accompanied by a troublesome cough. The discussion at this point is brief and covers minor illness only due to the detailed coverage offered in the related chapter on Respiratory illness in children.

Management of the Child

The illness is most likely to be managed at home and affect all the family with maybe only a visit to the GP and/or advice from organisations like NHS Direct as a health care intervention. The advice usually consists of the use of antipyretics such as paracetamol, rest and encouraging plenty of fluids, although hospital admissions may occur due to febrile convulsions, wheezy episodes and severe upper respiratory tract infections, which will require greater medical intervention.

Implications for the Healthcare Professional

General advice, if sought, will come from community staff, GPs and NHS Direct and/or primary care centres.

WWW

NHS Direct:
- http://www.nhsdirect.nhs.uk/

Asthma

Asthma is a chronic condition characterised by hyper-responsiveness of the airway due to inflammation. This results in the narrowing of the airway with associated cough and wheeze. The causative agents include genetic predisposition and environmental factors, including parental smoking, exposure to allergens in infancy and viral infection in infancy (Budd & Gardiner 1999). Chapter 28 provides much greater detail about the ever-increasing incidence of this illness. It will suffice in this section to give a brief introduction in relation to the specific needs of this age group.

Management of the Child

Attaching the diagnosis of asthma to the preschool child is controversial because at least one child in seven will have a wheezing episode before they reach the age of five. Assessment is difficult, although a diagnosis will require an accurate history of predisposing factors, incidence of wheeziness as well as auscultation and investigation via chest X-ray when a child presents with a wheezy episode initially. Peak expiratory flow rate (PEFR) is not a useful measure in this age group, who are unable cognitively to comply with the complex instructions, thus careful monitoring by parents in the form of a diary, if recurrent wheezing is becoming a problem, is an aid to diagnosis.

The mainstays of treatment and management are through the avoidance of triggers, i.e. allergens and smoking, use of inhalers 'preventers' and 'relievers' using the stepwise approach as advocated by the British Thoracic Society (BTS), which outlines the specific needs of the 2–5-year age group of children (BTS/SIGN 2003, 2004).

WWW

The British Thoracic Society:
- http://www.brit-thoracic.org.uk/

Implications for the Healthcare Professional

Nurses caring for children have a health education role to play, facilitated by the production of evidence-based guidelines that aid a consistent approach to health promotion. The National Asthma Campaign is an excellent source of information for healthcare professionals and parents/children alike. The outpatient clinic and dedicated asthma clinics, in the acute sector and in the community, ensure that very specific needs in relation to symptom management are offered to ensure that a child can live life to the full and not be restricted by the diagnosis of asthma.

WWW

The National Asthma Campaign:
- http://www.asthma.org.uk/

Croup (Laryngotracheobronchitis)

Again, the information offered here is supplemented significantly in Chapter 28. Croup has been defined as a 'swelling of the submucosa in the subglottic area' (Webster et al 1998). It can occur at any age, but is particularly common in the 6 months to 3-year age group. The infection is usually viral in origin and results in narrowing of the upper airway, presenting as hoarseness of voice, with a barking cough and inspiratory stridor. Any swelling in an already narrow airway will potentially cause respiratory distress (Box 41.2) and this is the case with croup, where the narrowest area, the cricoid cartilage, is affected.

Box 41.2

Signs of acute respiratory distress
- Increased respiratory rate
- Recession: intercostal, subcostal or sternal
- Inspiratory or expiratory noise: stridor or wheeze
- Grunting (usually only seen in infants)
- Accessory muscle use
- Flaring of the alae nasi
- Skin colour i.e. cyanosis
- Mental status i.e. agitation and/or drowsiness
- Increased heart rate

MANAGEMENT OF THE CHILD

The key to management is careful assessment of respiratory function as per the Advanced Life Support Group guidelines (ALSG 2001), i.e. airway, breathing and circulation (ABC) followed by a detailed examination of respiratory function. This involves ensuring that the child has a patent airway as a matter of emergency intervention, then proceeding to assess the extent of respiratory distress which includes respiratory rate, effort, pattern of breathing and airway resistance. Croup scoring systems are available to facilitate the assessment.

The potential diagnosis attached, due to the presenting symptoms, may be epiglotitis, although, because of the *Haemophilus influenzae* type b vaccination, this is very rarely seen today. The awareness of epiglotitis as a potential cause still has to be evident if planning to carry out throat inspection or take a throat swab especially for unvaccinated children.

Use of humidity is the mainstay of croup management though the evidence base for using this method of management is debatable (D'Amore & Campbell 2002). Its usefulness as a placebo means that it is still worth giving the advice to parents. All the advice offered on parent information internet sites as well as the leaflets given on discharge from hospital advocate the use of steam to produce humidity, i.e. by placing wet towels on radiators, as useful to alleviate symptoms. Any intervention that reduces stress and promotes relaxation in a child (and parent) who will be very distressed should be seen to be helpful. The use of steroid therapy is the key to manage croup. They reduce the inflammatory response and the steroids most commonly used are budenoside (via nebuliser) or dexamethasone (orally). Both have been found to be equally effective with minimal differences in the onset and duration of action (Chandler 2002). Which one used will largely depend on local guidelines and efficacy of use, i.e. dependent on the age of the child and his or her compliance with treatment.

Nebulised adrenaline is used in extremes cases, although the child must be ECG monitored because of the risk of transient tachycardia. This drug will be used to buy time until the child is transferred to a high-dependency environment (see Chapter 28).

The aims of care are to monitor and facilitate respiratory effort, promote rest, reduce pyrexia, promote intake of oral fluids and educate and support family (Chandler 2002).

Implications for the Healthcare Professional

The management of the child who comes into contact with A&E and/or paediatric assessment areas, which results in admission to hospital, will have an impact on the role of the children's nurse, who obviously has to have evidence-based guidelines to hand, as well as the nursing skills and competence to care for the child and family. This illness can be very frightening and the key to care is communication and sensitive management with the aim of early discharge and potentially a follow-up visit or phone call from a community children's nursing team.

Eating and Drinking

The infant stage of feeding is vital for future development, and the early childhood stage is no less important. A child's energy requirements and need for a consistent supply of protein, vitamins and essential minerals increase with rapid growth and high activity. Capacity for food is limited by the child's anatomy, i.e. size of stomach, so there is a requirement for nutrient-dense foods to meet growth requirements (Flanagan & Kennedy 1999). It is a critical time in relation to nutrition and habits developed now tend to continue through life.

Childhood obesity is of epidemic proportions in the USA and an estimated 17.6 million children under 5 have been classed as overweight worldwide (WHO 1997). The cause of this goes beyond the genetic make-up of an individual. In the UK, the prevalence of obesity in preschool children increased from 5.4% in 1989 to 9.2% in 1998 (Bundred et al 2001). Economic growth, modernisation and urbanisation have had an effect on our calorific intake and the types of foods we eat, which means that generally as a population we eat a diet with a higher proportion of saturated fats and sugars. The 21st-century diet, compared with that of the 1950s, provide children with less iron and fewer starchy foods, and more confectionary and soft drinks (British Nutrition Foundation 2003).

We also have a more sedentary lifestyle and participate in less physically demanding work generally, i.e. children even 20 years ago were walking to school whereas now they are driven everywhere. Today, children no longer play outdoor games, preferring the indoor activities like watching television and using a computer. The physical aspects of obesity will have significant effects on our health, notwithstanding the emotional and psychological effects on the child, who may develop a negative self-image and as a result low self-esteem (Strauss 2001) from the teasing and sometimes even bullying from peers and friends.

WWW

The British Nutrition Foundation's website contains useful resources for nurses and has a focus on education in primary and secondary schools:
- http://www.nutrition.org.uk/

Health eating advice for preschool children includes the advice that children up to the age of two should be offered relatively small volumes of food, full-fat versions of dairy products and should not be given starchy foods that are very high in fibre. Children aged one and above should be eating three meals a day with two in-between-meal snacks. From the age of two there should be a gradual introduction of low-fat dairy products for children who are growing well and eating a varied diet and by the age of 5 should be eating as per 'eating for health' plate model (SIGN 2003), which involves a balanced approach to eating from the five food groups: fruit and vegetables; bread, cereals and potatoes; milk and dairy products; meat, fish and alternatives; foods containing fat and foods containing sugar.

www

The British Dietetic Association offers information and resources useful for healthcare professionals, parents/carers and children alike, i.e. Eat 2b fit campaign (2003):
- http://www.bda.uk.com/

Economic factors add to the problems of society today and economically poorer families tend to have poor diets, which include high intakes of salt, sugar and dietary fat. They lack fruit, vegetables and iron. The effect of poverty and the impact of advertising, as well as fads and diets, all add to the increasing problem of obesity. As healthcare professionals, working in partnership with colleagues in education and social services sector, we have a major role to play in ensuring that parents get up-to-date nutritional advice and are aware of resources available to support families in need of financial help to feed their children.

A child may develop an allergy to food at any time during early childhood, i.e. peanut allergy. However, most milk-based allergies are developed during infancy and were discussed in Chapter 40. The focus in this section will be on the particular problem affecting this group of children, which fits into the title of nutritional deficiencies namely iron-deficiency anaemia.

Altered Growth or Failure to Thrive

'Altered growth' or the more recognisable term 'failure to thrive' is attached to a child who is failing to grow adequately – a definition at its most basic. Another definition is that of a child with a weight consistently below the 3rd or 5th percentile for age and/or a child who is failing to maintain a previously established pattern of growth (Wright 2000). This still simplistic definition belies the complexity of the syndrome, which involves not just monitoring nutritional intake but has to take note of the whole context – family and environment, economic, social, emotional and psychological factors. The primary focus is on weight and this, via developmental screening, is monitored closely during infancy and regularly during early childhood, which in itself is controversial, although accepted as stan-

dard practice in the UK. The constant monitoring of weight can be a cause of great worry to mothers in particular. The controversy is supported by recent changes in the percentile charts used, which responds to changes in UK reference data, reflecting the changes in our society with regards to whole populations of children, including children from ethnic minority groups, which means that children who are simply small in stature do not end up with a diagnosis of failure to thrive. Generally, the diagnosis is made in infancy so the discussion will stop at this point, though obviously the effects on the child and family will continue into early childhood.

NUTRITIONAL DEFICIENCIES

As already mentioned, the preschool child may experience nutritional deficiencies of many types and the key one to discuss here is the effect of iron deficiency, which causes anaemia. The particular groups of children affected are those from ethnic minority groups and socio-economically deprived toddlers (MacDonald 1999). Iron deficiencies impair psychomotor development and cognitive functions. The main causes of iron-deficiency anaemia include prolonged use of breastfeeding. Breast milk is the obvious nutritional source up to 6 months of age; however, the infant needs alternative sources of iron after 6 months. Other reasons include the early introduction of cows milk before the age of 1, and the fact that toddlers tend to be fussy eaters and eat small portions of food, drink lots of juice and are reluctant to eat meat (MacDonald 1999).

Management of the Child with Iron-deficiency Anaemia

The child will present with pallor, lethargy and impaired cardiopulmonary function (Belton & Hambridge 1991). There is evidence to support the fact that even with mild iron-deficiency anaemia the child will exhibit a decrease in responsiveness, decreased physical activity and attentiveness, thus delaying development. Once identified and diagnosed from history and blood tests the child will be treated with supplemental iron as well as promoting intake of iron-rich foods.

Scenario

A parent asks you to identify the food sources of iron, which her son, Edward, is likely to eat and ways of encouraging Edward to eat them. What is your response?

See the PowerPoint presentation for suggestions.

Implications for the Healthcare Professional

There have been suggestions, via a working group focused on the nutritional aspect of weaning (Department of Health (DoH) 1991a,b), to introduce screening for preschool children to ensure early treatment and guidance for children and parents experiencing this problem. However, no guidelines exist at present, although these would be very useful for children's nurses and all those involved in caring for children.

Health visitors will have a key role in assessing and monitoring a child's nutritional intake via diet history taken from parents, as well as educating generally about nutritional issues while undertaking other health checks during visits.

Another area to consider is the issue of food fortification, which does happen with the addition of vitamins and iron to foodstuffs such as cereals. There is a lack of accurate data on the utility of this intervention, although the evidence base supporting the use of iron-fortified formula in preventing iron-deficiency anaemia in infants and young children is more conclusive (MacDonald 1999).

As already mentioned, care has to be taken with storing iron preparations and the drug may cause abdominal upset and constipation.

Eliminating

Early childhood is when many new skills are learnt and one of the key areas involves the move from nappies to using the toilet via the process of toilet training. This usually happens between the ages of 2 and 3, with most children achieving full control by the age of 4 (Rogers 2002). It is a complex process, which involves a lot of practice – control of micturition involves coordination between several complex feedback loops running between bladder and the brain. The child needs to be aware of the need to pass urine, which has to take priority over other activities, of which there are multiple distractions at this age. The child has to perceive the signal correctly to be able to get to the toilet in time. There are also social issues to consider, i.e. sitting or standing as a gender issue. The whole process is complicated by clothing, the need to use toilet paper and then by having hands to wash. For this age group there will be no discussion in relation to encopresis and enuresis – the child is learning and mastering the art during these early years, although this does not mean that a child may have no problems within this activity of living. Health visitors have an important role in health education and support during the toilet training period, which will take place within the child's home in a safe environment. A variety of problems can affect a child in this particular age group, including the intestinal parasites, constipation (which may go hand in hand with the nutritional problems already mentioned) and

gastroenteritis. The subject area of gastroenteritis will serve as an example of a problem that can affect all ages but can have more severe consequences in the preschool child.

PowerPoint

Access the companion PowerPoint presentation for general parenting advice and hints and tips for successful toilet training.

Gastroenteritis

Acute gastroenteritis is characterised by sudden onset of diarrhoea and/or vomiting and includes a variety of symptoms including poor appetite, fever and abdominal cramps and can be defined as an increase in stool frequency and/or change in consistency of the stools (McVerry & Collins 1999). Many cases are caused by rotavirus as the usual suspect, though there can be bacterial and parasitic causes also.

PowerPoint

Access the companion PowerPoint presentation. Study the table summarising common intestinal parasites, including *Giardia*, which causes gastroenteritis. Having studied the table, you will note that not all parasites cause gastroenteritis.

The results of gastroenteritis can be serious in infancy and early childhood because any loss of fluid will affect fluid balance dramatically due to increased metabolic rate and the distribution of intracellular and extracellular fluid, which is different from adult fluid balance (Table 41.2). It is responsible for more than 1 billion cases and at least 4 million deaths per year worldwide. It can occur on average twice annually in child under 5 years of age, or three times if attending child care outside of the home (Prescilla 2003).

Activity

How do you assess the degree of dehydration the preschool child is experiencing on presentation either in the home, A&E or assessment area on a paediatric ward?
Answers on the PowerPoint presentation.

Management of the Child

Mild to moderate dehydration should be treated with oral rehydration solution for 3–4 hours with resumption of

Table 41.2 Summary of the Main Causes and Effects of Gastroenteritis in Children

Causative organism	Incubation period	Signs	Transmission	Additional points
Rotavirus	15–30 hours Once infected the illness can last more than a week, though usually 5–7 days	Severe diarrhoea: watery frequent stool Pyrexia Nausea and vomiting	Faecal oral route with secondary spread via respiratory route	Distinct seasonal pattern, i.e. winter months Mostly occurs in children aged 3–15 months
Adenovirus spp.	5–12 days and the illness usually lasts 5–12 days	Diarrhoea and also linked with an URTI	Person to person Faecal oral Aerosol	Seasonal pattern, i.e. winter months in cold weather
Hepatitis A	28 days and can last up to 4 weeks	Fever Malaise Nausea Jaundice		Children may have no symptoms Vaccination is available
Campylobacter	2–5 days typically and lasts 2–7 days usually with a spontaneous recovery	Pyrexia Abdominal pain Watery, profuse, foul-smelling diarrhoea, which may contain blood	Ingestion of contaminated food and mile (birds pecking milk bottle tops) Undercooked chicken and also carried in domestic animals	Seasonal pattern in that it usually peaks in the early summer
Salmonella spp.	6–72 hours and can last for days or weeks	Rapid onset of symptoms, which include nausea, vomiting and colicky abdominal pain Diarrhoea may contain blood and mucous	Undercooked poultry and eggs are the prime sources responsible Carried by poultry, pets and animals	Incidence increases July–October
Shigella spp.	2–4 days and is self-limiting lasting 3–5 days, though remains communicable for 1–4 weeks	Variable onset with high fever, cramping abdominal pain Watery diarrhoea with mucous and blood	Person-to-person contact indirectly via toilet flush, door knobs, etc.	Frequently affects children and incidence peaks in late summer
Escherichia coli	Variable depending on strain and self-limiting to 10 days	Gradual or sudden onset Diarrhoea is explosive and green and watery Pyrexia and abdominal distension	Personal to person via inanimate objects Undercooked meats	Summer
Escherichia coli 157	1–6 days, although can take 14 days	Haemorrhagic colitis, bloody diarrhoea and severe abdominal cramps		

Sources: Jones (2003), Lowe (2002), McVerry & Collin (1999), Prescilla (2003).

normal feeding following this. The administration of these solutions can be problematic, because children object to the taste of these solutions. The management of more severe dehydration will be dealt with on the basis of guidelines such as those supplied by the Advanced Life Support Group (ALSG 2000).

 WWW

PRODIGY guidance (Practical Support for Clinical Governance) – gastroenteritis:
- http://www.prodigy.nhs.uk/guidance.asp?gt=Gastroenteritis

Patient information leaflet:
- http://www.prodigy.nhs.uk/clinicalguidance/releasedguidance/webBrowser/pils/PL71.htm

PowerPoint

To feed or not to feed?

Access the companion PowerPoint presentation for more information relating to the management of mild–moderate gastroenteritis.

Implications for the Healthcare Professional

Health education relates to the issue of fluid management, although most parents realise that the prevention of dehydration is the way of managing the illness. Notifiable illnesses, such as salmonella, will need to be referred to the public health services and the importance of hand hygiene reiterated to all family members and contacts. The nurse working in the community will obviously need to be in possession of the assessment skills which would indicate, via information offered to parents, the point at which a child should be referred to the acute paediatric services for more intensive management i.e. intravenous fluids.

PowerPoint

Assessing the child presenting with gastroenteritis

Following (or in conjunction) with measurement of baseline observations and general assessment in relation to child's level of dehydration, what questions should you be asking of the parent/carer/child?

Many resources are available to help in the process of managing infection control in places such as nurseries and schools, as well as in the home. Teaching children and families how and when to wash their hands is a very basic but highly effective way of reducing the incidence of gastroenteritis.

 WWW

Many useful resources are available to help teachers in both schools and nurseries to teach infection control to preschool children and parents. Look at the 'Wired for Health' website:

- http://www.wiredforhealth.gov.uk/cat.php?catid=917

 WWW

The eMedicine website is a useful resource. It is medically orientated and American in origin, but provides useful information for all healthcare professionals:

- http://www.emedicine.com/ ped/index.shtml

WWW

Health Protection Agency:

- http://www.hpa.org.uk/

Information relating to salmonella infection:

- http://www.hpa.org.uk/infections/topics_az/salmonella/menu.htm

Personal Cleansing and Dressing

The preschool age child will be learning to wash and dress him- or herself under the supervision of parent or carers. It is an ideal time to check the integrity of the skin and identify any problems that can affect children of this age. This is the time when the child can learn about the importance of hand hygiene and develop good habits that will last a lifetime, i.e. brushing teeth and washing hands, information that will be reinforced at nursery and playgroups.

Dental Caries

An important, if often neglected area, is the affect of tooth decay on a child's development and growth. Dental caries are very easy to prevent and healthy teeth are a good indicator for future dental health (Ottley 2002). Generally, the incidence of tooth decay in the UK has decreased markedly, although there is little improvement in children from less advantaged areas. Children from lower social classes and ethnic minority populations are more likely have dental problems (Davies et al 2001). The younger a child is when he or she starts having the teeth brushed, the less the likelihood of decay (Hinds & Gregory 1995).

 Activity

The Department of Health NHS Plan (2000) national target was no more than one decayed, missing or filled tooth for 5-year-old children by 2003:

- Has the target been achieved?
- Do we promote dental hygiene in acute inpatient services?

It has been found in many studies that community nurses can be very effective as dental health educators (Blinkhorn & Davies 2001). The recommendation from this study was that dental advice, and a free dental pack, should be given at the 8-month hearing test and follow-up session. The basic and essential advice is to brush teeth twice a day with fluoride toothpaste. The preschool child should use toothpaste formulated for children, which has a lower fluoride content, because the child is unable to rinse and spit out the toothpaste effectively and will swallow most of it. Children only develop the manual dexterity to brush their own teeth properly at the age of 6, so the parent needs to assist and do the initial brush and maybe allow the child to finish off the process. Bottles are designed for babies not toddlers and, as discussed in the section on iron-deficiency anaemia, taking juice from a bottle put the teeth in danger of prolonged contact with sugar; a feeder cup should be used from 6 months of age. There is no need to dictate what to eat and not eat, and sweet things can be eaten as long as they are confined to eating times. Early visits to the dentist also help the process, so that children do not develop anxieties about going to the dentist (Ottley 2002).

WWW

British Dental Health Foundation:
- http://www.dentalhealth.org.uk/

Information about the use of fluoride:
- http://www.bda-dentistry.org.uk/advice/docs/ Fluoride-the%20facts.pdf

Eczema

The word eczema has Greek origins and means 'to boil over'. It describes red itchy skin, which develops into a rash of pustules, which eventually break down and leak serous fluid. It usually appears during the first year of life, although it can happen to adults and children at any point in their lives. The term 'atopy' is usually applied to childhood eczema, where the cause is inherited and results due to an immunological response (IgE) to environmental antigens. The areas most commonly affected are neck, flexures of the wrists and ankles, antecubital and popliteal areas (Elliott 1999).

Activity

Define the following dermatology terms, which you will come across in clinical practice: Blister, bulla, erythema, excoriation, papule, petechiae, pruritus, purpura, pustule, urticaria and vesicle.

Answers on the PowerPoint presentation.

MANAGEMENT OF THE CHILD

The basic management is that of easing the itching, maybe with the use of antihistamines, preventing scratching by cutting and filing of the child's nails, preventing infection by keeping nails clean and, most importantly,

keeping the skin well hydrated with the regular use of emollients. Topical steroids can be used to reduce inflammation and as an immunosuppressant. Night-time is particularly problematic, when damage due to scratching can be significant. This is the time when the use of antihistamines is useful as well as the use of wet-wrap bandages, which ensure that as well as cooling the skin affected areas are inaccessible to the child.

PowerPoint

Access the companion PowerPoint presentation for additional information regarding treatment and management of childhood eczema.

The overriding aim is to break the cycle of pruritus and scratching by removing the causative and aggravating factors with care. It has to be noted that special diets used to exclude some of these factors can cause major problems nutritionally and affect the child's growth and development.

IMPLICATIONS FOR THE HEALTHCARE PROFESSIONAL

The children's nurse will be a key information giver and provider regarding the protective basis of breastfeeding for any future children, and also for managing the effects of the house-dust mite, pollens, moulds and animal fur within the home. Caring for a child with a potentially severe and chronic illness can give the mother (as the usual prime caregiver) a burden of extra physical work The time spend bathing, dressing and nappy-changing a child who has the overwhelming need to scratch can be extraordinarily difficult. The diagnosis of atopic eczema also brings an extra burden of housework, as well as making meal times more difficult if a restricted diet is indicated (Elliott & Luker 1997).

The nurse needs to develop long-standing and effective partnerships with the child and family, especially in the more severely affected group of children, in whom chronicity is an issue. The nurse will have to be conversant in the arena of complementary medicine, as parents might be seeking to use alternatives such as Chinese herbal medicine, phototherapy and evening primrose oil. The nurse needs to take account of the fact that many of these treatments do not have a robust evidence base, and indeed, neither does the wet-wrapping technique. The nurse will also have a role in directing parents to seek the help and resources that support groups may have to offer and may also be able to help when the child is going through the transition of leaving the home environment and going to nursery and then on to school.

www

Visit some websites dealing with eczema and offering further information at:

- http://www.eczema.org/
- http://www.skincarephysicians.com/eczemanet/

The following link offers useful advice for starting school with eczema and is a highly visual and easy site to use generally:

- http://skincareworld.co.uk/libraryscw/Learning/ Articles/startingschool.htm

Scabies (*Sarcoptes scabiei*)

This parasite is a mite. Its name, which translated from the Greek is called the 'flesh cutter', sounds very dramatic but this is literally what this mite does as it burrows into the skin. Symptoms occur due to an allergic reaction to the waste products produced by the mite. The female mite will remain under the surface of the skin and lay eggs in the burrow, feeding on nutrients from the cells through which she has chewed. The active larvae will emerge through the burrow to invade the surrounding skin. It is quite difficult to diagnose because the rash displayed does look like an eczema type rash.

Statistically, this parasite affects the school-age child more frequently than the preschooler, although it warrants attention in this section because young children will come into contact with the infection due to family contact and via nursery and play groups.

The burrows are found between the fingers and on the anterior wall of the axilla. Scabies is contagious and spread in children by direct physical contact, although hand holding needs to be for 10 minutes or more. Mites can only survive a maximum of 3 hours away from the skin and they are difficult to catch from clothing or bed linen. This will hope fully reassure children's nurses that it is not easy to acquire the mite and prevent the over-reaction that many lay people and professionals may have when informed that a client has scabies.

PowerPoint

Access the companion Powerpoint presentation for:
- photographs of the scabies mite
- diagrammatic representation of the life cycle of the mite.

MANAGEMENT OF THE CHILD

The key symptom is intense itching, most commonly at night time. The itching is localised to the actual burrow sites, is burning in sensation and generalised. It can be mild to severe and occurs 4–6 weeks after infestation.

The treatment for scabies lacks a convincing evidence base and involves the application of scabicide over the whole body (Hadfield-Law 2001, Walker & Johnstone 2003). Permethrin is the treatment of choice in children. It is applied over the entire body surface and left to dry for 8–12 hours. It needs to be applied to cool dry skin, left for the correct time and washed off with plain, cool water followed by a bath. Following treatment, the rash can continue for 3–4 weeks. Sheets, clothes and fabric worn next to the skin should be washed in hot water and dried at high temperatures to kill the parasites.

IMPLICATIONS FOR THE HEALTHCARE PROFESSIONAL

The nurse needs to know how to treat scabies effectively, based on the limited evidence for efficacy, as well as ensuring that the treatment is undertaken correctly and all family members and close contacts are treated effectively. There is a wider public health issue and role in preventing outbreaks by limiting contacts, early diagnosis and health education. Pains should be taken to avoid scaring other parents and children and to take a reality check in relation to the infection. The infection can cause a lot of embarrassment to the sufferer and family members unnecessarily, and this is avoidable with education and support.

Head Lice

Head lice are small, six-legged wingless insects, grey–brown in colour and 1–3 mm long. They feed by sucking blood from the scalp of their host every 3–6 hours. The female louse lays about five eggs a day. These are smaller than pin heads and are laid on the hair shaft 1.5 cm from the scalp surface. The eggs hatch in about 7 days and the egg shells are left empty (nits). The young head lice (nymphs) take about 6–12 days to mature. The best places to find live lice are behind the ears and on the back of the head. The diagnosis can only be made on identifying a living, moving, head louse found in the hair (Blenkinsop 2003). Infestation is wide spread, especially in nurseries and schools. It is very irritating and if left untreated skin infections can occur.

PowerPoint

Access the companion Powerpoint presentation for:
- photographs of nits and head lice
- diagrammatic representation of the life cycle of the head louse
- health promotion and treatment advice.

MANAGEMENT OF THE CHILD

Treatment is with pediculicides on an individual-patient basis and following a 'structured mosaic' of treatments. This involves using the topical lotion in a structured way checking for effectiveness as you go along. If one fails you try a different class of insecticide from those available. The Cochrane review evaluating the effectiveness of pediculicides and/or wet combing methods was not conclusive (Dodd 2003), although further studies have been undertaken and are ongoing. The idea of 'bug busting' has become popular. This is a physical method of wet-combing using a fine-toothed comb on conditioned hair for 30 minutes every 3rd or 4th day over a 2-week period. The evidence base for the efficacy of all these treatments is questionable, although clinical guidelines do advocate the use of wet combing and, from a common sense point of view, the process does track the life cycle of the head louse, thereby in theory physically removing the infestation and the problem.

PowerPoint

Access the companion Powerpoint presentation for information on bug busting, what it is and how to do it.

IMPLICATIONS FOR THE HEALTHCARE PROFESSIONAL

There needs to be physical evidence of living lice before starting pediculicide treatment. Close contacts should be identified and treated at the same time. Nurses need to be aware of the local treatment policy because there is resistance to some products. As with the management of scabies, nursing advice will have to take account of the embarrassment and stigma children and families may experience. There is no need to keep children away from nursery because they will have had the lice for several weeks before diagnosis.

www

PRODIGY guidance on head-lice infestations is available at:
- http://www.prodigy.nhs.uk/guidance.asp?gt=Head%20lice

Quick reference guide:
- http://www.prodigy.nhs.uk/quickreferenceguides/QR%20HeadLice.pdf

Controlling Body Temperature

Children have a metabolic rate that is three times faster than that of an adult. The basal metabolic rate is related to the proportion of body surface area in relation to body mass, with obvious changes as body size increases. Thus young children have a higher metabolic rate and smaller body masses thus generating more heat with a smaller surface area from which to lose it (Casey 2000). Add to this the immaturity of temperature regulation centre (the hypothalamus) and it is clear, especially in this particular age group, that the children are particularly susceptible to temperature fluctuations. Thus an increase in body temperature is one of the most common symptoms of illness in children, whether caused by infection or head injury (where damage to the hypothalamus has been sustained). Body temperature is not just altered by environmental temperature but also by crying, playing and emotional upset (Wong 1997).

FEBRILE CONVULSIONS

A fever can be defined as an abnormal rise in body temperature usually above $37.5°C$ (Porth 1994), although it has to be remembered that child temperatures are higher than adult ones and the evidence base for defining what is 'normal' for a child's temperature is questionable (Mackowiak et al 1997).

Due to the influencing factors already detailed, it is not surprising that 3% children between the ages of 6 months and 3 years experience a febrile convulsion, which is caused by a rapid rise of temperature, most often caused by a bacterial or viral infection. Febrile convulsions can occur up to about the age of 7. There appears to be a genetic predisposition and convulsions can reoccur within the same period of illness or during future illnesses. Although frightening for parents and carers, febrile convulsions are usually benign with little risk of neurological damage, although some parents worry that their child may develop epilepsy in the future. The convulsions themselves usually last 1–2 minutes and are generalised in nature. If they do last longer (i.e. greater than 30 minutes) they may warrant further investigation, especially if the convulsion also has focal features and/or if the seizures recur in the same illness (Lissauer & Clayden 2001).

Management of the Child

The child with pyrexia will present with a variety of signs dependent on the stage of fever, i.e. shivering, feeling cold or hot and flushed and during the diaphoresis phase potentially shocked with cold, mottled extremities and general pallor (Casey 2000).

Although there is evidence to suggest that a fever has a therapeutic purpose (Casey 2000, Tortora & Grabowski 2002), because the high temperature will also restrict the growth and activity of the invading bacterial/viral micro-organisms, we do intervene to mechanically reduce temperature, the main aim being to promote comfort and alleviate the distress a high temperature may cause child and parent, as well as to prevent any further convulsions. These methods include the use of antipyretics such as paracetamol and ibuprofen, and the use of environmental interventions such as reducing clothing, making sure that the clothing that remains is loose-fitting and made of cotton, reducing the amount of bedding, using blankets and sheets rather than quilts, reducing room temperature by opening windows, using a fan (ensuring that the fan is directed away from the child and the effects do not cool the child too rapidly) and encouraging cool oral fluids (Huband & Trigg 2000).

The use of tepid sponging is still indicated in many textbooks, although the evidence base indicates that it does not significantly reduce temperature and may induce shivering, which will subsequently increase temperature rather than reduce it and may precipitate a crisis inducing a state of shock. A review of a limited number of studies by Watts et al (2003) concluded that there is only minimal clinical benefit from sponging in temperate climates, with the adverse affect of also causing discomfort to the child. The recommended rate of cooling of 0.5°C per hour can be more readily and comfortably achieved with the administration of antipyretics (Blumenthal 2000, Herder 1994). The evidence base supporting the use of antipyretics as a prophylaxis for febrile illness is not conclusive. Pursell (2000), having carried out a literature review of the major studies exploring the effectiveness of paracetamol and ibuprofen in reducing temperature and preventing reoccurrence of a further febrile convulsion, concluded that their usefulness should be considered in terms of promoting comfort alone. He argues that education about supportive care is of greater importance than obsessively administering paracetamol at regular intervals.

Implications for the Healthcare Professional

The advice resulting from the evidence base, in relation to the nursing care of a febrile child, is careful observation of the child and avoiding too frequent temperature measurement, which will exacerbate the anxiety of parent and child (Huband & Trigg 2000). However, it is generally accepted that temperature will be measured 1 hour after administration of antipyretics to ensure that they are having an effect and temperature reduction is not too dramatic. In supporting parents and carers, they should be advised that reoccurrence may occur and to ensure the safety of the child without restraint, i.e. in pram or chair. After the convulsion the child should be placed in the recovery position or on his or her side and someone should stay with child until he or she recovers. Advice will be offered regarding cooling methods and, in some cases, parents will need to be shown how to administer rectal drugs, i.e. diazepam and paracetamol.

The children's nurse needs to be aware of the normal ranges of temperature and how to use temperature-measuring equipment available in the clinical areas and at home. The nurse will also have to consider what additional nursing interventions will need to be undertaken, i.e. collection of specimens, so that the underlying cause of the febrile illness (e.g. urinary tract infection) can be identified and treated.

Infectious Diseases

CHICKENPOX

This illness is the classic preschool/early school years childhood illness. Chickenpox (varicella zoster) virus is spread by droplet from respiratory secretions and contact with skin lesions and contaminated objects. The incubation period is 2–3 weeks (typically 14–16 days). Infectivity is high 2 days before eruption of a macula rash and up to 5 days after the rash has become papular and developed into vesicles, where crusts have formed. Some children may display all three stages of the rash at the same time. The rash tends to spread from scalp or trunk to cover the whole of the body. Complications include secondary bacterial infections such as pneumonia, abscesses or cellulitis or even encephalitis with staphylococci or streptococci bacterial infections, although these are unusual in most children (Lissauer & Clayden 2001).

PowerPoint

Access the companion PowerPoint presentation for photographs of a child with chickenpox to aid identification of the rash in clinical practice.

Management of the Child

The essential management, usually at home, is to isolate the child from others. Calamine lotion may be applied to alleviate pruritus, the skin should be kept clean and pyrexia managed as discussed above. It is recommended that nails are kept short and children apply pressure to itchy areas rather than scratch them. The child should obviously be isolated from others during the infective stage. The illness will only cause significant complications to the immunocompromised or newborn child.

Implications for the Healthcare Professional

Health promotion via GP, practice nurse and/or health visitor is to ensure that parents do not give aspirin or any salicylates to treat symptoms because of the risk of Reye's disease and otherwise give basic advice in relation to symptom management.

MEASLES

It is worth mentioning measles as an illness within this section to reassert the nurse's role in promoting the uptake of MMR vaccination. We are more likely at this period of time to see outbreaks of measles infection where there is low coverage of vaccination. The introduction of the combined MMR vaccine, which was well received in 1988, means that cases of measles were reduced from over 26,000 in 1989 to 2,438 in 1999 with only 4.3 % cases confirmed [Public Health Laboratory Service (PHLS) 2002].

Measles, a notifiable disease, is caused by a virus and is spread through airborne droplets. A prodromal period of 2–4 days when the child is feverish, coughing, is tired and has conjunctivitis is followed by increases in temperature and sometimes Koplik's spots (white spots on a red background) appear in the buccal mucosa before the rash develops. The rash is maculopapular, starts at the hairline and progresses down the body. Three days later the rash becomes brownish and then fades. Complications include otitis media, pneumonia, croup, convulsions and encephalitis. Needless to say, as with most illnesses, the rate of complication is higher in this age group (Bedford 2003, Lissauer & Clayden 2001).

Diagnosis is confusing, and health professionals are now less experienced in diagnosis. However, the PHLS, to improve data collection, now issues saliva tests to confirm illness in suspected cases of measles, mumps and rubella.

PowerPoint

Access the companion Powerpoint presentation for photographs of a preschool child with measles.

Management of the Child

Most children with measles will be managed at home with symptomatic management of temperature (as above). Some children experience photophobia, so the common sense approach of dimming the lights is the best way to manage this situation.

Implications for the Healthcare Professional

The key area of nursing activity is in providing information about the MMR vaccine and encouraging evidence base discussion surrounding the facts about the safety of the vaccine, a debate no doubt that will continue for many years.

Scenario

A parent asks for your opinion as to whether she should give consent to the MMR vaccination:

- Reflect on your own feelings, beliefs and attitudes to the MMR vaccine.
- What effect has the media had on your role in advising parents to have (or not have) the vaccine?

Playing (and Working)

Play is an integral aspect of childhood and children in their early preschool years spend a lot of time engaged in play activities. Play is essential for development, as well as just giving pleasure to child and parent also. One skill learned is another game to be played (Sylva & Lunt 1984). Piaget considered that intelligence is closely linked with play. Through play the child has the opportunity to master and practise skills. The type of play engaged in changes through the developmental stages and thus any problems in development can be observed in play activities, thus stressing the importance of the role hospital play specialists and nursery nurses have when they undertake play and developmental assessments working as part of the multidisciplinary team. We should never undervalue opportunities to play with the children in our care, whether on the hospital ward or in the child's home, because it is a means of identifying in a non-stressful, non-invasive way whether developmental problems are evident.

Inequalities in health were highlighted in the DoH White Paper *Our healthier nation* (DoH 1999). One of the vehicles introduced by the Labour government to improve health inequalities is the Sure Start programme, which is targeted at disadvantaged children and focuses on improvement in the child's health as well as social and emotional development and ability to learn, which involves the use of play via play groups activity.

 www

Useful information about Sure Start:
- http: //www.surestart.gov.uk/

Expressing Sexuality

This is a time when boys and girls are starting to get the idea that boys and girls are somehow different. It is at the age of 2–3 years when children acquire gender identity. According to Kohlberg's cognitive developmental theory gender satiability is developed around their 4th birthday (Bukatko & Daehlar 2004). A child's identification of gender is based on physical features such as length of hair and clothing rather than on differences in genitalia, but in these pre-school years they will begin to prefer to play with same-sex children and to enforce gender-role norms. How much this is due to nature and how much to nurture, via the attitudes and behaviour of parents, peers and teachers, is debatable. This will affect their self-esteem and perception of self, as well as other factors relating to socialisation within specific environments. However, for the purposes of this chapter there are no specific health problems to be identified at this point so this brief discussion will suffice.

Sleeping

Sleep is essential for human well-being and functioning. The human circadian rhythm is cyclical, lasting 24 hours and consisting of sleep and wakefulness, which is reflected in periods of related activity and inactivity (Gustafasson 1992). Sleep is a time for growth and renewal and for the body to rest and replenish what has been utilised during the period of activity whilst awake. The activity of growth hormones is especially noteworthy with respect to the client group under consideration.

The sleep requirements of this age group are still substantial and are individually based and consist of a long period of night-time sleep and daytime naps, which is not surprising considering the activity of the child as well as the learning and growth that is taking place. Sleep is governed by our biological clock. While sleeping, growth hormones are actively functioning and developing. Sleep is a complex process that has two phases: rapid eye movement (REM) and non-rapid eye movement (NREM), which are cyclical in nature. REM sleep dominates a baby's sleep when the brain is growing and developing rapidly (Bennett 2003), which supports the theory that REM sleep promotes emotional healing and the growth and repair of brain tissue (Evans & French 1995). The obvious effects of sleep deprivation mean that growth will be affected, as will the other requirements of normal physiological functioning, such as cellular immunity and tissue repair, the reaction times and the attention span.

Whereas a newborn sleeps for 16–20 hours, a 3–18-month-old child will need 15–18 hours, including naps, and a 3-year-old will need approximately 11 hours of sleep, although there are individual variations.

Sleep deprivation leads to behavioural and family problems; it is not just the child who is sleep deprived, which can lead to family problems generally. The amount of sleep a child is getting or not getting is generally a major preoccupation of parents because of the effect it has on their coping ability. It can lead to disruption of family relationships, marital disharmony and to an altered parent/child relationship (Pritchard 1999). Persistent lack of sleep leads to other behavioural problems in this age group. Other sleep problems include night terrors, head banging and rocking and nightmares.

MANAGEMENT OF THE CHILD

The key is successful interaction between the parent and child. New sleep patterns can be learned, as can other behaviours, by giving the child cues, routine and consistency (Pritchard 1999). The use of 'transitional objects' for children aged 1–3 can help, i.e. blankets, teddies and other comforters. Naps are commonplace for this age group, although nursery and then school put a stop to this. Each situation has to be managed individually, with careful assessment, and will include an assortment of strategies such as developing certain night-time rituals, e.g. bath, stories and drinks. The environment should be calm, dark and at an ambient temperature.

The generic advice on many internet-based parental advice sites is the common sense approach to sleep, i.e. enjoy bedtime and its related routines, not to use going to bed as a punishment or to put the child to bed before he or she is tired. The lighting should be dimmed and everyone should talk in a quiet voice. The advice relating to a crying child is not necessarily to pick him or her up but to stay close. Use of the parental bed is not contraindicated as a short-term strategy for promoting sleep and alternative therapies may aid the process of falling asleep, e.g. lavender oil in the bath and listening to calming music. The use of positive reinforcement can also help, i.e. star charts and rewards.

 www

Visit a website offering advice to parents and healthcare professionals in relation to sleep problems and management:
- http://www.netdoctor.co.uk/health_advice/facts/childrensleep.htm

The Loughborough Sleep Research Centre.
- http://www.lboro.ac.uk/departments/hu/groups/sleep/ child.htm

IMPLICATIONS FOR THE HEALTHCARE PROFESSIONAL

Although specific disorders have not been discussed in this section, it is useful to consider the effect sleep deprivation can have in the home environment, never mind in the hospital sector, for the child and parent. Thus nursing considerations need to relate to how we ensure that parents and children get a good night's sleep on a hospital ward, as well as identifying and helping out with problems the parent may wish to discuss when the child is first assessed. Sleep generally is given a low priority during the assessment process, the focus being on the presenting problem itself.

Dying

Again this is not something we would associate with this age group. However, the effects of grief and bereavement may be an issue and children's nurses need to develop an understanding of how preschool children express feelings of sadness and happiness in general. Behavioural and emotional disturbances may go hand in hand with any of the health problems identified. We must not assume that in the 21st century, in a Western society, all children have a wonderful experience of early childhood.

Summary

This chapter is not an exhaustive account of the health problems a child may experience during early childhood through all the key areas have been covered at a level aimed to arouse interest and encourage further reading to develop an in-depth knowledge base with regard to this interesting time of life not only focusing on a physiological health-problems-based approach but promoting health and well-being to ensure a seamless transition from life at home and at nursery to starting school.

References

Advanced Life Support Group (ALSG) 2001 Advanced paediatric life support. The practical approach, 2nd edn. BMJ Publishing, Plymouth

American Academy of Pediatrics (AAP) 1996 Practice parameter: the management of acute gastroenteritis in young children. Pediatrics 97(3):424–435

Bedford H 2003 Measles: the disease and its prevention. Nursing Standard 17(24):46–52

Belton N, Hambridge K 1991 Essential element deficiency and toxicity. In: McLaren D et al (eds) Textbook of paediatric nutrition, 3rd edn. Churchill Livingstone, Edingburgh

Bennett M 2003 Sleep and rest in PICU. Paediatric Nursing 15(1):3–6

Blenkinsop A 2003 Nurse prescribers: head lice. Primary Health Care 13(8):33–34

Blinkhorn F, Davies K 2001 A role for health visitors in oral health promotion. National Dental Health Education Group Journal Spring:9–11

Blumenthal I 2000 Fever and the practice nurse: measurement and treatment. Community Practitioner 73(3):519–521

Bosworth C 1997 Burns trauma: management and nursing care. Baillère Tindall, London

British Nutrition Foundation (BNF) 2003 Online. Available at: http://www.nutrition.org.uk/

British Thoracic Society (BTS) and Scottish Intercollegiate Guideline Network (SIGN) 2003 British guidelines on the management of asthma: quick reference guide. Online. Available at: http://www.brit-thoracic.org.uk on the 05/06/04.

British Thoracic Society (BTS) and Scottish Intercollegiate Guideline Network (SIGN) 2004 British guidelines on the management of asthma – a national clinical guide: revised edition. Online. Available at: http://www.brit-thoracic.org.uk

Budd C, Gardiner M 1999 Paediatrics. Mosby, London

Bukatko D, Daehlar MW 2004 Child development: a thematic approach, 5th edn. Houghton Mifflin, Boston

Bundred P, Kitchiner D, Buchan I 2001 Prevalence of overweight and obese children between 1989 and 1998: population based series of cross-sectional studies. British Medical Journal 322:1240–1253

Casey G 2000 Fever management in children. Paediatric Nursing 12(3):38–42

Cernik K 1999a The developing child. In: Booth K, Luker KA (eds) A practical handbook for community health nurses: working with children and their parents. Blackwell Science, Oxford

Cernik K 1999b Caring within families. In: Booth K, Luker KA (eds) A practical handbook for community health nurses: working with children and their parents. Blackwell Science, Oxford

Chandler T 2002 Croup. Paediatric Nursing 14(7):41–47

Cork MJ 1997 The importance of skin barrier function. Journal of Dermatological Treatment 8:s7–s13

D'Amore A, Campbell Hewson G 2002 The management of upper airway obstruction in children. Current Paediatrics 12:17–21

Davies G et al 2001 Caries among 3-year-olds in Greater Manchester. British Dental Journal 190:381–384

Department of Health (DoH) 1991a Dietary reference values for food, energy and nutrients for the UK. HMSO, London

Department of Health (DoH) 1991b Weaning and the weaning diet. HMSO, London

Department of Health (DoH) 1999 Saving lives: our healthier nation. The Stationary Office, London

Department of Health (DoH) 2000 Modernising dentistry: implementing the NHS plan. HMSO, London

Department of Trade and Industry (DTI) 2001 Working for a safer world: 23rd annual report of the home and leisure accident surveillance system – 1999 data. HMSO, London

Dodd CS 2003 Interventions for treating head lice. Cochrane Review. The Cochrane Library, issue 3. Update Software, Oxford

Elliott B 1999 Managing atopic eczema: evidence and issues. In: Booth K, Luker KA (eds) A practical handbook for community health nurses: working with children and their parents. Blackwell Science, Oxford

Elliott B, Luker K 1997 The experiences of mothers caring for a child with severe atopic eczema. Journal of Clinical Nursing 6:241–247

Evans J, French D 1995 Sleep and healing in intensive care settings. Dimensions of Critical Care Nursing 4:189–199

Flanagan CM, Kennedy L 1999 Nutrition in childhood: advice and dilemmas. In: Booth K, Luker KA (eds) A practical handbook for community health nurses: working with children and their parents. Blackwell Science, Oxford

Flanagan M, Graham J 2001 Should burn blisters be left intact or debrided? Journal of Wound Care 10(1):41–45

Gowar J, Lawrence J 1995 The incidence, causes and treatment of minor burns. Journal of Wound Care 4(2):71–74

Greenberg ME 2003 Ascariasis. eMedicine Journal. Online. Available at: http://www.emedicine.com/ped/topic145.htm

Gustafasson U et al 1992 The relevance of sleep, circadian rhythm and lifestyle, related to holistic theory of health. Scandinavian Journal of Caring Sciences 6(1):20–23

Hadfield-Law L 2001 Dealing with scabies. Nursing Standard 15(31):37–42

Hall DMB, Elliman D (eds) 2003 Health for all children, 4th edn. Oxford University Press, Oxford

Hays W, Laws E 1991 Handbook of pesticide toxicity. Academic Press, San Diego, CA

Herder S 1994 Sponge baths for fever: a waste of nursing time. American Journal of Nursing 94(10):55

Hinds A, Gregory T 1995 National diet and nutrition survey: children aged 1½–4½. Vol. 2: report of the dental survey. HMSO, London

Holden C, English J, Hoare C et al 2002 Advised best practice for the use of emollients in eczema and other dry skin conditions. Journal of Dermatological Treatment 13:103–106

Huband S, Trigg E 2000 Practices in children's nursing; guidelines for hospital and community. Churchill Livingstone, Edinburgh

Jones S 2003 A clinical pathway for pediatric gastroenteritis. Gastroenterology Nursing 26(1):7–18

Laufer M 2003 Toxocariasis. eMedicine Journal. Online. Available at: http: //www.emedicine.com/ped/topic2270.htm

Lissauer T, Clayden G 2001 Illustrated textbook of paediatrics. Mosby, London

Lowe S 2002 An overview of gastrointestinal infections. Nursing Standard 16(49):47–52

MacDonald A 1999 Iron deficiency in infants and children. Primary Health Care 9(6):17–24

Mackowiak PA et al 1997 Concepts of fever: recent advances and lingering dogma. Clinical Infectious Diseases 25:119–138

Maw R 2000 Re-evaluating the ENT procedures. The Practitioner 244:608–617

McCrea S, Bates N 1999 Acute iron overdose: clinical features and management. Emergency Nurse 7(5):18–23

McCutcheon H, Fitzgerald M 2001 The public health problem of acute respiratory illness in childcare. Journal of Clinical Nursing 10:305–310

McVerry M, Collins J 1999 Managing the child with gastroenteritis. Nursing Standard 13(37):59–53

Northall F, Cullen G 1999 Pesticide poisoning: herbicides. Emergency Nurse 7(2):22–26

Ottley C 2002 Baby tooth care: a forgotten priority? Nursing Standard 16(18):40–44

Pickford M 2000 Prevention of poisoning. Primary Health Care 10(3):38–41

Porth M 1994 Pathophysiology: concepts of altered health states, 4th edn. Lippincott, Philadelphia

Prescilla RP 2003 Gastroenteritis. eMedicine Journal. Online. Available at: http://www.emedicine.com/ped/ topic834.htm

Pritchard P 1999 Sleep disorders in the preschool child: how the health professionals can help. In: Booth K, Luker KA (eds) A practical handbook for community health nurses: working with children and their parents. Blackwell Science, Oxford

Public Health Laboratory Service (PHLS) 2002 COVER programme: April to June. CDR Weekly 12:39

Pursell E 2000 The use of antipyretic medications in the prevention of febrile convulsions in children. Journal of Clinical Nursing 9:473–480

Reidpath DD, Glasziou PP, Del Mar C 1999 Systematic review of autoinflation for treatment of glue ear in children. British Medical Journal 318:1177

Rogers J 2002 Managing daytime and night-time enuresis in children. Nursing Standard 16(32):45–52

Roper N, Logan W, Tierney A 1996 The elements of nursing: a model for nursing based on a model of living, 4th edn. Churchill Livingstone, Edinburgh

Royal Society for the Prevention of Accidents (ROSPA) 2003 Fact sheet: child safety at home. Online. Available at: http://www.rospa.com.htm

Scottish Executive Health Department (SEHD) 2003 National guidance on managing head lice infection in children. SEHD, Edinburgh. Online. Available at: http://www.scotland.gov.uk

Scottish Intercollegiate Guidelines Network (SIGN) 2003 Diagnosis and management of childhood otitis media in primary care: a national clinical guide, 66. SIGN, Edinburgh

Strauss R 2001 Childhood obesity and self-esteem. Pediatrics 105:e15

Sylva K, Lunt I 1982 Child development: a first course. Basil Blackwell, Oxford

Taylor K 2001 The management of minor burns and scalds in children. Nursing Standard 16(11):45–51

Tortora GJ, Grabowski SR 2002 Principles of anatomy and physiology, 10th edn. Harper Collins, New York

Walker GJA, Johnstone PW 2003 Interventions for treating scabies: Cochrane methodology review. The Cochrane Library, issue 2. John Wiley, Chichester

Watts R, Robertson J, Thomas G 2003 Nursing management of fever in children: a systematic review. International Journal of Nursing Practice 9:S1–S8

Webster H et al 1998 Pulmonary system. In: Slota M (ed.) Core curriculum for pediatric critical care nursing. Saunders, London

Wolfram W 2003 Enterobiasis. eMedicine Journal. Online. Available at: http://www.emedicine.com/ped/topic684.htm

Wolkerstorfer A, Visser RL, De Waard van Der Spek FB et al 2000 Efficacy and safety of wet-wrap dressings in children with severe atopic dermatitis: influence of corticosteroid dilution. British Journal of Dermatology 143:999–1004

Wong D 1997 Whaley and Wong's essentials of pediatric nursing, 5th edn. Mosby, St Louis

Woodfield TA 1999 The acquisition of speech and language. Journal of Child Health Care 3(3):35–38

World Health Organization (WHO) 2003 Obesity and overweight. Global strategy on diet. Physical activity and health factsheet. WHO, Geneva

Wright C 2000 Identification and management of failure to thrive: a community perspective. Archives of Diseases in Childhood 82:5–9

Bibliography

NHS Centre for Reviews and Dissemination 1998 Preschool hearing, speech, language and vision screening. Effective Health Care 4(2). Online. Available at: http: //www.york.ac.uk/inst/crd/crdpublications.htm

NHS Centre for Reviews and Dissemination 2002 The prevention and treatment of childhood obesity. Effective Health Care 7(6). Online. Available at: http://www.york.ac.uk/inst/crd/crdpublications.htm

Scottish Intercollegiate Guidelines Network (SIGN) 2003 Management of obesity in children and young people. Quick reference guide: 69. SIGN, Edinburgh. Online. Available at: http://www.sign.ac.uk

World Health Organization (WHO) 1997 Obesity, preventing and managing the global epidemic: report of the WHO consultation of obesity. WHO, Geneva

Chapter Forty Two

42

Health Needs of Middle Childhood

Susan Hooton, Diane Scott

ABSTRACT

The purpose of this chapter is to provide the reader with an understanding of the world of the developing school child and the major health issues associated with this age group. For the purposes of this chapter, 'the middle childhood years' are defined as the primary/middle (in those areas of the country that have middle schools) school years: 5–12 years of age.

Learning Outcomes

- Consider theories of child growth and development.

- Relate common health and social care needs to child development.

- Outline major health promotion strategies and related issues.

- Consider common illnesses, disorders and hospitalisation.

- Consider the needs of the school-aged child in a practice setting (medical assessment unit).

- Enhance understanding of mental health and psychological well being of the middle-school-aged child.

The Social World of the School Child

The health and well being of children are inextricably linked to their parents' physical, emotional and social health, social circumstances and child rearing practices (American Academy of Pediatrics 2003 p 111)

In considering children's health, the need to consider the child's age, stage of development and social circumstances is of prime importance. The child's developmental stage will influence the way he or she perceives their world, the way that he or she interacts with others and his or her ability to adjust and adapt to changing health and social situations. Knowledge of child development therefore, provides vital clues for those working with children about the biological, psychological and social influences on a child's life, and the threats and dangers to children's health associated with everyday living. The better we understand the particular needs of children at varying developmental stages, the better we can provide care that will be acceptable and less frightening to the child.

Reflect on your Practice

Think of a child you have nursed recently and consider how his or her stage of development and understanding helped them to cope with their situation.

The National Service Framework (NSF) for Children (Deptartment of Health (DoH) 2003) contains standards for all groups working with children in health and social care settings and will be central in steering the way that services develop over the next ten years. This document enshrines the basic principle of making services suit the needs of children and states that the care we deliver to children must be genuinely 'child centred', wherever that care is delivered. For this to happen, those working with children across health, education and social care settings must ensure that children's wishes and experiences are taken into account and understand that children need very different support and facilities at different developmental stages.

Initially, the major influence on infants and very young children comes through the family members with whom the child most frequently comes into contact (Bukatko & Daehler 1998). As the child matures and starts attending nursery and school, the social circle of the child extends, providing new contacts and new challenges to the 'established order' within the child's life. For the middle-school-aged child, this extended social network widens to include school friends and others outside of the family.

Activity

- Placing the school child at the centre, map the range of social contacts that the average child will develop throughout their middle school years.
- What factors might influence the extent of this social network?

Many of these contacts will present new intellectual, cultural and physical interests and challenges for the school child; they may be involved in planning activities to help children perform and acquire new skills. Children will also find that as they mature, they have very different expectations placed on them, which will be formal and informal in nature (Bukatko & Daehler 1998).

The early primary school years see young children develop social skills such as sharing, turn taking and participation in group activities. It is the age where rules and rituals are learnt through play and structured activities, the need for conformity in middle school years being a central characteristic within the games that are so important to children (Bukatko & Daehler 1998, Piaget 1968). The later primary/middle school years are a time of gang membership and club membership with secret passwords and rituals that initiate and regulate the order of membership.

Schaffer (2004) proposes that children's groups usually adopt:

- routines
- customs to which members must conform
- distinct ways of greeting and dressing
- private jokes and verbal play routines
- agreed opinions about public and authoritative figures
- agreed opinions about popular music and sporting teams
- common values about what is right and wrong.

It is easy to see how a peer culture develops and how individual youngsters take on an individuality ascribed by their peers. Shaffer (2004) suggests this may conflict with and differ from the culture shared with adults and questions the assumption that young people acquire knowledge solely from adult family members, as 'peer collaboration' is clearly a central feature of maturity and knowledge acquisition.

Discipline is also acquired through group and team play and, increasingly, self-discipline must develop if children are to be included in group activities. Leaders are appointed who direct others and roles and rules are established which the school child will be expected to respect. The child is exposed to umpires, referees, school prefects and monitors and other figures of authority who will control and direct activity with authority.

However, not all school children adapt well to their changing world. Spender et al (2001) warn that many children will experience difficulty with these expectations and that not all school children are able to adapt to the challenges placed on them, often resulting in the child refusing to attend school. School refusal is a common phenomenon, which often presents with physical symptoms such as:

- nausea
- abdominal pains
- headaches
- diarrhoea
- panic attacks.

Interestingly, such symptoms often subside following the decision to allow a child not to attend school (Rutter 1999, Spender et al 2001). The 'peak times' for school refusal are at transition periods and are most commonly seen in 5- and 11-year-olds, when children start or change schools.

Spender et al (2001) also noted that up to 5% of school children will present with other disruptive or behaviour problems serious enough to cause dysfunction and referral. Conduct disorder is a well reported problem for many school children and is diagnosed when the young person can be assessed as displaying different types of misbehaviour, typically three from a prescribed list (Spender et al 2001) and may result, if untreated, in the child being excluded from school. This is an extremely undesirable situation as there are proven links between conduct disorder and childhood truancy which may result in future criminal activity (Mental Health Foundation 1999).

PowerPoint

Access the companion PowerPoint presentation (slide 1: Excellence in schools).

Between 5 and 12 years of age, children rapidly develop strength and balance. Exercise and physical activity is essential for the child's growing sense of coordination and for muscle and bone development. Much of the school child's exercise and physical activity will be experienced through school activities and physical education remains a key component of middle school curriculum. There is, however, much concern that school children in the 21st century engage in less physical activity than children of previous decades.

Activity

Make a list of popular playground games that promote activity. What are schools doing to:
- Promote such games?
- Prevent such games?
- What influences the trends in playground games?

It is suggested that school children are increasingly assessed on cognitive abilities such as numeracy and literacy skills, leaving less time in the curriculum for physical activity (Napier et al 2000). Also, social activity out of school appears to be restricted as school children become more technologically proficient and TV, video and computer games become all consuming. Although these technological games may keep young people occupied for great lengths of time, they certainly result in long periods of inactivity. In fact, obesity and other conditions associated with inactivity such as lethargy and constipation are increasingly prevalent within the middle school population.

The older school child enjoys being creative, enjoying puzzles and quizzes and is able to engage in complex games of fantasy. Stories are enjoyed and reading and numerical skills enable the child to understand more of the world about them. School children also have a developing interest in their bodies and their bodily functions, a factor that has been incorporated into health-enhancing activities. For example, this awareness of the natural interests of children has been successfully applied to teaching about health matters in school as well as leading to the creation of 'clubs' and summer schools for children learning how to cope with conditions such as diabetes and asthma.

Between 5 and 12 years, children have the ability to develop a strong sense of citizenship. This is a natural extension of them becoming able 'navigators' in the world outside of the home; they develop a strong sense of independence and justice and a developing sense of morality. Schaffer (2004) suggests that children develop morally through social and intellectual means, and friendships often act as 'peer sociometrics', providing a measure as to how well children are developing moral awareness. Moral development differs according to how well accepted children are by their peers and how well they engage with those around them. Schaffer (2004) lists characteristics demonstrated by popular children with a strong sense of moral awareness compared with rejected children and children who have suffered neglect and discusses the difficulties children experience internalising and externalising their individual experiences through interaction with their

peers. Such interactions are fundamental to the way that children start to formulate ideas about future intentions and career aspirations, largely based on the roles, opinions and expectations of those around them (Schaffer 2004, Piaget 1968).

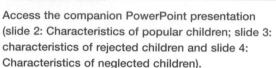

PowerPoint

Access the companion PowerPoint presentation (slide 2: Characteristics of popular children; slide 3: characteristics of rejected children and slide 4: Characteristics of neglected children).

Napier et al (2000) recognise the ways in which education and play are essential prerequisites to the school child in developing confidence and self-esteem. They adopt a constructivist stance in suggesting that school children play a very active role in their development and oppose views that child development is a passive process, shaped by adults. They assert that children are involved in constantly assessing themselves through their relationships and interactions with others as well as through their own social achievements. There is much evidence that personal attainments and mastery over the environment are important factors in developing confidence and self-reliance in childhood (Bukatko & Daehler 1998 pp 255–265, LaMontagne 1984, Napier et al 2000 pp 60–65) and that the establishment of self-concept is inter related with the development of self-esteem in childhood.

Napier et al (2000 p 65) suggest that self-concept and self-esteem are also essential elements in the central task of developing a sense of self-identity. They highlight studies that demonstrate a shift in perspective from the preschool child's (egocentric) emphasis on self-description towards the older school child's descriptions of self as compared with others, which happens at about 7 years of age. The fundamental links between physical, emotional and social development of the school-aged child and how this relates to and influences childhood health will underpin much that follows in this chapter.

The School Child and Health Promotion

The application of theories of child development to the health needs of school-aged children is vitally important to ensure successful implementation of health promotion strategies (Downie et al 1991).

Reflect on your Practice

- What are the major health campaigns aimed at school children?
- How do we decide what to target and what needs to be achieved?
- Who decides what to target?

PowerPoint

For middle-school-aged children, much health promotion activity is directed towards:

- road safety: link to PowerPoint presentation slide 6
- personal safety: link to PowerPoint presentation slide 7
- risks of sun bathing: link to PowerPoint presentation slide 8
- dental health: link to PowerPoint presentation slide 9
- nutrition: link to PowerPoint presentation slide 10.

Those involved in promoting health for the middle-school-aged child range from health advisors at government level and Strategic Health Authorities charged with improving the health of local populations and health economies, to individuals working directly with children such as school nurses, teachers, scout and guide leaders and health promotion specialists who might visit schools and organisations as part of the planned curriculum.

www

Learn about successful ways of presenting health promotion messages to children by visiting:

- http://www.comiccompany.co.uk

The government health strategy as outlined in *Our healthier nation* (DoH 1999) outlined the need to consider child health in the context of healthy families, healthy schools and healthy communities; realising the complex interdependence between children's health and the society in which they live. Schools are often seen to be ideally placed to improve children's health and all schools are expected to have policies for promoting health (World Health Organization (WHO) 2002).

Healthy living and personal and social education (PSE) are key components of the national curriculum, implemented in all schools. In fact, the concept of the health promoting school is now a key indicator against which schools are monitored.

Reflect on your Practice

- Make a list of factors that might identify a school as 'a health-promoting school'.
- How might children's services in hospitals learn from this initiative?

As they progress through school, children are increasingly able to take on board health promotion messages and

PowerPoint

Access the companion PowerPoint presentation (slide 5: Health-promoting schools).

to begin to take an active role in looking after themselves. The cognitive development of school children enables them to relate increasingly complex events and mental representations (Bukatko & Daehler 1998, Piaget 1968). They begin to understand cause and effect, which is classed as moving through the stage of 'concrete operations' between 7 and 11 years, towards the formal operational stage of the older school child who is able to reason hypothetically. The cognitive developmental theorist Piaget (1968) further suggests that school children now become less egocentric and better understand how they relate to others. Although Piagetian theories have received criticism over the years (see Shaffer 2004 p 190), many subsequent studies have confirmed his general claims about the sequence of children's developmental acquisitions and have refined and built on Piaget's early work to address weaknesses. According to Piaget, the older school child also has increased ability to classify, sequence, group and sort complex information and understand related concepts. This understanding will help application of health promotion messages for the older school child, as long as the individual abilities of each child are acknowledged within the process.

In agreement with Piaget, the constructivist child theorist Vygotsky proposes that children are active contributors to their own learning and development. Vygotsky stresses the importance of adults needing to understand the motivation behind each individual child's learning and accurately pick up the cues children send out to other individuals as a 'cooperative enterprise' (Shaffer 2004 p 201). Vygotsky places particular emphasis on:

- Interactivity between individual adults and children: as opposed to relying on age-related learning, which is the traditional Piagetian approach to understanding cognitive child development.
- Contextualising a situation and taking into account the social, historical, cultural and environmental factors that influence individual learning.
- Participation: the child participates and even drives events during learning encounters, as opposed to being a passive recipient.

Vygotsky's theories complement those of Piaget when considering how children might learn about their health and keeping healthy and how adults might more effectively deliver health promotion messages to children.

The concept of empowering children through health promotion activities has been prevalent in much of the UK health promotion literature for the past decade. Many school-aged children take responsibility for managing conditions such as asthma and diabetes and are fully able to self-manage their conditions, which is especially important in situations where parents are not always around, for example when the child is at school or during leisure activities.

Child health should not be seen as a privilege, afforded to certain groups of children. It is now well recognized, through the UN Convention (1989), that children have the right to live healthy lives and much work is directed towards addressing ongoing health inequalities in our society.

PowerPoint

Access the companion PowerPoint presentation (slide 11: UN Convention – children's rights).

The links between socio-economic disadvantage and poor child health are well recognised (Acheson 1999) as is the link between children who live in disadvantaged households and their increased exposure to domestic violence and to childhood accidents. The Children's National Service Framework (NSF) (DoH 2003), which sets out standards for the health and social care for all children in England, states that:

> *The improving picture of child health is marred by stark and persistent inequalities in health between children from advantaged families and those who are poor, across different ethnic groups, and across different parts of the country and different neighbourhoods.*

Successful health promotion strategies are multidimensional and must acknowledge the complex interplay of cultural, sociopolitical, economic and biological factors (Downie et al 1991). To improve the health of school children, the individual child's ability to take on board health messages and the relevance of those messages to the child's everyday 'reality' must be central to any health promotion activity.

The DoH (2003) has recognised the need to understand the nature of children's contact with health services and states that children and young people are frequent users of all types of health care, compared with adults. Children will be seen for routine health checks and immunisations during childhood, and are frequent visitors to Accident and Emergency departments, but the NSF acknowledges the central caring role of families when it states that '80% of all episodes of illness in childhood are managed by parents'. The pattern of attendance of children to health services is becoming better understood. The NSF states that 'a school child will present at the GPs up to two to three times per year and one quarter of all older children will attend an Accident and Emergency department'. What is less well understood, is how to optimise health-promoting opportunities for children, to reduce the incidence of childhood accidents and promote healthy growth and development.

Common Childhood Accidents

The middle-school-aged child has constantly developing and improving capabilities. School children become more adventurous in play, have increased mobility, and are generally allowed more freedom to travel alone (Bukatko & Daehler 1999). As children develop major developmental accomplishments, they come closer to danger and are extremely prone to accidents. In fact, the child's increasing sense of independence can be directly related to many of the major causes of accidents in childhood. Accidents remain the most common cause of death among children over five and road traffic accidents account for two-thirds of all fatal accidents among school-aged children (Department of Transport (DoT) 1992, 2000). The major causes of accidents to school children are:

- road traffic accidents
- falls
- head injury
- burns and scalds
- drowning
- poisoning
- bodily injury.

Minor soft tissue injuries, bruising and abrasions due to accidental injury are extremely common in middle childhood but the most common cause of severe injury and death is due to motor vehicle accidents, usually involving the child as a pedestrian. The DoT (2000) figures show that more than 5000 child pedestrians were killed or seriously injured on British roads that year, with many of these accidents being preventable.

PowerPoint

Access the companion PowerPoint presentation (slides 12 and 13: Department of Transport).

Wilson (1995) states that accident rates in childhood show distinct social class differences. She records that 'the chances of a child of unskilled manual parents being killed in a traffic accident are four times greater than those of a child of professional parents, and for a child of an unemployed head of household, they are seven times greater'.

She suggests that lack of supervision, lack of suitable play areas and lack of private transport are contributing factors, all of which are key indicators of social and economic disadvantage.

Trauma and Surgery

The major reasons for non-medical admissions to hospital for school children are either associated with trauma, often following an accident, or for planned surgery. Admissions to general surgical units might typically be due to:

- general trauma following accidents/falls
- head injury
- appendicitis
- surgical investigations
- lacerations
- dog bites/wounds
- non-complicated cosmetic surgery.

The Royal College of Nursing (RCN) Paediatric Nurse Manager's Forum report provides valuable information regarding the type of surgical admissions most commonly experienced in childhood (RCN 1999). It shows that the distribution of special surgical services across UK children's services is as follows (RCN 1999):

- orthopaedic (41.7%)
- ENT (38.2%)
- ophthalmology (7.2%)
- plastic surgery (5.5%)
- neurosurgery (2.4%)
- maxillofacial (2.0%)
- urology (2.0%)
- oral surgery (1.1%).

ORTHOPAEDIC CONDITIONS OF MIDDLE CHILDHOOD

Dearmun & Taylor (1995) suggest that there are usually two distinct groups of children admitted to the orthopaedic ward; those with unplanned, emergency admissions, usually following an accident, and those children with congenital or diagnosed mobility problems, who can be well prepared for hospital. However, the most common reason for a child referral to an orthopaedic surgeon is following a fracture.

As the developing child becomes more adventurous in play, more involved in competitive sport and is allowed more freedom, the incidence of musculoskeletal injuries increases dramatically. The 'weak link' in the school child's developing skeleton is described as being the growth plate or the epiphysis, making epiphyseal separations common, along with fractures of the child's long bones (Jones 1999). Most fractures are caused by blows applied to the skeleton, which result in breaking of the bone due to the excessive force. Jones states that because children's bones have different biochemical properties from adult bones, bowing, buckle fractures and greenstick fractures, which are incomplete fractures, are all common in childhood. Children's fractures heal more quickly, with quicker recovery of function and, increasingly, children with a fractured femur may find that they can have their traction at home, provided by a Hospital at Home team, to avoid lengthy hospital admissions and separation from family members.

Upper limb fractures of childhood are also common, usually occurring as a result of falling onto an outstretched hand, and most commonly occurring in school playgrounds and play areas. Fractures of the elbow are among the most unstable fractures and often need surgical fixing with plate insertions.

Certain orthopaedic conditions of childhood are more difficult to diagnose, such as the phenomenon of 'growing pains', which is a frequent complaint of school-aged children. It is stated that about 15% of children go through a period where they wake at night due to pains in their legs (Jones 1999). Although this condition affects many children and is acknowledged to be a painful condition, there are no specific clinical treatments apart from sympathetic management, involving heat application, simple stretching exercises, massage and reassurance.

DAY-CASE SURGERY

Many school children will find themselves being admitted to hospital as day patients, as much more childhood surgery is now delivered in day-case units. This is to be applauded because it means that children and their families spend much less time in hospital and children miss less school. Thornes (1991) published a comprehensive report advocating day-case surgery for children and identified twelve quality standards for the care of children undergoing day-case surgery. She upheld the principle of 'keeping children safely within their families, with the parents remaining the principal carers' thus reducing separation anxiety and family disruption.

However, the RCN Nurse Managers Report (1999) found an increasing number of children admitted to adult day-care units with few of Thornes' standards being met. Feasey (2000) undertook a study looking at the quality of care in children's day-case surgical units, across a wide range of ages and surgical procedures. She looked to investigate the experiences of parents taking their child home on the actual day of surgery. Her findings were that:

- Attendance at preadmission preparation clinics appeared to help reduce parental anxiety around the time of discharge.

- Parents responded positively to a follow-up telephone call on the day of discharge.

- The possibility of extending telephone follow-up service to medical admissions should be explored.

- Many families are not invited to preoperative preparation sessions, despite growing evidence of their success.

- Pain control following discharge requires further study.

- Families requiring overnight stay were grateful for this service.

- Information giving (oral and written) for parents and children is improving.

She concluded her study by stating that many more families now expect to take their children home on the day of surgery, placing greater demands than ever on day-case services, and the need to ensure safety for children and their families following discharge from hospital.

Scenario

Jack, aged 7, is to be admitted to the day-case ward for removal of a benign growth. Jack's family live a distance from the hospital and Jack's mum recently had twin daughters:
- Make a list of the advantages of day surgery from Jack's perspective.
- Make a list of the advantages of day surgery to Jack's parents.
- Are there disadvantages from either point of view?

PowerPoint

Access the companion PowerPoint presentation (slide 15: Advantages of day surgery).

Darbyshire's (2003) study of mother's experiences following day surgery confirmed many of the above points outlined by Thornes' earlier work. He concluded that, given the likelihood of even shorter inpatient stays for many children, due to worldwide political and economic factors the 'reality' of childrens' and parents' fears following discharge must be sought and taken into account.

Much work has been conducted on the specialist requirements of children in terms of the care they receive, the knowledge and skills of those providing care and the environment in which care is delivered. The Children's NSF (2003) sets out standards for the environment in which children should be nursed.

Reflect on your Practice

- Read the NSF Standards. How well does your hospital comply?
- Who has responsibility within the hospital for ensuring the standards are met?
- Have children been asked what they think of the standards?
- Should they be asked?

The DoH states that 'Care should be delivered in a safe, suitable and child-friendly environment'. Sadly, the RCN (1999) report found that more than 50% of the children admitted to non-paediatric areas are admitted to adult surgical inpatient areas that do not cater for the specific needs of children.

The Children's NSF has made a commitment to involve children directly in the care that they receive. This commitment has been followed through and strengthened in the 'Children Bill' (House of Commons 2004). The standards have resulted from consultation with children and respond to what children say they most want from hospitals and, as a result, there are standards on:

- environment
- diet and nutrition
- play and recreation
- education.

WWW

Learn about standards for children in hospital from the Getting the Right Start (NSF) website:
- http://www.doh.org.uk

   Access the Millennium Charter Standards for all sick children and families on the Action for Sick Children website:
- http://www.actionforsickchildren.org

   Standards for children's rights to play and education in hospital are available on the National Association of Play Staff website:
- http://www.nahps.org.uk

All these websites outline aspects of care that are important to children as service users but which may be sadly neglected if children are cared for in adult environments (DoH 2003).

The school child's growing ability to understand complex information and to understand relationships between health,

Evidence-based Practice

- Consider your working environment and make a list of the ways in which children are involved in making decisions about the care they receive.
- Can you find evidence that supports the need for children to be more fully involved in care decisions?

PowerPoint

Access the companion PowerPoint presentation
(slide 14: Involving children in care).

illness and treatment means that they can be involved in decisions regarding their care in quite complex ways.

Franck & Jones (2003) have produced a computer game designed to teach coping techniques for 6- to 12-year-olds undergoing venepuncture. Venepuncture is known to be one of the most distressing and worrying aspects of treatment for children (Cummings et al 1996, Franck & Jones 2003). In acknowledging that children need to be better involved in decisions regarding their care, Franck & Jones (2003) have built in a series of options for children to help alleviate pain and distress associated with venepuncture. Options range from the type of information the child requires, choice of therapeutic approach, such as whether to use breathing techniques, relaxation techniques or distraction techniques for pain control, and whether the child would like to rehearse the needle procedures in a safe and fun environment. This initiative demonstrates how understanding and matching the needs of school children to reflect their developmental abilities can result in a resource that helps children make decisions about how they want to manage their pain. Further examples of appropriately and directly involving school children in their care include:

- involvement in preadmission clinic activities
- involvement in care planning and goal setting
- choice around bed/cubicle/personal space
- choice around visiting/visitors
- choice around clothes to be worn for theatre
- choice around parents being in anaesthetic rooms
- choice around parents being in recovery rooms
- involvement in patient-controlled analgaesia (PCA)
- involvement in completing pain assessment charts.

Reflect on your Practice

How well does your clinical area provide the above choices for children and young people?

Assessment of the School Child in the Medical Unit

Due to the expansion of ambulatory care services, many children will now be admitted directly to the Medical Admissions Unit for assessment and treatment. In assessing the school-aged child who presents to the children's medical unit, the need to consider the age and stage of development continues to be highly significant. Obtaining an appropriate history, followed by a physical examination, are vital components in carrying out an accurate assessment and this requires a level of communication and trust not only with the parent or carer but, more importantly, with the child. Assessment should be carried out in a safe, suitable and child-friendly environment (DoH 2003). Increasingly, short-stay assessment and observation facilities are being developed and utilised in children's medical units, with a move to care on an ambulatory basis, where possible. Admission is only usually necessary for very young babies or children with signs of serious acute infection and homecare with support from, for example, Hospital at Home or community nursing teams is recommended.

Activity

You are helping to prepare a hot and anxious 6-year-old for a medical assessment by the consultant nurse. What do you need to consider to help to reassure the child and his father who is accompanying him?

PREPARATION FOR ASSESSMENT

The environment should be prepared according to the condition of the child, avoiding barriers such as desks and with age-appropriate toys or games. Personal details and the reason for assessment are communicated in advance from the referral source and the assessor should familiarise him- or herself with the details, addressing the child by name. Establishing a good rapport with the child and parent/carer from the outset is important. School-aged children generally have had enough contact with healthcare personnel that they can rely on past experiences to guide them (Barnes 2003).

The quality of past experiences may render a child wary or frightened during health assessment. A few minutes spent in determining what the child already knows or expects will happen to them is important. Time taken to reassure and explain to the child what will happen throughout the assessment process will help to overcome the fear of injury or embarrassment. The use of simple diagrams and teaching dolls is advocated to support this (Engel 1997). School-aged children are curious about the use and usefulness of equipment. A simple explanation about the purpose of equipment before using it can be reassuring, for example by telling the child 'I am going to listen to your heart beat through this stethoscope' and then allowing the child to handle and use the equipment.

Establishing a diagnosis rests on a traditional tripod of history, physical examination and investigations, with a carefully taken and properly recorded history as the clinical keystone (Barnes 2003, Engel 1997).

TAKING A HISTORY FROM CHILDREN AGED 9–12 YEARS

Increasingly, nurses are involved in undertaking health assessments of children. In some units nurse practitioners are trained to carry out initial assessments and should clarify their roles in the assessment process as they introduce themselves. Reassuring the family about the relevance of the information that they give and who has access to the information recorded is necessary at the start of the consultation. Throughout the assessment, information should be recorded accurately in a chronological order and following local hospital and NMC standards for record keeping. For example, the date and time of the assessment must be recorded, details of who is accompanying the child and who is giving the history and the record should be signed by the assessor.

Activity

What points need to be considered to promote effective communication during a medical assessment?

A broad opening statement such as 'tell me why you've come along to see us today?' helps to identify what prompted the referral and enables the child or parent/carers to discuss underlying concerns or worries. Open-ended questions used throughout the assessment encourages the child and parent/carer to tell their story and enable a more detailed history to be obtained. Age-appropriate language and the avoidance of jargon is important. School-aged children still think in concrete terms (Bukatko & Daehler 1998) but at a more sophisticated level than younger children, and throughout the assessment clarity should be sought as to whether the child has understood what has been said.

Children of school age are able to give their versions of events with parents' corroboration of certain points. Older children should be able to describe their own symptoms. Gill & O'Brien (2003) give an example of a child's description:

We saw a bright 10-year-old boy with a proven duodenal ulcer. He described his pain as being 'like a laser beam going through my stomach'. Brilliant.

The history should follow a logical sequence with details of the:

- Presenting complaint: this should include the onset and duration of the complaint, any previous episodes, aggravating or relieving factors and associated symptoms (Barnes 2003, Gill & O'Brien 2003).
- Previous medical history: previous notes should be obtained and reviewed prior to the assessment enabling a picture of the child's general health state to be obtained, where possible. Knowing the reasons for previous hospitalisation and response to illness helps in planning interventions for the current illness episode.
- Birth history: more relevant for the younger child but this may be important where the child is experiencing developmental or neurological problems.
- Feeding history: including details of appetite, likes and dislikes.
- Growth and development: growth pattern and whether normal milestones have been reached.
- Allergies: including the type of reactions.
- Immunisations: checking if the child is fully immunised or reasons for not being immunized.
- Medication: recording current prescription and non-prescription drugs, dose, frequency and duration of use.
- Infectious contacts: including anyone else with similar symptoms and exposure including recent travel.
- Social history: behaviour and temperament and particularly school progress and attainment.
- Family history: ages and health of immediate family members, family dynamics, familial illnesses and any congenital disorders.

PowerPoint

Access the companion PowerPoint presentation (slide 16: Medical assessment).

In eliciting the history, it is also necessary to establish what action or measures the child and family have already taken to try and cope with the illness. An attentive and empathic approach should be demonstrated during the assessment, the assessor listening carefully and picking up on what is not said as well as what is being said, from the child and parent. A good assessor is able to maintain appropriate eye contact, pick up on non-verbal cues and give encouraging gestures to aid communication. Respect for other cultures and the use of behaviour acceptable to that culture is necessary. Where possible, any underlying worries should be addressed throughout the consultation. An opportunity is provided to establish goals and to educate and support the child and family. When a child is referred for assessment children, parents/carers are concerned and broadly seek four degrees of information, which the assessor should address:

- What is it? What is wrong?
- What caused it? How did it happen?
- What will be the outcome?
- Will it happen again?

Throughout the assessment the assessor should observe the child, without staring or looking too closely, noting whether the child appears sick or generally well and noting particularly the interaction and relationship between the child and the parent/carer.

PHYSICAL EXAMINATION: SYSTEMS REVIEW

The child's age and stage of development must also be considered in the approach to examining each child. Each system of the body should be examined (Barnes 2003, Gill & O'Brien 2003). School-aged children, like younger children, can become suddenly unwell and exhibit acute symptoms. A detailed assessment should be used to detect those with serious illness or progressive signs of severe illness. An orderly systematic head to toe approach is advised but may be varied to suit the child.

The school-aged child, if able, should be allowed to stand on his or her own feet for part of the examination and the least distressing aspects of the examination should be performed first. Modesty is an issue and the assessor should have a good examination technique, exposing only the area to be examined and allowing the child to remove his or her own clothes as necessary. A gown should be provided to maintain some privacy. It is important to provide reassurance throughout the examination and when normal findings are made. The child's general appearance should be noted including the nutritional state and a record of the child's height and weight should form part of the assessment process. A standing height should be obtained. A wall-mounted stadiometer is recommended to get an accurate measurement, the child standing with heels, buttocks and shoulders against the wall. Weight should be estimated with the child on a standing scale in light garments, and read to the nearest 0.1 kg (Barnes 2003). The measurements should be plotted on an appropriate growth chart. Interval measurements, over a period of time should be used to establish a growth pattern.

PowerPoint

Access the companion PowerPoint presentation (slide 17: Measurements photograph).

Baseline observations should be recorded as part of the assessment process. Temperature measurement is particularly important assessing whether the fever correlates with the severity of the illness and for example, when a child presents with a fever, signs of local infection should be assessed.

There is a changing illness pattern, in the school-aged child from the young child. As body systems mature, e.g. the immune system becomes more competent, then infection can be localised and a more efficient antibody–antigen response produced (Rudolf & Levene 1999). The older the child, the more specific the symptoms will be and the greater the ability of the child to describe the symptoms, e.g. the site or nature of any pain. Physical signs, e.g. Kernig's sign in neck stiffness, are more specific in older children.

A variety of factors predispose children to develop acute illness, such as the development of common infections when first starting school, on coming into contact with other children. Signs of acute and potentially severe illness in school-aged children include (Rudolf & Levene 1999):

- toxicity: a high fever with marked flushing and possibly confusion
- severe pain: associated with pallor, tachycardia and immobility
- change in conscious level: always a sign of a severe illness
- shortness of breath and difficulty speaking
- dehydration
- any acute difficulty walking or unsteadiness of gait.

Discussion with a more experienced assessor should take place on finding any of the above signs.

COMPLETING THE ASSESSMENT

The child and parent/carer should be informed when the assessment is complete, providing the opportunity for them to ask any questions. Appreciation should be stated for their cooperation and the assessment findings should be shared with the child and family carer. Finally, the child and parent/carer should be informed about what will happen next and, where a treatment plan is commenced, this should be agreed with the child and family carer and recorded in the notes.

The Chronically Ill School Child

Certain groups of children will have prolonged contact with child health services throughout their childhood and into early adulthood. This includes children with chronic or enduring illnesses. The major chronic conditions of middle childhood are:

- asthma
- diabetes
- disability
- neurological conditions
- hyperactivity, attention deficit syndrome
- anaemia and blood disorders.

Early supportive interventions by the primary healthcare team are essential in providing support to children with chronic illnesses and their families. Children with multiple chronic conditions are known to be at increased risk of loneliness and social isolation leading to depression. Children's community nurses are well placed to work with chronically ill children and their families and to prevent unnecessary hospitalisation. Carter (2000) found that community children's nurses were found to employ high degrees of trust, flexibility, support, reflexivity and empowerment in their work with chronically ill school children. They were also found to be a much-valued resource for children and families wanting physical and psychological support. Jackson & Vessey (2000) discuss the impact of a chronic health condition on the general development of the school child. They suggest that a lack of physical stamina and school absences, which are often associated with chronic illness, may prevent children from participating in school and extracurricular activities. Such activities are known to contribute to widening social circles, gaining social skills and developing a sense of accomplishment and skills of self-sufficiency, leaving the chronically ill school child vulnerable in these aspects of development.

Children may also resist activities during which 'deformities' or disabilities may become exposed, to prevent embarrassment and ridicule, leading to withdrawal from mainstream activities and social isolation at school. Jackson & Vessey (2000) further highlight the need for school children with chronic illnesses to be given the skills, resources and opportunities to communicate information about their conditions to other school children, thereby removing the 'mystery and speculation' that often surrounds those who appear to be different.

Factors known to place children at greater psychological risk are:

- having a poor self-concept
- having a dysfunctional family
- living in isolated areas or in poverty
- taking medications that affect the child's psychological state
- enduring long-term mental health problems.

Although there are many risks presented to the chronically ill school child, there is also a growing awareness of how psychological problems in childhood can be alleviated by promoting resilience within the child and their family (Ray & Ritchie 1993, Rutter 1999).

PowerPoint

Access the companion PowerPoint presentation (slides 21 to 26: Risk and resilience factors).

Jackson & Vessey (2000) suggest that this is especially so for children with chronic ill health if 'therapeutic adherence' or compliance is to be achieved. This places particular demands on health professionals to work within the ethos of family-centred care and to communicate openly and honestly to school-aged children about their illnesses and to gradually and increasingly involve them in key decisions regarding their health care (Jackson & Vessey 2000). Parental compliance is, of course, essential because the child's condition will be predominantly managed at home. However, it is acknowledged that problems such as overprotection, parental guilt or despair or feelings of loss for the healthy child might adversely affect the child's adaptation and ability to manage their condition well socially.

Mental Health Problems in School Children

Since the publication of the Health Advisory Services (HAS) report *Together we stand* (HAS 1995), increased attention has been paid to children's and young people's mental health issues and the services that are provided for children and families. The report highlighted the increased incidence of mental health problems and disorders in children and young people and the need for improved services, and provided a framework to promote the commissioning of integrated and tiered services to cater for young people.

The Children's NSF (DoH 2003) acknowledges that in childhood, 'whilst physical health has improved, mental

Activity

What is mental health?
Attempt to write a definition of children's mental health.

health problems are on the increase'. Spender et al (2001) define mental health in children and young people as:

- a capacity to enter into and sustain mutually satisfying personal relationships
- a continuing progression of psychological development
- an ability to play and to learn so that attainments are appropriate for age and intellectual level
- a developing moral sense of right and wrong
- the degree of psychological distress and maladaptive behaviour being within normal limits for the child's age and context.

This definition has become universally accepted, across varying professions and reflects the HAS definition (1995) and the definition of young people's mental health as presented in the House of Commons report to the Health Select Committee into Child and Adolescent Mental Health (1997). Others have also attempted to define mental health in childhood.

PowerPoint

Access the companion PowerPoint presentation (slides 17 and 18: Department of Education and Skills).

Activity

Which definition do you prefer and why?

Spender et al (2001) state that 2–5% of children seen in primary care settings who are presented by their parents will have mental health problems as the main complaint. They state that hyperactivity, anxiety or behavioural problems are common overriding concerns. They further suggest that many children will initially present with physical problems, leading to a situation where it is difficult to tell whether the physical problems led to the psychological problems or vice versa. They provide the following list of risk factors to help with individual psychological assessment in children:

- chronic physical illness
- low intelligence
- damaged brain
- parental psychiatric disorder
- family disruption
- angry, bitter family relationships
- rejection by parents
- rejection by peers.

This form of assessment can be used very effectively with school children, who are able to engage in discussion, play and other activities which will all inform the initial mental health assessment.

Activity

- Make a list of individuals who are available to school-aged children with whom children might discuss mental health issues.
- Now rank in order the individuals who young people are most likely to seek out.

PowerPoint

Access the companion PowerPoint presentation (slide 19: Seeking out help and advice).

www

Learn more about children's and young people's mental health at:

- http://www.youngminds.org.uk

The Children's NSF (DoH 2003) emphasises the need to undertake appropriate mental health assessments on children and young people. It states that it is essential '. . . to ensure that staff have an understanding of how to assess and address the emotional well being of children, and are able to identify significant mental health problems'. It further states that all hospitals receiving and treating children and young people should have policies and liaison arrangements in place to deal with:

- management of overdoses
- acute psychiatric crisis
- direct clinical work
- complex cases
- child protection cases
- long term and life threatening diseases
- the death of a child.

It is therefore essential for those working with children with mental health problems in hospital settings to promote the mental well-being of school-aged children and to understand the social world of the child and the everyday worries and concerns that the child might have.

Bullying: Risk and Resilience

Many studies describe the harmful psychosocial effects of bullying in schools, identifying indicators of bullying as withdrawal, depression and suicidal ideation. Whitney & Smith (1993) found from their studies that roughly one in four primary school children and one in ten secondary school children are bullied at least once per term. Health-promoting schools will have policies to deal with aggression and bullying and encourage disclosure from children or their friends (WHO 2002).

Children who are different or withdrawn at school are known to be prime targets for bullying, placing school children with illnesses or disabilities at particular risk. Supervision and active promotion of resilience within all children are factors that reduce bullying (Social Services Inspectorate 1998, Whitney & Smith 1993). The Social Services Inspectorate reports highlight the particular social needs of disabled children at school. Few would dispute the move towards integrating children with special needs and disabilities into mainstream education, the benefits to both disabled and non-disabled children have been well discussed, however children with disabilities in mainstream schools need particular support. The Social Services Inspectors report (1998) states that there are 327,000 children under the age of 16 in England and Wales who have one or more disabilities. This figure is likely to rise with the number of infants now receiving early neonatal intervention. It is essential, therefore, that supportive mechanisms are in place for disabled children, children with learning difficulties and chronically ill children at school, and that the rights of all children to protection are upheld whilst children are apart from parents and other carers.

The Mental Health Foundation has identified a combination of factors that are known to promote resilience in children (Mental Health Foundation 1999) and have identified the following as 'protective' factors:

- friends
- supportive educational environment
- hobbies and social networks
- sense of humour
- communication skills
- religious and spiritual orientation.

Much of the present work on resilience has been informed by the work of Michael Rutter (1999).

PowerPoint

Access the companion PowerPoint presentation (slides 20 to 22: Risk factors and slides 23 to 25: Resilience factors).

Rutter observed that some children seem to cope better with life events than others facing the same challenges. He has conducted extensive research into defining and listing the 'protective factors' that promote resilience in children and young people, and help them cope better with adversity.

Mental Health and Social Disadvantage

There is much evidence linking social disadvantage with mental health problems in childhood, making clear the need for health and social factors to be considered together. However, certain groups of children remain vulnerable and are known to experience poorer physical and mental health outcomes as a direct result of their social circumstances.

Activity

Make a list of children who you consider to be particularly 'vulnerable' in today's society.

Your list will probably have included:

- 'looked after' children in local authority care
- children who have parents with mental illness
- children who care for relatives
- children living with domestic violence
- children living in poor/disadvantaged families
- children living in isolated communities
- children from minority ethnic backgrounds
- 'displaced' children (refugees)
- homeless youngsters.

Many of these youngsters will have additional health needs associated directly with their demanding social circumstances. Practitioners will have to find ways to access and to engage effectively with children and families in disadvantaged and isolated settings and will need particular skills in working with children and families to truly optimise child health for many children.

Summary

This chapter has attempted to present the major health issues and health problems of school-aged children. Emphasis throughout has been placed on the need to look at the individual child's developmental stage as a key factor to understanding and communicating central messages about health and well-being.

The need to gain an understanding of the child's family and social circumstances has also been stressed, as this so often enables us to gain a clearer picture of the child's everyday experiences and the barriers that many children face to living healthy lives. Thankfully, for the majority of school children, a visit to a health centre will be a pleasant experience and visits to hospital will be unusual and reduced to a minimum, with family and carers playing a central role.

The real challenges for us as a society, are about making the world a healthier and safer place for all children, to protect the most vulnerable of children and to enable families to care for their children in ways that promote physical, social and mental well being.

References

Acheson D 1999 Inequalities in health. HMSO, London

American Academy of Pediatrics (AAP) 2003 Foreword. Pediatrics 111(6):1541

Barnes K 2003 Paediatrics. A clinical guide for nurse practitioners. Butterworth Heinemann, London

Bukatko D, Daehler M 1998 Child development: a thematic approach, 2nd edn. Houghton Mifflin, New York

Carter B 2000 Ways of working: community children's nurses and chronic illness. Journal of Child Health Care 4(2):66–72

Cummings EA, Reid GJ, Finley GA 1996 Prevalence and source of pain in pediatric outpatients'. Pain 68(1):25–31

Darbyshire P 2003 Mothers' experiences of children's recovery. Journal of Child Health Care 7(4):291–312

Dearmun A, Taylor A 1995 Nursing support and care: meeting the needs of the child and family with altered mobility. In: Carter B, Dearmun AK (eds) Child health care nursing: concepts, theory and practice. Blackwell Science, Oxford, pp 500–514

Department of Health (DoH) 1997 Child and adolescent mental health services: report of the Health Select Committee proceedings. HMSO, London

Department of Health (DoH) 1999 Saving lives: our healthier nation. The Stationery Office, London

Department of Health (DoH) 2000 The NHS plan. The Stationery Office, London

Department of Health (DoH) 2003 Getting the right start: national service framework for children. Standards for hospital services. The Stationery Office, London

Department of Transport (DoT) 1992 Road accidents: Great Britain. HMSO, London

Department of Transport (DoT) 2000 The casualty report, UK government statistics service. HMSO, London

Downie RS, Fyfe C, Tannahill A 1991 Health promotion models and values. Oxford University Press, Oxford

Engel J 1997 Pediatric assessment, 3rd edn. Mosby, St Louis

Feasey S 2000 Quality counts: auditing day surgery services. Journal of Child Health Care 4(2):73–77

Franck LS, Jones M 2003 Computer-taught coping techniques for venepuncture: preliminary findings from usability testing with children, parents and staff. Journal of Child Health Care 7(1):41–54.

Gill D, O'Brien N 2003 Paediatric clinical examination made easy, 4th edn. Churchill Livingstone, London

Health Advisory Services (HAS) 1995 Together we stand: child and adolescent mental health services. HAS, London

Huston J, Woodward AA, Beasley SW 1999 Jones' clinical paediatric surgery: diagnosis and management, 5th edn. Blackwell Science, Oxford

Jackson PA, Vessey JA 2000 Primary care of the child with a chronic condition, 2nd edn. Mosby, St Louis

LaMontagne L 1984 Three coping strategies used by school aged children. Pediatric Nursing 10(1):25–28

Napier N, Banton R, Medforth N 2000 Children and assessment. In: Wyse D, Hawtin A (eds) Children: a multi-professional perspective. Arnold, London

Piaget J 1968 A theory of development. International encyclopaedia of the social sciences. Macmillan, New York

Ray LD, Ritchie JA 1993 Caring for chronically ill children at home: factors that influence parent coping. Journal of Pediatric Nursing 8(4):217–225

Royal College of Nursing (RCN) 1999 Children's services: acute health care provision. RCN, London

Rudolf M, Levene M 1999 Paediatrics and child health. Blackwell Science, Oxford

Rutter M 1994 Resilience: concepts and findings. Journal of Family Therapy 21:119–144

Schaffer R 2004 Introducing child psychology. Blackwell, Oxford

Social Services Inspectorate 1998 Inspection of services to disabled children and their families. The Stationery Office, London

Spender Q, Salt N, Dawkins J, Hill P 2001 Child mental health in primary care. Radcliffe Medical Press, Oxford

The Children Bill (2004) House of Lords. The Stationery Office, London

Thornes R 1991 Just for the day. Caring for children in the health services. British Paediatric Association, London

United Nations General Assembly 1989 Convention on the rights of the child. United Nations, New York

Whitney I, Smith PK 1993 A survey of the nature and extent of bullying in junior/middle and secondary schools. Education Research 35:3–5

Wilson M 1995 Children, health and families. In: Carter B, Dearmun AK (eds) Child health care nursing: concepts, theory and practice. Blackwell Science, Oxford

Child and Adolescent Mental Health: the Nursing Response

Michael Cooper

ABSTRACT

The aim of this chapter is to explore the issues of mental health in relation to childhood and the adolescent developmental tasks. The challenges facing adolescent health care will be explored with a particular consideration of the nursing response. The assumption is made that nursing is primarily an interpersonal activity and that for the nurse this is a starting point for successful interventions in adolescent health care. There are two central themes for this chapter. First, there is strong and growing evidence for the fundamental inter-relationship between physical mental and social health. Problems in adolescence in any of these areas indicate the likelihood of long-term adverse health and social consequences (Royal College of Paediatrics and Child Health (RCPCH) 2003). Second, is training and skills. In this chapter the case will be made that the children's nurse can make a significant contribution to the care of this client group in terms of physical and mental health. There are consistent and growing calls for better training and the support of specialist practitioners in adolescence and/or mental health.

Learning Outcomes

- Link childhood mental health and issues in adolescence.

- Review the nature of adolescence.

- Consider the impact of the adolescent developmental tasks on health behaviours.

- Be able to locate the young person in terms of their developmental tasks.

- Review the interpersonal and communication skills required when working with young people.

- Explore the nature of the therapeutic relationship.

- Identify nursing responses to young people with emotional problems and/or mental health issues.

- Locate appropriate resources to inform best practice with young people.

Introduction

This chapter is set within the context of both the *National service framework for children, standards for hospital services* (Department of Health (DoH) 2003) and the *National service framework for children, young people and maternity services* (DoH 2004). The earlier NSF advocates child-centred services that consider the whole child, not simply the illness. Seeing the whole child also means recognising that health protection and promotion, and disease prevention are integral to the young person's care in any setting. In exploring child-centred care it is recognised that the child exists within the context of a family, school, friends and local community. Further, children and young people have rights, and their treatment is a partnership. Respecting the role of parents is seen as a significant part of providing services for children. Prevention and health promotion are also seen as a fundamental question of attitude that looks beyond the immediate treatment of the presenting problem. This chapter seeks to explore those strategies involved in the promotion of mental health and opportunities for the prevention of health risk behaviours. The *National service framework for children, young people and maternity services* (DoH 2004) builds and develops the earlier work seeking to ensure that all children and young people get services that are age appropriate, accessible and that recognise that there needs are different. It is a national blueprint to ensure personalised child-centred health and social care services. It recommends that all staff working with children are able to recognise the contribution they can make to children's emotional well-being and that they understand their responsibilities for supporting children in difficulty.

Working with adolescents is a task many groups find challenging. In the foreword to the report *Bridging the gaps* (RCPCH 2003), David Hall reminds us that the British stand accused of 'not liking children'; he suggests perhaps we like adolescents even less. Generally, adolescents are considered to have needs that differ from both adults and children yet they are often nursed in environments that also contain either adults or children. If we add to this issues of emotional distress/mental health, things seem to move beyond the perceived areas of expertise or competence of many children's nurses (Norwich Union 2001). The picture may be complicated further by the nurse having to move quickly from the parents of a child who is seriously physically ill to an emotionally distressed, abusive, swearing, adolescent whose physical health may or may not appear to be seriously compromised. It is these dilemmas that this chapter wishes to address by providing information and educational resources, but more importantly some practical guidance on the interpersonal skills that might be helpful with this client group.

The Nature of Adolescence

It is commonly accepted that there are some dominant ideas about adolescence. It can be defined as a period in human development linked to biological markers, involving transitions (that can be seen as stages), in which the central task is establishing identity. It is suggested that universal definitions of adolescence should at best be restricted to describing adolescence as a 'period of transition' in which although no longer seen as a child the young person is not yet considered an adult. The World Health Organization (WHO) definition of adolescence states that the stage is commonly associated with physiological changes occurring with the progression from the appearance of secondary sexual characteristics (puberty) to sexual and reproductive maturity (WHO 1995). Dehne & Riedner (2001) suggest that these biological markers create problems because the falling age of onset of the menarche attributed to improved health means there is now a widening gap between the age of sexual maturity and the age at which sexual relations become legitimate. A central dilemma of the adolescent experience is that in some cultures physical maturity comes well before legal definitions of adulthood in terms of legal sexual behaviour, the right to vote, join the military, etc.

The combination of young people's relative inexperience in sexual matters and the social stigma attached to them being sexually active creates vulnerability that is only now being recognised and addressed (Dehne & Riedner 2001). However, adolescence is not characterized just a sexual dilemma, there is also vulnerability in relationships with peers, with adults and with organisations. It seems that adults don't know how to take adolescents seriously because they do not find it easy to understand their experience.

Activity

Although the biological triggers for puberty might be universal, how might the cultural ethnic values influence this process? What effect might economic and social factors have?

There is, however, a view that the dilemma of adolescence has been overplayed, in terms of a life stage that, by its very nature involved serious conflict and upheaval. More recent thinking suggests much less necessary difficulty and much more continuity between the child that was, through adolescence to the adult that will be. It is considered that normal adolescents negotiate this period of life transition with relatively little major disruption or sustained high-risk behaviour (Offer 1987, cited in Burt 2002).

Even if the more optimistic view of adolescence is taken, healthcare settings are likely to see more of those children involved in high-risk behaviours. These high-risk behaviours are also linked to the precursors of mental health problems, low self-esteem and dysfunctional families (British Medical Association (BMA) 2003).

The Developmental Tasks of Adolescence

A simple definition for adolescence, which acknowledges the developmental stages, is offered by the Registered Nurses Association of Ontario (RNAO) in its guidelines for nursing practice entitled *Enhancing healthy adolescence*:

The period of transition from childhood to adulthood that can be divided into early (11–14 years), mid (15–17 years) and late (18–21 years) (RNAO 2002a)

Individuals will negotiate these stages in their own time but, as a general principle, it is helpful to view adolescence in this way. There seems to be a significant degree of agreement that the stage models of the adolescent journey see personal identity as the focal concern (Kroger 1989, cited in La Voie 1994). These models take a stage approach, starting with the preadolescent, and continue the process of change through to post adolescence (La Voie 1994).

701

It is helpful to see the key adolescent task as a search for identity, that is, a sense of separate self but, as always, the self in relation to others. Adolescents are in search of an identity that will lead them to adulthood, they make a strong effort to answer the question 'Who am I?'.

Of the stage models, Erickson's psychosocial model is perhaps the best known. Erickson (1963) describes the adolescent task/crisis as identity versus confusion. He notes that the healthy resolution of earlier conflicts can now serve as a foundation for the search for an identity. If an individual has developed a sense of trust and a strong sense of industry then the search for identity will be easier. The adolescent must make a conscious search for identity. This is built on the outcome and resolution to conflict in earlier stages. If the adolescent cannot make deliberate decisions and choices, especially about vocation, sexual orientation, and life in general, role confusion becomes a threat.

Activity

How might our unresolved adolescent experiences influence our relationship with troubled young people?

Jacobs (1992) looks at adolescence in three stages:

- early adolescence and sexuality
- middle adolescence: authority and independence
- later adolescence: faith and responsibility.

In this model, early adolescence is linked to puberty and reinitiates issues of sexual identity and attitudes as part of the overall quest for personal identity. The young person may become very self-conscious and also very preoccupied with appearance and dress. The young person's changing physical appearance matters a great deal. This might evoke feelings of pleasure and confidence or strangeness and shame. Rivalry and competition are often important elements at this time as part of the adjustments within peer groups. However, rivalry is not confined to peer groups: just at the time the children are finding their sexual identity, their parents are conscious of imminent or present changes in themselves.

Jacobs talks of how a mother may be entering her menopause at the same time as the daughter achieves her menarche or a father may be aware of his spreading midriff and lack of muscular tone just as his son is reaching his peak of physical fitness. Even if that is not the case, parents in the UK will be made aware of their changing life position in what is a very youth-oriented culture. These changes in life positions for all family members are the context in which the young person's ambivalence towards his or her parents is acted out. On the one hand, the parent is still needed as an object of love and a protector but on the other there is a strong desire to push the parent away to find their own confidence and object of love. To both love and hate parents, who then may respond by being hurt or angry, can be a difficult conflict for the young person to contain and manage.

IMPLICATIONS FOR THE HEALTHCARE PROFESSIONAL

It is important to be mindful of the young person's need to assert him- or herself and of the adult response of meeting the challenge or setting the boundaries. This must be within a context of an acceptance of the young person and an understanding of what is motivating his or her behaviour. The limits must contain but not crush the young person's emotions and behaviour. It is important to recognise that although we (as nurses) may be appear to be the target of their discontent, it is likely that bigger issues are being acted out. These issues relate to their main developmental task of trying to assert who they are, within the context of ill health. Their illness has the potential to undermine their sense of independence directly through their own thoughts and beliefs. This might also be done indirectly and unwittingly through the actions of anxious parents and/or the collusion of nursing and medical staff.

This natural process of adolescence – separating from the parents as a way of increasing independence – may happen without much drama or may be very dramatic. Separation can be made easier if the young person can achieve a degree of financial independence. This might be quite a challenge if the young person is in continuing education, unemployed or unable to work through ill health. In the last stage, Jacobs suggests the concern is for the wider issues of their place in the wider society and their own transition into adulthood. For some there is concern about what is wrong with society and optimism about their proposed solutions. It is this stage that some of the compromises that underpin adult functioning are beginning to be made.

Coleman (1989) developed a 'focal theory' of adolescence, which suggests that at specific ages in adolescent different relationships come into focus, in the sense of being most prominent, or important. In early adolescence the concerns about heterosexual relationships are to the fore. In middle adolescence (15 years) the peer group becomes very important and in late adolescence (peaking at 17 years) conflicts with parents become central. Coleman (1989) added that there may well be overlap between the issues and that none of the issues are tied to a particular age or developmental level. A key idea that arises is that if the young person is able to deal with these issues one at a time it is easier to cope with the complex issues of adolescence. This would be why only a minority of young people are overwhelmed by the transitions of adolescence and might also link with Erikson's assertion that successful transition is linked to the success, or not, of earlier life stages. Therefore the more difficulties there have been earlier in life, the more likely adolescence will be a difficult time. During this process of individuation (separating out one's own identity), adolescents increasingly transfer their emotional attachment from parents to peers. Close peer friendships have a positive influence on adolescents' social and personality development and adolescents who perceive their peer friends as supportive have fewer psychological problems greater confidence and less loneliness (Hay & Ashman 2003).

Parental relationships remain important in terms of self-worth, particularly for those adolescents whose transition is well adjusted. Those who are more troubled tend to disregard parents and teachers as sources of self-esteem, preferring alternative audiences such as peers, as a change to the negative feedback from parents and school (Hay & Ashman 2003).

Activity

How might such knowledge about peer relationships influence our attempts to manage disruptive behaviour in a clinical setting?

What is significant from a nursing point of view is that we should take as much account of the adolescent's developmental stage as we would of the developmental stage of the younger child. If we want to be helpful and respectful, we need to go to where they are. This is the starting point of any helping relationship.

As nurses, we can begin to make progress in giving appropriate care only when we begin to understand how even the most undesirable of youthful behaviours usually represent (Burt 2002):

- the attempts of adolescents to complete these developmental tasks
- ambivalence about whether they want to move on to adulthood
- their perception that they may never complete the tasks successfully.

Peer Relationships

An understanding of the adolescent's developmental tasks will allow the nurse to focus caregiving in the most effective manner. The most important nursing intervention might be for the nurse to spend time with the young person's key friends, helping them accommodate the changed circumstances of the illness so that supportive peer relationships can be maintained. This in turn will enhance the

young person's self-concept and self-esteem, which will be needed in facing the difficult adjustments ahead. This strategy will also serve as a protective factor against emotional distress and the risk of mental ill health. This would support the idea of moving beyond pure medical thinking and embrace the concept of adolescent health (Bennett & Tonkin 2003).

Life span developmental theories tend to support these important ideas (Goosens & Marcoen 1999):

- They see the developing person as an active agent in his or her own development.
- Person and context are related: the individual must be seen within the context of their family their peer group and their developmental stage.
- Developmental readiness: i.e. adolescents will fare better if they are allowed more time to deal with important issues in their lives.
- 'Arena of comfort': this idea suggests that if adolescents feel comfortable in some environments then discomfort in other areas can be tolerated.

Activity

- How might the young person's sense of agency be influenced by ill health?
- Do the assessment strategies take into account the context of the person and their illness?
- Do the clinical procedures ensure space and the right information is being offered to help the young person accommodate the changes that are happening to them?
- How might the 'arena of comfort' concept be used in the planning of care?

When thinking of a holistic assessment process, it might be helpful to reflect on the interplay between the young person's illness and their transition through the adolescent developmental tasks. You might want to think of some questions you could ask during the assessment phase that might help you locate where the young person is in terms of their adolescent transition.

Issues of Sexuality, Gender Relationships and Physical Attractiveness

Sexuality might be seen as a taboo subject in that it is often an overlooked issue for those working with children and adolescents. Clearly, the reality is that children are exposed to issues of sexuality extensively within the popular media. Children and adolescents are aware of changes in their own bodies and those of their family and friends. There is a need to be sensitive to the young person's accommodation of his or her own sexuality in earlier adolescence, and their possible uneasiness with themselves in terms of sexuality. In middle adolescence we need to be aware of how younger nurses may be drawn by the young person into their peer network. They may want to see the nurse as a friend or identify with them, compete with them, or even reject them as a peer. The young person might develop intense feelings about individual nurses that may involve love and/or sexual attraction. It is worth noting that with the changing attitudes in society about the expression of sexuality means that we need to be aware of issues of primary sexual orientation, heterosexuality, homosexuality and/or bisexuality.

There is a need to keep the young person safe, and in some situations to keep staff safe as well. The issues arising out of nurses working with patients of the opposite gender are often underplayed, perhaps partly as an unconscious denial of the young person's sexuality. There is a significant trend for young women (led by their role models in popular culture) to suggest that some expression of bisexuality is cool. This could be followed by an increase in children of both sexes having sexual attraction towards nurses in what is a predominately female nursing work force.

Being ill can be a significantly challenge to the individuals confidence about their sexuality, personal appearance and thus self-worth. Studies show that awareness of sexuality and physical attractiveness significantly influenced females and males sense of self-worth (Hay & Ashman 2003).

Reflect on your Practice

In your experience, how are issues of young people's sexuality managed?

Factors that Influence Adolescent Health and the Healthcare Response

Key documents in this area are:

- *Bridging the gaps: health care for adolescents* (RCPCH 2003)
- *Adolescent health* (BMA 2003)
- *National service framework for children in hospital* (DoH 2003)
- *National service framework for children, young people and maternity services* (DoH 2004).

The factors that contribute towards health risk behaviours in children and young people are closely related to the factors that contribute to emotional distress and mental health problems.

There is strong and growing evidence for the fundamental inter-relationship between physical, mental and social health. Problems in any of these areas indicate the likelihood of long-term adverse health and social consequences (RCPCH 2003). These links mean that young people with health problems are likely to have a greater risk of presenting with mental health problems. It is important to note that most adolescents negotiate this period of life transition with relatively little major disruption or sustained high health-risk behaviour. Those who do experience major disruptions and who persistently engage in problem behaviours now have a significantly higher risk of health problems in later life. Thus successful intervention now has important payoffs in terms of future health problems prevented and future satisfying and productive lifetimes promoted (Burt 2002). There is a strong relationship between adolescent health and other aspects of adolescent life such as education, employment and housing. Interventions therefore should be multiprofessional and involve cooperation between health, education and social services (BMA 2003).

Most reports on adolescent health focus on health interventions in terms of health risks and protective factors. Key health risk factors identified by the BMA report *Adolescent health* (BMA 2003) include nutrition, exercise and obesity and smoking, drinking and drug use, mental health and sexual health. Similar health outcomes were selected for study in an Australian report, *Evidence-based health promotion no. 2: adolescent health* (Department of Human Services Victorian Government 2000). This systematic review identified six health outcomes: tobacco use, alcohol and drug use, sexual risk-taking behaviour, crime and antisocial behaviour, depression, and suicidal behaviour. There will be similar patterns in other industrially developed countries, although Australia has not identified obesity. Perhaps with sport and outdoors activity so embedded in the culture, the effects of overeating are mitigated by attitude, activity and exercise.

Research has shown that certain factors mitigate against health-risk behaviours:

- Within the individual: self-esteem, internal locus of control (feeling confident that one's own efforts will produce desired effects).
- Familial: absence of marital discord, family cohesion, and a good relationship with at least one parent.
- Environmental: having at least one good relationship with a significant adult figure other than one's parents (Burt 2002).

Activity

How might this information about mitigating factors in health-risk behaviours shape the priorities of nursing actions?

Factors that Increase the Likelihood of Health Risk Behaviours

The more positive the young person's self-esteem, the greater his or her sense of self-efficacy. Negative self-efficacy is linked with general unhappiness and past worries. The links are stronger for girls than boys but are significant for both. Negative self-efficacy and low self-esteem increase the possibility of health-risk behaviours. Poverty, family dysfunction or lack of parental involvement and support are the risk factors that consistently differentiate youth most likely to get in serious trouble from those who don't (Burt 2002).

Common antecedents to health-risk behaviours (Catalano & Hawkins 1995, cited in Burt 2002) are:

- extreme economic deprivation
- family conflict
- family history of the problem behaviour
- family management problems
- neighbourhood qualities that offer pervasive opportunities to engage in the problem behaviour (e.g. substance misuse) and that have a structure of disorganisation and low attachment identity.

It can be seen that the contemporary health problems of young people occur within the context of the physical, social cultural and political realities within which they live. Recognition by self-report that most adolescent health concerns were actually social and psychological in nature suggest that time has come to throw-off pure medical thinking and embrace the notion of adolescent health. What is needed is a holistic model of health care highlighting the multiplicity of human needs that may exist beyond and yet create the context of the presenting complaint (Bennett & Tonkin 2003).

IMPLICATIONS FOR HEALTHCARE PRACTICE

The above reinforces what has been said before: that the young person has to be seen in the context of his or her relationships with peers and family, and also within his or her social, economic, environmental and cultural parameters. Health-risks behaviours are unlikely to decrease just with the production of a health promotion leaflet and advice. However, if this is linked to a nursing style that demonstrates respect, and a genuine desire to seek to understand the individual, the impact is likely to be greater. Such a style is likely to promote self-efficacy and self-esteem and a move from a condition-centred to a child-centred approach (Beresford & Sloper 2003).

Childhood Mental Health

The idea that our early experiences shape our later lives is not new. The work of Freud and the psychoanalysis movement highlighted the importance of early life, and Bowlby (1988) and others made the link between problems in adolescence and childhood experiences. In early childhood our mental health is mediated in large part by our relationship with our primary caregivers. Illness can be seen as easier to define than health and is often described in diagnostic manuals. However, the question needs to be asked: what is mental health?

The definition in *Bright futures: promoting children and young people's mental health* (The Mental Health Foundation 1999) offers some indicators. This definition states that a mentally healthy child or young person is one who has the ability to:

- develop psychologically, emotionally, socially, intellectually and spiritually
- initiate, develop and sustain mutually satisfying relationships
- use and enjoy solitude
- become aware of others and empathise with them
- play and learn
- develop a sense of right and wrong
- resolve (face) problems and setbacks satisfactorily and learn from them.

It is as difficult to define mental health as it is health in general, but it is widely agreed that in children, mental health is indicated by (NHS Health Advisory Service 1995 p 15):

- a capacity to enter into and sustain mutually satisfying personal relationships
- continuing progression of psychological development
- an ability to play and to learn so that attainments are appropriate for age and intellectual level
- a developing moral sense of right and wrong
- the degree of psychological distress and maladaptive behaviour being within normal limits for the child's age and context.

Thinking about What Makes Us Mentally Healthy

The following are a list of attributes related to being mentally healthy. It might be helpful to spend a little time thinking about how your mental health is maintained and what factors contribute to your maintenance of these attributes.

- Self-esteem.
- Physical growth.
- Emotional growth.
- Resilience.
- Ability to make good personal relationships.
- A sense of right and wrong.
- The motivation to face setbacks and learn from them.
- A sense of belonging.
- A belief in my ability to cope.
- How to solve problems.

A useful definition of mental health (or psychiatric) disorder was given by Rutter and Graham (1968) as:

An abnormality of emotion, behaviour or relationships which is developmentally inappropriate and of sufficient duration and severity to cause persistent suffering or handicap to the child and/or distress or disturbance to the family or community.

In making a child psychiatric assessment five key questions are asked. Goodman & Scott, 1997.

- Symptoms: What sort of problem is it?
- Impact: How much distress or impairment does it cause?
- Risks: What factors have initiated and maintained the problem.
- Strengths: What assets are there to work with?
- Explanatory model: What beliefs and expectations do the family bring?

Strengths can often be seen in terms of protective factors that increase resilience in the face of stressors. It has been identified that certain factors increase the child's resilience in the face of stressors. Generally the interplay of risk and protective factors determines whether the child overcomes the stressors they face. In some situations the stressors can be so great or so many that they cannot be defended against.

RESILIENCE FACTORS

In the Child

- Being female.
- More intelligent.
- Easy temperament when an infant.
- Secure attachment.
- Positive attitude, problem solving approach.

- Good communication skills.
- Planner, belief in control.
- Sense of humour.
- Strong faith.
- Capacity to reflect.

In the Family

- At least one good parent–child relationship.
- Affection.
- Supervision, authoritative discipline.
- Support for education.
- Supportive relationship/marriage.

In the Environment

- Wider supportive network.
- Good housing.
- High standards of living.
- High school/college morale and positive attitudes with policies for behaviour, attitudes and antibullying.
- Schools/colleges with strong academic opportunities.
- Schools/colleges with non-academic opportunities.
- Range of sport, leisure opportunities.
- Appropriate relationships with adults.

Reflect on your Practice

Some factors effecting resilience cannot be influenced directly by nursing care. However, it might be helpful to consider those aspects of the children's ward environment that are likely to contribute to a young person's resilience.

Mental disorders can include (BMA 2003):

- emotional disorders, such as phobias, anxiety and depression
- conduct disorders
- hyperkinetic disorders, such as attention deficit disorder
- developmental disorders
- habit disorders
- eating disorders
- post-traumatic syndromes
- somatic disorders, such as chronic fatigue syndrome
- psychotic disorders, such as schizophrenia and drug-induced psychosis.

www

For a fuller account of child and adolescent mental disorders and latest evidenced-based findings, go to:

- http://www.focusproject.org.uk/finding-the-evidence

The Mental Health of Adolescents

The mental health of adolescents is extremely important not only in itself but also because of the strong links that it has with adolescent health-risk behaviours, violence and delinquency. In many senses, mental health is at the centre of adolescent health frameworks. Poor mental health can influence exercise patterns, obesity and body image, substance misuse and high-risk sexual behaviour.

Key Points

- Early adolescence (11–14): high rates of conduct and emotional disorders.

- Mid to late adolescence: peak time for the onset of depressive disorders and schizophrenia.

- Depressive symptoms: very common in adolescence. Most depressive disorders at this age are co-morbid with anxiety or slightly less common conduct disorder.

- Self-injury and self-harm: there is confusion over terminology with the incidence being given as 1:17 and possibly as high as 1:10. Deliberate self-harm is common in adolescent girls. The peak age for presentation is 15–24 for women and 25–34 for men.

- Eating disorders: e.g. bulimia and anorexia nervosa, disproportionately affect young females. This group has one of the highest death rates of all psychiatric illness.

- Attempted suicide: the rate of suicide is very low under 14 years old, attempted suicide begins to occur around 11 or 12 and increases rapidly in the early and mid teens. Young men are particularly at risk and are less likely than girls to show their distress beforehand.

INTERVENTIONS IN CHILD AND ADOLESCENT MENTAL HEALTH DISORDERS

Wider Interventions

Early intervention in adolescent mental health problems is essential to try and stop the deterioration of mental health, alleviate distress, and minimise the impact of mental health disorders on education and social development (BMA 2003). Such interventions might include.

- education about mental health problems
- first-line services to promote emotional well-being
- social skills training
- antibullying policies.

Child and Adolescent Mental Health Services

The Child and Adolescent Mental Health Service (CAMHS) offers four levels, or tiers, of interventions. Tier 1 represents early and preventative interventions through to tier 4, which represents tertiary services.

TIER 1

This primary level includes interventions by GPs, health visitors, school nurses, Social Services, voluntary agencies, teachers, juvenile justice workers, residential social workers. Non-specialists should:

- identify mental health problems early in their development
- offer general advice and in certain cases treatment of less severe problems
- pursue opportunities for promoting mental health.

TIER 2

Clinical child psychologists, paediatricians (especially community educational psychologists), child psychiatrists, community child psychiatric nurses/nurse specialists should be able to offer:

- training and consultation to other professionals
- consultation for professionals and families
- outreach to families and children requiring more specialist help but are unwilling to use specialist services
- assessment, which may trigger treatment in another tier.

TIER 3

A specialist service for more complex, severe and persistent disorders. It usually comprises a multidisciplinary team or service including child and adolescent psychiatrists, social workers, clinical psychologists, community psychiatric nurses, child psychotherapists, occupational therapists, art, music and drama therapists. The service offers:

- assessment and treatment of child and adolescent mental health disorders
- assessment for referrals to tier 4
- contributions to consultation and training at tiers 1 and 2
- participation in research and development projects.

TIER 4

Access to infrequently used but essential tertiary level services such as day units, highly specialised community teams and inpatients units for older children and adolescents who are severely mentally ill and at suicide risk. Providing:

- adolescent inpatient units
- secure forensic adolescent units
- eating disorder units
- specialist teams for sexual abuse
- specialist teams for neuropsychiatric problems (HMSO 1995).

THE NEED FOR INTERVENTION

- The prevalence of disorders is high: 10.4% of children, aged 5 to 15 years old, in England, Scotland and Wales, have been found to have a diagnosis of mental disorder based not just on symptoms but on evidence of distress or interference with personal function (Meltzer et al 2000).

- A significant rise in the prevalence of psychosocial disorders – depression, eating disorders, substance misuse, suicide and suicidal behaviour, crime and conduct disorders – in young people aged between about 12 and 26 years has been documented in developed Western countries, including Britain, since the end of the Second World War (Rutter & Smith 1995).

- Only a relatively small proportion of children with significant mental health problems and disorders find their way to specialist mental health services. This was found to be around 20% in the UK survey quoted above (Meltzer et al 2003). It is estimated that as many as 60–70% of children and adolescents who experience clinically significant difficulties have not had appropriate interventions at a sufficiently early age.

WHAT WORKS: PRIMARY PREVENTION

- The earlier in the child's life the prevention commences, the more likely it is to be effective.

- Prevention needs to be disorder, context and objective specific. Focused, highly structured, proactive programmes targeting risk factors rather than problem behaviours are more efficacious than generic unstructured ones, such as the provision of counselling or group discussion.

- There is good evidence that effective programmes have the following features in common:
  - Comprehensiveness: successful programmes include multiple components because no single programme component can prevent multiple high-risk behaviour.
  - System orientation: interventions should be aimed at changing institutional environments as well as individuals.
  - Relatively high intensity and long duration: successful programmes are rarely brief. Short-term programmes have, at best, time-limited benefits, especially with at-risk groups. Multi-year programmes tend to have an impact on more risk factors and have more lasting effects.
  - Structured curriculum: there is no clear indication as to the 'ideal curriculum' for preventive interventions, but proactive interventions should be directed at risk and protective factors rather than problem behaviours. In this way, multiple adverse outcomes may be addressed within a single programme.
  - Early commencement: this has been shown to be essential, and intervention during pregnancy brings additional benefits.
  - Specific to particular risk factors: it is unrealistic to hope that a generic preventive intervention will be able to reduce the risk for all psychological disorders. Prevention needs to be disorder, context and objective specific.
  - Specific training: there is less consistency in the literature on the qualifications required to carry out preventive work. Most studies in the UK use health visitors who have a statutory obligation to visit young children and their carers.
  - Attention to maintaining attendance: those families most in need of early prevention programmes are likely to need high levels of support to engage in an intervention, and continued assistance to maintain attendance. In experimental programmes, they are the most likely to drop out.

WWW

For a more detailed exploration see 'What works in promoting children's mental health: the evidence and the implications for Sure Start programmes' at:
- http://www.surestart.gov.uk.doc/0-34D33E.pdf

Promoting Emotional Well-being

It has been suggested that everyone in contact with young people should take the symptoms of emotional distress, behavioural difficulties and hyperactivity seriously, because they impair function and development and are unlikely to be transient. It was identified earlier that a significant number of professionals find working with adolescents difficult (BMA 2003). However, a key point of this chapter is that nurses can make a difference. In general, caring and protective relationships are potent protective factors against adverse outcomes: 'to hug is to buffer'. Connections with prosocial adults or mentors can be an important protective factor for young people at risk (Department of Human Services Victorian Government 2002). It is imperative to the promotion of child and adolescent health that nurses develop the skills that will enable them to successfully engage with the young person and ensure a nursing interaction that is rewarding both for the young person and the nurse.

Nurses often think they have not got the skills to work with young people with mental health problems or indeed any adolescents. There is sometimes confusion about what the task is. Clearly it is not therapy or counselling, that is for skilled therapists. However, there is a duty to promote health (physical and mental) by enhancing protective factors and intervening to reduce health risk behaviours. The therapeutic relationship the nurse enacts with the young person is the key intervention strategy.

WHAT DO YOUNG PEOPLE WANT?

When asked what they want, each time the feedback is similar: young people want more say and more prominent involvement in the main action (Bennett & Tonkin 2003). Young people have identified barriers to their effective use of services (RCPCH 2003).

- lack of information
- management of confidential issues
- lack of expertise and continuity of care
- failure to respect the validity of the young person's views
- being cared for alongside younger children or with a population they regard as elderly
- particular issues of access to services, disability, poverty, ethnicity, being looked after (in care) and sexual orientation.

The Healthcare Commission's first national survey of the young patient's experience was encouraging in that over 90% of respondents rated their care from excellent to good (Healthcare Commission 2004). Communication with staff was highly rated. The main concern was that young people wanted to be more involved in the decisions about their care. There was also a feeling that explanations about procedures, risks and benefits could be improved, and this supports previous work.

A consistent concern of young people is that they are not really listened to or taken seriously. There is a need for respect, a word that has strong currency with young people particularly the idea of being disrespectful. Respect is related to the young person feeling empowered in the relationship, being listened to and what they say being acted upon if appropriate (Ahmad et al 2003).

IMPLICATIONS FOR PRACTICE

As a starting point, we must be are able to work with the young person within the context of his or her developmental stage, i.e. in terms of their transition and what matters most to that individual right now: assessing the issues and the relationships that are in focus currently. A second important consideration might be the beliefs we bring to this relationship. What are our thoughts and feeling about adolescents generally and this young person in particular? When we are thinking about the young person we need to place him or her within the context of family and peers. Lastly, there is a need for an understanding of the nature of their illness and its unique interaction with their personhood.

Young people have identified certain key characteristics in adults who are approachable. The approachable adult (Lightfoot & Sloper 2002):

- is welcoming, and so makes the young person feel comfortable
- is interested in the young patient as a person, not just in the illness, and so is someone a young person can have an 'ordinary chat' with
- explains the things in a straightforward way
- can help the young person express his or her opinions
- will not patronise or judge the young person, but will take him or her seriously
- will take forward issues raised, with the relevant staff
- will mediate where there is conflict between patients and staff.

Young people can define their sense of well-being in terms of a continuum where feeling good and getting stressed are polarities of experience. In the report *Listening to children and young people* (Ahmad et al 2003), young people identified what made them feel good. Significant factors contributing to feelings of emotional well-being included: having people to talk to, personal achievement, being praised and generally feeling positive about oneself. Relationships with family or peers could contribute either positively or negatively to the sense of well-being.

Interpersonal Skills in the Helping Relationship with Young People

There is a powerful case for the provision of specialist units (Viner & Keane 1998) and/or specialist nurses (Needam 2000). Children's nurses often feel they do not have the skills to work with adolescents in general (Norwich Union 2001), let alone those with additional emotional or mental health problems. Some would go further and suggest that working with adolescents should be supported by a nurse specialist role in adolescent mental health. In *Bridging the gap* (RCPCH 2003) the RCPCH calls for additional training in adolescent health. The difficulty in this approach is that for each new problem or contemporary issue there are often the twin calls for more resources, and more training. Although not arguing against specialist support or additional training, it could be suggested that there is a danger of deskilling the existing nurses. It could be suggested that it would be better to think of key, core transferable skills, first, before considering the need of specialist skills.

If the description of the approachable adult outlined above is linked to what young people say they need to feel good, it could be argued that specialist skills are not required for most interactions. However, the professional nurse should have skills that go beyond lay care both in terms of the quality of their interactions and in terms of intentionality. Intentionality refers to the conscious and deliberate use of interpersonal skills to enhance the therapeutic nature of the interaction (Heron 2001).

Furthermore, children's nurses are already well acquainted with developmental stages so extending this concept into adolescence should not mean further extensive training. Whereas it is totally appropriate for children's nurses to be supported by adolescent health/mental health specialists, it is suggested that children's nurses can develop a therapeutic style that does allow meaningful engagement but that is not specialist or a specific therapy.

THE THERAPEUTIC STYLE OF THE NURSE

Nurses need to find a way of interacting that is more than 'having a chat' or the collecting of information for assessment but does not go as far as 'doing therapy'. Cooper & Glasper (2001) described such a process as a 'therapeutic encounter', describing it as:

A dynamic and sensitive interaction between what is known (professional knowledge) and what is 'yet to be known' (the young person's story) (Cooper & Glasper 2001 p 35)

Two key elements are identified.

1. The nurse's ability to have an internal ongoing reflective conversation (reflection in action).
2. The interaction is influenced by the belief systems of the nurse and the 'tribal stories' present in their working environment.

The reflective conversation will be monitoring the potential impact of the nurse's personal beliefs and the collective 'tribal stories' on the relationship they are forming with the young person. Cooper & Glasper (2001) give this example of extracts from tribal stories related to young people who self-harm:

Working with young people who self-harm often feels like it is a waste of time.
Our skills could be better used looking after someone who has a 'real illness'.
We are very busy here; there is not the time to give these people what they need.
They should be looked after somewhere else; this is not the place for them.
They are always manipulative; they tell lies.
We came into nursing to look after people with real illnesses, not these people.
Anyway, even if we had the time what could we say? If they are going to do it they will do it anyway!
Even if you do speak with her she won't answer, bet she will be back!

An example of a reflective 'self-conversation' when confronted by a young person who is rejecting care, swearing and being abusive might be:

Initial thoughts: *I find adolescents difficult when they are like this. They are so self-centred. I am having a hard shift. I don't need this. What about the other children and parents? They don't deserve this either.*
Initial formulation: *This young person needs to be told what the limits are.*

This preliminary assessment is likely to be reinforced by the tribal story (collective staff belief) that this young person is disruptive and either needs 'sorting out' or shouldn't be there in the first place. There is a tendency to see adolescents as being disruptive in an environment aimed at younger children (Norwich Union 2001). These collective beliefs might reflect the difficulty nurses have in finding the appropriate way to relate to these young people. Further reinforcement for this formulation might come from other parents and children's disapproval of the young person's behaviour. Another thing that might support this initial position is that, as a principle, it is good to set boundaries. The issue here, however, is the timing of such an intervention and whether it will inflame or calm the situation. The nurse needs to hold back the response and ask:

Reflective question: *What else should I be paying attention to in this situation?*

The first internal conversation is focused primarily on the nurse. There is a need to re-focus on the young person and to try and assess what is motivating their behaviour by exploring the following issues.

- What is the young person's underlying emotional state?
- What does he or she need?
- Is he or she trying to assert his- or herself?
- Is he or she feeling vulnerable and dependent, not grown up?
- Is he or she fearful for the future?
- How is the young person viewing me, my approach, my non-verbal communication?

This should lead to a reformulation:

Reformulation – new hypothesis: *This young person is scared. He/she is going for surgery tomorrow and wants help but is fearful about appearing childlike. He/she is probably angry about being ill, being with little children, and is not sure if we can be trusted. This uncertainty might be influenced by his/her previous attachment history and how reliable adults have been in the past. Has he/she had a secure base in times of trouble? Other factors influencing his/her behaviour will be his/her level of self-esteem and feelings of self-efficacy.*

SPECIFIC CORE COMMUNICATION SKILLS

Key communication skills make it more likely that the nurse will arrive at this more sensitive formulation. One of the key qualities central to all therapeutic communication is the ability to truly 'attend' to the other person. This is referred to as giving 'free attention'; this is the essential precursor of a second important quality 'active listening' (Egan 1990).

Free Attention

Heron (1975) describes giving free attention as:

A subtle and intense activity of being present for the client; it involves gaze, posture, facial expression, maybe touch. It has the qualities of:

– being supportive: out there with the client
– being expectant: waiting for the human being to emerge in ways that are meaningful to him or her and his or her fulfilment
– being non-anxious: the practitioner is free of claims and demands, of any harrying attitude towards the client.
It is always wider and deeper than the qualities of the client's speech, being attuned to his emerging potential as well as his actual behaviour.

Further, Heron (1975) suggests giving free attention is the *sine qua non* of all other sorts of interventions if they are to be truly and effectively human.

Egan (1990) identifies the following questions that nurses should ask when 'attending' a client:

- What are my attitudes towards this client?
- How would I rate the quality of my presence to the client?
- To what degree does my non-verbal behaviour indicate a willingness to work with the client?
- What attitudes am I expressing in my non-verbal behaviour?
- What attitudes am I expressing in my verbal behaviour?
- To what degree does my non-verbal behaviour reinforce my internal attitudes?
- In what ways am I distracted from giving my full attention to this client?
- What am I doing to handle these distractions?
- How might I be more effectively present for this person?

One of the tribal stories that have a basis in fact is that of the 'busy nurse'. It is certainly true that there are many demands on a nurse's time. Student nurses will often prefer to be busy because then they feel more 'nurse like'. So 'attending' is a skill that requires some practice and, more significantly, a belief that it is an important thing to do. However, once the skill is acquired it takes up far less time than might be at first imagined.

Active Listening

The second core skill is active listening. Egan (1990) suggests that listening carefully to what the client has to say seems:

. . . to be a concept so simple to grasp and so easy to do that one may wonder why it is given such explicit treatment here.

He suggests that it is amazing how often people fail to listen to one another. Certainly, young people often complain that they are not being listened to. Complete active listening involves four things:

1. Observing and reading the client's non-verbal behaviour: posture, facial expressions, movement, tone of voice, etc.
2. Listening to and understanding the client's verbal messages.
3. Listening to the whole person in the context of the social settings of life.
4. Tough-minded listening.

Points 1 and 2 can be understood from our life experience but it might be helpful to enlarge on what Egan means by items 3 and 4.

He refers to a 'people in systems' framework, which is the need to understand each client in terms not just in terms of a specific illness or problem but also with careful attention to his or her life setting, personal values, and biological and sociopsychological characteristics.

Tough-minded listening is about accepting that the client's feelings and visions of themselves, others and the world are real and need to be understood. However, clients' perceptions of themselves and their worlds are sometimes distorted. This does not mean that helpers challenge clients as soon as they hear any kind of distortion. Rather, they note gaps and distortions and challenge them if and when it is appropriate to do so.

Most communication theory will give lists of the factors that prevent effective listening. Egan (1990) identifies obstacles to listening and understanding clients:

- Inadequate listening: distracted, not giving our full attention.
- Evaluative listening: judging the merits of what is being said, comparing it to our own value system.
- Filtered listening: it is impossible to listen to others in an unbiased way, therefore the more self-knowledge we have the more we will recognise our particular filters.
- Knowledge as a filter, especially professional knowledge: we might be listening to validate a theory, maybe a diagnosis, rather than listening to the person.
- Fact-centred rather than person-centred listening: some assessment strategies might put us into a fact-centred approach.

Attending and active listening are the key vehicles for conveying respect to others. Studies show that young people work best with professionals who convey respect for them (Amhad et al 2003).

THE IMPORTANCE OF LISTENING TO THE STORY

Narrative theory is based on the supposition that, in large measure, people are the stories they tell themselves and that are told about them. Narratives can occur at different levels of social functioning. There are social and cultural narratives, interpersonal narratives and intrapersonal narratives. The narrative approach rests on the assumption that narratives are not representations of reflections of identities, lives and problems. Rather, narratives constitute identities, lives and problems. According to this position, the process of therapeutic re-authoring of personal narratives changes lives, problems and identities because personal narratives are constitutive of identity (Carr 1998). In short, this approach suggests we are the stories we tell about ourselves, and our told about us. Further our stories are embedded in and influenced by a wider social and cultural context.

Such an approach can have a number of implications for nursing practice. Within the context of these ideas we can explore nursing in terms of dominant discourses or stories. A discourse can be described in terms of:

Historically, socially, and institutionally specific structure of statements, terms, categories and beliefs that are embedded in institutions, social relationships and texts (Carr 1998)

If the assessment process reflected narrative theory, the approach would first seek the meaning the young person and his or her family gives to the events, rather than a professional system that seeks to impose meaning and explain behaviour.

 Reflect on your Practice

How much is the nursing task to explain, to inform, to understand, or to help the young person, make sense of things?

IMPLICATIONS FOR THE HEALTHCARE PROFESSIONAL

Nurses, when faced with the complex lives and backgrounds of young people with emotional disturbances, often feel powerless and think the situation is hopeless. Young people who come in with a history of repeated self-harm often provoke these feelings, accompanied sometimes by a degree of resentment. This may occur because the nurses fail to understand what the therapeutic task is. Clearly a life that has become so complex is hardly going to be turned around by an inpatient stay on a children's ward.

What we do know is that if the nurse can offer a secure, accepting base to the young person that is a positive experience. The other main therapeutic strategy is to listen non-judgementally and with care and compassion to the young person's unfolding story. This may not seem very active but it could be life enhancing for the young person.

One of the key ideas of narrative theory is the notion of 're-positioning', that is, taking up a different position in relation to the young person and or the problem. When we interact with young people and their families we are heavily influenced by a number of professional, personal and cultural discourses (tribal stories). A discourse is a dominant social and cultural story that can set the context in which an interaction takes place. Such discourse might relate to ideas as nursing, professionalism education, ethics and so on.

This can become problematic because instead of listening with a detached curiosity to what is being said and, through that process, really hearing the young person's story, his or her story can become 'entombed' with the professional narratives and belief systems. The client is then asked to enact a story told about them rather than his or her own story. To break out of our professional constructions and to reposition, it may be necessary to make an imaginative leap. We need to 'actively listen' in Egan's 1990 terms, repositioning ourselves so that we don't allow our professional knowledge and or personal prejudices to interfere with the flow of the young person's story.

Helping the Story Unfold

Belsher & Wilkes (1994) offer some key principles for working with adolescents. Although they were considering the work in terms of cognitive therapy, the principles can translate as general principles for working with young people.

Acknowledge the Adolescent's Narcissism

Narcissism refers to the tendency of adolescent patients to be somewhat egocentric in their interests and goals. This tendency should be seen as developmentally appropriate and can be used to develop the therapeutic relationship. Rather than using statements, questions can often be a good way of demonstrating we are listening. For example 'Would it be right to say you think . . . ?' acknowledges the young person as the best judge of his or her own views and will reinforce the feeling that he or she is being listened to. Unless there is a specific need for them, avoid levelling comments such as 'I have heard that before' or 'You're not the only one that feels like that'. In short, the young person needs to feel at the centre of his or her world, so it makes sense to start the therapeutic process from where he or she actually is. Another way nurses can affirm the adolescent's self-importance is to offer choices every time it is possible to do so. This would be responding to what the evidence

suggests adolescents want: more say and their views to be validated (RCPCH 2003).

Collaborative Empiricism

This is a central tenet of the cognitive therapy approach but again it can be adapted to general communication with adolescents.

To collaborate is to join with, to cooperate with, and this is a particularly useful position to take up with the young person. The nature of the nurse's specialist knowledge, life experience and health may lead the young person to feel in a one-down, less powerful position. Such a position would leave the young person very sensitive to the feeling of being patronised and more likely to want to assert him- or herself by being conflictual and oppositional, or through passivity and withdrawal. Another way that demonstrates collaboration is to be a voice for the young person, this links with young people's view that an approachable adult will take things forward on their behalf (Lightfoot & Sloper 2000).

Empiricism means giving value to factual data and evidence. To excessively confront or challenge the evidence for the position the young person holds would be very unhelpful and lead to resistance and conflict; it would be an inappropriate form of Egan's tough listening. However a genuine desire to see things from the young person's perspective by checking out the evidence he or she has for taking up his or her present position will demonstrate respect and help the young person's story become more coherent.

Adopt an Objective Stance

This means having the capacity of being able to be somewhat removed from the intricacies of the young person's situation. This is different from being disinterested or defensively detached from the situation. Objectivity is an important factor in all helping relationships but it is – perhaps – sometimes harder to maintain with young people. Their high levels of emotionality and tendency to see things in black and white terms can draw nurses into a parental role or encourage them to overidentify with the young person and into collusion. One of the ways to maintain a helpful objective stance is not to be drawn into the role of problem solver but rather to act as a facilitator of the young person's problem-solving skills. Collaborative empiricism can help objectivity in that both parties are working together to find the evidence necessary to support whatever is being explored, therefore neither should need an emotional investment in a particular position or belief. These positions or beliefs stand or fall on the basis of the evidence there is to support them.

Include Members of the Social System

This links with Egan's 1990 reminder that active listening involves listening to the person within the context of his or her social system. Young people are rarely in a position to make important decisions without reference to their parents and other adults in positions of authority. Further, their parents and peer group have a powerful effect on how they see themselves and, as such, can be helpful or unhelpful in terms of the young person's self-esteem.

Chase the Affect

To chase the affect is to pay particular attention to expressions and changes in emotional state. This means being sensitive to the verbal and non-verbal cues the young person gives and following them up: 'You seem to be thinking about something that has made you sad'. Such attention to the emotional expression is likely to convey empathy and a more accurate assessment of the overall situation leading to the most therapeutic response.

Socratic Questioning

This style of questioning and exploration promotes the young person to think about what he or she is saying and feeling. Again, any challenge to the young person's beliefs and assumptions must be made in a sensitive manner of genuine enquiry. The nurse must be seeking to understand the young person's world and thus help the young person become clearer about things. An example might be: 'When the doctor was talking to your parents about your illness what were you thinking?' or 'What did you feel like doing at that moment?'

Model for the Adolescent

This should be a subtle process in the relationship whereby the nurse models aspects of the behaviour that will be helpful. For example, if a nurse who wants to help the young person be more tolerant of younger children in the environment will model tolerance towards the young person.

The Therapeutic Relationship

The therapeutic relationship is grounded in an interpersonal process that occurs between the nurse and the young person. It is a purposeful, goal-directed relationship aimed at advancing the best interests of the client. The way we help (our style) seems to be at least if not more important than how we help (the model or theoretical approach we use). George (1997), in a review of the therapeutic relationship in nursing, identified Peplau as the first nurse theorist who stressed the nurse–patient relationship as a vehicle for achieving health. In the same paper, George (1997) highlights the research from psychotherapy that suggests the therapeutic relationship to be the variable most highly correlated with outcome, and points out that other research has shown the qualities of the therapist style as influential. The qualities of the therapeutic relationship include active

listening, trust, respect, genuineness, empathy and responding to client concerns. The requisite capacities for establishing a therapeutic relationship have been identified and defined as self-awareness, self-knowledge, empathy and awareness of boundaries and limits of the professional role (RNAO 2002).

REQUISITE CAPACITIES FOR ESTABLISHING THERAPEUTIC RELATIONSHIPS

Self-awareness

Self-awareness is the ability to reflect on one's subjective thoughts, feelings and actions. Thus, to be aware of any attitude being conveyed that could impede the therapeutic process and would react to counteract any potential negative effect on the client.

 Activity

You might want to consider an example from your own practice when you may have held an attitude or a view that impeded the therapeutic process.

Self-knowledge

With the development of self-knowledge, nurses are able to recognise that their own experience is shaped by nationality, race, culture, health, socio-economic conditions, gender, education, early childhood experiences and development, as well as relationships, accomplishments, beliefs, issues and concerns. By gaining self-knowledge nurses are able to differentiate between their own experience and values and those of the client. In this way, they are able to appreciate the unique perspective of the client (his or her story), are able to avoid burdening the client with their own issues and can prevent superimposing their own beliefs and preferred solutions on the client.

Empathy

Empathy is the ability of nurses to enter into the client's relational world, to see and feel the world as the client sees and feels it, and to explore the meaning it has for the client. Empathy involves nurses being able to attend to the subjective experience of the client and validate that their understanding is an accurate reflection of the client's experience.

Awareness of Boundaries and Limits of the Professional Role

Boundaries define the limits of the professional role. Nurses are obligated to place the client's needs before their own needs. Through self-awareness, nurses reflect on whether their actions are in the client's best interests. The supervision process should also be used to explore these issues. Sometimes, our own conscious or unconscious wishes make it hard to recognise boundary violations. Indications that boundaries may have been crossed include having special patients, spending extra time with patients, keeping secrets with clients and doing activities with clients that you do not share with colleagues.

WWW

For further exploration of these points visit the RNAO nursing guideline *Establishing therapeutic relationships*:

- http://www.rnao.org

THE SEQUENCE OF EVENTS IN THE RELATIONSHIP

For the sake of analysis, the therapeutic relationship can be seen in terms of a beginning, middle and end, although all three stages may occur in a single encounter.

The beginning can be seen as the process of engagement, formulating the working alliance. The middle is the working phase during which how the work is structured is important. The end can be seen as the disengagement phase or letting go.

Models of Helping

In her nursing model, Peplau (1952) describes three phases to the therapeutic relationship: orientation, working and resolution. In the beginning, both the nurse and the young person are strangers, each coming to the relationship with their own preconceptions of what to expect. These preconceptions will be based on their previous relationships, experiences, attitudes and beliefs. Peplau (1952) refers to the nurse and the client as being 'strangers' in this preorientation stage.

The Orientation Stage

In the orientation phase the parameters of the relationship are being established. The expectations of the young person and the nurse need to be explored and clarified. Consistency and listening are considered by clients to be critical at the beginning of a relationship. In this beginning stage, acceptance of the young person is important for the evolving relationship.

Activity

Are some young people and their families easier to accept than others? How can Stockwell's 1972 seminal

work *The unpopular patient* and subsequent research inform our practice on relationship building and patient acceptance?

The Working Phase

As the name suggests, this is the active phase where problems are identified and interventions decided on. How this is structured will depend on the helping model used, although the nurse should be involved in some key communication strategies. One of the common mistakes when working with distressed young people who are expressing negative or aggressive thoughts is to try to move them on to a more positive frame or want to offer alternative more constructive positions. Although this aim is laudable in itself the motivation is often to make the nurse feel more comfortable. Even if it is client focused, the timing is often wrong. One of the most important strategies, particularly with young people, is to validate the young person's thoughts, feelings and distress. This is not to collude with what in some cases might be a very distorted position (e.g. the anorexic stance) but to accept the young person's perspective and the distress caused by it. This working phase needs to be collaborative, led by the young person and facilitated by the nurse. The nurse needs to be the young person's advocate, ensuring that his or her views are considered in the overall care strategies.

The Resolution Phase

This final stage of the relationship is involved in completion of the relationship and endings. The process of ending is as important as the beginning but tends not to receive the same attention. It needs to be planned, talked about and should have been considered during the initial care planning: planning how and when the relationship should end. This is particularly important if the young person has a history of troubled or unreliable relationships. The nurse needs to be mindful of the experience of loss transition and change and the reactions of resistance, denial and ambivalence. While acknowledging the present, it may be helpful to be future orientated validating the young person's future plans.

Egan (1990), in *The skilled helper*, outlines one of the best known and most elaborated models of helping. It is important to remember that this model is designed for adults and that it would need to be sensitively adapted to the young person's developmental stage. It is also generally seen as a model of counselling. However, it could be argued that its structure allows it to adapt well to most helping situations. In its simplest form, the model has three stages:

- The present scenario (stage 1 the beginning stage): Helping the client identify, explore and clarify their problem situations and unused opportunities. Egan suggests that people can neither manage problem situations nor develop opportunities unless they identify and understand them.

- The preferred scenario (stage 2): Helping clients develop goals, objectives, or agendas based on an action-oriented understanding of the problem situation. Once clients understand either their problem situations or opportunities for development more clearly they may need help in determining what they would like to do differently. What things would look like if they were better than they are now?

- Getting there (stage 3): Help clients develop action strategies for accomplishing goals, that is, for getting from the present to the preferred scenario. Clients may know what they want to accomplish and where they want to go, but still need help in determining how to get there. This stage is the transition stage dealing with ways of moving from the present to the preferred scenario.

Egan envisages the model as a very active process in which the client needs to act on his or her own behalf right from the beginning of the process. This can be a challenge if the young person feels disempowered and not in control of life's circumstances.

 Activity

You might consider reading the chapter 'The overview of the model' in Egan (1990) *The skilled helper* and judge how useful it could be for your nursing practice.

DEVELOPMENT THEORY AND THERAPEUTIC STYLE

Aspects of developmental theory can be useful in an analysis of those qualities that help make a relationship therapeutic. Bowlby (1988) believed that the observation of normal development was relevant to psychotherapy and that, in getting a picture of what makes a good parent, we are likely to be in a better position to know what makes a good psychotherapist. This idea could be developed and extended to include the therapeutic style of all professionals in terms of their attachments and letting go of client/patient relationships. Adshead (1998) has outlined a number of ways in which professional carers act as attachment figures and utilise other aspects of developmental theory to achieve this.

Attachment Theory

Attachment theory holds that humans are essentially social animals who need relationships for survival and whose first relationships with primary care givers have unique characteristics. Attachment behaviour is any form of behaviour that results in a person attaining or maintaining proximity to an attachment figure, usually a caregiver. Such behaviour is most

obvious when people are frightened, fatigued or sick and is assuaged by comforting and care giving (Bowlby 1979a).

Previous attachment patterns will manifest themselves in any helping relationship and the helper is likely to be seen in terms of an attachment figure. The principle functions of any attachment figure are to provide a secure base and to modulate anxiety. In a helping situation both functions are achieved through an interactional process to which both the helper and the person helped contribute. Professional carers may be seen as providing the patient with a temporary attachment figure. The helper will provide a secure base.

Bowlby argues for the importance of the secure base, stating that:

Human beings of all ages are happiest and able to deploy their talents to best advantage when they are confident that, standing behind them, there are one or more trusted persons who will come to their aid should difficulties arise. The persons trusted, also known as attachment figure . . . can be considered as providing his (or her) companion with a secure base from which to operate (Bowlby 1979b p 103)

In childhood, the secure base is used as 'home' for what Bowlby calls 'a series of excursions', which continue throughout adulthood. As dependency decreases the excursions become longer, so that eventually the dependent individual can exist without anxiety away from the attachment figure. In the same way, within the helping relationship the professional carer provides a secure base from which the patient can make a series of excursions back to a level of optimal functioning.

It has been suggested that attachment figures simulate secure attachment by spending time in active reciprocal interaction (Rutter 1988). It seems that it is the quality of interaction more than the quantity that matters. In the first 3 months, mothers of secure infants respond more promptly when they cry, look, smile at and talk to their babies more, and offer them more affectionate holding. In the therapeutic relationship the degree of responsiveness of the helper is an important factor and mirrors the positive quality of earlier relationships as identified by Rutter.

Adshead (1998) suggested that the attachment figure can modulate anxiety in a number of ways: by acting as an effective container, by providing information and by providing consistent input. She suggests that the affective containment aspect of attachment can be seen as similar to the maternal containment function described by Bion (1962). The primary caregiver helps the baby to develop a capacity to think and tolerate anxiety by using his or her own mental processes to hold and digest the baby's internal projections. In this way, the baby's first cognitive and affective fragments are understood and contained, thus reducing anxiety. It is suggested that caregivers may be internalised cognitively and affectively by the person being helped in the relationship, and thus utilised to contain anxiety. At a conscious level, empathic listening may be experienced as soothing and comforting. Information giving and consistency, which help build trust, offer conscious containment of anxiety.

It is also possible to see the effective therapeutic environment in terms of Winnicott's (1987) phrase 'the holding environment' to denote not just the physical holding of the baby by the mother but the entire psychophysiological system of protection, support, caring and containing that envelops the child, and without which it would not survive physically or emotionally.

Again, with the unfolding of the young person's and family's narrative within the helping relationship there may be similarities with Stern's (1985) cross-modal attunement. In cross-modal attunement the mother follows the baby's babbling. Kicking, bouncing and so on with sounds or movements of her own that match and harmonise with those of the baby. In the use of accurate empathy and the ability to reflect back to the young person the sense that he or she has been seen and understood will create rhythms similar to those described in attunement.

WHAT CAN THE CHILD HEALTH NURSES DO?

Applying Theory to Practice

PowerPoint

When you have completed this section, compare your responses to the information on the companion PowerPoint presentation.

Scenario 1

Katie is 15 years old and has cystic fibrosis. She has been readmitted following a chest infection and weight loss. During her stay she seems to be increasingly introspective and sad.

Activity 1

How would you respond and why to Katie's question 'Look at me, who is ever going to want me like this?' Before referring to the PowerPoint presentation, you might want to at write down a response you might make and give a brief rationale for why you chose that response. It might be helpful to read the sections on core communi-cation skills, listening to and helping the story unfold.

Activity 2

What might be the developmental issues for Katie?

You might want to speculate by interpreting her situation in terms of the developmental model's outlined in the chapter.

Activity 3

What are the health risk factors in Katie's situation? It might be helpful to look again at the section on adolescent health and apply this to Katie's situation.

Activity 4

How might Katie's sense of agency be influenced by ill health?
It might be helpful to link this to issues of self-esteem and the developmental tasks.

Activity 5

What is the likely interplay between Katie's illness and her transition through the adolescent developmental tasks? When you have completed these activities, check your responses with a fuller account of the factors influencing Katie on the PowerPoint presentation.

Scenario 2

Shona is 13 years old and was admitted to the ward because of an overdose and continuing threats to self-harm. When the nurse first meets her she is taken aback by her physical appearance; Shona really looks as if she could be 18. This visual information comes on top of the narrative being told about her. She is sexually active, precocious and seductive in her manner. She declares in a dramatic way that she plans to take more tablets next time. Her relationship with her parents is different in that she acts as Mum's interpreter.

Activity 1

Reflect why at 13 you did not find yourself in Shona's situation. If you did have a troubled adolescence, identify those factors that allowed you to reach a point where you could successfully apply to train as a nurse.

Activity 2

Outline what this young person most needs from the nurse right now. Describe how it might be delivered and provide a rationale for the care given.

Activity 3

What factors in Shona's early development might have contributed to the situation she now finds herself in?

Activity 4

When listening to Shona's unfolding story, what elements of her story might indicate risk factors in terms of future self-harm?

Activity 5

Outline short- and long-term goals aimed at reducing Shona's health-risk behaviours linking the goals to the evidence base for practice.

Summary

The mental health of children and young people should be a central concern of the children's nurse. It may be helpful to refer to the key points below.

KEY POINTS

- There is strong and growing evidence for the fundamental inter-relationship between physical, mental and social health. Problems in adolescence in any of these areas indicate the likelihood of long-term adverse health and social consequences.

- It has been suggested that everyone in contact with young people should take the symptoms of emotional distress, behavioural difficulties and hyperactivity seriously, as they impair function and development and are unlikely to be transient.

- An understanding of the adolescent's developmental tasks will allow the nurse to focus care giving in the most effective manner.

- It is imperative to the promotion of child and adolescent health that nurses develop the skills that will enable them to successfully engage with the young person and ensure a nursing interaction that is rewarding both for the young person and the nurse.

References

Adshead G 1998 Psychiatric staff as attachment figures: understanding management problems in psychiatric services in the light of attachment theory. British Journal of Psychiatry 172:64–69

Ahmad Y, Dalrymple J, Daum M et al 2003 Listening to children and young people. Faculty of Health and Social Care, University of the West of England, Bristol

Bennett DL, Tonkin RS 2003 International developments in adolescent health care: a story of advocacy and achievement. Journal of Adolescent Health 33(4):240–251

Bion W 1962 Learning from experience. Heinemann, London

Bowlby J 1979a On knowing what you're not supposed to know and feeling what you're not supposed to feel. Canadian Journal of Psychiatry 24:403–408

Bowlby J 1979b The making and breaking of affectional bonds. Routledge, London

Bowlby J 1988 A secure base: clinical applications of attachment theory. Routledge, London

British Medical Association (BMA) 2003 Adolescent health. BMA Publishing, London

Burt MR 2002 Reasons to invest in adolescents. Journal of Adolescent Health 31(6) Suppl 1:136–152. Online. Available at: http://www.sciencedirect.com

Buston K 2002 Adolescents with mental health problems: what do they say about health services? Journal of Adolescence 25:231–242

Carr A 1998 Michael White's narrative therapy. Contemporary Family Therapy 20(4):485–503

Coleman JC 1989 The focal theory of adolescence: a psychological perspective. In: Hurrelmann K, Engel U (eds) The social world of adolescence: international perspectives. De Gruyter, Berlin

Cooper M, Glasper E 2001 Deliberate self-harm in children: the nurse's therapeutic style. British Journal of Nursing 10(1):34–40

Dehne KL, Riedner G 2001 Adolescence: a dynamic concept. Reproductive Health Matters 9(17):11–15

Department for Health (DoH) and Department for Education and Employment (DfEE) 1995 A handbook on child and adolescent mental health. HMSO, Manchester

Department of Health (DoH) 2003 National service framework for children, standards for hospital services. HMSO, London

Department of Health (DoH) 2004 National service framework for children, young people, and maternity services. HMSO, London

Department of Human Services Victorian Government 2002 Evidence-based health promotion: resources for planning, no. 2: adolescent health. Online. Available at: http://www.dhs.vic.gov.au/phd/0003097

Egan G 1990 The skilled helper: a systematic approach to effective helping. Brookes/Cole, California

Erikson EH 1963 Childhood and society, 2nd edn. Norton, New York

George L 1997 The psychological characteristics of patients suffering from anorexia nervosa and the nurses role in creating a therapeutic relationship. Journal of Advanced Nursing 26:899–908

Goodman R, Scott S 1997 Child psychiatry. Blackwell Science, Oxford

Goossens L, Marcoen A 1999 Relationships during adolescence: constructive vs. negative themes and relational dissatisfaction. Journal of Adolescence 22:65–79

Hay I, Asman AF 2003 The development of adolescents emotional stability and general self-concept: the interplay of parent, peers, and gender. International Journal of Disability, Development and Education 50(1):77–91

Healthcare Commission 2004 Patient survey report. Online. Available at: http://www.healthcarecommission.org.uk/assetRoot/04/00/81/84/04008184.pdf

Heron J 1975 Six-category intervention analysis. Human Potential Research Project, University of Surrey/British Postgraduate Medical Federation, University of London, pp 16–18

Heron J 2001 Helping the client: a creative practical guide, 5th edn. Sage Publications, London

Jacobs M 1998. The presenting past: the core of psychodynamic counselling and therapy. Open University Press, Buckingham

Kaplan LJ 1978 Oneness and separateness from infant to individual. Touchstone Simon & Schuster, New York, p 231

Kroger J 1989 Identity in adolescence: the balance between self and other. Routledge, London

La Voie JC 1994 Identity in adolescence: issues of theory, structure and transition. Journal of Adolescence 17:17–28

Lightfoot J, Sloper A 2002 Having a say in health: guidelines for involving young patients in health services development. SPRU, University of York, p 9. Online. Available at: http://www.york.ac.uk/inst/spru

Meltzer H, Gatward R, Corbin T et al 2003 Persistence, onset, risk factors and outcomes of childhood mental health disorders. Report based on the analysis of a three-year follow-up survey of the 1999 national survey of the mental health of children and adolescents in Great Britain commissioned by the Department of Health, the Department for Education and Skills and the Scottish Executive Health Department. The Stationery Office, London

Meltzer H, Gatward R, Goodman R, Ford T 2000 Mental health of children and adolescents in Great Britain. A survey carried out in 1999 by the Social Survey Division of ONS. The Stationery Office, London

Mental Health Foundation 1999 Bright futures: promoting children and young people's mental health. Mental Health Foundation Publications, London. Online. Available at: http://www.mentalhealth.org

Needham J 2000 The nurse specialist role in adolescent health. Paediatric Nursing 12(8):11–15

NHS Health Advisory Service 1995 Together we stand: the commissioning, role and management of child and adolescent mental health services. HMSO, London

Norwich Union 2001 The views of adolescents and nurses on the provision of health care in hospitals. Online. Available at: http://www.norwichunion.co.uk/health/literature/gen662_06_02_teenage%20 health.pdf

Peplau HF 1952 Interpersonal relations in nursing. Putnam, New York

Registered Nurses Association of Ontario (RNAO) 2002a Enhancing healthy adolescent development: nursing best practice guideline. RNAO, Toronto. Online. Available at: http://www.rnao.org

Registered Nurses Association of Ontario (RNAO) 2002b Establishing therapeutic relationships. RNAO, Toronto. Online. Available at: http://www.rnao.org

Royal College of Paediatrics and Child Health (RCPCH) 2003 Bridging the gaps: health care for adolescents. Council Report CR114. Online. Available at: http://www.rcpch.ac.uk

Rutter M 1988 Attachment and the development of social relationships. In: Rutter M (ed.) Scientific foundations of developmental psychiatry. American Psychiatric Press, Washington, DC, pp 267–279

Rutter M, Graham P 1968 The reliability and validity of the psychiatric assessment of the child. British Journal of Psychiatry 114:563–579

Rutter M, Smith DJ (eds) 1995 Psychosocial disorders in young people: time trends and their causes. John Wiley for Academia Europaea, Chichester

Stern D 1985 The interpersonal world of the infant: a view from psychoanalysis and developmental psychology. Basic Books, New York

Stockwell F 1972 The unpopular patient. Royal College of Nursing, London

Viner R, Keane M 1998 Youth matters: best practice for the care or young people in hospital. Caring for Children in the Health Services, London

Wilkes TCR, Belsher G 1994 Ten key principles of adolescent cognitive therapy. In: Wilkes TCR, Belsher G, Rush J, Frank E (eds) Cognitive therapy for depressed adolescents. Guilford Press, London

Winnicott DW 1987 In: Home is where we start from, essays by a psychoanalyst. Pelican Books, London

World Health Organization (WHO) 1995 Adolescent health and development: the key to the future. WHO Global Commission on Women's Health, Geneva

Caring for children with special needs

44 Chronic illness and the family 723

45 Caring for children with critical illness 739

46 Care of the child requiring palliative care 770

47 Children with learning disabilities 784

Chapter Forty Four

44

Chronic Illness and the Family

Barbara Elliott, Peter Callery, Julie Mould

ABSTRACT

This chapter focuses on the issues arising from childhood chronic illness for children's families. Specific concerns for children suffering from particular diseases have been covered in previous chapters so will not be addressed here. Rather, the general areas of health-related quality of life for children and parents, issues of self-management and the role of nurses working with families with a child with a chronic illness will be considered.

Learning Outcomes

- Define chronic illness and related concepts.
- Appreciate the range of chronic illnesses affecting children recognising common issues and concerns.
- Be aware of the concept of health related quality of life and its application in childhood chronic illness.
- Discuss the concept of self-management and its application in childhood chronic illness.
- Consider children's involvement in self-management.
- Consider the involvement of parents and other lay carers in self-management.
- Comprehend the range of nursing interventions employed in supporting children with chronic illness and their families.

Definitions of Chronic Illness

There are a number of different definitions of chronic illness but all recognise the protracted nature of the disease and the consequences for the individual's life. For example, chronic illness has been defined as: a condition that is long term and incurable or involves limitations in daily living requiring special assistance or adaptation in function (Perrin 1985). Eiser (1990) defines chronic diseases as those that affect children for extended periods of time, often for life, and which can be managed in terms of symptom control but not cured.

Children may be born with a chronic condition, such as cystic fibrosis, or develop one during childhood, such as asthma or diabetes. Every chronic condition that affects children has the potential to restrict their lives, and therefore the lives of members of their family, and make children feel different from their peers.

Key Features of Chronic Illness

- The symptoms interfere with many normal activities and routines.
- Medical treatment is restricted in its effectiveness.
- Treatment itself contributes to the disruption of daily living (Vessey 1999).

As with other areas of childhood illness, the sick child is no longer viewed in isolation but as an integral part of a family. Family-centred care is nowhere more important than in childhood chronic illness, when the family has to live with their child's illness and its repercussions for prolonged periods of time, if not the child's whole life. Enabling families to manage children's conditions on a day-to-day basis is an important goal of health care.

Many studies of the effects of chronic illness on children and their families have focused on specific diseases such as cystic fibrosis, diabetes, epilepsy and asthma. However, classifying patients according to diagnostic labels is perhaps not appropriate when examining the wider issues of the effects of chronic illness on children and families. It may be argued that the emotional demands of any chronic disease are more important predictors of adjustment than the specific demands of any particular disease, and there may be more variability in psychological, social and educational measures within diagnostic groupings than between them (Stein & Jessop 1989).

This chapter will therefore consider the general issues associated with childhood chronic illness using particular diseases to illustrate points raised.

Activity

Make a list of the different chronic diseases in childhood that you have encountered in the last 12 months. Consider the particular needs and problems of the children and their families. Discuss in your study group those problems/needs common to all or many of the children and their families and those which were disease specific.

Now reflect on the merits of grouping patients with the same diagnosis as a useful way of predicting their needs compared with the non-categorical approach of considering general issues of chronic illness.

Chronic illness is by definition persistent: children and their families must live with the illness for an extended period of time, possibly for the child's life. We have chosen not to use the term 'chronic disease' because this implies a medical perspective where the principal concerns are with the signs and symptoms of the condition and how these might be cured or at least treated. Instead, we use the term 'chronic illness' to focus attention on the experience of living with the symptoms and problems of the condition. Some problems can arise from the treatment, for example parents' concerns about the potential long-term effects of steroid use in asthma management. The outcome of treatments and other interventions, such as education about management, may be not cure but increased independence or better control of the illness.

INCIDENCE AND PREVALENCE

Information about the incidence, number of new cases of disease per unit of population in a defined period, and prevalence, number of new and continuing cases of disease, is limited. Statistics are more readily available for some chronic illnesses than others so overall rates are generally estimates. Cooper (1999 p 4) provides a useful table of the

incidence and expected survival rate of children with twelve chronic illnesses. There has been an increase in the incidence of certain diseases such as asthma and diabetes and an increase in the life expectancy of children with other chronic illnesses such as cystic fibrosis and cancer. Approximately one-fifth of children with chronic illness have more than one condition (Newachek & Stoddard 1994).

Completely new categories of chronic conditions are emerging as technology develops and childhood mortality rates improve. Preterm babies are surviving at earlier gestation and increasingly low birth weights. Organ transplants are enabling children to survive longer with previously fatal diseases and there are increasing numbers of ventilator-dependent children cared for both in hospitals and the community. There is obviously a wide range in the severity of chronic illness both within disease categories and between them. Some diseases, such as atopic eczema, may be common but not always perceived as an illness. This can bring further problems to children and their families as their experiences and needs may not be understood and even trivialised. A study of the prevalence of atopic symptoms in the UK found that almost half of the 12- to 14-year-olds surveyed reported one or more symptoms, itchy flexural rash, rhinoconjunctivitis or wheeze, and 4% reported all three (Austin et al 1999).

Children with chronic illness may not only have the symptoms of the disease and consequences of treatment to contend with but they also have increased rates of mental health problems and psychological difficulties (Vessey 1999). It has been suggested that an appropriate assessment tool to detect such problems should be added to routine paediatric outpatient assessments to aid detection and appropriate referral to child mental health services (Glazebrook et al 2003). The importance of recognising and effectively managing psychological well-being is also supported by evidence that adults with persistent chronic illness from childhood which limit their daily life suffer more depression and lower self-esteem than those with non-limiting conditions or healthy controls (Huurre & Aro 2002).

Seminar discussion topic

Watch the PowerPoint presentation, including the short video clip, on living with atopic eczema. Consider the physical, psychological and social implications of this disease for children and their families.

There is now a considerable amount of information about specific chronic diseases available on the internet. Some of this information is aimed at health professionals and other information is more suitable for parents and children. Certain internet sources are not particularly relevant to families and health professionals in the UK but others are becoming an important resource. Useful evaluations of the use of the internet are provided by Pandolfini et al (2000) and Pandolfini & Bonati (2002). The following activities will help you to assess the usefulness of some specific websites.

WWW

Access the websites for specific childhood diseases such as:
- http://www.cystic fibrosis.co.uk
- http://www.cftrust.org.uk
- http://www.eczema.org.uk
- http://www.diabetes.org.uk
- http://www.asthma.org.uk
- http://www.childrenfirst.nhs.uk/index.php

Compare the information found with that available on a generic site such as:
- http://www.kidshealth.org

Activity

Using a popular search engine such as Google, access internet sites related to five common childhood chronic diseases. Assess how useful they are for you as a nurse, parents and children. Do they have specific areas for children? How could they be improved?

CONCEPT OF HEALTH-RELATED QUALITY OF LIFE IN CHILDHOOD CHRONIC ILLNESS

To assess the effectiveness of interventions by nurses and other healthcare workers, it is necessary to use outcomes that are consistent with the focus on the experience of childhood chronic illness. Quality of life (QoL) is therefore an important concept in chronic illness. Measures of quality of life can either be generic or specific to particular diseases. The advantages of generic measurement would be that comparison could be made with healthy children. However, this is not practical with the instruments currently available: generic measures cannot detect differences that arise from the effects of particular illnesses, for example the effect of eczema on appearance. Therefore quality of life is usually measured in children with disease-specific instruments (Eiser 1997). For this reason we use the term 'health-related quality of life' (HRQoL) to recognise that the topics addressed relate to health-related aspects of quality of life.

A valid assessment of HRQoL could enable assessment of the impact of an illness and the effectiveness of treatments and other interventions, including education about management, often provided by nurses.

Assessment of HRQoL is particularly challenging in children. The development of instruments must take account of the 'response burden', that is, the 'extent to which issues of scale length or type of response need to be adapted for

children's language and cognitive skills' (Eiser & Morse 2001). Children must be able to read and understand questionnaires used to assess quality of life. It may be more appropriate to develop instruments that appeal to children's interests and do not demand high reading ages, for example computer games (Eiser et al 2000). It is also important to recognise that meaning of quality of life can be quite different for children and adults. Young children's quality of life is about having very shiny hair, lots of friends or running like a sports star rather than achievement of basic functional tasks (Eiser 1997). When adults rate children's quality of life their ratings are based on different frameworks to the children's ratings, and it might even be that very close parent–child agreement is indicative of poorer quality of life because childhood is about gaining autonomy and independence from parental views (Eiser 1997). As children develop 'any measure needs to have an in-built sensitivity to accommodate the normative changes that would be expected to occur during childhood' (Eiser 1997). It may therefore be necessary to ask different questions of children at different times in their lives and these questions may differ from those asked of parents when assessing quality of life. There are challenges for researchers to develop new approaches to quality of life assessment if they are to be child centred.

Evidence-based Practice

There is clear evidence that children's self-assessments differ from those of their parents:

In children younger than 11, children's global rating of change in symptoms correlated strongly with changes in quality of life but not with measures of airway calibre or asthma control, while parents' global ratings did not correlate with children's quality of life but showed moderate correlations with airway calibre and asthma control (0.50). In children over the age of 11, correlations with all clinical variables were higher for their own than their parents' global ratings (Guyatt et al 1997)

Therefore children's own views about their symptoms and their quality of life should be sought.

Practitioners should be careful to consider the way in which a measure has been designed and tested when deciding how to assess quality of life in children with chronic illness. Some questions that can help to decide on the appropriateness of a measure are:

- How have children's concerns been identified and integrated into the measure?
- Is the measure designed to make appropriate demands on children, for example, reading age and cognitive ability?

HEALTH-RELATED QUALITY OF LIFE FOR PARENTS

Chronic illness in childhood occurs in a social context in which a supportive relationship between parent and child is essential for successful management. The impact of childhood chronic illness on the lives of parents, the adaptation processes required and their needs have been the focus of a considerable amount of research in recent years (e.g. Canam 1993, Elliott & Luker 1996, Fisher 2001, Gibson 1995, Hentinen & Kyngas 1998, Hodgkinson & Lester 2002, Young et al 2002). There is an acceptance that parents are the main carers of children with chronic illness and considerable effort has been made in trying to understand the impact of this role on their lives and how healthcare professionals can support them in their role and facilitate successful coping. Better understanding of the experience of parenting a chronically sick child is thought to improve the relationship between health professionals and parents and ensure that care provided is appropriate and meaningful. Good relationships between health professionals and parents are considered to be beneficial both for children and parents. For example, a good relationship between doctors and mothers of children with atopic eczema was found to be the strongest predictor of adherence to skin-care treatment (Ohya et al 2001).

The emphasis on the inevitable negative impact of childhood chronic illness and disability has been criticised by some authors. It is not disputed that parenting a child with chronic illness is stressful at times but whether this causes distress in parents is being questioned. The focus of research and nursing literature on the tragedy of childhood illness and disability, parental stress, the burden of care and need for successful coping mechanisms is beginning to shift and the positive contributions to family life of children with disability is beginning to be recognised (Kearney & Griffin 2001).

Treatment of chronic illness may have a positive or negative impact on children's and parents' quality of life. Successful management of a disease may be at odds with children's or parents' experience of the illness and it is important that treatment outcome measures include consideration of patient and parent reported outcomes. International instruments to measure parents' experience of childhood chronic illness, and which can be used to determine the acceptability and efficacy of pharmaceutical treatment, have been developed (Whalley et al 2002).

It is essential that any quality of life instrument is developed from the perspective of those whose HRQoL it intends to measure. We have already suggested that a child's perspective of HRQoL may be very different from that of their parents. In the majority of cases, the HRQoL instrument is developed from the analysis of qualitative interviews with patients and parents (Henry et al 2003).

Analysis of these interviews provides information about the impact of the child's disease on the family and their experience of living with childhood chronic illness. A distinction must be made between instruments that use parents to assess their child's HRQoL and those that focus on assessment of the parents' HRQoL.

Evidence-based Practice

Instruments that purport to measure quality of life are frequently used in research studies that assess the impact of a disease on a child and/or his or her family. They may also be used to evaluate treatment strategies. It is essential therefore that they are tested for validity and reliability. They must also measure aspects of quality of life (QoL) that are important to those on whom the instrument is being used. Many of the instruments used today have been developed from qualitative interviews and tested on large numbers of patients and carers. Several adult QoL instruments have been adapted for use with children or parents as proxy participants. Comparisons between parent and child ratings of quality of life have been made, for example Vance et al (2001).

As well as influencing parents' HRQoL, the impact of chronic illness on families can be enormous. Efforts have been made to develop a scale to measure the impact of chronic illness on parents and families (Stein & Reissman 1980) and applied in specific diseases such as atopic eczema (Su et al 1996).

Within disease categories, parents' estimate of the severity of disease has been found to be the single strongest predictor of family impact of the disease (Balkrishnan et al 2003). It is important to recognise that it is the assessment of severity by the parents, and not by the professionals, that predicts the impact on the family. Chronic diseases considered as minor by health professionals may in fact have a greater impact on the family than other more serious diseases. For example, Su et al (1996) found that parents with children with moderate or severe eczema scored higher on the family impact score than parents with children suffering from diabetes. By contrast, assumptions of the negative impact on family life of children with severe disability are being challenged and the need for acceptance of the highly individual response of families must be recognised (Kearney & Griffin 2001).

Some of the issues assessed by the measures are considered below.

Emotional Responses

The emotional responses of parents to the diagnosis of chronic illness in a child are frequently linked to loss and grief. Parents may experience multiple losses, loss of their healthy child, loss of freedom and lifestyle, loss of confidence and support systems and potential loss of their child's life (Lowes & Lyne 2000). The grief reactions they may suffer have been studied in relation to many specific childhood diseases and are well documented in the nursing literature. For example, feelings of shock, anger, denial, sadness and frustration have been reported in parents of children newly diagnosed with diabetes (Hatton et al 1995). Time-bound theories of grief have been applied to parents of children with chronic illness, suggesting that they progress through a series of stages culminating in acceptance of their child's condition and resolution of their grief. Such theories have been challenged and an alternative model of 'chronic sorrow' has been suggested as representative of parents' experience of childhood chronic illness. Teel (1991) describes chronic sorrow as a recurring sadness interwoven with periods of neutrality, satisfaction and happiness suggesting that parents make a functional adaptation to childhood chronic illness but do not accept it. Lowes & Lyne (2000) provide a useful review of the literature on grief reactions to childhood chronic illness.

It must be remembered that diagnosis may also result in feelings of relief and hope, particularly if the parents have been concerned for sometime about their child's health. Parents may also be falsely accused of being in denial when they are trying to remain positive and optimistic about their child's condition. Kearny & Griffin (2001) quote a mother of a child with significant health problems:

I knew her condition was serious and her prognosis poor but to me she was my firstborn, beautiful child.

When a child has a chronic illness, Larson (1998) describes how the mother has to embrace the paradox between loving the child as he or she is and wanting to erase the disability; between coping with the incurability of the child's illness and looking for solutions; between maintaining hope for the child's future and struggling with negative information and their own fears.

Scenario

David is a third-year child branch student who is caring for a 6-month-old baby girl with cystic fibrosis. She has a chest infection but is otherwise well and her mother is delighted with her weight gain and achievement of normal development. David overhears the mother telling a friend that she doesn't think there is anything wrong with her baby and is considering stopping giving her medication because she is so well.

Consider how David might deal with this situation. How might he ensure that the mother recognises her baby's need for treatment but maintain her positive approach and delight in her child's progress?

Parental Health

Parental health and well-being may suffer as a consequence of caring for a child with chronic illness and, although not ill themselves, mothers in particular may suffer many of the consequences of chronic illness (Young et al 2002a). Mothers may experience stress in relation to caring for a chronically sick child and coping with the demands of the illness. Stress may be experienced in relation to decision making, the burden of care and accepting a change in identity (Hodgkinson & Lester 2002). Many research studies throughout the 1970s and 1980s explored the stress experienced by parents (in particular mothers) and the coping strategies they developed when dealing with chronic illness in a child (Faux 1998).

Financial Consequences

Parents of children with chronic illness may find it difficult to sustain full-time employment. Time off work to care for their child and attend hospital appointments, as well as the extra cost of childcare for a child with additional needs may make paid employment impossible. In addition, there are costs involved in bringing up and caring for a child with chronic illness that are extra to those for healthy children. A study of 273 parents who had responsibility for the day-to-day care of a severely disabled child found that it cost at least three times as much to bring up a child with severe disability from birth to 17 as to bring up a child without disability (Dobson & Middleton 1998). Additional costs result from clothing, bedding, laundry, food, equipment, furniture, transport, toys, toiletries and activities.

Scenario

Laura is a 6-year-old girl with atopic eczema. She requires frequent application of ointment to keep her skin hydrated. This makes her clothes greasy and sticky and she requires several changes of clothes each day. She can only wear pure cotton clothes next to her skin as man-made fibres irritate her. Her bedding needs to be changed every morning as it is soiled with skin cells, exudate and ointment.

Laura's condition deteriorates if she eats certain foods. Her mother has to prepare special food for her meals, much of which is wasted if Laura does not like it.

It is thought that house-dust mites contribute to Laura's skin condition so her parents have replaced the carpet in her bedroom with laminate flooring and her curtains with wooden blinds.

The benefits system in the UK recognises the additional costs involved in chronic illness and disability and parents can apply for a range of additional benefits. Some are extra amounts within existing benefits, such as the Disabled Child Premium in Income Support, and others are purely for disabled people such as Disability Living Allowance (DLA). However, for many families there is a considerable gap between their income and what they consider necessary to spend on their child (Dobson & Middleton 1998).

Children do not become eligible for certain benefits until they reach a specific age. For example, free nappies are available for children over 3 years old who are incontinent and children with mobility problems are eligible for the mobility component of DLA once they are 5 years old. Such age restrictions can seem unreasonable to parents and many may not be aware of their child's entitlements.

www

Access the website for disability benefits in the UK for current information about benefits:

- http://www.disabilitybenefits.co.uk

Activity

Consider a child with a chronic illness you have nursed recently. List the additional financial costs to the family involved in caring for their child. What help with these additional costs might the family receive?

Social Consequences

The role of being a parent of a child with chronic illness may compromise the ability to function adequately in other roles such as friend, professional, spouse or partner and parent of other children. Childhood chronic illness may make parents reluctant to leave the child to pursue social and leisure activities. In addition, the disease may produce additional caring needs and treatment regimens for parents, such as regular injections or physiotherapy, which may reduce the time available to meet their own social needs.

There is evidence that the nature of normal childcare, such as bathing, feeding and entertaining, may be changed when a child has a chronic illness and normally enjoyable tasks may become difficult and onerous. Parents of children with atopic eczema have described the constant struggle to keep their child entertained to distract them from scratching and the difficulties of bathing and nappy changing when skin is excoriated, itchy and sore (Elliott & Luker 1996). There is evidence to suggest that parents can feel particularly stressed in relation to their parenting skills when a child has a chronic illness and may be less efficient in disciplining their affected child (Daud et al 1993).

Restricted social activities may lead parents to perceive that they have less social support (Daud et al 1993). This is a concern as ongoing social support is crucial for the successful adaptation of parents to their child's chronic illness (Whyte 1994). Perceived social support has been found to be a predictor of family coping and a factor that influences the resilience of high-risk groups of families with a child with chronic illness (Tak & McCubbin 2002).

Marital Relationships

There is a belief that family dysfunction and marital problems frequently follow the diagnosis of chronic illness in a child. However, there is conflicting empirical evidence in this area and much anecdotal evidence to suggest that caring for a chronically sick child may bring parents closer together. Gender differences between mothers and fathers in how they cope with chronic illness in a child and from whom they receive their support have been reported (Katz 2002) and conflict may arise from these differences.

There are conflicting reports in the literature of the effects of caring for a chronically ill child on marital satisfaction and stability with some studies showing a negative effect and others finding no differences. Most studies of parents of children with chronic health problems report decreased marital satisfaction compared with parents of healthy children. A recent study by Contact a Family found that, whereas one-quarter of the 2000 parents studied felt that having a disabled child had brought them closer together, nearly half felt that it had caused problems in their relationships and almost 10% believed that it had lead to separation from their spouse or partner (Contact a Family 2004). Childcare responsibilities and decision making are likely to cause conflict and are the most frequently cited stresses of parents of children with chronic illness (Quittner et al 1998). However, a study that compared 94 married parents caring for a child with chronic illness with over 3000 married parents of well children found no differences in perceived marital quality or satisfaction between the two groups (Eddy & Walker 1999). Similarly, Katz & Krulik (1999) found no difference in levels of marital satisfaction between fathers of healthy children and those of children with chronic illness, although the latter group did experience a greater number of stressful life events and lower self-esteem.

Decreased marital satisfaction does not necessarily result in decreased marital stability. It is suggested that marital stability is a product of net outcomes (rewards minus costs), barriers to leaving the relationship and alternative attractions (Eddy & Walker 1999). When parents have a child with chronic illness there may be more strain on the relationship, resulting in fewer rewards and greater costs but the barriers to leaving are increased and opportunities for alternative attractions reduced. All children, whether sick or healthy, constitute important marital capital in that they increase the barriers to leaving a relationship for the majority of parents.

Siblings

The family context in which children with chronic illness live inevitably means that their well siblings are affected by the disease and its management. Within families, the relationship between siblings may be just as important as the parent–child relationship, if not more so. Brothers and sisters spend a considerable amount of time together and children can be very distressed by chronic illness in a sibling. They may supply considerable emotional, social and physical support to the sick child, thus being a source of help to their parents. However, well siblings have their own unique needs and may themselves make additional demands at a time when their parents' attention is focused on the sick child.

There is no question that some chronic illnesses result in well siblings being separated from the sick child and one or both of their parents on a regular basis and sometimes for prolonged periods. Their daily routine is disrupted and they may have fewer opportunities for social activities and interactions with their parents. The sick child frequently becomes the centre of attention and siblings may feel neglected and deprived of attention as their parents try to deal with problems without involving them (Drotar & Crawford 1985). Parents often believe that it is the well siblings who suffer the most through not receiving their fair share of attention.

However, the research literature in this area is contradictory as to the consequences of chronic illness for well siblings (Eiser 1993, Blubond-Langner 1996). There is a great deal of research literature reporting the negative effects of chronic illness on well siblings. A whole range of problems have been reported including somatic and psychosomatic disorders, school problems, increased accidents, behaviour problems including hyperactivity and antisocial behaviour, emotional problems, aggressiveness, withdrawal and poor social adjustment. At the other end of the spectrum are studies that indicate that chronic illness does not have a negative effect on well siblings, indeed there may be positive consequences. Empathy, compassion, coping and communication skills have been reported in well siblings, as well as an increased maturity, appreciation of their own health and increased family cohesion.

Explanations of why having a sibling with chronic illness results in some children experiencing positive outcomes and others negative ones have been sought and it is apparent that factors other than the disease alone are influential. A number of factors have been considered by various researchers and summarised by Blubond-Langner (1996). Factors such as age, birth order, gender, socio-economic status of the family, parents' marital situation, prior family problems, character of the disease and relationship with the sick child can all influence how a child copes with chronic illness in a sibling. It should be noted that much of the research to date has relied on parental, usually the mothers, reporting of the behaviour and health of their children, which may be influenced by many factors including the parents' own health and adaptation to their child's illness.

It is suggested that negative outcomes in well siblings should not be expected but that there should be an awareness of their unique relationship with the sick child and their individual needs. The adjustment of children to chronic illness in a sibling is best understood within the context of the family. Childhood chronic illness may be viewed as a stressor that, combined with other factors, may result in an increased risk of psychological problems for some siblings of sick children. The factors that mediate the effects of chronic illness on well siblings are poorly understood but it is believed that the quality of family functioning and relationships has both direct and indirect effects on siblings (Drotar & Crawford 1985).

Self-management in Chronic Illness

Self-management of chronic illness has the potential '. . . to allow people with chronic diseases to have access to opportunities to develop the confidence, knowledge and skills to manage their conditions better, and thereby gain a greater measure of control and independence to enhance their quality of life' (Department of Health (DoH) 2001). The more we focus on chronic illness rather than chronic disease, the more essential it is to recognise the expertise of the people living with the condition. However, there are important issues to consider when applying these ideas in childhood chronic illness. The first of these is who is the 'self' involved in self-management? Children cannot be seen in isolation because parents have legal and moral responsibilities for their care and protection. However, parents are proxies: their experience of the illness is different to their children's. Important differences emerge when children and their parents report symptoms or quality of life, or the impact of illness can differ between children and parents (Braun-Fahrlander et al 1998, Callery et al 2003, Renzoni et al 1999). To complicate matters further, the 'self' is not limited to one parent and one child. In addition to the adults in their family, children must deal with adult carers in other settings, for example at school. A variety of adults can contribute to the care of children in the absence of their parents, adding further elements to the 'self' involved in self-management.

The range of people involved in self-management will have differing objectives. Parents of children with asthma can judge asthma by its observable effects on their children's behaviour and its impact on parents' own lives, so that they may be most concerned about avoiding acute attacks (Callery et al 2003). They can accept a level of continuing symptoms and restriction of activity as 'tolerable' asthma. Children can be more concerned with the day-to-day effects of asthma and how these make them appear different to their peers (Callery et al 2003, Ireland 1997). Again, this can lead to acceptance of restriction of activity, for example to avoid appearing different by taking inhalers in public. These differences highlight the need to identify the objectives of children and of adult carers in planning self-management of chronic illness. Guidelines on asthma management stress the importance of individualisation of self-management plans (British Thoracic Society (BTS) & Scottish Intercollegiate Guidelines Network (SIGN) 2003). However, it appears that little attention has been paid to identification of children's objectives, concerns and experiences in self-management plans used in practice. In a survey of 47 UK centres using 30 self-management plans for school-aged children with asthma, only two plans had apparent space for inclusion of individualised objectives and 21 did not identify objectives even implicitly in the title (Milnes & Callery 2003). Only three plans were clearly addressed to the child, the remainder were impersonal (six), addressed to an adult carer through the child (twelve), principally to an adult carer (four), ambiguous (four) or open ended (one). These findings suggest a lack of consensus about the role that children should take in self-management of asthma.

It is important to understand the meaning of chronic illness to both child and parent, or other adult carer, because it influences the ways in which they respond to advice from health carers. Peak flow recording by children aged 5–16 years has been shown to be unreliable with the 'percentage of correct peak flow entries decreased from 56% to <50% from the first to the last study week ($P < 0.04$), mainly as a result of an increase in self-invented peak flow entries' (Kamps et al 2001). One response to such findings is to describe the behaviours as 'non-compliant' and to obtain more control over the process, for example by using electronic peak flow meters that would not record self-invented entries. However, an alternative approach is to seek to understand the perspectives of children and their adult carers to explain their reasons for behaving in this way in order to adapt advice to their needs. The differences between professional and family perspectives are highlighted by the different meanings attached even to apparently straightforward terms such as 'wheeze' by parents and professionals (Cane et al 2000, Young et al 2002).

Reflect on your Practice

Think about a consultation between a child, parent and nurse or doctor that you have observed. How much of the time did each of those involved speak? What was the nature of the talk when each was speaking? Were the child's objectives for treatment discussed? Did the child have opportunities to influence decisions about treatment and/or care?

Self-management education is effective in adults (Gibson et al 1999). The most recent review concluded that:

Educational programmes for the self-management of asthma in children and adolescents improve lung function and feelings of self-control, reduce absenteeism from school, number of days with restricted activity, number of visits to an emergency department, and possibly number of disturbed nights. Educational programmes should be considered a part of the routine care of young people with asthma (Guevara et al 2003)

The effect of education was most marked in children with severe asthma, when interventions were directed at individuals rather than groups and when interventions were based on peak flow recording. However, none of the studies included in this review assessed quality of life and other limitations in the study reports limited the conclusions that could be reached for various ages and other sub groups of children. Further research is required to identify the best way to provide education for different groups of children. More child-centred approaches to self-management, which incorporate the objectives and perspectives of children as well as their adult carers, might be the most promising way to improve the effectiveness of self-management education.

THE NURSE'S ROLE

Most children with a chronic illness are cared for by their parents at home. Caring for a child and family with a chronic illness requires the child, family, health professionals and voluntary organisations to work together to maintain optimal health, growth and development of the child.

On diagnosis few families realise the extent to which a chronic illness will change their lives (Eiser 1990) and adaptation to living with a chronic illness is a continual process. Components that predict the level of adaptation include the characteristics of the child, development stage, personality and coping style, family characteristics including family relationships, support and cohesiveness, other concurrent stresses on the family and the level and availability of social and service support (Edwards & Davis 1997). Facilitating families in this process of adaptation is a key role for nurses.

Nurses work with children with chronic illness and their families in a variety of roles. Hospital nurses may care for the child and family around the time of diagnosis and during periods of acute exacerbation of their illness. Community children's nurses may support the child and family at home helping them to incorporate care and treatment into their daily routine and manage the child's illness on a day-to-day basis. Health promotion and assessment of child development may be undertaken by health visitors. Many areas now employ nurses for specific diseases, such as cystic fibrosis and diabetes specialist nurses. These nurses use their specialist knowledge and expertise to support children and their families, and may also act in an advisory role for other nurses and health professionals involved in their care.

Professional Conversation

"
Julie is a clinical nurse specialist for children with cystic fibrosis.
"

I base my role as the Cystic Fibrosis Clinical Nurse Specialist (CNS) on four inter-related components:

- *clinical practice*
- *education*
- *research/audit*
- *change agent.*

Fifty per cent of my time is practice based, when I am able to utilise my skills and knowledge with children and their families in the home, school, outpatient and inpatient settings. I work as an autonomous practitioner and am expected to exhibit high levels of judgement, discretion and decision making in clinical care within my area of specialist practice.

Education is a major part of the role. Various teaching methods, delivered in a timely way and pitched at an appropriate level, are chosen to suit each individual child and family to enable them to gain knowledge and understanding of the disease and to deliver treatment and care in the home. As an educator, I can increase the knowledge and understanding of different health professionals either formally in the classroom or informally by working alongside them.

Through the utilisation of research to develop teaching packages and guidelines, I endeavour to improve the standards of care delivered to the CF children and their families. By auditing against these guidelines I can determine which areas require improving and which areas can be seen as good practice.

As a change agent I see myself in an ideal position to affect change not only directly with CF children and their families and other health professionals but also indirectly with the NHS Trust. Using resources innovatively can benefit the organisation and CF children and their families.

It is important that the CNS is seen as a role model and leader and a visible part of nursing practice. The CNS requires depth and breath of knowledge of their speciality and expertise in nursing care. This is gained through experience, further training and postgraduate qualifications.

If the child's chronic illness results in considerable disability and a number of services are involved to provide complex care then it is advisable for a key worker to be identified. For nearly 30 years legislation and policy guidance has recommended that children with disabilities, including those arising from chronic illness, are cared for by a multidisciplinary team coordinated by a key worker. In addition, research with families has repeatedly called for a single named person to help parents negotiate the maze of health and social service provision (Mukherjee et al 1999). This key worker must be able to cross boundaries easily between the different services that are provided to the children and their families in order to have full appreciation of their care and treatment. Mukherjee et al (1999) identified six elements that could form an appropriate model for key workers:

- proactive regular contact
- a supportive, open relationship
- a family-centred approach
- working across agencies
- working with families' strengths and ways of coping
- working for the family as opposed to working for an agency.

Despite the repeated endorsement of key workers both by legislation and families, they are frequently not part of the service provided to families with a child with chronic illness or disability (Ray 2002, Sloper & Turner 1992). A recent report from the Social Policy Research Unit indicates that key worker schemes remain patchy, with less than one-third of families with a severely disabled child in the UK having a key worker (Greco et al 2004). Few schemes have full-time or designated key workers, with the majority of professionals acting as key workers as a small part of their professional roles (Greco et al 2004). This can be problematic if the professional feels a responsibility for coordinating services but does not have the authority with the other professions involved so to do. Key workers remain an important aspect of care for children with chronic illness and disabilities requiring complex care provision and there is evidence that the number of key worker schemes across the UK is increasing (Greco & Sloper 2004). Nurses need to be aware of their roles with regard to both working as and working with key workers. Suggestions for implementing successful key working schemes are discussed by Mukherjee et al (1999).

Whether nurses are acting as key workers or simply involved in the care of a child with chronic illness either in hospital or the community they will be part of a team of health professionals. Team working and sound communication skills are fundamental to good nursing care of children and families. The following six factors may be helpful when caring for children with chronic illness and their families.

1. Finding Out

Prior to caring for a child and family with a chronic illness, it is necessary to have some background knowledge and to be aware of previous medical, nursing, social and psychological issues and interventions. Information can be gained by reading case notes and contacting the health professionals and other support agencies involved in the care of the child and family. Although not definitive, the following list shows the range of information nurses may learn about a child and family prior to even meeting or working with them:

- any problems antenatal, during labour, postnatal
- bonding
- type of disease (e.g. genetic)
- stage of illness and course disease is likely to take
- reaction to diagnosis
- reaction to illness
- operations
- frequency of hospitalisation
- respite care
- acute exacerbations of illness
- remission
- growth and development:
  - height, weight, head circumference, body mass index, nutrition
  - vision, hearing, speech, communication
  - breathing
  - mobility
  - elimination
  - sleep patterns
  - skin
- independence/dependence
- sexuality
- schooling
- family set-up
- support agencies involved
- doctors and other health professionals involved
- key worker
- coping strategies
- treatment

- competencies
- medications
- concordance
- behaviour
- normalisation
- parenting style
- ethnicity and family culture/beliefs
- finance/benefits
- transport.

This information gathering is crucial to the first part of any assessment to give the nurse a framework and knowledge to work with the child and family. Some of the information gathered may be based on another professional's subjective assessment so it is important that nurses remain non-judgemental at this stage.

Activity

During a clinical placement in the hospital or community, where you are involved in the care of children with chronic illness, select three children and look at their case notes. What picture and knowledge do you gain about these children and their families from the case notes alone?

2. Building up Relationships

Continuity of care is the main component in building-up a relationship with children with chronic illness and their families. It has been argued that parents with a child with disability need a professional approach from nurses, which acknowledges hope without labelling parents as unrealistic or in denial (Kearney & Griffin 2001).

Visiting children and their families at home is less formal than the hospital setting and the home environment makes it easier for them to discuss issues openly. When undertaking nursing interventions in the busy home environment there can be many distractions but these can provide useful information about the ongoing care and relationships. The children and family can communicate information and feelings that may have little to do with a current problem but have greater significance to their overall care.

It is important that nurses are mindful of the need to communicate effectively with children and their parents. The social position of children relative to adults means that communication between health professionals and children may be difficult and compromised by the influence of parents. Although parents have an important role in interpreting and facilitating communication between children and health professionals, they have been found to constrain communication and contribute to the marginalisation of children in encounters with health professionals (Young et al 2003). It is important, therefore, that nurses encourage children to communicate their needs effectively.

Nursing care of children with chronic illness does not always involve physical activities. Listening, seeing and feeling may be more appropriate actions. A positive attitude demonstrating an interest in the children and their families and not just the chronic disease is essential. Knowledge is gained by observation regarding habits of the family, such as smoking, safety in the home, cleanliness and hygiene, heating, availability of food, socio-economic status and extended family and support. There may be many opportunities for health promotion and advice can be given when appropriate.

Through regular, direct and/or indirect contact with chronically ill children and their families, nurses can assist them in adapting to meet the challenges of the chronic illness and reduce their feelings of being different. Parents of chronically ill or disabled children face a number of common tasks in adapting to their child's condition (Canam 1993):

- accept the child's condition
- manage the child's condition on a day-to-day basis
- meet the child's normal developmental needs
- meet the developmental needs of other family members
- cope with ongoing stress and periodic crises
- assist family members to manage their feelings
- educate others about the child's condition
- establish a support system.

Parents who are not completing these tasks may not have the knowledge, skills or resources necessary. The nurse can be influential in providing appropriate resources and therefore promoting effective coping strategies.

Coping strategies will vary from one family to another. Nurses should support children and their families during any life transitions or crises. By having a shared understanding of the issues nurses are in a position to listen to and value children and their families, raise their self-esteem and reassure them of their strengths. In this way nurses can facilitate children and families in their development of strategies for overcoming the difficulties and problems they are facing. Nurses must also acknowledge their own limitations in knowledge and expertise and refer to other services when appropriate.

By building up relationships nurses are in a position to form the second part of an assessment that embraces the child and family in totality and over time and a holistic therapeutic relationship can be developed. This relationship allows the child, family and nurse to discuss issues openly when fluctuations in the child's illness and family stability occur.

Activity

Compare and contrast the picture and knowledge you gained from the case notes of the three children in the previous activity with the picture and knowledge you gained from caring for them either in hospital or on home visits.

Consider how information gained from different sources can be used to form a holistic view of the child and family.

3. Education and Nursing Care

Chronic illness is dynamic. There may be acute exacerbations when hospitalisation is required, slow deterioration with new problems, and the need for palliative care in some cases. The dynamic nature of the illness means that children and their families need to be prepared in advance for possible changes in their child's condition and educated when changes occur in order to give the necessary care and treatment.

The term 'disease trajectory' is frequently used to describe the course of a disease and the work involved in its management. The disease trajectory is the developmental process involved in learning to live with a chronic disease and is characterised by stages through which an individual progresses to achieve responsibility for his or her disease management. For nurses to develop an understanding of chronic illness, it may be useful to view the illness in terms of stages with key triggers, which move individuals from one stage to the next. Such explanations provide neat frameworks for understanding illness behaviour and have been applied to a range of chronic illnesses, for example poliomyelitis (Davis 1963), diabetes (Thorne & Paterson 1999), juvenile rheumatoid arthritis (Frank et al 1998) and leukemia (Wills 1999).

There has been some questioning of the appropriateness of describing the development of childhood chronic illness in such a manner when there are so many individual differences and factors affecting the course and severity of individual illness experiences. However, understanding of disease trajectories for particular illnesses can help nurses prepare children and their families for changes in their condition and factors likely to affect its progression. Parents have a major responsibility for accurately diagnosing and managing changes in their child's condition and seeking assistance when appropriate. The vigilant monitoring of their child's condition, observing for complications and deterioration can be an onerous responsibility for parents (Ray 2002).

Families need education about the usual minor illnesses that occur in childhood as these may have a greater significance to children with chronic illness, for example they may be more vulnerable to infection. Information about the expected growth and development of their child is also important. Preparing families for changes in their child's condition aids them in developing strategies to adapt.

Although recognising that many children and families have detailed knowledge of their illness, nurses should never presume that they know everything about their illness. It is wise to explore their current knowledge and practical expertise regarding the illness before discussing new care and treatment. This helps clarify knowledge and identify any misconceptions held by children and families before new information is given. Information should be given clearly, concisely and honestly, based on the questions the family asks and on the context in which the conversation is held. Written information, videos, audiotapes, demonstrations, talking to other children and families can often reinforce any verbal information given.

Practical care can vary from basic nursing care, such as bed bathing, to highly technical care, for example, mechanical ventilation. Children and their families will inevitably be involved in such care but the level of their involvement should be negotiated on an individual basis. Nurses should negotiate care that has mutual aims and agree a plan of action with each child and family. Listening to their individual experiences helps nurses to plan interventions that are sensitive to the child and family's needs. Many treatment regimens are complex, time consuming and emotionally laden (Eiser 1990) and, consequently, it is important that nurses regularly review any practical care undertaken by the child and family to ensure that they are willing and confident to continue with such care.

A fundamental principle is that any care undertaken by children and their families at home must be negotiated, agreed and sometimes taught. Kirk (2001) found that parental obligations and the desire for discharge from hospital often made them naïvely accept responsibility for the care and treatment of their child at home, and that there was no effective negotiation. However, once they were at home, parents were in a more powerful position to negotiate their role and be assertive with professionals. They developed considerable expertise in caring for their child and became experienced in interacting with professionals (Kirk 2001).

Activity

When on clinical placement, ask the senior nurse to identify an appropriate child with a chronic illness to whom you can talk (under supervision) about his or her knowledge of their disease and what care and treatment they undertake at home.

With the senior nurse's agreement and supervision, ask parents caring for a child with a chronic illness what they know about the disease and what care and treatment they undertake at home.

Discuss the information gained with your mentor or the senior nurse.

4. Advocacy

Advocacy means influencing those who have power on behalf of those who have not (Teasdale 1998 p 10)

Patients, and child patients in particular, are vulnerable and lack power when they enter the healthcare system, and nurses may frequently find themselves in the position of acting as the patient's advocate. However, it must be recognised that whereas nurses are almost compelled to act as patients' advocates because of the expectations of their practice, this role can put unrealistic demands upon them (Gates 1994). Nurses should act as advocates in certain situations but their decision to do so should be based on clear understanding of the possible consequences of such action, and on their limitations. Independent advocates whom act on behalf of patients may be more appropriate than nurses in some circumstances, and nurses need to be aware of when it is appropriate to refer families to such services. Further discussion of advocacy in nursing is beyond the scope of this chapter and readers are recommended to refer to appropriate texts on the subject.

Nurses may have to act as advocates for those children with chronic illness and their families who lack the assertiveness, confidence and eloquence to represent themselves (Ellis 1995). In the early stages of a chronic illness a nurse may act as an advocate to interpret issues such as health service systems, medical terms, benefits and interaction with other professionals. As the child and family become more experienced in dealing with the chronic illness, and confident in asserting their needs, the advocacy role becomes less. Nurses can then empower children and their families by providing enough information and support to enable self-advocacy.

As the child moves into adolescence, the nature of family and peer relationships changes. Peer relationships become increasingly important during adolescence and it has been suggested that whereas family support remains important in practical aspects of the chronic illness, peers become more important in offering emotional support and companionship (La Greca et al 1995). However, chronic illness can have a negative effect on peer relationships, which may result in functional limitations, feelings of being different and social withdrawal (Kyngas 2000).

Conflict may arise within the family as the adolescent asserts his or her need for autonomy and independence and comes to terms with the restrictions imposed by the illness. Although such conflict is neither restricted to nor inevitable during adolescence, a number of studies have examined the issues facing adolescents with chronic illness. For example, Kyngas & Barlow (1995) found that adolescents with diabetes felt that adults could not perceive or understand their situation and that there was a worrying tendency of adolescents with poor metabolic control to lie about their level of management and self-care activities rather than be nagged by parents and health professionals. Non-adherence to treatment regimens may be problematic at this age and the result of feelings that their diagnosis is unjust (Hentinen & Kyngas 1992) or embarrassment in front of peers (Newton & Greene 1995).

The shift of care from the family to the adolescent is a period of great adjustment. The family may be protective and not want to 'let go' of the care and treatment it has given the child, often for years. Family anxiety and protectiveness may impede healthy adolescent development (Blum et al 1993). The adolescent needs to gain independence from the family but has to accept the responsibilities of self-care, which they may not want to undertake (Edwards & Davis 1997). Nurses working with this age group must make a careful assessment of developmental needs to determine the individual's readiness for self-management (Hentinen & Kyngas 1995).

5. Support

Nurses need to work with children's existing support networks and help them to develop new ones to ensure that they and their families feel adequately supported. Family, friends, teachers, youth workers and others provide social support to all children. When a child has a chronic illness these support systems may be reduced and new support networks may need to be developed in order to provide for the needs of the child and family. Ellerton et al (1996) compared the social support networks of children with a range of chronic illnesses with those of healthy children. Healthy children reported more support overall than children in the illness groups and children with spina bifida reported the smallest support networks and the fewest number of peers in their networks.

Families provide much practical support in managing children's chronic illnesses and dimensions of family support have been studied in relation to specific diseases. For example, Siarkowski (1999) reviewed the literature on childhood adaptation to insulin-dependent diabetes mellitus and found that family guidance and control produced better glycaemic control but that other dimensions of family support, such as warmth and caring, had no influence on glycaemic control. Friends are important in providing emotional and social support to children with chronic illness, particularly adolescents (Graetz et al 2000, LaGreca et al 1995).

School is an important source of support for children with chronic illness. The school should be responsive to the emotional, social and educational needs of a child and should be a place of safety and normality for the child (Edwards & Davis 1997). If appointed, the key worker should ensure that the school is aware of a child's illness and management. The school should take appropriate measures for children's individual needs and there should be one contact person at the school with whom the key worker can discuss each child and family's needs and concerns, and vice versa. As interventions in managing children with chronic illness are voluntary in many education settings, it is important that the school and staff feel supported, otherwise they may withdraw this voluntary care, which could restrict or deny such children an education in school (Watson et al 2002). Approaches that facilitate good communication between health professionals and school staff have been explored and joint meetings, shared documentation and local policies have been found to be beneficial (Mukherjee et al 2002). Problems in communication arise when the parent is used as the conduit for information, there are practical difficulties in arranging meetings and there is a lack of knowledge about professional roles (Mukherjee et al 2002).

Other professionals, whether employed by statutory or non-statutory agencies, have an important role to play in the support of children with a chronic illness and their families. The key worker or nurse together with the child and family identify issues that require referring to other agencies and coordinate services required. Services need to be planned in advance, not on a crisis basis, because of the lengthy processes involved in recruiting and training carers (Kirk 1999). It is frustrating to a family to find that services are not always designed and targeted to fit their child and family's needs. The key worker's knowledge of local, cultural, community-based services is essential.

Knowledge of national organisations for specific illnesses from which families can access information, raise funds for research and development and obtain help and support is important. Organisations for common chronic illnesses tend to have local branches. These provide support groups and can increase the availability of recreational and community-based activities. If the chronic illness is rare, a local branch may not be accessible and many families rely on postal mail, national support groups and the internet. These children and families are more vulnerable to isolation and lack of information, and often have to travel to tertiary centres for care and treatment. The latter can sometimes impose transport and financial constraints upon the family.

Contact a Family (available at: http://www.cafamily.org.uk) produces an excellent list of support groups all over the UK, and some overseas, for families with children with chronic illnesses. They link families who can provide support for each other and provide information about support groups.

Seminar discussion topic

The Cystic Fibrosis Trust campaigns to improve the clinical and social care of those affected by cystic fibrosis, as well as raising public awareness of the condition. It funds medical and scientific research aimed towards understanding, treating and curing cystic fibrosis. It also aims to ensure that people with cystic fibrosis receive the best possible care and support in all aspects of their lives. The Cystic Fibrosis Trust has established branches and groups throughout the UK to raise funds. The support service provides advice and information for those affected by cystic fibrosis, their families and their carers. More information about national and local activities can be obtained from:

- http://www.cftrust.org.uk

In your seminar group, discuss the range of activities undertaken by charities such as the Cystic Fibrosis Trust and how these activities can complement the work of statutory organisations. Consider resources provided locally as well as nationally.

6. Outcome

By implementing factors 1–5, nurses should have a broad picture of each child and family, which incorporates understanding of their:

- management of the illness
- integration of the child with chronic illness into family life
- quality of life.

Children and families with a chronic illness should be confident in their abilities to recognise early signs and symptoms of changes in the illness so that they can initiate interventions themselves or be able to contact the appropriate professional to prevent or minimise exacerbations of the illness and to reduce hospital admissions.

Nurses are in a prime position to observe and monitor children with chronic illness at home, in school and at clinic appointments so that growth and development, physical and social activity are optimally maintained for each child. Any concerns noted by nurses should be reported to the multidisciplinary team. Decisions made by the multidisciplinary team based on the information provided can be fed back to the child and family to negotiate and plan any necessary interventions.

Children with chronic illness can deteriorate slowly and exacerbations or complications of the illness can have a major affect and quicken the deterioration. Medical or surgical treatment cannot always return the children to their original health status. At this stage children may need to be hospitalised and interventions from professionals can become more complex. Families have to reorganise and manage their lives as their child's lifestyle changes. Using

factors 1–5, nurses must reassess each child and family and renegotiate care, treatment and support.

Activity

On your clinical placement, identify a child with chronic illness whose condition has worsened. Discuss with the nurse who is looking after this child and family the following:

- What care, treatment and support have been initiated for the child and family?
- Has the quality of life for the child and family changed? If so, to what extent?
- How do the child and family feel about these changes?

Summary

This chapter has considered the issues facing the families of children with chronic illness. Although it is important to recognise that each child with a chronic illness, and their family, is in a unique situation, common concerns and goals have been discussed, including health-related quality of life and self-management. Maintaining a reasonable quality of life for the whole family is important because this may help in strengthening their coping strategies. The range of nursing interventions employed with families and children has been explored, stressing the importance of a clear understanding of the illness and its effects on each individual child and their family. Building-up holistic therapeutic relationships to support children and families through the dynamic changes of chronic illness is an essential component of good nursing care.

References

Austin JB, Kaur B, Anderson HR et al 1999 Hay fever, eczema and wheeze: a nationwide UK study (ISAAC, international study of asthma and allergies in childhood). Archives of Diseases of Childhood 81:225–230

Balkrishnan R, Housman TS, Carroll C et al 2003 Disease severity and associated family impact in childhood atopic dermatitis. Archives of Diseases of Childhood 88:423–427

Blubond-Langer M 1996 In the shadow of illness: parents and siblings of the chronically sick child. Princeton University Press, Princeton, NJ

Blum RW et al 1993 Transition from child-centred to adult healthcare systems for adolescents with chronic conditions. Journal of Adolescent Health Care 14:570–576

Braun-Fahrlander C, Gassner M, Grize L et al 1998 Comparison of responses to an asthma symptom questionnaire (ISAAC core questions) completed by adolescents and their parents. SCARPOL-Team. Swiss study on childhood allergy and respiratory symptoms with respect to air pollution. Pediatric Pulmonology 25:159–166

British Thoracic Society (BTS) and Scottish Intercollegiate Guidelines Network (SIGN) 2003 British guideline on the management of asthma. Thorax 58:11–94

Callery P, Milnes L, Couriel J, Verduyn C 2003 Qualitative study of children's and parents' beliefs about childhood asthma. British Journal of General Practice 53:185–190

Canam C 1993 Common adaptive tasks facing parents of children with chronic conditions. Journal of Advanced Nursing 18:46–53

Cane RS, Ranganathan SC, McKenzie SA 2000 What do parents of wheezy children understand by 'wheeze'? Archives of Disease in Childhood 82:327–332

Contact a Family 2004 Relationships – no time for us. Online. Available at: http://www.cafamily.org.uk/relationships.html

Cooper C 1999 Continuing care of sick children: examining the impact of chronic illness. Mark Allen Publishing, Wiltshire

Daud LR, Garralda ME, David TJ 1993 Psychosocial adjustment in preschool children with atopic eczema. Archives of Diseases of Childhood 69:670–676

Davis F 1963 Passage through crisis. Bobbs-Merril, Indianapolis, IN

Department of Health (DoH) 2001 The expert patient a new approach to chronic disease management for the 21st century. DoH, London

Dobson B, Middleton S 1998 Paying to care: the cost of childhood disability. Joseph Rowntree Foundation, York

Drotar D, Crawford P 1985 Psychological adaptation of siblings of chronically ill children: research and practice implications. Journal of Developmental and Behavioural Paediatrics 6(6):355–362

Eddy LL, Walker AJ 1999 The impact of children with chronic health problems on marriage. Journal of Family Nursing 5(1):10–31

Edwards M, Davis H 1997 Counselling children with chronic medical conditions. The British Psychological Society, Leicester

Eiser C 1990 Chronic childhood disease. Cambridge University Press, Cambridge

Eiser C 1993 Growing up with a chronic disease: the impact on children and their families. Jessica Kingsley, London

Eiser C 1997 Children's quality of life measures. Archives of Disease in Childhood 77:347–354

Eiser C, Morse R 2001 Quality-of-life measures in chronic diseases of childhood. Health Technology Assessment 5(4):1–157

Eiser C, Vance YH, Seamark O 2000 The development of a theoretically driven generic measure of quality of life for children aged 6–12 years: a preliminary report. Child Care Health and Development 26:445–456

Ellerton M, Stewart MJ, Ritchie JA, Hirth AM 1996 Social support in children with a chronic condition. Canadian Journal of Nursing Research 28(4):15–36

Elliott BE, Luker K 1996 The experiences of mothers caring for a child with severe atopic eczema. Journal of Clinical Nursing 6:241–247

Ellis PA 1995 The role of the nurse as the patient's advocate. Professional Nurse 11(3):206–207

Faux SA 1998 Historical overview of responses of children and their families to chronic illness. In: Broome ME, Knafl K, Pridham K, Feetham S (eds) Children and families in health and illness. Sage, San Diego, CA pp 179–195

Fisher HR 2001 The needs of parents with chronically sick children: a literature review. Journal of Advanced Nursing 36(4):600–607

Frank RG, Thayer JF, Hagglund KJ et al 1998 Trajectories of adaptation in pediatric chronic illness: the importance of the individual. Journal of Consulting and Clinical Psychology 66(3):521–532

Garwick AW et al 1998 Families' recommendations for improving services for children with chronic conditions. Archives of Paediatric and Adolescent Medicine 152:440–448

Gates B 1994 Advocacy: a nurses' guide. Scutari Press, London

Gibson CH 1995 The process of empowerment in mothers of chronically ill children. Journal of Advanced Nursing 21:1201–1210

Gibson P, Coughlan J, Wilson A et al 1999 Self-management education and regular practitioner review for adults with asthma (Cochrane Review). The Cochrane Library. Update Software, Oxford

Glazebrook C, Hollis C, Heussler H et al 2003 Detecting emotional and behavioural problems in paediatric clinics. Child: Care, Health and Development 29(2):141–150

Graetz BW, Shute RH, Sawyer MG 2002 An Australian study of adolescents with cystic fibrosis: perceived supportive and nonsupportive behaviours from families and friends and psychological adjustment. Journal of Adolescent Health 26:64–69

Greco V, Sloper P 2004 Care co-ordination and key worker schemes for disabled children: results of a UK-wide survey. Child: Care, Health and Development 30:13–20

Greco V, Sloper P, Barton K 2004 Care coordination and key worker services for disabled children in the UK. Social Policy Research Unit, University of York, York

Guevara JP, Wolf FM, Grum CM, Clark NM 2003 Effects of educational interventions for self management of asthma in children and adolescents: systematic review and meta-analysis. British Medical Journal 326:1308–1309

Guyatt GH, Juniper EF, Griffith LE et al 1997 Children and adult perceptions of childhood asthma. Pediatrics 99(2):165–168

Hatton DL, Canam C, Thorne S, Hughes AM 1995 Parents' perceptions of caring for an infant or toddler with diabetes. Journal of Advanced Nursing 22(3):569–577

Henry B, Aussage P, Grosskopf C, Goehrs JM 2003 Development of the cystic fibrosis questionnaire (CFQ) for assessing quality of life in pediatric and adult patients. Quality of Life Research 12(1):63–76

Hentinen M, Kyngas H 1992 Compliance of young diabetics with health regimens. Journal of Advanced Nursing 17:530–536

Hentinen M, Kyngas H 1998 Factors associated with the adaptation of parents with a chronically ill child. Journal of Clinical Nursing 7:316–324

Hodgkinson R, Lester H 2002 Stresses and coping strategies of mothers living with a child with cystic fibrosis: implications for nursing professionals. Journal of Advanced Nursing 39(4):377–383

Huurre TM, Aro HM 2002 Long-term psychosocial effects of persistent chronic illness: a follow-up study of Finnish adolescents aged 16 to 32 years. European Child and Adolescent Psychiatry 12(2):85–91

Ireland LM 1997 Children's perceptions of asthma: establishing normality. British Journal of Nursing 6:1059–1064

Kamps AW, Roorda RJ, Brand PL 2001 Peak flow diaries in childhood asthma are unreliable. Thorax 56:180–182

Katz S 2002 Gender differences in adapting to a child's chronic illness: a causal model. Journal of Pediatric Nursing 17(4):257–269

Katz S, Krulik T 1999 Fathers of children with chronic illness: do they differ from fathers of healthy children? Journal of Family Nursing 5(3):292–315

Kearney PM, Griffin T 2001 Between joy and sorrow: being a parent of a child with developmental disability. Journal of Advanced Nursing 34(5):582–592

Kirk S 1999 Caring for children with specialised health care needs in the community: the challenges for primary care. Health and Social Care in the Community 7(5):350–335

Kirk S 2001 Negotiating lay and professional roles in the care of children with complex health care needs. Journal of Advanced Nursing 34(5):593–602

Krulik T 1980 Successful 'normalizing' tactics of parents of chronically ill children. Journal of Advanced Nursing 5:573–578

Kyngas H 2000 Compliance of adolescents with chronic disease. Journal of Clinical Nursing 9(4):549–556

Kyngas H, Barlow J 1995 Diabetes: an adolescent perspective. Journal of Advanced Nursing 22:941–947

La Greca AM, Auslander WF, Greco P et al 1995 I get by with a little help from my family and friends: adolescents' support for diabetes care. Journal of Paediatris Psychology 20(4):449–476

Larson E 1998 Reframing the meaning of disability to families: the embrace of paradox. Social Science and Medicine 47(7):865–875

Lowes L, Lyne P 2000 Chronic sorrow in parents of children with newly diagnosed diabetes: a review of the literature and discussion of the implications for nursing practice. Journal of Advanced Nursing 32(1):41–48

Milnes LJ, Callery P 2003 The adaptation of written self-management plans for children with asthma. Journal of Advanced Nursing 41:444–453

Mukherjee S, Beresford B, Sloper P 1999 Unlocking key working. Joseph Rowntree Foundation, The Policy Press, Bristol

Mukherjee S, Lightfoot J, Sloper P 2002 Communicating about pupils in mainstream school with special health needs: the NHS perspective. Child: Care, Health and Development 28(1):21–27

Newachek PW, Stoddard JJ 1994 Prevalence and impact of multiple childhood chronic illnesses. Journal of Paediatrics 124(1):40–48

Newton RW, Green SA 1995 Diabetes in the adolescent. In: Kelnar CJH (ed) Childhood and adolescent diabetes. Chapman and Hall, London, pp 367–374

Ohya Y, Williams H, Steptoe A et al 2001 Psychosocial factors and adherence to treatment advice in childhood atopic dermatitis. Journal of Investigative Dermatology 117:852–857

Pandolfini C, Bonati M 2002 Follow up of quality of public orientated health information on the world wide web: systematic re-evaluation. British Medical Journal 324:582–583

Pandolfini C, Impicciatore P, Bonati M 2000 Parents on the web: risks for quality management of cough in children. Pediatrics 105(1):e1

Perrin JM 1985 Introduction. In: Hobbs N, Perrin J (eds) Issues in the care of children with chronic illness. Josey-Bass, San Francisco, pp 1–12

Quittner A, Opipari L, Espelage D et al 1998 Role strain in couples with and without a chronic illness: associations with marital satisfaction, intimacy and daily mood. Health Psychology 17:112–124

Ray LD 2002 Parenting and childhood chronicity: making visible the invisible work. Journal of Pediatric Nursing 17(6):424–438

Renzoni E, Forastiere F, Biggeri A et al 1999 Differences in parental- and self-report of asthma, rhinitis and eczema among Italian adolescents. SIDRIA collaborative group. Studi Italiani sui Disordini Respiratori dell' Infanzia e l'Ambiente. European Respiratory Journal 14:597–604

Siarkowski AK 1999 Children's adaptation to insulin dependent diabetes mellitus: a critical review of the literature. Pediatric Nursing 5(6):627–639

Sloper P, Turner S 1992 Service needs of families of children with severe physical disability. Child: Health, Care and Development 18(5):259–282

Stein RE, Jessop DJ 1989 What diagnosis does not tell: the case for a non-categorical approach to chronic illness in childhood. Social Science and Medicine 29(6):769–778

Stein REK, Reissman CK 1980 The development of an impact-on-family scale: preliminary findings. Mediacal Care 18:465–472

Su JC, Kemp AS, Varigos GA, Nolan TM 1997 Atopic eczema: its impact on the family and financial cost. Archives of Diseases of Childhood 76:159–162

Tak YR, McCubbin M 2002 Family stress, perceived social support and coping following the diagnosis of a child's congenital heart disease. Journal of Advanced Nursing 39(2):190–199

Teasdale K 1998 Advocacy in health care. Blackwell Science, Oxford

Teel CS 1991 Chronic sorrow: analysis of the concept. Journal of Advanced Nursing 16:1311–1319

Thorne SE, Paterson BL 2001 Health care professional support for self-care management in chronic illness: insights from diabetes research. Patient Education and Counselling 42:81–90

Vance YH, Morse RC, Jenney ME, Eiser C 2001 Issues in measuring quality of life in childhood cancer: measures, proxies, and parental mental health. Journal of Child Psychology and Psychiatry and Allied Disciplines 42(5):661–667

Vessey J 1999 Psychological comorbidity in children with chronic conditions. Pediatric Nursing 25(2):211–214

Watson D et al 2002 Exploring multi-agency working in services to disabled children with complex healthcare needs and their families. Journal of Clinical Nursing 11:367–375

Whalley D, Huels J, McKenna SP, Van Assche D 2002 The benefit of pimecrolinmus on parents' quality of life in the treatment of pediatric atopic dermatitis. Pediatrics 110(6):1133–1136

Whyte DA 1992 A family nursing approach to the care of a child with a chronic illness. Journal of Advanced Nursing 17:317–327

Wills BSH 1999 The experiences of Hong Kong Chinese parents of children with acute lymphocytic leukaemia. Journal of Pediatric Nursing: Nursing Care of Children and Families 14(4):231–238

Young B, Dixon-Woods M, Findlay M, Heney D 2002a Parenting in crisis: conceptualizing mothers of children with cancer. Social Science and Medicine 55(10):1835–1847

Young B, Dixon-Woods M, Windridge KC, Heney D 2003 Managing communication with young people who have a potentially life threatening chronic illness: qualitative study of patients and parents. British Medical Journal 326(7384):305–309

Young B, Fitch GE, Dixon-Woods M et al 2002b Parents' accounts of wheeze and asthma related symptoms: a qualitative study. Archives of Disease in Childhood 87:131–134

Chapter Forty Five

45

Caring for Children with Critical Illness

Marion Aylott

ABSTRACT

The primary aim of this chapter and the companion PowerPoint presentation is to explore fundamental issues and key concepts for children's intensive care nursing practice. Children's intensive care combines aspects of many specialities, for example anaesthesiology, paediatrics, microbiology, cardiothoracic surgery and cardiology, into one integrated and unique whole to provide care for the most severely ill children. Children whose very existence is immediately threatened have many multiple aspects of care they require in common, regardless of underlying illness. Thus children who have suffered trauma, heart disease, severe infectious disease, devastating medical illness or are recovering from complex surgery all benefit from the collaborative practice of critical care to provide respiratory support, haemodynamic control and holistic support of the child and family. Therefore, this chapter gives a detailed account of these three nursing practice issues and will include a clinical scenario, which will provide opportunities to apply critical care knowledge gained in this chapter to a clinical situation.

Learning Outcomes

- Demonstrate an understanding of the key concepts of children's intensive care nursing.
- Explain the principles of respiratory and cardiovascular support within the intensive care setting.
- Consider the role of the children's nurse as part of the multi-professional team in helping to maintain respiratory support and haemodynamic control.
- Discuss the physical and psychological care of the child with critical illness and their family.

Glossary

Afterload:
The load against which the left ventricle ejects after opening the aortic valve.

Cardiac contractility:
Contractile capability of the heart.

Cardiac output:
The volume of blood that the heart pumps in 1 minute.

Central venous pressure:
A measure of pressure in the right atrium.

Chronotropic:
Agent that acts to increase heart rate.

Compensated shock:
Blood flow is normal or increased and may be maldistributed; vital organ function is maintained.

Compliance:
The ease with which the lungs and thorax expand during pressure changes.

Endotracheal intubation:
Insertion of endotracheal tube into the trachea either through a patient's nose or mouth and directly through the larynx between the vocal cords into the trachea to open and maintain airway.

Fibrosis:
Replacement of lung epithelium and elastic fibres with fibroplast scar tissue.

Frank–Starling's law:
An increase in preload leads to an increase in stroke volume.

FRC:

Functional residual capacity is the pool of air left in the lungs at the end of total expiration.

Heart rate:

The number of cardiac contractions that occur in 1 minute.

Hypoxia

An inadequate supply of oxygen.

Inotrope:

Agent that acts to improve myocardial contractility and enhance stroke volume.

Irreversible shock:

Inadequate perfusion of vital organs; irreparable damage; death cannot be prevented.

Minute volume

Amount of gas inhaled and exhaled in 1 minute.

PEEP/CPAP:

Positive end expiratory pressure, or continuous positive airway pressure, is the baseline pressure and controls functional residual capacity in the patient's lung.

PIP:

Peak inspiratory pressure indicates the maximum pressure that has occurred during the last ventilatory cycle.

Preload:

The load on the ventricle before ejection.

Shock:

Circulatory system failure to supply oxygen and nutrients to meet cellular metabolic demands.

Stroke volume:

The amount of blood ejected by both ventricles with each contraction.

Systemic vascular resistance:

The resistance against which the left ventricle must eject to force out its content with each beat.

Tidal volume:

The amount of gas or air breathed in or out in one breath.

Uncompensated shock:

Microvascular perfusion is compromised; significant reductions in effective circulating volume.

Introduction

A Paediatric Intensive Care Unit (PICU) is a specifically designed and equipped multidisciplinary healthcare specialty for the treatment of critically ill children from early infancy to adolescence (British Paediatric Association (BPA) 1993), which has been shown to be important in achieving the best possible outcomes for children (Pearson et al 1997). Nurses are an important element of the team of staff that cares for the critically ill child, and this is reflected by the high nurse:patient ratio – ideally 1:1 – that is characteristic of intensive care. To understand what criti-

cal care is, we must focus on the social context in which it occurs. Thus critical care is where care is critical (Coombs 2001). The role encompasses an independent as well as interdependent element. Although critical care nurses work one to one so that they can truly focus on each patient, they will contribute as part of a team when the need dictates. Additionally, nursing and therapeutic intervention in critical care extends beyond the patient. It includes the interface with technology, for example the lines, the monitors, the organ support machinery and the drains.

What is Critical Illness?

There are around 12,000 admissions each year to PICU in England, which averages approximately 120 in each Health Authority area (NHS Executive (NHSE) 1997a). Critical illness is a derangement in physiology with the potential to result in significant morbidity and mortality without prompt and appropriate invasive and therapeutic intervention (Hazinski 1999). There are, however, many differences in healthcare facilities available in PICUs across the UK relating to the case mix of patients admitted and the intensive care resources available in particular units. The variety of disease seen in any children's intensive care unit depends on the population from which it receives patients (Duncan 1998). For example, a hospital with a cardiac surgery programme will increase the number of patients that unit admits with that condition. Although a wide variety of disease may lead to critical illness, the fundamental interventions required are limited. The common pathway of deterioration in critical illness occurs as a result of progressive deterioration of respiratory and circulatory function with respiratory failure or shock as the pathophysiological expression with the final denominator being cardiopulmonary failure (Advanced Life Support Group (ALSG) 2001).

What Constitutes an Intensive Care Patient?

As we have seen, critical illness is characterised by acute loss of physiologic reserve but in many cases the course of illness is prolonged and often the underlying cause may be difficult to discern. Moreover, despite a child having a recognised critical illness there is great interpatient variability. In addition, until the very recent past children with critical illness were nursed in a range of settings including general adult intensive care units depending on geographical location. In Britain, paediatric intensive care developed in an ad hoc and fragmented way. Now, however, after 20 years of effort, Britain is moving towards a more integrated service.

Concerns about paediatric intensive care were first raised by the British Paediatric Association (BPA) in the

1980s, and again in 1993 when it published its report on paediatric intensive care. This report highlighted the fragmented configuration of paediatric intensive care provision, demonstrating that only 51% of children were cared for in paediatric intensive care units, 20% in adult intensive care units and 29% in children's wards (BPA 1993). Furthermore, only 36% of paediatric intensive care units provided a retrieval service. Concerns were also expressed regarding the lack of physical facilities, lack of education and training of both medical and nursing staff and poor staffing levels available to care for these critically ill children.

In 1996 an inquiry into the death of a child named Nicholas Geldard, who died in a paediatric intensive care unit in 1995 after inappropriate transport for management following a spontaneous cerebral haemorrhage, was published (Ashworth 1996). In response to this, the Department of Health (DoH) requested an inquiry into paediatric intensive care services with a view to developing a policy framework for paediatric intensive care (NHSE 1996). In 1997 *Paediatric intensive care: a framework for the future* was published (NHSE 1997a). This paper set out a strategy for developing and integrating the service for critically ill children within a geographical area and so centralise the skills and experience of medical and nursing staff. The central recommendations of this paper have been supported by others (Pearson et al 1997).

Today, children requiring intensive care are no longer cared for in general children's wards and centres that do not meet the standards as laid out by the NHSE framework document. Quality of paediatric intensive care is not only reliant on a centralised and standardised service but also – importantly – the effectiveness and appropriateness of treatment within a child- and family-orientated environment. To facilitate this, nurses working in paediatric intensive care units undertake a specifically designed, competency-based course to equip them with the knowledge, skills and understanding that underpins effective paediatric intensive care nursing practice.

 www

Read the DoH papers *Framework for the future* and *A bridge to the future* online:
- http://www.doh.gov.uk/nsf/paediatr.htm

Children are admitted to PICU when one or more body systems cannot maintain physiological homeostatic equilibrium without intensive therapeutic support. However, there are varying degrees of organ failure and levels of intensive support (NHSE 1997a,b).

 Activity

Analyse the categories of intensive care as defined by the DoH papers *A framework for the future* and *A bridge to the future*. Discuss in your learning group how these levels of care and facilities, including staff skills and expertise, compare with a general paediatric ward.

 Scenario

Introducing Daniel

The Badger ward paediatrician and nursing staff were concerned about the condition of 15-month-old Daniel, who weighed 13 kg and was developing increased respiratory distress since admission 4 hours earlier. Daniel had been admitted to Badger ward as a referral from his GP and was accompanied by his parents, Emma and Alan. Daniel had a 2-week history of an upper respiratory tract infection, which over the previous 2–3 days had worsened, with decreased appetite and fluid intake. Since admission to Badger ward, his respiratory distress had markedly increased. Initial treatment was directed towards alleviating his respiratory distress and included 30% oxygen via a head box and intravenous antibiotics. Despite this therapy there had been no evidence of improvement. The paediatrician contacted the PICU intensivist to review Daniel on Badger ward.

The paediatric intensivist and an experienced PICU nurse equipped with emergency bag and retrieval trolley responded immediately to this request. On assessment they found that Daniel was in obvious respiratory distress. He was irritable and reluctant to leave his mother's arms. His pulse rate was 180, respiratory rate 65 with grunting and sternal and intercostals chest recession. Inspiratory stridor and expiratory wheeze were readily audible and his tidal volume was decreased.

Daniel was transferred to PICU on the retrieval trolley on his mother's lap.

 Activity

Consider Daniel's situation and the DoH categories for intensive care. What was the rationale for Daniel's admission to PICU?

Relating back to Chapter 28, consider why the critical care team who assessed Daniel decided to transfer him to PICU in his mother's lap, without further intervention on Badger ward.

Scenario

On admission to PICU, additional vital signs were obtained:

- Daniel was awake and irritable and appeared exhausted
- respiratory rate had increased from 60 to 70
- his recession appeared pronounced
- oxygen saturation: 95%
- pulse rate had increased from 174 to 200
- radial and dorsalis pulses were weak and thready
- his skin was cool, dry and pale
- capillary refill: 4 seconds
- blood pressure: 90/60 mmHg
- he was conscious and responding to his mother
- blood glucose: 1.7 mmol/L
- axilla temperature: 38.5°C
- no skin rash noted
- an arterial gas was obtained: pH 7.25, pCO_2 7.6, pO_2 22, base deficit –3.

RAPID CARDIOPULMONARY ASSESSMENT

Recognition of potential respiratory failure, based on clinical evaluation of the child is vital (ALSG 2001). Intubation and ventilation of a child with potential respiratory failure will be considered if a child fails to improve after initial oxygen therapy or if further deterioration is observed. An individual must be able to support three specific functions:

- protect the airway
- adequately ventilate
- adequately oxygenate.

A failure to perform any one function will result in respiratory failure. Respiratory failure is defined as a major abnormality of gas exchange (Lissuer & Clayden 2001) and is an absolute indication for intubation and mechanical ventilation. However, not every patient who is intubated has a primary pulmonary pathology. Intubation and ventilation may serve to support the cardiovascular system. For example, for patients in cardiogenic shock the demands of the respiratory system may precipitate cardiovascular collapse. Supporting the patient with mechanical ventilation can reduce the demands on the heart, allowing it to recover. Intubation can also serve to protect the airway for those who cannot do it themselves, for example patients in coma as a result of a head injury. Moreover mechanical ventilation offers the option of hyperventilation for patients with intracranial hypertension.

Activity

Analyse the data collected during a rapid cardiopulmonary assessment of Daniel and arterial blood gas and list the factors that support the decision to intubate and ventilate.

RESPIRATORY SUPPORT

Intubation

Intubation and ventilation are always performed with caution, as anaesthetic agents as well as positive pressure ventilation will exacerbate hypovolaemia. Assessment of Daniel's perfusion indicates a degree of hypovolaemia therefore he was given 260 ml (20 mL/kg) of normal saline as an intravenous bolus with good effect observed by an improvement in his heart rate and perfusion. In addition, he was administered broad-spectrum intravenous antibiotics.

Intubation is a painful and unpleasant procedure and should never be performed on a conscious or semiconscious patient. Unless the child has completely collapsed, the medical practitioner, usually an anaesthetist or intensivist, will perform what is called rapid sequence induction. This means inducing anaesthesia and giving muscle relaxants. Common drugs used in this age group are morphine, midazolam and atracurium. When the drugs are being prepared for rapid sequence induction, equipment should be prepared and checked to be in good working order to ensure a safe procedure, as displayed in Fig. 45.1.

As the sedation and anaesthetic agent of choice is administered intravenously and the child starts to lose consciousness, the child will be preoxygenated with 100% oxygen using a bag-valve-mask device for at least 1–2 minutes. This ensures that the child is in optimum condition prior to the procedure of intubation. Once the child is assessed to be unconscious and bag valve mask ventilation is established the paralysing agent is administered intravenously. A nasogastric tube should be passed to empty gastric contents and left of free drainage thus preventing aspiration. It is also useful for decompression of gas accumulated in the stomach during bag-valve-mask ventilation. During the intubation procedure the medical practitioner may ask an assistant to apply cricoid pressure. This is external compression of the trachea to decrease the probability of aspiration and inflation of the stomach and also enhances visualisation of the glottis. Care must be taken to apply cricoid pressure symmetrically. Once the endotracheal tube is in place, observations are made to confirm that the tube is in the correct position. This is done by:

- observing for bilateral chest movement with ventilation
- auscultation using a stethoscope to ensure breath sounds heard clearly over the anterior and posterior chest and in both axillae
- confirming that there are no breath sounds over the stomach
- confirming that O_2 saturations are improving
- confirming that the heart rate is stable and within normal limits.

Action	Rationale
Suction apparatus with appropriate size suction catheter.	Relatively small amounts of mucus accumulation, oedema or airway obstruction can reduce airway patency or obscure view of the vocal cords for intubation.
Assemble appropriate sized and working bag valve mask device.	To ensure effective ventilation.
Positioning to achieve optimal airway patency is essential to bag valve mask. A shoulder roll may be used to help extend the neck and position the airway in a neutral position (nose perpendicular to the ceiling). An airway adjunct may also be used if head position is difficult to maintain	A child under the age of 2 years has a large, heavy head with prominent occiput, short chubby neck and a large tongue. Furthermore, sedation and CNS dysfunction will exacerbate these effects.
Assemble appropriate sized and working laryngoscope and blade. Check adequate illumination from bulb.	A straight laryngoscope blade is better in younger children as it is used to pick up the floppy epiglottis. A curved laryngoscope blade is better in older children who have a stiff epiglottis where the blade is placed in the vallecula.
Assemble the correct size endotracheal tube (ETT) plus one a size above and one size below.	The narrowest part of the airway in a child under 8 years is at the level of the cricoid cartilage which is cone-shaped. An ETT may pass through the vocal cords easily in the young child but be too large to pass through the cricoid cartilage. Select the correct size uncuffed tube carefully using a broselow tape, a recognised chart of the formula; $$\frac{Age + 4}{4}$$ For the child under 2 years: Age / Kg / ETT Newborn / 3.5 / 3.5 3 months / 6.0 / 3.5 1 year / 10 / 4.0 2 years / 12 / 4.5
Assemble ETT with introducer if wanted.	The practitioner intubating may request an introducer. This makes the tube more 'stiff' which makes intubating easier. When inserting the introducer take care to ensure that it does not protrude beyond the tip of the ETT itself as this may cause tissue trauma to the trachea. Many bend the top of the introducer over the connector after checking for profusion as a further safety mechanism.
Assemble tape ready cut to secure ETT in place.	This enables stability of the ETT in place. Various methods of securing an ETT exist. Find out how your PICU prefers to secure an ETT.
Stethoscope.	To confirm ETT placement prior to the formal confirmation of a chest X-ray.

Fig. 45.1 • The action and rationale for preparation prior to intubation.

The endotracheal tube is then secured in place and a chest X-ray ordered for formal confirmation of tube placement.

Scenario

Daniel was intubated with a size 4.5 mm endotracheal. Initial ventilation parameters were:
- respiratory rate: 30
- inspiratory time: 0.8 seconds
- tidal volume: 180 mL
- PEEP: 5 cmH$_2$O.

Synchronised mandatory ventilation (SIMV) mode was selected; resultant peak inspiratory pressure (PIP) was 28 cm H$_2$O. Analgesia and sedation were maintained with continuous infusions of morphine and midazolam, respectively.

MECHANICAL VENTILATION: PHYSIOLOGICAL PRINCIPLES AND EFFECTS

Mechanical ventilatory support is the major supportive treatment used in critical care. A mechanical ventilator is simply a machine used to replace or supplement the natural function of breathing. It is usually a temporary measure until the patient can breathe adequately without help. Ventilation is simply the movement of gas into and out of the lungs. To safely and effectively provide care for intubated infants and children receiving assisted ventilation it is necessary to have an understanding of the fundamental physiological principles of lung function and the physiological effects of assisted ventilation in terms of both gas exchange and pulmonary mechanics and an appreciation of the particular disease process leading to the need for assisted ventilation.

Ventilation and Perfusion Relationship

The primary function of the lungs is to enable gas exchange between inspired air that reaches the alveoli and the blood of the pulmonary capillaries. This process of gas exchange is crucial for homeostasis and is interdependent with the circulatory system's prime role of blood transport. To enable adequate gas exchange it is crucial that oxygen and carbon dioxide move between air and blood by simple diffusion across the alveolar surface. More specifically, there is a balance between ventilation (V) and perfusion (Q). However, it is more complicated than this. V and Q are not evenly distributed throughout the lung (Hazinski 1999). Figure 45.2 illustrates how V increases from apex to the base of the lung and Q increases from apex to base relatively more than perfusion. During normal quiet breathing in an upright position the bases of the lung receive about 50% more ventilation than the apices. This is due to:

- gravity
- variations in airways size (remember Poiseuille's law, Chapter 4)
- variations in alveolar elastic properties (surfactant – to be discussed later).

If oxygen is not delivered to alveolar capillaries, or the alveolar surface is damaged, oxygen and/or carbon dioxide elimination may be impaired, V and Q are not balanced and respiratory failure ensues. In a single lung unit V and Q must be matched to allow gas exchange (Fig. 45.3).

Mechanical ventilation is an attempt to normalise the patient's ventilation–perfusion ratio. However, perfusion is determined by:

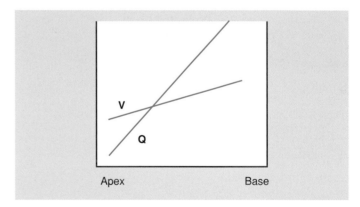

Fig. 45.2 • The ventilation (V) and perfusion (Q) relationship.

Fig. 45.3 • A simple illustration of V and Q mismatch.

- the amount of oxygen in the blood
- the oxygen binding capacity of haemoglobin
- cardiac output.

Therefore, when a patient is being ventilated, therapeutic interventions must also be taken to optimise perfusion through ensuring there is a sufficient delivery of inspired oxygen, concentration of haemoglobin and cardiac output. We will look at cardiac output in more detail later.

THE MECHANICS OF BREATHING

Three factors affect the mechanics of breathing:

- force (pressure)
- displacement (volume)
- rate of displacement (flow), which comprises compliance and resistance.

These factors are all interrelated:

Pressure = Volume ÷ (Compliance + Resistance)
i.e. Pressure = Volume ÷ Flow

During normal inspiration the mechanical contraction of the inspiratory muscles causes the thoracic cage to enlarge in volume. This increased volume causes a pressure gradient between the lungs and the atmosphere. This pressure differential is enough to cause an in-rush of air into the lungs. The work that the inspiratory muscles perform represents the negative pressure applied. Figure 45.4a shows the changes in airway pressure in the mouth during spontaneous quiet breathing. Airway pressure during inspiration is negative, allowing air to enter the lungs, and is positive during expiration. Also, there is normally a brief pause, when airway pressure remains at atmospheric pressure. Figure 45.4b shows the upper airway pressures (measured at the mouth) during mechanical ventilation. In artificial ventilation, the ventilator must provide the inspiratory pressure provided by the inspiratory muscles in normal respiration. This is done by creating a positive intrapulmonary pressure whereby air is pushed out of the ventilator into the lungs of the patient, thus raising the pressure in the airways relative to atmospheric pressure. This resultant increase in intrapulmonary pressure forces the lungs to expand. It is important to remember that artificial ventilation fundamentally alters normal airway pressures. This fact accounts for most of its benefits and complications.

In the equation Pressure = Volume ÷ (Compliance + Resistance), compliance and resistance are assumed to remain constant and is illustrated by (a) in Figure 45.5. However, this is not the case in cardiopulmonary illness. With stiff lungs (reduced compliance) patients tend to take rapid, small breaths, to minimise elastic workload as in Fig. 45.5b. With high airway resistance, for example in asthma, patients take large slow breaths (Fig. 45.5c). As can be seen in Fig. 45.5, the inspiratory lung volume is low in both. Thus, their combined effect is a greater load presented to the ventilator. Pressure, volume and flow change over time in illness, therefore they are considered variable. From the equation of motion, the ventilator must control one of these variables. A mechanical ventilator will control airway pressure, inspired volume or inspired flow.

But wait . . . there is more to compliance. To achieve compliance, alveolar lung units have an important lung property

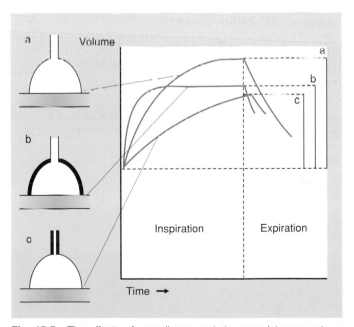

Fig. 45.5 • The effects of compliance and airway resistance on lung volume. (a) The effect of normal compliance; (b) the effect of reduced compliance; (c) the effect of increased airways resistance.

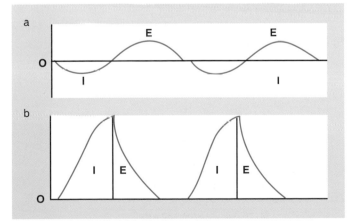

Fig. 45.4 • Changes in airway pressure during (a) normal spontaneous breathing versus (b) artificial mechanical ventilation.

– they are elastic. They can be expanded by small forces and return to their resting state. Two components are responsible for their elastic behaviour:

● Elastic tissue consisting of elastic and collagen fibres embedded in alveoli walls and around bronchi.
● The surface tension reducing effect of surfactant increases compliance.

Thus less pressure is required to inflate alveoli (Martini 1998). The lung contains a foamy phospholipid fluid commonly known as surfactant. Pulmonary surfactant is produced by type I and II alveolar pneumocytes, and is responsible for decreasing the surface tension of the lining fluid within the bronchial tree. Without surfactant, pulmonary airways become unstable and have decreased compliance. Surfactant decreases the surface tension of the alveoli in order to aid the diffusion of gases (Martini 1998). A reduction in production of surfactant will directly affect gas exchange. General causes of reduced surfactant production are:

● acidosis
● hypoxia
● hyperoxygenation
● pulmonary oedema
● atelectasis.

To help understand this concept, think about blowing up a balloon. At first it is difficult and then there is a 'give' and the balloon inflates easily. This occurs in the same way in the lungs. The greatest workload in the respiratory cycle is in early inspiration where the pressure–volume curve is relatively flat (Fig. 45.6).

Once the steep part of the pressure–volume curve (PVC) (the P_{flex}) is reached, the lung suddenly inflates easily; this is the inflection point. The PVC is flattest at low lung volumes and consequently the work of breathing is highest. If the lungs were left filled with air so that the rest-

ing state is at or above the inflection point, the work of breathing is reduced considerably. Going back to our analogy, this is like letting a balloon deflate incompletely and then re-inflating it. This is the basis for positive end expiratory pressure (PEEP), which is a continuous constant pressure of gas delivered to prevent alveolar collapse (PEEP will be discussed in more detail later).

Finally, the last physiological mechanism we must consider is closing volume. In health, the lungs dangle downwards in the pleural cavity supported by a vacuum of negative pressure. As you would expect, the magnitude of this negative pressure is greater in the apices than in the bases. The effect of this is to splint the airways open at the end of the tidal volume (normal expiration) – the expiratory reserve volume (ERV) (McChance & Heauther 2002) (Fig. 45.7). Apical alveoli are more inflated at rest than basal. But during inspiration, because the latter are at a steep part of the pressure–volume curve, the gas turnover (see Fig. 45.6) is greater. However, in illness, further confounded by upper airway compromise and especially when lying supine, there is a tendency for distal, particularly basal airways to collapse in expiration. This is known as the closing volume. If this is not addressed by delivering PEEP through the ventilator, eventually the closing volume will impinge on and begin to exceed functional residual capacity (FRC) and atelectasis (alveolar collapse) will occur at the end of quiet expiration.

As we have seen, artificial ventilation is unlike normal ventilation. Positive pressure ventilation can be injurious to the lungs, which were designed as a negative pressure circuit receiving oxygen at 21%. Moreover, artificial ventilation is most often required by patients with underlying lung or cardiovascular pathology which makes the lung tissue even more susceptible to ventilator-induced lung injury and cardiovascular complications.

Evidence-based Practice

Evidence has been mounting since the late 1980s that mechanical ventilation can cause and exacerbate lung tissue injury (Dreyfus et al 1985, Kolobow et al 1987). Although most of this evidence has originated from animal studies, clinical reports support this concern (Bohn 1998):
● oxygen toxicity
● barotrauma (pressure)
● volutrauma (shearing forces)
● insufficient humidification.

VENTILATION: LESSONS LEARNED

Accumulating evidence has revealed that high oxygen concentrations, high inflation pressures, large tidal volumes

Fig. 45.6 • Alveolar compliance and the pressure–volume curve.

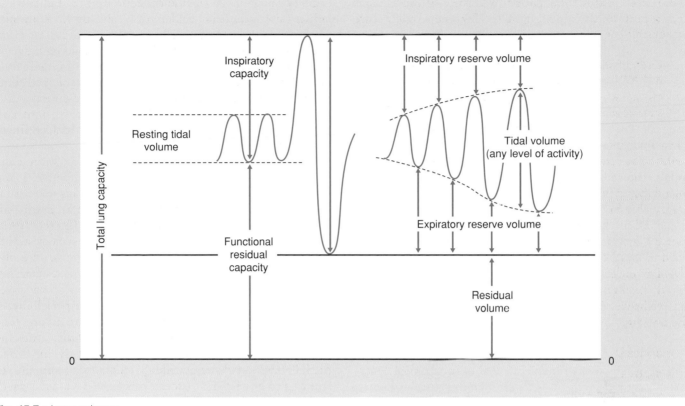

Fig. 45.7 • Lung volumes.

and low PEEP ventilation strategies are damaging to the lungs:

- Oxygen in supraphysiological concentrations is injurious to the lung, particularly in concentrations over an FiO_2 of 0.60 (Robb 1997a).

- Positive pressure ventilation is non-physiological and causes pulmonary injury. The higher the pressures used, the greater the injury. This is referred to as barotrauma and is typically associated with excessive airway pressures leading to extra-alveolar air and also includes pneumothorax, pneumomediastinum, pneumoperitoneum and subcutaneous emphysema. What exactly qualifies as a dangerous pressure is not known (Bohn 1998).

- Volutrauma is lung injury secondary to alveolar overdistension. It is manifested by disruption of the alveolar capillary membrane and alterations in gas exchange. The propensity for volutrauma is related to the volume of lung available and to regional differences in compliance. In, for example, pneumonia where lung volume is significantly diminished and compliance is reduced, the risk of volutrauma is increased (Kerr 1997).

- Shearing forces caused by repeated expansion of collapsed alveoli is injurious to the lung by causing the release of inflammatory mediators independent of over-

distension or oxygen concentration (Bohn 1998). The concept of 'shear' injury along with the increase in dead space to tidal volume ratio prevents the use of high rates to compensate for small tidal volumes/low pressures.

STRATEGIES TO REDUCE LUNG INJURY

In response to these findings, respiratory experts have espoused the use of lung protective ventilator strategies (Kerr 1997). One strategy is to use sufficient PEEP to raise FRC above closing capacity without compromising cardiac output and as a consequence oxygen delivery. This strategy keeps alveolar units on the steep part of the compliance curve (see Fig. 45.6). Higher levels of PEEP help to maintain:

- alveolar recruitment (the 'open lung' approach)
- reduce V/Q mismatch and progressive hypoxemia
- achieve lower tidal volumes (4–8 mL/kg).

Thus, higher levels of PEEP lead to reduced end inspiratory volumes preventing shear/stretch injury.

Another strategy advocated is the use of pressure-limited ventilation and increasing mean airway pressures by permissive hypercapnia and hypoxemia (Reynolds et al 1993).

There is no research evidence to dictate what acceptable oxygen or carbon dioxide levels are. The general philosophy is that an acceptable level is determined by what intensivists are willing to do to get there considering the research findings available regarding the causation of lung injury. For example, if an oxygen saturation of 95% can only be achieved through using a PEEP of 12 cmH_2O and a FiO_2 of 1.0 (100%) this is not acceptable in the light of the best available evidence. Both high PEEP and high inspired-oxygen concentrations are injurious to the lung. However, if achieving a carbon dioxide level of 5.4 kPa results in a peak pressure of 30 cmH_2O, this might be acceptable as this carbon dioxide level is acceptable. In general (Parker et al 1993):

- peak pressures greater than 35 cmH_2O are not acceptable
- the upper limit for an acceptable FiO_2 is 0.60
- the upper PEEP limit is 15 cmH_2O.

It is recognised that these limits are arbitrary in nature and no study has ever demonstrated what safe limits are (Hill 1997). These limits are made by intensivists in the context of the patient's clinical situation and expected clinical course. Thus the overall goal of mechanical ventilation is not to achieve a target blood gas value but to maximise oxygen delivery while minimising pulmonary injury.

Inhaled nitric oxide (iNO) was originally thought to be the 'magic bullet' for improving V/Q mismatch in severe respiratory failure (Tibballs 1998). Given its ability to vasodilate blood vessels, be delivered as a gas (act on blood vessels that perfuse ventilated alveoli: selective pulmonary vasodilatation) and its short half-life (no systemic hypotension), it was studied with great interest. However, although iNO does improve oxygenation in acute respiratory distress syndrome, it does not improve outcome. It has more of a beneficial effect in patients with pulmonary hypertension, especially neonates with persistent pulmonary hypertension of the newborn or post-operative cardiac patients.

There are options, beyond adjusting the ventilator, which have implications for nursing. Body positioning affects ventilation/perfusion (V/Q) matching and therefore arterial oxygen levels. Accumulation of secretions and atelectasis can occur in the dependent regions of the lungs, therefore regular position changes will help to avoid problem areas developing. Position can also affect a child's FRC. A reduction in FRC will make a child more vulnerable to atelectasis and allow more rapid hypoxia. It is important to consider which positions may help to optimise oxygenation and this is a multi-professional decision made in consultation with a respiratory physiotherapist. It is well established that atelectasis develops in the dorsal areas of the lung when patients are in a supine position for any extended period of time (Ganong 2001). 'Prone positioning' a patient can help re-expand these collapsed areas, improve alveolar ventilation and hence gas exchange (Ball et al 2001). Additionally, the chest wall has a more favourable compliance curve in the prone position. Most patients will usually have improved oxygenation when prone and can tolerate being prone for 20 hours at a time, with regular pressure relief. It has not been established that prone positioning improves mortality but it can be useful in the patient that is difficult to oxygenate.

In normal circumstances the upper airway warms and humidifies air, so that it reaches core temperature and 100% saturation just below the carina. This process is known as gas conditioning (Williams et al 1996). During gas conditioning inspired air is also cleaned and filtered of foreign particles by the mucociliary transport system, which extends from the nasopharynx towards the bronchioles (Estes & Meduri 1995). Thus, gas conditioning optimises gas exchange and protects delicate lung tissue. The placement of an endotracheal tube bypasses this defence mechanism and the gas exchange function of the lung. The placement of the endotracheal tube physically shifts the conditioning, and heat and moisture recovery functions, further down the airway which would not normally be required to give up heat and moisture.

Hence in the intubated patient, the mucociliary transport system is the sole remaining mechanical defence system. The mucociliary transport system's function depends on the:

- thickness of the mucus
- depth of the aqueous layer
- cilia beat frequency.

If the temperature of inspired gas is less than core temperature the beat frequency of the cilia will reduce and the gas will be heated to a suboptimal temperature causing the relative humidity of the gas to be reduced. Less than optimal humidification results in a compromised mucociliary transport and pooling of mucus in the lower airways thus restricting gas exchange and being an ideal site for bacterial colonisation (Centers for Disease Control (CDC) 1994). Furthermore, the gel layer will lose moisture and become thicker. If suboptimal humidification is allowed to continue, cell damage might occur and the process of gas conditioning will move deeper into the lung. Increased thick mucus and reduced clearance of secretions from small airways results in reduced airway patency and lung compliance (Williams et al 1996). Thus the nurse must ensure that inspired gases are maintained at core temperature and humidity. Effective humidification will also maximise lung defence by reducing exposure to contaminants invading the airways by increasing clearance of contaminants by suctioning.

Activity

To ensure patency of the airways, the nurse must ensure that active humidification is set to administer inspired gas at 37°C and 100% relative humidity in the lungs to assist lung clearance of secretions from the endotracheal tube by suctioning using an evidence-based technique. Trauma, infection and cardiopulmonary compromise are well-documented adverse events associated with a poor technique:

- Read the review by Pollard (2001).

CARDIOVASCULAR COMPLICATIONS: LESSONS LEARNED

Mechanical ventilation through its delivery of positive intrathoracic pressure has an adverse effect on the heart. Consequently, patients require close assessment and monitoring of their cardiovascular function. Increasing intrathoracic pressure decreases venous return to the right side of the heart and subsequently to the left side of the heart (Robb 1997b). Therefore patients may need additional fluid volume to maintain cardiac output. The nurse must be mindful to observe cardiovascular parameters in relation to ventilator airway pressure. Decreased cardiac output due to positive pressure ventilation is often ameliorated by fluid administration. The degree of cardiac compromise may often limit the amount of PEEP that a child can tolerate and hence what the intensivist is willing to use.

MODES OF VENTILATION

The goals of assisted ventilation are to achieve adequate gas exchange while at the same time minimising damage to the lungs or interference to the circulation. The review of the risks and side effects of positive pressure ventilation possibly goes some way towards explaining why there are quite so many modes of ventilation available today.

This chapter will now turn to a brief synopsis of the common approaches to ventilation based on physiological principles. It is by no means exhaustive or complete, and is not intended to be. For a more exhaustive discussion of management issues surrounding mechanical ventilation of the sick child refer to one of the major intensive care texts, such as the *Manual of pediatric critical care* (Hazinski 1999).

Ventilators (Fig. 45.8) deliver gas to the lungs using positive pressure at a certain rate. The amount of gas delivered can be limited by time, pressure or volume. The duration can be cycled by time, pressure or flow. The basic terms used with ventilators are:

- Peak inspiratory pressure (PIP): indicates the maximum pressure that has occurred during the last ventilatory cycle.
- Positive end expiratory pressure (PEEP): is the baseline pressure and controls functional residual capacity (FRC).
- Pressure above PEEP (PAP).
- Mean airway pressure (MAP).
- Inspiratory time (Ti): shown in seconds.
- Expiratory time (Te): shown in seconds.
- Tidal volume (Vt): amount of gas delivered with each breath.
- Minute volume (MV): amount of gas breathed in or out over 1 minute = Vt × Rate.
- Continuous positive airway pressure (CPAP).

Note: CPAP is equivalent to PEEP, except the term is usually used when referring to patients who are not intubated but on what is called nasal CPAP (NCPAP).

The common ventilation modes illustrated in Fig. 45.9 are:

Fig. 45.8 • A ventilator (top) and a close-up of the control panel (below).

- **Assisted control mode (AC):** the ventilator will guarantee that the patient receives a set tidal volume or peak airway pressure with every breath. The patient can breathe 'above' the set rate but will receive full support regardless of their effort.

- **Intermittent mandatory ventilation (IMV):** the ventilator supports breaths only at the set rate and interval. Breaths 'above' the set rate are not supported.

- **Synchronised intermittent mandatory ventilation (SIMV):** the ventilator synchronises an IMV 'breath' with the patient's effort. If, for example, the set rate is 10, then every 6 seconds the patient will receive a machine triggered breath. In between those 10 breaths, the patient is free to breathe but those breaths are not supported. These breaths can be supported if a 'pressure support mode' is added.

- **Pressure support or pressure control mode (PS/PC):** the ventilator supplies pressure support but no set rate. A patient needs to generate a certain amount of work to trigger it. Additionally, a patient has to breathe through an endotracheal tube that is almost always narrower than their own airway and ventilate the increased dead space imposed by the ventilator circuit. A patient may not be able to generate adequate tidal volumes for these reasons. To compensate for this increase in the work of breathing, pressure support is given.

Irrespective of mode, whenever a breath is supported by the ventilator, the limit of the support is determined by a preset pressure or volume. Thus, if volume is set, pressure varies and conversely, if pressure is set, volume varies according to the patient's lung compliance.

In continuous positive airway pressure (CPAP), PEEP is elevated baseline airway pressure (Fig. 45.10). The two terms 'PEEP' and 'CPAP' are used interchangeably and can lead to confusion. They are in fact the same thing. The con-

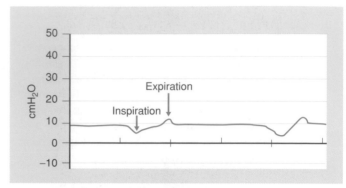

Fig. 45.10 • CPAP – pressure wave.

cept of PEEP is that a pressure is applied at the end of expiration to maintain alveolar recruitment and can, therefore, improve oxygenation and ventilation. Airway pressure is kept positive and not allowed to return to atmospheric. PEEP is usually set at between 4 and 10 cmH$_2$O, which is usually enough to ensure that the patient receives sufficient tidal volume (Pearson 2002). It can also stent open areas of trachea malacia (abnormal softening) and thereby improve ventilation and oxygenation even if these areas in of themselves do not participate in gas exchange. A great advantage is that CPAP can be delivered non-invasively either by nasal prong or mask (Fig. 45.11).

As ventilator technology has advanced, newer modes have been developed such as, pressure-regulated volume control (PRVC), volume support, inverse ratio (IRV), airway-pressure release ventilation (APRV) and high-frequency oscillatory ventilation (HFOV). Some are variations of volume or pressure modes and some are completely unrelated to conventional mechanical ventilation. It is important to recognise that none of these modes has yet been shown to be better than another or to reduce mortality for any disease.

Ventilator Settings

The initial settings prescribed and set by the intensivist for both volume and pressure are similar. Except in volume control a tidal volume is set at usually 8–10 mL/kg and in pressure control the peak airway pressure is set. The starting peak airways pressure is set at what is needed to adequately inflate the patient's chest and generate breath sounds and is usually 15–20 cmH$_2$O above PEEP. The starting breath rate is usually one that would be physiologically appropriate for the age of the patient. Immediately after intubation patients are usually placed on a FiO$_2$ of 1.0 and are weaned down as long as the oxygen saturations remain acceptable. PEEP is usually set at 5 cmH$_2$O and then increased as needed to achieve acceptable oxygen saturations with a FiO$_2$ less than 0.6 (Pearson 2002) (Fig. 45.12).

Fig. 45.9 • Ventilator modes.

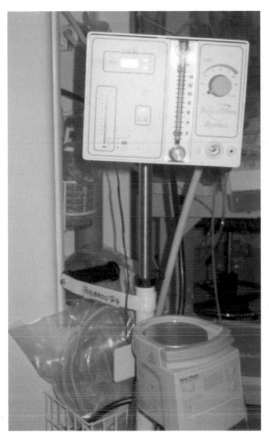

Fig. 45.11 • CPAP driver.

RESPIRATORY ASSESSMENT AND MONITORING OF THE VENTILATED CHILD

Clinical observation of the ventilated child is mandatory. Generally it is the intensive care nurse who observes, assesses, communicates, monitors, analyses and interprets data in order to effectively care for the critically ill child 24 hours a day (Fig. 45.13). In addition to the usual respiratory and cardiovascular observations discussed in Chapter 4, the critical care team must observe adaptation of the ventilator to the child and the degree of harmony between these two partners.

This is achieved by: observing the child's work of breathing and spontaneous chest movement against ventilator induced chest movement; regular 3–4-hourly blood gas analysis (as often as quarter-hourly if the child is unstable); constant cardiorespiratory observation; monitoring and hourly recordings together with ventilator observations. 'Monitoring' is a term usually reserved for automatic visual display of patient data such as temperature, pulse, respiration and blood pressure (Fig. 45.14). A continuous monitoring system, with safety alarm limits set, providing a minute-by-minute accurate picture of the child, means that effective decision making is carried out in 'real time' and at the 'right time' (Wheatley 2001). In the critical care environment the capabilities and complexity of modern technology are used to their best advantage. Deciding what needs to be monitored is complex but fundamentally essential in the care of the critically ill patient.

Activity

Figure 45.12 presents a simple paradigm to help explain how medical practitioners decide which ventilation parameter to alter based on the results of an arterial blood gas. Use the figure to determine what parameters might be altered by the intensivist in response to the arterial blood gas below taken 4 hours after Daniel was intubated and ventilated:
- pH 7.56, pCO_2 3.2, pO_2 20.0, base deficit –5
- Oxygen saturations were 100%.

Activity

Analyse your local intensive care observation chart and note the breadth of data that is collected at least hourly.

Consider the similarities and differences between data you would collect on a child receiving oxygen therapy on a children's medical ward.

To affect oxygenation adjust:	To affect ventilation adjust:
• FiO_2 • PEEP • Ti • Te • PIP	• Rate • Vt
PEEP, Ti & PIP affect mean airway pressure (MAP)	Alveolar ventilation is determined by the expired minute volume (Vt x rate)

Fig. 45.12 • Simple paradigm to explain likely ventilation setting changes.

Fig. 45.13 • Nursing assessment.

Fig. 45.14 • A monitor.

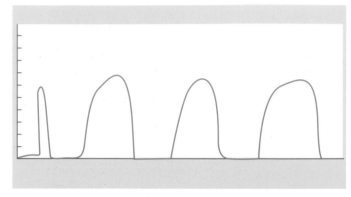

Fig. 45.16 • End tidal CO_2 showing on a caprogram display.

In addition to the respiratory monitoring techniques covered in Chapter 4, the nurse observing the ventilated child will monitor end tidal carbon dioxide ($ETCO_2$) and record ventilation parameters, which are analysed in the light of the child's vital signs, pulse oximetry and arterial blood gas results in collaboration with the medical team (Fig. 45.15).

Capnography is the measurement of carbon dioxide (CO_2) in each breath of the respiratory cycle. The capnograph displays a waveform of CO_2 (measured in kPa or mmHg) and it displays the value of the CO_2 at the end of exhalation, which is known as the end tidal CO_2 (Fig. 45.16). The capnograph sensor is placed between the endotracheal tube and the breathing circuit.

ETCO_2 provides a non-invasive method of evaluating ventilation and is helpful in assessing placement of the endotracheal tube. CO_2 is exhaled through the trachea and not usually from the oesophagus and so the measurement of CO_2 in the expired air distinguishes tracheal from oesophageal intubation. Provided the patient has a stable cardiac status and stable body temperature, an $ETCO_2$ with a normal capnograph trace approximates to the partial pressure of CO_2 in arterial blood ($PaCO_2$) (normal $PaCO_2$ is approximately 5.3 kPa) (Bhende 2001). The arterial PCO_2 is normally 0.3–0.7 kPa higher than the $ETCO_2$ reading and thus can be used to reduce the frequency of blood gas analysis required.

Figure 45.17 illustrates the different components of the capnograph trace. The first phase occurs during inspiration. The second phase is the onset of expiration, which results in a rapid increase in CO_2. The third phase, the expiratory plateau, occurs as the CO_2 is exhaled from all the alveoli. The highest point (4) of the plateau is known as the $ETCO_2$ and marks the end of expiration. Phase four is the onset of inspiration. If the waveform does not return to the baseline during inspiration this indicates that re-breathing of exhaled gas is occurring and is accompanied by a rise in $ETCO_2$ reading. Sudden loss of the capnograph, that is a decrease to zero, should alert the clinician to a catastrophic event such as oesophageal intubation, total obstruction, or ventilator malfunction. An exponential decrease of $ETCO_2$ can be seen due to loss of pulmonary blood flow as in cardiac arrest or sudden hypotension for example. A gradual decrease in $ETCO_2$ indicates decreased production such as in hypothermia. Rising $ETCO_2$ can be seen either due to increased CO_2 production, such as in sepsis, malignant hyperthermia, or due to decreased CO_2 elimination when there is decreased alveolar ventilation (Bhende 2001).

Fig. 45.15 • Ventilator board.

Scenario

One hour after intubation, the nurse noted that Daniel's heart rate was 145, blood pressure 130/92, respiratory rate 30 and oxygen saturation 100%. Ominously, the $ETCO_2$ that had been reading 5.6 kPa had increased to 9.7 kPa.

Professional Conversation

"
Michael, a registered children's nurse new to PICU, summons his mentor for help and records this learning episode in his reflective diary.
"

Trouble-shooting

If after intubation or at any time during ventilation therapy a child's condition deteriorates the pneumonic 'DOPE' is a useful tool to help make a systematic patient assessment and perform appropriate interventions when waiting for the arrival of the intensivist who had been asked to attend Daniel. Is the deterioration as a result of:

- **D** = displaced tube?
- **O** = obstructed tube?
- **P** = pneumothorax?
- **E** = equipment?

Assess A: the airway first – is the tube still in? Is it in the right position? The endotracheal tube was still at 13 cm at the lips. Had the endotracheal tube not been in place it would have been removed and bag–valve–mask ventilation instituted.

Assess B: breathing next – is the chest rising? Had the chest not been seen to rise with ventilation Daniel would have been disconnected from the ventilator and bag valve inflations given to eliminate the ventilator circuit as the problem. 'Bagging' by hand can also allow the facilitator to gauge compliance.

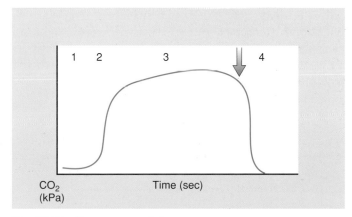

Fig. 45.17 • The capnograph trace.

Are breath sounds present and equal? Changes in breath sounds? Endotracheal tubes can become obstructed with secretions or be dislodged especially if the patient moves (or is moved)? Need for endotracheal tube suction? Mucus plugs can block lower airways as easily as they can obstruct the endotracheal tube. A suction catheter was placed through the endotracheal tube to be certain that it was patent and to rule out obstruction by mucous plug. It was patent and suction did not return any abnormal secretions. The chest rise appeared to be symmetrical bilaterally and breathe sounds were unchanged on auscultation. We noted the increasing blood pressure and administered sedation. Despite these actions the problem persisted.

The entire ventilatory circuit from the level of the endotracheal tube back to the ventilator was checked to find that the tubing was kinked thus restricting flow in the circuit. The tubing was repositioned to relieve the obstruction and Daniel's $ETCO_2$ started to decrease immediately back to its previous level. If this had not revealed a problem and the child's vital signs were stable we would have considered the potential of malfunction of the $ETCO_2$ device.

Extubation

As discussed earlier, children require respiratory support for many pulmonary and non-pulmonary problems. In the majority of cases, intubation and mechanical ventilation are necessary until the underlying cause of the respiratory failure is improved or resolved. The focus of management and care is thus facilitating the resumption of spontaneous ventilation that is 'weaning'. Weaning is essentially the transfer of demands from the ventilator to the child. It is important to assess the individual child's ability to handle the increased demands that extubation will place upon the child. In practice the critical care team is always weaning the child by progressively reducing ventilator support settings as the child's condition improves thus minimising the adverse effects of ventilation. Progressive reduction of rate, FiO_2 and PEEP demands that the child does more and is guided by arterial blood gas results. A child is usually ready to be extubated when he or she:

- is able to protect his or her own airway
- has a FiO_2 of less than 0.35
- is breathing at a comfortable physiological rate
- is receiving an pressure support that is just enough to compensate for the added work of breathing imposed by a ventilator circuit and ETT
- requires a PEEP less than 5 cmH₂O (Pearson 2002).

Haemodynamic Control

Scenario

On admission to PICU, additional vital signs were obtained:

- Daniel was awake and irritable and wanting to remain in Emma's lap
- respiratory rate: 70
- marked sternal and intercostals recession
- oxygen saturation: 95%
- heart rate: 200
- radial and dorsalis pulses: weak and thready
- skin was cool, dry and pale
- capillary refill: 4 seconds
- blood pressure: 90/60 mmHg
- he was conscious and responding to his mother Emma
- he appeared exhausted
- blood glucose: 1.7 mmol/L
- axilla temperature: 37.5°C
- no skin rash noted
- an arterial gas was obtained: pH 7.25, pCO₂ 7.6, pO₂ 22, base deficit −3.

In our scenario, Daniel is admitted to PICU and a rapid cardiopulmonary assessment was undertaken by the admitting critical care nurse which was documented as above. You will note from the data collected that there are signs and symptoms of cardiovascular instability for example marked tachycardia, poor perfusion (capillary refill >2 seconds), hypoglycaemia and a reduced level of consciousness. In reality, Daniel's cardiovascular status would have been managed almost simultaneously with his respiratory failure by the critical care team following a systematic ABC approach. However, for the purposes of this chapter respiratory support and haemodynamic control has been artificially separated for ease of presentation and to facilitate learning in a step-by-step approach.

HAEMODYNAMIC PRINCIPLES

The management of critically ill patients is based on knowledge of fundamental physiological variables. Monitoring of the haemodynamic status of these patients has developed from the non-invasive monitoring of a single parameter to the more invasive technological monitoring of multiple parameters we see today. This allows a comprehensive analysis of haemodynamic status enabling healthcare practitioners to not only provide effective treatment but importantly to anticipate deleterious events and intervene proactively in advance.

Haemodynamics refers to the forces, such as preload and afterload that affect the circulation of blood throughout the body. Critical care nurses assess the stability of these factors when they take a blood pressure or palpate a pulse. Although

the interaction of these forces is quite complicated, the concepts can be more easily understood by substituting the word, 'stretch' for preload and 'resistance' for afterload. Preload and afterload are closely related. Put simply, they reflect the heart's effectiveness in managing blood flow out of its chambers that is cardiac output. This chapter will now turn to a more detailed explanation and discussion of the determinants of cardiac output introduced above.

CARDIAC OUTPUT

Cardiac output (Fig. 45.18) is defined as the volume of blood pumped by the heart in 1 minute, and is represented by the equation:

$$\text{Cardiac output (CO)} = \text{Stroke volume (SV)} \times \text{Heart rate (HR)}$$

Stroke volume (SV) is the amount of blood pumped by the heart in one contraction. Thus, an increase in SV or HR causes an increase in cardiac output and conversely a decrease in SV or HR results in a decrease in cardiac output. An adequate cardiac output is essential to supply oxygen and nutrients to major organs and peripheral tissues. For example, a reduction in cardiac output may diminish blood flow to the brain and result in an altered level of consciousness. Alterations in heart rate, contractility, preload and afterload can affect cardiac output.

WHAT IS CONTRACTILITY?

Contractility is the force generated by the heart during each contraction. The contractility of the heart can be influenced by what is known as the preload. Preload is the force that stretches the contractile muscle fibres, the myofibrils, of the resting heart. This 'stretch' is determined by the amount of blood present within the left ventricle prior to contraction. The greater the volume of blood in the left ventricle, the greater the stretch on the myofibrils the greater the contractile force and thus, the greater the preload. An adequately filled and stretched left ventricle should briskly contract to eject blood. However, there is a point where the stretch (fill) is insufficient and cardiac output is diminished. Likewise there is a point where the stretch (fill) is too extreme that output is diminished. This

Fig. 45.18 • Determinants of cardiac output.

relationship between preload (stretch) and contractile force is explained by the Frank–Starling mechanism (Fig. 45.19).

Starling's mechanism states that, up to a point, the more the myofibrils are stretched in diastole, the more forcefully the heart contracts in the next systole. A simple analogy is an elastic band. If we apply a moderate stretch to the elastic band it will 'ping' back with moderate force. Likewise, if we apply a strong stretch to the elastic band it will 'ping' back with greater force. However, if we repeatedly provide too great a force to the elastic band it will very quickly lose its elasticity and fail to do its task. It is much the same with the myofibrils in the heart, if over-burdened, they will eventually fail; this is represented in Fig. 45.19. It must be remembered, however, that children, particularly under the age of 8 years have insufficient myocardial contractile proteins to significantly increase contractility and are therefore largely dependent on an increase in heart rate to maintain cardiac output.

Stroke volume is affected by preload, contractile force and afterload. As discussed, preload is the amount of blood delivered to the heart during diastole but this is in turn dependent on venous return. Venous return can be affected by variable venous capacitance known as afterload, which can increase or decrease blood return to the heart (preload).

UNDERSTANDING AFTERLOAD

Afterload is the resistance against which the heart must pump. When the heart overcomes resistance, the blood can be ejected. Sources of resistance include blood pressure (BP), systemic vascular resistance (SVR), and the condition of the aortic valve.

Blood pressure (BP) = Cardiac output (CO) ×
Systemic vascular resistance (SVR)

When there is arterial vasoconstriction, as in shock or aortic valve narrowing as in aortic stenosis, the ventricle has to create a greater amount of pressure, or afterload to overcome that resistance. A useful analogy is that it is akin to opening a door against a strong wind.

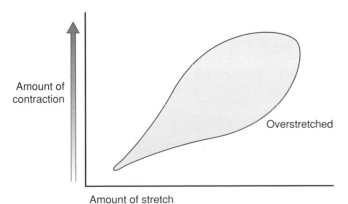

Fig. 45.19 • The Frank–Starling mechanism.

WHAT IS SHOCK?

The body's cells require a constant supply of oxygen and nutrients and elimination of carbon dioxide and waste products. These needs are fulfilled by the circulatory system in conjunction with the respiratory system, central nervous system and gastrointestinal system. The ultimate goal of this integrated control of the circulation is to maintain blood flow to the tissues to the optimum extent. Normally the body can compensate for some reduction in tissue perfusion through a variety of compensatory mechanisms. However, when compensation fails, shock develops. Shock has been defined as '. . . a complex clinical syndrome that is the body's response to cellular metabolic deficiency' (ALSG 2001 p 111). It is characterised by inadequate delivery of oxygen and metabolic substrates to meet the metabolic demands of the tissues that is a state of imbalance, and a threat to homeostasis (Fig. 45.20).

Metabolism in normal conditions is aerobic. In contrast, metabolism in poor perfusion states is anaerobic and although glucose is broken down into pyruvic acid, there is not enough oxygen present to metabolise it and pyruvic acid accumulates along with other metabolic acids (Marieb 2002). Anaerobic metabolism uses glycogen and fat for energy leading to a build up of lactic acid and carbon dioxide. Shock occurs first at cellular level resulting in generalised cellular hypoxia (starvation) and widespread impairment of cellular metabolism. This process if unchecked leads to cell death; tissue death; organ failure; system failure; and ultimately death (ALSG 2001).

Using a well-known analogy (ALSG 2001) (Fig. 45.21), the characteristics of shock involve dysfunction of the body's:

- pump (heart)
- fluid volume (blood)
- container (blood vessels).

Inadequate tissue perfusion can result in derangement of any of these components. The heart is the pump of the circulatory system. Put simply, it receives blood from the venous system, pumps it to the lungs to be oxygenated and then pumps it to organs and peripheral tissues. When the heart 'fails' the output is reduced. The amount of blood pumped around the body by the heart is dependent on:

Fig. 45.20 • Homeostasis.

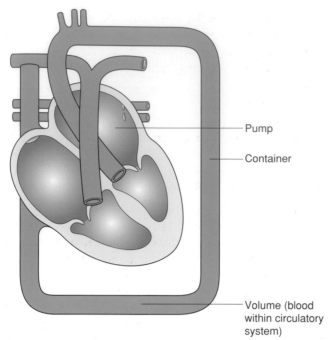

Pump

Container

Volume (blood within circulatory system)

Fig. 45.21 • Pump, container and fluid analogy.

- heart rate
- ability to empty the heart, which depends on:
  - contractility
  - resistance to flow and blood pressure
- ability to fill the heart which depends on:
  - amount of blood returning for re-circulation
  - filling pressures versus compliance.

Blood is the fluid of the cardiovascular system. Blood is a viscous fluid that is thicker, more adhesive and slower moving than water. As the cardiovascular system is essentially a closed system, an adequate volume of blood must be present to fill the system. Blood transports oxygen, carbon dioxide, nutrients, hormones, metabolic waste products and heat.

The blood vessels which include arteries, arterioles, capillaries, venules and veins, serve as the container for the cardiovascular system. This container provides a continuous, closed, pressurised pipeline that moves blood under the control of the autonomic nervous system, which delivers haemoglobin saturated with oxygen to diffuse into cells at end organs. The vessels regulate blood flow to different areas of the body by adjusting their size and re-routing blood through the microcirculation. Contraction of venous circulation increases preload and SV, but contraction of arterioles increases afterload and BP. The microcirculation is responsive to local tissue needs. Capillary beds can adjust size by opening and closing pre and post capillary sphincters to supply undernourished tissue or bypass tissue with no immediate needs. Therefore, blood flow is dependent on peripheral resistance, which in turn is dependent on internal diameter, length of the vessel and blood viscosity.

Tissue perfusion is dependent on the circulatory system, consisting of pump, container and fluid. But equally as important are conditions for optimal uptake, effective oxygenation and utilisation of oxygen in the body (Hazinski 1999). The conditions are:

- Adequate concentration of oxygen – ideally 97–100% of haemoglobin is saturated with oxygen.
- Oxygen diffuses across the alveolar–capillary membrane.
- Adequate number of haemoglobin molecules attached to red blood cells to enable transport of oxygen.
- Adequate and efficient off-loading of oxygen at tissue–cellular level.

These conditions are often referred to as the 'Fick principle'.

In summary, it can be seen that shock is a cellular state of imbalance resulting in inadequate tissue perfusion and can be caused by either one or a combination of the following components (Fig. 45.22):

- An inadequate pump:
  - inadequate preload
  - inadequate contractile strength
  - inadequate heart rate.
- An inadequate fluid volume:
  - insufficient fluid volume.
- An inadequate container:
  - excessive dilation without increase in fluid volume
  - excessive SVR.

Stages of Shock

The three recognised stages of shock (ALSG 2001) are commonly identified as:

- compensated shock
- decompensated shock
- irreversible shock.

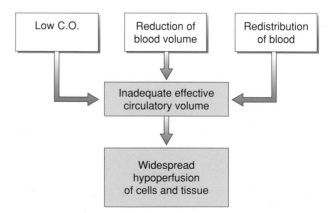

Fig. 45.22 • Common pathway.

Compensated Shock

In the initial stage, cardiac output and perfusion are decreased and the body acts to defend itself and preserve major organs by way of a series of reflex mechanisms involving the central nervous system and neurohormonal systems. These reflex compensatory mechanisms occur in the macrocirculation, in the kidney and the microcirculation. For this reason, this stage is often referred to as 'compensated' shock. These subtle indicators make shock difficult to detect at this stage especially in children who, as a result of usually young healthy major organs, are efficient compensators.

Decompensated Shock

If untreated, shock will progress to 'decompensated shock' where compensatory mechanisms fail and shunting of blood to vital areas becomes ineffective resulting in severe hypoperfusion. A loss of autoregulation of the microcirculation and increased capillary permeability causes reduced blood volume to the right side of the heart and reduced cardiac output. This in turn reduces blood pressure, which reduces coronary artery perfusion. Myocardial oxygen demand then exceeds myocardial oxygen supply. Imbalance of arterial blood supply to the myocardium causes arrhythmias, muscle ischaemia, and a self-perpetuating cycle of reduced cardiac output and cardiac failure occurs. This prolonged loss of cardiac output also:

- Reduces cerebral blood flow.
- Causes renal tubules to become ischaemic.
- Prolonged vasoconstriction causes ulceration of the stomach wall allowing bacteria and toxins to cross into the bloodstream.
- Bilirubin is not metabolised by the underperfused liver and waste products build up.
- Cell death causes release of enzymes from the pancreas, which depress the myocardium.
- Ischaemia of alveolar cells inhibits surfactant production in the lungs causing alveolar collapse, atelectasis, and reduced pulmonary compliance leads to acute respiratory distress syndrome (ARDS).
- Increased pulmonary vascular permeability causes interstitial and intra-alveolar oedema.

Irreversible Shock

The final stage of shock, sometimes also referred to as the 'refractory stage' is a profound condition where vital organs falter as a result of being starved of oxygen for too long:

- Hypotension is unresponsive to drugs and fluids.
- Severe hypoxaemia is unresponsive to oxygen therapy.
- Anuria and build-up of toxic waste as the renal system fails.

- Liver causes hyperglycaemia and build-up of waste products and allows no metabolism of drugs.
- Pancreatic dysfunction further affects myocardial contractility, haematologically.
- Multiple emboli form, intravascular clotting and severe coagulopathy.
- Neurologically, there is reduced response to stimuli and sympathetic stress response due to failure of the medulla causing circulatory failure and death eventually occurs.

Early Recognition of Shock

Early recognition of shock is essential. The outcome of children once in de-compensated shock is, in general, very poor (Pearson 2002). Early recognition of the child in compensated shock and prompt and appropriate intervention as a result has been shown to reduce mortality and secondary morbidity. As already stated, the early indicators of shock are subtle and difficult to detect largely because children who as a result of usually young healthy major organs are efficient compensators. To recognise the initial body response to a loss of cardiac output, the nurse must be fully cognisant of the compensatory mechanisms used by the cardiovascular system. In addition, a thorough knowledge and understanding of the pathophysiology of different types of shock together with a high index of suspicion facilitates recognition of these subtle signs and symptoms. It is to a physiological description of the compensatory mechanisms of shock that this chapter now turns.

Shock: Compensatory Mechanisms

Young children are able to maintain a normal cardiac output and thus remain normotensive until vascular and cardiac decompensation is imminent (Partrick et al 2002). To recognise the initial signs of shock a high index of suspicion can help to raise your awareness of the subtleties of compensation. Ask yourself 'is this child at risk?' For example:

- Has the child got a history of diarrhoea, vomiting and decreased oral intake?
- Has he or she had surgery recently?
- Has he or she got allergic symptoms and recent exposure to a known allergen?
- Has he or she got a congenital heart defect?

The cardiovascular system is regulated by many feedback control loops and as a result, its responses are not simple. At the onset of shock, during the compensatory stage, the systemic and microcirculatory system work together and their activities tend to remain coordinated (Martini 1998). There is a combination of neural, hormonal, chemical and humoral mechanisms for defending cardiac output.

Mean arterial blood pressure (MAP) is sensed by baroreceptors located in the aortic and carotid bodies which monitor the circulation closely for changes in blood pressure. These receptors control arterial pressure mainly by adjusting heart rate and arteriolar vessel radius. Baroreceptors respond to small changes in vascular tone and pressure and message the sympathetic nervous system (SNS) to decrease vagal tone which increases heart rate and decreases coronary artery resistance thus improving myocardial oxygen supply (Fig. 45.23). MAP is also the basis for autoregulation by the heart, lungs and brain.

Autoregulation is the automatic adaptation of the radius of an arteriolar vessel in an organ to maintain constant blood flow over a wide range of mean pressures to protect functioning of that organ (Darovic 1995). Arterioles are the primary sites that contribute to systemic vascular resistance (SVR). In addition, in the microcirculation, adrenergic control of the arterioles is a major determinant of blood flow into the capillaries. The adrenal gland in response will increase catecholamine release. Catecholamines consist of adrenaline and noradrenaline which are endogenous vasoconstrictors which cause added vasoconstriction in an added attempt to improve cardiac output (McCance & Heuther 1994). Catecholamines also enhance cardiac contractility and heart rate. Constriction of blood reservoirs such as the skin, skeletal muscle, liver and spleen disgorge blood to be shunted from the capillary beds to flow directly from arterioles into the venous system thus increasing circulating blood volume (Figs 45.24 and 45.25). This arteriovenous shunting helps to redirect blood flow to vital organs. Arteriovenous shunting is one reason why blood pressure data alone are not a reliable indicator of peripheral tissue perfusion (Epstein 1997).

Renin production is increased as a result of decreased renal perfusion, which leads to angiotensinogen production eventually yielding angiotensin which is a potent vasoconstrictor. Antidiuretic hormone (ADH) is released from the posterior pituitary gland another potent vasoconstrictor which prevents the elimination of water. The continued failure of the kidneys to eliminate and excrete hydrogen ions causes a metabolic acidosis and consequent decrease in blood pH which in-turn further impairs myocardial function and cardiac output. Aldosterone is released stimulated by ADH causing sodium reabsorption in the renal distal tubules and as water follows sodium helps to conserve both sodium and water. Retained sodium assists in the reabsorption of tissue fluids (see Fig. 45.24). Decreased mean arterial pressure leads to arteriolar constriction, which together with decreased pressure in capillaries leads to decreased hydrostatic pressure that, due to reabsorbed sodium, is less than osmotic pressure assists increased reabsorption of fluid 15 mL/kg/hour from the tissues (Prior 1999).

Chemoreceptors located locally in tissue beds sense the hypoxia due to the now inadequate blood flow to the tissues as a result of systemic circulation constriction and cause further vasoconstriction (Marieb 2002). The cells become starved of oxygen. Tissue begins to metabolise anaerobically and the patient becomes acidotic. Respiratory function during shock is very important in compensation. In response the body begins to hyperventilate in order to blow

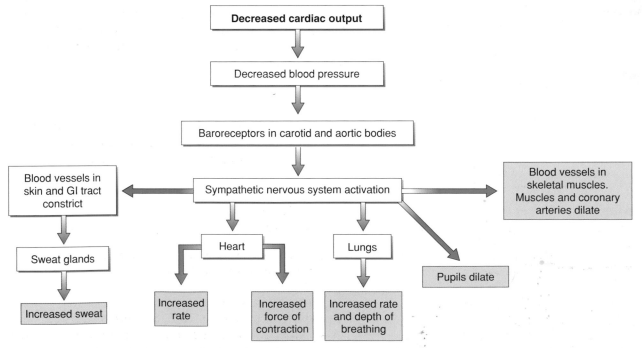

Fig. 45.23 • Neural compensatory mechanism.

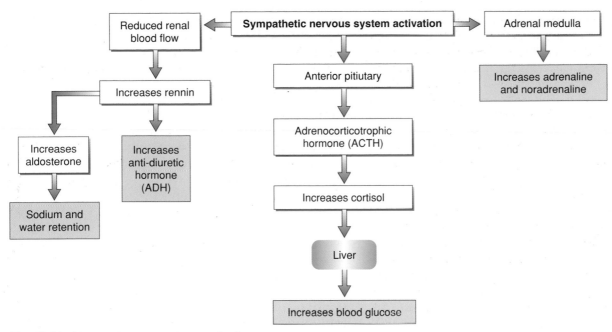

Fig. 45.24 • Hormonal compensatory mechanism.

off excess carbon dioxide resulting in respiratory alkalosis (see Fig. 45.25). This hyperventilation will also help to improve venous return (pump model).

In summary, the mechanisms for restoring cardiovascular homeostasis are:

- Redistribution of blood flow: attempt to preserve perfusion to vital organs.

- Augmentation of cardiac output:
  - increased heart rate
  - increased peripheral resistance.

- Restoration of intravascular volume: arteriovenous shunting.

These protective mechanisms will eventually cease to function and circulatory failure will ensue if not recog-

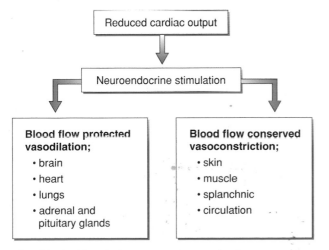

Fig. 45.25 • Chemical compensatory mechanism.

nised and intervention initiated aggressively (Edwards 1998). Again, blood pressure is not the key to deciding whether or not a child is in shock, although it does help to decide whether they are in compensated or decompensated shock. Much of the body's response revolves around the maintenance of normal aerobic metabolism and thus maintenance of viable cell function and measurement of the degree of tissue oxygenation in vital organs. The body's compensatory mechanisms are beneficial in the early stages but these homeostatic mechanisms soon become counterproductive. Nurses play a major role in recognising shock and play a direct role in influencing timely and appropriate intervention in conjunction with medical colleagues.

Types of Shock

Any reduction of blood volume by whatever means (pump, container, fluid) can cause shock. Shock is classified according to the causes to three classes (Table 45.1):

- hypovolaemic
- cardiogenic
- distributive.

It is important to be aware that more than one type of shock may be present at the same time.

Hypovolaemic Shock

This is the most common form of shock in children (Maill et al 2003). It is caused by a loss of intravascular volume. The decrease in blood volume may be caused by:

Table 45.1 Classification and causes of shock

Classification	Clinical causes	Primary mechanism
Hypovolaemic	Circulating fluid volume loss	Exogenous blood, plasma, fluid or electrolyte loss
Cardiogenic	Pump failure	Myocardial ischaemia Cardiac arrhythmias Cardiac failure
Distributive	Increased venous capacitance and extra-cardiac obstruction of blood flow	Massive inflammatory response, e.g. septic and anaphylactic shock

- external blood loss, e.g. haemorrhage.
- internal blood loss, e.g. ruptured spleen.
- severe dehydration as a result of:
  - vomiting
  - diarrhoea
  - excessive plasma loss, e.g. burn
  - excessive diuresis, e.g. diabetic ketoacidosis.
- third space loss, e.g. peritonitis.

Activity

Hypovolaemic shock is a volume problem:
- What signs and symptoms would you expect to see in a child in hypovolaemic shock?

A child's body can tolerate a loss of 20–25% circulating volume prior to a drop in blood pressure and cardiac output. In hypovolaemic shock the body attempts to maintain circulation despite the deficit.

Cardiogenic Shock

Cardiogenic shock is caused by an inability of the heart to pump sufficient blood. Inadequate function of the heart may be caused by heart failure that is weak cardiac contraction, from any cause. Cardiac output falls despite normal or elevated blood volume and cardiac pressures. Examples include:

- myocardial ischaemia
- arrhythmia
- congenital heart disease
- cardiomyopathy due to drug toxicity.

A major difference between cardiogenic and other types of shock is that pulmonary oedema secondary to heart failure is most usually present (McCance & Heuther 2002).

Activity

Cardiogenic shock is a pump problem:
- What signs and symptoms would you expect to see in an affected child?

Distributive Shock

Distributive shock is a container problem and is caused by excess vasodilatation causing loss of afterload and SVR. Examples are:

- neurogenic shock (rare)
- anaphylactic shock e.g. bee sting, peanuts
- septic shock.

Neurogenic shock occurs due to widespread and massive vasodilation due to imbalance of the parasympathetic (overstimulation) and sympathetic (understimulation) stimulation of vascular smooth muscle. Interruption of the sympathetic nervous system, which normally maintains muscle tone, results in persistent vasodilation. This overwhelming vasodilation results in pooling of the blood in the peripheries resulting in poor perfusion of the heart, brain and kidneys. The individual will have warm, dry skin and a slow heart rate. Neurogenic shock for example may be caused by trauma of the spinal cord and medulla above T6, which is extremely rare in children due to their immature anatomy and physiology (Maill et al 2003).

Anaphylactic shock is the widespread immune and inflammatory response (Hazinski 1999). The pathological response is similar to that of neurogenic shock that is vasodilation, increased vascular permeability causing peripheral oedema causing relative hypovolaemia and smooth muscle constriction leading to bronchoconstriction and dyspnoea. Individuals present with an almost immediate response to inciting antigen with any combination of the following; Cutaneous manifestations such as urticaria, erythema, pruritis, angioedema; respiratory compromise with stridor, wheezing, bronchorrhea, respiratory distress and varying degrees of circulatory collapse with tachycardia, vasodilation, hypotension.

Septic Shock

Septic shock is classified as a distributive shock. However, it is a combination of problems with the pump, container and fluid and is characterised by a:

- loss of preload
- loss of afterload/SVR
- loss of contractility.

Septic shock is the most common cause of death in PICU (Pearson 2002). A well-known cause of septic shock is meningococcal septicaemic which has a fatality rate of 50%

if the patient is already in shock when they first receive medical help (BMA 2002). A purpuric rash known as purpura fulminans is usually seen in meningococcal disease and constitutes a medical emergency.

 WWW

Link to this British Medical Association website and study the photographs of the non-blanching purpuric rash usually seen in meningococcal septicaemia:
- http://www.meningitis.orgdocs/GPleaflet

The terms sepsis, severe sepsis and septic shock are used to identify the continuum of the clinical response to infection (Bone et al 1997). An uncontrolled body system response to infection can rapidly escalate to severe sepsis and septic shock is causing acute organ dysfunction and ultimately death (Hazinski 1999). Although bacterial infection is the most common cause, fungal, viral and protozoa infections may also cause septic shock (Dolan 2003).

Whatever the initial cause of the infection, patients with septic shock have an overwhelming inflammation followed by a common pathway consisting of a systematic inflammatory cascade activated by inflammatory mediators (toxins) (Bone 1996). These mediators stimulate the release of cytokines, which act to amplify the inflammatory response and leads to systemic endothelial damage. Exposure of tissue and presence of cytokines stimulate the coagulation cascade. Coagulopathy leads to intravascular thrombus formation. In addition diffuse endothelial injury leads to vasodilation and increased capillary permeability resulting in extravasation of protein rich fluid and hence oedema (Gosling et al 1996). Therefore there is progressive vasodilation and maldistribution of blood flow, which ultimately causes organ hypoperfusion. A substance known as myocardial depressant factor (MDF) is secreted from white blood cells in response to endotoxin. MDF depresses the myocardial contractile function and results in ventricular dilatation thus further compromising cardiac output (Pathan et al 2004). To further complicate matters, in response to the pro-inflammatory mediators, excessive anti-inflammatory mediators are also released which then cause immunosuppression.

The clinical manifestations of septic shock depend on where the child is in the inflammatory response trajectory (Collins 2000). In the early phase of septic shock the child has a hyperdynamic circulatory state, often referred to as 'warm shock'. The initial mediators of inflammation lead to a marked reduction in SVR due to vasodilation and cardiac output increases. The child's heart rate increases, their pulses are 'bounding' and their skin is described as warm, dry and well perfused. In this situation a child is normotensive but may have a widened pulse pressure as vasodilation decreases diastolic blood pressure (DBP) and increased cardiac output raises systolic blood pressure (SBP). A progression from warm to cold shock occurs as hypovolaemia and ventricular dysfunction occur. This progression can be rapid in small children because of their limited ability to maintain the increased cardiac output (Butt 1998). In response to a fall in cardiac output, catecholamines are released causing vasoconstriction. Increasing vasoconstriction compromises oxygen delivery and leads to anaerobic metabolism and lactic acid production. Acidosis in the capillary beds causes the arterioles to dilate and the venules to constrict causing pooling and stasis of blood. Hypotension develops as intravascular volume is further depleted from ongoing capillary leak and progressive myocardial depression occurs (Fig. 45.26). If the cycle of depleted intravascular volume, poor tissue perfusion, impaired oxygen utilisation, exhausted metabolic energy supplies and myocardial dysfunction is not broken, the child will progress to vascular collapse, irreversible multiple system organ failure and death (Butt 1998).

 Activity

Septic shock is a pump, container and fluid problem:
- What signs and symptoms would you expect to see in a child in 'cold' shock?

Haemodynamic Monitoring

Haemodynamics is the state of the circulatory system as it relates to the perfusion of the body's tissues. Haemodynamic instability occurs when there is inadequate perfusion (global or regional) to support normal organ function. It has long been recognised that the physiological response of the patient to a stress or disease process will very largely determine the outcome (Webster 1999). It is important, there-

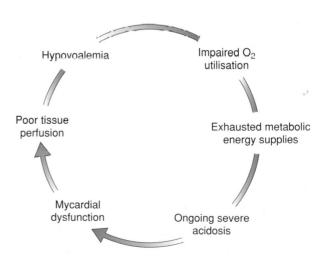

Fig. 45.26 • Pathophysiological cycle.

fore, to monitor the physiological responses of patients since this not only allows the assessment of physiological reserve but will also give a baseline against which the effectiveness of any applied treatment can be judged. Basic knowledge of the principles or monitoring and correct interpretation of data is important since a failure to do so can result in significant morbidity or indeed mortality of the patient. In the critically ill and haemodynamically unstable patient tissue oxygenation is determined by measuring components of cardiac output such as heart rate, arterial blood pressure, central venous pressure, arterial oxygenation and haemoglobin. In complex situations such as septic shock pulmonary artery pressure monitoring may also be used. This chapter will now introduce you to the concepts of arterial blood pressure and central venous pressure monitoring.

Arterial blood pressure (ABP) is measured by a catheter commonly placed in the radial, brachial or tibial artery and which is kept patent using a continuous infusion of intravenous heparin saline, 1 unit per mL at between 0.5–2 mL/hour depending on the size of the child. Arterial pressure is measured at its peak, which is the SBP, and at its trough, which is the DBP. The SBP is determined by the stroke volume, contractility, systemic arterial resistance and preload. The SBP is a clinical indicator of afterload. The DBP is affected by systemic arterial resistance and heart rate. Systemic mean arterial pressure (MAP) is defined as the mean perfusion pressure throughout the cycle.

$$\text{Mean arterial pressure (MAP)} = \text{Systemic vascular resistance (SVR)} \times \text{Cardiac output (CO)}$$

Pulse pressure is the difference between systolic and diastolic pressure and is normally about 40 mmHg. An increased pulse pressure may be the result of increased SV or contractility and is common during fever and anaemia. An acute decrease in pulse pressure may indicate an increase in SVR, decreased SV or decreased intravascular volume (McGhee & Bridges 2002). In summary, because of the multiplicity of factors that contribute to ABP, interpreting changes in arterial pressure and its components (SBP, DBP, MAP and pulse pressure) as indicative of any single factor may lead to an erroneous assessment of a patient's condition. Furthermore, however, numerically satisfactory ABP or MAP values are not necessarily related to adequate perfusion and organ system function. For optimal management of critically ill patients, ABP data must be integrated with information gained from clinical assessment of patient's status. This is particularly important in the management of the critically ill child. Children have significant physiological reserve and compensatory mechanisms and therefore may display an appropriate ABP for age even with significant circulating volume loss (Partrick et al 2002).

Central venous pressure (CVP) is measured by a catheter placed in the right atrium attached to a transducer which amplifies the energy signal and displays its wave form onto a monitor using a similar set-up to an arterial line as described above. Venous pressure is a term that represents the average blood pressure within the thoracic vena cava near to the right atrium. Thus, determination of the CVP provides a direct measurement of the changes in the pressure of blood returning to the heart. CVP is a useful tool for assessing the volume status of a patient. Since veins dilate and collapse passively depending on how much blood (volume) they contain, the pressure of blood in large veins depends directly on the patient's 'volume status'. The more fluid in the venous system the higher the central venous pressure is. A normal CVP is 2–8 mmHg in the self-ventilating patient (Darbyshire 1998). CVP is influenced by a number of factors including:

- cardiac output
- respiratory activity
- contraction of skeletal muscles (particularly legs and abdomen)
- sympathetic vasoconstrictor tone
- gravity.

A decrease in cardiac output either due to decreased heart rate or loss of heart contractility results in blood backing up into the venous circulation (increased venous volume) as less blood is pumped into the arterial circulation. The resultant increase in thoracic blood volume increases CVP. An increase in total blood volume as occurs in renal failure or with activation of the renin–angiotensin–aldosterone system will increase venous pressure. Venous constriction elicited by sympathetic activation of veins, or by circulating vasoconstrictor substances, for example, catecholamines, decrease venous compliance, thereby increasing venous pressure. It is important to remember that increased intra-thoracic pressure associated with positive pressure ventilation causes a reduction in CVP.

Treatment of Shock: Always Starts with ABCs

Airway needs will vary depending on the aetiology of shock, from no intervention to aggressive intervention. In our scenario, Daniel was assessed to be in respiratory failure and was immediately intubated and ventilated. However, sometimes a patient can be in shock but be breathing adequately and oxygenating well. Given the knowledge that shock syndrome causes excessive oxygen demand, it is advised that these patients are always given 100% oxygen via a non-rebreathe bag regardless of good saturations (ALSG 2001). Often, these patients ultimately need intubation and respiratory support to help them compensate for profound metabolic acidosis.

Scenario

On admission to PICU, Daniel's circulatory assessment found:

- heart rate: 200
- radial and dorsalis pulses: weak and thready
- skin was cool, dry and pale
- capillary refill: 4 seconds
- blood pressure: 90/60
- prior to intubation, 20 mL/kg normal saline was given rapidly

Daniel had progressed rapidly to respiratory failure accompanied by signs and symptoms of shock. He exhibited marked tachycardia, cold extremities with delayed capillary refill and poorly palpable peripheral pulses; these are suggestive of hypovolaemia. However, Daniel's history of upper respiratory tract symptoms and fever suggested an infectious aetiology. The rapid deterioration to a shock state from what earlier in the day appeared to be a seemingly benign prodrome in an otherwise healthy child made the critical care team suspicious that this might be sepsis. Therefore, unless an alternative diagnosis is very clear, a third-generation cephalosporin antibiotic is given as soon as a blood culture is taken (ALSG 2001). As is often the case, the precise aetiology of Daniel's illness was not clear. Despite this, the clinical findings indicated the need for prompt intervention.

Activity

Refer to Chapter 23 in ALSG (2001) *Advanced paediatric life support: a practical approach*, where techniques for achieving vascular access are described.

Antibiotic therapy, although essential in addressing the underlying cause, does not treat septic shock as severe sepsis involves a disturbance in the immune system response to the original infection. Additionally, antibiotics do not directly improve tissue perfusion or the associated delivery of oxygen and nutrients. Furthermore, oxygen therapy is of limited benefit because the primary problem is not inadequate oxygenation but inadequate transport of oxygenated blood. Remember that in severe sepsis a patient has excess coagulation and inflammation and impaired fibrinolysis with disruption of the endothelial layer. The endothelial wall disruption includes markedly increased capillary permeability and venodilation. The venodilation that occurs causes a relative hypovolaemia. Therefore, treatment of septic shock must be aimed at recovering function at microcirculatory level in order that dysfunctioning organs can begin to function again.

Circulation

Irrespective of aetiology, initial shock therapy is directed at restoring circulating blood volume and perfusion. Fluid resuscitation is the mainstay of initial haemodynamic management. Optimal cardiac output is dependent upon volume, heart rate and contractile fibres in the myocardium achieving the appropriate amount of stretch. Therefore, replacing lost volume will support cardiac output by increasing preload, thus enhancing cardiac muscle stretch and subsequent contraction, the optimum effect of the Starling mechanism. Thus a simple fluid bolus helps to improve a patient's haemodynamic status.

If not already available, vascular access should be obtained as quickly as possible once a 'shock state' is recognised. The UK Resuscitation Council (2002) recommends that medical practitioners make three peripheral intravenous attempts over a maximum of 90 seconds and progress to immediate placement of an intraosseous needle if unsuccessful. Replacement must be made using a fluid bolus of 20 mL/kg of isotonic fluids given within a 10–20-minute period. Normal saline is the solution of first choice because it is ubiquitously available and carries minimal risks. However, repeated administration of iso-oncotic crystalloid solution boluses can lead to extravasation of fluid from the intravascular to the interstitial space especially in situations where there is increased capillary permeability, for example in septic shock. In these circumstances colloids may be administered as they have an important effect on the intravascular space. When infused, the osmotic colloid pressure on the intravascular space increases. As a result, fluid is drawn from the interstitial space into the intravascular space. Therefore, the blood is rehydrated by osmosis (Alderson et al 2001).

Activity

Read Docherty & McIntrye (2002), which includes a simplified interpretation of the arguments and discussion offered in the Cochrane Review (Alderson et al 2001).

Activity

Daniel is given 20 mL/kg normal saline over 10 minutes. His circulation should then be re-assessed:

- What will you assess, why and how?

Scenario

Despite a transient improvement after an initial bolus of 20 mL/kg normal saline with a heart rate of 130 and capillary refill of 3–4 seconds, Daniel requires further fluid therapy. After 60 mL/kg (3 × 20 mL/kg boluses) Daniel remains pale with a heart rate 160, SBP 70 mmHg, capillary refill of 5 seconds and pulse oximetry that is not picking up. A central line has been inserted and Daniel has a CVP reading of 4 mmHg. He is started on dopamine at 4.0 mcg/kg/min and dobutamine at 10 mcg/kg/min administered via the central venous line.

A 5 mL/kg bolus of 10% dextrose in addition to maintenance fluids commenced has improved his blood glucose from 1.7 to 4.2 mmol/L.

As severe sepsis worsens, the benefits of fluid therapy are reduced, mainly because fluid therapy alone cannot address the cellular problem of increased capillary permeability as seen in severe sepsis. The fluid bolus has little effect on CVP. The widespread endothelial damage, vasodilation and capillary permeability are so great that pressure cannot be developed in the system. Because myocardial depression and vasodilation may be features of the patient's septic shock, inotropic agents may be valuable in restoring adequate perfusion. An inotrope is an agent that improves myocardial contractility and enhances stroke volume.

Activity

Refer to the UK Paediatric Formulary *Medicines for children*, 2nd edn (RCPCH 2003) and review the actions, dosage and side effects and nursing implications for the administration of the following inotropic agents: adrenaline, noradrenaline, dopamine and dobutamine.

In patients with no significant improvement after two or three fluid boluses, particularly if sepsis is expected, inotropic agents are used to maintain arterial pressure. The agents most commonly used are catecholamines. Dopamine and dobutamine are both catecholamines but have different profiles as they activate different specific receptors. Their main course of action is through adrenergic receptors:

- α: peripheral vasculature stimulation: vasoconstriction
- β_1: myocardium stimulation: inotropy and chronotropy
- β_2: lungs and peripheral vasculature stimulation: smooth muscle relaxation (vasodilation and bronchodilation).

Dopamine is the gold standard as the initial vasopressor support of septic shock because of its versatility and its activation of dopamine receptors, thus possibly protecting the kidneys and preventing acute renal failure due to tubular necrosis. Dopamine, a precursor of adrenaline (epinephrine), administered as a continuous infusion, affects preload by causing vascular constriction or dilation through its effect on the sympathetic nervous system. Dopamine acts on α, β and dopamine receptors. Low-dose dopamine, 2 mcg/kg/min to 4 mcg/kg/min, has peripheral vasodilating effects but causes little or no increase in force of myocardial contraction (positive inotropy). However, low-dose dopamine may help to maintain splanchnic circulation and promote renal perfusion via dopamine receptor action. Dopamine affects β receptors at 5–10 mcg/kg/min and α receptors at >10 mcg/kg/min. If unable to meet haemodynamic goals with dopamine, medical practitioners will have a low threshold for switching or adding other agents such as adrenaline, noradrenaline and dobutamine, which have been shown to be beneficial in the hemodynamic support of septic shock. Dobutamine, a synthetic catecholamine, is also administered as a continuous intravenous infusion and acts primarily on β-1 receptors. Dobutamine increases myocardial contractility (inotropic effect) and heart rate (chronotropic effect) and therefore increases stroke volume. It also causes peripheral vasodilation decreasing afterload. Overall dobutamine improves cardiac output.

Monitoring the Child in Shock

Seminar discussion topic

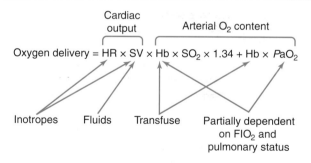

Shock is an altered state of tissue perfusion severe enough to induce derangements in normal cellular function. Neuroendocrine, hemodynamic and metabolic changes work together to restore perfusion. Treatment of shock is primarily focused on restoring tissue perfusion and oxygen delivery while eliminating the cause. The general goal is to maximise oxygen delivery and minimise oxygen demand and thereby enhance perfusion:

- Haemodynamic goals:
  - mean arterial pressure > 60 mmHg
  - heart rate within normal parameters
  - central venous pressure > 8 but < 15 mmHg
  - capillary refill < 2 seconds.

- Organ perfusion goals:
  - CNS: improved sensorium
  - skin: warm, well perfused
  - renal: urine output > 1 mL/kg/hour
- Oxygen delivery adequacy:
  - arterial oxygen saturation > 95%
  - Hb concentration > 10 g/dL
  - lactate < 2 mmol.

Work with colleagues to determine the implications for nursing in working collaboratively to achieve these goals.

Family-centred Critical Care

The hospitalisation of a child with a life-threatening illness constitutes a major stress experience for both the child and parents endangering the child's and the parent's biological, social and psychological integrity. Infants and children admitted to intensive care (Fig. 45.27) require immediate stabilisation and life support that is frightening, invasive and likely to alter the appearance of the infant or child with an uncertainty about outcome. Nurses must be knowledgeable of the impact this phenomenon has on children and their families and the factors influencing their adjustment to this stressful experience to assist children and their families in developing positive, adaptive coping mechanisms. Contemporary health care, assessment of need at the level of the client group has become increasingly important (DoH 1999) and is hoped will enhance quality of care.

Evidence-based Practice

Studies of adult patient recollection of intensive care experience are plentiful and report disturbing accounts of hallucinations, inability to communicate, pain, anxiety and memory of vivid details relating to intensive care procedures and mechanical ventilation (Granberg et al 1996). Playtor et al (2000) provide the only research data of children's experiences. They investigated 44 children's recollections, aged between 4 and 16 years of their intensive care experience using semi-structured interviews. Only 15% of the recollections were negative. More specifically: no child treated with neuromuscular blocking agents remembered any period of paralysis; six children complained of a lack of sleep, of these, three complained about the noise and the other three complained of pain/discomfort; eight children remember feeling frightened; eight remember being thirsty; two had negative recollections of the nasogastric tube and one child had negative recollections of the endotracheal tube. Following discharge, two children experienced dreams but only one of these children described the dreams as frightening.

Reflect on your Practice

What strategies do you think could be used to address these negative experiences for children in practice?

Much research has been carried out in an endeavour to understand parental experiences of intensive care. Therefore, the needs of family members of the critically ill child are well established, although maternally biased. A critique of this literature reveals that positivistic studies, which attempt to quantify parental feelings and experiences, dominate the literature with the majority being American (Noyes 1998). The perceived needs of American parents can be expected to differ from those of British parents for a number of reasons, for example the differing healthcare delivery systems and philosophies, healthcare professional education and training and the culture and expectations of parents (Temmink et al 2000), which are arguably not transferable to a British population. Therefore, we will focus on the results of British research.

British positivistic researchers were concerned with the question 'What are the most important needs and stressors of parents of children on intensive care?'. They consistently demonstrate the importance of certain features of the parents' stressor experience, such as, uncertainty about the child's condition, the environment and parental role alteration and establish the parental need for information, reassurance and support and to be near their child (Farrell & Frost 1992, Haines et al 1995, Heuer 1993). These researchers also defined variables that impacted on these stressors, for example, parental gender (Heuer 1993) and acuity of illness and need for intervention (Haines et al 1995). These studies clearly demonstrate that a child's need for intensive care is a major stressor and that parents have a hierarchy of concerns

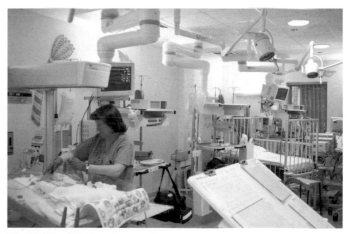

Fig 45.27 • PICU environment.

analogous with a hierarchy of needs (Maslow & Lowry 1998), that is, that the level of technological intervention has an impact on the nature of the stressors experienced. However, it is suggested that the use of scales in principle are inappropriate for the investigation of parental experience as they fail to establish any knowledge of parental situational meaning construction or a comprehensive understanding of parental needs (Aylott 2002). Understanding parental experience is a question of quality and nature rather than quantity. Subjectivist research using a qualitative methodology through its open-minded exploratory approach aims to understand the complex world of this lived experience from the point of view of the parents who lived it (Aylott 2000, Noyes 1999, Place 1997). These studies ask 'What is it like to have a child in intensive care?'

Place (1997) in his ethnographic study of children's intensive care, offers a sensitive analysis of the relationship between the parent, their new parent role and their child's altered appearance. Place describes how the body is 'technomorphic', that is, revisable by connection to technological artifacts which in turn has an impact on social interaction, self and identity. He also makes a distinction between what he calls 'child data' that is what is happening within the body and 'data child' which is the physical manifestation of the body through its connection to surrounding technological artifacts such as monitors reading vital signs. The 'child data' and 'data child' explicate each other. In intensive care healthcare professionals and parents are all concerned to maintain the integrity of the 'technomorphic' body, which forms a key dimension in the interactions between health carer, child and parents.

Noyes (1999) conducted an exploratory study to elicit mother's lived experiences of their children's intensive care crisis and coping utilising a symbolic interactionism perspective (a philosophical perspective which views human experiences as an emergent process in which meaning arises from the interactions between subject and object). She reports on the impact of the initial shock and crisis, the child's appearance and the implications of being resident. Noyes (1999) demonstrated that mothers whose children are undergoing intensive care are in crisis and are vulnerable at this time and recommends that nurses proactively seek to address the psycho-emotional needs of parents prior to and immediately after admission and deliver family-centred care. Furthermore, this has long term implications as mothers' stress-related symptoms and perception of their families as dysfunctional after discharge from hospital has been shown to persist as long as 6 months after a child's illness event (Board & Ryan-Wenger 2002).

Aylott (2000) conducted an exploratory study of parents' experience of their child's extracorporeal membrane oxygenation (ECMO) utilising a grounded theory approach.

ECMO is an invasive technique that oxygenates blood outside the body, obviating the need for gas exchange in the lungs, and, if necessary, provides cardiovascular support. Children that require this treatment are extremely sick. Parents described: the horror of critical illness that was acute and sudden with a telescoped trajectory offering little chance to reflect and prepare for the experience; a sense of loss, an alienation of the mundane, which had altered significance from everyday life 'taken for granted-ness'; how the boundaries between their child's body and other technologies became blurred as the body was colonised and extended to include both the child and the technological elements; how understanding 'child data' as described by Place (1997) became important in communicating with staff and gaining 'control' and involvement in their child's care. This was also described as therapeutic in dealing with cognitive dissonance about the child's outward appearance once stabilised despite the internal disorder and disease.

These studies (Aylott 2000, Noyes 1999, Place 1997) are useful in showing that parents' accounts are more than 'stories about' they are importantly ways of 'seeing as'. Negotiation and partnership are important concepts as a means of cultivating parent trust in staff, maintenance of hope and their ability to cope. Although the clinical picture may vastly constrain physical involvement in their child's care, parents wish to challenge and collaborate in decision making and sometimes in procedures. This is in essence family-centred care.

Family-centred care moves beyond the rhetorical theoretical recognition of the centrality of the child and family in health care. A family focused multiprofessional critical care team views the child and family as a unit to be cared for and organises care delivery around them as a unit as opposed to the more traditional patient-centred model (Henneman & Cardin 2002). However, providing family-centred care in a critical care setting is not a simple endeavour and is often misconceived as a list of interventions, for example open visiting. Family-centred care is a philosophical approach to care that recognises the needs of the family as well as the important role that they play during a child's critical illness therefore it should be more accurately referred to as family-centred critical care in this setting. Although providing family-centred critical care means that the critical care team recognise their responsibility to help the family, as well as the child, survive the crisis of an illness and have an obligation to endeavour to meet their fundamental needs, it is important to stress that meeting a child's needs should always be the priority for both the child's family and the critical care team (NMC 2002).

Research has indicated the fundamental needs of the family of the critically ill child as the need for honest and open information, the need for reassurance and support and the need to be in partnership with healthcare professionals regarding their child's care. These needs need to be ascertained from individual families and from individuals within a family and interpreted accurately. Thus it is important that nurses receive clarification about what these needs are and entail whilst at the same time recognising their dynamic nature. Empowering child and family participation in experiences that enhance control and independence and build on their strengths in the critical care environment demands advanced effective communication skills of the nurse and multi-professional team and the establishment of therapeutic relationships under stressful conditions.

Research indicates that it is important to a child's family that they are assured that their child is receiving the best possible care (Aylott 2000). Several investigators document the benefits of family presence during invasive procedures and resuscitation which includes knowing that everything possible was being done for their child; reducing anxiety and fear; feeling of being comforting and helpful to their child and the staff; sharing critical information about their child and the child's condition; maintaining the child–family relationship; closure on a life shared together; and facilitating the grieving process in the critical care environment and later at home (Eckle & MacLean 2001, Jarvis 1998, Meyers et al 2000, Sacchetti et al 2000). Adult patient studies indicated that having family present provided comfort, helped with coping and pain control, maintained the family bond, and reminded health providers that the patient was a person with a family who deserved dignity, and respect (Redley & Hood 1996, Robinson et al 1998) (Table 45.2). This has stimulated discussion about this controversial topic in both professional and consumer literature (Goldstein et al 1997, Powers & Rubenstein 1999, Rosenczweig 1998, Sacchetti et al 2000).

Although many family members and healthcare providers support the option of family presence, family members frequently are not given the option to remain with their child during invasive procedures and resuscitation efforts. This separation during treatment occurs for a variety of reasons. Health professionals express concern that: the event may be too traumatic for the family; clinical care might be impeded; family members might become too emotional or out of control; staff may experience increased stress with family present; unit rooms are too crowded, staff are focused on the child and may not be available to assist family members; the shortage of nurses; and the risk of increased liability (Eckle & MacLean 2001, Jarvis 1998, Meyers et al 2000, Rosenczweig 1998). Yet, families reported that they would be present again if a similar event occurred (Meyers et al 2000). In addition, investigators reported that there were no adverse psychological effects among family members and the operations of the emergency care providers was not disrupted when the option of family presence was used (Meyers et al 2000, Robinson et al 1998, Sacchetti et al 2000).

Table 45.2 Advantages and disadvantages of family presence during invasive procedures and resuscitation

Advantages	Disadvantages
Holistic approach: acknowledges role of family	Family may disrupt procedure/resuscitation efforts
Child/family bond facilitated	Healthcare staff perceive that they may not be able to show emotion
Family can observe efforts of healthcare team	
Family see that all that can be done is done	Fear of litigation due to lack of understanding
Imagination is more fearsome than reality	Observer effect may inhibit staff performance
Reduce litigation because of openness	May cause psychological damage to family
Family can provide comfort	Long term effects on family unit not known
Families perceive that they are participating in procedure/resuscitation	Increases stress of staff involved
	Child's privacy may be violated
Facilitates bereavement process	Resuscitation efforts may be unnecessarily prolonged
Facilitates relationship between family and staff	Interference of procedure/resuscitation
	Distraction of focus from child
	Family anger/violence towards staff

Activity

Analyse the evidence-based proposed advantages and disadvantages of family presence during resuscitation listed in Table 45.2. Consider the question:
- 'Do the advantages of allowing parents to be present during their child's resuscitation outweigh the potential disadvantages?'

Interestingly, parental presence at resuscitation has been fully supported by the UK Resuscitation Council since 1996, despite the controversy and in advance of much of this research. Every critically ill child is a member of a family system and is usually the major source of support for the child during times of stress, crisis and decision making. Research studies have shown that most families want the option to be present during invasive procedures, during their child's medical procedures and at the time of their child's death.

Summary

Topics for this chapter were chosen because of their importance to children's morbidity and mortality and their prevalence as problems in intensive care. This three-part chapter has considered the respiratory support, haemodynamic control and family-centred critical care required by a child with life-threatening illness on a paediatric intensive care unit. It demonstrates the principles of intensive care, which require that nurses apply specialist evidence-based knowledge and skills in the direct provision of care to manage a dynamic and rapidly evolving illness process in collaboration with medical and allied profession colleagues. The challenge is to provide this technologically sophisticated care in a compassionate environment and facilitate in depth interaction between the critically sick child and their family.

References

Advanced Life Support Group (ALSG) 2001 Advanced paediatric life support: the practical approach, 3rd edn. British Medical Association, London

Alderson P, Schierhout G, Roberts I, Bunn F 2001 Colloids versus crystalloids for fluid resuscitation in the critically ill. The Cochrane Library, issue 4. Update Software, Oxford

Ashworth W 1996 Inquiry into the care and treatment of Nicholas Geldard. North West Regional Health Authority, Manchester

Aylott M 2000 Parents' experience of their child's extra-corporeal membrane oxygenation: a qualitative study. Nursing in Critical Care 5:228–235

Aylott M 2002 Interviewing as therapy: researching parents' experiences of their child's life threatening illness requiring ECMO. Nursing in Critical Care 7(4):163–170

Ball C, Dams J, Boyce S, Robinson P 2001 Clinical guidelines for the use of the prone position in acute respiratory distress syndrome. Intensive and Critical Care Nursing 17:94–104

Bhende MS 2001 End-tidal carbon dioxide monitoring in pediatrics – clinical applications. Journal of Postgraduate Medicine 47:215–218

Board R, Ryan-Wenger N 2002 Long-term effects of pediatric intensive care unit hospitalisation on families and young children. Heart and Lung: the Journal of Acute and Critical Care 31(1):53–66

Bohn D 1998 New ventilation strategies. In: Duncan A (ed.) Paediatric intensive care. BMJ Books, London, pp. 41–91

Bone RC, Grodzin CJ, Balk RA 1997 Sepsis: a new hypothesis for pathogenesis of the disease process. Chest 112(1):235–243

British Medical Association (BMA) 2002 Meningococcal meningitis and septicaemia: guidance notes. Meningitis Research Foundation, London

British Paediatric Association (BPA) 1993 The care of critically ill children. Report of the Multidisciplinary Working Party on Paediatric Intensive Care. BPA, London

Butt W 1998 Management of septic shock in children. In: Duncan A (ed.) Paediatric intensive care. BMJ Books, London, pp. 236–266

Centers for Disease Control (CDC) 1994. CDC guidelines. Respiratory Care 39(12):1191–1236

Collins T 2000 Understanding shock. Nursing Standard 14(49):35–39

Coombs M 2001 Critical care: where care is critical. Nursing in Critical Care 6(3):111–114

Darbyshire P 1998 Making sense of central venous pressure monitoring. Nursing Times 84(6):36–38

Darovic GO 1995 Hemodynamic monitoring: invasive and non-invasive clinical application. WB Saunders, Philadelphia

Department of Health (DoH) 1999 Making a difference: strengthening the nursing, midwifery and health visiting contribution to health and healthcare. HMSO, London

Docherty B, McIntrye L 2002 Nursing considerations for fluid management in hypovolaemia. Professional Nurse 17(9):545–549

Dolan S 2003 Severe sepsis – a major challenge for critical care. Intensive & Critical Care Nursing 19:63–67

Dreyfus D, Basset G, Soler PS, Saumon G 1985 Intermittent positive-pressure hyperventilation with high inflation pressures produces pulmonary microvascular injury in rats. American Review of Respiratory Diseases 132(4):880–884

Duncan A 1998 Paediatric intensive care. BMJ Publishing, London

Eckle N, MacLean S 2001 Assessment of family-centered care for pediatric patients in the emergency department. Journal of Emergency Nursing 27(3):238–245

Edwards S 1998 Hypovolaemia: pathophysiology and management options. Nursing in Critical Care 3(2):73–82

Epstein O 1997 Clinical examination. Mosby, London

Estes R, Meduri G 1995 The pathogenesis of ventilator associated pneumonia: 1 mechanisms of bacterial translocation and airway inoculation. Intensive Care Medicine 21:365–383

Farrell M, Frost C 1992 The most important needs of parents of critically ill children: parent's perceptions. Intensive and Critical Care Nursing 8:130–139

Ganong WF 2001 Review of medical physiology, 20th edn. Lange Medical Books, New York

Goldstein A, Berry K, Callaghan A 1997 Resuscitation witnessed by relatives: has proved acceptable to doctors in paediatric cases [letter]. British Medical Journal 314:144–145

Gosling P, Bascom JU, Zikria BA 1996 Capillary leak, oedema and organ failure: breaking the triad. Care of the Critically Ill 12(6):191–197

Granberg A, Bergbom-Endberg I, Lundberg D 1996 Intensive care syndrome: a literature review. Intensive and Critical Care Nursing 12:173–182

Haines C, Perger C, Nagy S 1995 A comparison of the stressors experienced by parents of intubated and non-intubated children. Journal of Advanced Nursing 21:350–355

Hazinski MF 1999 Manual of pediatric critical care. Mosby, New York

Henneman EA, Cardin S 2002 Family-centred critical care: a practical approach to making it happen. Critical Care Nurse 22(6):12–19

Heuer L 1993 Parental stressors in a paediatric intensive care unit. Paediatric Nursing 19(2):128–131

Hill N 1997 Complications of non-invasive positive pressure ventilation. Respiratory Care 42:432–442

Jarvis AS 1998 Parental presence during resuscitation: attitudes of staff on a paediatric intensive care unit. Intensive and Critical Care Nursing 14:3–7

Kerr M 1997 Paediatric ventilatory care. In: Morton MS (ed.) Paediatric intensive care. Oxford University Press, Oxford, pp. 109–151

Kolobow T, Moretti MP, Fumagalli R et al 1987 Severe impairment in lung function induced by high peak airway pressure during mechanical ventilation: an experimental study. American Review of Respiratory Diseases 135(3):312–315

Lissuer T, Clayden G 2001 Illustrated textbook of paediatrics. Mosby, London

Maill L, Rudolf M, Levene M 2003 Paediatrics at a glance. Blackwell Science, Oxford

Marieb E 2002 Essentials of human anatomy and physiology, 7th edn. Benjamin Cummings, San Francisco

Martini FH 1998 Fundamentals of anatomy and physiology. Prentice Hall, New Jersey

Maslow AH, Lowry R 1998 Towards a psychology of being. John Wiley, London

McCance K, Heuther S 2002 Pathophysiology: the biological basis for disease in adults and children. Mosby, London

McCance KL, Heuther SE 1994 Pathophysiology: the biological basis for disease in adults and children, 2nd edn. Mosby Year Book, St Louis

McGhee BH, Bridges MEJ 2002 Monitoring arterial blood pressure: what you may not know. Critical Care Nurse 22(2):60–78

Meyers TA, Eichhorn DJ, Guzzetta CE et al 2000 Family presence during invasive procedures and resuscitation: the experience of family members, nurses, and physicians. American Journal of Nursing 100(2):32–42

NHS Executive (NHSE) 1996 Paediatric intensive care. NHSE, Leeds

NHS Executive (NHSE) 1997a Paediatric intensive care: a framework for the future. Report of the National Co-ordinating Group on Intensive Care to the Chief Executive of the NHS Executive. NHSE, London

NHS Executive (NHSE) 1997b Paediatric intensive care: a bridge to the future. Report of the Chief Nursing Officer's Taskforce to the Chief Executive. NHSE, London

Noyes J 1998 A critique of studies exploring the experiences and needs of parents of children admitted to paediatric intensive care units. Journal of Advanced Nursing 28(1):131–141

Noyes J 1999 The impact of knowing your child is critically ill: a qualitative study of mother's experiences. Journal of Advanced Nursing 29(2):427–433

Nursing and Midwifery Council (NMC) 2002 Code of professional conduct. NMC, London

Parker JC, Hernandez L, Peevey K 1993 Mechanisms of ventilator induced lung injury. Critical Care Medicine 21:131–135

Partrick DA, Bensard DD, Janik JS, Karrer M 2002 Is hypotension a reliable indicator of blood loss from traumatic injury in children? The American Journal of Surgery 184(6):555–559

Pathan N, Hemingway CA, Alizadeh AA et al 2004 Role of interleukin 6 in myocardial dysfunction of meningococcal septic shock. The Lancet 363(9404):203–209

Pearson G 2002 Handbook of paediatric intensive care. WB Saunders, London

Pearson G, Shann F, Barry PW et al 1997 Should paediatric intensive care be centralised? Trent versus Victoria. The Lancet 349:1213–1217

Place B 1997 The constructing of bodies of critically ill children: an ethnography of intensive care. In: Prout A (ed.) Childhood and the body. Macmillan, London, pp. 135–143

Playfor S, Thomas D, Choonara I 2000 Recollection of children following intensive care. Archives of Disease in Childhood 83:445–448

Pollard C 2001 Endotracheal suction in the infant with an artificial airway. Nursing in Critical Care 6(2):76–82

Powers KS, Rubenstein JS 1999 Family presence during invasive procedures in the pediatric intensive care unit. Archives of Pediatric Adolescent Medicine 153:955–958

Prior FGR 1999 Plasma colloid osmotic pressure in the critically ill. Care of the Critically Ill 15(5):167–172

Redley B, Hood K, 1996 Staff attitudes towards family presence during resuscitation. Accident and Emergency Nursing 4(3):145–151

Resuscitation Council UK (1996) Should relatives witness resuscitation? Resuscitation Council UK, London

Reynolds EM, Ryan D, Doody D 1993 Permissive hypercapnia and pressure controlled ventilation as a treatment of severe adult respiratory distress syndrome in a pediatric burn patient. Critical Care Medicine 21:468–475

Robb J 1997a Physiological changes occurring with positive pressure ventilation: part one. Intensive and Critical Care Nursing 13:293–307

Robb J 1997b Physiological changes occurring with positive pressure ventilation: part two. Intensive and Critical Care Nursing 13:357–364

Robinson S, MacKenzie-Ross S, Campbell-Hawson G et al 1998 Psychological effect of witnessed resuscitation on bereaved relatives. Lancet 352:614–617

Rosenczweig C 1998 Should relatives witness resuscitation? Canadian Medical Association Journal 158(5):617–620

Royal College of Paediatrics and Child Health (RCPCH) 2003 Medicines for children, 2nd edn. RCPCH, London

Sacchetti A, Carraccio C, Leva E et al 2000 Acceptance of family member presence during pediatric resuscitations in the emergency department: effects of personal experience. Pediatric Emergency Care 16:85–87

Temmink D, Francke AL, Hutten JBF et al 2000 Innovations in the nursing care of the chronically ill: a literature review from an international perspective. Journal of Advanced Nursing 31(6):1449–1458

Tibballs J 1998 Clinical aspects of nitric oxide therapy. In: Duncan A (ed.) Paediatric intensive care. BMJ Books, London, pp. 196–235

Webster NR 1999 Monitoring the critically ill patient. Journal of the Royal College of Surgeons 44:386–393

Wheatley I 2001 How can patient monitoring provide an effective tool to augment clinical judgement in the critical care environment? Nursing in Critical Care 6(3):145–147

Williams R, Rankin N, Smith T et al 1996 Relationship between the humidity and temperature of inspired gas and the function of the airway mucosa. Critical Care Medicine 24(11):1920–1929

Chapter Forty Six

46

Care of the Child Requiring Palliative Care

Jayne Price, Marisa McFarlane

ABSTRACT

The primary aim of this chapter is to examine the holistic needs of the child requiring palliative care in the context of the family. Palliative care for children has evolved as a specialist sphere of practice that can be delivered to children and their families within a variety of settings. Throughout the course of this chapter and the companion PowerPoint presentation, the biopsychosocial and spiritual care needs of children with life-limiting illness, and of their families, will be examined within a partnership approach to caring.

Learning Outcomes

- Recognise the development of the philosophy of caring and the specialist sphere of paediatric palliative care from a historical perspective.

- Examine the components that contribute to the philosophy of palliative care.

- Appreciate the importance of a family-centred and multidisciplinary approach to care of a child with a life-limiting illness.

- Understand the biopsychosocial and spiritual needs of the life limited child and his or her family.

- Appreciate the needs of the family in bereavement.

Introduction

The death of a child causes a devastating loss to families and communities and in turn leads to one of the most profound and long-lasting of griefs. The death of the child defies the natural order of events (Brewis 1995). Knowing that a child is going to die poses a particular challenge for parents and professionals (Armstrong-Dailey 1990). Over recent years, the care of children and young people with life-limiting illnesses has been the subject of growing interest and has evolved as a specialist sphere of practice – paediatric palliative care. It is imperative to recognise that palliative care services for children are organised differently than palliative care services for adult patients. Given the degenerative nature of many of the life-limiting illnesses of childhood, palliative care services are traditionally involved with the child and family from an early stage, often over a long period of time (Hynson and Sawyer 2001).

The need for care can be unrelenting and can lead to social deprivation and stress for the family (Farrell 1996), and burn-out in staff regularly caring for this specific client group (Costello and Trinder-Brook 2002).

The Evolution of Paediatric Palliative Care

The hospice movement was born out of a desire to improve care for dying people. It had become accepted that the modern medical establishment was not fully addressing all the needs of dying people and their families. By the early 1980s there were over 60 hospice-type services. The need for expansion of services was identified from simply providing care for adult cancer patients and in 1982 the first Children's Hospice was opened in Oxford. Helen House developed from the special friendship between Sister Frances Dominica and a child called Helen, who had a life-limiting illness. Through this relationship, Sister Frances recognised the need of respite care and practical support for other families in similar situations. Her vision was for a haven where this practical support and respite care could be delivered. Helen House provided a 'home from home' where families could share the caring, providing them an environment where practical help, friendship and quality time were offered. This was to 'blaze a trail in the provision of hospice care for children and young people' (Worswick 2002 p 160). The number of children hospices grew in conjuction with the development of 'hospice-at-home teams'. The growth generated an appraisal into the care delivered to children with life-limiting illnesses and their families and, in 1995, a group of representatives from existing children's hospices met to formulate guidelines for good practice within children hospices. From this the benefit of meeting together to share ideas and experiences became obvious. Hence the Association of Children's Hospices (ACH) was established as an official charity in 1998 (Price et al 2005).

 WWW

Visit the Association of Children's Hospice (ACH) website. Establish the purpose of ACH and the services it provides for children and their families:

* http://www.childhospice.org

The holistic philosophy of hospice care has since permeated into a variety of settings and should not be viewed as being restricted to a children's hospice setting. This being so, it is now referred to as paediatric palliative care. Future developments need to continue within this speciality. These should include strategic research and educational developments locally, nationally, and internationally as we move forward in the contiual provision of care based on the best evidence (Price et al 2005).

Paediatric Palliative Care: A Distinct Speciality

Palliative care for children and young people with life limiting conditions is an active and total approach to care, embracing physical, emotional, social and spiritual elements. It focuses on enhancements of quality life for the child and support for the family and includes the management of distressing symptoms, provision of respite and care through death and bereavement (ACT and RCPCH 2003 page 9)

The above definition highlights the different attributes that contribute to the philosophy of palliative care for children. This care can be delivered in a variety of settings, hospital, hospice or home. The ACT Charter outlines the needs of children and families and can be viewed on the companion PowerPoint presentation.

 WWW

Visit the Association for Children with life-limiting illness (ACT) website. Read 'The guide to the development of children's palliative care services' (2003) – click on publications:

* http://www.act.org.uk

At least 15,000 children require palliative care in the UK (ACT and RCPCH 2003) and a wide range of conditions renders their need for this type of care. Four broad groups of children have been identified as likely to require this unique type of care whose needs can change over time (ACT and RCPH 2003):

* Group 1: life-threatening conditions for which curative treatment may be feasible but can fail. Palliative care may be necessary during periods of prognostic uncertainty and when treatment fails for example cancer, irreversible organ failures of heart, liver and kidney.

* Group 2: conditions where there may be long periods of intensive treatment aimed at prolonging life and allowing participation in normal childhood activities but premature death is still possible, e.g. cystic fibrosis, muscular dystrophy.

* Group 3: progressive conditions without curative treatment options, where treatment is exclusively palliative and may commonly extend over many years, e.g. Batten's disease, mucopolysaccharidosis.

* Group 4: conditions with severe neurological disability that may cause weakness and susceptibility to health complications and may deteriorate unpredictably, but are not considered progressive, e.g. multiple disabilities such as brain or spinal cord injuries and including some children with severe cerebral palsy.

Reaction to a Life-limiting Illness

The diagnosis of a life-limiting illness rocks the most stable of families. It is the start of a journey that can resemble a roller-coaster ride: the ups and downs along the uncertain road of the illness trajectory. Many factors affect the psychological impact of facing a life-limiting illness. These include the age and cognitive development of the child, the duration and type of treatment, the prognosis or time frame expected, the degree of disruption to normal routine and education, the degree to which body image may be affected and the potential separation from siblings and main caregivers.

Judd (1996) notes the overall reaction to the diagnosis of a life-limiting illness is similar to that of bereavement. The child is grieving for the 'normal' life they may feel they have lost and the family is grieving the loss of their 'normal' child. The family needs support at the time of diagnosis and afterwards (Royal College of Nursing (RCN) 1999).

Kubler-Ross (1970) identified five reactions to dying; these can equally be applied to a diagnosis of a life-limiting or life-threatening illness. These are denial, anger, bargaining, depression and acceptance. The child and the family may experience a multitude of different feelings at different times and there is no set way for how the individual may feel at any particular time. Regardless of the type of feelings being experienced at any particular time, the child and family require cohesively planned care and support from an experienced team who are responsive to individual need.

Palliative care provision for children must therefore be tailored to the individualised needs of the children and their families and include a wide array of agencies and services within the NHS and outside to ensure a holistic quality care is delivered (Act 2003).

The Team Approach to Paediatric Palliative Care

The need for a multi-agency approach to paediatric palliative care is essential in the provision of seamless care to children and their families (ACT 2004). This approach must encompass a partnership centred round the individual needs of the child and family. The family includes parents, siblings and the wider family circle.

Clear, concise communication is a fundamental component of successful team working. Each team member has a role to play, must share the identical goals of care and respect the individual roles of team members and also the family. A cohesive package is required with clarity of roles in order that conflicting information is avoided. Team variance can create an environment where confusion is present. The healthcare professional must function effectively and efficiently on an individual basis and as part of the team. The palliative care package for the child and family whether in hospital, home or hospice should have an identified key worker. This worker will coordinate the care and ensures a seamless package is provided, that clarity of roles is ensured and good communication is maintained (ACT 2003). In the community the key worker is usually a CCN, palliative care nurse, hospice or Macmillan nurse.

The team will be made up of different professionals, depending on the individual family and their circumstances. Each team member must ensure that the holistic needs are identified and addressed:

- social worker
- pharmacist
- dietitian
- occupational therapist
- physiotherapist
- teachers
- psychologist
- music therapist
- hospital consultant
- GP
- aromatherapist/reflexologist
- hospital chaplain, minister, priest
- charitable agencies/voluntary organisations
- nurses (hospital/hospice and community)
- play specialist.

The assessment, planning, implementing and evaluation of plans of care including symptom control for children with a life-limiting illness need to be multidisciplinary (ACT 2003).

Holistic Care of the Child and Family

It is important to remember that, if carefully considered and managed, the care delivered to the child and the family surrounding and following the death of their child can have a positive effect on their memories (Davies 1997). This highlights to the nurse his or her professional responsibility to both the child and family in ensuring that the individual needs are met in a sensitive and holistic manner.

The care should be assessed, planned, implemented and evaluated using a collaborative partnership approach to care and should address the holistic needs of the child and family.

It is important to remember that quality of the remaining time is imperative. Therefore, the child has certain rights when approaching death in assuring quality in this period.

Gardner (1977) outlines the rights of the dying child:

- To know the truth about the probable outcome of their illness or, as most children have already worked it out for themselves, to affirm the truth.
- To share thoughts about dying – not just the probability of death but the many questions that follow.
- To live as full and normal a life as possible.
- To participate in the process of dying. To have a say whether treatment continues or not and in whether to die in hospital, at home or in hospice.

PSYCHOLOGICAL CARE

The family requires time to come to terms with the fact that the child's life is limited or that death may be imminent. Family members need to be empowered with information to enable them to make decisions about care and the desired place of death. Parents will have many questions about the impending death of their child:

- what symptoms will he or she get?
- what can be given for it?
- who will help and support us?
- how long will it be?
- how will we cope?
- what shall we say to the child?
- what about his or her brothers and sisters?

The nurse needs to ensure that, where possible answers are given, reassurance is offered and that time is permitted in order that they can assimilate information before they can discuss the change in circumstances with their child. Parents will need support in order to do this and are more likely to be open and honest with their child if adequate support is provided (Bluebond-Laugner 1992). The family will have options but may require guidance when making a decision. Parents may also need advice about how to discuss the situation with siblings and strategies about involving siblings and preventing sibling isolation and resentment occurring may also be necessary.

Scenario

David is eight. His 11-year-old sister Clare was diagnosed with a brain tumour 2 years ago. This did not respond to treatment and she is now approaching death. Clare is being cared for at home and is unable to leave the house.
Consider the changes David might be experiencing:
- in his family life and routine
- in his relationship with his parents
- in his own emotions.
What strategies could these parents use to prepare David for Clare's imminent death?

The emotional responses of the family impact on the care and support they give their child. It is common for parents to experience anger, guilt and blame. Mothers appear to express their feelings more freely than fathers and it is often assumed by healthcare professionals that fathers can cope (Hill 1996). It is essential that the nurse ensures that the needs of the father are also addressed.

Improvements and developments within community services have led to many families choosing their own home as the place where they want their child to be nursed. Where appropriate, the child or young person should be included when the family considers the choice of where the child should be nursed. All their options should be outlined and again they may require time to discuss and make a decision (Brown 2002).

Activity

List the advantages and disadvantages of caring for a dying child in his or her own home.

An honest and truthful approach has been identified as one of the rights of the child and is viewed as an essential component of effective communication in quality palliative care. The understanding children have of death evolves gradually. The nurse must have a knowledge of the child's developmental stage and their concept of death so that he

or she can communicate effectively with the dying child (Chesterfield 1992).

It is understandable that parents want to protect their child from harm and distress. A situation of mutual pretence can arise where both the child and the parent pretend to be unaware of the situation to protect each other (While 1989). However, if the child is to be an integral component of the partnership approach, he or she needs to be armed with the same information and knowledge as the family.

The nurse must accept that honesty can be extremely painful and that sensitivity must be central to this. In certain situations, some parents may still wish to withhold the truth from their dying child in an attempt to protect the child. This can be a difficult situation for the healthcare professional, who must respect the family's right. However, the nurse must inform the family that if the child asks a member of the nursing staff outright, that the nurse will not lie. Swaffield (1985) identified that many of the children whose parents had chosen not to tell them of their impending death were aware of it anyway.

Scenario

John is an 11-year-old boy in the terminal stage of his illness. His parents want him to know the truth about his impending death. They think he probably knows but ask his named nurse to tell him. What would you do if you were that nurse?

Again, it is important to re-iterate that individuality is the key in palliative care. However, the named nurse in this particular situation endeavoured to facilitate and support the parents in their decision. She sat down with John and, holding his hand, asked him if there was anything he wanted to talk about or if there were any questions he wanted to ask. He simply asked 'Can you please make sure I am not in pain?' He did know.

Truth telling and talking to the dying child can cause the nurse to face an ethical dilemma, especially if it contravenes the family's wishes. Other ethical dilemmas in palliative care include feeding and fluids in the child facing death. This can also cause distress for families and raise ethical issues for staff.

PowerPoint

Access the companion PowerPoint presentation and look at the case study.

Lansdown (1994) identifies four key components of effective communication with children about death. It is important that the nurse gives these due attention and consideration:

- The age and cognitive ability of the child are instrumental in the care process and a good knowledge of this is essential when the nurse is managing the care process of the child receiving palliative care.

- The value of appreciating the existing communication system within the family.

- The realisation that effective communication can reduce anxiety.

- The choice of the medium communication most readily used by the child.

Helpful advice when talking to children about death

- Listen carefully to what the child is saying.

- Only answer specific questions posed.

- Avoid long and complicated answers that may confuse the child.

- Let the child set the pace.

- Use simple language.

A wide range of verbal and non-verbal communication strategies can be used when communicating with life-limited children. Touch, play, art and the therapeutic use of story telling are important strategies in palliative care, aiding the child in expressing their concerns, fears and feelings (Done 2001). These strategies are also useful in aiding siblings to express their feelings and are useful media for preparing them for the impending death. Play is widely recognised as the language of the child and as such play is an important communication medium for the child. Play specialists in both the hospital and community have expert training to enable them to fully implement play packages in order to maximise benefit to the child and family (Price and Spence 2004).

 www

Go online to the Jessie's fund (music therapy) website and examine the purpose and value of music therapy in the care of children with life-limiting illness:
- http://www.jessiesfund.org.uk

Music therapy is becoming increasingly used in the care of children with life-limiting illnesses.

Charitable organisations have a role to play in the psychological well-being of children with life-limiting illnesses and their families for example organisations such as Make-a-Wish, Dreams Come True and Dial A Dream. Wishes granted are wide ranging and can give the family happy memories, which can comfort them in dark days.

Families and children can gain much psychological and social support from groups where they meet with other families whose children have the same condition. They also have

 www

Go online to the Make-a-Wish and Starlight Foundation websites and familiarise yourself with the mission statements of the charities and the ways in which they have in the past helped children and families. Read the personal stories of wishes that have been granted:
- http://www.make-a-wish.org.uk
- http://www.starlight.org.uk

experts and counsellors to assist the child and family in developing family and personal coping strategies. Examples of these groups are Contact-a-family, React and other local support groups.

SYMPTOM CONTROL FOR CHILDREN

It is essential to recognise that the symptoms experienced by children are rarely simply physical events. Symptoms should be regarded as more often a complex experience with physical, psychological, social and emotional components (Brady 1996). It must be recognised that assessment regardless of the symptom is an ongoing process, which permits choice and flexibility when circumstances for the child and family change (DoH et al 2000).

Assessment includes extracting and assimilating verbal information. With some children this is not possible, for example, the preverbal child, the unconscious child and the child with special needs. In other children a variety of tools of assessment will be utilised, that is a combination approach using verbal and non-verbal indicators. Families should be welcomed as partners in all stages of the nursing process, parents should feel they have a choice and be in control of the situation (Vickers & Carlisle 2000).

Adequate symptom control is viewed as the ultimate aim of palliative care regardless of the setting in which it is delivered. Symptoms experienced vary depending on the child and specific diagnosis.

 www

Visit the Association for Children with Life-limiting Illness (ACT) website and read the paper entitled 'Guide to the assessment of children with life-limiting conditions' – click on 'publications':
- http://www.act.org.uk

Negotiation with and open lines of communication between the child, family and nurse are essential in achieving optimum symptom control.

The child's stage of development must be central to assessment and management of symptoms. Combinations of pharmacological and non-pharmacological interventions should be utilised.

Parents and other family members should be encouraged to continue involvement in their child's care even as the child's condition deteriorates. Continual assessment of the needs of the parent and their coping is required, as is the necessary support.

The nurse must consider that symptoms that may not be disturbing the child can be very distressing to parents.

Scenario

Carol, an 8-year-old girl, was in the terminal stage of her illness trajectory; she was unconscious, settled and comfortable. Her parents were by her hospital bed and very involved with her care. A few days before her death, Carol developed noisy respirations. This caused her parents great distress and they found it extremely frightening. This symptom was managed by administering a hyoscine patch, which was placed behind Carol's ear. Explanations and reassurance was provided for the parents. The noise was reduced and parental anxiety was eased.

This scenario illustrates the importance of involving the parents, consideration for their needs and recognising that they suffer alongside their child.

Many symptoms are managed by the administration of medication to the child. A number of routes of administration can be used and the chosen route depends on the age, condition of the child and any access devices that the child may have in place.

The oral route is usually first choice for administration of medication in child, many drugs are available in elixir form. The child and family should be involved in decisions about the preferred format.

Intramuscular injections should be avoided in children where possible. Many children at this stage in illness may have a central line in position, which provides a useful alternative route for administration. Some children may have a nasogastric tube in place and this can be utilised successful for administration of medication. Infusions can be given subcutaneously via syringe drivers (McNeilly et al 2004) or via an existing central venous catheter.

Rectal preparations are available for many drugs; they should be avoided in children with low platelet counts and repeated use can cause soreness in children.

The focus of complementary therapies in palliative care is on symptom control. Buckle (2003) discusses the value of aromatherapy and massage in children's palliative care. These techniques can aid in promoting communication with children, reducing anxiety, enhancing relationships and enhancing quality of life in terms of symptom management. Other types of complementary therapies include reflexology, guided imagery and hypnotherapy. These therapies can be used in conjunction with conventional medicine. As with all interventions the child's welfare must be paramount and underpin all care delivered.

The most frequently occurring symptoms experienced by children and interventions are identified in Table 46.1. Other symptoms which a child could experience include bleeding, infection, anorexia, and muscle spasm.

WWW

Refer to Rainbow Children's Hospice guidelines – basic symptom control in paediatric palliative care at
• http://www.rainbows.eazytiger.net/symptom.htm

ACT has a discussion forum which brings together those working within paediatric palliative care both nationally and internationally – this is a very good forum for sharing practice experiences about symptom control and other issues. Information on this is available at http://www.act.org.uk – click on 'networking' and then 'Paedpalcare'.

SPIRITUAL CARE

Many families have established sources for spiritual support and these will continue during the palliative phase of the illness. The nurse must ensure that the spiritual needs of the child and family are addressed. Spiritual needs can occur independently of religion needs. Spiritual care should include the uniqueness of the child and family, and should address their needs, values and beliefs. Some families who have previously had little or no religious faith or belief may wish to have contact with a minister as they face the death of their child. The child him- or herself might want to discuss ideas, views and fears from a spiritual stance. Some adolescents may wish to talk, discuss and plan the arrangements for their funeral with the minister before their death. If this is their wish, it is important that they are given the opportunity to do so. Anger 'against God' can be common in some parents whose child is dying – the minister may be a channel by which they can vent their anger and a professional who may help and facilitate them working through their feelings and emotions.

For some families, to have their child baptised may be important at this time and should be facilitated. Children and families should be given the opportunity, time and privacy to perform any religious acts that may provide them comfort, for example lighting a candle (obviously safety must be paramount).

We are now living in a very wide and diverse cultural society. It is essential that all members of the multidisciplinary team caring for the child recognise the individuality of each child and family and recognise, respect and accept any specific beliefs of rituals surrounding death and beliefs of death.

THE SOCIAL NEEDS OF THE CHILD AND FAMILY

Caring for a child with a life-limiting illness has emotional, psychological and social effects on the child and family.

Financial burdens can grip families who have care for a child with life-limiting illnesses. The child's illness could necessitate one or both parents giving up work to care for the child. Families may be unaware of the help they are entitled to, which can include income support, care allowances and travel and other grants. A social worker will be able to advise, direct and assist the family in this area. Voluntary agencies may also provide help assistance with household chores. For example, CLIC Sargent Cancer Care for children Northern Ireland provides a family support service whereby volunteers help with ironing, cleaning, etc. to allow the parents to spend more time with the sick child and siblings.

Other organisations may be able to offer holidays for the complete family unit in purpose-built facilities. The multi-disciplinary team should work together in ensuring that the family is aware of the availability of services and their entitlement.

The child's education is an important part of maintaining a quality life for the child with a life-limiting illness. Its importance is twofold. First, education is an essential way of the child continuing to develop to his or her potential. Second, it allows continuing integration with peers. As the child's condition changes, his or her educational needs will need to be re-assessed to see how best they can be addressed. Hospitals and hospices have teachers as part of the multidisciplinary team and home tutors can also be available if the child is unable to attend his or her own school (DoH 2004).

Table 46.1 Symptom Management in Children's Palliative Care

Symptom	Possible causes/ exploration	Pharmacological management	Non-pharmacological management	Comments/ special notes
Pain Pain is most feared by parents whose child is approaching death (Goldman 1998) grow and develop	Pain is multifaceted made up of physiological, emotional, spiritual and social aspects, each of these elements require consideration, as does the fact that the child continues to	Analgesia should be selected for the type of pain being experienced Keep analgesia simple initially and gradually progress as necessitated by the specific need of the child. (See WHO pain ladder on Evolve website) A variety of routes can be used oral, rectal, subcutaneous or IV infusion. The IM route should be avoided in children as this can cause much distress and psychological trauma	These include guided imagery, relaxation, distraction therapy and positioning of the child Careful explanations and parental presence may have a positive affect in reducing fear and anxiety and thus may reduce the intensity of the pain experienced	Assessing and managing total pain is a priority when caring for the child and family Refer to pain assessment chapter (Chapter 17) Pain diaries can be very useful for parents and healthcare professionals
Nausea and vomiting	Can be as a result of constipation, raised intracranial pressure (ICP) (Brady 1994), and anorexia or as a side effect of opioid therapy	A wide range of antiemetics are available. Antiemetics act on different sites so it is essential to recognise the potential cause of the nausea and vomiting in order that the correct antiemetic is selected. First-line antiemetics are classed as maxalon, haloperidol and cyclizine (Twycross and Back 2004). If vomiting and nausea are not resolved combinations that work on different sites can be used in combination effectively. Dexamethasone can be added to first line to enhance efficacy	Avoid strong odours Increase oral intake Offer small amounts of food Good oral hygiene Distraction techniques including play	These drugs can be given orally often in elixir or tablet form Certain antiemetics come in melt form that can provide a useful alternative for children If the oral route is not suitable for a particular child, then rectal or subcutaneous routes can be used Many antiemetic drugs are compatible with opiates and can be added to syringe drivers and administered with analgesia

Table 46.1 Symptom Management in Children's Palliative Care—cont'd

Symptom	Possible causes/ exploration	Pharmacological management	Non-pharmacological management	Comments/ special notes
Respiratory symptoms: including cough, dyspnoea, congestion, respiratory distress, grunting	The cause of the respiratory symptom and the severity of the problem is dependent on the nature of the underlying disease. Children with neurodegenerative disease and cystic fibrosis are most likely to experience problems related to the respiratory system in the terminal stage of illness	Diazepam to reduce the anxiety associated with breathlessness, simple linctus for an irritating cough and hyoscine can be used successfully for the management of excessive secretions. Laboured respiration and grunting may occur in the latter stages of illness when death is imminent, the child is normally in a deep unconscious state. Parents require explanation and reassurance during this stage. Rectal diazepam may alleviate this. Oxygen therapy and nebulised bronchodilators may be useful. Morphine can assist in easing dyspnoea	Appropriate positioning of the child may also ease this symptom propping the child upright to permit optimal lung expansion. The physiotherapist may be of assistance and some gentle physiotherapy may help loosen secretions. Oral-pharyngeal suctioning as needed. Use a fan to circulate air. Use relaxation and deep breathing exercises. Keep the room well ventilated	Breathlessness can be increased by anxiety. Anxiety can exacerbate the physical symptoms. Anxiety of parents clearly affects the worries of the child (Rodin 1983)
Constipation	Constipation can result due to inactivity, dehydration, an obstruction (e.g. tumour involvement), nerve involvement or as a side affect of medication (e.g. opiates)	Where possible, the aim of treatment should be to avoid it in the first place. If the child does develop constipation a variety of laxatives can be selected. Oral aperients should be used in the first instance and hopefully if they are successful the use of rectal treatments can be avoided	Encourage fluid intake. Encourage increased activity if appropriate given child's condition. Enlist the help and support of the family who will be able to give information to the nurse about the child's normal bowel movements. Provide privacy and maintain dignity during defecation	A laxative should be prescribed and administered at the commencement of opiate therapy
Symptoms of central nervous system (fits, agitation, twitching and restlessness)	Children with neurodegenerative conditions or brain tumour may suffer seizures. Twitching and agitation may be caused by electrolyte imbalance, hypoxia and opiates. Altered sleep pattern and depression can also lead to agitation	Rectal diazepam is particularly useful and effective for children having a fit. Midazolam can be added into the syringe driver to address the agitation, which can be experienced in the late terminal stages of life in children	Non-pharmacological interventions for agitation should include calm, reassuring, open communication to the child and the use of relaxation, guided imagery or massage	If the child who is prone to a fit is being cared for at home the families should have a supply of diazepam and be taught how to administer them. The family should also be taught seizure management strategies to maintain their child's safety

Continued

Table 46.1 Symptom Management in Children's Palliative Care—cont'd

Symptom	Possible causes/ exploration	Pharmacological management	Non-pharmacological management	Comments/ special notes
Skin problems/ pruritus	Children who are facing death are prone to this as a result of a decrease in oral intake and medication such as opiates Children who have biliary, renal or hepatic disease would also be prone to this skin irritation Children who have been on or are on steroids may be predisposed to skin problems, as their skin can be thinned and papery in appearance Skin breakdown can occur as a result of reduced mobility and also due to a decrease in the child's nutritional intake	Skin care products can manage skin irritation and Piriton administered orally or intravenously may help ease discomfort	Avoid harsh soaps, which may dry the skin Avoid the use of highly perfumed bath/shower products and moisturising products Keep fingernails short and discourage scratching Keep the child cool and dress child in cotton clothing	Dry skin and pruritus are more common in children than breakdown of skin areas Regular assessment of a child's skin condition should be carried out to establish if any change has taken place Regular and accurate assessment of the child's skin integrity should be carried out and recorded. The parents or main caregivers should be educated as to how to carry this out Mobility should be encouraged as the child's condition dictates. If the child is confined to bed then their position should be changed 2-hourly. Air mattresses can be obtained by nursing staff (either hospital or community)

Adapted from Rainbow Childrens Hospice Guidelines (2005) and Goldman (1998)

RESPITE CARE

Respite care is an instrumental part of palliative care for children and young people. Caring for a child with a life-limiting illness is both physically and emotionally draining for the family (Maguire 2001). The care may involve 24-hour devotion of the parent to the sick child. It is essential that the family is offered some time away for the physical and emotional exhaustion that the tasks of caring can cause. Parents and families willingly undertake very complex care at home when their child has a life-limiting illness. Their ability to cope will decrease and their level of stress will increase unless they receive regular respite care. Judd (1994 p 218) defines respite care as:

Complementary, flexible care in the home or home from home setting with appropriate medical and nursing support, offering parents or carers an interval of relief.

As with all other aspects of palliative care for children and families, the need and type of respite care required needs to be tailored to the individual family. Several types of respite provision can be offered:

- Planned respite care in the child's own home: this involves children's community nurses, trained care assistants or nursery nurses who carry out the care normally undertaken by the family in the child's own environment.

- Planned respite care in the home of another family: this type of respite is usually only appropriate when the care of the child is not usually medically complex. Some families will accept more complex children with appropriate training.

- Respite care in a residential setting: for those children and families who meet the criteria set by children's hospices one or two weeks respite can be offered. The whole family may take a break together in purpose-built, family-centred environments where the siblings can receive special care and attention. Other residential settings may be available through social services or voluntary organisations.

The range or respite provision offered is limited in certain parts of the UK (Thurgate 2005) however with an increase in the profile of the needs of children with life-limiting illness, and their families, new services continue to be developed in an attempt to meet the increasing demand.

Care of the Child Following Death

The need for parental support and advice is never greater than at the time when the death occurs. Even if the death has been expected, the parents' reactions at the time of death are unpredictable. Parents who have just lost their child will usually require guidance from the healthcare professional. The professional must therefore be aware of the relevant issues and be knowledgeable and informed about the options facing the family at this sad time.

- Time and privacy should be given to parents when decisions have to be made.
- Families should be able to stay with their child for as long as they wish and be encouraged to hold, cuddle, wash and dress their child if desired.
- Families should be prepared for how the child's appearance will change after death and the possible noises the body may make.
- Cultural and religious beliefs and practices should be adhered to.
- Families should be given the opportunity to talk through procedure and not merely given the written information.
- Written booklets are useful to back up verbal information and guide parents to further support networks (Davey 1995).
- The family might want a handprint or lock of hair to keep – consent should be obtained from the family.
- Families should be given time to spend with their child; this may include siblings. They should never feel rushed or hurried.
- Parents should be informed of their choices regarding taking their child home following a planned death in hospice or hospital (Whittle & Cutts 2002).

Bereavement Care

The death of a child is a uniquely traumatic experience for a parent (Rando 1985, Brewis 1995). The grieving process following such a loss is complex and multifaceted. The def-

inition of palliative care cited at the outset of this chapter includes bereavement support as one of the essential components that comes under the umbrella of palliative care. This section therefore examines the needs of a family following the death of their child and the nurse's role in bereavement care.

Activity

Consider the factors that may affect an individual's grief.

At this stage it seems appropriate to clarify the terms that are commonly used here. Hindmarch (1994) suggests that:

- bereavement is what happens
- grief is what one feels in reaction to the bereavement
- mourning is what one does to express grief.

The devastation caused by a child's death is far reaching, affecting parents, siblings, grandparents, wider family circles, healthcare professionals and communities. Rando (1986) identifies that the loss of a child to a parent can seem like a physical loss that is that they have lost a part of themselves, the loss of their role, loss of hopes, dreams and their identity as protector. Klass (1988) identifies two central features of parental grief following the death of their child. First, is that it represents to the parent a loss of self and, second, that is represents a loss of competence. Barbara Schatz (1986) maintains that as a bereaved mother not only did she lose part of herself but also the family unit because it was had irrevocably changed. She also highlighted that a mother of an only child loses her role as a mother. Schatz also identifies that bereaved mothers experience sensory deprivation. She believes that learning to live without one's child is a life-long task for a mother:

> At each milestone in her own life and that of her family she is cognizant of the fact that one of her children is missing. A part of each bereaved mother grieves for ever (Schatz 1986 p 309)

Worden (1991) describes the process of mourning as a series of tasks linked to stages. He identified four stages with inherent tasks, which the mourner must work through to resolve one's grief:

- to accept the reality of loss
- to work through the pain of grief
- to adjust to an environment in which the deceased is missing
- to emotionally relocate the deceased and move on with life (the task of resolution).

However, this staged approach can be seen as providing a very rigid approach to grief work, although it does permit individuality, moving in and out of different stages and overall provides a very prescriptive framework. Goldman (1998) states that the progress through phases of grief is not straightforward or only in one direction.

Barbara Schatz (1986) raises the issues with the theory that indicates a stage of acceptance or resolution. She claims that a bereaved mother may never reach this stage and may never finish grieving:

I will live the rest of my life without one of my children. I will think of that child during the sad times in my life and wish they could be with me in the hard (Schatz 1986 p 313)

It is important to recognise that Worden's grief work does not necessarily state that the stages are experienced sequentially or that any time limit can be applied. Uniformity is not part of the grieving process. There are no rules in grief and both parents are likely to respond in different ways.

Evidence-based Practice

Feely & Gottlieb (1988) identified that mothers' response to grief was characterised by more despair, anger, isolation, guilt and depersonalisation than fathers' grieving. The study also identified that mothers were more likely to discuss their feelings with other people, unlike fathers, who are more likely to keep busy, take on more work and enlist in outside activities. This leads to the conclusion that mothers express their grief in terms of feelings and fathers are more inclined to intellectualise their grief.

It is essential, however, not to stereotype the results to the grief of all mothers and fathers.

Activity

Consider some roles that may negatively affect fathers when dealing with their grief. Check below.

William Schatz (1986) identified the following male roles as negatively affecting the way he dealt with his grief following the death of his son:

- The role of being strong, a macho man always in control of his emotions.
- The role of competing and winning in a crisis and being the best.
- The role of being protector of family and possessions.

- The role of being the family provider.
- The role of being problem solver, fixing things or finding someone who can.
- The role of controller.
- The role of self-sufficient standing on his own two feet.

The nurse who is coordinating the bereavement care of a family should be aware of these issues and patterns of grief.

Siblings require particular attention during the period leading up to the death of the child as mentioned earlier and following the death through bereavement. Following the death, even though it may have been expected is a time of great turmoil, interruption and uncertainty for the siblings. The age and cognitive development will obviously affect their understanding. Children have very definite needs in bereavement. They require information, reassurance, time to express their feelings and the need to be involved (Brown 2002). Children need also to have some type of routine maintained, this coupled with support from the adults around them, may be difficult as the parents are struggling to deal with their own loss and feelings. Parents may need help from the healthcare professional in coordinating the bereavement care to gain an insight into patterns of childhood grief and suggestions as to how the child may be helped through the process.

Fox (1988) has outlined four tasks for grieving children:

- To understand or begin to make sense out of what is happening.
- To grieve and express emotional responses to loss.
- To commemorate in some formal or informal way the life of the person who has died.
- To learn how to integrate the loss into one's life to continue with everyday activities of living and loving.

Children can be helped in bereavement by having a momento of the person who has died. This way the child is provided with a tangible reminder of the person who is gone, is reminded of their existence and reassured that life does go on. This could be a favourite toy, photograph, another item of value to the child who has died or even a selection of items in a designated memory box. A number of resources are available to help children experience a healthy grieving process (see the list of books available for children on the companion PowerPoint presentation).

Parents are often anxious about siblings attending the funeral. On one hand, they want to protect them and on the other the parent may feel unable to cope with their own feelings and the feelings of the child. Children should be involved in discussions about this, should be given information beforehand about what they should expect at the service and their wishes and opinions should be listened to. If they do wish to attend, it may be appropriate for another adult to be assigned to look after them during the service (Black 1998). If they do not attend they should be told as soon afterwards what happened and be given the chance to visit the grave.

It can be very helpful if children are involved in bereavement support groups, which enable the child to work through their grief and to see that they are not alone. Many children's hospices run groups such as these. With support and guidance from family and professionals, the child will learn to adapt to their loss and live their own life.

www

Visit the Winston's Wish website and investigate ways in which this organisation helps support bereaved children.
• http://www.winstonswish.org.uk

It is also important to remember the extended family circle and community that may be affected by the death of the child. Grandparents not only lose their grandchild but also have the added burden of 'losing' their own child who is consumed with grief. Many grandparents may experience 'survivor guilt' and could ask 'Why am I still living when my grandchild is dead?'

The wider community is also affected by the death of a child and it is important that the healthcare professional coordinating the bereavement follow-up ensures that contact is made with the child's school. Teachers may feel uncertain how to support the other pupils and staff at this time and usually welcome advice at how to manage the grief and commemorate the child who has died.

The bereavement component of the palliative care may be coordinated and provided by a community children's nurse, Macmillan nurse, hospice nurse or other identified healthcare professional. The individual family should dictate the frequency of visits and type of support required. Contact may well decrease as the family develops coping strategies. The nurse may have to refer a parent to a psychologist or bereavement counsellor if they feel that the individual concerned needs further specialist bereavement support (Dunne 2004). Many hospitals and hospices hold annual remembrance services, which are important to families. Other ways organisations can assist with remembering the child are inclusion in the book of remembrance and sending cards and flowers on specials dates, for example the first anniversary of the child's death.

THE NEEDS OF THE HEALTHCARE WORKER

Care of dying children is undoubtedly stressful for all those involved in the care package. It may be that the nurse has developed a close therapeutic relationship with the child and his or her family over – in some situations – a lengthy period of time.

The death of a child may lead to extreme guilt, anger, sadness and perhaps the feeling that the healthcare worker has failed the child and family. Avoiding burn-out requires careful self-stress management strategies and awareness of the needs of others in the team. All members of the team must be remembered: porters, domestic assistants and student nurses also can develop a bond with the child and family and can sometimes be overlooked when a death occurs. It is important to remember that you may be a healthcare professional but that also you are a human being with real feelings and emotions. It is essential to recognise our feelings and pain at a loss and deal with this. An 'ostrich approach' is dangerous and ignoring one's own needs can have a detrimental effect in the long term. Organisations such as Child Bereavement Trust offer support and training for healthcare workers in this area.

Evidence-based practice

Costello & Trinder-Brook (2000) carried out a study examining the experiences of 44 children's nurses who cared for dying children in hospital. Positive experiences highlighted by nurses included being able to give support to grieving parents, feeling they could give the child individual attention, controlling pain and other symptoms as well as providing follow-up care after death. Negative experiences that came out of the study included poor staffing and skill mix, sudden death, emotional attachment to the child and involvement with the family. The study indicated that the death of the child in hospital has a major impact on the nurse and also highlights the importance of preparing nurses for the emotional impact that the death of a child will have.

Activity

List some organizations that help bereaved families (a full list of names of these and contact details are found on the companion PowerPoint presentation).

Reflect on your Practice

Reflect on ways that you have seen or consider may be useful strategies for staff coping with death of a child.

HELPFUL TIPS FOR ADDRESSING NEEDS OF THE HEALTHCARE PROFESSIONAL AFTER THE DEATH OF A CHILD

- Nurses should be informed of the death of a child even when they are off duty.
- Regular support group meetings and clinical supervision may be beneficial for staff caring for dying children.
- An open secure environment where feelings can be discussed and shared.
- Regular social activities and nights out for the team.
- Services of psychologist if required.
- Flexibility and understanding for other team members: it may be important for some to attend the funeral to say their final goodbye. This should be facilitated when possible.
- Individual strategies: listening to music, sports activities and retail therapy may help.

Summary

Palliative care is multifaceted and addresses holistic care needs at different stages of the illness trajectory.

Quality palliative care for the child or young person requires a cohesive partnership approach, centred on the family with a collaborative multidisciplinary focus to care. Nurses play a key role in the team approach and are required to identify and address the needs, fears and anxieties of the child and whole family circle with good communication being fundamental.

KEY POINTS

- Palliative care for children can be delivered in a variety of care settings and has developed as a distinct speciality.
- The child and family should be central to decisions about the care delivered.
- The multidisciplinary team should address holistic needs of the child.
- Honest and simple responses are important in communicating to children about death.
- Parents and siblings need much support and information as death approaches.
- It is important to remember that for a parent who has lost a child bereavement is a long, complicated and very individual process.
- Nurses need to recognise that caring for children and families facing death is extremely stressful. They should be aware of the importance of developing their own personal management strategies.

Acknowledgements

Thanks go to: Patricia McNeilly, Teaching Fellow, Queen's University, Belfast; David Thomas, Paediatric Oncology Outreach Nurse, Leeds; the staff of Horizon House (Children's Hospice), Northern Ireland; the Paediatric Macmillan Team, Royal Belfast Hospital for Sick Children; Staff Nurse Paul Carlin, Children's Haematology Unit, Royal Belfast Hospital for Sick Children.

References

Armstrong-Dailey A 1990 Children's hospice care. Pediatric Nursing 16(4):337–339

Association for children with a life-threatening illness (ACT) 2003 Assessment of children with life-limiting conditions and their families – a guide to effective care planning. ACT, London

Association for children with a life-threatening illness (ACT) and Royal College of Paediatrics and Child Health (RCPCH) 2003 Guide to development of paediatric palliative care services, 2nd edn. ACT/RCPCH, London

Association for children with life-threatening illness (ACT) 2004 Integrated multi-agency care pathways for children with life-limiting conditions. ACT, London

Black D 1998 Bereavement in childhood. British Medical Journal 316:931–933

Brady M 1994 Treatment of common symptoms in paediatric care. CME Bulletin, Palliative Medicine 1(3):63–68

Bluebond-Laugner M 1992 Children and death – directions for the 90s. New Jersey University Press, New Jersey

Brady M 1996 Symptom control in dying children. In: Hill L 1996 Caring for dying children and families. Chapman Hall, London.

Brewis E 1995 Issues in bereavement – there are no rules. Paediatric Nursing 7(9):337–339

Brown E 2002 (ed.) The death of a child: care for the child, support for the family. Acorns childrens Hospice Trust, Biruvaghaur

Buckle S 2003 Aromatherapy and massage – the evidence. Paediatric Nursing 15(6):24–27

Chesterfield P 1992 Communicating with dying children. Nursing Standard 6(20):30–32

Costello J, Trinder-Booker A 2000 Children's nurses' experiences of caring for dying children in hospital. Paediatric Nursing 12(6):28–32

Davey N 1995 Paediatric bereavement care. Paediatric Nursing 7(9):24

Davies C 1997 When a baby dies. Nursing Times 93(8):28–29

Department of Health (DoH) et al 2000 Framework for the assessment of children in need and their families. The Stationery Office, London

Department of Health (DoH) 2004 National service framework for children, young people and maternity services. Ill child (standard 6). The Stationery Office, London.

Done A 2001 The therapeutic use of story telling. Paediatric Nursing 13(3):17–20

Dunne K 2004 Grief and its manifestations. Nursing Standard 18(45):45–51

Farrell M 1996 The role of a children's hospice. Paediatric Nursing 8(4):6–8

Feeley N, Gottlieb LN 1988 Parents coping and communication following their infant's death. Omega 19(1):51–67

Fox SS 1988 Good grief: helping groups of children when a friend dies. Cited in: Langton H (ed.) 2000 The child with cancer – family centred care. Baillière Tindall, London

Gardner G 1977 The rights of dying children: some personal reflections. Psychotherapy Bulletin 10:20–23

Goldman A (ed.) 1998 Care of the dying child. Oxford University Press, Oxford

Hill L 1996 Caring for dying children and families. Chapman Hall, London

Hinchmarch C 1994 On the death of a child. Radcliffe Medical Press, Oxford

Hynson JL Sawyer SM 2001 Paediatric palliative care: distinctive needs and emerging issues. Journal of Paediatric Child Health 37:323–325

Judd D 1994 Give sorrow words – working with a dying child, 2nd edn. Whurr Publishers, London

Klass D 1988 Parental grief, solace and resolution. Springer, New York

Kubler-Ross E 1970 On death and dying, Tavistock Press, London

Landsdown R 1994 Communication with children. In: Goldman A (ed.) Care of the dying child. Oxford University Press, Oxford

Maguire H 2001 Developing a hospice service in Northern Ireland. Paediatric Nursing 13(8):19–21

McNeilly P Price J McCloskey S 2004 The use of syringe drivers: a paediatric perspective. International Journal of Palliative Nursing 10(8):399–402

Price J Spence N (2004) Play in the community–quality care for the child with cancer. Cancer Nursing Practice 3(8):31–34

Price J McNeilly P McFarlane M 2005 Paediatric palliative care in the UK: past, present and future. International Journal of Palliative Nursing 11(3):124–126

Rainbow Children's Hospice 2005 Guidelines – basic symptom control. Online. Available at: http://www.rainbows.carytiger.net/symptom.htm

Rando AT (ed.) 1986 Parental loss of a child. Research Press, Illinois

Royal College of Nursing (RCN) 1999 Supporting parents when they are told of their child's health disorder or disability: guidance for nurses, midwives and health visitors. RCN, London

Schatz BD 1986 Grief of mothers. In: Rando AT (ed.) Parental loss of a child. Research Press, Illinois

Schatz WH 1986 Grief of fathers. In: Rando AT (ed.) Parental loss of a child. Research Press, Illinois

Swaffield F 1985 Protecting the parents? Nursing Times 31:51–52

Thurgate C 2005 Respite for children with complex health needs: issues from the literature. Paediatric Nursing 17(3):14–18

Twycross R, Back I 1998 Nausea and vomiting in advanced cancer. European Journal of Palliative Care 5(2):39–45

Vickers J, Carlisle C 2000 choices and control: parental experiences in pediatric terminal home care. Journal of Pediatric Oncology Nursing 17(1):12–20

While A 1989 The needs of dying children and their family. Health Visitor 62:176–78

Whittle M, Cutts S 2002 Time to go home: assisting families to take their child home following a planned hospital or hospice death. Paediatric Nursing 14(10):24–28

Worden JW 1991 Grief counselling and grief therapy. Tavistock Press, London

Worswick J 2000 A house called Helen – the development of hospice care for children. Oxford University Press, Oxford

Useful Websites

http://www.act.org.uk – the Association for Children with Life-threatening conditions and their families

http://www.hospice-spc-council.org.uk

http://www.make-a-wish.org.uk – Make-a-wish organisation

http://www.ach.org.uk – Association of Children's Hospices

http://www.chionline.org – Children's Hospice International

http://www.jessicsfund.org.uk – Jessie's Fund (music therapy)

http://www.calamily.org.uk – Contact a family

http://www.dial-a-dream.co.uk – Dial a Dream

http://www.reactcharity.org

Chapter Forty Seven

47

Children with Learning Disabilities

Victoria Jones, Ruth Northway

ABSTRACT

In nursing, more than one-third of all the people we come into contact with are disabled in some way (Disability Rights Commission and Department of Health (DoH) 2004). People experience disability in many different ways, one of which is in the form of the intellectual impairment that is currently termed 'learning disability'. In virtually all areas of children's nursing there will be children and young people who have been labelled as having a learning disability. They may have additional health needs and require the support of a range of professionals and different agencies. Parents and other family members also require this support and it is important that it is provided in a coordinated manner.

Learning Outcomes

- Understand the importance of considering the child before their impairment.

- Define 'learning disability' and identify the factors that can give rise to learning disabilities.

- Understand the ways in which the presence of a learning disability can impact on the lives of children and their families.

- Appreciate the role of the nurse in supporting children with learning disabilities and their families in the context of an interprofessional and interagency approach to care.

Introduction

It is essential that children with learning disabilities are regarded as children first and that their needs are met as well as those of the rest of the family. Their needs are the same as for any other child but in addition their special needs must also be addressed (Lindsay 1998 p 51)

This quote makes some very important points, which form the basis of this chapter. First, it stresses that children with learning disabilities are children first. Second, it recognises that they have additional needs and that their families may have additional needs. This chapter will, therefore, focus on identifying some of these additional needs and suggest some ways in which children's nurses can work together with the child, his or her family, and other professionals to ensure that these needs are both recognised and met.

It is also important to say that this chapter is written from the perspective of a social model of disability. In the past, society (which includes nurses and other members of the healthcare professions) tended to view disability and disabled people in terms of a medical or individual model of disability. This approach has meant that disabled people were viewed as not being able to do things because of their disability. In contrast, the social model of disability argues that whereas some people may have certain impairments (such as a visual, mobility or intellectual impairment) what actually prevents them from taking a full role in society is a range of physical, social, psychological and economic barriers. In other words, it is these barriers that disable them. This different view of disability has important implications for the way in which we respond to the needs of disabled people (Northway 1997). This chapter will therefore consider both the nature of the impairment that children and young people with learning disabilities are assessed as having as well as the barriers that they and their families may face. The emphasis when considering the nature of professional support should thus be on the identification and (where possible) removal of these barriers.

A final point, which it is important to stress, is that children and young people with learning disabilities, and their families/carers, are not a homogenous group. For example, their social circumstances, personal resources, cultural background and environmental circumstances will vary. In addition, the area in which they live may determine the support services available to meet their needs. This means that we must be wary of generalising and should seek to understand the particular circumstances of each child and his or her family.

The Nature of 'Learning Disabilities'

TERMINOLOGY AND LABELLING

Activity

- Write a list of all the words you have heard being used to refer to someone who has a learning disability. Try to put them into two columns – positive terms and negative terms as we perceive them today.
- Which ones have been used in legislation?
- Make a list of terms you are not sure about. Try to investigate them.

Some groups of people who have been given the label 'learning disabilities' have indicated that, if they must have a label at all, 'people with learning difficulties' is the most acceptable term for others to use for them. They emphasise that people with learning difficulties are people first and intellectually impaired second. Recent guidance from the government (Department of Health 2001) reinforces this distinction but uses the term 'learning disability' to refer to the same group of people. The government goes on to reject the term 'learning difficulty' because it is used in legislation to refer to a group of people with a wider range of educational needs. The term 'learning disability' is thus the current term that is used to refer to individuals and groups of people who would previously have been referred to as having a 'mental handicap' or being 'mentally subnormal'. Such terms are no longer used because they are viewed as having negative connotations.

The term 'learning disability' is a label applied to individuals and groups for many different reasons (e.g. to organise service provision, define a condition, or explain a delay in achieving developmental milestones). Throughout history, people who currently are labelled as having learning disabilities have had many labels applied to them. These tend to reflect the overarching social and economic climate of the day, dominant theoretical perspectives and the lan-

guage incorporated into the law of the time (Gates & Wilberforce 2003). For example, the 1983 Mental Health Act replaced the term 'subnormal' with the terms 'mental impairment' and 'severe mental impairment'. Both the Act and these terms are still in use today in legal situations. To understand the nature of learning disability we therefore have to take account of the social and historical context. Different theoretical perspectives have been used to try to understand and explain the nature of learning disabilities. These include sociological, psychological, medical and anthropological perspectives (Gates & Wilberforce 2003).

Activity

- Make a list of some of the ways that being labelled as 'learning disabled' could be helpful. Then make a list of some of the ways having a label could be detrimental. It may help to think about how we label other people and things.
- Consider how, in your role as a nurse, you can make best use of labels and terminology for all your clients whilst avoiding some of the negative impacts associated with being labelled.

Being labelled as having a learning disability can have negative consequences due to prevailing social attitudes. Others can view the person with a learning disability as being different and difference in this context is viewed negatively. They can have low expectations of people with learning disabilities and stereotype them as having a range of negative characteristics. This then has an impact on the life experiences of the person to whom the label is applied. For example, if they are viewed as not being able to learn they will not be provided with educational opportunities and, because they have not been given the chance to learn, their educational development will be delayed. The original view of others (that the person cannot learn) is thus reinforced. Social attitudes thus become one of the barriers that disable people who have impairments.

Having a label or a diagnosis can, however, also bring some benefits. For example, unless you are assessed as having a particular condition or need you may be unable to access certain services and support mechanisms. An example of this might be access to additional educational support in the classroom, which can only be accessed after assessment and diagnosis as having a learning disability.

Labels and diagnoses can also be seen to be of benefit to service planners and service providers. Epidemiological and demographic studies (which rely upon the identification, collation and quantification of certain characteristics) are used as a basis upon which to decide priorities for service development. Similarly, criteria are often applied by services to decide who should (and who should not) be able to access their service. They may thus serve as criteria for rationing of limited resources.

Formal criteria have been developed to 'identify' people who fit into the group of people labelled as having learning disabilities. These can be grouped under cognitive, social functioning and developmental approaches.

COGNITIVE FUNCTIONING APPROACH

Despite there being a lot of disagreement about exactly what intelligence is, and whether we can establish fair and equal ways to measure it, intelligence has been used as a factor to determine if someone has a learning disability since the early 1900s (see Gross (1991) for a critical discussion).

The intelligence quotient (IQ) is a standardised figure that makes it possible to compare how an individual performs against other people in the population when taking a test of their cognitive ability. IQ is worked out using the following formula:

$$\frac{\text{Mental age (test result)}}{\text{Chronological age (actual age)}} \times 100 = IQ$$

The World Health Organization (WHO 1993) refers to IQ measurements to distinguish the degree of impairment experienced by people with learning disabilities. In this way a child's learning disability may be described as being:

- mild
- moderate
- severe
- profound.

SOCIAL FUNCTIONING APPROACH

This refers to the ability of an individual to adapt to the demands made by society and to hold roles in their community. For example, the ability of a child to meet his or her social needs in a classroom setting (communication, self-help, independence and relationships.) However, measuring the degree of social functioning of an individual is difficult. If we refer back to the social model of disability it can be seen that the extent to which the child can function is going to be influenced by the degree to which appropriate supports are in place. For example, how many of us would find that our social functioning was impaired if we were unable to wear one form of support, namely our glasses or contact lenses? Similarly, a child may have some degree of intellectual impairment but his or her ability to be independent in a classroom setting may depend on the extent to which picture symbols are used to indicate where key facilities (such as the toilet) are. Additionally, many

people who might have an element of impaired social functioning might not have a learning disability; some may also have physical or mental health needs that impair their social functioning. It is also important to take account of the age of the child and what would normally be expected in terms of their social development.

Reflect on your Practice

Think about the situation of children with learning disabilities in the context of a children's ward in which you have worked. How could their social functioning have been improved in this context?

THE DEVELOPMENTAL APPROACH

The WHO (1993) refers to social functioning/ability in its current definition of learning disability, but also introduces a further element, namely the period during which the impairment occurred:

Learning disability is a state of arrested or incomplete development of mind, which is especially characterised by impairment of skills manifested during the developmental period . . . (WHO 1993)

This distinguishes a learning disability from other forms of impairment of social and cognitive functioning that may arise later in life, such as those that result from brain injury or dementia.

COMBINING APPROACHES

What tends to happen is that the cognitive, social and developmental approaches are combined when seeking to provide a definition of learning disabilities and when seeking to determine whether an individual has learning disabilities or not. This can be seen in the current definition used by the DoH (2001 p 14) in the White Paper *Valuing people*, which states:

Learning disability includes the presence of:
– a significantly reduced ability to understand new or complex information, to learn new skills (impaired intelligence), with;
– a reduced ability to cope independently (impaired social functioning);
– which started before adulthood, with a lasting effect on development.

Factors that can Give Rise to the Presence of a Learning Disability

A learning disability can result from a single causative factor or from multiple interacting factors. Of all people who are labelled as having a learning disability it is often only possible to identify the specific causative factor for less than half. This figure, however, has increased in recent years due to advances in genetics.

Watson (1993) identifies four stages at which learning disabilities may occur. These are preconceptual, prenatal, perinatal (the first 28 days of life), and postnatal (28 days onwards). At each stage factors relating to heredity and the environment can exert an influence. Some causative factors are:

- Preconceptual: this might include the fact that genetic characteristics of the parents may give rise to an increased risk that the child will inherit a particular condition. In addition, the health of the mother may give rise to increased risks.

- Prenatal: this might include, for example chromosomal anomalies, genetic disorders, infection, irradiation, immunological and toxicological damage, maternal malnutrition.

- Perinatal: this might include, for example, difficult or abnormal labour, birth injury, prematurity and gestational disorders.

- Postnatal: this might include, for example, malnutrition of the child, sensory and social deprivation, blood chemistry imbalances, infection, ingestion of toxins and cerebral trauma.

Although it may be possible to identify key factors to explain the presence of a learning disability in some children it is often difficult to try and relate their level of cognitive or social functioning to one cause as it would be impossible to know the many other factors which may have had a chance to influence their performance.

In addition the link between the causative factor and the effects this has on the individual are often unclear. For example, in the case of children who have Down syndrome, the causative factor is known (i.e. trisomy 21) but exactly how this brings about the characteristic features of the syndrome is not so certain. It does, however, tell us that because the child has Down syndrome they are more likely to have certain health conditions such as cardiovascular problems, leukaemia, hypothyroidism and sensory impairments (NHS Health Scotland 2004). That is not to say that all children with Down syndrome will have these problems, but rather that they have an increased risk.

It is therefore unhelpful to apply a 'cause and effect' model that raises the risk of implying or offering a prognosis for a child that may be wholly inaccurate. Indeed, such an approach may even serve to deny children the opportunity to be the individuals that, both genetically and socially, we all are.

www

For information on specific conditions and syndromes, along with details concerning inheritance patterns visit the web site of the organisation Contact a Family:
- http://www. cafamily.org.uk

The Incidence of Learning Disability

The difficulties in determining precisely who might be considered to have a learning disability have been outlined above. Despite these difficulties, however, it is possible to try and identify how many people have a learning disability. For example, the DoH (2001) stated that in England alone about 1.2 million people have a mild learning disability. A further 210,000 people have a severe or profound disability and of these it is thought that approximately 65,000 are children or young people.

The prevalence of moderate and mild learning disability is generally higher among deprived and urban populations. The incidence of severe and profound learning disabilities, however, does not vary across regions or socio-economic groups but the number of people with severe learning disabilities is expected to increase by up to 10% in the next decade (DoH 2001). This is due to:

- Greater life expectancy.
- Increasing numbers of children with complex and multiple disabilities surviving to adulthood.
- A significant rise in the number of children with autistic spectrum disorders.
- A greater incidence in the number of children with profound disabilities born to some families of South Asian heritage.

These last three factors have clear implications for children's nurses with regard to the skills and competencies needed to work effectively with learning disabled children and their families. There will also be implications for those managing and developing services, who will need to ensure they can meet the needs of this expanding population.

The Impact of Learning Disability on the Child and the Family

When considering the impact of learning disability on the child and his or her family, it is important to consider a number of different aspects from initial diagnosis and growing up through to transition to adult services. An understanding of each of these aspects is important if children's nurses are to provide an effective service to children with learning disabilities and their families. In addition it is important to consider the health needs of children with learning disabilities since children's nurses have a key role to play in identifying such needs and in ensuring that they are met. In thinking about the impact of a child with learning disabilities on the family it is important, however, to remember that this impact can be positive and that where difficulties do arise these can often be the result of a lack of support or inappropriate service provision (Maxwell & Barr 2003). As SCOPE notes:

> . . . many of the difficulties that ensue when a child has a disability are largely a result of the way society responds to that fact rather than being an inherent part of the disability itself (SCOPE 1999 p 28)

This is clearly linked to an understanding of disability based on the social model. Barriers that can negatively affect the child with a learning disability and their family thus need to be identified and eliminated.

Activity

- Read the paper written by Maxwell & Barr (2003) for an excellent overview of the experience of one mother of a young person with Down syndrome over the early years of his life. Although this is one mother's account, it clearly highlights a range of issues that are evident in the wider literature.
- When reading the article, try to identify some of the barriers which the child, the mother and the rest of the family have experienced.
- What helped the family and what caused them additional difficulties?

Initial Diagnosis

Receiving the news that your child has a learning disability can be a difficult process. However, it can also be a point from which parents can begin to plan the future (Dobson et al 2001, Maxwell & Barr 2003). Crucial to this process is the manner in which concerns regarding the child's development are shared with the family since problems occur when a carefully considered and planned approach is not taken (SCOPE 1999).

Unfortunately, there are many examples of parents receiving the news in an insensitive and inappropriate manner. In addition, it is not uncommon for parents to express concerns regarding their child only to have them dismissed or not taken seriously by professionals (SCOPE 1999). In its report *Right from the start*, SCOPE (1999) highlights

the very difficult nature of the process and identifies that parents were sometimes told 'too little too late' or 'too much too soon'. As a result of its findings, SCOPE has undertaken a programme of work that seeks to improve this process. In its template for good practice, the key principles are identified as valuing the child and respecting the parents (SCOPE 2003). The key practice framework stresses the need for preparation, who should be present, tuning into the parents, the next steps (practical help and information), as well as the need for support for professionals.

WWW

Read online the work undertaken by the SCOPE 'Right from the start' project. How is information given to parents in your clinical area? Can you see any ways in which it could be improved?

- http://www.rightfromthestart.org.uk

Having received the diagnosis, parents are then faced with the prospect of telling other people. Maxwell & Barr (2003) provide the example of when Virginia Maxwell and her husband were told by other people that their son was 'a gift from God' but that a family member also told them that 'he was from the devil' and that they were being punished for their sin. Such reactions from others give an indication of some of the difficulties that parents will face over and above having to adjust to the diagnosis themselves.

Growing Up

In a study undertaken in 1998, Dobson et al gathered information by the use of questionnaires and diaries with 182 parents of severely disabled children (Dobson et al 2001). They found that the parents of disabled children spent almost twice as much as the parents of non-disabled children, resulting in many families having additional financial concerns. However, the project's original aim – to explore the financial implications of raising a severely disabled child – was expanded when it was recognised that the financial costs constituted only one element of the data that was analysed. The families reported a lack of emotional and practical support in raising their children and referred to a process of 'adjustment' in their family life.

For many families of disabled children, other factors also come into play. The experience of being stared at, being the topic of professional conversations and not feeling like a typical family were themes in Dobson et al's (2001) findings. Many parents felt that their family was viewed as both 'different' and as the victim of a personal tragedy. This denied them the 'emotional and social worth' attributed to most families. They concluded that it is vital that practitioners, services and policy makers make use of the expertise of parents to ensure the appropriate provision of services and efficient use of resources, which will benefit the whole community. Unfortunately, however, the knowledge and experience which parents have concerning their children with learning disabilities is not always valued by others (Maxwell & Barr 2003).

WWW

Read the Dobson et al (2001) report and other Joseph Rowntree Foundation research findings at:
- http://www.jrf.org.uk

Families have highlighted that relevant and accessible information is one of the aspects of services they most value (Sloper & Mitchell 2000). The policy context in health provision emphasises patient involvement in decision making but, despite this, it is an area many parents feel poorly served. *Valuing people* (DoH 2001) thus states that, under the 'Quality protects' programme, children's social services will:

> *. . . provide more and better information for families and increase the availability of key workers and other measures designed to improve coordination (DoH 2001 section 3.5)*

Sloper & Mitchell (2000) worked with families to identify quality criteria for information. They interviewed 27 parents who cared for children with a range of disabilities. They also consulted a group of practitioners working in both health and social care settings. This relatively small number of participants could be a reason to limit the extent to which it is possible to generalise from the findings of the study. However, to try to combat this the research was designed to recruit parents who made use of a range of services and were based in the north of England and practitioners who were selected from the south. They concluded that a three-tiered approach combining directories, in-depth booklets and local information key workers was the ideal way to meet the information needs of families. They also highlighted that quality presentation and clear information about the roles of different agencies were critical considerations in developing information for families of disabled children.

Parental access to information is essential when considering issues such as which school their child should attend. For example, it is current policy that children with learning disabilities should have their educational needs assessed, that educational placement should ensure that these needs are met and that appropriate support mechanisms are in place. Wherever possible, the child should be educated alongside non-disabled peers in mainstream schools. However, some parents feel that their child would not receive appropriate support to meet their additional needs within mainstream schools. Likewise, there are others who, faced with the offer of an educational placement within a special school, argue their child's right to placement in mainstream education and stress the responsibility of the Local Education Authority to provide such a placement along with any additional support required.

Provision of information concerning the options available and the mechanisms in place to challenge decisions that they are not happy with is crucial to parents in such situations. For further information concerning educational provision for children with a learning disability and for information concerning the debates surrounding integrated and segregated education, see Dickinson & Dickinson (2003).

It is important to remember that the presence of a child with learning disabilities within the family has an impact not only on the parents but also on siblings. Some work has

Seminar discussion topic

Examine the arguments for and against inclusive education. What are the philosophies that underpin these approaches?

been undertaken with siblings (see, for example, Burke & Montgomery 2000, Evans et al 2001).

Burke & Montgomery suggest that their pilot work indicates that having a disabled brother or sister can bring both benefits and disadvantages. Included in the latter is the fact that siblings may be asked to take on caring tasks. In addition, where the learning disability is due to an inherited genetic disorder then this may affect their future decisions concerning children of their own (Maxwell & Barr 2003). However, the provision of support groups can assist in promoting positive interaction with their learning disabled sibling as well as increasing self-esteem (Evans et al 2001). It is therefore important that, when working with families, all family members are considered.

Transition to Adult Services

Reflect on your Practice

Mrs Lewis is the mother of a 16-year-old girl with profound and multiple disabilities. She has been a frequent visitor to the children's ward over a number of years because her daughter has experienced a range of health problems. During this period of time you have got to know her well. During the most recent visit, however, she had appeared very concerned about the future. She said that at school they had been making plans for what would happen after her daughter left school but that she was very worried.

Given that planning is taking place for her daughter's future what do you feel might be causing Mrs Lewis's current anxiety? What might be the role of the children's nurse in addressing some of her concerns?

The transition from children's services to adult services can be a time of great stress for families. Although it is a process that should be carefully planned, research suggests that it can be a 'rather abrupt affair' (Ward et al 2003). The research undertaken by Ward et al revealed that often parents and young people were told at one outpatients appointment that their next contact with services would be with adult services. Even when families did report that transition planning had taken place, more than half stated that transfer to adult health services had not been considered at all. On a more positive note the researchers indicate that 18% of respondents felt that transfer of responsibility for health had been addressed well. They suggest that this indicates that such planning can be undertaken effectively. To improve the situation they argue that health must be addressed as part of the wider process of transition planning and that health professionals who know the child must be involved in this process (Ward et al 2003). This has clear implications for children's nurses as well as for those working in adult services. Effective supports and services need to exist (NHS Health Scotland 2004).

The Health Needs of Children with Learning Disabilities

NHS Health Scotland (2004) state that, compared with the rest of the population, people with learning disabilities have:

- a higher number of health needs and more complex health needs
- a higher level of unmet health needs
- a different pattern of health needs. The types of health needs they experience can differ and some are specific to people with learning disabilities.

As has already been noted, people with Down syndrome, for example, are at increased risk of having certain health problems (NHS Health Scotland 2004). In addition, children with learning disabilities have an increased

✚ Evidence-based Practice

NHS Health Scotland (2004) has undertaken a major review of the evidence concerning the health needs of people with learning disabilities. This document both reviews the evidence regarding health needs across the lifespan and makes recommendations for the development of more responsive services. For further information visit:
- http://www.healthscotland.com

prevalence of epilepsy (with children with severe and profound learning disabilities having a greater prevalence), are at increased risk of visual and sensory impairments, and there is a reported high prevalence of mental ill health and problem behaviours (NHS Health Scotland 2004). However, although we know that the health needs of people with learning disabilities can be greater, and that some people have additional needs as a result of their specific impairment, these needs often go unnoticed and unmet. Over the past 20 years it has been increasingly recognised that people with learning disabilities have undetected and unmet health needs (Howells 1986, NHS Health Scotland 2004, Wilson & Haire 1990). As a result it is suggested that people with learning disabilities die as a result of preventable conditions (Barr et al 1999).

Before reading further, look at the case scenarios below.

◆ Scenario

Jenny

Jenny is a 12-year-old girl who has severe learning disabilities. She lives at home with her parents and is a frequent visitor to her local children's ward as she has regular and severe epileptic seizures. She is currently in the ward for a review of her medication following a particularly severe seizure. When she had the seizure she was at home and had been found in the living room lying on the floor. When she recovered from the seizure she seemed very disorientated but did not appear to have otherwise injured herself as she got to her feet and started to walk around. While she was on the ward it was noticed that when she was assisted to bath she would wince whenever her left hip was touched. She was X-rayed and she was found to have sustained a fracture during her seizure, which had not previously been detected.

Simon

Simon is a 15-year-old boy with mild learning disabilities. It has been suggested that he may suffer from autistic spectrum disorder. He is normally very active but he does not enjoy being in close contact with other people. However, he does appear to have good understanding of what other people say to him and, when his mood allows, he is able to converse with others. He is currently in hospital following appendectomy. When he was brought into the ward he was very withdrawn and obviously in pain but did not want anyone to go near him. His mother said that she had noticed him getting less active over the past couple of days and had tried to get him to tell her what was wrong. However, each time she did this he just got agitated and went to his room. Eventually, however, he had become so unwell that she took him to their GP. Their regular GP was away and so they saw a locum who appeared very hurried, did not take the time to examine Simon because he was uncooperative, and said that she thought that it was just to do with his condition (meaning his autism and learning disabilities). His mother then took him to the emergency department at the hospital where they (eventually) diagnosed him as having appendicitis. He has now been on the ward for a couple of days following his operation but the nurses are worried that he is not recovering as well as they would expect and they suspect that he is in pain. However, although he appears to understand what they say to him they cannot get him to tell them what is wrong. He is also beginning to display what they feel is strange behaviour. Although most of the nurses are trying very hard to meet Simon's needs, one nurse on the ward says that children like Simon shouldn't be on general wards – they should be looked after in specialist areas. In addition, another parent on the ward has complained to the ward staff about his behaviour, also believing that he shouldn't be on the ward.

Consider each of the above scenarios – what barriers did these young people face in relation to having their health needs met? What could have been done to overcome these barriers?

www

For further information concerning autistic spectrum disorders please visit the website of the National Autistic Society:
- http://www.nas.org.uk

In reading through the above scenarios you will, hopefully have identified a number of key barriers that are commonly faced by people with learning disabilities in relation to their health care needs. These include:

- Communication: people with learning disabilities can find it difficult to communicate to others that they feel unwell. They may not be able to use verbal communication methods or they may have a limited vocabulary, which makes it difficult in a healthcare system which often relies upon the ability of the patient to describe their symptoms. Sometimes communication can take the form of what is perceived as 'difficult' behaviour and, unfortunately, this can be attributed to the fact that a person has a learning disability rather than that they may be unwell or in pain. It is not just people with learning disabilities, however, that have communication difficulties. Sometimes healthcare professionals also lack the skills required to communicate effectively with people with learning disabilities. They may use medical jargon, complex sentences, or be unable to understand augmentative forms of communication such as Makaton (a form of sign language).

- Time: determining whether someone with a learning disability has a health problem can be a long and complex process due, for example, to the communication difficulties outlined above and to other factors such as the fact that procedures may have to be introduced more slowly. However, within the healthcare system pressures of work can mean that time is not always made available for this process. This can result in health needs not being identified.

- Diagnostic overshadowing: what this means is that any change in behaviour or health need is viewed as part of the person's learning disability. This then means that professionals and services can fail to respond since they view it as not being amenable to change. This is clearly shown in the scenario where a locum GP said that Simon's difficulties were due to the fact that he has learning disabilities and autism.

- Negative attitudes: thankfully, these are relatively rare. Nonetheless, they are still prevalent among some members of society and also among nurses and other professionals. Negative attitudes and discrimination may not be as explicit as in the case study above. However, negative perceptions concerning the quality of life of children with learning disabilities may lead to a reluctance to offer certain forms of life-saving or life-enhancing treatments, such as adequate pain control.

A number of things can be done to overcome some of these barriers. For example, all health professionals need to be aware of the additional health needs that people with learning disabilities may experience, thus making them more alert to the possibility that they can occur and overcoming the potential for diagnostic overshadowing. Health professionals need to develop their skills in communicating with people with learning disabilities including the development of skills in augmentative forms of communication. The way in which services are structured also needs to be examined so that additional time is made available when children with learning disabilities require examination or treatment. Finally negative attitudes, wherever they are found, need to be challenged. It is only by doing so that children with learning disabilities will be able to exercise their right to health care on an equitable basis with other children.

Working Together

The Chief Nursing Officer's *Review of the nursing, midwifery and health visiting contribution to vulnerable children and young people* (DoH 2004) notes that care is often fragmented 'between health, social care and education, between the hospital and between nurses, midwives and health visitors'. Because children and young people with learning disabilities clearly come within the group of children who are considered to be potentially vulnerable this fragmentation is a source of concern. Collaborative working is required if appropriate support is to be provided for families of children with learning disabilities. An important step towards this is to understand the role of some of the professionals who might be involved.

THE ROLE OF THE LEARNING DISABILITY NURSE

The learning disability nurse is one of the professionals who might be involved with children with learning disabilities and their families (for further information see Jenkins et al 2003).

Over many years there has been a great deal of debate as to the role of the specialist learning disability nurse. In 1995, the then Chief Nursing Officer for England commissioned a review of the role. In the report which resulted the following were identified as key roles for learning disability nurses (Kay et al 1995):

- assessment of need
- health surveillance and health promotion
- developing personal competence
- the use of enhanced therapeutic skills
- managing and leading teams of staff
- enhancing the quality of support
- enablement and empowerment
- coordinating services.

Each of these roles may be seen as being relevant to working with children with a learning disability. For example, nurses may be able to undertake specialist assessments of behavioural needs and work with families to develop their confidence and competence in managing their child's behaviour. In other instances they may work with young people with learning disabilities in relation to sexual health promotion (Atkinson 2002). They might also be involved in the assessment of risk in relation to epilepsy and the development of appropriate management plans with families (O'Brien & Loughran 2004). As a coordinator of care, and due to their experience of working with people with learning disabilities across the lifespan, learning disability nurses may also have much to offer at the point of transition from children's to adult health services.

Activity

For further information concerning the role of the learning disability nurse, see Turnbull (2003).

Current policy advocates that people with learning disabilities, including children, should use generic health services wherever possible and receive specialist support (if required) to access such services. However, in some areas this has meant that the role of learning disability nurses in working with children has reduced over the past two decades. Not all children with a learning disability will require the support of a learning disability nurse and some may only require such support for a short period of time. However, others with more complex physical and/or behavioural needs may require support on a more continuous basis. In such instances it is important that the skills, knowledge and experience of the learning disability nurse are recognised and their involvement in working with children and families is actively sought. Indeed the Chief Nursing Officer's report (DoH 2004) argues that integrated children's teams should 'routinely' be seeking the involvement of learning disability nurses.

COLLABORATIVE WORKING

Scenario

Louise

Louise is a 7-year-old who enjoys doing things with her family and who likes visiting her local fast-food shop for a milkshake. She also has very complex needs. She has severe learning disabilities and cerebral palsy. She has mobility problems and needs to use a wheelchair. She also has difficulties with swallowing.

Shaun

Shaun is a 14-year-old boy who likes doing all the things that other teenagers like to do. He spends each Saturday going to his local football club along with his dad and other mates and enjoys playing his music too loud in his bedroom. Shaun has moderate learning disabilities and also has epilepsy. Recently he has started to become very moody and argumentative. Only last week he lashed out at his younger sister. His family is getting very worried about his behaviour.

Reflect on your Practice

Think about the two scenarios above:
- Which professionals might be involved with Louise, Shaun and their families at the moment?
- Is this likely to change over the next 5 years?
- What support might the learning disability nurse offer?
- What support might the children's nurse or school nurse offer?

- What difficulties could there currently be in relation to coordinating support to these two families?
- How might some of these be overcome?

The range of needs experienced by children with learning disabilities and their families means that no one profession is going to be able to provide all of the support required (Bollard 2003, Kay et al 1995). There has been much discussion and debate concerning the need for multi-professional and interprofessional working but, unfortunately, this does not always translate into effective service provision. Kerr (2001) identifies two key interfaces that need to be carefully managed in relation to children and young people with learning disabilities:

- The interface between services for children and those for adults.
- The interface between the range of agencies and professionals involved in the lives of people with learning disabilities.

Bollard (2003) distinguishes between multi-professional and interprofessional working, arguing that the former does not require interaction between the professionals involved whereas the latter implies interaction. This is what is required if coordinated services are to be provided for children with learning disabilities and their families.

Interaction, collaboration and partnership do, however, need to extend beyond the need for professionals to work together with professionals. For services to really make a positive impact children and young people along with their families and carers all need to be viewed as important members of the team.

Summary

This chapter has explored the nature of learning disability, its effect on the child and their family, and the ways in which nurses can work together with the child, their family, and other professionals to ensure that needs are identified and met in an appropriate and timely manner.

Finally, when attempting to think about children and families who have 'learning disability' it may help to remember the following points:

- Children with a learning disability are children first. They have the same needs as other children but also have additional needs.
- A learning disability is a permanent condition. However, people with learning disabilities grow and develop as individuals just like everyone else but generally at a slower pace.

- People with learning disabilities have the same human rights as non-learning disabled people.
- Some people are born with a learning disability, some acquire a learning disability as the result of an injury or illness.
- Some people with learning disabilities also have a physical or sensory impairment but many do not. Some are also at increased risk of certain health conditions.
- Children with a learning disability need to be seen in the context of their family and support provided to all family members. Professionals need to be aware of the significance of key stages in the child's life such as initial diagnosis, commencing school and transition to adult services.
- People with learning disabilities have dreams and aspirations like all other people and many of them may be achievable if they are offered appropriate support by the multidisciplinary team and their communities.

Men and women with learning disabilities can be parents, employees, Olympic athletes, husbands and wives. Some have driving licences, GCSEs and teaching qualifications. A few have climbed to Everest's base camp. For others, their greatest triumph may be smiling or some act of self-determination. As it is for all children, it is impossible to know what kind of a person a child with a learning disability will be when he or she grows up. For this reason it is of paramount importance to remember that they are children and young people first, with a disability second, and will continue to grow and develop throughout their lives. It is simply that, due to impairment, these stages may take longer. The failure to recognise this in the past has contributed to making the experience of learning disability more limiting than it might otherwise be. Nursing practitioners, as members of the multidisciplinary team, can play a key role in minimising the negative impacts a learning disability may have on an individual and their family and in promoting quality of life for all.

References

Atkinson S 2002 It's great to grow up. Learning Disability Practice 5(10):28–30

Barr O, Gilgunn J, Kane T, Moore G 1999 Health screening for people with learning disabilities by a community nursing service in Northern Ireland. Journal of Advanced Nursing 29(6):1482–1491

Bollard M 2003 Inter-professional working: its relevance and importance to learning disability practice. In: Jukes M, Bollard M (eds) Contemporary learning disability practice. Quay Books, Salisbury, pp 20–30

Department of Health (DoH) 2001 Valuing people. A new strategy for learning disability for the 21st century. DoH, London

Department of Health (DoH) 2004 The chief nursing officer's review of the nursing, midwifery and health visiting contributon to vulnerable children and young people. The Stationery Office, London

Dickinson D, Dickinson L 2003 Compulsory school education. In: Gates B (ed.) Learning disabilities. Toward inclusion. Churchill Livingstone, Edinburgh, pp 107–123

Disability Rights Commission and Department of Health (2004) You can make a difference – improving hospital services for disabled people. The Stationery Office, London

Dobson B, Middleton S, Beardsworth A 2001 The impact of childhood disability on family life. York Publishing Services, York

Gates B, Wilberforce D 1993 The nature of learning disabilities. In: Gates B (ed.) Learning disabilities. Toward inclusion. Churchill Livingstone, Edinburgh, pp 3–19

Gross RD 1991 Psychology: the science of mind and behaviour. Hodder and Stoughton, London

Howells G 1986 Are the medical needs of mentally handicapped adults being met? Journal of the Royal College of General Practitioners 36:449–453

Jenkins R, Mansell I, Northway R 2003 Specialist learning disability services in the UK. In: Gates B (ed.) Learning disabilities. Toward inclusion. Churchill Livingstone, Edinburgh, pp 349–367

Kay B, Rose S, Turnbull J 1995 Continuing the commitment. The report of the Learning Disability Nursing Project. Department of Health, London

Lindsay M 1998 Signposts for success in commission and providing health services for people with learning disabilities. Department of Health, London

Maxwell V, Barr O 2003 With the benefit of hindsight. A mother's reflections on raising a child with Down syndrome. Journal of Learning Disabilities 7(1):51–64

NHS Health Scotland 2004 Health needs assessment report: people with learning disabilities in Scotland. NHS Scotland, Glasgow

Northway R 1997 Disability and oppression: some implications for nurses and nursing. Journal of Advanced Nursing 26:736–743

O'Brien D, Loughran S 2004 Risk assessment and epilepsy. Learning Disability Practice 7(3):12–17

SCOPE 1999 Right from the start. Looking at diagnosis and disclosure – parents describe how they found out about their child's disability. SCOPE, London

SCOPE 2003 Right from the start template. Good practice in sharing the news. SCOPE, London

Sloper P, Mitchell W 2000 User friendly information for families with disabled children: a guide to good practice. York Publishing Services, York

Turnbull J (ed.) 2003 Learning disability nursing. Blackwell Science, Oxford

Ward L, Mallett R, Heslop P, Simons K 2003 Planning for health at transition. Learning Disability Practice 6(3):24–27

Watson D 1993 Causes and manifestations of learning disabilities. In: Gates B (ed.) Learning disabilities. Toward inclusion. Churchill Livingstone, Edinburgh, pp 21–40

Wilson J, Haire B 1990 Health care screening for people with mental handicap living in the community. British Medical Journal 301:1379–1381

World Health Organization (WHO) 1993 Describing developmental disability. Guidelines for a multiaxial scheme for mental retardation (learning disability). WHO, Geneva

Useful Websites

http://www.doh.gov.uk/learningdisabilities/new.htm

http://www.communityliving.org.uk

http://www.viauk.org/

http://www.valuingpeople.org.uk/

http://www.bild.org.uk/

As the subject of this book is children's and young people's nursing, all entries within the index refer to this unless otherwise stated. Publications and legal cases are entered in italics. Page numbers suffixed by t refer to tables or boxed material; those suffixed by f refer to figures. *vs.* indicates a comparison.

Aberdeen Children's Hospital 10
absence fit 356
accidental poisoning, early childhood
    667–668
accidents, middle childhood *see* middle
    childhood, health problems
acetylcholine 509
Acheson, Donald 34 35
acquired rubella 661–662
Action for Sick Children (ASC)
    contribution to quality of care 64,
        242–243
    foundation 14
active listening 141, 711–712
acupuncture, analgesia 272t
acute illnesses, middle childhood 695
acute lymphoblastic leukaemia 501–502
acute myeloid leukaemia 501
acute pain *see* pain; postoperative pain
acute renal failure (ARF) 416–418
    diagnosis 417
    hyperkalaemia 417
    management 417–418
    prognosis 418
adaptive immune response 477
addiction, definition 270
Addison's disease 543
Adelaide Children's Hospital (Australia)
    10
Adelaide Children's Hospital (Ireland) 9
adenoidectomy 281–282, 285f
    standing orders 295t
adenotonsillectomy 282
adenoviruses 449t
    gastroenteritis 676t
administration routes, drugs *see* drug
    administration routes
admission *see* hospital admission;
    hospitalisation

adolescents 193–195, 701–705
    assertion 702
    chronic illness 734–735
    consent issues 320
    developmental tasks 701–702
    'focal theory' 702–703
    gender relationships 703–704
    growth 188–195
        body mass 193
        brain development 195
        breast development 194
        cardiovascular system 193
        facial proportions 192–193
        growth spurt 195
        head 192 193
        hormones 193, 193f, 195f
        respiratory system 193
        sexual maturation *see below*
        skeletal system 189
        skin 193
        stages 193–195
        teeth 189–190
    hospital accommodation 124
    interaction with
        adults, approachability of 709
        application 717–718
        'chase the affect' 714
        collaborative empiricism 713
        interpersonal skills needed *see*
            interpersonal skills
        modeling behaviour 714
        narcissism acknowledgement 713
        objectivity 713
        social system inclusion 713–714
        Socratic questioning 714
    long-term adverse health behaviours
        704
        affecting factors 705
    low self-esteem 705

    malignant disease survival 502
    mental health 707
    nature of 701
    parental relationships 703
    peer relationships 703
    physical attractiveness 703–704
    sexual maturation
        boys 194–195, 195f
        girls 194, 194f
        menarche 194
    sexuality 703–704
    stressors 131–132, 200–201
    therapeutic relationship 714–718
        attachment theory 717
        boundary awareness 714–715
        development theory 716–717
        empathy 714
        models of helping 715–716
        orientation phase 715
        resolution phase 715–716
        self-awareness 714
        self-knowledge 714
        working phase 715
adrenal function disorders 542–545, 542t
    acute adrenocortical insufficiency
        543–544
    chronic adrenocortical insufficiency
        (Addison's disease) 543
    congenital adrenal hyperplasia 542–543
    phaeochromocytoma 544–545
    primary hyperaldosteronism 544
adrenal gland 542f
    hyperplasia 542–543
adrenal insufficiency 543–544
    causes 544t
adrenaline, croup management 673
adrenocortical insufficiency
    acute (adrenal crisis) 543–544
    chronic (Addison's disease) 543

adrenoleucodystrophy, genetic testing 910
adults
    attitudes to children 5–6
    child interest in 25
Advanced Life Support Group
    choking guidelines 668
    respiratory function assessment
        672–673
advanced paediatric life support (APLS)
    570–571
advanced trauma life support (ATLS)
    570–571
advocacy 229, 312–313
    nurses' role in chronic illness
        734–735
Advocating for Children (2000) Royal
    College of Paediatrics and Child
    Health (RCPCH) 229
afterload 755
    definition 739
age-appropriate strategies
    illness understanding 134
    informed consent 227
age of child, hospitalisation effects 122
Age of Legal Capacity (Scotland) Act
    (1991) 226
aggravating stressors 198
aggressive behaviour, adolescents 131–132
airway
    chest assessment and examination
        426, 427f
    obstructions 292
airway pressure 745f
airway resistance 426, 426f
    breathing 745–746, 745f
    neonates 172
alcohol misuse, sources of stress 305
Alder Hey children's hospital *see* Royal
    Liverpool Children's Hospital
aldosterone, shock compensatory
    mechanisms 758
alleles, genes 607
allergic rhinitis, glue ear 670
allergies
    eczema 645
    prevalence 236
alliances and boundaries, families 30–31
Allitt, Beverly 41–42
Alma Ata declaration 110
alopecia, malignant disease 492
altered body image, psychosocial
    development 158
alveoli 424, 424f
    toddlers 184
ambiguous genitalia 543
ambulances, appropriate use 354
ambulatory care 331
    origins 7
    psychological trauma 64
American Pain Society 270
anaemia, iron-deficiency 674–675
anaerobic metabolism, shock 755
anaesthesia
    emergency 291
    epidural 268, 269t

induction 289–291
    local *see* local anaesthesia
    topical, emergency department use
        361t
anaesthetic mask, child's view 289f
anaesthetic room, parents presence 293
anaesthetist's duty, informed consent 286
analgesia 267–270
    administration routes 267
    analgesic ladder 267, 267f
    cardiovascular problems 473
    drugs 267–271, 268t
        misconceptions 270–271
    emergency department methods 361,
        361t
    nurse-controlled *see* nurse-controlled
        analgesia (NCA)
    patient-controlled *see* patient-
        controlled analgesia (PCA)
    stomatitis 497
    subcutaneous 270
    see also pain, management
anaphylactic shock 760
androgen, excess production 542
aneuploidy, chromosomes 616
angiocardiography, cardiac
    catheterisation 472
anions 394, 394t
    anion gap 395
anorexia, malignant disease treatment 498
anorexia nervosa 707
anti-D antibodies, neonatal jaundice 633
anti-smoking advice, malignant disease
    survivors 502
antibiotics
    advent of 62
    atopic eczema management 646
    genitourinary problems 407
    otitis media 670
    shock treatment 763
antibodies *see* immunoglobulin(s)
antidiuretic hormone (ADH) 536
    shock compensatory mechanisms 758
antiepileptic drugs 526–527
antigen-presenting cells (APCs),
    gastrointestinal tract 480
antihistamines, atopic eczema
    management 647, 678
antipyretic drugs, fevers/pyrexia 681
anxiety
    family response, reduction 66
    role confusion 26
    separation 63–64
    transmission from adult to child
        71–72
apnoea of infancy 435, 651
    infectious causes 435
apocrine glands 478
appendicectomy, laparoscopic 283, 288f
appendicitis, acute 283
appetite loss, malignant disease 498
arginine vasopressin *see* antidiuretic
    hormone (ADH)
Armstrong, George 7, 62, 331
Arnold–Chiari malformations 528

aromatherapy, analgesia 272t
art
    stress assessment by 204
    therapy, hospitalisation preparation
        73
arterial blood pressure *see* blood
    pressure
arteries
    embryonic development 463
    transposition 467
arthritis
    acquired rubella 662
    cystic fibrosis complications 452
    septic 658
artificial feeding techniques, complex
    motor disability 383
artificially-acquired active immunity 654
artificially-acquired passive immunity 653
aspirated foreign body 435
assent 225–226, 228
    definition 217
assertion, adolescents 702
assessment 89–103
    appropriate tools or devices 97
    auditing/recording practice 101–103
        information governance 102–103
        information management 101–102
        parent held records 102
        record content 102
    clinical decision making 91
    clinical judgement 91
    clinical process 90–92, 90f
    clinical reasoning 90–91, 91f
    communication technology 94
    conceptual models 90
    context of care 91–92, 92f
        interpersonal context 91–92
        philosophical context 92
    decision making 99–100
    diagnostic reasoning 91
    evaluation and outcomes 100–101,
        101t
    family responsibility, extent of 93
    focus of 95–96
    focused assessment 97–99
        tools and methods 97–99
    generalised frameworks 96–99
    instruments 98
    language choice 92
    nature of 89–90
    nursing assessment 96–97
        disease-focused models 95
        functional health patterns 97b
    nursing diagnoses 91
    nursing process model 90
    nursing specialist roles 96
    planning care 99
    practice 94–101
    principles applied 92
    problem solving 90
    scope and priority 97
    by telephone *see* telephone health
        assessment
assisted control mode (ACM),
    mechanical ventilation 750

Association of British Paediatric Nurses (ABPN) 13
Association of Chief Children's Nurses (ACCN) 45
Association of Sick Children's Hospital Nurses 13
Association of Spina Bifida and Hydrocephalus (ASBAH) 530
asthma 438–440, 672
  aetiology 438
  assessment 444–443, 672
  care scenario 444–443
  evidence-based research 211–215
  exacerbation, stressful life events 203
  life-threatening 439
  management 439–440
  middle childhood 696
  oxygen saturation 440
  prevalence 438
  response 438–439, 439f
  severe 439
  trigger avoidance 672
astrocytomas 521
at risk register 304
atonic fit 356
atopic eczema 643–645, 644t
  assessment 644
  breastfeeding 643
  development 643
  family history 644
  features 644–645
  localisation 643
  management 645–647
    antibiotics 646
    antihistamines 647
    corticosteroids 646
    family needs 645
    inflammation 646
    pruritus control 646
    secondary infections 646
    skin hydration 646
    wet-wrap dressings 647, 647b
  physiology 643–644
  signs/symptoms 644b
  skin features 643–644
    thickening (lichenification) 645
  sleeping 643
atresia of bowel 280
atria, embryonic development 462
atrial septal defects 468
atrioventricular valve, development 463
attachment, development of 24
attachment theory 14, 62–63
  adolescents, therapeutic relationship 717
Atwell, John 37–38
audit/auditing
  assessment see assessment
  clinical see clinical audit
Audit Commission, emergency care teams 358
auscultation, cardiovascular problems 470–471

autoimmune liver disease, cystic fibrosis complications 452
autoinflation, glue ear 671
autonomic nervous system (ANS) 507
autonomy 225
  ethics 311–312
autosomal dominant inheritance 614, 615f, 616t
autosomal recessive inheritance 615, 616t
autosomes 607, 614
avascular necrosis, fracture complications 562
AVPU scale 431

B lymphocytes 479, 484
babies and toddlers (1–24 months) 176–185
  1 month 176–177
  1 year 182
  3 months 178–179
  6 months 179–181
  6 week check 177–178
  8 months 181–182
  18 months 183
  consent issues 319
  normal observations 185
  relationship with mother figure 24
  see also early childhood; infancy/infants
Babinski reflex 176
baby walkers, dangers 587
back posture
  3 months 179f
  6 months 179, 180f
bacteria
  commensal skin flora 478
  immune system avoidance 485
  see also individual species
Bacteroides fragilis 482
balanitis xerotica obliterans (BXO) 416
Barnett v Chelsea and Kensington HMC (1968) 326–327
baroreceptors, blood pressure 470
barotrauma, PEEP/CPAP 747
barriers, immune system see immune system
basic care, complaints 48
bath scalds 586
bed rest 62
  complications 568
Bedford Fenwick, Mrs E. 12
bedtime routines 648
behaviour
  aggressive, adolescents 131–132
  changes, hospitalisation 122
  modeling, adolescents, interaction with 714
  social see social behaviour and play
behavioural indicators
  maltreatment 306
  pain 266, 266t
behavioural problems
  middle childhood 687
  vulnerability 34

beliefs and values, family functioning assessment 29
Belt-up School Kids (BUSK) 584
benchmarking 216, 247
Bendall, Eve 15
beneficence 312
benefits system, in chronic illness 728
bereavement
  communication 142–143
  complaints 49
  early childhood 683–684
  loss of a parent 199–200
bereavement care 779–781
  community 781
  extended family 781
  healthcare workers 781
  male roles 780
  siblings 780–781
  see also palliative care
best interests 322, 324
Better care for the seriously injured (2000) 358
Bifidobacterium 482
biliblankets 633
bilirubin, neonatal jaundice 632–633
biological control, cultural assessment 59–60
biotherapy 496
birth, physiological changes 170
Black, Douglas 34
Black report (DHSS 1980) 34, 123
blame, inherited conditions 612
blame culture 116
blood gases, arterial 425t
blood glucose monitoring, type 1 diabetes 548
blood pressure 470t
  3–12 months 185
  cardiovascular problems 470
  circulation 430–431
  diastolic see diastolic blood pressure (DBP)
  fetal 170
  monitoring 762
  neonates 173
  systolic see systolic blood pressure (SBP)
  see also mean arterial blood pressure (MAP)
blood profiling 512
body, water composition see water composition, body
body fluid and electrolyte imbalance 389–404
  assessment 399–402
  biochemical investigations 399–402
  body fluids 389–390
  cardiac arrest 402
  dehydration 396–399
    see also entries under dehydration
  fluid loss, behavioural response 395f
  homeostasis 395–396
  survival time without water 390
  therapeutic strategies 402

body fluid and electrolyte imbalance
(*Continued*)
  water composition, body 389–393
    see also entries *under* water
      composition, body
body image, malignant disease treatment
  499
body positioning, lung injury reduction
  748
body temperature
  early childhood 680–681
  febrile response 487
  measurement, hypothermic neonates
    625
  middle childhood 695
  neurological dysfunction 516
  normal variations 431t
  regulation, neonates 624
  respiratory illness 431
Bolam test 321, 326
Bolitho v City and Hackney (1988) 326
bone
  cancellous 559
  compact 559
  development 560t
  fractures 562–566
    repair and bone healing 560
    see also fractures
  growth, formation and reabsorption
    560
  joints 560
  remodelling 560, 561f
  skeletal muscle 561–562
  spongy 559
  structure 559–560, 559f
bone age 167
bone marrow aspirates 496
Booth Hall Children's Hospital 9
Bordetella pertussis see pertussis
  (whooping cough)
bottlefed babies, stools 173
Botulinum toxin, complex motor
  disability 380
boundary awareness, adolescents,
  therapeutic relationship 714–715
bowel atresia 280
Bowen, Jaymee 312
Bowlby, John
  hospitalisation effects 33, 108
  nurse education 14
  theory of attachment 62–63
Braille, information for hospitalisation
  70
brain
  anatomy 509
    brain stem 509
    cerebral hemispheres 509
  development
    adolescence 195
    neonates 175–176
  traumatic injury 530–532
    aetiology 530
    classification 530–531
    long term outcomes 531–532

non-progressive 511t
    presentation 531
    treatment and management 531
  brain stem 509
    gliomas 521
  brain tumours 520–523
    aetiology 520–521
    classification 521
    diagnosis 522
    long-term outcomes 523
    presentation 521–522
    treatment and management 522–523
breast development, adolescence 194
breast milk
  infection, as source of 628
  protective properties 481, 628
'breast milk jaundice' 633
breastfeeding 637
  atopic eczema 643
  food intolerance 640
  stools 173
breath sounds 429–430
breathing *see* respiration
A Bridge to the Future (1997) 43
*Bridging the Gaps: health care for
  adolescents* (2003) 43
Bridging the Gaps (CCHS 1993) 40
*Bright futures: promoting children and
  young people's mental health* 705
The Bristol Inquiry (2000) 44, 592–593
  reforms, resulting from 123, 248
Bristol Royal Infirmary 44
  consent for major heart surgery 314
  information provision 321
  see also The Bristol Inquiry
British Medical Association (BMA),
  research guidelines 314
British Orthopaedic Association 358
British Paediatric Surveillance Unit
  (BPSU), inflammatory bowel
  disease 454
British Thoracic Society, asthma
  management guidelines 440
brittle bone disease *see* osteogenesis
  imperfecta
bronchioles 424
bronchiolitis 435–436
  assessment and care scenario
    440–442
bronchopneumonia 437
bronchospasm 438
brown fat 172, 624
budesonide, croup management 673
bulimia 707
bullying, middle childhood 697–698
Bunnell Davis, John 7, 106
burns, early childhood *see* early
  childhood, health problems

C-reactive protein (CRP) 483, 486
cachexia, malignant disease treatment
  498
calamine lotion, chickenpox 681
calcium, bone, role in 560

Calman–Hine report (1995) 491
Cambridge splint, developmental
  dysplasia of hip (DDH) 574
Campylobacter, gastroenteritis 676t
Campylobacter jejuni, diarrhoea 449t
cancellous bone 559
cancer 490–491
  see also malignant disease
cancer-related fatigue (CRF) 498–499
cannulation 289
capillary refill, respiratory illness 431
capnography, mechanical ventilation
  assessment/monitoring 752, 752f,
  753f
'Captain Chemo' 494
cardiac arrest, body fluid loss 402
cardiac catheterisation 472
cardiac contractility 754–755
  definition 739
  see also Frank–Starling's law
cardiac cycle 465–466
  output 466
  phases 466
cardiac failure, congestive *see* congestive
  cardiac failure
cardiac murmurs 471
cardiac output 754
  definition 739
  determinants 754f
cardiac transplantation 468
cardiogenic shock 760, 760t
cardiopulmonary assessment, rapid,
  critical illness 742
cardiopulmonary resuscitation (CPR)
  apnoea of infancy 651
  parental presence 364
cardiovascular problems 460–475
  classification 467
  diagnostic assessment and evaluation
    469–472
    auscultation 470–471
    blood pressure 470
    cardiac catheterisation 472
    chest radiography 471
    echocardiography 471–472
    electrocardiography 471
    inspection 469
    palpation 469–470
  mechanical ventilation complications
    749
  nursing considerations 472–473
    positioning of child 472
  origin and extent determination
    466–468
  therapeutic intervention 473
cardiovascular system
  5 years to adolescence 193
  cardiac cycle 465–466
  developmental changes 464–465
    endocardium 465
  heart, normal size and position
    464
  myocardium 464–465
  pericardium 464

embryonic development 460–464
  atria 462
  chamber and vessel concordance 463–464
  valves 463
  ventricles 462–463
  heart features, electrophysiology 465
  neonates 172–173
The Care of Sick Children. A review of the Guidelines in the wake of the Allitt Inquiry 42
Care of the Next Infant (CONI) scheme 650
care partnerships, emergency departments 365
care pathways 99
care planning, assessment 99
care plans 99
Carey, S 150–151
Caring for Children in the Health Services (CCHS) 37–40
  standards 37
Carlile Review (2002) 35, 284, 290
carrier(s)
  genetic testing 607
  genetics 607
carrier population, immunisation 118
casein, cow's milk allergy 453
castration anxiety 160
catecholamines
  shock compensatory mechanisms 758
  shock treatment 764
cations 394, 394t
causation of foreseeable harm 327
cell-mediated innate immunity 482–483
central nervous system (CNS) 507
  infections 511t
  palliative care 777t
  see also brain
central venous pressure (CVP)
  definition 739
  monitoring 762
Centre for Health Information and Promotion (CHIP) 70, 599
Centre for Health Information Quality (CHIQ) 596, 601–602
  assessment of information providers 604
  information production 599
cephalic tetanus 655
cerebral hemispheres 509, 509f
cerebral oedema 390–391
  rebound 403
cerebral palsy 372
  gastro-oesophageal reflux 446
  studies 376
cerebral perfusion pressure (CPP) 513
cerebrospinal fluid (CSF) 510, 510f
cerebrovascular studies, cerebral dysfunction 512
certainty, genetic counselling 619
changes in children's nursing 5–6
Chapman, Lester 298–299
charitable dispensaries 7

charities, palliative care 774
Charter for Children in Hospital (1984) 243
'chase the affect,' adolescents, interaction with 714
chemotherapy 494–495
  brain tumour, neurological dysfunction 522–523
CHEOPS (Children's Hospital of Eastern Ontario) pain scale 263t
Chester v Afshar 321
chickenpox 681–682
  nephrotic syndrome complications 409
child abuse 200
  causation theories 304
  see also maltreatment
Child Accident Prevention Trust (CAPT) 582
Child and Adolescent Mental Health Services (CAMHS) 707–708
Child and Family Court Advisory and Support Service (CAFCASS) 317
child development, assessment 23–29
A child eye view 74
Child Health in the Community (1996) 41
Child Health Rights: Implementing the United Nations Convention on the rights of the Child Within the National Health Service (1995) 42
child maltreatment *see* maltreatment
child poverty 45
child protection
  Children Act (1989) 298
  children as researchers 238–239
  children's nurse, role 297 308
  emergency department assessment 365
  helplines and websites 307
  issues 224 225
  key concept definitions 298–304
  Laming report 335
  National Health Service Direct, referral of at risk 335
  research 218
  United Nations Convention on the Rights of the Child 273, 299
Child Protection Conference 307
Child Protection Register 304, 307
child-resistant containers, medicines 588–589
child restraint systems 584–585
Child Surveillance Programme 582, 587
childhood
  changing concepts 4–6
    influential writers 5
  definition 298
  early *see* early childhood
  middle *see* middle childhood
childhood illnesses, non applicable to adults 223
children

adults, physical differences between 222–223
developmental differences 223–224
growth and development *see* growth and development
legal definition of 222
physical growth 188–195
social differences 224
The Children Act (1989) 3–4, 40
  child protection 298
  children's rights 137
  play, importance 67
  refusal of treatment 323–324
  'significant harm' 300, 307
The Children Act (2004), agency cooperation duties, introduction 328
The Children Act (Scotland) (1995) 3–4, 298
Children and Young Person's Act (1933) 322
Children Bill (2004) 298
Children First: A Study of Hospital Services (1993) 41
  Accident and Emergency services for children 354
children in need 305–306
The Children (Northern Ireland) Order (1995) 298
The Children's Charter (1996) 43
Children's Commissioner for Wales report (2003) 593
Children's Commissioners 4, 206, 328
Children's Hospital of Philadelphia 10
children's hospitals
  establishment 7 8
  growth 8–10
Children's Memorial Hospital (Canada) 10
Children's National Service Framework 690
children's rights 136–137, 298–299
  breaches, contemporary examples 313 314
choking, early childhood 668
Chomsky, Noam, language acquisition/development 155
chromosomes 616–617
  abnormalities 616–617, 617t
    deletions 617t
    microdeletions 617t
    number alterations 616
    structural alterations 616–617
    translocations 617, 617f, 617t
  aneuploidy 616
  autosomes 607, 614
  examination 616, 616f
  homologous 616
  polyploidy 616
  sex *see* sex chromosomes
chronic illness 723–738
  adolescents 734–735
  definitions 723
  disease trajectory 733

chronic illness (*Continued*)
  education 153
  health-related quality of life
      (children) 725
    assessment 725
    treatment effects 726
chronic illness 723–738
  health-related quality of life (parents)
      726–729
    disease severity estimates 726
    emotional responses 726–727
    financial consequences 727–728
    marital relationships 728–729
    parental health 727
    sibling effects 729
    social consequences 728
    treatment effects 726
  incidence and prevalence 724–725
    changing rates 724
  internet resources 724–725
  middle childhood 695–696
  outcome 736
  self-management *see* chronic illness,
      self-management
  severity 724
  support 735–736
    national organisations 735
    professional 735
    schools 735
chronic illness, self-management
      729–736
  educational programmes 730
  helper range 729–730
  nurses' role 730–736
    advocacy 734–735
    background information 732
    communication 732–733
    on diagnosis 730–731
    educational role 733–734
    formality (lack of) 732
    key worker schemes 731–732
    practical care 734
    relationship building 732–733
    support role 735–736
chronic renal failure (CRF) 418–419
  clinical features 418
  diagnosis 418
  dialysis 419
  management 418–419
  transplant 419
chronotropic agents, definition 739
circle of Willis 510
circulating blood volume (CBV) 392
circulation
  blood pressure 430–431
  capillary refill 431
  changes at birth 170
  chest examination 430–431
  skin perfusion and body temperature
      431
  vital signs 430
circulatory system 461
circumcision 280–281, 283f, 415–416
citizenship, middle childhood 688

cleansing, early childhood 677
Climbié Inquiry *see* Victoria Climbié
      Inquiry
clinical audit 248–252
  conducting 249–251
  cycle 251f
  definition 249
  improving care, examples 251–252
  principal stages 249–251
  role 242–255
clinical decision making 99–100, 318
  assessment 91
  clinical judgments *vs.* 92t
  postoperative pain algorithm 261f
clinical governance 243, 245–247
  benchmarking 216, 247
  Bristol Inquiry, importance following
      314
  definition 245
  key activities 246f
  key features 246
  National Health Service Direct Online
      595–596
  temple model 245f
  user involvement 247
clinical judgement, assessment 91
clinical negligence scheme for trusts 605
clinical process, assessment 90–92, 90f
clinical psychologists, hospitalisation 74
clinical reasoning, assessment 90–91,
      91f
clinical trials *see* research, trials
closing volume, breathing 746
Clostridium tetani see tetanus
clotting cascade 486
clubfoot 575
coeliac disease 451–453
  aetiology 451–452
  complications 452
  diagnosis 452
  management 452
cognitive development 147–152
  delay 200
  middle childhood 689–690
  novice to expert shift theory 150–151
  Piagetian 147–151
    concrete operational stage (7–11)
        148
    critiques of 149–150
    formal operational stage (11–12)
        148
    important observations 160
    influence 149–150
    key concepts 148
    preoperational stage (2–7)
        147–148
    propositional operations 148
    reflective abstraction 148
    sensory motor stage (birth to 2
        years) 147
  zone of proximal development
      (Vygotsky) 151–152
  see also psychological development
cognitive perception, of pain 259

colds (coryza), early childhood, health
      problems 671
collaborative empiricism, adolescents,
      interaction with 713
collaborative working, learning
      disabilities 792–793
collagen 486
colloids, shock treatment 763
colon *see* intestine; large intestine
combined course, SRN and RSCN 15
commercially produced health
      information 596
Commission for Health Improvement
      (CHI) *see* Commission for
      Healthcare Audit and Inspection
      (CHAI)
Commission for Healthcare Audit and
      Inspection (CHAI) 253–254
  audit tool 65
  complaint investigation 46–47
  foundation 239
  information quality 604
  standards monitoring 124
Commission for Patient and Public
      Involvement in Health (CPPIH)
  foundation 239
  preparation programmes 66
  public involvement 247
Commission for Social Care Inspection
      45
Committee of the Central Health
      Services Council 33, 35–36
Committee on Child Health Services
      (1976) 36–37
common colds (coryza), early childhood,
      health problems 671
communicating hydrocele 279
communication 127–145, 224
  bereavement 142–143
  with children and their families, pain
      management 273
  children's understanding of health and
      illness 133–134
    age-appropriate strategies 134
  complaints 48
  cultural assessment 58
  development, early childhood
      670–671
  difficulties in families 30
  disability 137–138
  in healthcare context 134–136
  hospitalisation preparation 74
  imparting expert information
      140–141
  learning disabilities, health needs 791
  life-limiting illness 137–138
  listening 141
  nurses' role in chronic illness 732–733
  ongoing communication 139–140
  painting 134f
  palliative care 773–774
  with parents 138–141
  play 132–133
    dolls 133

drama 132
painting 132
puppets 132
storytelling 132–133
serious diagnosis 139
siblings 141–142
communication skills 127–132
1–2 years 130
2–5 years 130
13–adulthood 131–132
family-centred care 81
LEARN model framework 81
middle childhood 130–131
'company they keep' hypothesis 131
neonates 128–130
imitation 128–130
intersubjective companion space 128
National Health Service Direct nurses 334
Nursing Mutual Participation Model 81
pre-birth 127–128
community
bereavement care 781
hospitalisation preparation 72–73
community children's nursing services 108–109
development 13–14
district nursing 106–107
health visiting 107–108
history 104–105
children's hospital introduction 105–106
provision 110f
public health role 110–112
range of nursing services provided 111
school nursing 108
specialist pathways 110
community support, hospitalisation 117
compact bone 559
'company they keep' hypothesis 131
compartment syndrome 562 564
compensated shock 757
definition 739
see also shock
compensation recovery 327
competencies, children's nurses 16
competency for consent 226
parents of questionable competency 320
complaints 45–52
basic care 48
bereavement 49
communication 48
disappointment 48
evaluation 50–51
front line management 49–50
handover 48
investigation 46–47
lessons learned 50, 50f
nursing practice 48–49
outcome 50–51

pathway 50, 50f
procedure stages 46–47
published cases 51–52
complaints manager 46
complement 483, 483f, 485
complementary therapies
atopic eczema management 678
hospitalisation preparation 73
palliative care 775
complex interventions 212–213
children's perspectives 215
research, phases of development 215
complex motor disability 371–388
artificial feeding techniques 383
gastronomy 384
assessment and intervention 378–386
communication 382–384
eating and drinking 382–384
mobility 379–382
Roy adaptation model (1976) 379
Botulinum toxin 380
causes 372
definition 372
drooling 383
equipment used 374–375
adapted tricycle 381f
adaptive seating 382, 382f
communication symbols 386f
feeding equipment 384f
postural control walker 380f
powered wheelchairs 380
prone stander 381f
impact 374–376
information sources 374
long-term management 379–380
medical models 372–373
orthopaedic surgery 380
physiotherapy 379–380
play 384
postural control 379–380
registers 374
services
aims 376–377
expectations 377–378
experiences 377
social models 372–373
standards 378
surveys 375t
World Health Organisation (WHO) perspective 373
compliance, respiratory 745–746, 745f, 746
definition 739
concepts of health/illness 152–154
applications 153–154
misconceptions 153–154
concrete operational stage (7–11), Piagetian cognitive development 148
confidence, development, middle childhood 688
Confidential Enquiry into Maternal and Child Health (CEMACH) 253

Confidential Enquiry into Maternal Deaths (CEMD) 253
Confidential Enquiry into Stillbirths and Deaths in Infancy (CESDI) 253
confidentiality
National Health Service Direct 335
older children's concerns 143
research 218
Confidentiality: protecting and providing information (GMC 2004) 250
conflict between parents 325
conflict situations
communicating with children and families 325
communication 141
congenital rubella 662
congestive cardiac failure 468–469
compensatory mechanisms 469
fluid retention 473
therapeutic intervention 473
conjunctivitis 480
conscience development 25
consciousness, assessment, neurological dysfunction 514–516
consent
freely given 320–321
informed see informed consent
for organ retention, Royal Liverpool Children's Hospital (Alder Hey) 313 314
consent forms, older children, surgery 286
Conservation of Resources Theory 202
constipation 456–457
causes, organic 456t
diagnosis 457
malignant disease treatment 498
management 457
palliative care 777t
urinary tract infection 406
consumer health information 593–596
commercially produced information 596
The Help for Health Trust 593–594
information kiosks 596
internet services 594
National Health Service direct online 594–596
patient organisations and self-help groups 594
telephone services 594
television services 596
consumer opinion, parental information 71
context of care, assessment see assessment
continuous intravenous morphine infusions 268–269
continuous positive airway pressure (CPAP) see PEEP/CPAP
continuous quality improvement (CQI) 244
controversial treatment, consent 325–326

convulsions 355–357
convulsive epilepticus 357
Coombs test, neonatal jaundice 633
coping strategies
　chronic illness and disability 138
　hospitalisation *see* hospitalisation,
　　family responses
　stress/stressful events 198, 201–202
Coram, Thomas 6, 105–106
core competence statements, genetic
　counselling 618b
coronal synostosis 524f
corporal punishment 298–299
cortical bone 559
corticosteroids
　atopic eczema management 646, 678
　croup management 673
　malignant disease 498
　radiotherapy induced swelling 523
Corynebacterium diphtheriae 654, 654b
cough reflex 480
　neurological assessment 516
counselling, genetic *see* genetic
　counselling
couple subsystem, family alliances 30
Court, Donald 36–37
Court Commission 107
Court of Appeal 322
Court report 36–37, 109
cows' milk allergy 453, 640
cows' milk intolerance 640, 640t
cranial surgery, postoperative care,
　immediate 518–519t
cranial vault remodelling 281
craniofacial surgery 281, 283f
craniopharyngiomas 521
craniosynostosis 523–525
　aetiology 523
　long term outcomes 525
　presentation 524–525
　treatment and management 525
　types 524f
creatinine 395
Creutzfeldt–Jakob disease 326
cricoid pressure, intubation 742
criminal liability 327–328
crisis
　coping with, inherited conditions 612
　psychosocial development 23
critical care, family-centred *see* family-
　centred critical care
critical illness 739–769
　definition 740
　glossary 739–740
　haemodynamic control 754–765
　rapid cardiopulmonary assessment
　　742
　respiratory support *see* respiratory
　　support
　see also intensive care
Crohn's disease 455t
croup (laryngotracheobronchitis) 434,
　672–673
　management 673

cryptorchidism 415
cultural aspects, surgery 287
cultural expectations, family
　communication 30
cultural safety 59–60
culture 54–60
　assessment 58–60
　　biological control 59–60
　　communication 58
　　environment 58–59
　　social organisations 58
　　time 58
　defining 54–56
　disrespect 57
　ethnicity 55–56
　ethnocentrism 56–57
　sterotyping 57
culture shock 57–58
Cumberledge, Julia 109
Cumberledge report (DHSS 1986)
　110–111
Cushing's reflex 516
Cushing's syndrome 555f
　care scenario 554–556
CWILTED triage enhancement 359
cyanotic cardiovascular lesions 467
cycle helmets 585
cystic fibrosis 448–451
　diagnosis 450
　gastrointestinal function 450
　genetic testing 617, 910
　management 450–451
　patterns of inheritance 615
　respiratory function 450
cytokines 479, 483–484, 484f, 485
　blood circulation changes 485–486
　macrophage release of 485f
　septic shock 761

Dandy–Walker syndrome 528
Data Protection Act, National Health
　Service Direct 335
day-case surgery, middle childhood
　691–693
daycare services 64
deafness, infants 129–130
death
　care following 779
　early childhood 683–684
　see also bereavement
decision making 99–100, 318
　see also clinical decision making
decision support system, National
　Health Service Direct 334, 337
Declaration of Helsinki 227–228, 315
decompensated shock 757
dehydration 396–399
　assessment and biochemical
　　investigations 399–402
　assessment and care principles
　　397–399
　causes 396
　definition 396
　hypothermic neonates 625

neonates 173, 625
percentage calculation 403
types 396–397
weight loss 396
delayed union, fracture complications
　562
deliberate harm 328
dendritic cells 484
denial, separation anxiety 63–64
dental caries, early childhood 677–678
dental defects, cystic fibrosis
　complications 452
dental eruption, toddlers 184
depression, role confusion 26
depressive symptoms, adolescents 707
Der Struwwelpeter 6
dermatitis
　atopic *see* atopic eczema
　inflammatory response 486
　see also eczema
despair, separation anxiety 63
detachment, seperation anxiety 63–64
development 168–170
　assessment 169–170
　interlinked aspects 170t
　measurement 169
　rate differences 169
　see also growth and development;
　　*specific systems (e.g. cognitive
　　development)*
development theory, adolescents,
　therapeutic relationship 716–717
developmental dysplasia of hip (DDH)
　573–574
　treatment 574
developmental milestones 170
developmental psychology *see*
　psychological development
developmental stages 223
　Erikson, Erik *see* psychosocial
　　development
　Freud, Sigmund *see* Freud, Sigmund,
　　personality development theory
　Piaget, Jean 223, 223t
　see also cognitive development
developmental status, hospitalisation
　effects 122
dexamethasone 523
　croup management 673
diabetes mellitus 545–554
　education 551–552
　　developmental work 215
　incidence 545–546
　maturity onset diabetes of the young
　　(MODY) 553–554
　middle childhood 696
diabetes mellitus, type 1 diabetes
　546–552
　adolescence 551
　assessment and diagnosis 546
　care and management 546–551
　　blood glucose monitoring 548
　　diet 548
　　exercise 548–549

insulin dosages and regimes
546–548
needle phobia 547–548
complications 549–551
chronic 550–551
diabetic ketoacidosis 549–550
hypoglycaemia 548, 549t
education 551–552
diabetes mellitus, type 2 552–553
diabetic ketoacidosis 203
type 1 diabetes 549–550
type 2 diabetes 553
diabetic mothers, infants of,
hypoglycaemia risk 626
diagnosis, learning disabilities 788
diagnostic genetic testing 607
see also genetic testing
diagnostic overshadowing, learning
disabilities, health needs 791
diagnostic reasoning, assessment 91
dialysis 419
Diana, Princess of Wales Community
Child Nursing Teams 14
diaries and journals, research interviews
232
diarrhoea 447–448
acute, fluid therapy 402–403
acute infectious 447
causative organisms 449t
blood chemistry, abnormalities 399t
dehydration 396
diastolic blood pressure (DBP) 470,
470t
septic shock 761
see also blood pressure
diathermy
adenoidectomy 282
circumcision 280–281
operation procedures 291
diet(s)
advice, early childhood 673–674
elimination, food allergies 645
ketogenic, epilepsy 527
lacto-ovovegetarian 642t
lactovegetarian 642t
macrobiotic 642t
type 1 diabetes mellitus 548
weaning 639
see also nutrition, infancy
dimercaptosuccinic acid (DMSA)
scanning, genitourinary problems
407
diphtheria 654
signs/symptoms 654b
dipstick testing, urine 406–407
direct inguinal hernia 278–279
disability
communication 137–138
middle childhood 696
Disability Living Allowance
(DLA) 728
Disabled Child Premium in Income
Support 728
disabled children

vulnerability 34
vulnerability to abuse 305
disappointment, complaints 48
DISCERN, appraisal tool 601
discharge 293–294
information, paediatric emergency
assessment units (PEAU)
350–351
discipline acquisition, middle childhood
687
disease prevention, research studies 236
disease trajectory, chronic illness 733
disempowerment, family centred care
81–82
disimpaction, constipation 457
dispensaries
charitable 7
mortality rate reduction 7
origins 6–7
dissent 217
distraction 68
analgesia 272t
theatre reception 288
distraction method, hearing assessment
181–182
distributive shock 760, 760t
district nursing 106–107
divorce 27, 199–200
DNA 613
Do Not Attempt Resuscitation (DNAR)
326
dobutamine, shock treatment 764
doctors and nurses play sets 68
documentation, pain management 273
dolls, hospitalisation preparation 68, 73,
133, 135f
domestic violence, sources of stress 305
dominance, genetics 607, 614
Donaldson, Liam 313, 318, 320
dopamine, shock treatment 764
Doppler percutaneous flow probe 470
double blinding 233
Down syndrome
gastro-oesophageal reflux 446
genetic basis 616, 617f
learning disabilities 787
plastic surgery 326
Draft Standard on Child Protection 225
drama, communication tool 132
dressing, early childhood 677
drinking, complex motor disability
382–384
nursing assessment 383, 383t
nursing intervention 383–384
drooling, complex motor disability
383
drowning 586
drug administration routes
analgesia 267
palliative care 775
drug dosage, safety see medication
administration, safety
drug metabolism 223
drug misuse, sources of stress 305

Duchenne muscular dystrophy 372
ductus arteriosus, patent 468
duress 320–321
duty of care 326
DVD films, hospitalisation preparation
70
dysfunctional communication, children
131

early childhood
bereavement 683–684
body temperature control 680–681
cleansing 677
communication development
670–671
death, effects of 683–684
dressing 677
egocentricity 666–667
elimination 675
motor skill acquisition 666
nutrition see nutrition, early childhood
physiological changes 183–184
playing 682
sexuality 682–683
sleeping 683
early childhood, health problems
665–685
accidental poisoning 667–668
asthma see asthma
burns/scalds 668–669
fluid loss 669
management 669t
choking 668
dental caries 677–678
eczema 678–679
see also eczema
environmental safety 666–667
accident incidence 667
fevers/pyrexia 680–681
gastroenteritis 675–677, 676t
oral rehydration solutions 675–676
glue ear 670–671
autoinflation 671
grommet insertion 671
head lice 679–680
mobilising 670
non-accidental injury 670
Roper–Logan–Tierney model 666,
666b
scabies 679
sleep deprivation 683
upper respiratory tract infections
671–672
epiglottitis 673
signs/symptoms 672b
see also individual diseases/disorders
early psychological traumas 33
eating, complex motor disability
382–384
nursing assessment 383, 383t
eating disorders, adolescents 707
eccrine glands 478
echocardiography 471–472
ecomaps 20–21, 22–23, 22f

economic aspects, nutrition, early childhood 674
eczema 643–647, 678–679
  allergies 645
  atopic *see* atopic eczema
  food allergies 645
  irritants 645
  management 678
education 14–16
  diabetes, nurses role and responsibilities 551–552
  inherited conditions 612
  nurse 14
  nurses' role in chronic illness 733–734
  origins of 10–14
  palliative care 776
Education Act (1944) 108
educational needs, learning disabilities 789
educational programmes, chronic illness, self-management 730
educative play 67
egocentricity, early childhood 666–667
eight-month check 181–182
Electra complex 160
electrocardiography (ECG) 290, 471t
  cardiovascular problems 471
electroencephalogram (EEG), cerebral dysfunction 512
electrolytes
  functions and regulatory systems 394–396
    plasma reference values 394t
    requirements 394t
  imbalance *see* body fluid and electrolyte imbalance
electromyography (EMG), cerebral dysfunction 512
elimination, early childhood 675
elimination diets, food allergies 645
Ellerton and Merriman 65
emergency anaesthetics 291
emergency assessment units *see* paediatric emergency assessment units (PEAU)
emergency department management 353–367
  care teams 357–358
  environment 358
  family-centred care 364–366
  fits, convulsions and seizures 355–357
  medicine administration and safety 361–364
    see also medication administration, safety
  national picture 353–354
  nurses roles 358
    nurse practitioner 366
  observations 366
  pain
    recognition and assessment 360–361
    relief 361, 361t

play, role of 366
respiratory failure 360
transportation 354–355
treating children and adults together 354
triage 358–360
wound management 366
emergency intubation 289
emotion interpretation ability, young children 130
emotional abuse, definition 301
emotional contagion, hospitalisation 71–72
emotional difficulties, vulnerability 34
emotional life, families 30
emotional responses, parents, chronic illness 726–727
emotional well-being, mental health 708–709
empathy, adolescents, therapeutic relationship 714
empiricist psychological perspective 147
  language acquisition/development 155
employment overseas 15
empowerment 78, 591–605
  definition 591–592
  family centred care *see* family-centred care
  patient-centred care 592–593
encephalitis, acquired rubella 662
end-of-life issues 324–325
endocardium 465
endocrine disorders 535–557
  adrenal function 542–545, 542t
    see also entries under adrenal function disorders
  endocrine system physiology *see* endocrine system
  gonads 545
  thyroid function *see* thyroid function disorders
  see also diabetes mellitus
endocrine system 535–545
  gland types 535, 536f
  hypothalamus 535–536
    hypothalamic hormones 536f
  neonates 173
  pituitary gland 536–540
    see also entries under pituitary gland
endoscopic injection therapy, vesicoureteric reflux 412
endotracheal intubation, definition 739
English National Board for Nursing and Midwifery (ENB) 43
enmeshment, family functioning 31
enteral feeding
  neonates 628–629
  preterm infants, mucosal immunity 481
environment, genetic interactions 308
environmental control, cultural assessment 58–59
ependymomas 521
epidurals 268, 269t
epiglottitis 434–435

early childhood 673
Haemophilus influenzae 658
epilepsy 525–527
  aetiology 525–526
  classification 526
  fits 355
  incidence 525f
  long term outcomes 527
  presentation 526
  syndromes 526
  treatment and management 526–527
epiphyseal fractures 564f
equipment misuse 306
Erickson model, adolescent development 702
Erikson's stages, psychosocial development *see* psychosocial development
Escherichia coli
  diarrhoea 449t
  gastroenteritis 676t
  neonatal sepsis 478
  urinary tract infection 405
Escherichia coli 157, gastroenteritis 676t
The Essence of care 51, 247
  benchmarking toolkit 216
  paediatric emergency assessment units (PEAU) 349
ethics 309–316
  four principles 311–312
  genetic testing 620–621
  pain management 273
  palliative care 773
  predictive genetic testing 621
  unethical practices in the past 310
ethnicity 55–56
ethnocentrism 56–57
European Commission, research 235
European Convention for the Protection of Human Rights and Fundamental Freedoms (1950) 317
European Convention on Human Rights, article 8 325
European Convention on the Rights of the Child (1989) 5
European Court of Human Rights 325
European Health Council's Resolution on Paediatric Medicinal Products 235
Every child matters (DfES 2003) 44, 299
evidence-based practice
  benchmarking 216
  categorisation of evidence 212–213
  child protection and confidentiality 218–219
  complex intervention research 215
  critical appraisal issues 216–219
  ethical considerations 212, 216–219
  experimental research 212
  formulating questions 211–212

guidelines, research with children
    217–218
    minimising bias 212–213
    randomised controlled trials 214–215
    research foundation 235
    researcher role conflict 218
    systematic reviews 213–214
    types of evidence 213–215
examination syllabus, compilation
    12–13
experimental treatment, consent
    325–326
expert information, communication
    140–141
    guidelines 140–141
expiratory reserve volume (ERV),
    breathing 746
expiratory time (Te) 749
expressivity
    genetics 607
    inherited conditions 615–616
extended family, bereavement care 781
extracellular fluid 391–392
    interstitial fluid 392
    intravascular fluid compartment 392
extubation ('weaning'), respiratory
    support 753
eyes
    infection barriers 480
    neonates 172

fabricated or induced illness (FII) 306
face, legs, activity, cry, consolability
    (FLACC) 262, 263t, 265t
faces pain scale 262, 263f, 263t
facial proportions, 5 years to
    adolescence 192–193
failure to thrive (FTT)
    nutrition, early childhood 674–675
    see also nutrition, infancy
falls 587
families
    communication 30
    concerns 114–115
    defining 19
    development assessment 23–29
    diagram 20–22, 21f
    emotional life 30
    functioning, assessment 29
    life cycle theory 27–29
    nursing 18–32
    stress 201
        coping 202
        sources 305
    structure assessment 20–23
        ecomaps 20–21, 22–23, 22f
        genograms 20–22, 21f
    systems theory 19–20
    understanding system 19–20
    working with 18–32
family-centred care 77–88
    challenges 85–86
    communication skills 81
    as a concept 78–80

continuity 81
    definitions 78–80
    disempowerment 81–82
    emergency departments 364–366
    empowerment 81–83
        competencies 83
        outcomes 82
        process 82–83
        relationship building 83
    family expertise 86
    frameworks 78–80
        functional 79–80
        hierarchical 79–80
        holistic 79–80
    historical perspectives 62
    individual family variation 78
    negotiating care 83–85
        assessment 84
        evaluation 85
        implementation 85
        planning 84–85
    ongoing evaluation 81
    practice continuum tool 80–81, 80f
        equal status 80
        nurse-led care, family involvement
            80
        nurse-led care, family participation
            80
        nurse-led care, family partnership
            80
        nurse-led care, no family
            involvement 80
        parent-led care, nurse-consulted
            care 80
    professional and legal issues 86–87
        negligence 86
        nursing documentation 86
family-centred critical care 765–767
    advantages 767t
    'child data' vs. 'data-child' 766
    definition 766–767
    disadvantages 767t
    grounded theory approaches 766–767
Family Division of the High Court 317
family history, atopic eczema 644
family information nurse (FIN) 599
family information service 599
Family Law Reform Act (1969) 320,
    323
family rights breaches, contemporary
    examples 313–314
family tree (genograms) 20–22, 21f
farm injuries 587–588
fat embolism, fracture complications
    562
fatal maltreatment 302
fatigue, malignant disease treatment
    498–499
febrile response 486–487
    see also fever
Female Genital Mutilation Act 2003
    319
femoral derotation, developmental
    dysplasia of hip (DDH) 574

Fenwick, B. 12
fetal blood pressure 170
fetal origins hypothesis 236
fever
    early childhood 680–681
    febrile response 487
fibrosis, definition 739
Fick principle 756
field block, emergency department use
    361t
financial assistance, foundling hospitals
    and dispensaries 7
financial concerns
    learning disabilities 788
    palliative care 776
financial consequences, chronic illness
    727 728
fine movement see vision and fine
    movement
fire-related deaths 583
A first class service: quality in the new
    National Health Service (DoH
    1998) 239, 243
Fit for the Future (1976), Accident and
    Emergency services for children
    353
fits see seizures
FLACC (face, legs, activity, cry,
    consolability) 262, 264t, 265t
flaccid paralysis, poliomyelitis (polio)
    657
fluid loss, burns/scalds 669
fluid replacement therapy, shock
    treatment 763–764
'focal theory,' adolescents 702–703
focus groups, research 232–233
focused assessment see assessment
follow-on milks 638
fontanelle 174, 178
food allergies
    early childhood 674
    gastrointestinal problems 448–457
    infancy see nutrition, infancy
food fortification, nutrition, early
    childhood 675
food intolerance
    breastfeeding 640
    infancy see nutrition, infancy
foramen ovale, patent 468
foreign languages, hospitalisation
    preparation 70
formal operational stage (11–12),
    Piagetian cognitive development
    148
formula, nutrition, infancy 637–638
Foundation for Sudden Infant Death
    (FSID) 650
Foundling Hospital, Hatton Gardens,
    establishment 6, 105–106
foundling hospitals, origins 6–7
fractures 562–566
    complications 562–564
    holding methods 565–566
    middle childhood 691

fractures (*Continued*)
neurovascular observations 564–565
open, classification 572t
repair 560
traction 566–569
see also entries under traction
treatment 565
types 562, 563f, 564f
Framework for the future (1997) 365
Frank–Starling's law 755, 755f
definition 739
see also cardiac contractility
Fraser guidelines 311
free attention 711
freely given consent 320–321
Freud, Sigmund, personality
development theory 159–160
id, ego and superego 159
relevance to research 223, 223t
stage 1, oral stage (birth to 1 year)
159
stage 2, anal stage (1–3 years)
159–160
stage 3, phallic stage (3–6 years)
159–160
stage 4, latency period (6 to puberty)
160
stage 5, genital stage (puberty
onwards) 160
frozen watchfulness 306
fruit juices, weaning 639
functional framework, family-centred
care 79–80
functional health patterns 97
nursing assessment 97b
functional residual capacity (FRC),
definition 740

gag reflex 516
Gallows traction 566, 567f
gas conditioning, lung injury reduction
748
gastritis 283
gastro-oesophageal reflux 446–447
gastroenteritis
dehydration 396
early childhood *see* early childhood,
health problems
see also diarrhoea
gastrointestinal motility, neonates 627
gastrointestinal problems 445–459
diarrhoea 447–448
food allergies 448–457
malabsorption 448–457
vomiting 446–447
gastrointestinal tract
infection barriers 480–482
neonates 173
gastronomy, complex motor disability
384
gastroschisis 279–280, 281f
gate control theory 257
Gaudian, C. 68
Geldhart, Nicholas 43

gender differences, adolescent stressors
200
gender relationships, adolescents
703–704
gender roles 24–25
General Nursing Council (GNC) 12–13
generalised assessment 96–99
tools 97
see also assessment
generalised tetanus 655
genes 613
alleles 607
definition 607
environment interactions 308
genetic counselling 617–620
certainty 619
core competence statements 618b
information need 619
skills 619
see also inherited conditions
genetic diseases *see* inherited conditions
genetic testing 617, 618b
adrenoleucodystrophy 910
carrier 607
cystic fibrosis 617, 910
definition 607
diagnostic 607
ethical issues 620–621
increase in 608–609
predictive *see* predictive genetic
testing
presymptomatic 607
genetics
alterations 614
carriers 607
DNA 613
dominance 607, 614
expressivity 607
genes *see* genes
genome 608
genotype 608
heterozygosity 608, 616
homozygosity 608, 616
inheritance 614–615
karyotype 608, 616, 616f
multifactorial conditions 608
mutations 614
nucleotides 613
penetrance 608
phenotype 608
recessive 614
see also chromosomes; inherited
conditions
Genetics White Paper 609
genitourinary problems 405–422
acute renal failure (ARF) 416–418
antibiotic therapy 407
chronic renal failure 418–419
circumcision 415–416
cryptorchidism 415
diagnostic problems 406
education 407–408
hypospadias 413–414
investigations 407

nephrotic syndrome 408–410
nursing considerations 407
phimosis 416
poststreptococcal glomerulonephritis
(PSGN) 410–411
prevention 407–408
urinary tract infection *see* urinary tract
infections
urine collection 406
urine testing 406–407
vesicoureteric reflux 411–412
Wilms' tumour (nephroblastoma)
412–413
genograms 20–22, 21f
genome 608
genotype 608
germ theory 115
German measles *see* rubella
*Getting the right start: national service
framework for children* (2003), care
partnerships 365
giardia 449t
Gillick competency 225–226
parental refusal 320
research purposes 217, 228
*Gillick v West Norfolk and Wisbech
AHA* (1986) 311, 320
Glasgow Coma Scale (GCS) 391, 514,
514t
Adelaide Scale 515
James' adaptation 515
polytrauma 570
Glasgow Hospital for Sick Children 10
Glass, David 325
glial cells 508
global developmental delay,
hospitalisation preparation 73
glomerulonephritis, poststreptococcal *see*
poststreptococcal
glomerulonephritis (PSGN)
glucocorticoid hormones, hypoglycaemic
neonates 626
gluconeogenesis, hypoglycaemic
neonates 626
glucose 395
glue ear, early childhood *see* early
childhood, health problems
glycogenolysis, hypoglycaemic neonates
626
'good enough parenting' 300
Government Response to the House of
Commons Health Committee
Reports on Children and Young
People (1197) 42–43
Gow, Peggy 38
graduated extension and fading, bedtime
routines 648
gram-negative bacteria, complement
483
granulocyte colony stimulating factor
(GCSF) 496
grasp reflex 176
Graves' disease 541
care scenario 554

Great Ormond Street Hospital for Children *see* Hospital for Sick Children (Great Ormond Street)
grommet insertion, glue ear 671
gross negligence manslaughter 327–328
group B haemolytic streptococcus *see* *Streptococcus* group B haemolytic
'growing pains,' middle childhood 691
growth and development 165–168
    assessment 167–168
        percentile charts 168
    changes in shape and proportion 168
    factors affecting 164
    height and weight gain trends 185
    hospitalisation effects 122
    measurement 165–167
        bone age 167
        head circumference 167
        length/height 165–166
        skinfold thickness 167, 167f
        surface area 167
        weight 165 166
    pattern of growth 165
    rates 165f
        normal 540t
    velocity, babies and toddlers (1–24 months) 176
    see also development
growth hormone deficiencies 537–540
    biosynthetic somatrophin 539
    care and management 539, 539t
    child and family resources 539–540
guided imagery, hospitalisation preparation 73
guidelines
    asthma management 440
    choking 668
    imparting expert information 140–141
    psychosocial development assessment 20
    research 314
Guiding physicians in biomedical research involving human subjects 310
guilt
    inherited conditions 612
    psychosocial development 158
gut-associated lymphoid tissue (GALT) 481

haemodynamic control 754–765
haemodynamic monitoring, shock 761–762
haemoglobin, sickle-cell disease 614
Haemophilus influenzae 658–659
    diagnosis 658
    epidemiology 658
    management 658
    pathology 658
    vaccination 658–659
Haemophilus influenzae B 434
handover

complaints 48
information repetition 48
handwashing policies 478
Harlow, Harry 63
Hart v Brown 325
head
    5 years to adolescence 192–193
    circumference 167
    positioning
        3 months 178, 178f, 179f
        6 months 179, 180f, 181f
        babies and toddlers (1–24 months) 176, 176f
        neonates 174, 175f
head lice, early childhood 679–680
health
    assessment by telephone *see* telephone health assessment
    children's conceptions *see* concepts of health/illness
    child's understanding of 133–134
    concepts 152–154
    inequalities 34, 45
    misconceptions 153–154
    needs, learning disabilities *see* learning disabilities
    policy *see* health policy
    promotion, middle childhood 688–690
Health Commission 45, 253
Health for all children 582
health information, consumer *see* consumer health information
Health of the Nation (DoH 1992) 110
health policy 33–53
    complaints 45–52
        see also complaints
    inequalities 34
    reviews 34–35
        government response 34–35
    role 34
    variations 35, 36
    see also specific policies
health promotion
    immunisations 653
    middle childhood 688–690
    sexual, malignant disease survivors 502
health-related quality of life
    chronic illness *see* chronic illness
    studies 230–231
Health Service Circular 34
Health Service Commissioner 47–48
health visiting
    history 107–108
    primary care support 118
health visitors, sudden infant death syndrome (SIDS) 650
healthcare research, involving children 222–241
    advocacy and best interest 229
    areas/models of involvement 237–238
    child protection issues 224–225
    children not as small adults 222–224

competency 226
conduction methods 229
critiquing research papers 235–236
design and methodologies 230
difficulties 238–239
evidence-based practice 235
extent of involvement 239–240
focus groups 232–233
Government support 239
informed consent issues 225–226, 227
origin of disease and prevention 236
quality of life studies 230–231
randomised controlled trials 233
reasons for 234
research interviews 231–232
as researchers 236–237
risk *vs.* benefits 228
unlicensed and 'off-label' medicines 234
US *vs.* EU perspectives 234–235
volunteering 227, 228
vulnerability and autonomy 225
write and draw method 232
see also research
healthcare workers, bereavement care 781
hearing and speech 180
    1 month 177
    1 year 182
    3 months 179
    6 months 180
    18 months 183
    assessment, 8-month check 181–182
    neonates 172
heart
    developmental changes 464–465
    electrophysiology 465
    embryonic and fetal, development *see under* cardiovascular system
    embryonic development 460–464
    murmurs 471
    normal range 465t
    normal size and position 464
    transplantation 468
heart failure, congestive *see* congestive cardiac failure
heart rate 430f
    definition 740
    infants 465–466
    neonates 172
heat
    loss, neonates 624
    regulation, neonates 171
height
    measurement 165–166, 166f
        gain trends, babies and toddlers 185
    middle childhood 695
Help for Health Trust 593–594
Helsinki Declaration 310
hepatitis A, gastroenteritis 676t
hernia
    inguinal *see* inguinal hernia
    repair 278–279

heterozygosity, genetics 608, 616
Hi-Quality Key, assessment tool 601
hierarchical framework, family-centred care 79–80
High Court, Family Division 317
hip
  assessment, babies 178
  developmental dysplasia (DDH) 573–574
'hip click,' developmental dysplasia of hip (DDH) 573
hip spica cast, nursing care 574–575
histamine 486
history inconsistencies 306
history of children's nursing 3–17
history taking
  middle childhood 694–695
  open-ended questions 694
  paediatric emergency assessment units (PEAU) 348
  respiratory illness 432
'holding on' 24
holistic framework, family-centred care 79–80
home care schemes, emerge of 13–14
homeostasis 395–396, 755f
homologous chromosomes 616
homozygosity, genetics 608, 616
honesty, palliative care 773
Horder Report 14–15
horizontal stresses, families 29
hormones
  growth and development 165t
    adolescence 193, 193f, 195f
  see also individual hormones
hospices 771
  see also palliative care
hospital-acquired infections 478
hospital admission
  intensive care, criteria 740
  preadmission programmes 205, 287
  traumatic memories 205–206
  unexpected, effect on siblings 121
  see also hospitalisation
Hospital for Sick Children (Edinburgh) 9–10
  children's outpatient department 109
Hospital for Sick Children (Great Ormond Street)
  early history 62
  foundation 7–8
  mission statement 312
Hospital for Sick Children (Toronto) 70
  telephone consultation 336
hospital play corners 72
hospital welfare 14
hospitalisation
  effect on child development 33–34
  family response see hospitalisation, family responses
  nature of 120, 123
  preparation 65–72
    play 133

  psychological see hospitalisation, psychological preparation for
  recovery promotion 134
  as stressor 205–208
  see also hospital admission
hospitalisation, family responses 114–126
  age of child 122
  coping strategies 114–118
    community support 117
    'family wisdom' 115–117, 116t
    primary care support 117–118
    socioeconomics 116
  developmental status of child 122
  informed consent 124
  parental concerns 120–121
  planned vs. unplanned 123–124
  psychological reactions 120–122
  siblings 121
  socioeconomic class 123
  statistics 115
  ward choice 124
hospitalisation, psychological preparation for 61–76, 65–72
  attachment theory 62–63
  community preparation 72–73
  daycare services 64
  definition 61
  historical perspectives 61–64
  importance 64–65
  initiatives 61
  materials 69–71
  maternal deprivation 63–64
  parents 71–72
  practitioner perspectives 74
  preparation programmes 66–67
    distraction 68–69
    dolls 67
    information 69
    play 66
    visual materials 69–71
    written material 69–71
  recognition 61
  specific preparation needs 73
  surgery 284
  variation in child needs 72
house fires 585
House of Commons Health Committee reports (DoH 1997) 42–43
Human Fertilisation and Embryology Act 1990 319
Human Genome Project 608–609
Human Growth Foundation 540
human papillomavirus (HPV), circumcision 416
Human Rights Act (1998) 4–5, 310–311
  article 3 311
  breaches 317
  end of life issues 324
Human Tissue Act (1961) 313
humidity, croup management 673
Hutt, Jane 35
hyaline cartilage 560

hydrocele 279
  communicating 279
hydrocephalus 528–530
  aetiology 528
  classification 528
  diagnosis 528
  long-term outcomes 530
  presentation 528
  treatment and management 528–530
hyperaldosteronism, primary 544
hyperbilirubinaemia, hypothermic neonates 625
hypercapnia, permissive, lung injury reduction 747–748
hyperglycaemia, type 2 diabetes 553
hyperkalaemia 402
  acute renal failure (ARF) 417
hyperlipidaemia, nephrotic syndrome 408
hypernatraemia
  dehydration 397
  hypothermic neonates 625
hyperpituitarism 537
hypertension, chronic renal failure 419
hyperthyroidism 541–542
hypervolaemia 397
hypnosis, analgesia 272t
hypoalbuminaemia, nephrotic syndrome 408
hypoglycaemia
  neonatal see entries under neonates, health problems
  type 1 diabetes 548, 549t
hyponatraemia 390
  dehydration 397
  water intoxication 397
hypopituitarism 537
hypospadias 281, 284f, 285f, 413–414
  causes 414
  complications 414
  postoperative care 414
  surgery 414
hypotension, septic shock 761, 761f
hypothalamus 535–536
  hypothalamic hormones 536f
hypothermia, neonatal see entries under neonates, health problems
hypothyroidism 540–541
hypovolaemia 392
hypovolaemic shock 759–760, 760t
hypoxemia, permissive, lung injury reduction 747–748
hypoxia
  definition 740
  neonates, hypoglycaemia risk 626

ibuprofen, fevers/pyrexia 681
identity, formation in adolescence 25
identity search, adolescent development 702
identity status 25–26
'if only syndrome' 48–49
Ilizarov frame 569f
illness

acute, middle childhood 695
causation categories 116, 116t
children's conceptions *see* concepts of health/illness
child's understanding of 133–134
chronic *see* chronic illness
concepts 152–154
life-limiting *see* life-limiting illnesses
minor, chronic 733–734
misconceptions 153–154
severity assessment, respiratory illness 436f
as stressor 205–208
imagery, analgesia 272t
imaging techniques, cerebral dysfunction 512
imitation, neonatal communication skills 128–130
immanent justice, Piagetian cognitive development 149
immune system 476–489, 653–654
　active immunity 653–654
　　artificially-acquired 654
　　naturally-acquired 653–654
　　see also immunisation
　barrier mechanisms 477–482
　　eyes 480
　　gastrointestinal tract 480–482
　　respiratory tract 479–480
　　skin 477–479
　　urogenital tract 482
　immediate response 477–484
　　see also innate immunity
　inflammatory response 484–487
　　see also inflammatory response
　passive immunity 653
　　artificially-acquired 653
　　naturally-acquired 653
　successful pathogens 485
　see also immunity
immunisation 118, 651–662
　health promotion aspects 653
　importance of 651–653
　lack of 652, 652t
　　nonattendees 652
　recommended 653t
　see also vaccination/vaccines
immunity
　establishment of 476
　innate *see* innate immunity
　neonates 629
　see also immune system
immunoglobulin(s) 478–479, 483
　gastrointestinal tract 481
　immunoglobulin A (IgA) 481
　immunoglobulin E (IgE), atopic eczema 644
　immunoglobulin G (IgG) 483
　immunoglobulin M (IgM) 483
　neonates 174, 629
　respiratory tract 480
imprinting theory 62–63
inadequate feeding, failure to thrive (FTT) 643

indirect inguinal hernia 278–279
individuality, palliative care 773
infancy/infants
　consent issues 319
　definition 637
　eczema *see* atopic eczema
　examinations
　　6-week check *see* six (6)-week check
　　8-month check 181–182
　health problems 637–664
　　eczema *see* atopic eczema; eczema
　　immunisation *see* immunisation
　　nutrition *see* nutrition, infancy
　massage, hospitalisation preparation 73
　parental recognition 149
　recumbent length 165, 166f
　sleep/rest 647–651
　　apnoea of infancy 651
　　beneficial effects 648
　　physiology 647–648
　　routines 648
　　see also sudden infant death syndrome (SIDS)
　see also babies and toddlers (1–24 months); neonates; preterm infants
infections
　malignant disease 497
　mortality rates 476
　neonates *see* neonates, health problems
　risk, respiratory illness 423
infectious diseases, early children's hospitals 7
infertility, cystic fibrosis complications 452
inflammation, atopic eczema 646
inflammatory bowel disease (IBD) 454–455
inflammatory response 484–487
　febrile response 486–487
　gastrointestinal tract 481
　mediators 486
　pain 486
　protective properties 486
　respiratory tract 480
　signs 484
inflection point, breathing 746
information
　giving
　　consumer health information growth 593–596
　　empowering families *see* empowerment
　　families 597–599
　　kiosks 596
　hospitalisation preparation 69
　learning disabilities 789
　local, production of 599–600
　quality, improvement 600
　repetition, handover 48
　writing patient information leaflets 600–605

accuracy 605
availability 604
clarity 603
linking to national strategy 604–605
relevance 602–603
style 600–601
informed consent 225–228
　competent person, giving 319
　controversial or experimental treatment 325–326
　definition 217t
　forms of 319
　freely given consent 320–321
　Helsinki Declaration 310, 321
　issues 225–226
　Nursing and Midwifery Council stance 226
　obtaining valid consent 319
　organ retention 314
　perioperative setting 284–286
　questionable competency, parents 320
　refusal of treatment 321
　research 227–228
　treatment 318–319
infringement of rights 4
inguinal hernia 280f
　direct 278–279
　indirect 278–279
inhalation, mechanism of 425
inhaled nitric oxide, lung injury reduction 748
inherited conditions 607–622
　accepting the condition 610
　　siblings 610
　crises effects 612
　education 612
　emotional effects 612
　　blame 612
　　guilt 612
　examples 615t
　expressivity 615–616
　impact of 609–613
　　on parents 610
　incidence 612
　management of 610
　normal developmental needs 611
　patterns of inheritance 614–615
　　autosomal dominant 614, 615f, 616t
　　autosomal recessive 615, 616t
　　mitochondrial DNA 615–616
　　X-linked inheritance 615, 615f, 616t
　penetrance 615–616
　stress effects 612
　support systems 612
　see also genetic counselling; genetics
injury prevention 581–590
　3 E's strategy 581
　drowning 586
　falls 587
　farm injuries 587
　house fires 585
　playground injuries 588

injury prevention (*Continued*)
poisoning 588–589
practitioner role 582–583
advocate for children 582
child surveillance programme 582–583
working with other organisations 583
risk factors 583–584
personality 584
social gradients 583–584
road traffic accidents 583–585
scalds 585–586
innate immunity 477–484
barrier mechanisms 477–482
cell-mediated mechanisms 482–483
humoral defence mechanisms 483–484
inotropic agents
definition 740
shock treatment 764
inspiratory time (Ti) 749
Institute of Child Health 34
instrument nurse, legal responsibility 291
insulin, dosages and regimes, type 1 diabetes 546–548
integrated care pathway 99
'integrated stress and coping framework' 199
intelligence quotient (IQ), learning disabilities 786
intensive care
admission criteria 740
design 770
family presence 364–365
levels of care 365
parental experiences 765
see also critical illness
interactionist psychological perspective, language acquisition/development 155–156
Interdepartmental Committee on Physical Deterioration (1904) 108
interleukins (IL) 485
intermittent mandatory ventilation (IMV), mechanical ventilation 750
International Association for the Study of Pain (IASP) 256–257
International Classification of Functioning, Disability and Health (2002) 373
International Classification of Impairments, Disabilities and Handicaps (1980) 373
International Conference on Harmanisation (ICH) 229
Guideline for good clinical practice 223, 227
International League Against Epilepsy (ILAE) 355
seizure classification 526, 526f

International Society of Paediatric Oncology (SIOP), Wilms' tumour (nephroblastoma) 413
internet
child friendliness of care 94
chronic illness 724–725
hospitalisation preparation 70
quality of advice 117
interpersonal context of care, assessment 91–92
interpersonal skills 710–714
active listening 711–712
free attention 711
narrative theory 712
re-positioning 713
reformulation 711
therapeutic style 710–711
interstitial fluid 392
intersubjective companion space, neonatal communication skills 128
intestine
atresia 280
neonates 173–174
see also large intestine
intracellular fluid 390–391
intracranial pressure (ICP) 513f
hyponatraemia 391
raised 512–513
intramuscular injections, palliative care 775
intravascular fluid compartment 392
intubation, respiratory support 742, 743f, 744
invasive procedures, parental presence 364
INVOLVE 237–239
iron-deficiency anaemia 674–675
irreversible shock 757
definition 740
irritants, eczema 645
isonatraemic dehydration 396–397
It's all in the zap 495

jaundice, neonates 173, 632–634
non-physiological 633–634
physiological 627, 632–634
joints 560
Jolly, J. 64–65
Just for the Day (CCHS 1991) 39
justice 312

kangaroo care 635
karyotype 608, 616, 616f
Kennedy, Ian 44, 314, 321
Kennedy report 124
ketogenic diet, epilepsy 527
key performance standards (KPS), research 237
key worker schemes, nurses' role in chronic illness 731–732
kidney transplant 419
Kidscape 199

labelling, learning disabilities *see* learning disabilities
lactase 453
lacto-ovovegetarian diets 642t
Lactobacillus 482
lactoferrin, breastmilk 481
β-lactoglobulin, cow's milk allergy 453
lactose intolerance 453–454, 641
lactovegetarian diets 642t
lambdoid synostosis 524f
Laming report, child protection, confidentiality issues 335
Lamprill, J 233
Langerhans cells 479
language
acquisition/development 129, 154–156
delay 200
empiricist psychological perspective 155
interactionist psychological perspective 155–156
nativist psychological perspective 155
practical applications 156
appropriateness 121
focus groups 233
choice, assessment 92
see also hearing and speech
laparoscopic appendicectomy 283, 288f
large intestine
atresia 280
commensal bacteria 481–482
laryngospasm 289
laryngotracheobronchitis *see* croup
leaflets, hospital preparation 70
LEARN model framework 81, 84
learning disabilities 511t, 784–794
causative factors 787
pre-/peri-/postnatal 787
cognitive functioning approach 786
developmental approach 786
growing up 788–789
educational needs 789
financial concerns 788
information 789
view of 788–789
health needs 790–791
communication 791
diagnostic overshadowing 791
negative attitudes 791
time 791
impact of 787–788
incidence 787
initial diagnosis 788
intelligence quotient (IQ) 786
labelling 785–786
benefits 785–786
negative consequences 785
service planners 785–786
service providers 785–786
social functioning 786

social model 784–785
terminology 785–786
transition to adult services 789–790
working together 791–793
collaborative working 792–793
nursing role 792
learning disability nurses 792–793
Learning to listen report (DoH 2003) 239
legal actions, limitations 327
legal incompetence 310
legal issues 317–329
family-centred care 86–87
legal system 317–321
Legg–Calve–Perthes' disease 575–576
'letting go' 24
leucocyte esterase 407
leukaemia
acute lymphoblastic 501–502
acute myeloid 501
diagnosis 492
investigations 496
lichenification, atopic eczema 645
lies, childhood communication skills 131
life-limiting illnesses
communication 137–138
reaction to 771 772
see also palliative care
life stressors, social responses and coping 198–202
limitless ability 25
listening 141
Listening to Children: Children, Ethics and Social Research (1995) 42
liver, neonates 174
liver disease/dysfunction, cystic fibrosis complications 452
Liverpool Infant Distress Scale, neonatal pain assessment 630
lobar pneumonia 437
local anaesthesia 268
emergency department use 361t
local authority child protection registers 304
local research ethics committees (LRECs) 217, 315
localised tetanus 655
Lorenz, Konrad 62–63
loss of a parent 199–200
low self-esteem, adolescents 705
lower respiratory tract infection 437 438
lumbar puncture
cerebral dysfunction 512
leukaemia 496
lung
growth, toddlers 184
injury reduction, ventilation *see* mechanical ventilation
structure 424, 424f
volumes 425
breathing 747f
lung surfactant

breathing 746
respiratory distress syndrome 631
lymph 392
lymphatic system, toddlers 184
lymphocytes
B lymphocytes 479, 484
breastmilk 481
T lymphocytes *see* T lymphocytes
lysozymes 479
breastmilk 481
salvia 481
tears 480

macrobiotic diets 642t
macrophages 479, 484–486
breastmilk 481
Makaton system 386f
make believe play 186–188
malabsorption, gastrointestinal problems 448–457
male roles, bereavement care 780
malignant disease 490–506
diagnosis
confirmation 493–494
informing child 493–494
pre-diagnosis 491–492
reaching a diagnosis 492–493
illness trajectory 491–501
diagnosis and treatment *see above/below*
discharge 500
palliative care and death 501
psychological care 499–500
relapse/recurrence 501
remission 500–501
malignancy, definition 490–491
shared care 491
survival 502–503
adolescents 502
siblings 503
treatment
commencement 494–496
side effects 496–499, 502
see also specific treatment types
malnutrition, mortality rates 477f
maltreatment 297
causation theories 304
definitional problems 299 301
fatal 302
identification 301
morbidity causes 44
National Commission of Inquiry into the Prevention of Child Abuse's definition 301
non-fatal 302–303
official statistics 304
prevalence 302–303
professional responsibilities 305–307
recognition 306
referral 306–307
risk factors 305
scale of problem 302–303
social class bias 305

theories of 304
undetected cases 305
malunion, fracture complications 562
Manchester and Salford Sanitary Reform Association 107
Manchester triage system 358–359
manslaughter, gross negligence 327–328
Marcia, James 25
marital relationships, parents, chronic illness 728–729
massage, analgesia 272t
maternal deprivation 63–64
maternal hormones 171, 173
maternal nutrition, alterations 236
maternity services 45
maturation, definition 165, 169
mature minor, consent issues 320
maturity onset diabetes of the young (MODY) 553–554
Maxwell's six dimensions of quality 243–244
McCubbin's resiliency model 201
McMaster model, family functioning 29
mean airway pressure (MAP) 749
mean arterial blood pressure (MAP)
monitoring 762
shock compensatory mechanisms 758
measles 659–660, 682
complications 659
diagnosis 659
epidemiology 659
notification rate 652t
prevention 659–660
see also measles, mumps and rubella (MMR) vaccine
treatment 659
measles, mumps and rubella (MMR) vaccine 660, 661, 662, 682
safety of 652
side effects 660
Meath Children's Hospital 9
mechanical ventilation 744–745
assessment/monitoring 751 753
capnography 752, 752f, 753f
cardiovascular complications 749
lung injury reduction 747–748
body positioning 748
gas conditioning 748
inhaled nitric oxide 748
permissive hypercapnia 747–748
permissive hypoxemia 747–748
modes of 749–751, 750f
assisted control mode (ACM) 750
intermittent mandatory ventilation (IMV) 750
pressure support/control mode (PS/PC) 750
synchronised intermittent mandatory ventilation (SIMV) 750
settings 750
shearing forces 747
trouble-shooting 753

mechanical ventilation (*Continued*)
  ventilation-perfusion relationship 744–745, 744f
  see also respiratory support; *specific ventilation modes*
meconium 173
medical models of disability 372–373
medication administration, safety 361–364
  accuracy 362
  calculations 363–364
  dosage confirmation 362–363
  route 363
  side effects 363
  units used 362
  weight of child 362
medication misuse 306
medicines
  accidental poisoning 667–668
  poisoning risk 588
medulloblastomas 521
melanin levels, neonates 171
memory T cells, gastrointestinal tract 480
menarche, adolescence 194
  critical weight of onset 195
meninges 510
meningitis, *Haemophilus influenzae* 658
meningococcal septicaemic, septic shock 760–761
mental health 700–719
  adolescents 707
  assessment
    questions 706
    resilience factors 706
  children 705
  emotional well-being 708–709
  intervention 707–708
    necessity 708
    primary prevention 708
  middle childhood *see* middle childhood, health problems
  types 706
  young peoples' needs 709
Mental Health Act 1983 323–324
mental illness
  adolescents 200
  sources of stress 305
  treatment refusal 323–324
metabolism, toddler 184
methicillin-resistance *Staphylococcus aureus* (MRSA) 478, 485
metopic synostosis 524f
micro-organisms, commensal skin flora 478
microdeletions, chromosome abnormalities 617t
micturating cystourethrogram (MCU), genitourinary problems 407
middle childhood 188–195
  bullying 697–698
  citizenship 688
  cognitive development 689–690
  confidence development 688

developmental stage 686
  health promotion 688–690
  motor skills development 687–688
  physical activity 688
  self-esteem development 688
  social world 686–688
    discipline acquisition 687
    self-discipline acquisition 687
    skills development 687
middle childhood, health problems 686–699
  accidents 690–691
    social class *vs.* 690–691
  acute illnesses 695
  assessment 693–695
    height 695
    history taking 694–695
    physical examination 695
    preparation 693–694
    self-treatment 694
    temperature 695
    weight 695
  behavioural problems 687
  chronic illness 695–696
  mental health 696–697
    assessment 697
    social disadvantage 698
  motor vehicle accidents 690
  psychological problems 696
  school refusal 687
  socioeconomics 690
  surgery 691–693
    day-case surgery 691–693
    orthopaedic conditions 691
    venepuncture 693
midwife, primary care support 117–118
Midwives Act (1902) 12
Milburn, Alan 297, 313
milk feeds *see* nutrition, infancy
mineral oils, constipation 457
mineralocorticoids 542
minimal burden 228
minimal check, bedtime routines 648
Minister for Children 206
minor illnesses, chronic illnesses 733–734
minute volume (MV) 749
  definition 740
mitochondrial DNA, inherited conditions 615–616
mobile phones, child friendliness of care 94
mobility, complex motor disabilities 379–382
  nursing assessment 380–381, 381–382t
  nursing interventions 382
modeling behaviour, adolescents, interaction with 714
models of helping, adolescents, therapeutic relationship 715–716
Moncrieff, Alan 14–15
Monro–Kellie doctrine, raised intracranial pressure 512

Moos, R H 199
moro reflex 176, 176f
Mother Care for Children in Hospital 64
motor disability, complex *see* complex motor disability
motor function assessment
  6-week check 178
  8-month check 181
motor neuron 508f
motor skills, acquisition/development 170
  early childhood 666
  middle childhood 687–688
motor strength, consciousness assessment 515
motor vehicle accidents *see* road traffic accidents
moulding, neonates 174
movement, fine *see* vision and fine movement
MRSA 478, 485
mucopolysaccharides, saliva 481
mucus, infection barriers 480
multicultural Britain 54
multiple attachments 63
mumps 660–661
  complications 661
  prevention 661
    see also measles, mumps and rubella (MMR) vaccine
  signs/symptoms 660
  treatment 660
murder 328
muscle, skeletal 561–562
muscle biopsies, cerebral dysfunction 512
music therapy
  hospitalisation preparation 73
  palliative care 774
mutations 614
Mycobacterium tuberculosis 437
mycoplasma, pneumonia 437
myelination of nerves
  neonates 175
  toddlers 184
myocardial depressant factor (MDF), septic shock 761
myocardium 464–465
myoclonic fit 356

nail bed pressure, consciousness, assessment 515
narcissism acknowledgement, adolescents, interaction with 713
narrative theory 712
nasopharynx 424
National Association for the Welfare of Children in Hospital (NAWCH) *see* Action for Sick Children (ASC)
National Children's Bureau 218
National Children's Hospital (Ireland) 8–9

National Commission of Inquiry into the Prevention of Child Abuse 301–303
National Confidential Enquiries 253
National Confidential Enquiry into Perioperative Deaths (1989), emergency care teams 357
national curriculum, hospitalisation advice 121
National Health Service *see* National Health Service
National Health Service Act 107
National Institute for Clinical Excellence (NICE)
  asthma management guidelines 440
  consciousness assessment 515
  standards, identification 124
National Institute for Health (NIH) 234
national organisations, chronic illness support 735
National Paediatric Neuroscience Benchmarking group, consciousness assessment 515
National Patient Safety Authority (NPSA) 253
National Service Framework (NSF) 224
  disabled children 378
  information quality 604
National Service Framework for Children 44–45, 124, 248–249, 314
  Accident and Emergency services for children 354
  children's rights 206
  clinical governance 314
  healthcare demands in society 334
  information giving 593
  research 234–235
  standards 65–66
National service framework for children, standards for hospital services, mental health 700
National service framework for children, young people and maternity services, mental health 700–701
National Service Framework for Standards in Diabetes (2001) 552
National Society for the Prevention of Cruelty to Children (NSPCC) 297–298, 302
National Triage Scale 359
National Working Group on Child Protection and Disability 305
nativist psychological perspective 147
  language acquisition/development 155
natural killer (NK) cells 482
naturally-acquired active immunity 653–654
naturally-acquired passive immunity 653
nature-nuture debate 146–147
nausea

malignant disease treatment 497
  palliative care 776t
needle phobia, type 1 diabetes 547–548
negative attitudes, learning disabilities, health needs 791
negative eugenics 620
neglect, definition 301
negligence 326–327
  family-centred care 86
Neonatal and Paediatric Pharmacists Group statement, unlicensed medicine research 234
neonatal units, environment 634–635
neonates 170–176
  appearance 171
  cardiovascular system 172–173
  endocrine system 173
  eyes 172
  gastrointestinal system 173
  genitalia and breasts 171
  head positioning 174, 174f, 175f
  hearing 172
  immune system 174
  intestine 173–174
  measurements 170–171, 171f
  neurological system 175–176
  postoperative pain management 292
  reflexes 175
  renal system 173
  reproductive system 174
  respiratory system 172
  sepsis, causative organisms 478
  skeleto-muscular system 174, 174f, 175f
  skin 171
  small for gestational age (SGA), hypoglycaemia risk 626
  temperature 172
  thermoregulation 171–172
neonates, health problems 623–636
  attachment 634–635
  care issues 634
  hypoglycaemia 174, 626–627
    clinical signs 626–627
    definition 626
    gluconeogenesis 626
    management 627
    risk, infants at 626
    sequelae 627
  hypothermia 624–625
    cold stress 625
    definition 624
    heat loss 624
    hypoglycaemia risk 626
    management 625
    neutral thermal environment (NTE) 625
    rewarming 625
    temperature measurement 625
    temperature regulation 624
  infection 627, 629–630
    immunity 629
    nursing care 629–630
  nutrition 627–629

    feeding 628
    growth and development 627–628
    requirements 628
  pain 630
  parents 634
  prewarming equipment 624
  respiratory problems 631–634
    clinical signs 631
    jaundice *see* jaundice
    management principles 632
    meconium aspiration syndrome 632
    persistent pulmonary hypertension of the newborn (PPHN) 632
    pneumonia 632
    respiratory distress syndrome 631
    transient tachypnoea of the newborn (TTN) 631
neonatorum tetanus 655
neoplastic disorders 511t
nephroblastoma *see* Wilms' tumour (nephroblastoma)
nephrotic syndrome 392, 408–410
  complications 409
  diagnosis 408–409
  hyperlipidaemia 408
  hypoalbuminaemia 408
  medical treatment 409
  minimal change nephrotic syndrome 408
  nursing management 409–410
  pathology 408
  prognosis 410
nerve myelination 508
nervous system
  blood supply 510
  brain anatomy 509 510, 509f
  cells 508–509
  embryology 508, 508f
  malformations *see* neurological dysfunction
  neuron regeneration 510
  protection and coverings 510
  role, structure and function 507–511
  ventricular system 510
  see also brain
neurocutaneous disorders 511t
neurofibromatosis, patterns of inheritance 616
neurogenic shock 760
neuroglycopenia, hypoglycaemic neonates 627
neuroimaging, cerebral dysfunction 512
neurological dysfunction 507–534
  conditions, management
    brain tumours 520–523
    craniosynostosis 523–525
    epilepsy 525–527
    hydrocephalus 528–530
    traumatic brain injury 530–532
    see also individual conditions
  conditions, range 511–512, 511t
  disorders, range of 511–512
  principles of care 512–520

neurological dysfunction (*Continued*)
  cranial surgery, postoperative
    518–519t
  diagnostic procedures 512
  emotional and psychological needs
    519–520
  neurological assessment 513–516,
    515t
  neurosurgery 516–519
  raised intracranial pressure
    512–513
  rehabilitation 520
  unconscious child 516, 517t
  verbal component 515t
neuromuscular disorders 511t
neuron 508
  regeneration 510
neurotransmitters 509
neurovascular observations, fractures
  564–565
neutral thermal environment (NTE),
  neonates 625
neutropenia, malignant disease 492,
  496–497
neutrophils 482, 484, 486
New National Health Service: Modern
  Dependable (DoH 1997) 243
Newcastle Royal Victoria Hospital 62
National Health Service
  executive, clinical audit 248
  introduction of 13
  quality framework 243f
  reforms 243
National Health Service 24 332
National Health Service Cancer Care
  Plan (2000) 491
National Health Service Clinical
  Assessment System (National
  Health Service CAS) 341–342
National Health Service Direct 117,
  330–345, 594
  aims 332–333
  call volumes 334
  child protection responsibilities 335
  child specific care 333–336
  computerised decision support system
    334, 337
  confidentiality 335
  Data Protection Act 335
  decision to call 340
  development 331–333
  digital TV services 595
  ethical dilemmas 342
  informational databases 341–342, 342f
  journey through 340f
  nurses
    communication skills 334
    competency-based assessment 336
    shortage 336
    training and assessment 337
  strengths and challenges 332–333,
    333t
  work with other services 335
  see also telephone health assessment

National Health Service Direct Online
  332, 594–596
  clinical governance 595–596
National Health Service Modernisation
  Agency 100, 247
National Health Service Performance
  Assessment Framework 244
The National Health Service plan (DoH
  2000) 51, 239, 247
  information giving 594–595, 601
National Health Service Research
  Support Unit 238
Nightingale, Florence 11–12, 62, 107,
  242
nitric oxide, inhaled, lung injury
  reduction 748
nitrite 407
nitrous oxide, emergency department
  use
  361t
nociception, neonates 630
non-accidental injury
  early childhood 670
  see also child abuse
non-fatal maltreatment 302–303
non-maleficence 312
non-paralytic aseptic meningitis,
  poliomyelitis (polio) 657
non-rapid eye movement (NREM) sleep
  648, 683
non-shivering thermogenesis 171
  neonates 624
non-specific immunity *see* innate
  immunity
non-steroidal anti-inflammatory drugs
  (NSAIDs) 268t
  emergency department use 361t
non-therapeutic treatment, consent
  325–326
non-union, fracture complications
  562
noradrenaline
  neonates 172
  neurotransmitters 509
normative play 67
North American Society for Paediatric
  Gastroenterology and Nutrition
  (NASPGN), mineral oils and
  constipation 457
*North Glamorgan National Health
  Service Trust v Walters* 327
North West Clinical Practice
  Benchmarking Group 216
North West Paediatric Benchmarking
  project 247
Novo Pen 547f
NSPCC, partnership with National
  Health Service Direct 335
nucleotides, genetics 613
numerical pain rating scale 262, 263f
Nuremberg Code 227–228, 309
nurse-controlled analgesia (NCA) 267,
  269–270
  postoperative 292

nurse practitioners role, emergency
  department management 366
Nurses, Midwives and Health Visitors
  Act (1974) 15
nurses, role and responsibilities
  child maltreatment 305–307
  diabetes education 551–552
  disability services 377
  disabled children, communication
    with 385
  emergency department management
    358
  informed consent, surgery 286
  pain interventions 271
  *see also specific nursing roles (e.g.
    instrument nurse)*
Nurses Registration Bill, unification 12
nursing
  definition 95
  diagnoses, assessment 91
Nursing and Midwifery Council (NMC),
  NMC Code of Professional
  Conduct (2002) 86–87, 311
  child protection issues 307
  consent issues 226
nursing assessment *see* assessment
Nursing Council of New Zealand 54,
  59–60
nursing documentation, family centred
  care 86
Nursing Mutual Participation Model 81
nursing process model, assessment 90
nutrition, early childhood 673–674
  dietary advice 673–674
  economic aspects 674
  failure to thrive (FTT) 674–675
  food allergies 674
  food fortification 675
  nutritional deficiencies 674–675
  obesity 673
  weaning 675
nutrition, ill neonates *see entries under
  neonates, health problems*
nutrition, infancy 637–643
  failure to thrive (FTT) 642–643
    assessment 642
    inadequate feeding 643
  food allergies
    cows' milk allergy 640
    eczema 645
    elimination diets 645
    food intolerance *vs.* 641, 641t
  food intolerance 640–641
    cows' milk intolerance 640, 640t
    diagnosis 640
    food allergy *vs.* 641, 641t
    foods to avoid 640
    lactose intolerance 641
    management 640–641
    soya-based formula 640
  milk feeds 637–638
    calculations 638
    follow-on milks 638
    formula 637–638

weight gain 638
see also breastfeeding
vegetarian diets 641–642
  deficiencies 641, 642t
  nutritional adequacy 642
  weaning 641–642
weaning 638–639, 639t
  diet 639
  fruit juices 639
  timing 638–639
  vegetarian diets 641–642
nutritional adequacy, vegetarian diets 642
nutritional deficiencies, nutrition, early childhood 674–675

obesity
  nutrition in early childhood 673
  type 2 diabetes 552
object permanence 147
  Piagetian cognitive development 149
Objective Pain Scale (OPS) 264t
objectivity, adolescents, interaction with 713
observation of children, settings 196
obstructive sleep apnoea 282
  standing orders 295t
oedema *see specific anatomic regions (e.g. cerebral oedema)*
oedipal phase 160
off label medicine research 234
OFSTED 45
old wives tales 115
ombudsman 47–48, 51
omphalocele 279–280
ongoing communication 139–140
open-ended questions, history taking 694
operating room
  child's eye view 284, 289f
  flow through rooms 288–293
operation procedures 291–292
opioids 267, 268t
  addiction 270
  emergency department use 361t
  intravenous infusion 268–269
OPS (Objective Pain Scale) 264t
oral disorders, feeding problems 628
oral drug administrations, palliative care 775
oral hydration solution (OHS) 402
oral hygiene, malignant disease 497, 498t
oral rehydration solution (ORS)
  diarrhoea 448
  gastroenteritis 675–676
oral ventilation, feeding problems 628
organ donation, potential backlash 313
orientation phase, adolescents, therapeutic relationship 715
oropharynx 424
orthopaedic disorders 558–577
  bone biology 559–562
  see also bone

developmental dysplasia of hip (DDH) 573–574
discharge planning 576
hip spica cast 574–575
middle childhood 691
osteogenesis imperfecta *see* osteogenesis imperfecta
Perthes' disease 575–576
polytrauma 570–571
talipes (clubfoot) 575
orthopaedic surgery, complex motor disability 380
osteogenesis imperfecta 571–573
  classification 572t
  description 571–572
  nursing care 573t
  treatment
    medical 572
    surgical 572–573
osteomyelitis, *Haemophilus influenzae* 658
osteosarcoma 496
otitis media 671
  glue ear 670–671
Our healthier nation 689
Our inheritance, our future 609
outpatient department, hospitalisation preparation 72
overcrowding 34
overdependence, family functioning 31
overseas employment 15
oxygen requirement, neonates 172
oxygen saturation
  asthma 440
  measurement 429, 429f
  monitoring 290
oxygen therapy, shock treatment 763

paediatric emergency assessment units (PEAU) 346–352
  admission rates 350
  conditions encountered 348t
  discharge and follow-up care 350–351
  history taking 348
  nurses
    role 347
    skills developed during practice 349t
  observation 349–350
  referral and admission 347–349
  telephone health assessment 347
  waiting times 349
paediatric operating room environment 284
pain
  acute 257
    management 256–277
    unrelieved 258
    see also pain, management; postoperative pain
  adult-child differences 257, 258t, 260t
  age-specific perceptions 260t
  analgesic drugs 267–271

assessment 261–262
  asking child 262
  neonates 630
  scales 98
  tools, emergency department 360
  tools for neonates 265–266t
  tools for non-verbal child 262
  tools for verbal child 262, 263–264t
behavioural indicators 266, 266t
definition 256–257
history, taking of 260–261, 262t
ill neonates *see entries under* neonates, health problems
intervention evaluation 271
malignant disease treatment 498
management 259–267, 273
  children's views 258–259
  communication 273
  documentation 273
  effective, reasons for 257–259
  multidisciplinary team involvement 271
  nurses responsibility 271
  parental involvement 271
  see also analgesia
non-drug methods 271, 272–273t
palliative care 776t
pathways 257
physiological indicators 266, 267t
postoperative *see* postoperative pain
relief *see* analgesia
see also postoperative pain
painting, communication tool 132, 134f
palliative care 770–783
  evolution of 770–771
  holistic care 772–779
  physical needs 774–775, 776–778t
    CNS symptoms 777t
    complementary therapies 775
    constipation 777t
    drug administration routes 775
    nausea and vomiting 776t
    pain 776t
    parental concerns 775
    pruritus 778t
    respiratory symptoms 777t
    skin problems 778t
    verbal communication 774
  psychological care 772–774
    charities 774
    communication 773–774
    ethics 773
    honesty 773
    individuality 773
    music therapy 774
  respite care 778–779
    definitions 778
    own home 778
    residential 778–779
  social needs 775–776
    educational needs 776
    financial concerns 776

palliative care (*Continued*)
  as specialty 771
  spiritual care 775
  team approaches 772
  see also bereavement care
palmar sweating 171
palpation
  cardiovascular problems 469–470
  chest examination 428
pancreatic enzymes, neonates 173
pancreatin, cystic fibrosis 450
paracetamol 267f, 268t
  fevers/pyrexia 681
paralysis, flaccid, poliomyelitis (polio) 657
paraphimosis 280
parathyroid hormone (PTH), bone, role in 560
parent
  loss of, stress 199–200
  records held by 102
parent-held records 102
  content 102
  malignant disease 491
parental anxiety, reduction 291
parental concerns
  hospitalisation 120–121
  palliative care 775
parental consent 217
parental knowledge, child illness 120–121
parental preparation, hospitalisation 71–72
parental presence programme, bedtime routines 648
parental psychopathology 200
parental refusal
  hospitalisation preparation 71
  treatment 321–322
parental relationships, adolescents 703
parental responsibility 318
  discharged child 71
Parental Responsibility Agreement 226
parental subsystem, family alliances 30–31
parenteral nutrition, neonates 629
parenting role, support 306
Parents Staying Overnight in Hospital with their Children (CCHS 1988) 38
Paris Children's Hospital 10
parliamentary commissioner 47
Parson's sick role 119–120
partial (focal) fits 355
partnership, care process 93, 94t
passive immunity, neonates 174
patent ductus arteriosus 468
patent foramen ovale 468
patent processus 279
Patient Advice and Liaison Service (PALS)
  complaints 46–47
  information giving 597
  public involvement 247
  role 239
  user involvement 247, 249·

Patient and Public Involvement Forums (PPIFs) 239, 597
patient-centred assessment 97
patient-centred care, empowerment 592–593
patient-controlled analgesia (PCA) 267, 269
  postoperative 292
patient-held records, malignant disease 491
Patient's charter 599
The patients charter -services for children and young people (DoH 1996), Accident and Emergency services for children 354
patients rights, surgery 287
Pavlik harness, developmental dysplasia of hip (DDH) 574
PDCA cycle: Plan, Do, Check and Act 244
peak inspiratory pressure (PIP) 749
  definition 740
pediculicides, head lice treatment 680
PEEP/CPAP 746, 749, 750, 750f
  barotrauma 747
  definition 740
peer relationships, adolescents 200, 703
penetrance
  genetics 608
  inherited conditions 615–616
Penmate 547f
percentile charts, growth assessment 168
percussion, chest examination 430, 430f
pericardium 464
perinatal factors, learning disabilities 787
perioperative nurse responsibility, privacy, operating theatre 286
perioperative settings, ethics and law 284–287
peripheral circulation, neonates 173
peripheral nerve block, emergency department use 361t
peripheral nervous system (PNS) 507
peritonitis, nephrotic syndrome complications 409
permethrin, scabies treatment 679
permissive hypercapnia, lung injury reduction 747–748
permissive hypoxemia, lung injury reduction 747–748
personality development 156–161
  Freud, Sigmund's theory *see* Freud, Sigmund, personality development theory
Perthes' disease 575–576
pertussis (whooping cough) 433, 654–655
  complications 655
  nursing care 655
  re-emergence 654–655
  signs/symptoms 655
  spread 655

phaeochromocytoma 544–545
phagocytosis 483, 486
pharmacogenetics, definition 608
phenotype, genetics 608
philosophical context of care 92
phimosis 280
  genitourinary problems 416
phototherapy treatment, jaundice, neonates 634
physical abuse, definition 301
physical activity, middle childhood 688
physical attractiveness, adolescents 703–704
physical examination, middle childhood 695
physiological change, psychological status 65
physiological indicators
  maltreatment 306
  pain 266
physiotherapy, complex motor disability 379–380
Piagetian psychological perspective, research relevance 223, 223t
PICO framework 211–212
Pierre–Robin syndrome 628
pituitary gland 536–540
  anterior, hormones 538f
  disorders 537, 538t
  growth hormone deficiencies *see* growth hormone deficiencies
  posterior 536–537
Planetree model, patient-centred care 592
plasma 392
plaster casts 565–566
  developmental dysplasia of hip (DDH) 574
plastic surgery, Down's Syndrome 326
Platt report *see Welfare of Children in Hospital* (1959)
play
  classification of types 67
  communication 132–133
  complex motor disability 384
  early childhood 682
  historical aspects 5
  hospitalisation preparation 67
  role of 25
  stress assessment 204
  therapeutic *see* therapeutic play
playground injuries 588
pneumonia 437
Poiseuille's law 426
poisoning 588–589
  accidental, early childhood 667–668
poliomyelitis (polio) 656–658
  epidemiology 657
  eradication of 656–657
  pathology 657
  signs/symptoms 657
  vaccination 657–658

polymorphonuclear leucocytes (PMNs)
482
polyploidy, chromosomes 616
polytrauma 570–571
orthopaedic definitive care 571
Population Investigation Committee 34
positive end expiratory pressure (PEEP)
see PEEP/CPAP
positive eugenics 620–621
Post-registration Education Project
(UKCC 1993) 109
postanaesthetic care unit (PACU) 292
discharge 292–293
postcode healthcare 312
posterior fossa syndrome 522
postnatal factors, learning disabilities
787
postoperative pain
decision-making algorithm 261f
management 292
children's perceptions 258–259
see also pain
postoperative recovery, parents presence
293
poststreptococcal glomerulonephritis
(PSGN) 410–411
diagnosis 410–411
management 411
pathophysiology 410
prognosis 411
signs and symptoms 410
posture
1 month 176–177
1 year 182
3 months 178
6 months 179
18 months 183
complex motor disabilities 379–380,
380f
supine see supine posture
practice continuum tool, family centred
care 84
praise and rewards, hospitalisation 74
preadmission programmes 205
surgery 287
preconceptual factors, learning
disabilities
787
predictive genetic testing 607
ethical issues 621
impact of 910
pregnancy, previous sudden infant death
syndrome 650
preload, definition 740
premature discharge, paediatric
emergency assessment units
(PEAU) 350
prenatal factors, learning disabilities 787
preoperational stage (2–7), Piagetian
cognitive development 147–148
preoperative stress reduction 66
preparation, hospital admission see
hospitalisation, psychological
preparation for

Preparing your child for hospital: a
parent's guide 207
preschool children 186–188
growth and development 186–188
2 years 186
3 years 186–187
4 years 187–188
see also early childhood
presentation delays 306
pressure above PEEP (PAP) 749
pressure support/control mode (PS/PC),
mechanical ventilation 750
presymptomatic genetic testing 607
preterm infants
enteral feeding, mucosal immunity
481
hypoglycaemia risk 626
prewarming, neonatal equipment 624
primary health care 104–113,
108–109
community children's nursing see
community children's nursing
services
definition 104
history 104–105
hospitalisation support 117–118
primary health care team (PHCT)
108–109
hospital preparation 72
primary prevention, mental health
intervention 708
privacy issues, surgery 286
problem solving
assessment 90
communication 141
family functioning assessment 29
profession-centred models of care 93
programming 236
progressive degenerative disorders 511t
Prohibition of Female Circumcision Act
(1985) 319
Project 2000 15
projection 24
Promoting better health (DoH 1988)
110
prone stander, complex motor disability
381f
propositional operations, Piagetian
cognitive development 148
protein intake, chronic renal failure 418
protest, separation anxiety 63
prothrombin levels, neonates 173
Providing Trained Nurses for the Sick
and Poor in London and Elsewhere
107
pruritus
atopic eczema 646
palliative care 778t
Pseudomonas aeruginosa, cystic fibrosis
450
psychological care, palliative care see
palliative care
psychological development 146–163
nature-nuture debate 146–147

empiricist psychological perspective
147
observations, truth and understanding
160–161
see also cognitive development
psychological problems
middle childhood 696
stressful life events 203
surgery 284
psychological traumas, early 33
psychosexual development, psychosocial
development 158
psychosocial development
altered body image 158
assessment 19–23
practice guidelines 20
undertaking 20–23
Erikson's stages 23–27, 23f, 156–158
important observations 161
links to other developmental theories
and care delivery 157–158
relevance to research 223, 223t
stage 1 (trust vs. mistrust) 23–24,
157
stage 2 (autonomy vs. shame and
doubt) 24, 157, 159
stage 3 (initiative vs. guilt) 24–25,
157–158, 160
stage 4 (industry vs. inferiority) 25,
158
stage 5 (identity vs. role confusion)
25, 158
family 27
guilt 158
individual 23–29
personality development, Freud see
Freud, Sigmund, personality
development theory
psychosexual development 158
role confusion 158
value of assessment 26–27
variation 23
puberty
identity formation 25
physical changes
boys 195f
girls 194f
public health 104–113
community children's nursing see
community children's nursing
services
history 104–106
migration from countryside 105
pulmonary circulation 461
pulmonary plethora 467
pulse pressure, monitoring 762
pupil reaction, consciousness assessment
515
puppets, communication tool 132
pyrexia, early childhood 680–681

quality
as concept 243–244
cycle of improvement 244f

quality (*Continued*)
  ensuring 242–255
  Maxwell's six dimensions of 243–244
quality of life
  definition 230–231
  malignant disease 494
  measures 98
Queen's Institute for District Nurses 107
Queen's Medical Centre (Nottingham) 66
questions, mental health assessment 706

radiography, chest, cardiovascular problems 471
radiotherapy 495
  brain tumour, neurological dysfunction 522
  long term development 523
raised intracranial pressure (RICP) 512–513
randomised controlled trials 214–215, 233
rapid eye movement (REM) sleep 648, 683
Rathbone, William 106
Raytec swabs 282
re-positioning, interpersonal skills 713
recessive characteristics, definition 608
recognition of mother, neonates 635
record accuracy 327
Redfern, Michael 44
Redfern report 313
reflective abstraction, Piagetian cognitive development 148
reflexes, neonates 175
reformulation, interpersonal skills 711
refusal of treatment 321–324
  adolescents with deeply held convictions 323
  children 322–323
  conflict between parents and doctors 324–325
mentally ill child 323–324
  parents 321–322
register
  creation of 12, 13t
  inclusion on part 15 15
  percentage of children's nurses 15, 16t
  supplementary 12–13
Registered Sick Children's Nurses (RSCN)
  direct-entry, demise of 36
  direct-entry programme 15
  training 9
registration, origins 10–14
regression, hospitalisation 122
Reid, John 45
relationship building, nurses' role in chronic illness 732–733
relaxation, analgesia 272t
remarriage 27

renal failure
  acute *see* acute renal failure (ARF)
  chronic *see* chronic renal failure (CRF)
renal system, neonates 173
renin, shock compensatory mechanisms 758
Res Ipsa Loquitur 327
research
  American and European perspectives 234–235
  child-led methodologies 229
  child protection 218–219
  children as researchers 218, 236–238
    difficulties 238–239
  conduction of 229, 314–315
  confidentiality 218
  design and methodology 230
  disease prevention 236
  ethics 217–218
  future 219–220
  government support 239
  guidelines 217–218
  historical aspects 219–220
  interviews 231–232
  involvement 237–238
    extent of involvement 239–240
  necessity 234
  papers, critique 235–236
  quality of life 230–231
  refusal 228
  rights, protection, children and families 314–315
  risk *vs.* benefit 228
  role conflict 218
  trials
    malignant disease 494
    randomised controlled 214–215, 233
  see also healthcare research, involving children
Research Governance Framework for Health and Social Care
  role 227–228, 315
  volunteer involvement 237
resilience factors, mental health assessment 706
resiliency model, McCubbin's 201
resolution phase, adolescents, therapeutic relationship 715–716
respiration
  airway pressure 745, 745f
  airway resistance 745–746, 745f
  chest assessment and examination 426–430, 427f
  closing volume 746
  compliance 745–746, 745f, 746
  expiratory reserve volume (ERV) 746
  inflection point 746
  lung volumes 747f
  mechanics of 745–746
  nervous control 425
  onset of 170
  surfactant 746

respiratory depression
  opioids 270
  postoperative neonates 292
respiratory distress, neonatal 625
respiratory failure
  definition 742
  emergency management 360
respiratory illness/problems 423–444
  anatomy and physiology *see* respiratory system/tract
  chest assessment and examination 426–432
    airway 426, 427f
    breathing 426–430, 427f
    circulation 427f
    disability 431–432
    history taking 432
  hospital admission 423
  infection 433–438
    locations 433f
    lower tract 437–438
    risk 423
    upper tract 433–436
    see also specific conditions
  management 432–433
  morbidity 423
  neonates *see entries under* neonates, health problems
  terminology used, respiration patterns 432f
respiratory rate 429–430, 429f
  febrile response 487
  neurological dysfunction 516
respiratory support 742–744
  extubation ('weaning') 753
  intubation 742, 743f, 744
    cricoid pressure 742
  see also mechanical ventilation
respiratory symptoms, palliative care 777t
respiratory syncytial virus (RSV) 423
respiratory system/tract
  5 years to adolescence 193
  anatomy and physiology 424–426
    airway resistance 426
    breathing, nervous control 425
    lung volumes 425
    infection barriers 479–480
    neonates 172
    toddler 184
respite care, palliative care *see* palliative care
responsibilities, role in childhood 24
resuscitation
  cardiopulmonary *see* cardiopulmonary resuscitation (CPR)
  family presence 364
resuscitation status 324
rewarming, hypothermic neonates 625
rhinitis, allergic, glue ear 670
The Right Start; the National Service Framework for Children, Young People and Maternity Services (DoH 2004) 45

risk analysis 48
road traffic accidents 583–585
  middle childhood 690
Robertson, James
  hospitalisation effects 33, 62, 108
  nurse education 14
  seperation anxiety 63–64
role confusion 26
  psychosocial development 158
role models 25
rooting reflex 175, 175f
Roper–Logan–Tierney model
  dehydration 399
  early childhood 666, 666b
von Rosen splint, developmental dysplasia of hip (DDH) 574
rotaviruses 449t
  gastroenteritis 675, 676t
Royal Belfast Hospital for Sick Children 72
Royal College of Nursing (RCN) 95
  emergency nursing 358
  Research in Child Health (RiCH) Group 216
  standards of care project 243
  telephone consultation 336
Royal College of Paediatrics and Child Health (RCPCH)
  Advocating for Children (2000) 229
  emergency care teams 357–358
  paediatric emergency assessment units (PEAU) 346
  research with children guidelines 217, 219, 314
  research with unlicensed medicines 234
Royal College of Surgeons, emergency care team recommendations 357 358
Royal Commission on the Health of Towns 105
Royal Hospital for Sick Children, Glasgow 311
Royal Liverpool Children's Hospital (Alder Hey) 44
  organ retention 313–314
The Royal Liverpool Children's Inquiry (2001) 44, 313
Royal Manchester Children's Hospital 8–9
Royal Universal Dispensary 7
rubella 661–662
  acquired 661–662
  clinical manifestations 661–662
  congenital 662
  diagnosis 662
  epidemiology 661
  pathology 661
  prevention see measles, mumps and rubella (MMR) vaccine
  treatment 662
  vertical transmission 662

Safeguarding children (DoH 1999) 305
Safety -a universal concern for everybody 583
sagittal synostosis 524f
saline, shock treatment 763
saliva, protective properties 481
salivary glands, babies and toddlers 185
Salmonella
  diarrhoea 449t
  gastroenteritis 676t
Salter's osteotomy, developmental dysplasia of hip (DDH) 574
Sanitary Reform Associations 106
Sarcoptes scabiei (scabies) 679
scabicides 679
scabies, early childhood 679
scalds 585–586
  early childhood see early childhood, health problems
Schloendorff v Society of New York Hospital (1914) 318
school age children, consent issues 319
school-based preparation programmes 72
school environment, stress 199
school nursing 108
school phobia 199
school playing fields 45
school refusal, middle childhood 687
schooling, malignant disease, treatment 502
schools, chronic illness support 735
SCOPE, learning disabilities 788
Scottish Intercollegiate Guidelines Network (SIGN) 250
seat belts 584–585
sebaceous glands 479
  neonates 171
secondary infections, atopic eczema management 646
Seeking consent: working with children (DoH2001) 225–226
seizures 355–357
  acute, management 356–357, 357t
  generalised 355–356
  see also individual types of seizure
self-awareness, adolescents, therapeutic relationship 714
'self-conversations' 710–711
self-discipline acquisition, middle childhood 687
self-esteem
  low, adolescents 705
  middle childhood 688
self-harm/self-injury, adolescents 707
self-knowledge, adolescents, therapeutic relationship 714
self management, education on, asthma 214–215
semiological seizure classification 526
separation, loss of parent 199–200
separation anxiety 207
  stages 63–64
separation theories 14

septic arthritis 658
septic shock 760–761
  clinical manifestations 761
  cytokines 761
  diastolic blood pressure (DBP) 761
  inflammation 761
septicaemia, malignant disease 497
Serious Case Reviews 225, 302
serious diagnosis, communication of 139
serotonin 486
serum 392
service planners, learning disabilities 785–786
service providers, learning disabilities 785–786
sex chromosomes 614
  definition 608
  numerical abnormalities 616
sex-roles 24–25
sexual abuse, definition 301
sexual health promotion, malignant disease survivors 502
sexual maturation
  boys 194–195
  girls 194
sexuality
  adolescents 703–704
  early childhood 682–683
shared patient record 94
Sheffield Free Hospital for Sick Children 9
Shigella
  diarrhoea 449t
  gastroenteritis 676t
shock 755–765
  anaphylactic 760
  compensated 739, 757
  compensatory mechanisms 757–759
    chemical 759, 759f
    hormonal 758–759, 759f
    mean arterial blood pressure 758
    neural 758, 758f
  decompensated 757
  definition 740
  early recognition of 757
  haemodynamic monitoring 761–762
  irreversible 740, 757
  monitoring 764–765
  pump, container and fluid analogy 755–756, 756f
  septic see septic shock
  stages 571t, 756–757, 756f
  treatment 762–764
    antibiotics 763
    catecholamines 764
    dobutamine 764
    dopamine 764
    fluid replacement therapy 763–764
    inotropic agents 764
    oxygen therapy 763
  types 759–761, 760t
    anaphylactic 760
    cardiogenic 760, 760t
    distributive 760, 760t

shock (*Continued*)
hypovolaemic 759–760, 760t
neurogenic 760
septic *see* septic shock
uncompensated 740
short gut syndrome 280
siblings
bereavement care 780–781
chronic illness effects 729
communicating with 141–142
effect of hospitalisation 121
infant communication skills 129
inherited conditions, effects of 610
subsystem, family alliances 31
sick role 119–120
sickle-cell disease
genetics 614, 614f
haemoglobin effects 614
*Sidaway v Board of Governors of the
Bethlam Royal Hospital and the
Maudsley Hospital* (1985) 321
sign language, young children 130
silo bag, gastroschisis 280, 282f
sinusitis, early childhood, health
problems 671
six (6)-week check
motor function 178
vision 177–178
skeletal muscle 561–562
skeletal system
5 years to adolescence 189
babies from 6 weeks 178
development 560t
function 559
skeletal traction 566–567
skills development, middle childhood
687
skin
5 years to adolescence 193
hydration, atopic eczema management
646
infection barriers 477–479
commensal micro-organisms 478
malignant disease treatment 499
neonates 171
perfusion, respiratory illness 431
problems, palliative care 778t
toddler 184
skin traction 567f
application 568
skinfold thickness 167, 167f
skull, sutures 510
sleep
atopic eczema 643
babies from 6 weeks 178
deprivation, early childhood 683
early childhood 683
non-rapid eye movement (NREM)
648, 683
rapid eye movement (REM) 648, 683
slings traction 567
sloughing, infection barriers 479
small for gestational age (SGA)
neonates, hypoglycaemia risk 626

smoke detectors 583, 585
Snow, John 105
social behaviour and play
1 month 177
1 year 182
3 months 179
6 months 181
social consequences, chronic illness
effects 728
social exclusion, sources of stress 305
social functioning, learning disabilities
786
social models of disability 372–373
social organisations, cultural assessment
58
Social Services, maltreatment referrals
306–307
social support, adolescents 200
social system inclusion, adolescents,
interaction with 713–714
Society of Medical Officers of Health
34
socioeconomics
child maltreatment 305
hospitalisation 116
middle childhood 690
unnecessary deaths 36–37
Socratic questioning, adolescents,
interaction with 714
sodium levels, chronic renal failure 418
somatic nervous system (SNS) 507
Southampton Children's Hospital 9, 62
day surgery unit 109
soya-based formula
food intolerance 640
lactose intolerance 641
Specific Issue Order 321
speech *see* hearing and speech
Spence, James 62
spina bifida 372
spinal cord pathways 257f
spinal metastasis 522
spinal muscular atrophy 372
spiritual care, palliative care 775
splitting, feelings 24
spongy bone 559
stair gates 587
standard of care, breach 326
Standing Medical Advisory Committee
of Central Health Services, casualty
departments 353
standing orders 293, 295t
Staphylococcus aureus
methicillin-resistance (MRSA) 478,
485
skin flora 478
Staphylococcus epidermidis, neonatal
sepsis 478
startle reflex 176
status epilepticus 356–357
management principles 357t
Statutory Rules and Orders of the Local
Government Act (1992) 107
step reflex 176, 176f

sternal rub, consciousness, assessment
514–515
steroids *see* corticosteroids
sterotyping 57
stomach acid secretion
babies 481
neonates 173
stomach capacity
neonates 173
toddlers 184
stomatitis, malignant disease treatment
497
storytelling 70
communication tool 132–133
Strategy Discussion, child maltreatment
307
*Strengthening accountability, involving
patients and the public: practice
guidance of the Health and Social
Care Act* (DoH 2001) 236–238
streptococcal infections
pneumonia 437
poststreptococcal glomerulonephritis
(PSGN) 410–411
Streptococcus group B haemolytic
neonatal sepsis 478
respiratory illness 433
Streptococcus mutans 481
stress 197–210
adolescent stressors 200–201
assessment 204–205
in healthcare context 203–205
child abuse 200
childhood responses 199
coping 201–202
capacity, predisposing factors 202
family environment 202–203
family stress 201
illness and hospitalisation 205–208
impact 203
life stressors, social responses and
coping 198–202
loss of parent 199–200
parental psychopathology 200
protective factors 201
school environment 199
stressful events 198
measurement problems 198
Stress Impact Scale (SIS) 203–204
stress inoculation 72
stress-point intervention by nurses
(SPIN) 73
stress-point preparation 69
stressors 305
adolescent 200–201
see also stress
stroke volume 754
definition 740
factors 755
infants 465–466
subcutaneous analgesia 270
substance misuse 306
suck and swallow reflex, neonates 627
suck reflex 159, 175f

suction diathermy, adenoidectomy 282
sudden infant death syndrome (SIDS)
    649–650, 649t
    at-risk children 649–650
    discovery 650
    epidemiology 649
    home care 650
    hospital arrival 650
    later pregnancies 650
    preventive strategies 649–650
suicide attempts, adolescents 200, 707
supine posture
    3 months 178, 178f
    6 months 179, 180f
supplementary register 12–13
supplements (nutritional), neonates 628
support, nurses' role in chronic illness
    735–736
support systems, inherited conditions
    612
supraorbital pressure, consciousness,
    assessment 515
supraventricular tachycardia 474
Sure Start programme 116
    health aspects 110
    new services 305
surface area measurement 167
surgeons duty, informed consent 286
surgery 278–296
    cancer 495–496
    children's need for 278–283, 279t
    ethic and law 284–287
    family, role of 283–284
    middle childhood see middle
        childhood, health problems
    patients rights 287
    preadmission programmes 287
    privacy 286
    psychological trauma 284
Sutherland, T. 69
swallow reflex 480
sympathetic nervous system, febrile
    response 487
synchronised intermittent mandatory
    ventilation (SIMV), mechanical
    ventilation 750
systematic reviews 213–214
systemic circulation 461
systemic vascular resistance
    definition 740
    shock compensatory mechanisms 758
systolic blood pressure (SBP) 431f, 470,
    470t
    septic shock 761
    see also blood pressure

T lymphocytes 479, 484
    memory, gastrointestinal tract 480
tachypnoea, fluid requirement increase
    396
talipes (clubfoot) 575
tears, infection barriers 480
technology-dependent children, surveys
    375t

teddy bears, hospitalisation preparation
    133
Teenage Cancer Trust 499
Teencancer 499
teeth
    5 years to adolescence 189–190
    brushing 677–678
    see also entries beginning dental
telephone health assessment 330–345
    consultation 336–343
        factors affecting progress 338f
    electronic resources 339
    nurse skills 339
    paediatric emergency assessment units
        (PEAU) 347
        following discharge 351
    variables
        caller 338
        nurse 338
        system types 337
telephone triage 336
    see also National Health Service
        Direct; telephone health
        assessment
television health services 596
television shows, hospital based 71
Telling Concerns report (2003) 593
temperature see body temperature
temple mode, clinical governance 245f
Temple v South Manchester Health
    Authority (2002) 327
tenotomy, developmental dysplasia of
    hip (DDH) 574
tepid sponging, fevers/pyrexia 681
testes, assessment in babies 178
testicular cancer, cryptorchidism 415
tetanus 655–656
    complications 656
    management 656
    pathology 655
    signs/symptoms 655, 656
    vaccination 656
textures and pressure, surgery
    preparation 73
theatre reception 288–289
therapeutic play 67, 207
    programmes 66
therapeutic research 228
thermal stimulation, respiration 170
thickening of skin, atopic eczema 645
Thomas splint traction 566, 567f
thoracic surgery, support 472–473
'three mountains experiment,' Piagetian
    cognitive development 149
thromboembolism, nephrotic syndrome
    complications 409
thyroid function disorders 540–542
    hyperthyroidism 541–542
    hypothyroidism 540–541
thyroid gland 541f
tidal volume (Vt) 749
    definition 740
time
    cultural orientations 58

learning disabilities, health needs
    791
tissue necrosis factor (TNF), type 2
    diabetes 552
toddler/preschooler post-operative pain
    scale (TPPPS) 264t
toddlers see babies and toddlers (1–24
    months); early childhood
Together we stand 696–697
toilet training 675
tolerance, opioids 270
tonic clonic fit 356
tonic fit 356
tonsillectomy 282
    standing orders 295t
tonsillitis 282, 286f
    dehydration 487
    inflammatory response 486
tooth brushing 677–678
    see also teeth
topical anaesthesia, emergency
    department use 361t
Tort of Negligence 326
total body water (TBW) 389, 390f,
    391f
total quality management 244–245
touch, analgesia 272t
Townsend v Worcester and District HA
    (1995) 327
toxoids 654
TPPPS (toddler/preschooler post-
    operative pain scale) 264t
trachea 424
traction 566–569
    developmental dysplasia of hip
        (DDH) 574
    external fixation 569, 569f
    internal fixation 568–569, 568f
    nursing care 567–568
        bandages 568
        position of patient 567, 568
transcellular fluid 392–393
transcultural nursing 54
transcutaneous electric nerve stimulation
    (TENS) 273t
transfusions, in utero, jaundice 633
transgenerational stresses, families 29
transitional objects, sleeping in early
    childhood 683
translocations, chromosomal 617, 617f,
    617t
transportation, to emergency
    department 354–355
trauma deaths 364–365
traumatic memories, hospital admission
    205–206
triage 358–360
    categories 359t
    CWILTED triage enhancement 359
    Manchester triage system 358–359
    National Triage Scale 359
    telephone 336
triangle mark, health information quality
    596

tricycle, adapted, complex motor disability 381f
trust, mistrust *vs.* 123
tuberculosis 438
tumour(s) 490–491
    see also malignant disease
tumour necrosis factor alpha (TNF–α) 485
Turner syndrome, genetic basis 616
Tuskegee syphilis study 310
type 1 diabetes *see* diabetes mellitus
type 2 diabetes *see* diabetes mellitus

U-bags 406
ulcerative colitis 455–456
    Crohn's disease, differences between 455t
ultrasonography, genitourinary problems 407
United Nations Convention on the Rights of the Child (1989) 3, 136, 310–311
    article 12 (respect of child's views) 206, 219, 229
    article 13 (freedom of expression) 219, 237
    child protection 273, 299
    disabled children 376–377
    legal aspects 317
uncompensated shock, definition 740
understanding, health and illness 133–134
unexpected admissions, effect on siblings 121
UNICEF Child Friendly Hospital Initiative 273, 311
United Kingdom Central Council for Nursing, Midwifery and Health Visiting (UKCC) 15, 109
Universal Dispensary for Children 10–11
    origins 7
University Hospital, Southampton 599
unlicensed medicine research 234
upper respiratory tract infections 433–436
    early childhood *see* early childhood, health problems
urea 395
urea and electrolyte (U&E) assay 395, 401
urinary tract infections
    Escherichia coli 405
    susceptibility 405–406
    vesicoureteric reflux 411
urine
    testing and collection 406–407
    voiding, neonates 173
urogenital tract
    infection barriers 482
    see also genitourinary problems
US Centre for Disease Control 310
Utting, William 34

Utting report 34

vaccination/vaccines 118, 654
    Haemophilus influenzae 658–659
    MMR *see* measles, mumps and rubella (MMR) vaccine
    poliomyelitis (polio) 657–658
    tetanus 656
    see also immunisation
vagal nerve stimulation, epilepsy 527
varicella zoster virus (chickenpox) 681–682
VAS (Visual Analogue Scale) 264t
vascular neurological disorders 511t
vasoconstriction
    hypothermic neonates 624–625
    shock compensatory mechanisms 758–759
vasodilation, inflammatory response 484
vasopressin *see* antidiuretic hormone (ADH)
vegan diets 642t
vegetarian diets, infants *see* nutrition, infancy
veins, embryonic development 463
venepuncture, middle childhood 693
ventilation 289
    mechanical *see* mechanical ventilation
ventilation-perfusion relationship, mechanical ventilation 744–745, 744f
ventricles, embryonic development 462–463
ventricular failure, congestive cardiac failure 469
ventricular hypertrophy 465, 467
ventricular septal defect (VSD) 463, 467, 468
ventricular shunts
    complications 529t
    hydrocephalus 528–529
    position 529f
ventriculoperitoneal shunts, hydrocephalus 528–529
verbal abuse, childhood communication skills 131
verbal communication, palliative care 774
verbal descriptor scales, pain, emergency department 360
vernix caseosa 171, 479
vertical stresses, families 29
vertical transmission, rubella 662
vesicoureteric reflux 411–412
    endoscopic injection therapy 412
    follow-up 412
    investigations 411
    management 412
    pathology 411
    urinary tract infection 411
vicarious liability 327
Victoria Climbié Inquiry 44, 328
    health professionals, role 297–298

videos, hospitalisation preparation 70
vincristine 498
virtual tours, hospitalisation preparation 70
viruses, avoidance of immune defences 485
Visintainer and Wolfer 65
vision and fine movement
    1 month 177
    1 year 182
    3 months 179
    6 months 180
    18 months 183
vision assessment
    6-week check 177
    8-month check 181
visual analogue scale (VAS), pain assessment 262, 264t
visual material, hospitalisation preparation 69–71
vital signs, circulation 430
vitamin and mineral absorption, neonates 174
vitamin K, neonates 173
vocal fremitus, chest examination 428
Voelcker, Arthur Frances 12
Volkman's ischaemic contracture 565
volutrauma 747
vomiting 446–447
    causes 446t
    see also specific conditions
    dehydration 396
    investigations 448t
    malignant disease treatment 497
    palliative care 776t
von Rosen splint, developmental dysplasia of hip (DDH) 574
vulnerability 225
Vygotsky, Lev 147
    cognitive development 151–153
    language acquisition/development 155

Wales, planned children's hospital 9, 15
walking, development of 169
ward visits, preparation 67
Warnock review (1978) 108
water, biological functions 393–396
    children's requirement 393t
water composition, body 389–393, 390f
    body fluid compartments 390–393, 391f
        extracellular fluid 391–392
        intracellular fluid 390–391
        transcellular fluid 392–393
    body fluids 389–390
    fluid loss, behavioural response 395f
    fluid requirement 393t
    homeostasis 395–396
weaning
    diets *see* nutrition, infancy
    nutrition, early childhood 675
weight
    5 years to adolescence 193
    gain, nutrition, infancy 638

loss, dehydration 396
measurement 166, 166f
  gain trends, babies and toddlers 185
middle childhood 695
The Welfare of Children and Young People in Hospital (1991) 40–41
Accident and Emergency services for children 353–354
Welfare of Children in Hospital (1959) 35–37
  early ignorance of 242
  hospitalisation, effects 14, 33
  key recommendations 108–109
  practice change following 64–65
well telly clinic 72
West, Charles 7–8, 10–11, 106
wet-combing, head lice treatment 680
wet-wrap dressings, atopic eczema management 647, 647b, 678
What to do if you're worried a child is being abused (DoH 2003) 301,

Where the Children? (CCHS 1987)

findings and recommendations 37–38
whooping cough *see* pertussis (whooping cough)
Williamson and Butler 232
Wilms' tumour (nephroblastoma)
  considerations 413
  genetic alterations 412–413
  presentation and diagnosis 413
  prognosis 413
  treatment 413
Wilsher v Essex AHA 326–327
withdrawal symptoms, opioids 270
women's roles 27
Wood, Catherine Jane 11, 37, 106
word choice, hospitalisation preparation 69
working phase, adolescents, therapeutic relationship 715
Working together to safeguard children (DoH 1999) 301
World Health Organisation (WHO)
  disability perspectives 373
  disease elimination goals 651–652
  learning disability definition 786

poliomyelitis eradication programme 656–657
quality and clinical audit 242, 245
quality of life 230
World Injury Control Conference (1989) 583
wound management, emergency departments 366
write and draw method, research interviews 232
written information, hospital preparation 69–71, 207

X-linked inheritance, inherited conditions 615, 615f, 616t

Yacoub, Magdi 313
Young people as researchers — a learning resource pack 238
Youth Matters. Evidence-based best practice for the care of young people in hospital (1988) 43
youths *see* adolescents

Zaadi dolls 68